Textbook of
CLINICAL
ELECTROCARDIOGRAPHY

Textbook of
CLINICAL
ELECTROCARDIOGRAPHY

SECOND EDITION

SN Chugh

MD MNAMS FICP FICN FIACM FIMSA FISC
Professor and Unit Head in Medicine
and Incharge Endocrine and Metabolism
Pt. BD Sharma PGIMS
Rohtak

2006

JAYPEE BROTHERS
MEDICAL PUBLISHERS (P) LTD
New Delhi

Anshan

Tunbridge Wells
UK

First published in the UK by

Anshan Ltd
in 2006
6 Newlands Road
Tunbridge Wells
Kent TN4 9AT, UK

Tel/Fax: +44 (0)1892 557767
E-mail: info@anshan.co.uk
www.anshan.co.uk

ISBN 1 904798 667

British Library Cataloguing in Publication Data
A catalogue record for this book is available from the British Library

Printed in India by Gopsons Papers Ltd., A-14, Sector 60,Noida

to
my parents,
wife Dr Kiran Chugh,
son Dr Anshul Chugh
and
daughter Ashima Chugh (med. student)

Preface to the Second Edition

The overwhelming success to the First Edition of *Textbook of Clinical Electrocardiography* has encouraged me to bring out coloured Second Edition of this book. The new edition has provided me a further opportunity to alter the previous text and to add new topics. The ECGs in this edition have been coloured with full explained legends. Though no new chapter has been added but few topics have been revised and up dated. The book is rewritten concisely to reduce the bulk of this book.

The basic aim of this book remains unchanged, namely to describe the text extensively followed by ECG illustrations. The introduction of colour throughout the book has provided an additional opportunity to beautify the tables and figures as well as making increased use of coloured photographs.

Throughout this edition, emphasis is placed on the explanation of ECG with text. The main emphasis is laid on chapters on 'Conduction Defects and Arrhythmias' where ECG is considered as gold standard for the diagnosis.

The book is intended for the postgraduate students and clinicians for clinical practice. It is also useful for the students who intend to pursue further study in cardiology.

I am thankful to M/s Jaypee Brothers Medical Publishers Pvt Ltd., who has taken sincere efforts to publicise the first edition of this book and made it a success. The new coloured second edition is excellent proof of their efficiency and proficiency indicating the status and standard of the publisher. I congratulate them for this edition also.

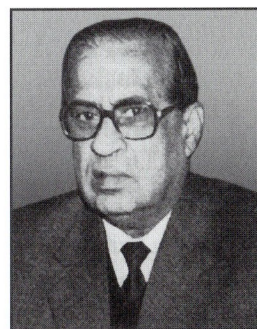

SN Chugh

Preface to the First Edition

It is a tedious and unpleasant task to write a book. Nobody would take up this challenging job unless or until there are good reasons or compulsions to do so. The electrocardiography though a basic bed-side investigation and a gold standard for diagnosis of rhythm and conduction disturbances, is a neglected subject in the field of cardiology. Postgraduate students of medicine acquire the knowledge only from the books of electrocardiography available in the market. The market is flooded with books on the subject of electrocardiography; some are deficient in illustration while others are lacking in material and substance.

With vast expansion in the field of electrocardiography, two aspects have received much attention in recent time such as stress and ambulatory electrocardiography. Similarly with recent expansion in the indications of pacemakers it has become a well accepted therapeutic option. Hence a physician/student has to face such patients in the hospital or in clinical practice. Therefore one must acquire a thorough knowledge about these two aspects of electrocardiography.

I am presenting the first edition of the book. I have taken care of the difficulties of the students/physicians and have tried to cover most of the aspects concerned with electrocardiography. The unique aspect of this edition is that it covers certain chapters which are not discussed in details in certain standard textbooks of electrocardiography.

I have included an additional chapter on pre-arrest arrhythmias and cardiac resuscitation based on recommendations made by European Resuscitation Council endorsed by British Resuscitation Council.

SN Chugh

Acknowledgements

I became too tired and bored while writing this book, and many times thought to defer it. I am thankful to my residents who did not let me down and constantly inspired me to complete the formidable task. They helped me a lot in proof-reading and making necessary corrections.

I am thankful to my colleagues, Dr HK Aggarwal and Dr Harpreet Singh, both Associate Professors in Medicine, Dr Sanjeev Nanda, Associate Prof. of Paediatrics, and Dr K Laler, Lecturer and Head of Cardiology for timely help and suggestions.

It is my privilege to thank M/s Jaypee Brothers Medical Publishers (P) Ltd, New Delhi and their team for bringing the first edition of this book. I admire their patience and tolerance during this period. I appreciate the adventure and labour put by them in preparing excellent diagrammatic illustrations.

Note to Readers

Dear Colleagues/Students

To write a book is a herculean task and to face criticism thereafter is disgusting. One must remember that "To err is human". The omission and commission in interpretation of ECG is unavoidable because of great degree of normal variations. It is not surprising to note that two physicians may not have same opinion on a single ECG.

I request my colleagues and students that it being a single handedly written book, may have certain omissions, but I have tried to depict in the ECG whatever I have written in the text. A great degree of care has been exercised in interpreting the ECGs, still any deficiency or error found may be taken in good spirit and I may be excused for that. Any suggestions on any aspect of this book will be entertained with thanks.

SN Chugh

Contents

SECTION ONE
Physiological Mechanisms Governing Electrocardiographic Deflections

1. Fundamentals of Electrocardiography 3
2. The Electrode and the Lead System 7
3. Action Potentials and Waveforms 13
4. The Cardiac Vector and the Electrical Axis 25
5. The Electrical Rotation of the Heart 40

SECTION TWO
The Electrocardiogram

6. Normal Electrocardiogram 49
7. Normal Electrocardiographic Variants in Adults 67

SECTION THREE
Chamber Hypertrophy or Enlargement

8. Atrial Hypertrophy/Enlargement 75
9. Ventricular Hypertrophy/Enlargement 87

SECTION FOUR
Conduction Defects

10. Intracardiac Conduction Defects 107
11. Sinus Node Dysfunction 111
12. Atrioventricular (AV) Blocks 122
13. Bundle Branch Blocks 135
14. The Fascicular Blocks or Hemiblocks 154
15. The S_I, S_{II}, S_{III} Syndrome 167

SECTION FIVE
Stress Electrocardiography

16. Stress Electrocardiography 173

SECTION SIX
Continuous Ambulatory Electrocardiographic Recording

17. Continuous Ambulatory Electrocardiographic Recording 197

SECTION SEVEN
Coronary Artery Disease

18. Myocardial Ischaemia 207
19. Myocardial Infarction 225

SECTION EIGHT
Congenital and Heredofamilial Disorders

20. Congenital Heart Disease 285
21. Heredofamilial Prolonged Q-T Syndromes 313
22. Accelerated Conduction or Pre-excitation 316
23. Hypertrophic Cardiomyopathy 330

SECTION NINE
Acquired Heart Disease

24. Rheumatic Heart Disease 339
25. Myocarditis and Cardiomyopathies 355
26. Pericarditis 366
27. Acute Pulmonary Thromboembolism (Acute Cor Pulmonale) 374
28. Chronic Obstructive Pulmonary Disease (COPD) and Chronic Cor Pulmonale 380
29. Systemic Hypertension 389

SECTION TEN
The Disorders of Cardiac Rhythm

30. Basic Physiopathologic Considerations. 397
31. Sinus Rhythm and Its Manifestations 407
32. Abnormal Atrial Rhythm (Atrial Arrhythmias or Dysarrhythmias) 412
33. Atrioventricular (AV) Nodal Disturbances 430

34. Paroxysmal Supraventricular Tachycardias 440
35. Ventricular Arrhythmias/Dysarrhythmias 448
36. Reciprocal Rhythm and Reciprocal Tachycardia 478
37. Atrioventricular Dissociation 491
38. Parasystole 498
39. Ventricular Aberrancy or Aberrant Intraventricular Conduction 503
40. Escape Rhythm 521
41. Ventricular Fusion Beats 527
42. Ventricular Capture Beats 530

SECTION ELEVEN

Artificial Pacemakers

43. Artificial Pacemakers 535

SECTION TWELVE

Miscellaneous Disorders

44. Heart in Endocrine Disorders and Injuries 557
45. Drugs, Poisons and the Heart 564
46. The Electrolytes and the Heart 582
47. Heart in Cerebrovascular and Neuromuscular Disorders 591

Appendices

A. Cardiac Drugs—Oral and Intravenous 599
B. Normal 12-Lead Surface ECG and Its Variations in Adults 607
C. Analysis of an Arrhythmia. 609
D. Proforma for ECG Reporting. 611
E. The ABCs of Cardiopulmonary Resuscitation 613

Index 619

Physiological Mechanisms Governing Electrocardiographic Deflections

SECTION ONE

1

Fundamentals of Electrocardiography

- *The electrocardiogram—An introduction*
- *The Einthoven concept*
- *Anatomy and physiology of conduction tissue*
- *The modes of activation of the heart*

THE ELECTROCARDIOGRAM— AN INTRODUCTION

Definition

The graphic representation of the electrical events of the heart on a paper, recorded from the body surface electrodes placed at some distance displaying the electrical activity in waveforms in different planes, is called *'electrocardiogram'*.

Electrical Activity

The electrical activity of the heart depends on the generation of action potentials through the heart muscle by electrical stimulation. The heart muscle possesses an intrinsic property of excitability and conductivity. The electrical potentials generated in the heart propagate through the specialised conducting tissue in a waveform in a co-ordinated manner. Therefore, the electrical activity generated in the sinoatrial (SA) node-the pacemaker, spreads through the conduction pathways, i.e. atria, then to atrio-ventricular (AV) node, bundle of His and its branches, the Purkinje system and ultimately to the ventricles resulting in an electrocardiographic complex consisting of P-QRS-T during one beat of the heart. The electrical events are followed by mechanical

events in the heart; hence, co-ordinated function called electro-mechanical events.

Usefulness of Electrocardiogram (ECG)

The ECG is a graphic recording of electrical potentials generated in the heart. It does not represent mechanical events. The ECG should be considered as a laboratory test only and is not a *sine-quanon* of any heart disease diagnosis. A patient with organic heart disease may have normal ECG; while on the other hand, a perfectly normal healthy individual may show non-specific changes on ECG. Therefore, on the basis of normal ECG, no assurance of the absence of the disease may be given to any one. The ECG should be analysed and interpreted in the light of clinical findings. In general, a physician who is looking after the patient is the most qualified person to interpret the ECG correctly. The ECG interpreted by someone else other than the treating physician may, sometimes, be erroneous and misinterpretation may be sent based on the findings of ECG. The ECG is useful in the following conditions;

1. Chamber hypertrophy and dilatation. (atrial and/or ventricular hypertrophy and dilatation)
2. Myocardial ischaemia and infarction.

3. Arrhythmias. It serves as a gold standard for diagnosis.
4. Myopericardial disease or pericarditis.
5. Conduction disturbances at various stages from the SA node to Purkinje system.
6. Systemic illnesses affecting the heart.
7. Effect of drugs and monitoring the drug therapy such as quinine, quinidine and procainamide.
8. Electrolytes disturbance specially hypo and hyperkalaemia; and hypo and hypercalcaemia. Both are important cations for the heart.
9. Detection of efficacy of various cardiac intervention procedures, i.e. angioplasty, bypass surgery, etc.
10. Continuous ambulatory electrocardiography helps in evaluation of symptoms related to daily activity.

What does an ECG complex indicate?

An ECG complex of P-QRS –T indicates the total electrical events that occur during one beat. The P wave represents the total electrical activity of the atria. The QRS-T complex represents the electrical events of the ventricles, i.e. both electrical activation (depolarisation) and recovery (repolarisation).

What does an ECG complex record?

On ECG, the magnitude and direction of the electrical impulse recorded on the body surface is a resultant action potential produced within the myocardial cells due to depolarisation and repolarisation processes occurring at that point of time after passing through the cancellation of opposing forces from the other cells. Normally, an individual cell is excitable but its activity does not reach to the surface because the opposing cancellation forces make it a weak electrical potential; but cumulative effect of a group or groups of cells can make the electrical potential reproducible on the surface as resultant electrical force or potential which is recorded as *deflections* or waves. The signals recorded on the surface don't specify their sites of origin, because a given vector (resultant force) at the body surface cannot be accounted for innumerable combinations of cellular signals at their sources in the heart.

EINTHOVEN THEORY OF ELECTRICAL ACTIVITY

In 1902, Einthoven recorded an electrical current from the human heart by a galvanometer. He postulated the concept that human body represents as a larger volume conductor having the source of electrical activity at the centre. As an extension of this hypothesis, the net electrical activity at any instant in the cardiac cycle may be viewed as originating from a polarised point source at a theoretical *'electrical center'* of the heart. Since this equivalent dipole would have direction and magnitude, one might extend this pattern into a sequence of instantaneous vectors recordable from the body surface.

ANATOMY AND PHYSIOLOGY OF CONDUCTION TISSUES OF THE HEART (FIG. 1.1)

Sinoatrial (SA) node: It is the intrinsic natural pacemaker of the heart. It is located in the upper part of the right atrium. There are three internodal-connecting pathways present in atrial musculature which fan out from SA node and converge at AV node. There is an additional interatrial pathway called *Bachmann's bundle*, which transmits the sinus impulse to the left atrium.

Atrioventricular (AV) node: The three internodal (anterior, middle and posterior) conducting pathways

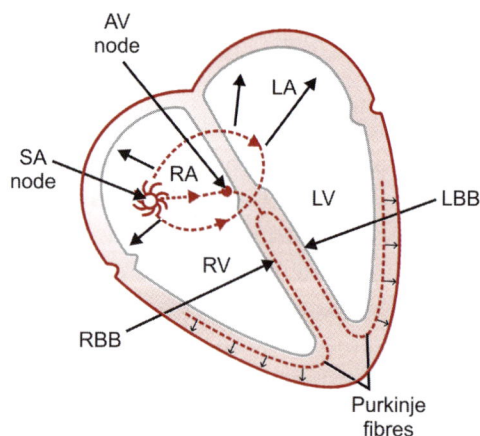

Fig. 1.1: Conduction system of the heart and spread of excitation wave from SA node to the ventricles is represented by arrows

SA node	=	Sinoatrial node
AV node	=	Atrioventricular node
RBB	=	Right bundle branch
LBB	=	Left bundle branch

meet at AV node which acts as a *'way station'*. At AV node, the impulses are slowed down and a normal physiological delay occurs, that allows time to the atria to contract and to pump blood to the ventricles (a mechanical event).

Bundle of His: After normal physiological delay in AV node, the impulse enters a short pathway called *'Bundle of His'* which runs for a short distance and splits into right and left bundle branches.

Right bundle branch (RBB): It conducts impulses to the right ventricle. It divides into smaller branches and forms a network of conducting fibres called *Purkinje system*. The Purkinje fibres arborise with fibres from the left bundle branch to complete the Purkinje conduction system. The Purkinje fibres from right bundle branch conduct impulses to the right ventricular muscle cells.

Left bundle branch (LBB): The left bundle divides shortly after its origin into two fascicles (anterior and posterior) that supply the left ventricle. These fascicles supply their respective areas of the ventricles, i.e. anterior supplies the anterosuperior surface and posterior supplies the posteroinferior surface of the left ventricle.

Both the anterior and posterior fascicles branch to form Purkinje fibre system and conduct impulses through this system to the left ventricular wall, thus, completing the process of electrical excitation which is repeated cyclically at an average rate of 72 beats in a minute (bpm).

The right ventricle is activated slight ahead of left ventricle because right bundle branch is activated before the left, but contraction of both the ventricles is synchronous and instantaneous.

APPLIED PHYSIOLOGY

The P wave

The P wave of ECG complex indicates an atrial depolarisation (an electrical event) which proceeds when AV valves are closed. Spread of electrical excitation to AV node ultimately results in opening of AV valves and discharge of blood from atria to the ventricles. The contraction of atrial muscle to pump blood is a mechanical event, hence, P wave represents an electrical event preceding the mechanical event.

The QRS Complex

The QRS complex of ECG indicates ventricular depolarisation, which is followed by recovery, i.e. repolarisation in which there is reversal of activation process resulting in inscription of ST segment and T wave. Occasionally a small deflection due to delayed or secondary repolarisation is seen as a 'U' wave, which is prominently visible in hypokalaemia. Normally it is so small that either it is not seen or seen rarely. Its significance is not fully defined.

With arrival of an electrical depolarisation wave in the ventricles, the ventricles contract forcing the AV valves to close and semilunar valves to open so as to pump the blood into aorta and pulmonary circulation. Therefore, this electro-mechanical systole started by the electrical activation of ventricles (QRS complex) is followed physiologically by a mechanical event (cardiac contraction); and in this way, a cardiac cycle is completed in each beat and P-QRS-T complex is recorded during each beat.

MODES OF ACTIVATION OF THE HEART (ATRIA AND VENTRICLES, FIGS 1.2A AND B)

Both the atria of the heart are thin-walled structures not equipped with specialised conduction system, are activated longitudinally and by contiguity, i.e. the excitation wave from SA node spreads to the whole chamber, each fibre, in turn, activating the adjacent fibre.

Activation of both the ventricles occurs through the specialised and highly efficient conduction system, which transmits supraventricular impulses from the endocardial to the epicardial surfaces through the terminal ramifications of Purkinje system. Excitation, is therefore, transverse through the ventricular myocardium, and this activates the whole chamber near-synchronously.

The two modes of activation, i.e. longitudinal occurring in the atria and transverse occurring in the ventricles, have following differences and clinical significance (Table 1.1).

SECTION ONE

Table 1.1: Modes of activation of atria and ventricles	
Longitudinal activation	*Transverse activation*
• Occurs in the atria • Proximal parts are activated first followed by distal parts. • This type of activation favours potential Out-of-phase state. • It is easy to induce fibrillation in atria due to this type of activation which results in asynchronous state. • The longitudinal activation does not reflect the thickness of the atrial wall, thus atrial hypertrophy cannot be reflected electrocardiographically.	• Occurs in the ventricles • It results in activation of all parts simultaneously, hence, it is sequential. • This favours potential In-phase state. • This type of activation results in fibrillation of ventricle due to synchronous or near-synchronous state. • The transverse mode of activation indirectly reflects the thickness or transverse bulk of the ventricular wall, thus hypertrophy of the ventricles can be reflected and expressed electrocardiographically.

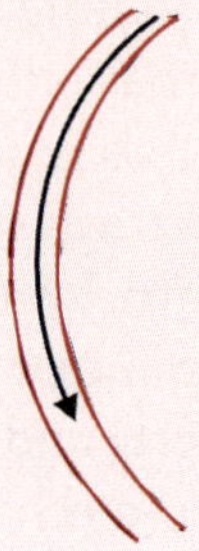

Fig. 1.2A: Longitudinal activation of atrial wall

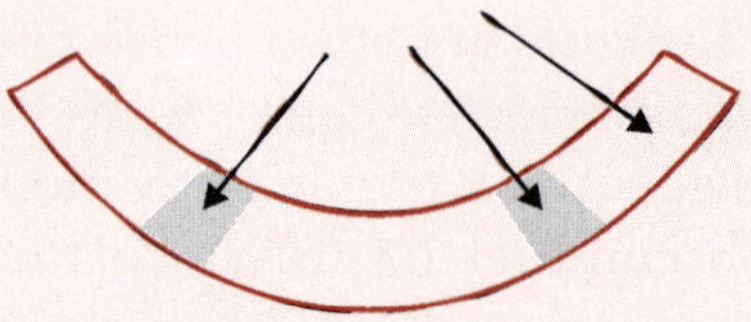

Fig. 1.2B: Transverse activation of ventricular wall

Suggested Reading

1. Cranefield PF: The conduction of the cardiac impulse. Mount Kisco, NY: Futura Publishing Company Inc, 1975.
2. Einthoven W: Selected papers on Electrocardiography. Snellen, A (Ed). Leiden, University Press, 1977.
3. Fisch C: Electrocardiography of arrhythmias, Philadelphia: Lea and Febiger, 1989.
4. Fisch C: Evolution of clinical electrocardiogram. *J Am Coll Cadiol* **14**: 1127, 1989.
5. Fozzard HA, Das Gupta DS: Electrophysiology and the electrocardiogram. *Mod Concepts Cardiovas Dis* **44**: 29, 1975.
6. Fye WB: A history of origin, evolution and impact of electrocardiography. *Am J Cardiol* **73**:937, 1994.
7. Fye WB: Disorders of heart beat. A historical overview from antiquity to mid – 20th century. *Am J Cardiol* **72**: 1055, 1993.
8. Horan IG: Manifest orientation. The theoretical link between the anatomy of the heart and clinical electrocardiogram. *J Am Call Cardiol* **9**:1049, 1987.
9. Lewis T: The mechanism and graphic registration of the heart beat. London, Shaw and sons, Ltd. 228, 1920.

SECTION ONE

2

The Electrode and the Lead System

■ *The electrodes*
■ *The lead system and its classification*
■ *Chest lead system*
■ *Orientation of different leads*
■ *Continuous monitoring system*
■ *Special lead system*

THE ELECTRODES

The ECG lead system is composed of five electrodes; four for limbs (one to each limb) and one for the chest which is shifted at various sites on the precordial region. The identification of electrodes is done either by the colour of electrode (colour coding system) or by the label on the electrodes as RA (right arm), LA (left arm), LL (left leg) and RL (right leg). The right leg electrode is an inactive ground electrode for all the leads (Fig. 2.1). The leads (RA, LA, LL and RL) are attached to their respective electrodes.

THE LEAD SYSTEM

A 12 leads electrocardiogram is standard and conventional because it records the electrical activity of the heart from 12 different views in two planes, i.e. frontal and horizontal. Each lead provides deflection depending on the resultant electrical force of the impulse. The frontal plane leads are called I, II, III, aVR, aVL, aVF and horizontal plane leads are called precordial leads that include V_1 to V_6.

Classification of Lead System

The routine ECG consists of 12 leads – I, II, III, aVR, aVL, aVF and V_1-V_6.

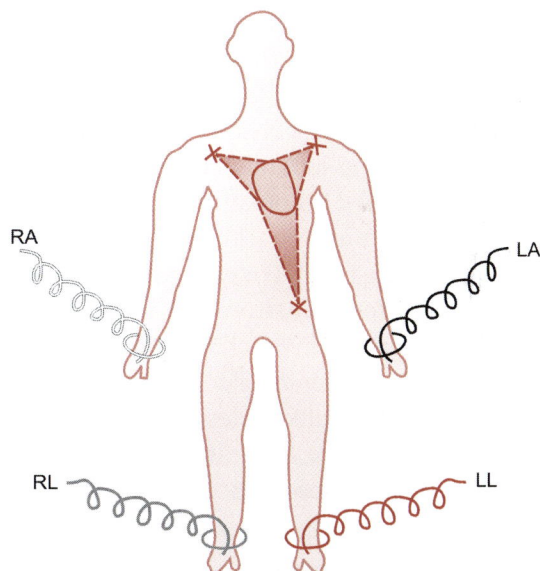

COLOUR CODING SYSTEM OF LIMB ELECTRODES

- White - Right arm (RA)
- Black - Left arm (LA)
- Green - Right leg (RL)
- Red - Left leg (LL)

Fig. 2.1: Limb electrodes: They are placed above the wrists and ankles or alternatively on shoulders and lower abdomen near the junction of each limb with the trunk. In amputated limb, it is placed above the amputation stump. RA = Right arm, LA = Left arm, RL = Right leg, LL = Left leg

The leads are classified into two groups;
1. Limb leads, i.e. bipolar and unipolar
2. Chest or precordial leads.

1. Limb Lead System

A. Bipolar limb leads: The limb electrodes are placed on the right arm (RA), left arm (LA), left leg (LL), and right leg (RL). The right leg (RL) electrode acts as an earth or neutral electrode (Fig. 2.1). These limb electrodes actually record the electrical impulses generated from the heart and transmitted to right shoulder (RA), left shoulder (LA) and left groin (LL), therefore these electrodes can be placed anywhere below these points. The colour coding of the electrodes is given in the box (Fig. 2.1). The bipolar leads I, II, III requires two electrodes at a time to record tracing. Out of these two electrodes, one acts as positive and other as a negative. Bipolar electrodes record the net potential generated from these two electrodes as illustrated in the Figure 2.2A.

B. Unipolar limb leads (Fig. 2.2B): The same bipolar limb leads are used to form unipolar limb leads, i.e. aVR, aVL, aVF; where the letter 'a' stands for augmented, which means the electrical forces in these leads are enlarged in response to electrically created negative center. The letter 'V' stands for unipolar. These leads are called unipolar because they use only one electrode at a time to record the electrical forces generated from the heart. For each unipolar lead, the specific electrode is positive (+) in reference to electrically created negative center in the machine and these leads give augmented electrical forces.

The bipolar limb electrodes used to form each unipolar limb leads are given in the box along with the diagrammatic representation.

2. Chest electrodes and chest leads: These are unipolar chest leads formed by a chest electrode which is moved at six different positions or by six different chest electrodes (Fig. 2.3) placed at different positions to record the electrical forces in reference to centrally created electrically negative center. These leads are designated by the letter 'V' as V_1, V_2, V_3, V_4, V_5 and V_6. Similar to unipolar limb electrodes, each unipolar chest electrode is the positive (+) electrode, which records the heart's electrical forces in relation to negative center.

It is important to place the chest electrodes in their proper positions (Fig. 2.3) for accurate recording of the chest leads, especially when serial tracings are being taken.

Placement of chest electrodes (Fig. 2.3): They are placed as follows;

V_1 = Fourth intercostal space, right sternal border
V_2 = Fourth intercostal space, left sternal border
V_3 = Midway between V_2 and V_4
V_4 = Fifth intercostal space, left midclavicular line
V_5 = Fifth intercostal space, anterior axillary line
V_6 = Fifth intercostal space, mid-axillary line.
V_7 = Fifth intercostal space, posterior axillary line
V_8 = Fifth intercostal space, posterior scapular line
V_9 = Fifth intercostal space, left border of the spine

NB: Leads V_7-V_9 conventionally are not taken except under special circumstances.

Right sided chest leads (V_{3R-9R}) placed in the same location as left sided chest leads (V_3–V_9) can also be recorded if needed. V_{2R} is then represented by lead V_1 and V_2 represents V_{1R}.

$3V_{1-9}$: These leads are recorded one space higher, i.e. in 3rd intercostal space. The same terminology can be used for leads taken at other inter-spaces $2V_{1-9}$, $6V_{1-9}$, etc.

Significance of recording different chest leads. The conventional chest leads V_1-V_6 are recorded routinely, while right sided chest leads (V_{3R}, V_{4R}, V_{5R}, V_{6R}) are recorded under special circumstances as follows;
1. V_{3R} or V_{4R} are recorded for right sided events such as acute pulmonary embolism, right ventricular infarction, right ventricular hypertrophy, etc, to define right ventricular epicardial complex (rS) if it is not visible in conventional lead V_1.
2. The chest leads on right side ($4V_{3-6}$) are recorded in a patient with dextrocardia to define left ventricular epicardial complex (qRS) as conventional leads V_1-V_6 will show right ventricular epicardial complex in this condition.
3. Leads taken one space higher, i.e. 3rd intercostal space is indicated in high lateral wall infarction,

A

RA ⊖ —I→ ⊕ LA
LL

Lead I

RA ⊖ —II→ LA
⊕ LL

Lead II

RA LA ⊖
III
⊕ LL

Lead III

B

RA ⊕ LA
LL

Lead aVR (RA electrode is ⊕)

RA LA ⊕
LL

Lead aVL (LA electrode is ⊕)

RA LA
⊕ LL

Lead aVF (LL electrode is ⊕)

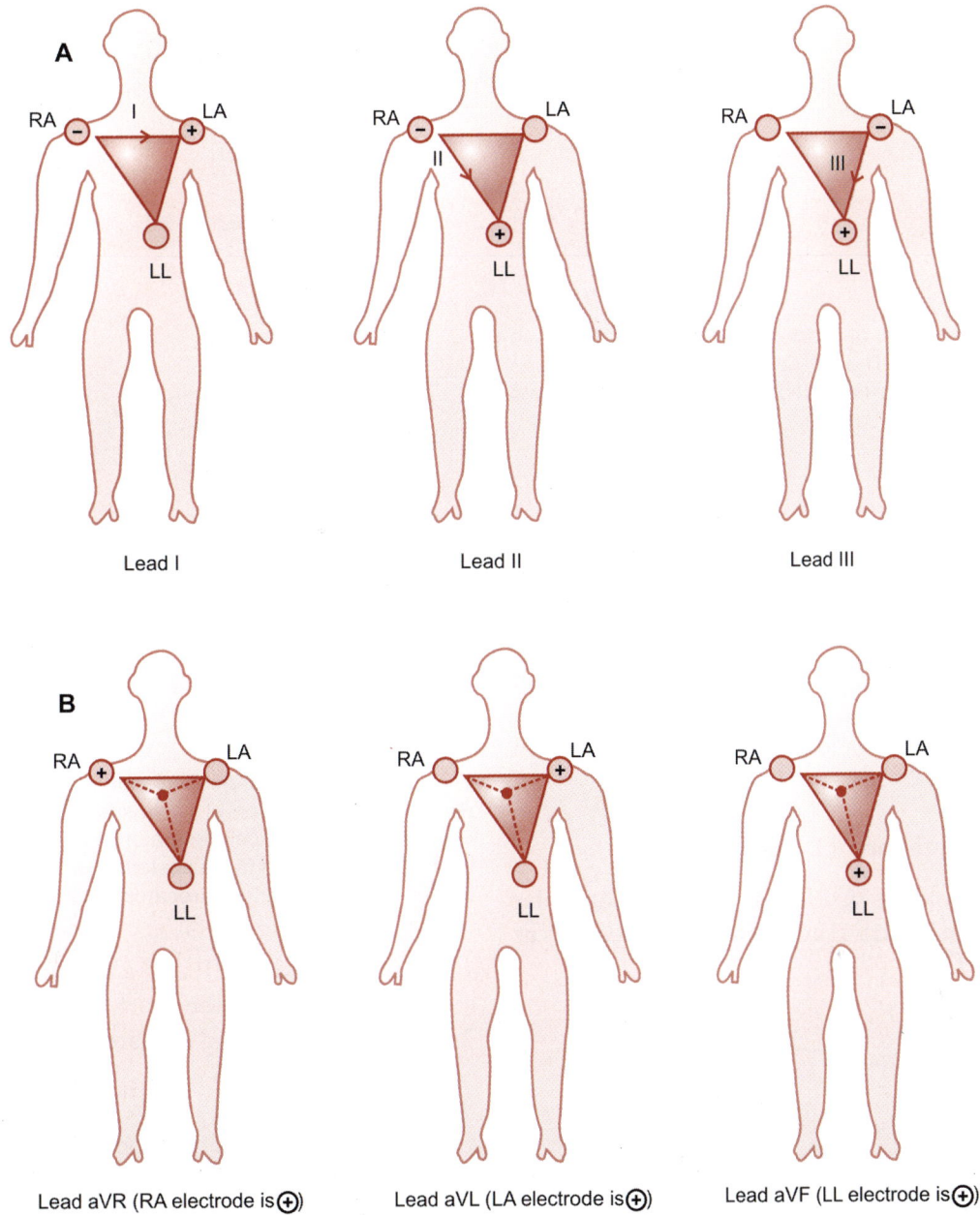

Fig. 2.2: Limb lead system.
A. Bipolar limb leads (I, II and III). They record electrical potential difference between two electrodes one designated as (+) and other designated as (–). The arrows show direction of flow of current between two electrodes
Lead I : LA electrode is positive and RA electrode is negative
Lead II : LL electrode is positive and RA electrode is negative
Lead III : LL electrode is positive and LA electrode is negative
B. Unipolar limb leads (aVR, aVL and aVF)

when infarction pattern is not seen in precordial leads (V_1-V_6) but is seen in leads I and/or aVL.

Lead axis: When the paired electrodes are oriented in any particular direction, the theoretical straight line joining the electrodes is known as the *axis* of that lead or lead axis. This is different from the electrical axis of the heart, which is discussed in later chapter. A lead so placed will detect and transmit any change in the

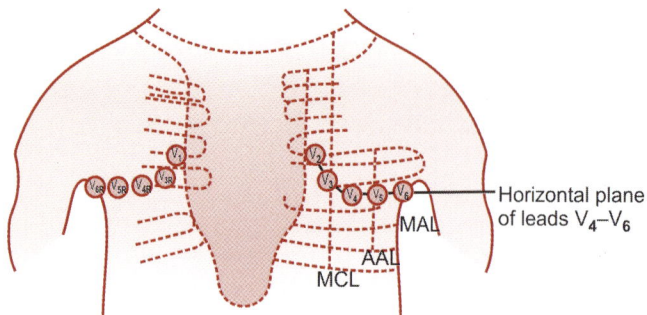

Fig. 2.3: The placement of six chest electrodes (V_1 to V_6) on the anterior chest wall. The V_{3R-9R} all placed on the right side in the same location as left sided V_3 to V_9. The lead V_1 will become V_{2R}

electrical potential which occurs between its electrodes.

The 12 leads electrocardiogram consisting of three limb leads (I, II, III), three unipolar augmented leads (aVR, aVL, aVF) and six chest leads (V_1-V_6) record the net electrical forces generated in the heart and recorded within electrical field of the heart. The 12-lead system is diagrammatically represented in Figure 2.4.

Arbitrary Orientation of Different Leads

The orientation of the ECG leads to the left ventricular 'cone'-the main electrical generator of the heart, is as follows (Fig. 2.5).

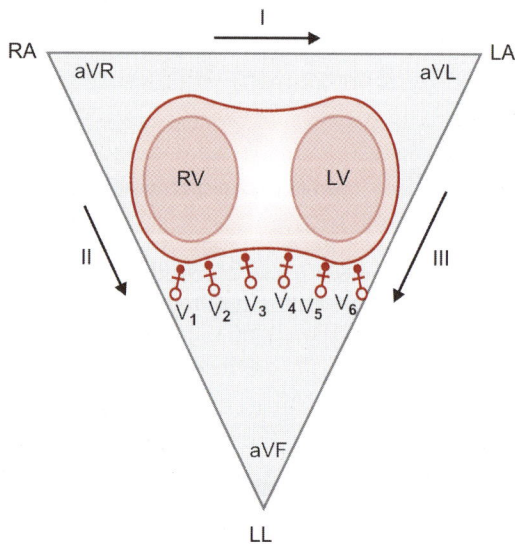

Fig. 2.4: Diagrammatic representation of 12 leads of the electrocardiogram to complete the lead system

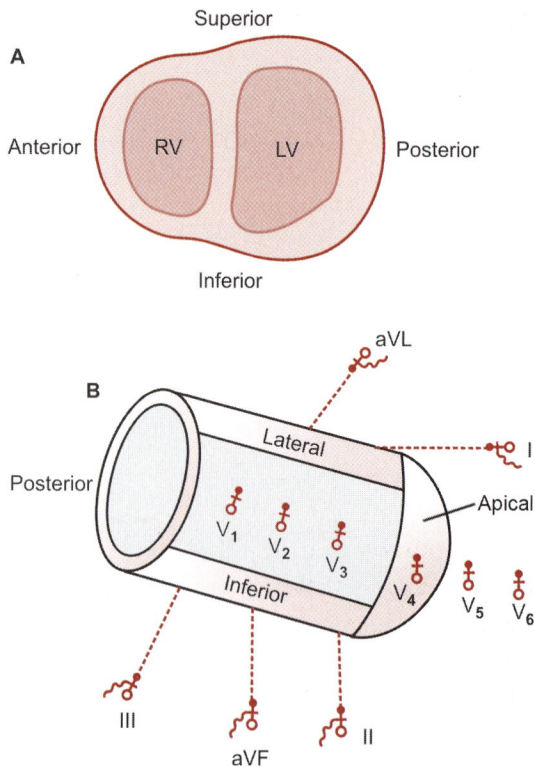

Fig. 2.5: Diagrammatic representation. **A**. cross-section through ventricles **B**. orientation of various leads to the left ventricle cone-the main electrical generator of the heart. There is no lead which is oriented to the posterior wall of the heart, i.e. this area is unrepresented electrocardiographically

1. Standard leads II, III and aVF are oriented to the inferior surface of the heart.
2. Standard leads I and aVL are oriented to high and superior left lateral wall.
3. Lead aVR is oriented to the cavity of heart, hence, records all the negative complexes. Lead V_1 also tends sometimes to be oriented to the cavity of the heart.
4. Leads V_1-V_6 are oriented to the anterior wall of the heart. They are further subdivided into:
   i) Anteroseptal leads; V_1 to V_4.
   ii) Apical leads; V_5-V_6.
   iii) Lateral leads; leads I and aVL. These are also called high lateral oriented leads because if ECG changes are limited to these leads only, the ECG is repeated one space higher-up to record the changes.
   iv) Leads I, aVL, V_5 and V_6 are called high lateral and superior oriented leads.

v) Leads V_1 and V_2 are called right oriented or right precordial leads.

vi) Leads V_3 and V_4 are called interventricular septum or transitional zone leads.

vii) Leads V_4-V_6 are called left precordial or left oriented leads.

CONTINUOUS MONITORING SYSTEM USED IN CCU (CORONARY CARE UNIT)

In a hospital, bedside continuous monitoring of ECG is done in critically ill patients. One or more leads may be monitored. A three electrode monitoring system is employed in which one electrode acts as a positive (+), other acts as negative (-) and third acts as earth or ground electrode (Fig. 2.6). One limb lead at a time (I, II or III) may be recorded by placing the electrodes in their respective positions while keeping the earth electrode stationary usually just underneath the right clavicle.

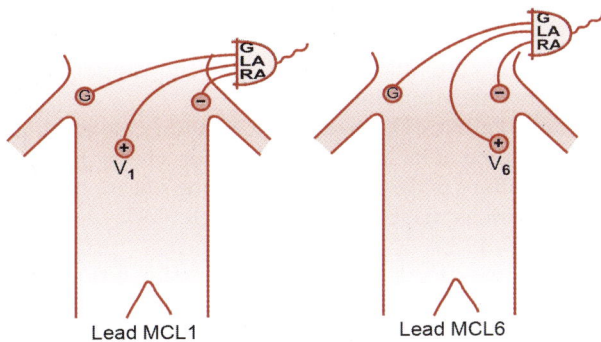

Lead MCL1   Lead MCL6

Fig. 2.6: Three leads monitoring system. Modified chest leads MCL1 and MCL6 are created by placing the positive electrode (LA) in the appropriate precordial position, the negative electrode (RA) is placed under the left clavicle, and the ground electrode (G) is kept underneath right clavicle

A. The three electrodes monitoring system

In this system, chest leads may be created for continuous monitoring as follows;
- Put the positive electrode in appropriate chest electrode location anywhere between V_1 to V_6 positions.
- Put negative electrode under left clavicle
- Earth or ground electrode is put underneath right clavicle.

This is termed as modified chest leads (MCL) system in which we can record any chest lead by just placing the positive electrode in the respective position of that lead.

B. The five electrodes monitoring system

In this system, all the four electrodes (RA, LA, LL, RL) are placed in their respective positions. The fifth electrode being placed on the chest in the desired V_1 through V_6 position. Using this system, any one or more leads of the 12 leads electrocardiogram may be monitored on the bedside. This is actually akin to a bedside ECG monitoring with the help of ECG machine.

SPECIAL OR UNCONVENTIONAL LEADS FOR RECORDING ATRIAL ACTIVITY FROM BACK OF THE HEART

The P waves represent atrial activity. Sometimes, P wave may not be seen on conventional leads, hence, special leads has been designed or used for recording them. These leads are called unconventional leads or special leads, created for a more adequate assessment of atrial activity. These include.

1. **Lewis lead:** This is created or modified lead I, in which right arm (RA) electrode is placed in 2nd right intercostal space near to right sternal border. Left arm (LA) electrode is placed in right 4th intercostal space near to right sternal border.

2. **Oesophageal leads:** Anatomically oesophagus is situated in the posterior mediastinum, posterior to the heart. Any electrode placed in the oesophagus will be in close contact with the heart than through the chest or limb electrode. Therefore, it will give excellent display of atrial activity (P wave).
- An oesophageal wire (V lead) is placed inside the nasogastric tube or a specially designed nasogastric tube with an electrode embedded in a gelatinous capsule on its tip; and the tip is advanced 25-30 cm in order to place it close to the atria. (Fig. 2.7). The record from V lead will give detailed information of P waves.

Intra-atrial leads: Specially designed electrode wire (V lead) may be used for this purpose; which is

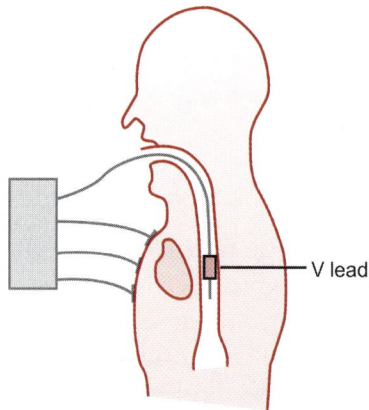

Fig. 2.7: Oesophageal leads depicted are used to magnify P waves. The V lead is attached to a special wire or nasogastric tube with an exploring electrode on the distal tip (embedded in a gel cap). The tip is advanced into the oesophagus until it is positioned behind the atria. Since the recording electrode is in close proximity to the atria, P waves appear larger than usual on the ECG

advanced into the right atrial cavity through jugular or subclavian or temporal vein. The record from 'V' lead gives good display of atrial activity (P waves).

Suggested Reading

1. Barr RC, Spach MS, Herman-Giddens: Selection of the number and positions of measuring locations for electrocardiography. *IEEE Trans Biomed Eng* **18**:125, 1971.
2. Brody DA, Coeland DG: The principles of oesophageal electrocardiography. *Am Heart J* **57**:3, 1959.
3. Burger HC, van Millan JB: Heart vector and leads I, II and III. *Br Heart J* **8**:157, 1946.
4. Damato AN et al: Recording of specialised condition fibers CAV nodal, His bundle and right bundle branch in man using an electrode catheter technique. *Circulation* **39**:435, 1969.
5. Frank E: Determination of the electrical centre of ventricular depolarisation in the human heart. *Am Heart J* **46**:670, 1955.
6. Goldberger E: Unipolar Lead Electrocardiography, 2nd ed: Philadelphia: Lea and Febiger, 1950.
7. Hammill SC, Pritchett EL: Simplified oesophageal electrocardiography using bipolar recording leads. *Ann Intern Med* **95**:14, 1981.
8. Helm RA, Chou T: Electrocardiographic leads. *Am J Cardiol* **14**:317, 1964.
9. Helm RA: An accurate lead system for spatial vector-cardiography. *Am Heart J* **53**:415, 1957.
10. Helm RA: The vectocardiographic derivation of sacalar leads. *Am Heart J* **46**:519, 1953.
11. Horan L, Flowers N, Brody D: Principal factor wave forms of the theoretic QRS complex. *Circulation reference* **15**:131, 1964.
12. McFee R, Parungao A: An orthogonal lead system for clinical electrocardiogrphy. *Am Heart J* **62**:93. 1961.
13. Shaw M et al: Oesophageal electrocardiography in acute cardiac care. Efficacy and diagnostic value of a new technique. *Am J Med* **82**:689, 1987.
14. Sodi-Pallares D, Bisteni A, Medrano GA, et al: The activation of the free walls in the dog's heart: In normal conditions of the free walls in the dog's heart: In normal conditions main left bundle branch block. *Am Heart J* **49**:587, 1955.

3

Action Potentials
and Waveforms

- Action potentials and waveforms; various states of membrane action potential and recording of depolarisation and repolarisation as waveforms
- The genesis of P wave (atrial depolarisation wave) and its recording in various leads
- Ventricular activation complex; the genesis of QRS in different leads
- Intrinsicoid deflection or ventricular activation time (VAT)
- Physiology of R wave progression

CHARGED OR POLARISED OR RESTING MEMBRANE

Normally at rest, the membrane is said to be charged or polarised due to the presence of positive (+) charge outside the membrane of cardiac cells; while inside of the membrane is less positively charged or said to be negative (-). The outside positive (+) charge is due to sodium (Na^+) ions and calcium (Ca^{++}) ions. The less positive or negative charge (-) inside the membrane is due to potassium (K^+) ions. The potential difference due to these charges is called 'action potential'. These cations are unable to cross the membrane at rest. Inside the cell, the cation (K^+) dominates, and at rest keeps the membrane positively charged on outside and negative charge inside. This movement of ions in the resting stage of muscle is called *phase 4* of action potential.

Depolarisation : When a stimulus, say electric current is applied to the resting cell, it gets electrically activated and flow of ions occurs, i.e. sodium moves inside the cell through fast channels and calcium moves through slow channels and make the inside of the cell as electrically positive (+), while flow of potassium from inside to outside makes the outside surface of the cell electrically negative (-). This reversal of polarity is called *depolarisation or phase zero (0) of the*

action potential. During depolarisation, the muscle is activated to contract (mechanical event). Depolarisation, is an electrical process that can be recorded on the ECG in waveforms. Therefore, P wave on the ECG indicates atrial depolarisation, while QRS complex indicates ventricular depolarisation of phase 0 of the action potential (Fig. 3.1).

Repolarisation: Action potential has five phases (0,1,2,3,4) out of which, phase 1,2, and 3 occur during repolarisation. Immediately after depolarisation (Phase 0), the repolarisation occurs simultaneously during which muscle cells try to return to their previous resting phase after passing through the process called *repolarisation*, which can be recorded on the ECG as waveforms or segments. The ST segment and T wave on ECG represent repolarisation, which includes three phases (1,2,3) of action potential. The aim of repolarisation is to bring the cell back to resting state so that process can be repeated again. The three phases of repolarisation are diagrammatically represented in the Figure 3.2.

GENERATION OF ACTION POTENTIAL IN PACEMAKER CELLS

Pacemaker cells have an intrinsic property to generate pace. Pacemaker cells in SA node or at other sites do not need the stimulus for activation, which is required

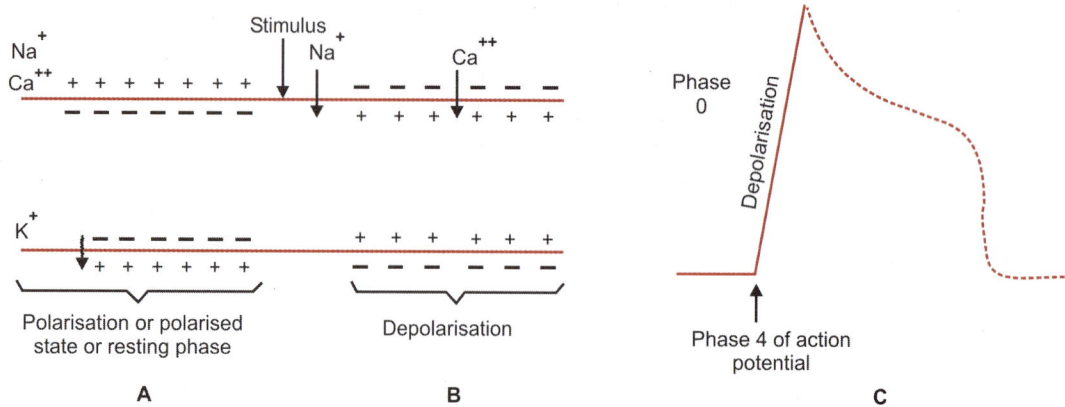

Fig. 3.1: Action potential: **A:** Indicates polarised or charged membrane of muscle cell at rest, i.e. positive (+) charge outside and negative (-) inside; called stage 4 of action potential. **B:** Indicates negative charge outside and positive inside; called 0 phase of action potential. **C:** Indicates resting action potential (phase 4) and action potential during activation (phase 0) on action potential curve

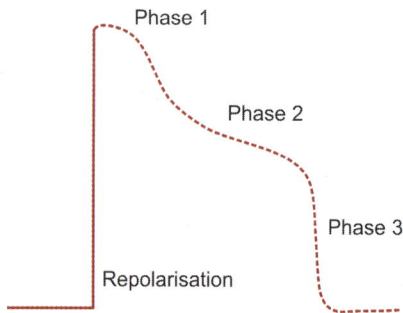

Phase 1: The fast sodium channels close suddenly, while, slow Ca^{++} channels remain open

Phase 2 (Plateau phase): Inflow of calcium to the cell is balanced by outflow of K^+ from the cell. This phase correlates with the ST segment on ECG

Phase 3: Now calcium channels also close but slow K^+ channels remain still open, which continuously leaks to outside. This phase correlates with T wave on ECG

Fig. 3.2: Phases of repolarisation on action potential curve. The inside of the cell changes from positive (+) back to its negative (−) charge

only by cardiac muscle cells. Due to this intrinsic property, they are capable of initiating spontaneous depolarisation. During resting phase 4, potassium flows out of the cells and there is simultaneous movement of sodium from outside to inside the cells-a phenomenon not seen in cardiac muscle cells. Due to this movement of cations, a critical voltage threshold is reached when calcium ions start moving

inside the cells leading to bringing of automatic depolarisation (Phase 0) as shown Figure 3.3.

The repolarisation of pacemaker cells is similar to cardiac muscle cells. The depolarisation is followed by repolarisation and the cycle is completed and repeated again.

Clinical Importance of Action Potential

The action potential forms the basis of classification of various antiarrhythmic drugs. Pacemaker cells are called *slow cells* because they are depolarised by

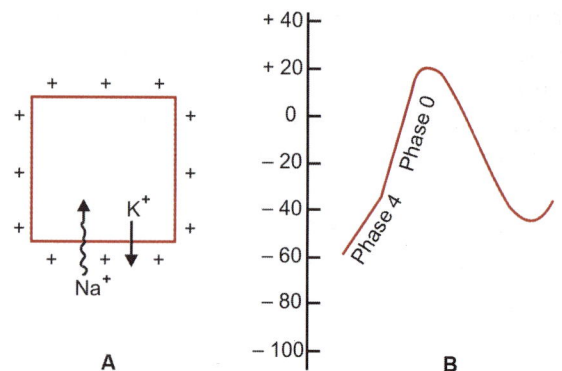

Fig. 3.3: The pacemaker cell: **A:** During resting phase 4, K^+ leaks to the outside, and Na^+ leaks to the inside of the cell. **B:** When a critical voltage threshold is reached, depolarisation (Phase 0) starts as Ca^{++} enters the cell through slow channels.
Note: The pacemaker cells are different than cardiac muscle cells. They do not need stimulus for depolarisation because they have inherent property of spontaneous depolarisation

movement of calcium from outside to inside through slow channels. The cardiac muscle cells are called *fast cells* because they are depolarised by rapid movement of sodium from outside to inside through fast channels. The various antiarrhythmic drugs act on these channels or may act at different phases of action potential to slow or retard the process of depolarisation and repolarisation, thus, used to prevent or treat the arrhythmia. The class IV antiarrhythmic drugs-calcium channel blockers, as the name suggests, block slow calcium channels and slow the heart rate. On the other hand, class I antiarrhythmic drugs block the fast sodium channels in the muscle cells, hence, are effective to suppress the ectopic focus or impulses. Based on the mechanism of action, the antiarrhythmic drugs are classified into 4 groups (see the box).

Classification of antiarrhythmic drugs based on their mechanism of action

Class	Mechanism of action
I	Block sodium channels
II	Block beta receptors
III	Block K^+ channel and multiple phases of action potential
IV	Block slow calcium channels (calcium channel blockers)

Recording of Depolarisation and Repolarisation as Waveforms

Depolarisation dipole: During depolarisation, there is change of charge across the muscle cell of the heart. The outside positive (+) charge changes to negative (-) and inside charge becomes positive (+). As both these charges move across the cell, a dipole is created called *depolarisation dipole*. This dipole consists of a positive charge and a negative charge. The positive charge of the dipole leads the activation wave. When an electrode is placed adjacent to the cell, this dipole can be recorded as a waveform or deflection.

Upright (positive) and downward (negative) deflections: An upright (positive) deflection is recorded if positive charge moves towards the electrode. A negative (downward) deflection is recorded if charge is moving away from the electrode. Hence, the direction of the waveform depends on which part of the dipole is facing the electrode and which part is away from the electrode (Fig. 3.4).

Repolarisation: During repolarisation (recharging) of the muscle cell, the outside charge changes from negative to positive. As this electrical process moves, a pair of opposite charges forms a repolarisation dipole which is opposite to depolarisation dipole. It is hereby stressed that it is the negative charge that leads the wave of repolarisation, therefore, if this dipole moves towards the electrode, a downward deflection is produced, because it is negative charge which is moving towards the electrode (Fig. 3.5). This is in contrast to the depolarisation dipole in which positive charge was moving towards the electrode, hence, positive deflection was produced.

RECORDING OF DEPOLARISATION AND REPOLARISATION AS WAVEFORMS (P-QRS-T COMPLEX) ON ECG

The recording of depolarisation and repolarisation of atria and ventricles in waveforms is presented as diagram (Fig. 3.6). The waveforms are given in the box.

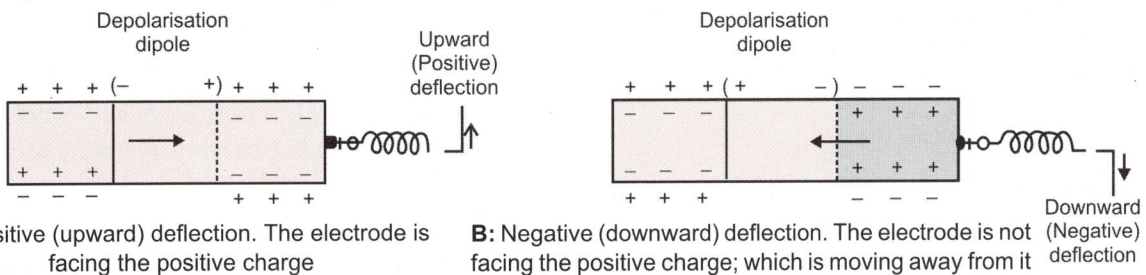

A: Positive (upward) deflection. The electrode is facing the positive charge

B: Negative (downward) deflection. The electrode is not facing the positive charge; which is moving away from it

Fig. 3.4: Depolarisation dipole and its recording as positive (upward) and negative (downward) deflections. An electrode placed adjacent to a muscle records depolarisation either as positive or negative deflection depending on the location of the electrode in relation to depolarisation. A depolarisation dipole is a moving pair of charges with positive charge leading the way
A: A positive deflection is recorded on ECG when depolarisation dipole moves towards the electrode
B: A negative deflection is recorded on ECG when depolarisation dipole is moving away from the electrode

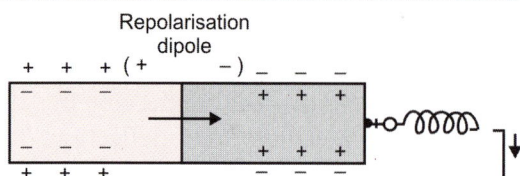

Fig. 3.5: A repolarisation dipole. In this process, a pair of charges move but negative charge leads the activation front of dipole. If this negative charge moves towards the electrode, a negative or downward deflection is produced as shown by an arrow. This repolarisation dipole brings back the depolarisation deflection to the baseline.

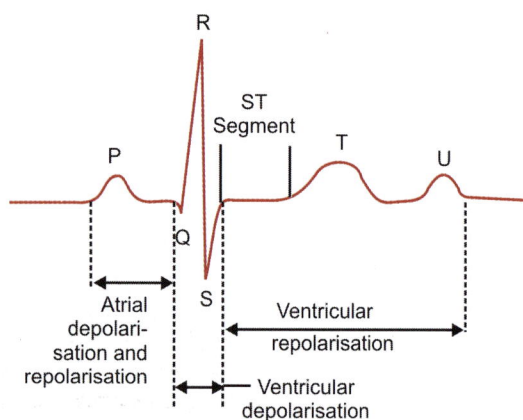

Waveforms of Electrocardiogram

The P wave: It is an upward positive deflection and represents atrial depolarisation wave.
The Pa or Ta wave: A minimal downward deflection, which is not seen on surface ECG, indicates the atrial repolarisation. This wave gets burried in PR segment.
The QRS complex: It represents ventricular depolarisation.
The T and U waves: These waves represent ventricular repolarisation.

Fig. 3.6: The normal P – QRS – T complex representing depolarisation of atrial and ventricular muscles cells

ATRIAL DEPOLARISATION WAVE (ATRIAL COMPLEX–P WAVE)

The Genesis of P Wave

The P wave represents the wave of atrial depolarisation which spreads from the SA node situated in the right atrium through both the atria to AV node via internodal conduction system. The P wave normally precedes QRS complex. It is said to be positive if it shows upward deflection above the baseline, and negative if it shows downward deflection. It is said to

be biphasic if an initial positive deflection is followed by a terminal negative deflection. It is normally positive in leads I, II, aVF and V_4 through V_6 because positive charge flows towards these electrodes. It is usually negative (below the baseline) in aVR as charge moves away from this electrode. The leads III, aVL and V_1 to V_3 may show upright or biphasic P wave because positive charge initially moves towards these electrodes but gets deflected away from them immediately, leading to a positive and a negative deflection respectively.

The P wave vector: The normal frontal plane P wave vector is directed to the region of +45° to +60°. It is oriented leftwards and superior-inferior direction, with the result the P wave is always upright in leads I, II, III, aVF, and V_3 to V_6. This is the reason why these leads are considered best for P wave analysis especially leads II and aVF. It may be upright or inverted in lead III and aVL depending on the mean frontal plane axis, i.e. if P wave vector lies between 0° to +30° (left axis deviation of P wave), it will produce an inverted P wave in lead III and, if P wave vector lies between +60° to +90° or more (right axis deviation of P wave), it will produce an inverted P wave in lead aVL. Depending on the anterior orientation of P wave axis on the horizontal plane, the upright or negative P wave is produced in V_1 and V_2 (Fig. 3.7). Biphasic P wave means initial positive and terminal negative deflection, can normally be seen in lead V_1.

The Ta wave is negative deflection due to atrial repolarisation, can be seen best in those leads which show good P wave, i.e. leads II, III and aVF. These Ta waves, if present, distort the PR segment. Most often, however, the Ta wave is not visible on 12 lead ECG as it merges with PR segment.

The P wave is always upright in leads I, II, aVF and V_3-V_6, upright or biphasic in leads V_1-V_2 and negative in aVR. Depending on mean frontal plane P wave axis, it may also get inverted in leads III, and aVL.

VENTRICULAR ACTIVATION COMPLEX (DEPOLARISATION)

Genesis of QRS Complex

It takes place in the following steps.

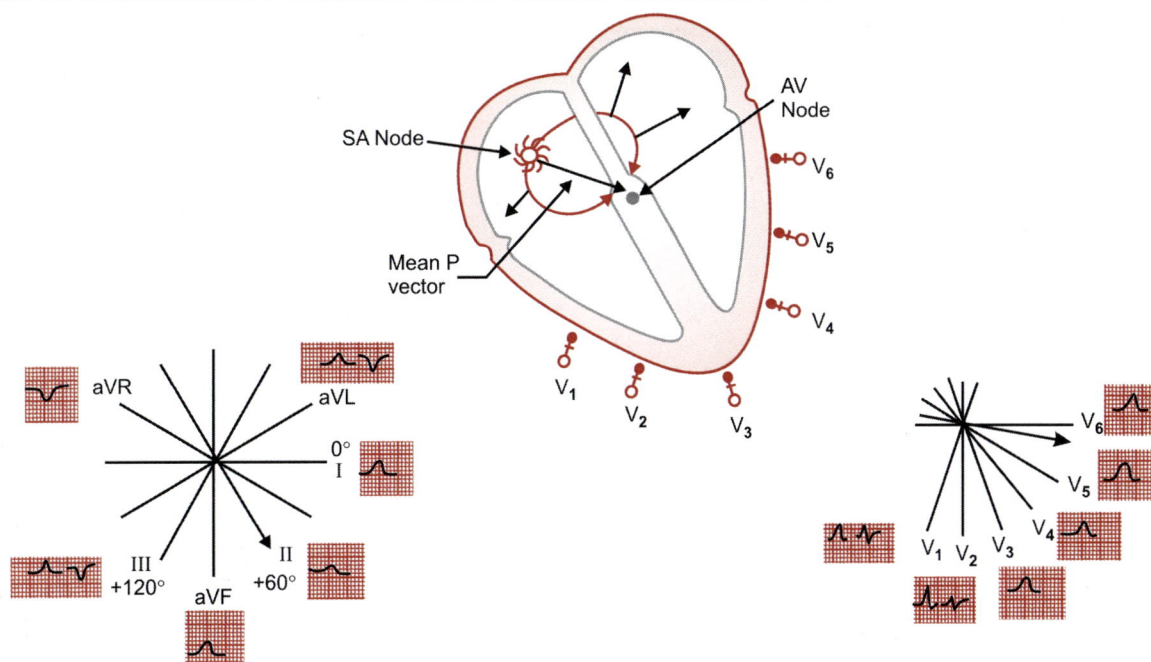

Fig. 3.7: Recording of normal P waves in different leads depending on the mean P wave vector on frontal and horizontal plane. As P wave vector normally is oriented to +45° to +60° (Facing positive pole of lead II, aVF), upright P waves are recorded in leads I, II, and aVF. Lead III will record an inverted P wave if mean frontal plane P wave vector is between 0° to +30° (left axis deviation of P wave); and lead aVL will record a negative P wave if mean frontal plane vector lies between +60° to +90° or more (right axis deviation of P wave); otherwise upright P wave will be recorded in these leads. Depending on the degree of anterior orientation of P wave vector on horizontal plane, the leads V_1 and V_2 will record positive or biphasic P wave. The lead V_3-V_6 normally have upright P

i) *Septal depolarisation* (Fig. 3.8): Activation of the ventricles begin with endocardial region of the septum from the left spreading transversely to the right (Fig. 3.8). It is opposed by a smaller activation force which occurs synchronously from right to left. The large left to right (L→ R) force dominates, hence, septum gets activated from left to right normally by this force called *septal force* or *septal vector*. This vector is of short duration and of small magnitude, produces a small q wave in leads I and V_5-V_6 and r wave in leads V_1-V_2. This septal vector may be oriented inferiorly or superiorly – in latter instance, a q wave will be recorded in aVF (Fig. 3.8).

ii). *Dominance of left ventricle and activation of both ventricles (right as well as left, Fig. 3.9)*
The wave of excitation after depolarising the interventricular septum spreads through the bundle branches to the ventricles and activates its free walls. The activation is transverse from the endocardial to epicardial surface. During the activation, two

opposing forces act; one from the left ventricle which is large , dominant and is directed from right to left; and the other is from the small thin right ventricle which is directed from the left to right. These forces occur synchronously and oppose each other. Since the left ventricle being dominant due to its muscle mass, its force counteracts the small left to right force of right ventricle, hence, the net or resultant vector of these two main forces, in addition to various small forces, is directed from right to left resulting in activation of both the ventricles and right ventricle is activated ahead of left ventricle. Therefore, this vector will produce R wave in leads I, V_5 and V_6 (Fig. 3.9).

The morphology of QRS complexes in leads II, III, aVL and aVF will depend on the frontal plane QRS axis. The lead V_1 has a small r wave and a large S wave (rS complex) and R:S ratio is < 1 normally. As one advances from V_1 to V_6, the R wave becomes larger and S wave becomes smaller with the result that the leads V_5 and V_6 have dominantly R wave with a small s wave (qRs complex).

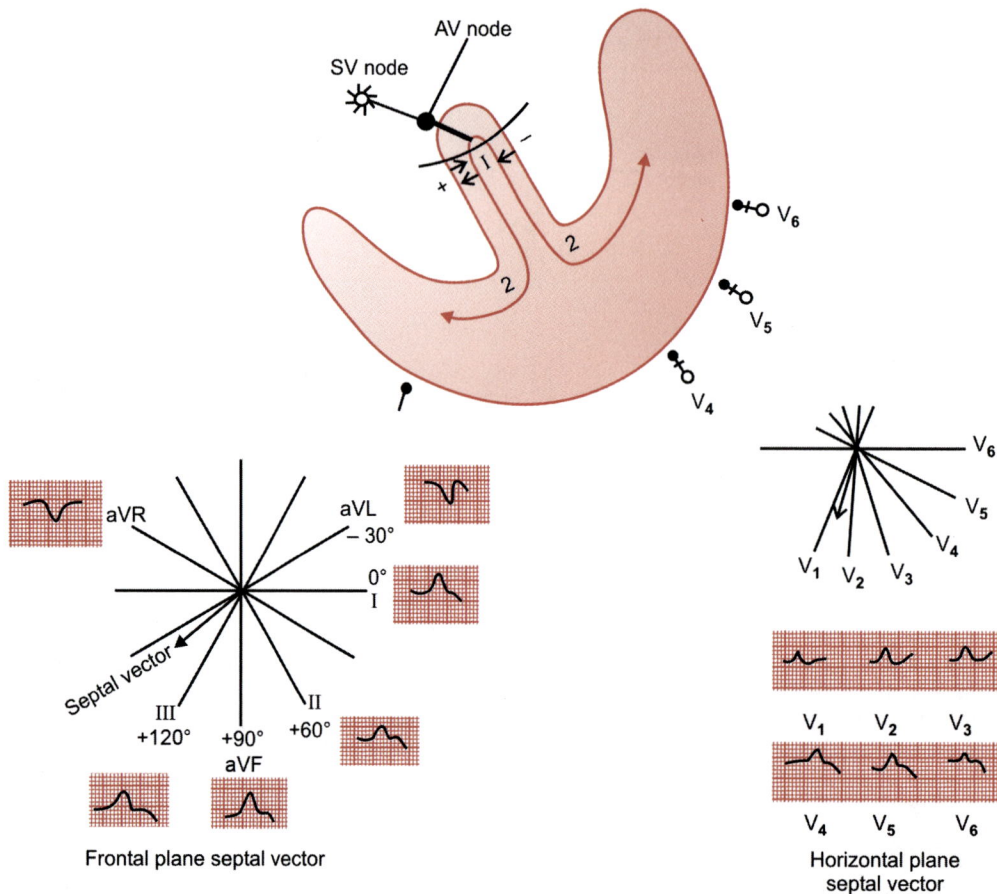

Fig. 3.8: Depolarisation of septum from left to right. The mean septal vector is oriented right and anteriorly resulting in positive deflection (r wave) in V$_1$-V$_2$ and negative deflection (q wave) in leads I, aVL, V$_5$-V$_6$

Resultant vector is a force which reflects the resultant electrical activity of several synchronous electrical vectors (forces) travelling in different directions. The mean QRS force is directed to the left, inferiorly and somewhat posteriorly, leads to inscription of R wave in V$_5$-V$_6$ and S wave in leads V$_1$-V$_2$.

iii) Activation of posterobasal portions of the heart, pulmonary conus and uppermost part of interventricular septum: The late mean QRS vector is oriented to the right producing a small s wave in leads I and V$_5$- V$_6$ (Fig. 3.10). Thus, a qRs complex is recorded normally in these leads. In 5% cases of normal adult population, it is directed anteriorly leading to terminal r´ wave in V$_1$-V$_2$ called rsr´ complex.

Activation of posterobasal parts of the heart leads to inscription of S wave in leads V$_4$-V$_6$ and occasional r´ wave in leads V$_1$-V$_2$.

iv) Ventricular repolarisation: Ventricular repolarisation produces an isoelectric ST segment and, T and U waves. The T waves may be upright or inverted depending on the mean T wave vector which is oriented to the left, inferiorly (0° to +90°) on frontal plane and slight anteriorly on horizontal plane. As result of this, upright T waves occur in leads I, II and aVF and inverted T waves in aVR. The mean frontal plane T wave axis is in the same direction as that of QRS, hence, the polarity of T wave in leads III and aVL will depend on the frontal plane axis like QRS.

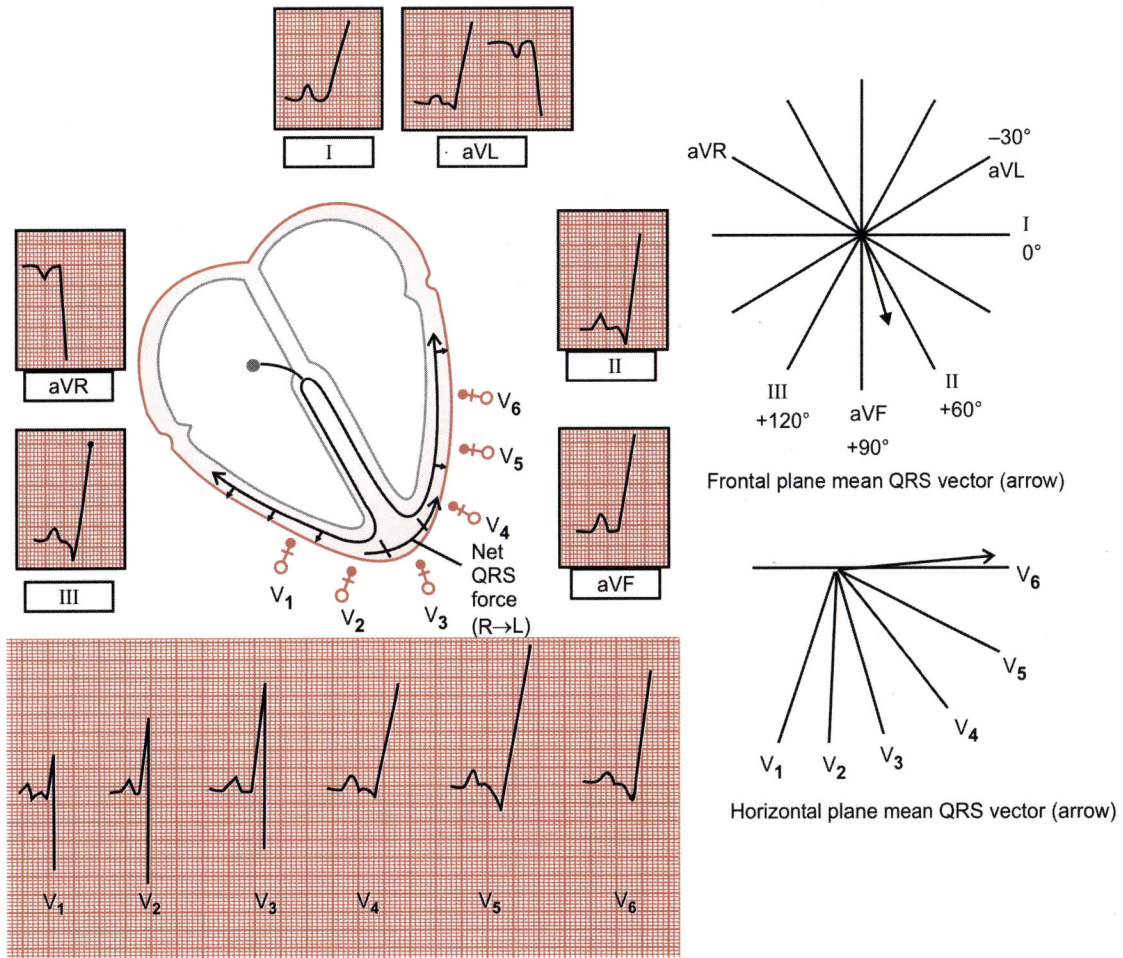

Fig. 3.9: The activation right and left ventricles by major QRS forces. The mean QRS force is directed to left, inferiorly and somewhat posteriorly registering R wave in leads I, V_5-V_6

In the same way as in QRS, if T wave axis lies between 0° to +30°, then T wave will be inverted in lead III; and if T axis is between +60° to +90° or more, then T will be inverted in lead aVL. The direction of T wave in lead V_1 depends on how much the T wave vector is oriented anteriorly, hence, it may be upright or inverted in lead V_1 but is upright from V_2-V_6. The different directions of T wave with orientation of T wave vector on frontal and horizontal plane are diagrammatically represented in Figure 3.11.

Ventricular repolarisation normally leads to inscription of isoelectric ST segment, upright T wave and U waves in all the leads except aVR.

Types of QRS Complex (Fig. 3.12)

Following three types of QRS complexes are seen in 12 lead surface electrocardiogram.

i) Right ventricular epicardial (rS) complex
ii) Left ventricular epicardial (qRs) complex
iii) Cavity complex (QS complex)

Right Ventricular Epicardial Complex

A lead oriented to the right ventricle (right epicardial lead) such as lead V_1 or lead V_2, will first face the resultant septal vector which is towards it, hence, a small r wave will be registered as an initial upward deflection (Fig. 3.12). This is followed by the large resultant vector of left ventricular free wall which is from right to left and is directed away from right oriented or epicardial leads resulting in a large downward deflection called S wave. Thus, right oriented or right epicardial leads (V_1 or V_2) will register rS complex normally (Fig. 3.12). Occasionally, a second positive deflection that corresponds to S wave of

SECTION ONE

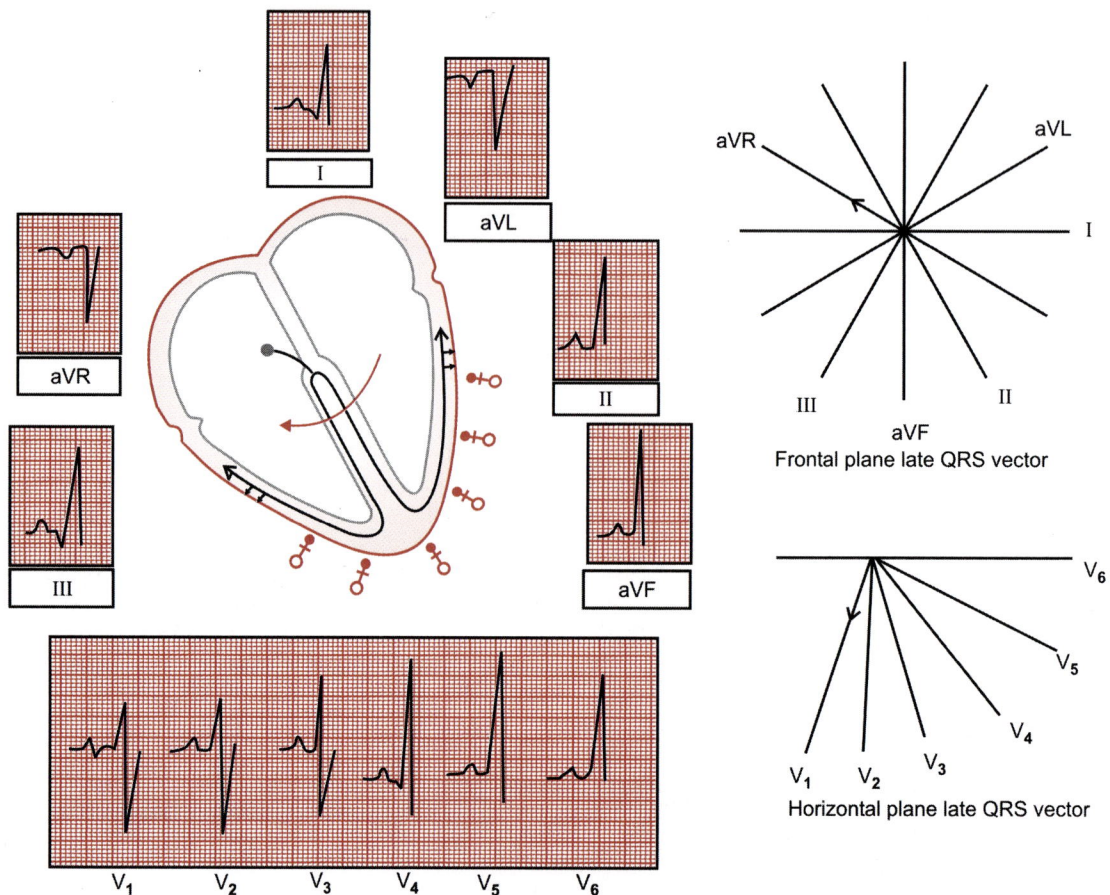

Fig. 3.10: Activation of posterior and basal portions of the heart including pulmonary conus and uppermost part of interventricular septum. The late QRS vector is oriented rightward, superiorly and anteriorly as shown by arrows. The late force produces a S wave in the different leads (I, V_4-V_6) thus completing the process of ventricular depolarisation

qRS complex may be produced resulting in rSr´ (or rsr´) pattern in V_1.

Left Ventricular Epicardial Complex

A left oriented lead such as lead V_5 or lead V_6, aVL and standard lead I, first sense the septal vector which is moving away from them, hence, will register a small initial downward deflection- a small q wave. This is followed by the large resultant vector of the left ventricular free wall which is from right to left, hence, moving towards the positive pole of these leads, thus, they will register a large positive deflection called R wave. A left ventricular epicardial complex registered by left oriented leads is a qR complex. The qR complex will normally be seen in standard lead I, aVL and V_5 to V_6 (Fig. 3.12). The terminal S wave recorded in left

precordial leads (V_5-V_6) is due to activation of posterobasal portions of the heart. Therefore, left ventricular complex may have qR or qRs pattern. Conventionally, the left ventricular complex is called as qR complex rather than qRs complex because usually no wave is recorded in right precordial leads that corresponds to s wave of left precordial leads.

The transition zone: It is a zone of electrocardiographic transition between complexes recorded by right oriented leads (rS) and that recorded by left oriented or epicardial leads (qR). This zone may be seen in one or more than one leads. The ventricular activation complex of leads V_1 and V_2 is usually rS and that of V_5 and V_6 is qR, hence, transition zone lies in mid-precordial leads V_3 or V_4. The complex in transition lead or transition zone is blend of right and left

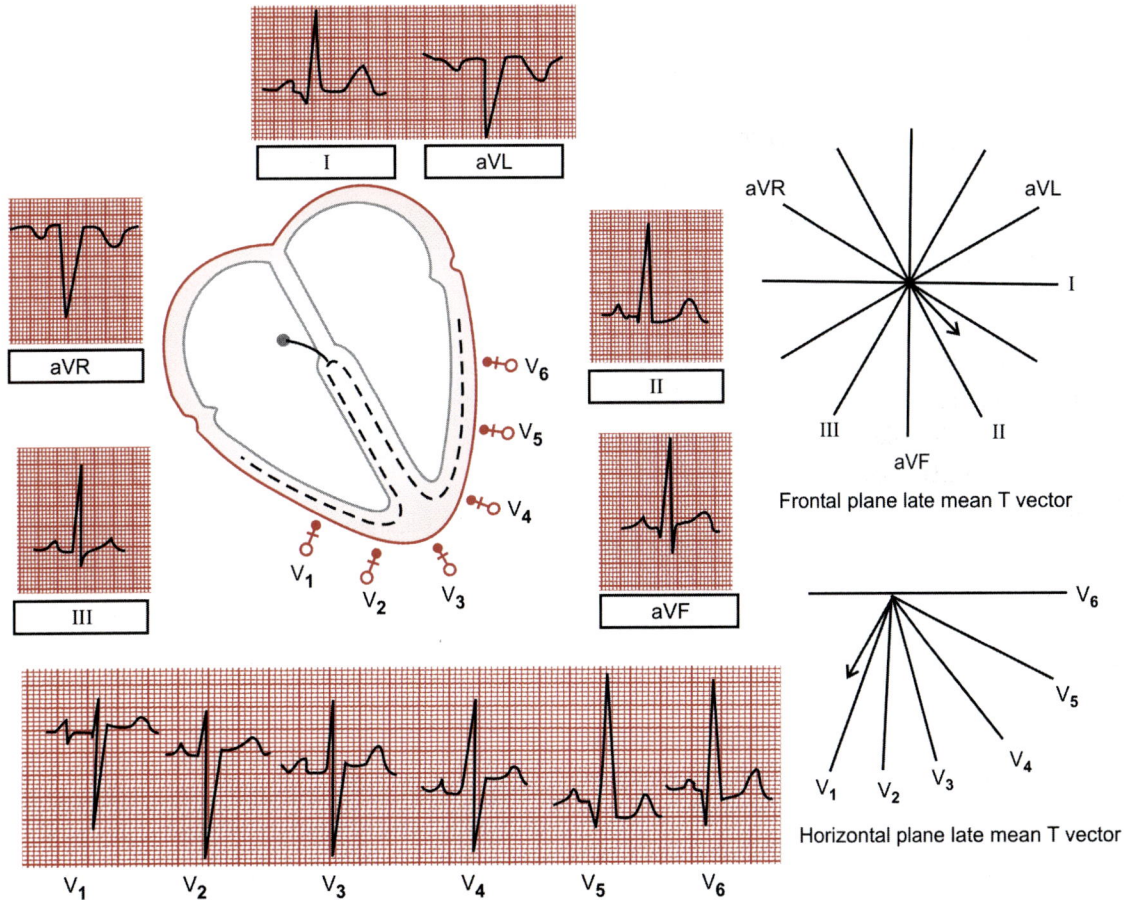

Fig. 3.11: Process of repolarisation producing ST segment and T wave in different leads. The mean T vector is directed to the left, inferiorly and anteriorly producing T inversion in aVR and aVL (both leads show cavitary pattern)

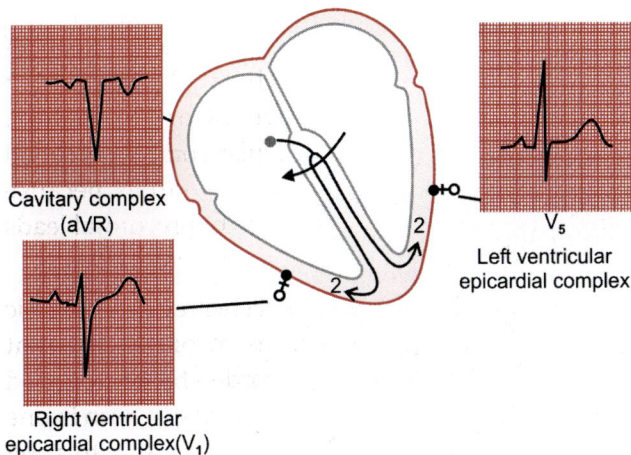

Fig. 3.12: Diagrammatic illustration of basic ventricular activation and genesis of three types of complexes, right ventricular epicardial complex (rS) seen in lead V_1 and V_2, left ventricular epicardial complex (qRs) seen in V_5 and V_6 and a cavitary complex (QS) seen in aVR

epicardial complexes, i.e. RS complex (R and S waves are large and equal in amplitude). The significance of transition zone lies in determination of electrical rotation of the heart on horizontal axis. Clockwise rotation is said to be present if transition zone shifts towards patient's left and reader's right, i.e. lead V_5 and, in counterclockwise rotation, it is shifted towards patient's right and reader's left, i.e. towards lead V_1.

The Cavitary Pattern and the Cavitary Lead

In a lead oriented to the cavity of the heart (cavitary lead), both atrial and ventricular vectors are directed away from that lead, so, the lead normally registers all negative deflections (inverted P, negative QRS and inverted T). The lead aVR is a cavitary lead where negative deflections of P, QRS and T wave are normally seen (Fig. 3.12).

SECTION ONE

THE INTRINSIC OR INTRINSICOID DEFLECTIONS

When an electrode is placed over the chest overlying left ventricle, a qR complex is recorded. The beginning of the R wave, theoretically represents the cardiac activation front reaching the muscle immediately beneath the electrode. It is also assumed that the apex of the R wave represents the time when all the left ventricular muscle mass from the endocardial to epicardial surface beneath the electrode has been depolarised, hence, the distance between the beginning of R wave to its top is called intrinsic or intrinsicoid deflection and in matter of time, it is called the *ventricular activation time (VAT)*.

Since the electrodes are not in direct contact with the myocardium, but are placed some distance away on the chest wall (chest leads) or even more remotely, for example standard leads I and aVL, so the deflections recorded on 12 lead surface ECG are not true deflections, hence, the intrinsic deflection being not true is called *'intrinsicoid deflection'*. In electrocardiography, it refers to ventricular activation time which means the time taken by the impulse to travel from endocardium to epicardium of a ventricle.

Normally, the VAT is measured from the beginning of QRS complex to the top of R wave in case there is positive QRS deflection or to the top of S wave if QRS is negative, i.e. lead V_1 (Fig. 3.13). The normal VAT is 0.03- 0.05 second in left oriented and 0.02–0.03 second in right oriented leads. The VAT will be increased due to thickness of free walls of ventricles (ventricular hypertrophy) or delayed conduction through bundle branches (bundle branch blocks) or through its fascicles (fascicular blocks). It is an important but most neglected measurement in electrocardiography.

THE PHYSIOLOGY OF R WAVE PROGRESSION

The R wave progression is a gradual increase in the height (amplitude) of R wave in the chest or precordial leads from V_1 through V_6 on ECG provided that chest leads have been placed at appropriate positions on the precordium. Incorrect placement of electrode or electrodes may make normal ECG interpretation as an abnormal one.

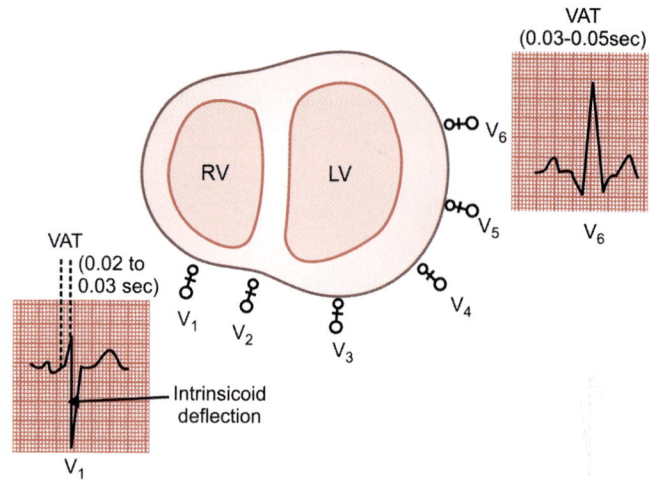

Fig. 3.13: Diagrammatic illustration of intrinsicoid deflection (the ventricular activation time, i.e. VAT) of ventricle;
Lead V_1 – a right oriented lead
Lead V_6 – a left oriented lead

Physiologically, the left ventricle is thicker (has more muscle mass) than right ventricle which is approximated to be three times, thus, depolarisation of left ventricle contributes to majority of QRS complex deflection. Since left ventricle lies to the left and behind the right ventricle, therefore, to understand about the R wave progression, one should remember how the electrical impulses are conducted through the ventricles. To repeat it once again the ventricular depolarisation starts with initial activation of interventricular septum from left to right (L→R), therefore, right sided chest leads (V_1 & V_2) face the initial electrical force, hence, record initial r wave, while corresponding to it a small q wave is recorded in leads V_5 and V_6 (left sided leads). The inferior oriented leads II, III and aVF record a small q wave due to superior orientation of QRS vector. This is immediately followed by activation of lower portion of right side of the interventricular septum and adjacent free-walls of the ventricles. A rapid endocardial to epicardial propagation of impulses occurs through both the ventricles. In normal heart, the greater mass of left ventricle predominates and the magnitude and direction of electrical forces (vectors) reflect this fact.

During normal depolarisation, the sequence of instantaneous QRS vectors rotate from rightward and anterior to leftward, posterior and inferior, therefore,

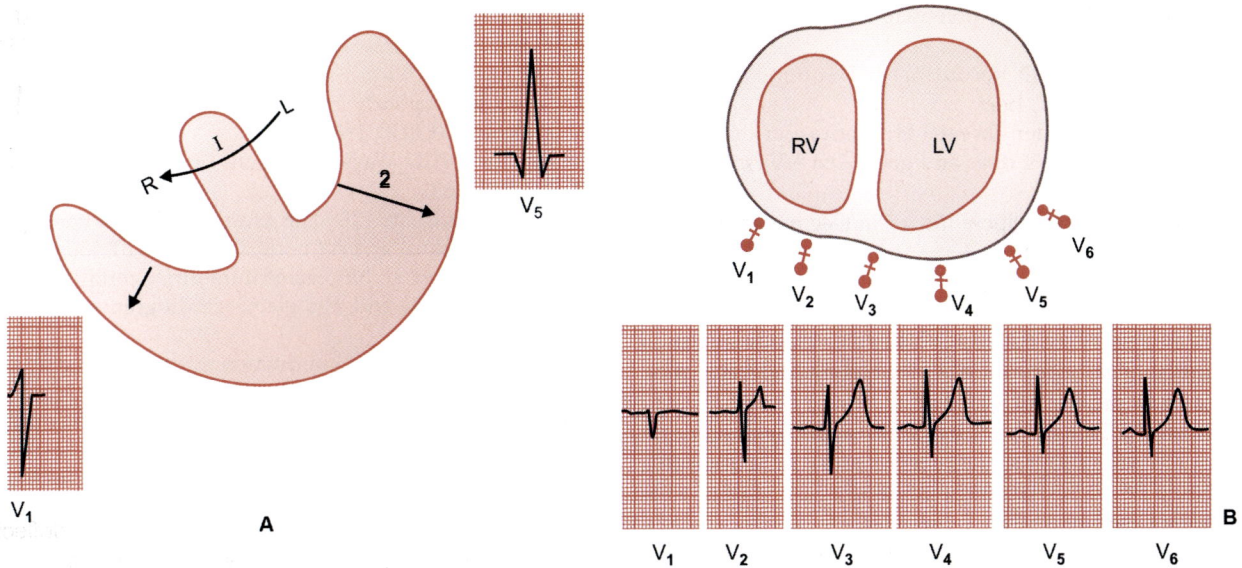

Fig. 3.14: Progression of R wave: **A:** Depolarisation of septum from left to right (L→R) produces r wave in V_1 and 'q' wave in V_5 or V_6. The remaining QRS deflection represents both right and left ventricular depolarisation, therefore, shift of the mean electrical force (vector) from rightward, anterior to leftward, posterior and superior records big 'R' wave in V_5-V_6 and corresponding deep S wave in lead V_1 or V_2. **B:** Normally, height of R wave progressively increases as one moves from lead V_1 towards V_6, a phenomenon called 'R wave progression'

the left sided chest leads (V_5-V_6) record maximum height of R wave due to maximum electrical activity of left ventricle being towards the positive pole of these electrodes. The right sided leads (V_1 or V_2) record corresponding deep S wave due to movement of electrical force away from them. The intermediate or mid-precordial leads (V_3 or V_4) show equiphasic deflections, i.e. equal R and S, hence, called *transitional leads* and underlying zone is called *transition zone*. Lastly, the posterobasal portion of both the ventricles is stimulated leading to small s wave in V_5 & V_6 due to movement of forces away from them and secondary rudimentary r´ wave in V_1 or V_2 due to movement of forces towards these leads again which is usually not seen (Fig. 3.14).

Thus, one can say that normally height of R wave progressively increases in chest leads as one moves from V_1 toward V_6, a phenomenon called 'R wave progression'. The transition zone lies in mid-precordial leads (V_3 or V_4).

Reversed progression of R wave or non-progression of R wave is usually abnormal (Fig. 3.15).

Clinical Significance

1. Reversed progression of R wave refers to tall R wave in right precordial leads, is seen in right ventricular hypertrophy/dominance.
2. Non-progression or a poor progression of R wave is seen in extensive anterior myocardial infarction.
3. Low voltage of QRS complexes where R wave progression is not clear cut, should not be interpreted as poor progression of R wave.

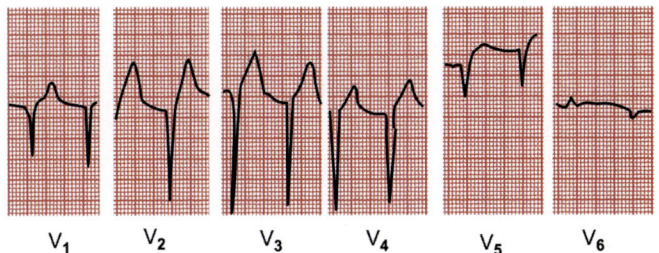

Fig. 3.15: Non-progression of R wave in the precordial leads

Suggested Reading

1. Burchell HB, Essex HE, Pruitt RD: Studies on the spread of excitation through ventricular myocardium 11. The ventricular septum. *Circulation* 6:161, 1952.

2. Cranefield PF: Action potentials and arrhythmias. *Circ Res* **41**:415, 1977.

3. Damato AN et al: Recording of His bundle activity. *Circulation* **39**:287, 1969.

4. Durrer D, Vander Tweel LH: Excitation of the left ventricular wall of dogs and goat. *Ann NV Acad Sci* **65**:779, 1957.

5. Geselowitz et al: Dipole theory in electrocardiography. *Am J Cardiol* **14**:301, 1964.

6. Hoffman BF, Cranefield P: The physiological basis of cardiac arrhythmias. *Am J Med* **37**:670, 1964.

7. Holsinger JW Jr, Wallace AG, Sealy WC: The identification and surgical significance of atrial internodal conduction tracts. *Ann Surg* **167**:447, 1968.

8. Horan LJ, Flowers NC: Limitations of the dipole concept in electrocardiographic interpretation. In Schlant RG, Hurst JW (Eds): Advances in Electrocardiography. New York: Grune and Stratton Inc, 1972.

9. Horiba M: Stimulus condition in atria studied by means of intracellular microelectrode I. That in Bachmann's bundle. *Jap Heart J* **4**:333, 1963.

10. Ipolito TI, Blie JS, Fox TT: Massive T wave inversion. *Am Heart J* **48**:88, 1954.

11. Jacobson D, Schrise V: Giant T wave inversion. *Br Heart J* **28**:768, 1966.

12. James TN, Sherf L: Specialised tissues and preferential condition in the area of the heart. *Am J Cardiol* **28**:414, 1971.

13. James TN: The connecting pathways between SA node and AV node and between right and left atrium in the human heart. *Am Heart J* **66**:498, 1963.

14. James TN, Sherf L, Urthaler F: Fine structure of bundle branches. *Br Heart J* **36**:1, 1974.

15. Kishida H, Cole JS, Surawicz B: Negative U wave: A high specific but poorly understood sign of heart disease. *Am J Cardiol* **40**:2030, 1982.

16. Marriott HJL: Ways and means of conduction. *Chest* **55**:93-94, 1969.

17. Merideth J, Titus JL: The anatomical atrial connections between sinus and AV node. *Circulation* **37**:556, 1968.

18. Millar RN et al: Studies of intra-atrial conduction with bipolar atrial and His electrocardiograms. *Br Heart J* **35**:604, 1973.

19. Sherf L: The atrial conduction system. Clinical implications. *Am J Cardiol* **37**:814, 1976.

20. Sodi-Pallares D et al: The activation of interventricular system. *Am Heart J* **41**:569, 1951.

21. Titus JL: Normal anatomy of human cardiac conduction system. *Mayo Clin Proc* **48**:24, 1973.

22. Truex RC: Anatomical considerations of human AV junction. In Dreifus LS, Likkoff W (Eds): *Mechanisms and Theory of Cardiac Arrhythmias*. New York: Grune & Stratton, 1966, 333.

23. Watanabe Y: Purkinje repolarisation as a possible cause of U wave in electrocardiogram. *Circulation* **51**:1030, 1975.

24. Wit AL, Rosen MR, Hoffman BF: Electrophysiology and pharmacology of cardiac arrhythmias. Relationship of normal and abnormal electrical activity of cardiac fibres to the genesis of arrhythmias. *Am Heart J* **88**:515, 1974.

25. Wit AL, Rosen MR: Pathological mechanisms of cardiac arrhythmias. *Am Heart J* **106**:798, 1983.

26. Zips DP, Jalife J (Editors): Cardiac electrophysiology and arrhythmias.Grune & Stratton, 1985.

4

The Cardiac Vector and the Electrical Axis

■ *The cardiac vector, the electrical axis, the electrical field of the heart and axial reference systems*
■ *Determination of mean manifest electrical axis of QRS on hexaxial reference system*
■ *Causes of axis deviations and their pathogenesis*
■ *The significance of QRS-T angle*
■ *Determination of P wave and ST segment axis and their abnormalities*

Cardiac Vector

The representation of a force by a graphic description of its direction and magnitude is called *'vector'*. The term 'cardiac vector' designates all the electromotive forces of the cardiac cycle. A vector has magnitude, direction and polarity. In electrocardiography, a vector may be projected into a two-dimensional plane as a scalar vector or considered in three dimensional plane as spatial vector. It may be used to represent instantaneous forces in sequence of the cardiac cycle. At any given instant during depolarisation and repolarisation, electrical potentials are propagating in many directions in space. Over 90% of these potentials are cancelled by opposing forces and only net force is recorded. This net electrical force at a given instant is called *'instantaneous vector'*. The mean or dominant direction of all these instantaneous vectors for a given portion of the depolarisation – repolarisation sequence (e.g. QRS complex) is called *'mean vector of QRS or mean QRS axis*. Mean, maximum and instantaneous vectors are most commonly applied to the analysis of QRS complex. The same principles can be applied for analysis of vectors of P wave, ST segment and T wave. The mathematical symbol of a vector is an arrow (→) pointing in the direction of the net potential (positive or negative); the length of the arrow indicates the magnitude of the electrical force.

Electrical Axis

It means the direction of the net electrical force in the heart. An arrow (→) that has both direction and length can be used to indicate the axis.

The lead axis: Each lead has a positive (+) and a negative (-) pole, the location of these poles is called polarity of the lead. A hypothetical line joining the poles of a lead pointing the direction of ventricular depolarisation is called axis of that lead. The orientation of each lead is different in relation to heart. The total QRS axis can be built up by analysing each of the lead axes.

THE ELECTRICAL FIELD OF THE HEART

The heart is situated in the centre of its electrical field. The intensity of the field decreases with the increase in the distance from the centre, thus, electrical intensity recorded by an electrode progressively diminishes when the electrode is moved progressively away from the heart. With distances greater than 15 cm away from the heart, the decrement in intensity of the electrical field is hardly noticeable. Consequently all electrodes placed beyond 15 cm from the heart, for example, an electrode whether placed 20 cm or 30 cm or 40 cm from the heart will record the same electrical potential. Using this principle, Einthoven deliberately placed limb electrodes as far away from the heart as possible, i.e. on the extremities—right arm, left arm, and left leg. These electrodes are thus considered to be equidistant from the heart.

AXIAL REFERENCE SYSTEMS

1. Triaxial Reference Systems

A. Standard limb leads (I, II, III) triaxial reference system.
B. Unipolar limb lead (aVR, aVL, aVF) triaxial reference system.

A. *Standard limb leads triaxial reference system*

The lead axes of the three limb leads form an equilateral triangle with the heart as the centre (Fig. 4.1). The Einthoven triangle and the lead axes form the triaxial reference system (Fig. 4.2). Each standard lead axis is separated from the other by 60°.

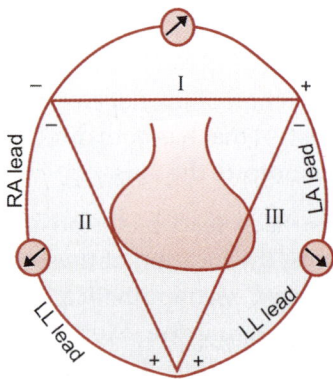

Fig. 4.1: The Einthoven triangle
- RA (right arm) → LA (left arm) = Lead I
- RA (right arm) → LL (left leg) = Lead II
- LA (left arm) → LL (left leg) = Lead III

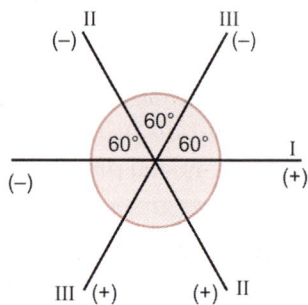

Fig. 4.2: The triaxial reference system. The lead axes of the Einthoven triangle redrawn to form the triaxial reference system

The three lead axes thus bisect each other forming a triaxial system with each of the axis separated from one another by 60°. Note the polarity and orientation of the lead axes remain the same (Fig. 4.3).

B. *Unipolar limb lead triaxial reference system*

A unipolar limb lead is made up of a positive (+) pole attached to one of the limbs and a negative pole (-) which is created by attaching the three wires of all the three electrodes to a central terminal, the potential of that terminal will be zero at all times. Each unipolar limb lead thus consists of positive potential at one of the limb electrodes and negative potential at zero is located in the centre of the heart (Einthoven triangle) which is equidistant from all its apices. The axis of unipolar limb lead is, thus, a hypothetical line drawn from the right shoulder (aVR), left shoulder (aVL) and left leg (aVF) to the centre of Einthoven triangle (Fig. 4.4). These three unipolar lead axes also form a triaxial reference system with the axes 60° apart.

2. Hexaxial Reference System

A hexaxial reference system is evolved when the triaxial reference system of standard leads and triaxial reference system of the unipolar limb leads are combined and superimposed on each other. The triaxial system formed by the unipolar limb leads is superimposed in such a way that it bisects the angles (60°) of the triaxial system of standard leads, thus, a hexaxial reference system divides the frontal plane into 6 equal intervals of 30° each (Fig. 4.4). This hexaxial reference system is used for graphing the mean manifest frontal plane electrical axis.

How to Label the Hexaxial System?

By an irrational convention, all the degree in the upper hemisphere of hexaxial reference system are labelled as negative degrees and all the degrees in lower hemisphere are labelled as positive degrees. Thus commencing from the positive end of standard lead I axis which is labelled as 0°, and progressing counterclockwise, the leads will be successively at -30°, -60°, -90°, -120°, -150° and -180°. Progressing clockwise from the same point (lead I axis at 0°), the successive leads will be at +30°, +60°, +90°, +120°, +150° and +180° (Fig. 4.5).

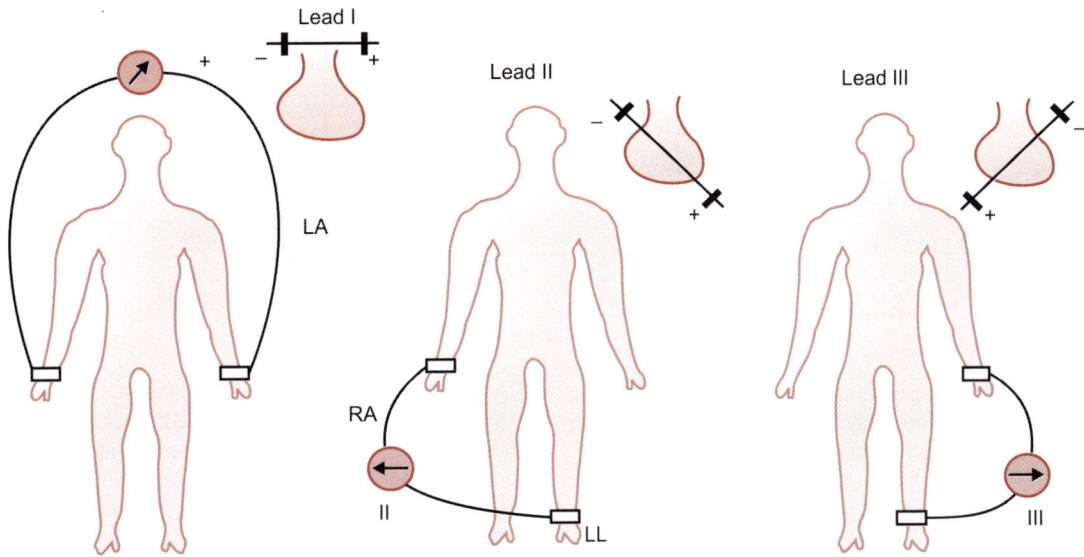

Fig. 4.3: The standard lead axes making the Einthoven triangle. The orientation and polarity of lead axes remain same

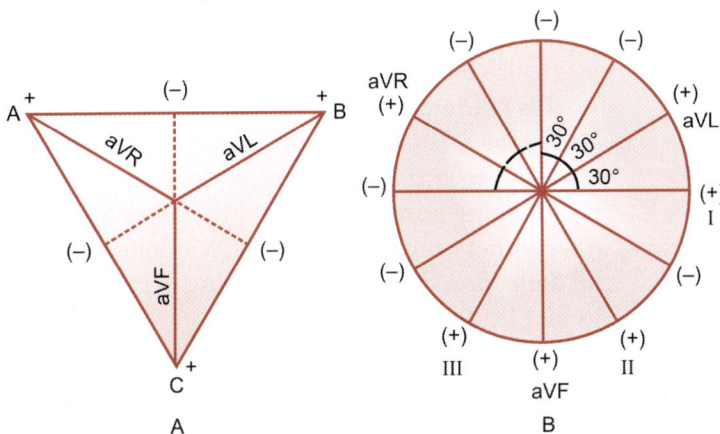

Fig. 4.4: Axial reference systems: **A:** The triaxial reference system formed by three unipolar limb leads. **B:** Hexaxial reference system formed by a combination and superimposition of two triaxial reference systems, i.e. one triaxial system formed by unipolar and the other by bipolar limb leads. Each lead axis is, thus, separated from its two neighbouring axes by 30°

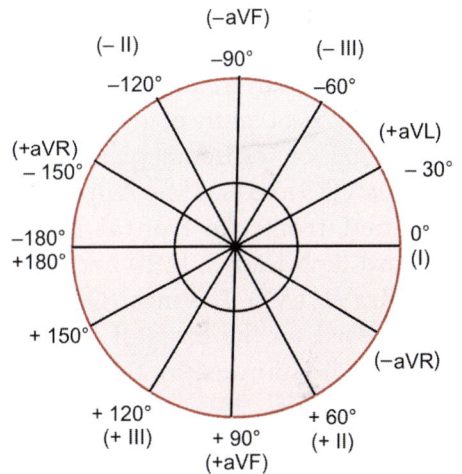

Fig. 4.5: Conventional labelling of hexaxial reference system.
NB: The positive and negative units on the hexaxial system must not be confused with positive poles of the lead axes. From the hexaxial reference system, it has become clear that positive poles of standard leads (I, II, III, aVR, aVL and aVF) axes lie from -30° to +120° with an exception that negative pole of aVR is located at +30°

SECTION ONE

VENTRICULAR DEPOLARISATION, INSTANTANEOUS QRS VECTORS AND THE MEAN MANIFEST ELECTRICAL AXIS

Ventricular Depolarisation, Instantaneous QRS Vectors

Earlier, it has been discussed, how the ventricles are depolarised. The initial activation of septum creates

(Fig. 4.6) a resultant septal vector which is directed from the left to right (vector I), followed by synchronous activation of both ventricles from the endocardial to epicardial surface through the free walls of the ventricles starting from the apex to the base of heart (Fig. 4.6. vectors 3, 4, 5). The larger free wall vectors dominate on the left side (left ventricle), hence, vectors 3, 4 and 5 of left ventricle (driving forces) dominate

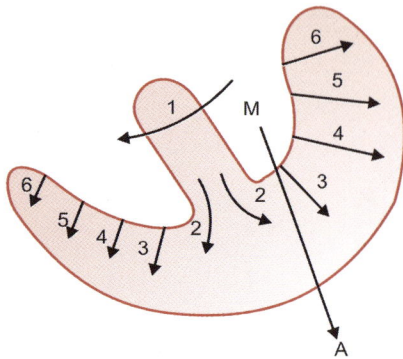

Fig. 4.6: Diagrammatic representation of six instantaneous QRS vectors. M→A represents the mean or dominant direction of these forces called 'mean frontal plane QRS axis'

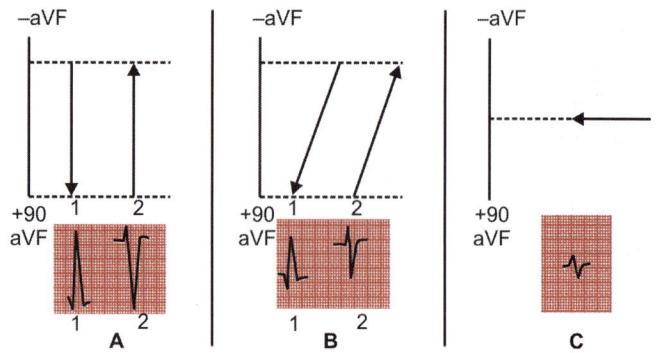

Fig. 4.7: Diagram illustrating the effect of different orientations of vectors on lead aVF. **A:** Cardiac vector is parallel to aVF and is directed towards its positive pole, hence, a large positive or upward deflection is recorded labelled as I; and if it faces the negative pole of that lead, a negative deflection labelled as 2 will be seen. **B:** The vector is obliquely placed and faces the positive pole of that lead, then positive deflection (1) of lesser magnitude than if it would have been parallel will be recorded. The deflection is negative (2) if it is towards negative pole. **C:** The vector is perpendicular to lead aVF, hence, it will record either a very small or a nil complex or a small equiphasic complex

over the right vectors which oppose them (opposing force), hence, resultant vectors derived from driving forces (left ventricle) and opposing force (right ventricle) are directed dominantly to the left. The mean of all these vectors (1,2,3,4 and 5) is called '*mean vector*' and is expressed on ECG as mean QRS vector as shown in figure by a single arrow (M→A). This, in fact is the electrical centre of gravity. The direction of mean QRS axis on the frontal plane is known as *mean frontal plane* QRS axis (see M→A in the Fig. 4.6) and is determined from the frontal plane six leads (3 standard limb leads I, II, III and 3 unipolar limb leads aVR, aVL, aVF). This mean QRS axis is graphed and expressed on the basis of hexaxial reference system, which is formed by these six conventional frontal plane leads.

Mean Manifest Electrical Axis

Determination of Mean Manifest Electrical Axis on Hexaxial Reference System (Frontal Plane)

Before graphing the electrical axis, one should know:

1. That if a cardiac vector travels parallel to a particular lead; it will make greatest deflection on that lead; and if the vector is directed towards the positive pole of that lead, it will produce positive (+) or upward deflection. However, if it is directed to the negative pole (-) of that lead, the deflection will be downward or negative.
2. That if the vector is at right angle or perpendicular to a particular lead, then that lead will record either a small or nil complex or an equiphasic QRS complex (positive and negative deflection are small and equal).

It is evident from these statements that if two leads axes are at right angle to each other, then one lead will record the maximum deflection due to vector being parallel to it, and the other lead will have either small equiphasic QRS deflections or nil deflection since the vector being perpendicular to that lead (Fig. 4.7).

3. That if the vector is obliquely oriented to a lead (Fig. 4.7B) and it faces the positive pole of that lead, then it will record upward deflection of lesser magnitude than if it would have been parallel to that lead (compare A&B of Fig. 4.7).

NB: The net positive or negative deflection in any lead is obtained by subtracting the smaller deflection from the larger deflection of the same lead. For example, in the case of a qR complex, the negative 'q' wave is 2 mm and positive R wave is 6 mm, the net deflection will be (6-2) 4 mm positive. Similarly we can calculate net deflection in 'rS' complex or any other complex.

Determination of Frontal Plane QRS Axis with the Help of an Electrocardiogram

CASE 1: When there is an equiphasic QRS or a very small QRS in one of the six limb leads (Fig. 4.8) then, axis can be calculated by perpendicular method.

Perpendicular method: The mean QRS axis is perpendicular to the lead with equiphasic QRS deflections. For this one should remember the followings:

Lead I and aVF are perpendicular to each other.
Lead II and aVL are perpendicular to each other.
Lead III and aVR are also perpendicular to each other.

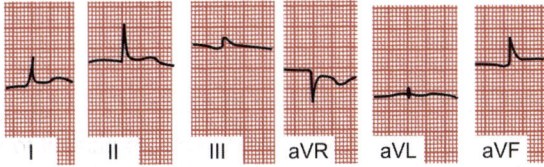

Fig. 4.8: The electrocardiogram (standard leads) showing an equiphasic QRS in lead aVL (squared), hence the QRS axis on frontal plane is perpendicular to lead aVL, i.e. towards positive pole of lead II which shows largest positive deflection of QRS

Method

i. Examine all the six frontal plane leads (standard leads I, II, III and unipolar leads aVR, aVL and aVF).
ii. Determine the most equiphasic QRS deflection or a very small QRS deflection. This is seen in lead aVL (Fig. 4.8).
iii. Based on the principle of deflection, it is evident that QRS axis must be perpendicular to aVL (since principle of deflection states that QRS axis is perpendicular to that lead which shows an equiphasic QRS deflection). Since by placement of leads in hexaxial system, lead II is perpendicular to aVL, hence, axis must be parallel to it and it must show maximum positive deflection as axis faces the positive (+) pole of lead II.
iv. Inspect lead II for confirmation of the fact stated above. Now since lead II shows dominant large positive QRS (Fig. 4.8), therefore, mean QRS axis is directed towards positive pole of lead II.
v. Reference to hexaxial reference system (Fig. 4.5), the positive pole of lead II is situated at +60°. Thus, mean manifest QRS axis of the electrocardiogram is directed at +60°.

CASE 2: How to calculate QRS axis when there is no lead with an absolutely equiphasic deflection but two adjacent leads have equal either positive or negative QRS deflection—An application of bisector method.

When QRS deflection is not entirely equiphasic in any of the six limb leads, but is either equally negative or positive in two adjacent leads; in such a situation; the axis lies midway between the two lead axes. This is demonstrated with the help of an ECG (Fig. 4.9) and axis is calculated by bisector method.

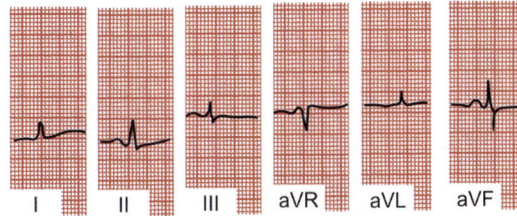

Fig. 4.9: The electrocardiogram shows six leads of frontal plane. Note the leads II and aVF (adjacent leads) have more or less equal deflections. The mean frontal plane QRS axis is +75° by bisector method discussed below

Bisector Method

Imagine by placing the hexaxial reference system with all six lead axes on the top of the body (Fig. 4.10). The positive end of lead I is at 0° and aVL at -30°. Both are directed to the left and lateral side of the heart. These leads are called lateral limb leads. The positive end of the lead II is at +60°, III at +120° and aVF at +90°; are directed downwards and reflect the inferior side of the heart. These leads are called inferior limb leads. There is one exception, i.e. positive end of aVR is directed towards the right side of the body. The negative end of aVR is at +30°, lies between positive ends of leads I and lead II, hence, is adjacent to either of the leads (Fig. 4.10).

Method

i. Inspect all the six leads provided at a glance. There is no lead which shows an equiphasic deflection or complex.
ii. Select two adjacent leads with equal positive or negative deflection. Leads II and aVF have equal positive deflection. Based on the principle of deflection, if two adjacent leads record the same pattern of either positive or negative deflection, then mean QRS axis lies in-between these two adjacent leads, i.e. towards positive pole if net deflection is positive (+) and towards negative pole if net deflection is negative (-) respectively. Therefore, in this case (Fig. 4.9), the mean axis

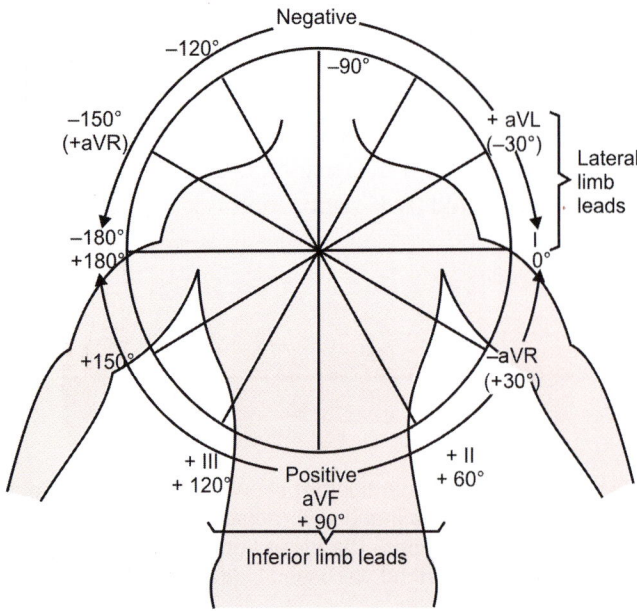

Fig. 4.10: Hexaxial reference system (diagram) with all six leads in position. Leads I and aVL are directed laterally (lateral limb leads) and leads II, III, aVF are directed inferiorly (inferior limb leads)

lies between positive poles of lead II (+60°) and aVF (+90°). Since there is no lead which has positive pole in between leads II and aVF, the leads II and aVF have equal positive and negative deflection and net deflection in both the lead is positive, therefore, mean frontal plane QRS axis lies between the positive pole of lead II and positive pole of aVF.

iii. Reference to hexaxial system, positive pole of lead II lies at +60° and positive pole of aVF lies at +90°, therefore mean manifest QRS axis is (60+90 ÷ 2) = +75°.

Note

1. The lead aVR is a exceptional lead on hexaxial system as its negative pole is interposed between positive poles of adjacent leads I and II, therefore, if aVR is selected as an adjacent lead, which is usually not, then its negative deflection must be equal to positive deflection in an adjacent selected lead for an application of bisector method.

2. Sometimes, out of three adjacent leads, two nonadjacent leads may show equal positive or

negative deflections, then also bisector method is applied which is directed to the lead interposed between two leads. For examples, out of leads, II, III and aVF, leads II and III (nonadjacent leads) have equal positive deflection, then applying bisector method, the mean axis will be towards positive pole of lead aVF (interposed lead) which can be confirmed by its maximum positive deflection.

Case 3: How to calculate QRS axis when neither there is any lead with equiphasic deflection nor there are any two adjacent leads with equal deflections (positive or negative)- an application of adjustment method.

There can be a situation, when there is neither an equiphasic complex in any frontal plane leads, nor there are two adjacent leads with equal positive or negative deflection, then axis is calculated by adjustment or approximation method (Fig. 4.11).

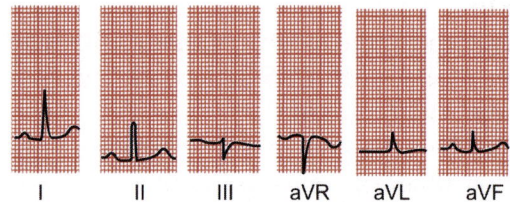

Fig. 4.11: The electrocardiogram depicting the six leads of frontal plane. Note there is neither an equiphasic nor a small QRS nor equal QRS complexes in two adjacent leads. The mean QRS axis is +10° by adjustment method (discussed below)

Adjustment Method or Approximation Method

i. Inspect all the six leads. There is no lead with nil or a very small or an equiphasic QRS complex. Also, there are no two adjacent leads with equal QRS deflections. Here, adjustment method has to be applied to get approximate mean frontal plane QRS axis.

ii. Examine the leads to find out a lead with a maximum positive deflection and a lead with maximum negative deflection. Here in the Figure 4.11 lead I has maximum positive deflection and lead aVR with maximum negative deflection. It gives an indication that mean frontal QRS axis lies between positive pole of lead I and negative pole of lead aVR. Note that positive pole of lead I lies on both sides of 0° (i.e. +0° to - 0°).

iii. Reference to hexaxial system (Fig. 4.10), lead I has more positive deflection than negative deflection of aVR, which means the mean frontal plane QRS axis is more aligned towards the positive pole of lead I (+0°) and less towards negative pole of aVR (+30°).

iv. Keeping in view the more positive deflection of lead I than negative deflection of lead aVR, the axis does not lie exactly in between them (0+30 ÷ 2 = 15°), but is more towards lead I, hence, it is more than 0° and lies near to +15°. Thus the approximate mean axis of QRS is +10°.

Alternative method: In this method, the net magnitude and direction of the QRS complexes in any two adjacent leads out of the three standard leads are plotted along the axes of the two adjacent standard leads selected. The net positive deflections are plotted along the positive pole of the leads and net negative deflections along the negative poles. The net deflection is calculated by subtracting the negative deflection from the positive.

The axis of each lead is divided into equal parts; and 1 mm deflection equals one part or one division. The net deflection of the two leads are represented by points, e.g. 1 mm = one point. Perpendicular lines are drawn from the last points in such a way that they intersect at some point. A line drawn from the centre of the reference system to the intersection of perpendiculars represents the approximate mean QRS vector (Fig. 4.12) and its angle represents the axis of the QRS complex in the frontal plane. Nowadays, this method is rarely employed. The Figure 4.12 demonstrates the calculation of axis of Figure 4.11 by alternative method.

> *By applying the same principle on various components of ECG, we can calculate the mean axis of P wave, ST segment and T wave.*

Other Methods for Determination of Axis

Quadrant Method

Consider the axial wheel of hexaxial reference system as a four-quadrant pie. The normal axis points towards

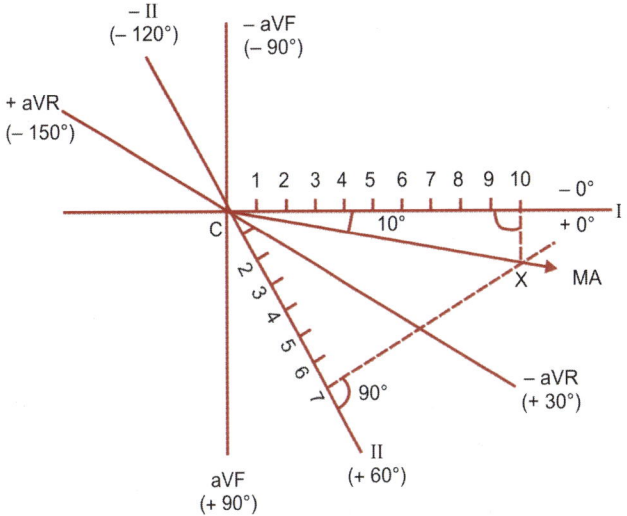

Fig. 4.12: Calculation of mean QRS axis of Figure 4.11 by alternative method (diagram). Note lead II has net positive deflection of 7 mm and lead I has net positive deflection of 10 mm. Ten points are marked at equidistant along the positive pole of lead I in such a way that each point represent 1 mm. Seven points of equal distance are marked along the positive pole of lead II. The perpendiculars drawn at points 10 of lead I and from point 7 of lead II intersect at X. Join X with centre C. The line MA (mean axis) represents mean axis of QRS

the left lower quadrant. If QRS points to the left upper quadrant, it is termed as *'left axis deviation'* and if it points to the right lower quadrant, it is termed as *'right axis deviation'* taking the normal axis as between 0° to +90°. If QRS axis points towards right upper quadrant (reader's left side), then it is termed as 'extreme right axis or extreme left axis deviation' or indeterminate axis or axis with no man's land'.

The quadrant method is easiest and quickest way to determine QRS axis. It does not give accurate measurement, but gives rough idea of the axis. By placing it inside the one of the four quadrants in the axial wheel, we can estimate the axis within seconds by this method.

The leads that need to be examined are leads 1 and aVF because they are perpendicular to each other. For sake of example, leads 1 and aVF are drawn along the approximate axis in the quadrant (Fig. 4.13). The following steps need to be examined;

1. *Examine lead I*: If the QRS is predominantly positive, the direction of force is towards positive pole of lead I or somewhere within left upper or lower quadrant. If the QRS is dominantly negative,

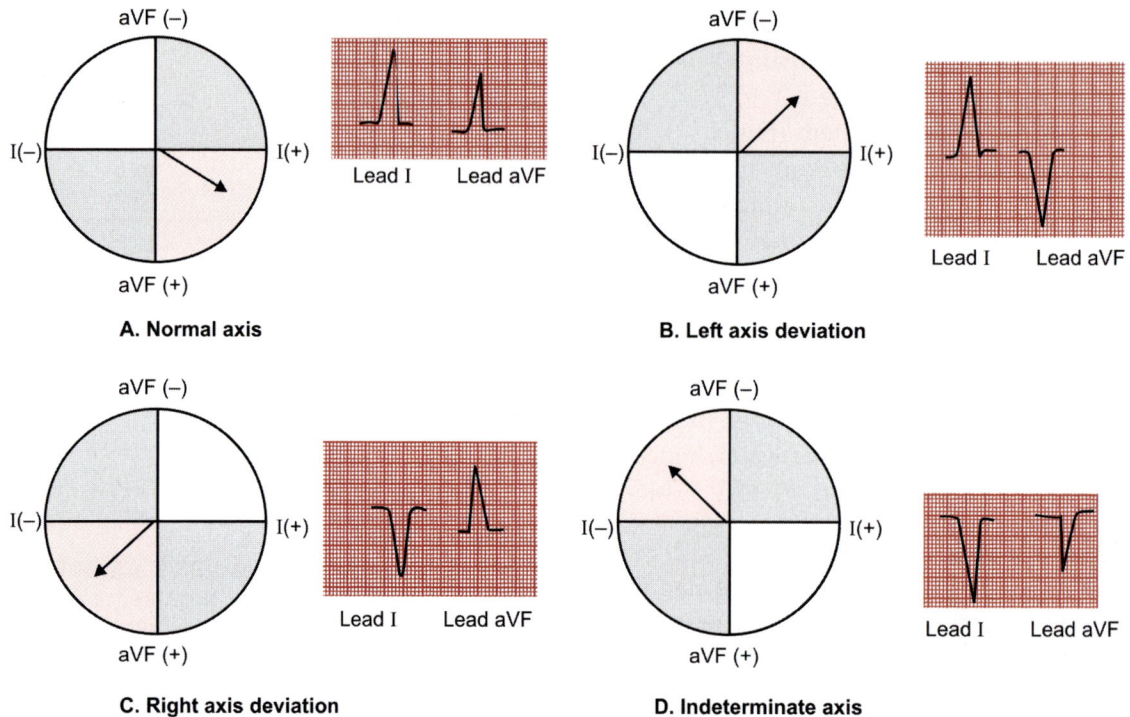

Fig. 4.13: Normal axis and axis deviation estimation by quadrant method (diagram)

the direction of the force is away from negative pole of lead I and it lies somewhere within right upper or right lower quadrant.

Shade the two quadrants corresponding to the direction of electrical force in lead I.

2. *Examine lead aVF:* Apply the same method as described for lead I and shade the corresponding quadrants depending on the direction of the force in aVF. If QRS is positive in lead aVF, shade the lower two quadrants, and if predominantly negative, shade the upper two quadrants.

The final estimate of QRS is located in the single double shaded quadrant that overlaps (Fig. 4.13).

Visual Impression Method

This gives an instantaneous rough estimate of abnormal axis deviation. In this method, two leads, i.e. lead I and III are selected. Put the QRS complex of lead III just below the lead I. If the major deflection of the two leads is pointing towards each other, then there is abnormal right axis deviation, and if the two complexes are parting away from each other, then it is left axis deviation (Fig. 4.14).

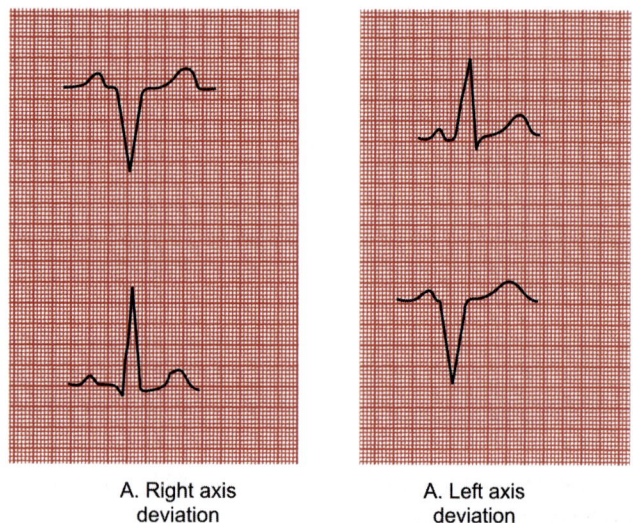

A. Right axis deviation   A. Left axis deviation

Fig. 4.14: Rough estimate of abnormal QRS axis by visual impression method

AXIS DEVIATION

The normal mean frontal plane QRS axis is usually directed to the left and inferiorly. In the earliest days of electrocardiography, the normal axis was considered between 0° and +90°, but now the normal

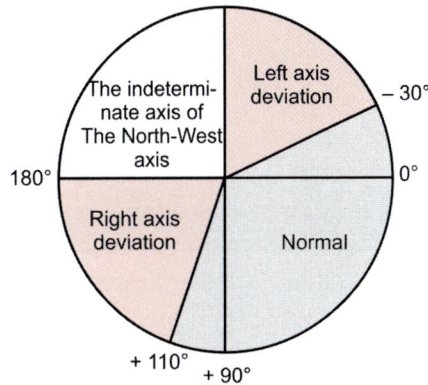

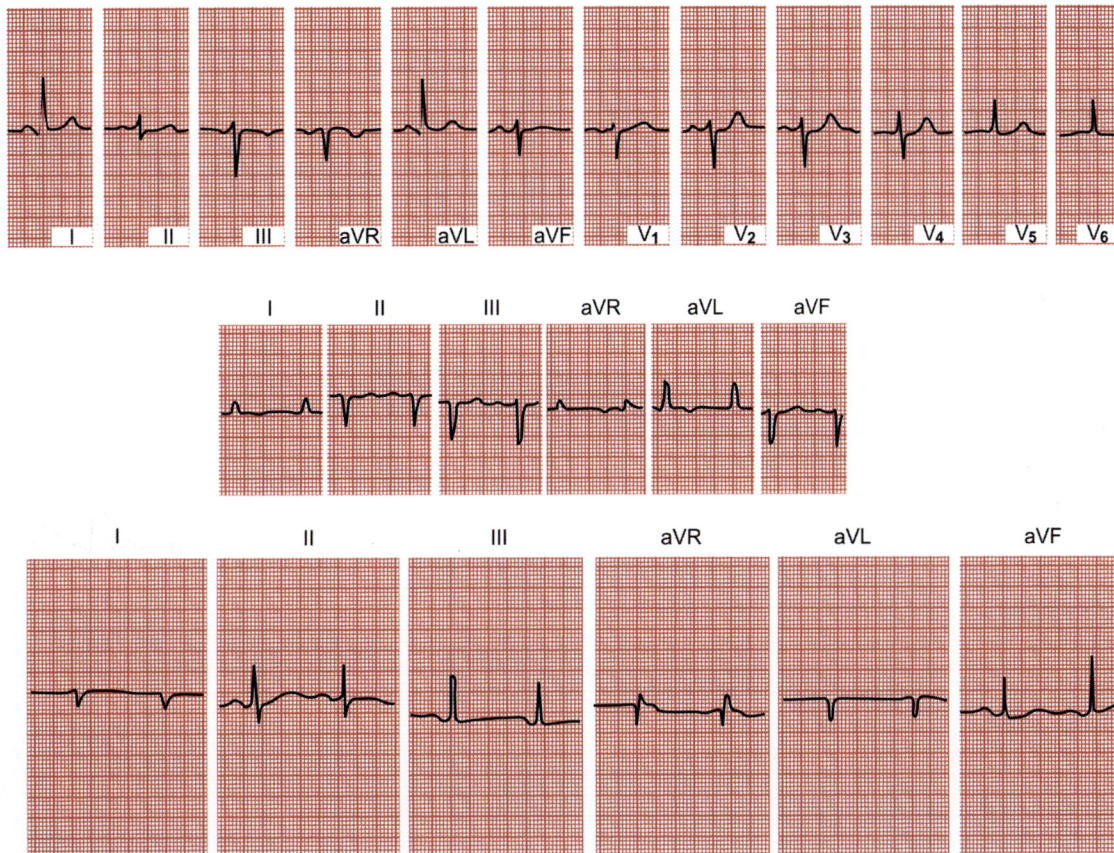

Fig. 4.15: The illustration of normal and abnormal frontal plane QRS axis

A – by diagram and B – the electrocardiogram (1 to 3) showing deviation of axis and normal axis.

1. The electrocardiogram showing normal axis of -15°. The major deflection in lead I and aVL is positive and equal, hence, axis is $0° + (-30°) \div 2 = -15°$.
2. The electrocardiogram shows abnormal left axis deviation.
3. The electrocardiogram shows abnormal right axis deviation.

acceptable variation of the axis is −30° to +110° (Fig. 4.15). The deviation of axis from normal is called *axis deviation* and it represents an abnormal direction of ventricular depolarisation. The axis between −30°

and -90° is termed as *"left axis deviation"* and between +110° and +180° as *"right axis deviation"* and both are considered as abnormal. Nowadays, left axis deviation between 0° and −30° is considered as a variant of normal due to horizontal heart position and right axis deviation between +75° and +110° represents normal vertical heart.

The Causes of Axis Deviation and Its Mechanism

The abnormal axis deviation beyond –30° to +110° or 0° to +90° (if both are considered as normal) and their causes with mechanism of production are given in the Table 4.1. In absolute terms the axis deviation between -30° and -90° is considered as abnormal *left axis deviation*. The axis deviation between +110° and +180° is considered as abnormal *right axis deviation*.

Calculation of QRS Vector on Horizontal Plane

The spatial representation of ventricular depolarisation is presented in the Figure 4.16. Six or seven instantaneous vectors in the sequence of depolarisation are also indicated by arrows in spatial orientations. These spatial vectors take origin from the centre

Table 4.1: Causes of axis deviation and their pathogenesis	
Cause	*Mechanism*
Left axis deviation (LAD)	
1. *Inferior wall infarction*	In infarction, axis tends to deviate away from the infarcted zone, hence, QRS forces are directed upwards and to the left in inferior wall infarction.
2. *Left anterior hemiblock*	Left anterior hemiblock means delayed conduction through anterior division of left bundle branch, therefore, conduction will proceed through the posterior division predominantly, resulting in shifting of QRS axis upwards and to the left.
3. *Left ventricular hypertrophy*	Predominantly QRS forces are shifted upwards and to the left due to increase in the muscle mass of the left ventricle as a result of its hypertrophy.
4. *Pacing from the apex of right or left ventricle*	When the heart is paced from the apex of either right or left ventricle, then the QRS forces are directed upwards and to the left and resulting in left axis deviation. But it is frequently directed superiorly and to the right resulting in indeterminate axis-also called axis deviation to north-west region.
5. *Ventricular tachycardia* with focus in left ventricle	Same, as above.
6. *Emphysema*	Usually, axis is towards right superior quadrant (indeterminate axis or axis in north-west region) but occasionally it may be left axis deviation, the reason is uncertain.
7. *Wolff-Parkinson-White (WPW) syndrome*	In WPW syndrome, if pre-excitation is from right lateral or postero- septal bypass tract, then, QRS axis will be directed upwards and to the left leading to left axis deviation.

NB: The effect of obesity and pregnancy has been analysed on the ECG. It has been found that obesity does not shift the axis beyond -30° left which is considered as a variant of normal axis due to horizontal heart position in this condition. Similarly, Schwartz and Schamroth found normal axis in pregnant women at full term. Thus, pregnancy is also not associated with left axis deviation or any significant change in QRS axis.

Right axis deviation (RAD)	
1. *Right ventricular hypertrophy*	Due to increase in thickness of right ventricle, the dominant QRS forces get oriented to the right and inferiorly leading to, a tall R wave in leads III, V_1 and V_2 with deep S wave in lead I. There is an associated large or tall P wave(P-pulmonale) due to concomitant right atrial hypertrophy.
2. *Anterolateral myocardial infarction*	Anterolateral myocardial infarction results in right axis deviation due to shift of QRS forces away from the infarcted area, i.e. away from the left lateral and superior wall of the left ventricle. The mean QRS will point to the right and inferiorly resulting in right axis deviation.
3. *In certain types of WPW syndrome*	If excitation in WPW syndrome is from the left lateral or left postero-septal bypass tract, the mean frontal plane QRS axis is directed to the right and inferiorly leading to right axis deviation.
4. *Left posterior hemiblock*	When conduction is interrupted or delayed in postero-superior division of left bundle branch (left posterior hemiblock), the activation of left ventricle will proceed through the anterior division of left bundle branch resulting in a mean frontal axis which is directed to the right and inferiorly.

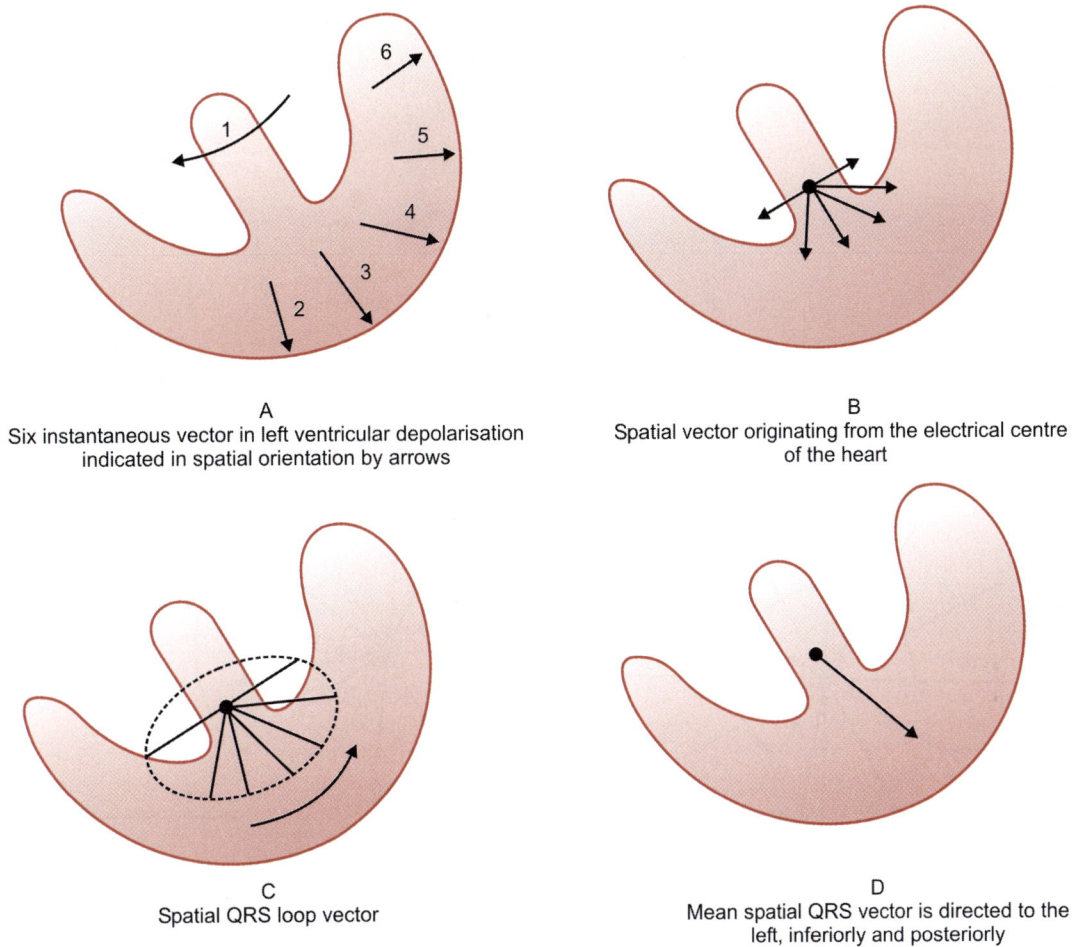

A
Six instantaneous vector in left ventricular depolarisation indicated in spatial orientation by arrows

B
Spatial vector originating from the electrical centre of the heart

C
Spatial QRS loop vector

D
Mean spatial QRS vector is directed to the left, inferiorly and posteriorly

Fig. 4.16: Construction of mean spatial QRS vector (diagram).
It is directed to the left and inferiorly

of the heart. If a line is drawn through the terminations of all spatial vectors, it produces a spatial QRS loop called *'loop vector'*. The mean spatial QRS vector is average of all instantaneous vectors and is directed to the *left, inferiorly* and *posteriorly* (Fig. 4.16).

Calculation of QRS Vector on Both Frontal and Horizontal Plane

The frontal plane, horizontal plane and mean QRS vector of the given electrocardiogram (Fig. 4.17) has been demonstrated below. For calculation of frontal

Explanation

Analysis of QRS vector on frontal plane (I, II, III, aVR, aVL, aVF)	*Analysis of QRS vector on horizontal plane (V$_1$, V$_2$, V$_3$, V$_4$, V$_5$, V$_6$)*
The electrocardiogram (diagram) reveals that net QRS voltage is larger in lead aVF than lead II and almost equiphasic in lead I. Therefore, mean QRS axis is almost perpendicular to lead I or for that matter towards positive pole (+90°) of aVF. But positive deflection is more in aVF than lead II, hence, mean axis is oriented toward aVF than lead II, hence, it is approximated to be around +80°.	The ECG (diagram) shows that transition zone (equiphasic zone) lies between lead V$_3$ and V$_4$. The spatial vector, according to law of deflection lies perpendicular to axis midway between the vectors of the leads V$_3$ and V$_4$. Therefore, as shown in hexaxial system of horizontal plane tracing of (Fig. 4.17B) the mean QRS axis is perpendicular to the bisector of vectors of leads V$_3$ and V$_4$.
The QRS axis is oriented to the left and posteriorly.

SECTION ONE

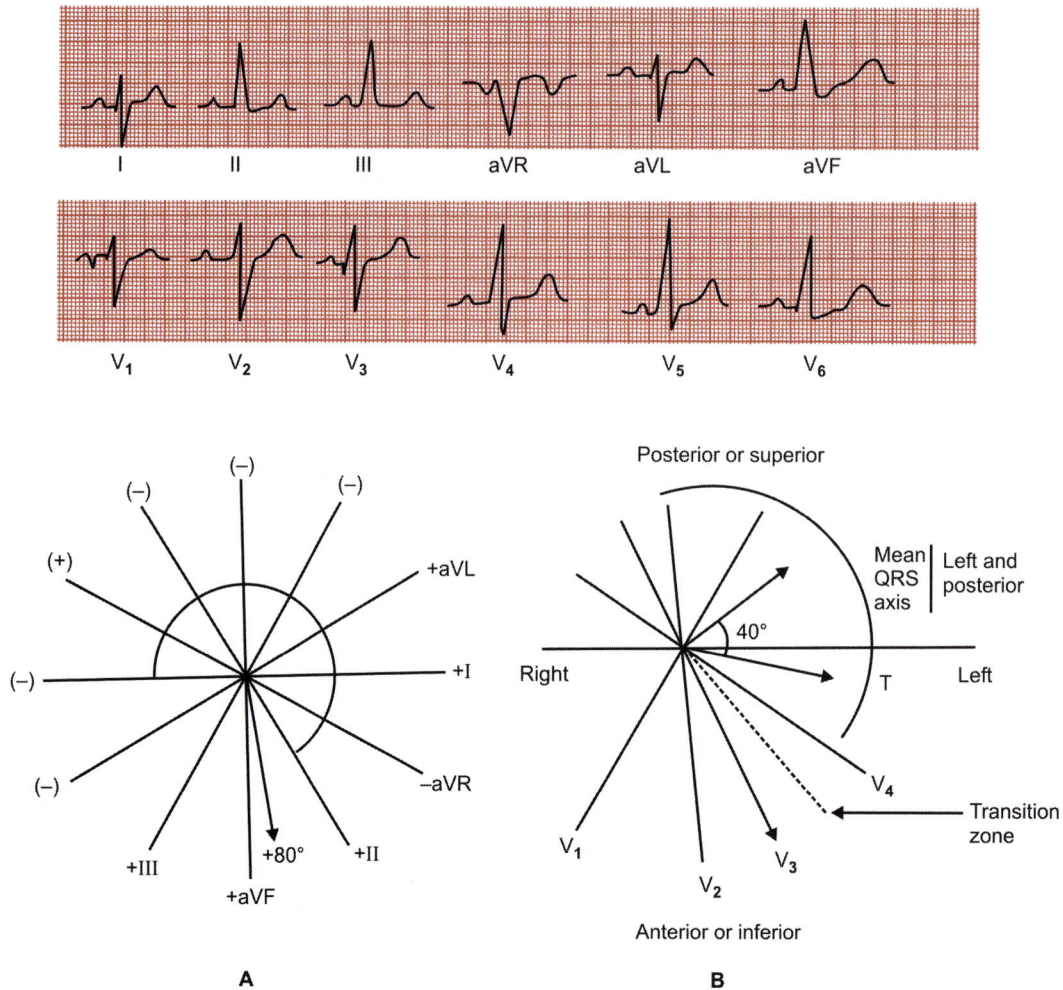

Fig. 4.17: The electrocardiogram drawn shows mean QRS axis of the +80° on frontal plane and it is directed to the left and posteriorly on horizontal plane
A: Diagram for calculation of mean QRS in frontal plane.
B: Diagrammatic representation of orientation of QRS and QRS – T angle on horizontal plane.

plane vector, leads I, II, III, aVR, aVL and aVF are analysed and for horizontal plane precordial leads V_1-V_6 are analysed.

Mean QRS Vector of the Given Electrocardiogram

When informations gathered from analysis of QRS vector on horizontal plane is added to the informations gathered from frontal QRS axis, it is apparent that mean QRS vector of ECG is oriented to the left, inferiorly and posteriorly which is normal QRS axis.

The T Wave Axis and QRS-T Axes Angle

Similar principle may be applied to the analysis of mean T wave axis which is normally oriented to the same general direction as the QRS axis. T wave axis is shown by arrow (→) as it lies towards lead I (T is taller than inverted in aVR-adjacent lead) and the QRS-T angle is 40° (labelled) in Figure 4.17B.

The mean frontal T wave axis is similarly oriented to the mean frontal plane QRS axis. The T wave axis must be considered in its relation to QRS and not in isolation. The angle between QRS axis and T wave axis (QRS-T axis angle) normally does not exceed 45°

on the frontal plane and 60° in the horizontal plane. When angle is more than 60° in horizontal plane, the ECG is considered to be abnormal and the disease is usually present. Indeed, in most cases, the QRS – T angle does not exceed 45° in any plane which is considered to be its upper limit.

Significance of QRS – T Angle

While assessing the significance of QRS – T angle, it must be remembered that the T wave axis is always directed away from the region of pathology or disease, i.e. strain, ischaemia or infarction. Thus, causes of wide QRS –T angle include;

1. *In cases of left ventricular hypertrophy and strain (LV strain).* Due to systolic overload of left ventricle as result of hypertension, aortic stenosis or due to any cause, the T wave axis gets directed to the right i.e. away from the strained left ventricle, hence, T wave is inverted in leads V_5, V_6, I and aVL (left ventricular leads).
2. *In case of right ventricular hypertrophy and strain.* In systolic or pressure overload of right ventricle due to pulmonary stenosis, cor pulmonale, mitral stenosis or due to any other cause; the T wave axis is directed to the left, i.e. away from the strained right ventricle, hence, T is inverted in leads V_1 and V_2.
3. *In case of myocardial ischaemia due to coronary artery disease (CAD).* The T wave axis is directed away from the diseased region of the left ventricle with consequent development of wide QRS –T angle on frontal plane.
4. *In fully developed acute myocardial infarction.* The T wave axis is directed away from the infarcted zone or region, thus, in inferior wall infarction (represented by leads II, III & aVF, also called inferior leads), the T wave axis is directed superiorly and to the left due to wide QRS – T angle (>60°), thereby resulting in negative or inverted T waves in leads II, III and aVF, positive or upright T waves in leads I and aVL and an equiphasic or isoelectric T wave in aVR. In anterolateral myocardial infarction, the T wave axis is to the right and inferiorly, away from the infarcted anterolateral zone, thereby resulting in positive or upright T wave in standard leads II, III and aVF, a negative or inverted T in standard

leads I and aVL and precordial leads V_5-V_6 and an equiphasic T wave in lead aVR.

Determination of P Wave Axis

This is explained with the help of diagram of 6 frontal plane leads of an ECG. This is calculated as follows:

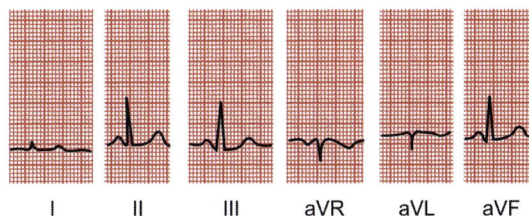

Fig. 4.18: Calculation of P wave axis of an on ECG on frontal plane. The P wave axis on frontal plane is +60° (Read the text for calculation)

1. Examine all the six standard leads. Find out the lead with most equiphasic P wave deflection or an isoelectric or negligible deflection of P wave. This is seen in lead aVL of the figure (Fig. 4.18). Based on the principle of deflection, P wave axis must be perpendicular to lead aVL.
2. Reference to hexaxial system, the lead II and aVL are perpendicular to each other. To confirm the above observation, examine the lead II again, which shows the most positive P wave deflection. This confirms that P wave axis is directed to the positive pole of lead II. Thus, since lead II positive pole is situated at +60° of hexaxial reference system, the P wave axis of given ECG is +60°.

Normal P wave axis: Normal P wave axis is in the region of +40° clockwise to +60° (Fig. 4.19). The abnormality of P wave axis (Fig. 4.19) and the associated conditions are discussed below.

ST Segment Axis

The normal ST segment in all the leads is usually isoelectric, hence, has no manifest axis; if it is deviated above or below the baseline, then it may produce measurable axis.

Deviation of the ST segment is determined by applying the same principles as used for QRS, T and

SECTION ONE

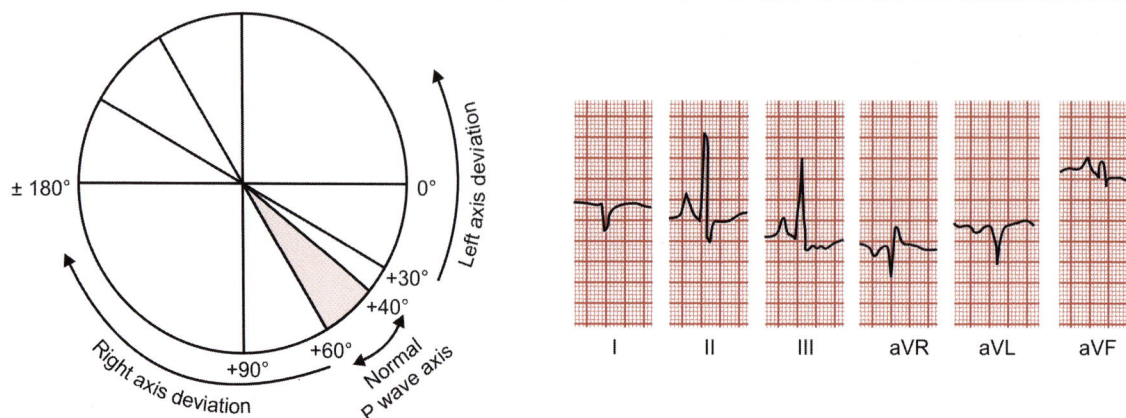

Fig. 4.19: A: Diagram showing range of normal P wave and abnormal P wave axes.
B: The right axis deviation of P waves. The ECG (standard leads) shows tall P waves in leads II, III and aVF. The P is inverted in aVL and tallest upright P wave in lead III indicates that mean P wave axis lies between negative pole of aVL (+150°) and positive pole of lead III (+120°) hence, P wave axis is + 135° (right axis deviation)

ABNORMAL P WAVE AXIS AND ASSOCIATED CLINICAL CONDITIONS

Range of P wave axes	Clinical conditions
+60° to +90° clockwise	If P wave has this axis then it is called 'P pulmonale' and is seen in; • chronic cor pulmonale • Pulmonary embolism • Pulmonary stenosis • Pulmonary hypertension
−40° clockwise to +60° or +70°	This axis deviation of P wave is seen in congenital heart disease, hence, called 'P' congenitale. This is commonly seen in Ebstein's anomaly. • P wave axis between -30° clockwise to +45° is seen in left atrial hypertrophy.
−80° to −90° counterclockwise	It is associated with retrograde activation of atria by the impulses conducted through or originating in AV node. It is seen in right-sided bypass tract of WPW syndrome.
−90° counterclockwise to −150°	It is associated with retrograde conduction from left-sided bypass tract of WPW syndrome. This P wave axis falls in north-west region called indeterminate axis.
+120° clockwise to +150° (rightward P wave axis)	It occurs in mirror image dextrocardia or due to reversed arms electrodes (technical dextrocardia). In both the conditions, mean frontal QRS axis is directed to the right. The difference lies in QRS pattern of chest leads. In mirror image dextrocardia, the QRS pattern is reversed from V_1 to V_6. In technical dextrocardia (reversed arms electrodes only), the QRS pattern is normal from V_1 to V_6.

P wave. Steps are again repeated as follows with the help of an ECG.

1. Examine all the frontal plane leads (Fig. 4.20) and find out the most equiphasic ST segment or an isoelectric ST segment. This lies in aVR of given electrocardiogram.

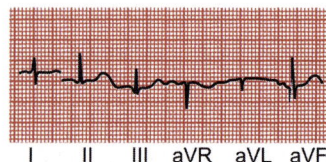

Fig. 4.20: Determination of ST segment axis on frontal plane. The ST segment axis is +120° (Read the text)

2. Based on the principle of deflection, the ST segment axis is perpendicular to aVR lead.
3. According to hexaxial reference system, lead III is perpendicular to lead aVR, the positive pole of which is situated at +120°.
4. Now inspect lead III which has maximum upright ST segment. This confirms that ST segment axis is directed to the positive pole of lead III which is situated at +120°. Thus mean ST segment axis is + 120°. If lead III shows maximum ST segment depression, then the axis is oriented to the negative pole (-60°) of lead III in that situation, lead aVL (adjacent lead) with positive pole at -30° will show upward ST segment of greater magnitude.

Abnormality of ST Segment Axis and Associated Conditions

The mean ST segment axis deviation above or below the baseline is seen in patients which coronary artery disease. The mean manifest frontal plane axis of ST segment is directed towards the surface of injury. Thus:

1. *In inferior wall infarction.* The ST segment axis is directed inferiorly and to the right, this will result in positive deflection or raised ST segment in standard leads II, III and aVF (inferior limb leads), depressed or negative ST segment in standard leads I and aVL (anterior leads facing the opposite negative charge) and an equiphasic or isoelectric ST segment in lead aVR (Fig. 4.21).

2. *In anterolateral myocardial infarction.* Just reverse to what has been discussed above in inferior wall infarction, will occur due to orientation of ST segment axis to the left and superiorly (–30° to –60°). Consequent to this axis, elevation of ST segment occurs in leads I and aVL and depression of ST segment is seen in leads II, III and aVF and biphasic or isoelectric ST segment in aVR and sometimes, may also be seen in lead II (Fig. 4.22).

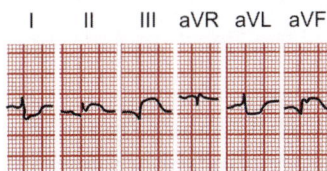

Fig. 4.21: The ST segment axis in inferior wall infarction. This is directed to the right and inferiorly. Note the ST segment elevation in leads II, III and aVF and ST depression in leads I and aVL

3. *Pericarditis*. In pericarditis, the brunt of the superficial myocardial injury occurs around the apex, hence, mean manifest frontal plane axis is directed to the apex, namely in the region of +30°.

The abnormal ST segment axis in different clinical situations is diagrammatically represented in Figure 4.22.

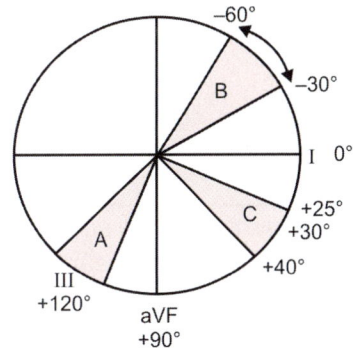

Fig. 4.22: Diagrammatic illustration of ST segment axis in:
A. Acute inferior wall myocardial infarction (around +120°)
B. Anterolateral myocardial infarction (–30° to –60°)
C. Acute pericarditis (around +30°)

Suggested Reading

1. Bachman S, Sparrow D, Smith LK: Effect of aging on the electrocardiogram. *Am J Cardiol* **48**:513, 1981.
2. Browne KF, Prystowsky E, Heger JJ et al: Prolongation of QTc in man during sleep. *Am J Cardiol* **52**:55, 1983.
3. Burckhardt D, Raeder E, Miller V et al: Cardiovascular effects of tricyclic and tetracyclic antidepressants. *JAMA* **239**:213, 1978.
4. Burger HC, Van Millaan JB: Heart-vector and leads. *Br Heart J* **9**:153, 1947.
5. Friedman HM: Diagnostic electrocardiography and vector cardiography. New York: McGraw Hill Bool Co, 1985.
6. Giardina E, Bigger JT, Glassman AH et al: The electrocardiographic and antiarrhythmic effects of imipramine hydrochloride at therapeutic plasma concentration. *Circulation* **60**:1045, 1979.
7. Grant RP, Estes EH Jr: Spatial vector electrocardiography.The clinical characteristics of ST segment and T vectors. *Circulation* **3**:182,1951
8. Hermann HC, Kaplan LM, Bierer BE: QT prolongation and torsade de pointes ventricular tachycardia poduced by tetracyclic antidepressant agent metaprotiline. *Am J Cardiol* **51**:904,1983.
9. Lipman BS, Massie E, Kleiger RE: Clinical Scalar Electrocardiography. 6th ed. Year Book, 1972.
10. Schwartz DB, Schamroth L: The effect of pregnancy on frontal plane QRS axis. *J Electrocardiol* **12**:279, 1979.
11. Zack PM, Wiens RD, Kennedy HL: Left axis deviation and adiposity. The US Health and Nutrition Examination Survey. *Am J Cardiol* **53**:1129, 1984.

SECTION ONE

5

The Electrical Rotation of the Heart

- ■ *General aspects and types of rotation*
- ■ *Positions of the heart evolved due to its rotation on anteroposterior axis*
- ■ *Rotation of heart around horizontal axis—clockwise and counterclockwise rotation*
- ■ *Effect of deep respiration on the rotation of the heart*

SECTION ONE

The electrical axis is not synonymous with the anatomical position of the heart. In electrocardiography, one speaks of heart position in reference to a pattern of ECG resulting from the spread of excitation wave. Therefore, the position of heart or rotation of heart should be viewed as differences in electrical emphasis or electrical distribution and direction rather than anatomical changes in the heart position.

Types of rotation: Theoretically, heart is thought to rotate around two hypothetical axes.

Anteroposterior Axis

The anteroposterior axis, theoretically, runs through the interventricular septum from the anterior to the posterior surface of the heart. The rotation on this axis occurs on frontal plane (Fig. 5.1) and is reflected in frontal plane leads (I, II, III, aVR, aVL and aVF). This type of rotation represents different heart positions as discussed below.

Longitudinal or Oblique Axis

The longitudinal or oblique axis runs through the interventricular septum from the apex to the base. Rotation around this axis is viewed from below the heart looking upwards towards the apex (Fig. 5.2).

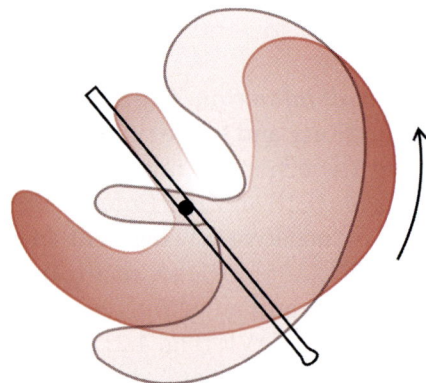

Fig. 5.1: Rotation around the anteroposterior axis (diagram)

The rotational effect is reflected in chest leads (V_1 to V_6). Rotation on this axis is called *clockwise or counterclockwise* depending on the shift of the transition zone.

POSITIONS OF THE HEART

1. Rotation of the Heart on Anteroposterior Axis

Rotation on anteroposterior axis results in different positions of heart in reference to electrocardiography. This is the most significant of the rotational patterns seen on the ECG. In the interpretation of ECG, one should determine the voltage, electrical axis, heart

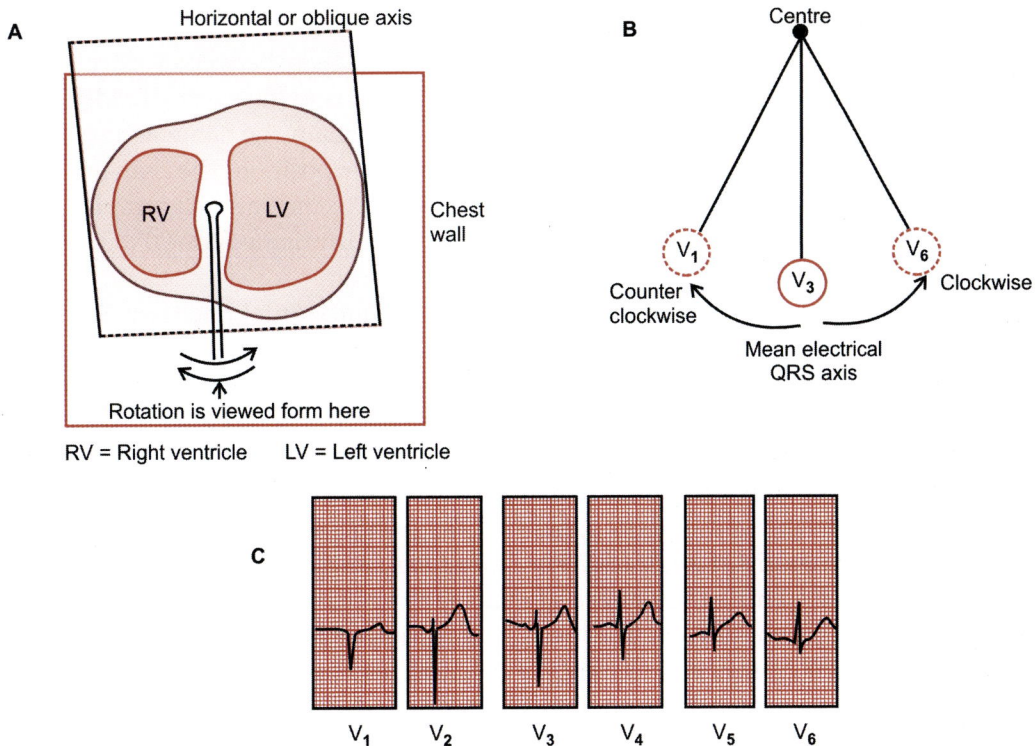

Fig. 5.2: A: Diagrammatic representation of the heart with apex removed to show rotation around horizontal or oblique axis
B: Clockwise and counterclockwise rotation
C: The ECG showing no rotation of the heart

rate, rhythm and electrical rotation of the heart to determine its position. The rotation on this axis is expressed in the unipolar extremity leads and their resemblance to the patterns seen on the right ventricular epicardial lead (V_1) and left ventricular epicardial lead (V_6).

Various Positions of the Heart

There are 5 subdivisions of this rotation resulting in vertical, horizontal, intermediate, semivertical and semihorizontal heart positions.

i) **Vertical position** (Figs 5.3 and 5.4): In vertical position of the heart, the main body of the left ventricle is oriented to standard leads II and aVF, which record left ventricular epicardial (qR) complex, and leads I and aVL record the right ventricular epicardial (rS) pattern. The lead aVR records right ventricular cavity pattern (QS or rS).

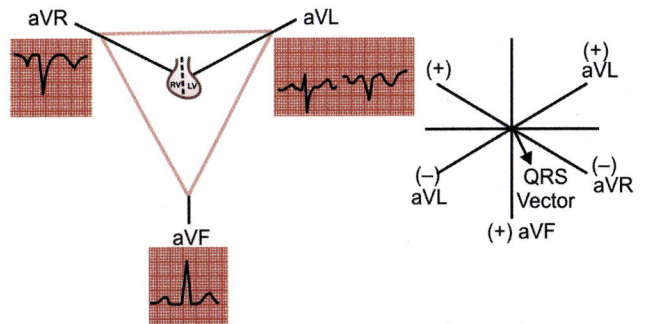

Fig. 5.3: Vertical heart position (diagram): The mean QRS axis is oriented to the left and anteriorly (+80°), hence, major upward deflection is seen in aVF and major downward deflection in aVL and aVR

ii) **Horizontal position:** (Figs 5.5 and 5.6): The position of the heart in electrical field due to horizontal rotation is such that left ventricle faces lead aVL and right ventricle faces aVF. The major upward deflection occurs in aVL producing qR pattern; and aVF records major downward

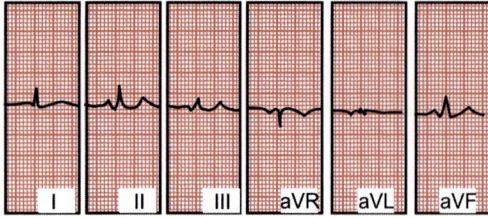

Fig. 5.4: Vertical heart position. The ECG shows qR (left ventricular epicardial complex) in aVF and rS complex (right ventricular epicardial complex) in aVL

deflection (rS), the pattern resembles right ventricular epicardial complex.

iii) **Intermediate heart position** (Figs 5.7 and 5.8): This is midway position between vertical and horizontal. The heart in this rotation occupies such a position that left ventricle faces leads aVL and aVF, hence, qR (left ventricular epicardial pattern) is recorded in both these leads. The lead aVR records either left ventricular or right ventricular cavity complex (rS or QS).

iv) **Semivertical position:** The heart occupies a position midway between vertical and intermediate positions in the electric field. The lead aVR and aVF remain the same as in vertical and intermediate position. The change occurs in lead aVL which records a small complex because the QRS vector is oriented to +90°, i.e. perpendicular ($\perp$) to aVL.

v) **Semihorizontal position:** The heart occupies a position midway between intermediate and horizontal positions. The lead aVR and aVL remain the same as in horizontal heart position. The lead aVF records a small complex because QRS is oriented to +0° ($\perp$) to aVF.

To summarise, the vertical and horizontal heart positions are still in use in electrocardiography, though actually so called a horizontal heart position is an expression of left QRS axis deviation; while so called vertical heart position is really an expression of an inferior and rightward directed QRS axis. The others

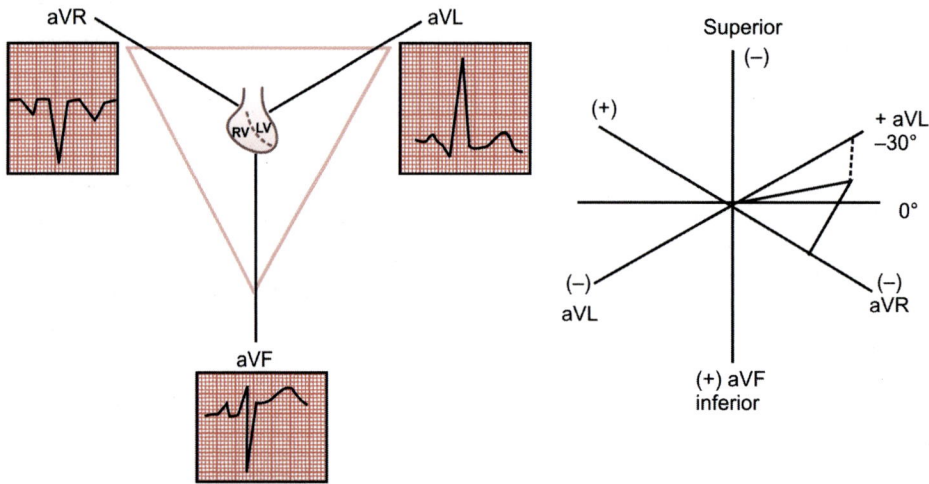

Fig. 5.5: Horizontal heart position (diagram): The mean QRS vector on hexaxial system is oriented to the left and superiorly (0 to –30°) leading to major upward deflection in aVL(qR)-resembling left epicardial complex pattern (V_6), and major downward deflection (rS) in aVF-resembling right ventricular epicardial complex (V_1). The lead aVR records all downward deflections due to cavity pattern

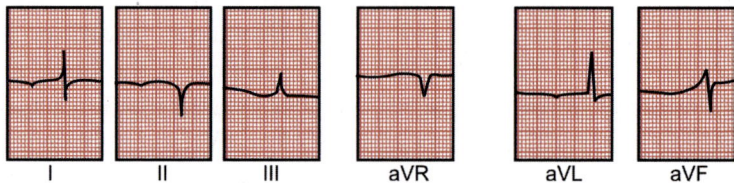

Fig. 5.6: Horizontal heart position: The ECG shows qR complex in aVL and rS complex in aVF

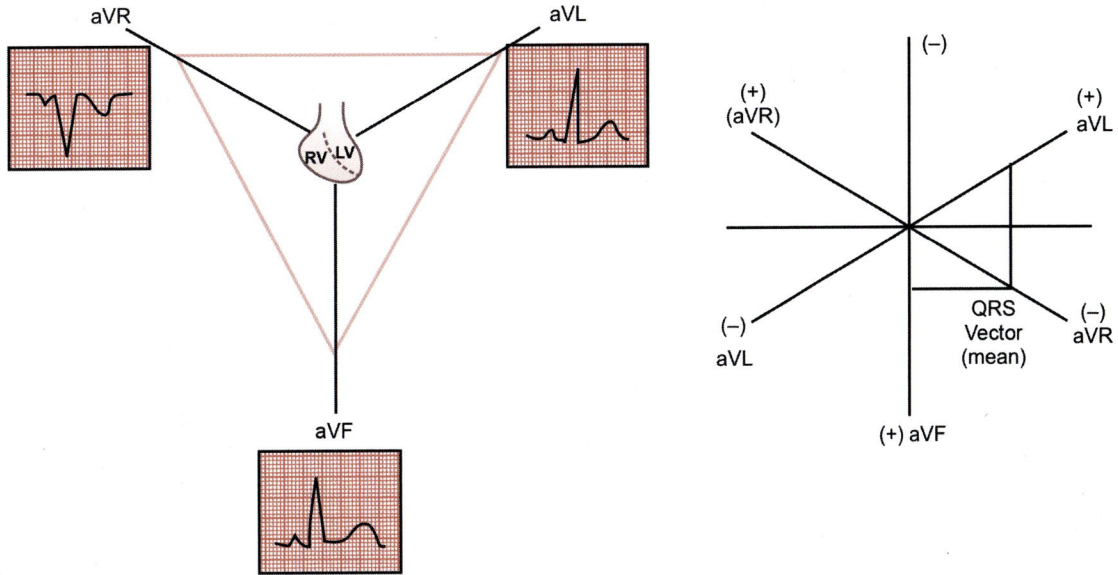

Fig. 5.7: Intermediate heart position (diagram): The mean QRS vector is oriented to the left and inferiorly between aVF (+90°) and aVL(-30°). This gives mean QRS axis of +30°. Since +30° axis is along the negative pole of aVR, hence, aVR shows negative deflection (QS) and leads aVL and aVF have positive deflections.

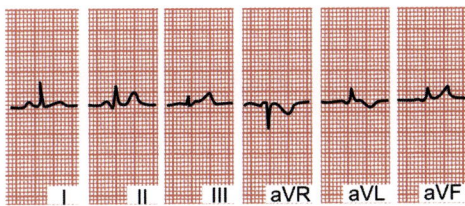

Fig. 5.8: Intermediate heart position. The ECG shows mean frontal plane axis of +30°. The leads aVL and aVF record qR complex while aVR shows major downward deflection

positions though have been described but are not much of significance.

2. Rotation Around Horizontal or Oblique Axis

Rotation on long (horizontal or oblique) axis occurs either clockwise or counterclockwise. The direction of rotation is viewed from the inferior surface of the heart looking upwards from below the diaphragm. The rotation is diagnosed from the precordial leads (V_1 through V_6). For rotation, first, find out the transition zone, i.e. leads having equal upward and downward deflections, which, normally lies in mid-precordial lead or leads, i.e. V_3 and V_4 (Fig. 5.2).

1. Clockwise Rotation

In this rotation, transition zone is shifted to the patient's left or reader's right, so that, the transition

complex (equal upward and downward deflections) is seen now in lead V_5 or V_6 (Fig. 5.9B). No such anatomical shift, however, occurs. The interventricular septum lies parallel to the chest wall at virtually all times. In this rotation, right ventricle occupies more anterior position and left ventricle is pushed behind or is hidden behind right ventricle, hence, all chest leads (V_1 to V_6) may record right ventricular epicardial complex (rS or RS). The change in the electrical pattern is thus brought about by a change in the direction of dominant horizontal QRS force-in an analogous fashion to the QRS axis deviation on the frontal plane.

2. Counterclockwise Rotation

In counterclockwise or anticlockwise rotation, the position of the ventricles is reversed. The left ventricle tends to occupy anterior position and right ventricle goes behind in such a way that transition zone is shifted rightwards towards V_1, hence, V_2 may record left ventricular (qR) epicardial complex (Fig. 5.10). The lead V_1 may have either rS or the transition complex (RS). If transition complex (RS) is seen in V_1 then right ventricular epicardial complex (rS) will be seen in lead V_4R if recorded.

SECTION ONE

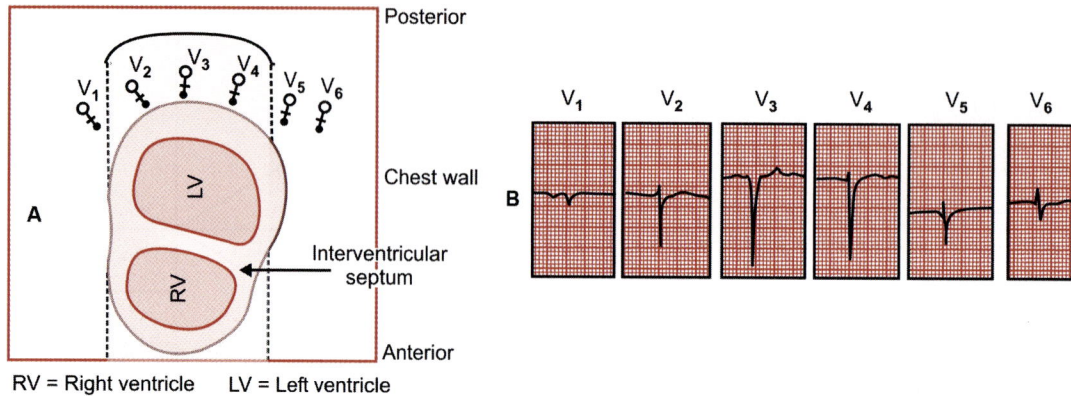

Fig. 5.9: A: Diagrammatic illustration of clockwise rotation: The transition complex is seen in V_5. Lead V_6 has RS pattern indicating that left ventricular epicardial complex has not been recorded. The left ventricular complex will be seen in any lead from V_7 to V_9 if recorded. **B:** The electrocardiogram (V_1-V_6) shows clockwise rotation of heart. Note right ventricular epicardial complex (rS) is persisting upto V_6. The transition zone (R=S) also lies in V_6

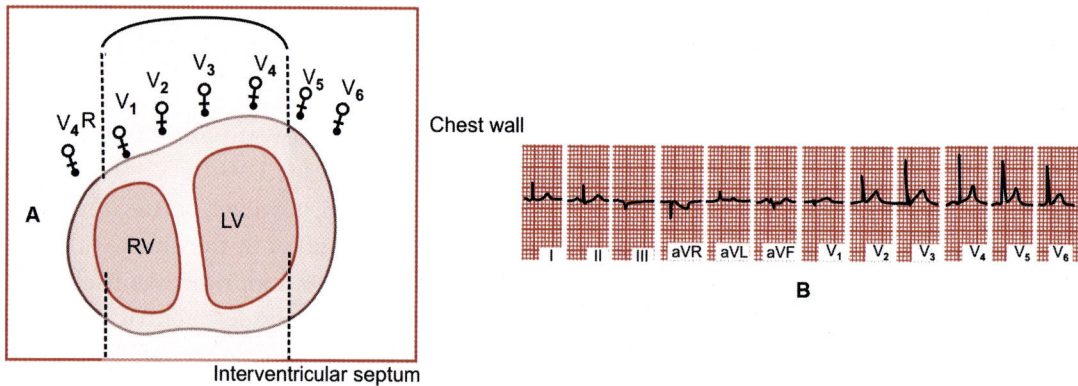

Fig. 5.10: A: Counterclockwise rotation (diagram): The left ventricular epicardial (qR) complex is seen in lead V_2 and the transition zone in lead V_1 (equal upward and downward deflections). The right ventricular epicardial complex (rS) is seen in V_{4R} (as shown).
B: The electrocardiogram (V_1-V_6) shows counterclockwise rotation. Note the followings;
1. Transition zone displaced to the right between V_1 and V_2
2. Left ventricular complex (RS) in V_2
3. Left axis deviation in standard leads

EFFECT OF DEEP RESPIRATION ON THE ROTATIONAL PATTERNS

Both phases of respiration (inspiration and expiration) can alter the appearance of ECG complexes in different leads. With deep inspiration, the heart becomes more vertical and rotates clockwise. With expiration, the heart becomes more horizontal and rotates counterclockwise. Variations in stroke volume of right and left ventricles during inspiration and expiration may also play a role in these ECG changes to some extent (Fig. 5.11). It is customary to record leads III and aVF after deep inspiration if there is a small initial insignificant 'q' wave which may disappear with deep inspiration (Fig. 5.11).

Suggested Reading

1. Daugherty JD: Change in the frontal plane QRS axis with changes in the anatomical position of the heart. *J Electrocardiol* **3**:299, 1970.
2. Daugherty JD: The relation of frontal plane QRS axis to the anatomical position of the heart. *J Electrocardiol* **3**:267, 1970.

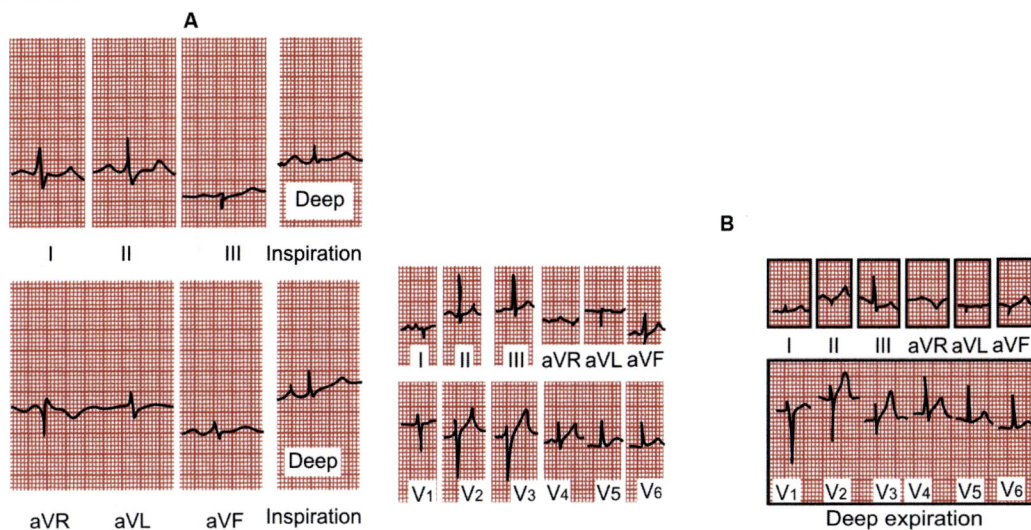

Fig. 5.11: The effect of respiration on rotation of heart.
A: The effect of deep inspiration on ECG. The frontal phase QRS axis is around + 85° and heart position is vertical. There is improvement in voltage in lead III. The q wave, if present may disappear.
B: The effect of deep expiration. It is not customary to record these leads after deep expiration. Mean frontal plane axis has shifted from +85° to + 65°. There is increase in voltage from V_4-V_6 during expiration. This is due to rotational effect of phases of respiration on position of heart changing it from vertical to semivertical during expiration

3. Daugherty JD: The relation of frontal QRS axis to age and body built. *J Electrocardiol* **3**:285, 1970.
4. Grant RP: The relationship between the anatomical positions of the heart and the electrocardiogram. A criticism of unipolar electrocardiography. *Circulation* **7**:890, 1953.
5. Johnston FD, Ryan JM, Bryant JM: The electrocardiogram and the position of the heart. *Am Heart J* **43**:306, 1952.
6. Report of Committee on Electrocardiography, American Heart Association. *Circulation* **35**:583, 1967.
7. Report of Committee on Electrocardiography, American Heart Association. *Circulation* **52**:11, 1975.

SECTION ONE

The Electrocardiogram

SECTION TWO

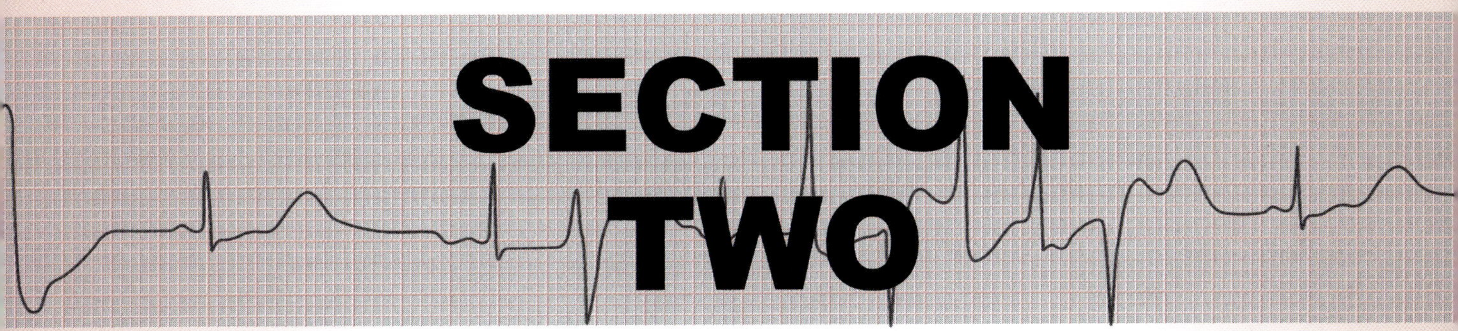

6

Normal Electrocardiogram

- *The electrocardiographic paper, standardisation, calculation of heart rate, natural pacemakers and their discharge rates and pre-requisites for good ECG recording*
- *Intervals (P-R, QRS, QT or QTc), segments (PR segment, ST segment) and junctions (R-S junction)*
- *Voltage measurement*
- *The electrocardiogram of infants and children*

The Electrocardiographic (ECG) Paper (Fig. 6.1)

The electrocardiographic paper is a graph paper with horizontal and vertical lines at 1mm distance, that intersect to form large and small squares. A heavier or dark line is present after every 5 mm. Horizontal measurements indicate units of time while vertical measurements reflect voltage. One small square on vertical measurement equals to 1 mm, represents 0.1 millivolt (mV) and on horizontal measurement (width) represents 0.04 second. Each large square is equal to 5 mm, reflects 0.5 mV (height) and 0.20 second width (Fig. 6.1). After 5 big squares, the dark line of 5th big square extends on to upper white border, acts as a time marker of 1 second (5 small squares × 0.04 sec × 5 big squares = 1 second).

Speed of the Paper

In routine practice, the standard speed of ECG paper is 25 mm per second. A faster speed of 50 mm/sec is occasionally used to visualise wave deflections better.

Standardisation of ECG

Standardisation of ECG means to adjust the voltage of QRS in order to make its interpretation easier. Standardisation is adjusted to increase or decrease the size of QRS complex. The ECG is standardised for

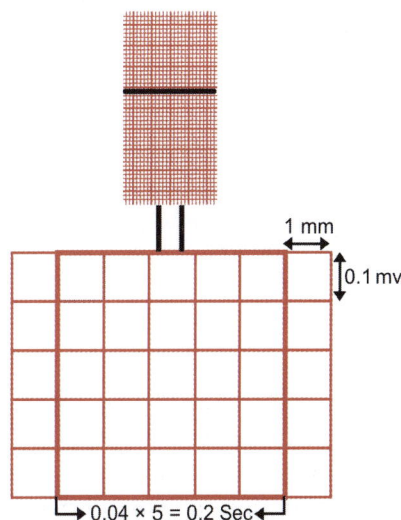

Fig. 6.1: The ECG paper. The width of each small square is used to calculate intervals of time; each equals to 0.04 second. Each large square equals to (5 × 0.04 sec) = 0.2 second. The height of each square is used to assess the voltage; each small square equals to 0.1 mV and a large square equals to 0.5 mV

accurate measurement of voltage in vertical direction. A special signal is inscribed in the recording and is seen in the beginning of the record called *'standardisation'*. The standard signal is 1 mV deflection, equals 10 mm in height (Fig. 6.2).

1. **Normal or full standardisation:** A 10 mm (1 mV) upward deflection from the baseline is called *'full or normal standardisation'* or standardisation 1.

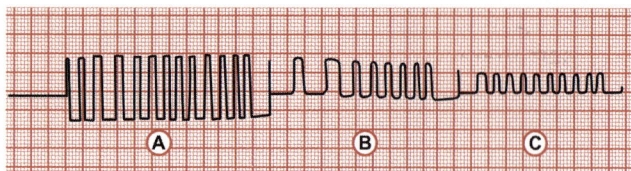

Fig. 6.2: The electrocardiographic paper and 1 mV calibration signals
A: Double standardisation 2 cm = 20 mm = 1 mV
B: Normal standardisation 1 cm = 10 mm = 1 mV
C: Half standardisation 0.5 cm = 50 mm = 1 mV

2. **Half standardisation**: Occasionally, when the voltage or height of QRS deflection is extremely high touching the upper or lower white border of the graph above or below with normal standardisation; such as in hypertrophy of one or both ventricles, then voltage is reduced to half (5 mm or 0.5 mV)–called '*half standardisation (Std 1/2)*'. For calculation of voltage of a complex, it has to be multiplied by 2 because here one big square (5 mm) equals 1 mV.

3. **Double standardisation**: If the waveforms are too small and make the interpretation difficult, then *double standardisation* is done. At double standardisation, a box of 2 mV in height is recorded which equals 4 large (20 small) squares. At double standardisation, 20 mm equals 1 mV (Fig. 6.2).

Variations during Standardisation

Undershooting (overdamping) or overshooting (underdamping) may occur when writing stylus is either too firm or too loose on the plateform or writing edge of ECG paper, so that its excursions are somewhat retarded (undershooting) or are too free to produce spikes on the inscribed signal (overshooting).

1. **Overdamping or undershooting**: During normal standardisation (Fig. 6.3A) two clear cut right angles are observed; one at the junction of the end of upstroke of inscribed signal with horizontal part and the other at the junction of downstroke with baseline. One can say that the normal inscribed signals is a box in the form of perfect rectangle with respect to baseline. In overdamping due to rigid or firm stylus, these two right angles get blunted or become rounded of (Fig. 6.3B). Due to overdamping, the electrocardiographic deflections may be diminished in amplitude and a small s wave may in fact disappears and ST segment appears as elevated-called pseudoelevation (Fig. 6.4).

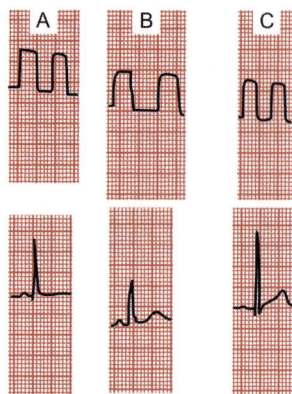

Fig. 6.3: Variations during standardisation
A. Normal standardisation
B. Overdamping
C. Underdamping

2. **Underdamping or overshooting** (Fig. 6.3C): The overshooting of the upswing and the downswing of the recording stylus which is too loose or not pressed firmly, results in sharp 'spikes' at the corners of the inscribed signal box, called underdamping (Fig. 6.3C). Due to underdamping, the deflection may be inscribed more rapidly resulting in a fractionally narrower complex. Secondly the deflection gets increased in amplitude and a S wave, in fact, may become exaggerated.

HEART RATE

It is defined as number of beats per minute (bpm). On ECG, heart rate usually implies ventricular rate which means the number of QRS complexes in a minute. Normally, each QRS is preceded by a P wave, hence, heart rate also refers to atrial rate (the number of P waves in a minute). Therefore, on ECG, both ventricular and atrial rates can be calculated if there

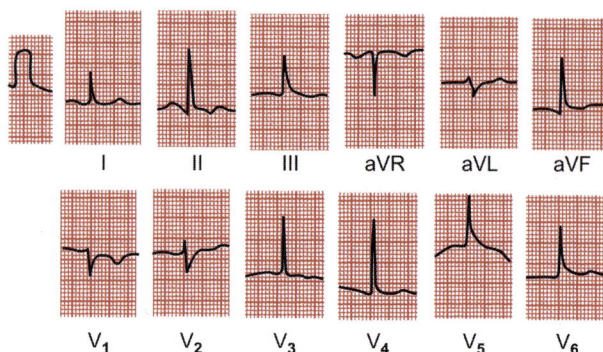

Fig. 6.4: Overdamping of stylus producing pseudoelevation of ST segment

is dissociation between atria and ventricles and their rates are unequal. Normally, there is no dissociation, hence, both atrial and ventricular rates are equal.

Calculation of Heart Rate on ECG

Whether you calculate ventricular rate or atrial rate, three methods are usually employed depending on the regularity or irregularity of the heart rhythm.

i) If rhythm is regular, then following methods may be used;
a) 1500 method
b) R-R method

a) **The 1500 method**: The method is called 1500 method because one minute on ECG covers 1500 small squares (1 big square = 0.2 sec; 5 big squares = 1 second; 60 big squares = 1 minute). This method is used to calculate the heart rate when rhythm is regular. On ECG paper, there is a time marker in the form of a darkline on white upper border, count the number of QRS complexes in-between 12 such lines and multiply it by 5 to get the heart rate in one minute or count in-between 30 such lines and multiply it by 2.

b) **R-R method**: Count the number of small squares between two consecutive QRS complexes in any lead. Dividing 1500 by number of small squares that you have counted, gives the heart rate (ventricular rate) per minute. Thus; *ventricular rate per minute = 1500 ÷ No.of small squares between two adjacent QRS complexes.* For example, if the distance, between two adjacent QRS is 15 small squares, then heart rate will be 1500 ÷ 15 = 100/

min (Fig. 6.5). To save time, students can make a chart that can be used for at-a-glance calculation of heart rate.

For rapid calculation, find out two consecutive R waves whose peak falls on the lines irrespective whether dark or light. Then count down the number of big squares and the remaining small squares between them. The big squares are multiplied by 5 and the remaining small squares are just added to it, gives the total number of small squares between two adjacent QRS complexes. Dividing 1500 by number of small squares that you have counted, gives the heart rate. This is similar to 1500 method.

ii) If rhythm is irregular, then heart rate is calculated by
a) Six second method. (This gives approximate heart rate).

Six second method: Provided that the heart rate is irregular and the 1500 method or R-R interval method cannot be applied, the six second method is used to calculate the heart rate. This is easiest but least accurate approach for calculating the heart rate. In this method, simply count the number of QRS complexes occurring within 6 seconds remembering that 5 big squares are equal to 1.0 sec for which a time marker in the form of a darkline on the upper white border is provided. In other words, count QRS complexes in 30 big squares or within 6 dark lines on upper white border, which equals to 6 seconds. Multiplying the result by 10, gives the approximate heart rate of that patient in one minute (Fig. 6.6).

Lead II

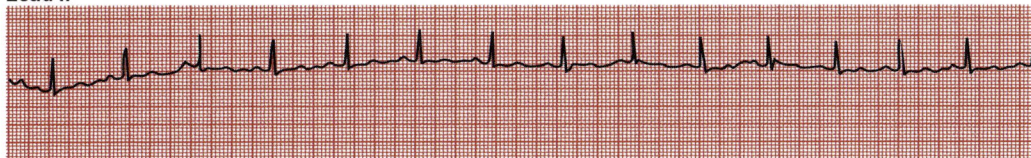

Fig. 6.5: Calculation of heart rate by R-R method: The distance between two successive QRS (R-R interval) is 15 mm, hence, heart rate is 1500 ÷ 15 = 100 /min and is regular

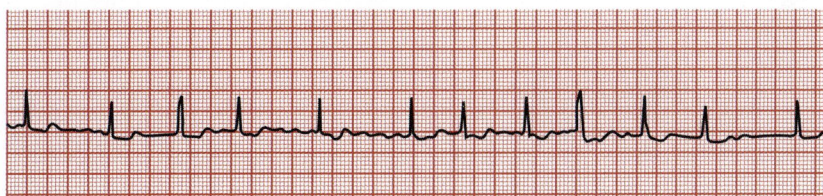

Fig. 6.6: The calculation of heart rate on ECG by six second method. The number of QRS complexes in 6 seconds are 9, hence, heart rate is 11 × 10 = 110/min and is irregular

SECTION TWO

NATURAL PACEMAKERS AND HEART RATES

The heart has an intrinsic property to generate pace. The dominant pacemaker is sinoatrial node (SA node) situated in the right atrium. The SA node independently starts the electrical impulse which is propagated. The ability to initiate the impulses spontaneously is called *automaticity*.

Subsidiary Pacemakers

Other potential pacemaker sites in the heart are;
   i) Atria
   ii) Atrioventricular (AV) node
   iii) Ventricles

   These subsidiary pacemakers sites remain dormant when SA node sets the pace. All these sites have automatic pacemaker cells, which can also initiate impulses independently, usually at a slower rates than the SA node. Normally, SA node being the fastest sinus pacemaker dominates the subsidiary pacemakers and does not allow them to generate pace.

   These lower (subsidiary) pacemakers generate the impulses when SA node fails to generate the impulses. The rhythm that these subsidiary pacemakers provide is called '*escape rhythm*'. These lower escape pacemaker sites act like electrical backup that fire at slower rates.

   The intrinsic property of pacemakers to generate the impulses becomes slower and slower from SA node to atria, AV node and ventricles (Fig. 6.6A), therefore, the rate of discharge of various pacemakers may be written as;

SA node > Atria > AV node > Ventricles

   The rate of discharge of various pacemakers are given in the information box on page 397. When SA node fails to generate the pace, and if AV node or junction takes up the activity of the pacemaker, then rhythm produced is called '*junctional or nodal rhythm*'. When both SA node and AV node fail to generate the impulses, then one of the ventricles takes up the function of the pacemaker and sets the pace of heart at slowest rate of 15-40 beats / min (bpm). The rhythm thus produced is regular and called '*ventricular escape rhythm or idioventricular rhythm*'. This rhythm is typically seen in AV dissociation and complete (third degree) heart block.

Pre-requisite for Good Electrocardiogram Recording

Artifacts and technically poor records will be obtained if following precautions are not followed.
1. The ECG should be recorded with the patient lying comfortably on a bed large enough to support the whole body. The patient must be fully relaxed. It is better to explain the procedure in advance to an apprehensive patient so as to allay anxiety or fear. The technically good record of ECG is depicted in Figure 6.7. Muscular motions and twitchings can alter the record (Fig. 6.8).
2. Good contact must exist between the skin and the electrode. While applying a chest electrode, attention must be paid to put the electrode on clear skin free of hair or by making space by displacing the hair so that they do not interfere. Poor contact will result in suboptimal record (Fig. 6.9).
3. The ECG machine must be properly standardised so that 1 millivolt (mV) will produce a deflection of 10 mm. Incorrect standardisation will produce inaccurate voltage of the complexes which can lead to faulty interpretation.

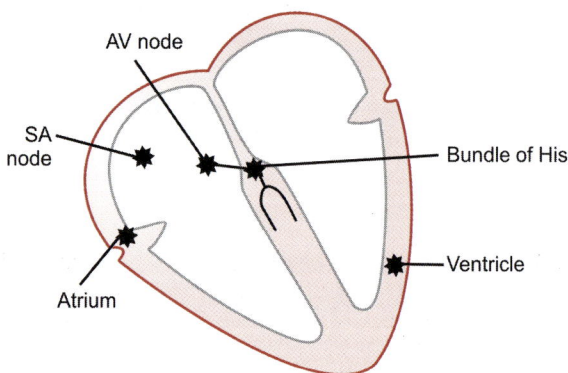

Fig. 6.6A: Pacemaker sites in the heart (diagram)

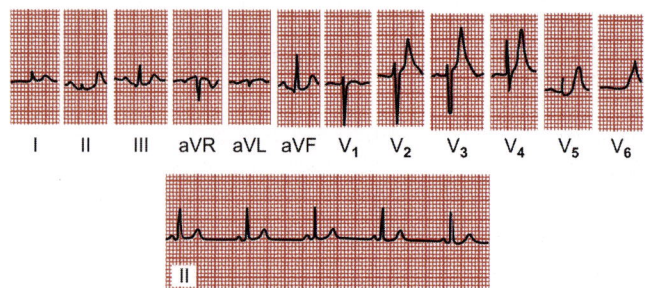

Fig. 6.7: Technically good record of electrocardiogram

A

Simultaneous recording

B

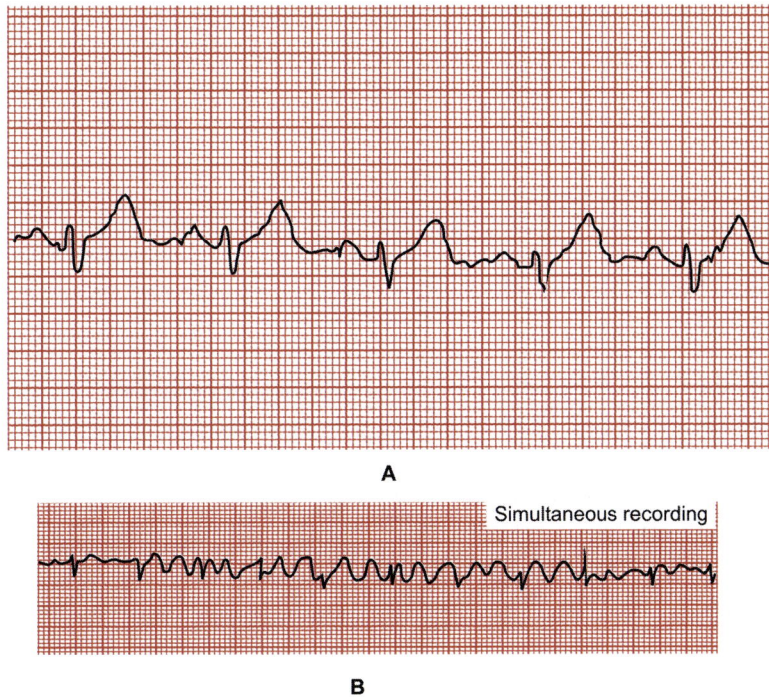

Fig. 6.8: The effect of muscular contractions/tremors
A: The artifact due to strong muscular contractions or tremors producing irregular distortions of the baseline and deflections.
B: The ECG lead II shows motion artifact. The first complex is normal followed by motion artifact observing both rhythm and morphology of P-QRS-T complex

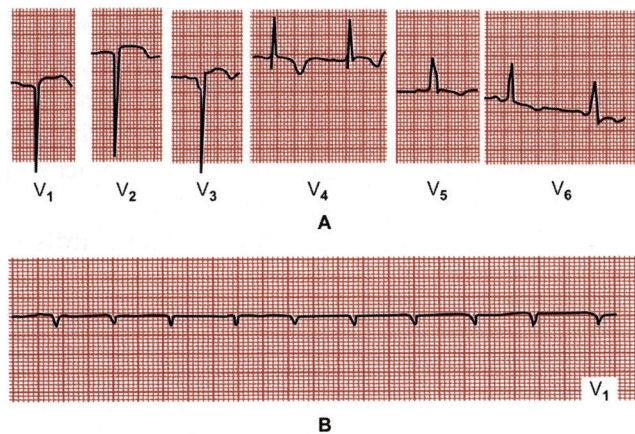

V$_1$ V$_2$ V$_3$ V$_4$ V$_5$ V$_6$

A

V$_1$

B

Fig. 6.9: Suboptimal record due to poor contact between skin and the electrode.
A: The artifact is seen in lead V$_6$ involving P-QRS-T complex. There is suboptimal recording of inverted T in the same lead
B: Suboptimal graph (lead V$_1$) recording very small complexes. This was due to scratching of skin on anterior chest wall leading to poor contact between skin and exploring electrode.

The patient and the recording machine must be properly grounded to avoid alternating current interference.

4. An electronic equipment in contact with the patient, e.g. an electrically regulated heater or electrically regulated infusion pump or suction machine can produce artifacts on the ECG (Figs 6.10A and B).

THE NORMAL ELECTROCARDIOGRAM IN ADULTS

A 12 lead normal electrocardiogram consists of 3 standard leads (I, II, III), 3 unipolar leads (aVR, aVL, aVF) and 6 chest or precordial leads (V$_1$ through V$_6$).

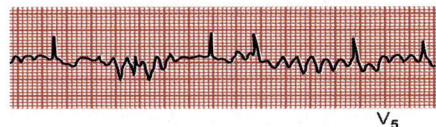

V$_5$

Fig. 6.10A: The effect of suction on electrocardiograph simulating atrial flutter. The lead V$_5$ shows fluttering of the baseline and electrocardiographic deflections. The ECG was recorded during suction in an unconscious patient. The artifact was suspected due to fluttering of electrocardiographic deflections which disappeared after cessation of suction

SECTION TWO

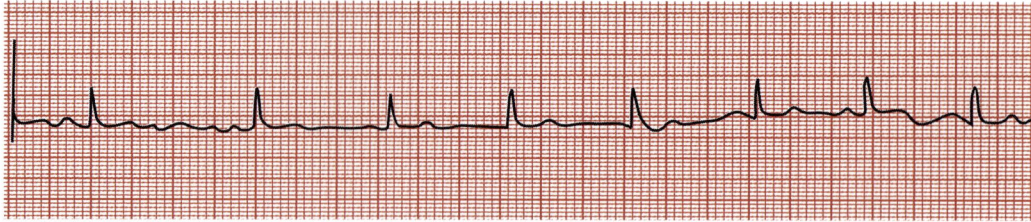

Fig. 6.10B: Effect of muscular contraction simulating atrial flutter recorded from a patient with IV drip in Rt arm. The artifact was suspected in first two complexes which settled down. The drip was removed and lead II was repeated which was perfectly normal

Electrophysiologically, there are three major events that occur during each cycle, i.e. atrial event (depolarisation and repolarisation), ventricular depolarisation and ventricle repolarisation. The electrocardiographic deflections or waveforms/ complexes inscribed during these events have already been discussed in Chapter 3 (Action Potential and Waveforms).

NORMAL COMPONENTS OF AN ECG COMPLEX (Fig. 6.11)

1. Waveforms: P-QRS-TU
2. Angle: QRS-T angle
3. Segments: PR, ST, TP
4. Junction: QRS – T junction called J point
5. Intervals: P-R, QRS, QT (QTc), P-P, R-R.

The Normal P Wave

It is produced by atrial depolarisation. It is normally upright in leads I, II, aVF and V_2-V_6. Depending on the frontal plane axis, it may be upright or flat or biphasic in leads III and aVL (Fig. 6.12). It is always inverted in aVR. Depending on its orientation in chest leads, it may be normally upright or biphasic or flat or inverted in lead V_1 and sometimes in lead V_2 also.

The P Wave Characteristics

The characteristics of normal P wave are given in the box.

NORMAL P WAVE
- **Shape** - rounded
- **Height and width** - 2 to 2.5 mm
- **Duration**- 0.08 to 0.10 sec but not greater than 0.11 sec
- **Visibility** – It is best seen in leads II, III and aVF because normal P wave vector is directed towards the positive poles of these leads
- **P wave axis:** It has between + 40° to + 60°.

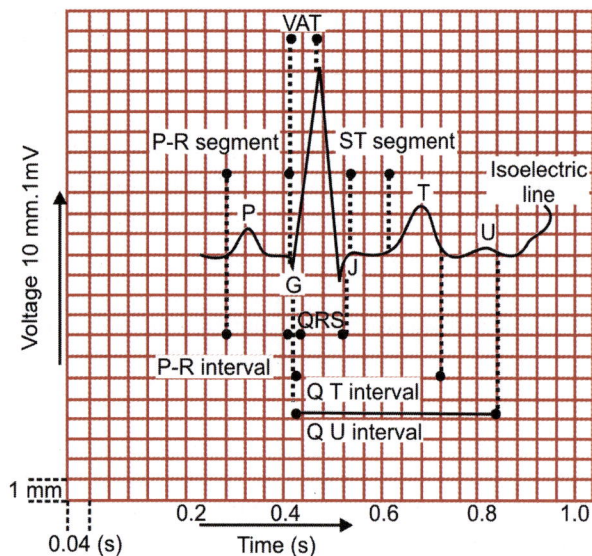

Fig. 6.11: Normal electrocardiogram showing waveforms, segments, junctions and intervals

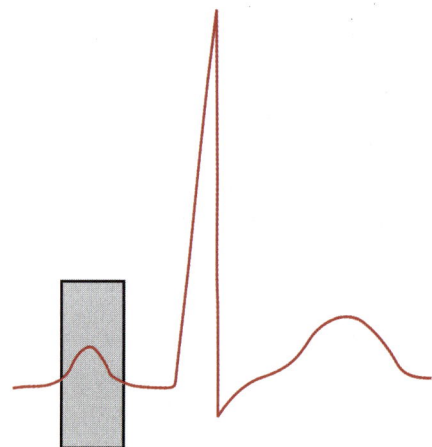

Fig. 6.12: The P wave in frontal plane leads (diagram)

The Normal QRS-T Complex/Deflection

The QRS complex represents ventricular depolaris-ation and T wave represents ventricular repolarisation (Fig. 6.13).

Characteristics of Normal QRS Complex

The normal QRS is positive in all leads except aVR. It is equiphasic in lead (V_3 or V_4). It has following characteristics (Fig. 6.14).

i) Height is less than 25 mm in any lead.

ii) Width or duration of QRS is 1 to 2.5 mm or 0.04 to 0.10 seconds.

iii) Intrinsic or intrinsicoid deflection. This is also called ventricular activation time (VAT). Normally it should not exceed 0.03 sec in right oriented leads, (V_1 or V_2) and 0.05 sec in left oriented leads (V_5 or V_6). This is shown in diagram (Fig. 3.13).

The normal QRS complex has smooth limbs with no notchings or slurrings. Exception to this is the presence of a small notching on QRS in lead III or aVL due to occurrence of the frontal plane transition zone in one of these two leads. The mean QRS duration is 0.09 sec but it ranges from 0.04 to 0.10 sec. The QRS duration > 0.10 sec, is abnormal.

A normal q wave on frontal plane does not exceed 0.03 second. Normally, it is 0.01 sec in duration and 0.05 mV or less in magnitude. A 'q' wave of more than one small square of ECG paper (>0.04 sec) is considered as an abnormal. A normal q wave is seen in leads I, aVL and V_5-V_6.

Since lead I is oriented towards left ventricle, it will record a left ventricular epicardial complex (qR) similar to lead V_6 (Fig. 6.14), but of less amplitude because V_6 is more proximal or closer to electrical impulses of the heart.

A small terminal 's' wave may manifest in two or in all the three standard leads (I, II, III) simulating S_I, S_{II}, S_{III} syndrome and when this occurs, then lead V_5 and V_6 will also record S waves. The large S wave in leads I, II and III (S_I, S_{II}, S_{III} syndrome) is usually abnormal (Read Chapter 15).

The left oriented precordial leads (V_5-V_6) record a qR complex (left epicardial complex). The small r wave of right epicardial complex (rS) is larger than q wave of left epicardial complex (qR). These initial deflections are due to septal depolarisation forces. A

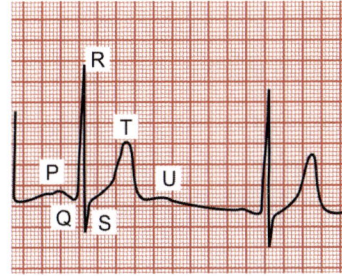

Fig. 6.13: The electrocardiogram (lead V_5) showing normal P-QRS-TU characteristics

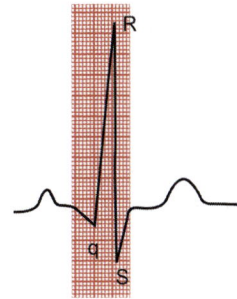

Fig. 6.14: Normal QRS complex (lead V_5). A q wave is the initial negative deflection followed by an upright R wave, which is first positive wave, and then, S wave occurs as first negative deflection after R wave

NB: Deflection means inscription of a wave above or below the baseline, it is termed as negative if it is below the baseline and termed positive if inscribed above the baseline

relatively tall r wave may uncommonly occur in lead V_1 as a normal variant; when this occurs, the amplitude of R wave will not exceed the amplitude of S wave in the same lead (R< S). Relatively large R wave or R wave equal to S wave may normally be seen in lead V_1 in children < 10 yrs of age.

The transition zone (the lead which records equiphasic qRS complex, i.e. RS complex) commonly manifests normally in lead V_3 or V_4. Usually the lead V_3 is called transition lead on horizontal plane axis. Transition zone in precordial leads means a transition between right ventricular epicardial complex (rS) and left ventricular epicardial complex (qR).

The amplitude of R wave gradually increases normally as one proceeds from V_1 towards V_5, so that, lead V_5 has invariably a taller R wave than lead V_6. This is called normal progression of R wave in precordial leads. Obese persons, mesomorphic individuals, thick persons, women with heavy breasts will tend to have low voltage of QRS-T complexes normally.

Factor Governing QRS Complex

These are given in the box.

Factors Affecting QRS Amplitude

Electrical force: More the electrical force generated in the left ventricle, more will be the height of R wave.

Distance between the electrode and the ventricle: Lesser the distance, larger will be the deflection. Since the chest or precordial leads are nearer to the ventricles, hence, record more QRS-T deflections than the frontal plane leads.

Body built: A thin person will tend to have large ECG complexes than an obese person.

Frontal plane QRS: If frontal plane QRS is directed to the positive pole of a lead, then that lead will show a large QRS deflection. For example, if QRS axis is +60°, i.e. towards the positive pole of lead II, then there will be a large deflection of QRS in lead II.

Age: As a whole, there may be less amplitude of QRS in old persons but, otherwise, leads I and aVL may show large deflections than other frontal plane leads due to shift of QRS axis leftwards in old age.

Progression of R Wave in Precordial Leads

Normally, the height of the R wave increases and depth of S wave decreases as one advances from lead V_1-V_6, the mechanism of which has already been discussed in Chapter 3 (see Fig. 3.15).

Abnormalities of R Wave Progression

1. Poor R wave progression (Fig. 6.15)
2. Early transition (Fig. 6.16)

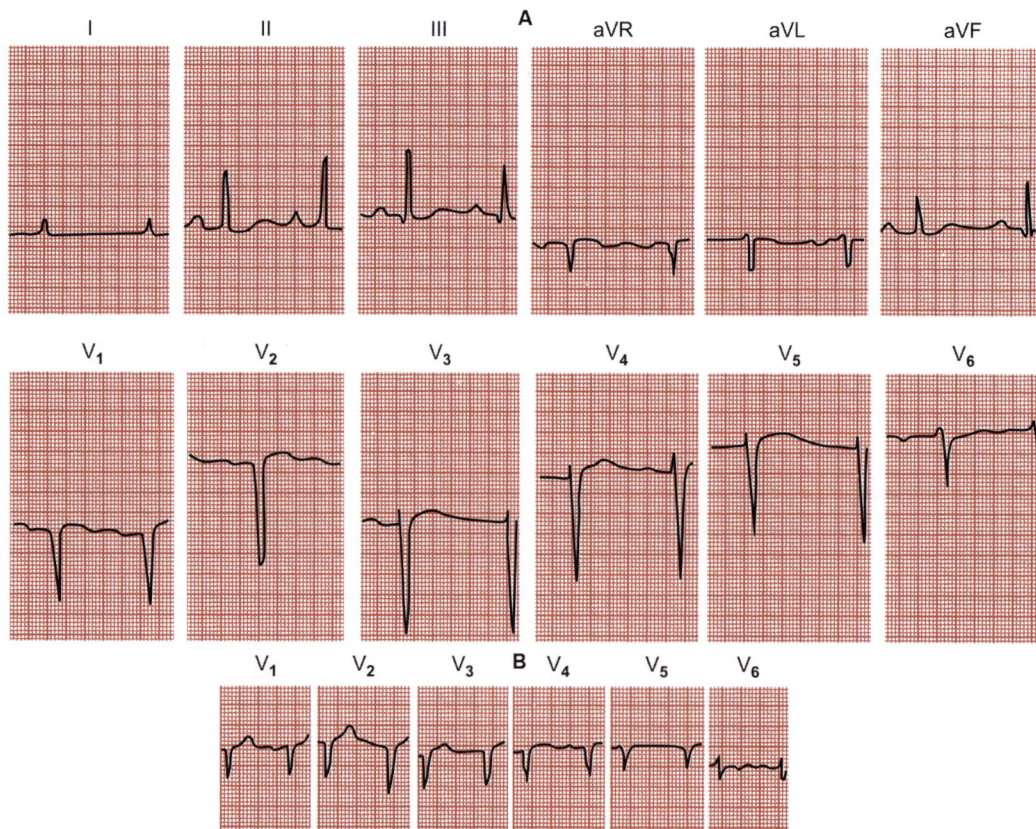

Fig. 6.15: Progression of R wave in precordial leads (V_1-V_6)
A: Poor progression of R wave from V_1-V_6 in a patient with chronic obstructive pulmonary disease (COPD). A small r wave is constantly present (rS complex) from V_3-V_6
B: Nonprogression of R wave in old anterior wall infarction (V_2-V_6). A small r is present in V_1 but disappeared due to infarction in leads V_2 to V_5 (QS complex) and there is a small r wave again in V_6 (height of R wave is reduced due to infarction)

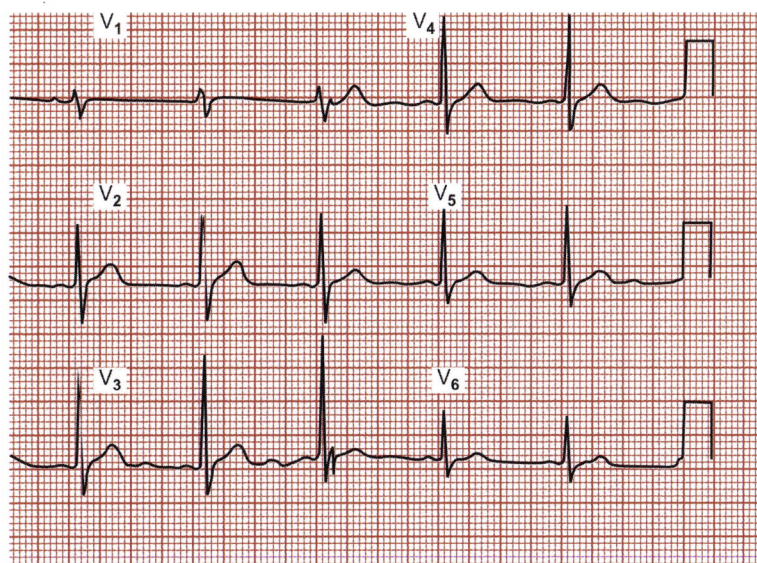

Fig. 6.16: Early transition: The ECG recorded from a normal young adult. Note the large R more than S in V_2 while r in V_1 is less than S wave, hence, transition zone is shifted towards V_1

1. **Poor 'R' wave progression (PRW):** Poor R wave progression is said to be present when R wave of QRS complex does not become predominantly positive by lead V_4 or R wave in V_1 to V_3 remains small and does not increase progressively in size. It is seen in anterior or anteroseptal myocardial infarction, sometimes in left ventricular hypertrophy and other cardiac diseases such as cardiomyopathy or lung diseases such as chronic obstructive pulmonary disease (COPD).

2. **Early transition:** Early transition is said to occur when QRS complex become predominantly positive earlier than expected normally, i.e. in lead V_1 or V_2. This may be found in posterior myocardial infarction, right ventricular hypertrophy or as a normal variant in infants.

Incorrect placement of electrode may cause R wave progression abnormal

The QRS Deflection with their Nomenclature (Fig. 6.17)

The QRS deflections represent ventricular depolarisation. The ensuing deflections of an ECG complex are labelled in an alphabetical sequence as P-QRS-TU.

The Q wave: An initial downward deflection after the P wave is termed Q wave.

The R wave: An initial upward deflection after the Q wave is R wave. If Q wave is absent, then R wave follows the P wave after P-R interval.

The S wave: The negative deflection following R wave is termed S wave.

Depending on the amplitude of deflection, these are denoted by *capital* or *small* letters; if it is equal to or more than 5 mm, it is noted by a capital letter, if it is less than 5 mm then it is denoted by small letter. Thus a small r wave followed by a large S wave is termed as *rS complex*. A complex with a large R and S

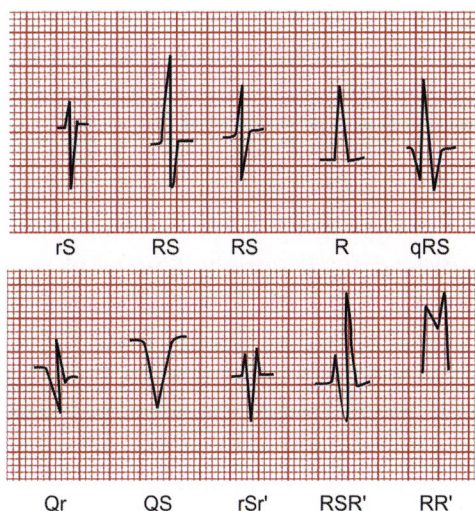

Fig. 6.17: QRS deflections and their nomenclature

of equal or more or less equal amplitudes is termed as *RS complex*; if both are less than 5 mm, then it is written as *rs complex*. A large R wave (>5 mm) followed by a small S wave (<5 mm) is written as *Rs complex*. A single wave complex, which is completely positive, is termed as *R wave complex*. A complex with a small initial negative deflection followed by a large tall upward deflection, which in turn, is followed by a relatively large terminal downward deflection is written as *qRS*; a deep and wide initial downward deflection followed by a small terminal positivity is written as *Qr complex*. A complex with complete negativity is written as *QS complex*. A second positivity following R deflection is written as (r´). Thus, an *rS complex* followed by a small terminal positivity is written as *rSr´ complex*; when this terminal second positivity is large, the complex is written as *rSR´*. When the deflection is positive and notched, the complex is written as *RR´*.

The Normal T Wave (Fig. 6.18)

The T wave normally is a positive deflection with blunt apex and asymmetric limbs that follows QRS complex. The T wave amplitude tends to diminish with age. The T wave is taller in athletes. Since mean T wave vector is to the left, inferiorly and somewhat anteriorly, hence, it is upright in leads I, II and aVF and is inverted in aVR. The polarity of T wave in leads III and aVL depends on the position of the heart and mean frontal plane T axis similar to QRS, i.e. if mean frontal plane T axis is between 0° to +30°, the T wave is inverted in lead III; if it lies between +60° to +90° or more, then the T wave becomes inverted in aVL instead of lead III.

Depending on anterior orientation of mean T wave vector, the T is normally either upright or inverted in lead V_1 but is upright in all other precordial leads (V_2-V_6). If T is upright in V_1, it is of lesser amplitude than T wave of lead V_6. If upright T wave of lead V_1 is either equal or larger than T wave of lead V_6 ($TV_1 \geq TV_6$), it indicates a potential presence of a cardiac disease provided other factors such as an incorrect placement of electrodes and woman with heavy breasts can be excluded. Tall or relatively tall T waves are not infrequently seen in mid-precordial leads.

The inverted T wave in leads V_1 to V_3 occurs in infancy and childhood due to right ventricular

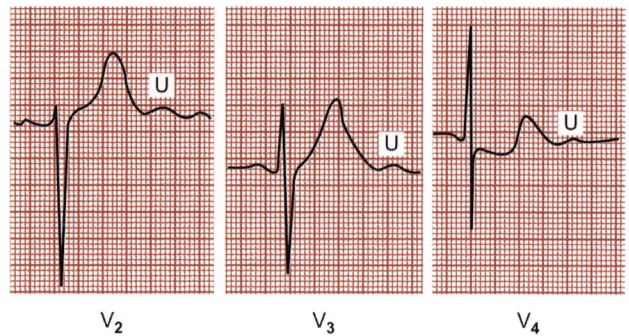

Fig. 6.18: The normal T and U waves. The ECG leads (V_2-V_4) show normal T and U waves which are normally best seen in mid-precordial leads

dominance (juvenile pattern), occasionally be seen in adults called persistent juvenile pattern .

The repolarisation wave or T wave is usually an upward deflection in all leads except aVR. It is usually inscribed in the same direction as the QRS complex. It has relatively blunt apex or nadir.

The Normal U Wave (Fig. 6.18)

The normal U wave is a small, shallow, rounded upward deflection which is inscribed immediately after T wave, is best seen in mid-precordial leads (V_2-V_4) if present. It is less than 1mm in amplitude but may occasionally be as high as 2 mm especially in athletes. It is more prominent in precordial than frontal plane leads. It has same direction as the T wave. It may not be visible in certain normal persons It becomes prominent in hypokalaemia. It represents delayed ventricular repolarisation. The genesis and significance of 'U' wave is not well defined.

The Normal QRS-T Angle (Fig. 6.19)

The normal T wave axis on the frontal plane has more or less same direction as that of QRS. The angle between QRS and T axes on the frontal plane is called '*QRS-T angle*', which is normally of 15° to 40° but does not exceed 60° in any circumstance, however, some authorities believe 45° as the upper limit of the normal.

Significance of QRS-T angle. The QRS-T angle becomes wide in a large number of conditions including anterior myocardial infarction. Wide QRS-T angle occurs in certain disorders which have already been discussed in Chapter 4.

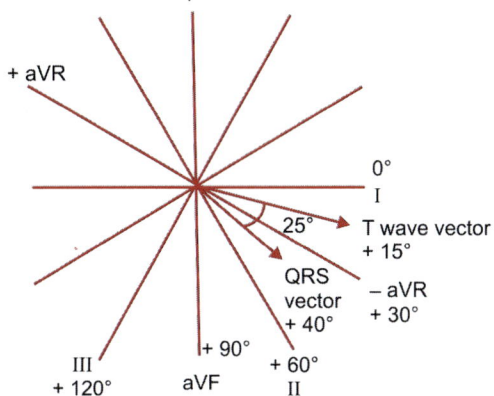

Fig. 6.19: Normal QRS-T angle of 25° drawn (diagram). The mean QRS axis is +40° and T wave mean axis is +15°

THE NORMAL ELECTROCARDIOGRAPHIC INTERVALS

1. The P-R interval
2. The QRS interval
3. The QT or QTU, QTc and QTd intervals
4. The P-P interval
5. The R-R interval
6. The JT interval

1. The P-R Interval (Figs 6.20 and 6.21)

It is interval between the beginning of the P wave to the beginning of Q wave of QRS complex or R wave of QRS complex if Q wave is not seen. It actually represents the time taken by the impulse to travel from SA node to atria, then to AV node with its physiological delay, and passage of impulse through bundle of His and its branches. It ends with the beginning of depolarisation of the ventricles. The characteristics of normal P-R interval and pathological conditions associated with variations in P-R interval are give in the box.

The P-R interval and its abnormalities

Normal duration is 0.12–0.20 sec. The P-R interval varies with the heart rate. Rapid heart rate shortens it, while slow heart rate prolongs it. Normally it is less than 0.12 sec. in infants. At heart rate of 60 bpm, P-R interval of 0.22 sec may be regarded as normal.

Short P-R interval (< 0.12 sec) indicates an accelerated conduction through an accessory pathway that bypasses AV node (WPW syndrome) or seen in atrial or nodal ectopics. Certain drugs (steroids) also shorten it.

Long P-R interval (> 0.20 second): Lengthening of P-R interval occurs in various conduction blocks or delayed depolarisation of atria due to drugs, hypertrophy or atrial dilatation. P-R interval is also lengthened if conduction through AV node is delayed by diseases or antiarrhythmic drugs (digitalis, bet ablockers, calcium channel blockers). If sinus is sick or lazy (sick sinus syndrome), the P-R interval may get prolonged.

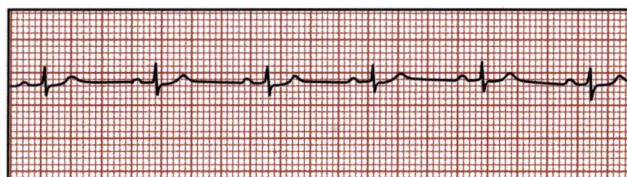

Fig. 6.21: The ECG lead II shows normal P-R interval of 0.22 sec of a heart rate of 60/min

2. The QRS Interval (Fig. 6.22)

It is measured from the beginning of QRS to its endpoint called 'J' point. The QRS also includes intrinsicoid deflection or ventricular activation time

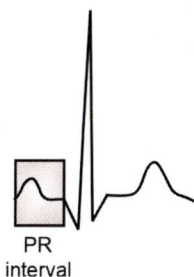

Fig. 6.20: Normal P-R interval

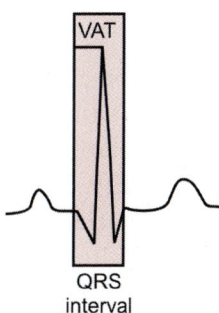

Fig. 6.22: The QRS interval: It is measured from the beginning of QRS to its end-point-the J point (an iso-electric point where S wave returns to the baseline and forms starting point of ST segment)

SECTION TWO

(VAT), thus it actually refers to time taken for complete depolarisation of both the ventricles from endocardial to epicardial surfaces. The normal characteristics of QRS complex have already been discussed.

Widening of QRS complex: The QRS complex is said to be widened if its duration exceeds 2.5 mm or 0.10 sec. The causes of widening of QRS are given in the Table 6.1 and mechanism and type of widening of QRS is shown in Figure 6.23.

Table 6.1: Causes of widening of QRS
1. Bundle branch blocks or fascicular blocks
2. Intraventricular conduction delay
3. Aberrant conduction within the ventricles such as supraventricular impulse(s) with aberrant conduction or with premature ventricular complexes (VPCs), idioventricular rhythm and ventricular tachycardia
4. Early and abnormal activation of the ventricles through an accessory pathway or bypass tract

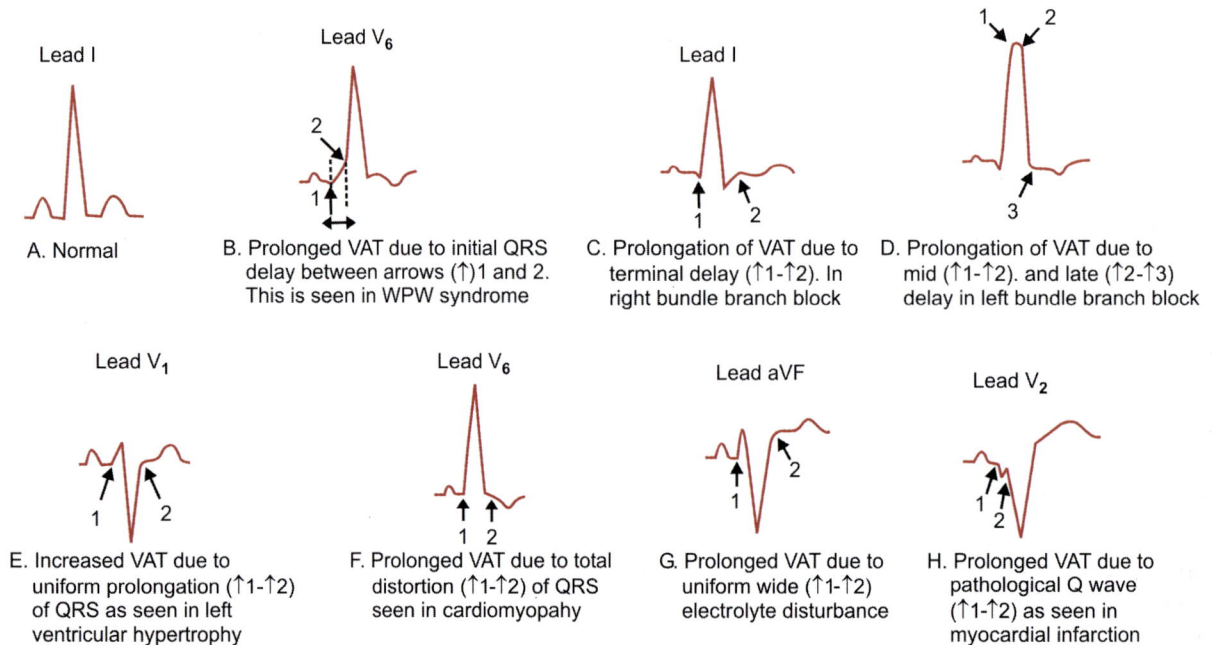

A. Normal

B. Prolonged VAT due to initial QRS delay between arrows (↑)1 and 2. This is seen in WPW syndrome

C. Prolongation of VAT due to terminal delay (↑1-↑2). In right bundle branch block

D. Prolongation of VAT due to mid (↑1-↑2). and late (↑2-↑3) delay in left bundle branch block

E. Increased VAT due to uniform prolongation (↑1-↑2) of QRS as seen in left ventricular hypertrophy

F. Prolonged VAT due to total distortion (↑1-↑2) of QRS seen in cardiomyopahy

G. Prolonged VAT due to uniform wide (↑1-↑2) electrolyte disturbance

H. Prolonged VAT due to pathological Q wave (↑1-↑2) as seen in myocardial infarction

Fig. 6.23: Mechanism of widening of QRS and prolongation of VAT in different pathological conditions as compared to normal

The ventricular activation time (VAT): This is also called intrinsicoid deflection which has already been discussed. It is measured from the beginning of the Q wave to the top of the R wave. It should not exceed 0.03 sec in leads V_1-V_2 and 0.05 sec in leads V_5-V_6 (Fig. 6.24).

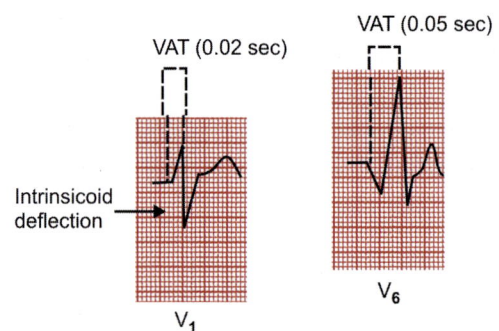

Fig. 6.24: Normal ventricular activation time in right (V_1) and left (V_6) precordial leads

3. The QT Interval (Figs 6.25 and 6.26)

The interval from the beginning of QRS complex to the end of T wave is called QT interval. It is sum total of the time taken by depolarisation and repolarisation of the ventricles. The total electrical activity of the ventricles is reflected in QT interval. It is variable in different parts of the ventricles, but the QT interval measured on the surface electrocardiogram represents the total longest interval of QT.

The QT interval shortens with tachycardia and lenghtens during bradycardia. In other words, the QT changes with change in R-R interval; the latter represents the heart rate. Therefore, for meaningful expression, the QT must be corrected for heart rate-

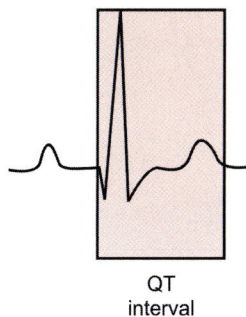

Fig. 6.25: The QT interval (diagram): It is measured from the beginning of QRS to the end of T wave (shaded area)

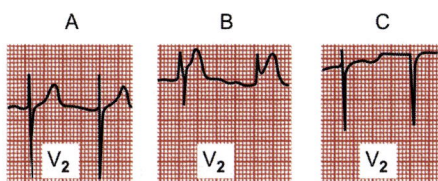

Fig. 6.26: The QT and QTc interval.
A: Normal, **B:** Short, **C:** Prolonged

called corrected QT (QTc) interval. The QT interval is corrected for what it would be at a rate of 60 bpm.

Corrected QT (QTc) by Bazett's formula = $\dfrac{QT \text{ interval in sec}}{\sqrt{R\text{-}R \text{ interval in sec}}}$

Measurement of QT: It is measured in seconds from the beginning of Q wave to the end of the T wave. It is difficult to measure sometimes because it is difficult to delineate the beginning and end of the interval. It is customary to measure it in the lead having 'q' wave such as leads I, II, aVL, V_5 or V_6 so as to avoid error of ignoring the initial part of QRS. Similarly, the end point of T wave may be difficult to find out, but if U wave is present, then it becomes easy as the dip between T and U wave becomes the end point of T wave.

The characteristics of QT or QTc are given in the box.

> **CHARACTERISTICS OF QT OR QTc**
> *Normal range of QTc* is 0.35 to 0.43 sec (Mean 0.39+0.04 sec)
> *Variation:* Physiological variation is due to age, sex and heart rate
> It is longer in females, in old age and during slow heart rate
>
> *Corrected QT (QTc)* is measured to obviate the effect of heart rate on QT. It is less than 0.40 sec. in males and less than 0.45 sec in females.

> ### Q-T INTERVAL—UPPER LIMITS OF NORMAL (in seconds)
>
> | HR/min | Men and children | Women |
> |--------|------------------|-------|
> | 40 | 0.49 | 0.50 |
> | 45 | 0.47 | 0.48 |
> | 50 | 0.45 | 0.46 |
> | 55 | 0.43 | 0.43 |
> | 60 | 0.42 | 0.42 |
> | 65 | 0.40 | 0.41 |
> | 70 | 0.39 | 0.39 |
> | 75 | 0.38 | 0.38 |
> | 80 | 0.37 | 0.37 |
> | 85 | 0.36 | 0.36 |
> | 90 | 0.35 | 0.36 |
> | 95 | 0.35 | 0.36 |
> | 100 | 0.34 | 0.35 |

Relation of Heart Rate (R-R interval) to QT and QTc (Tables 6.2 and 6.3)

1. The QT interval is corrected for what it would theoretically be at a rate of 60 bpm, because at this rate, the R-R interval is 1.0 second and, since the

Table 6.2: QTc derived from different heart rates associated with constant QT interval (0.39 sec)			
HR/min	R-R/sec	QT/sec	QTc/sec
50	1.20	0.39	0.36
55	1.10	0.39	0.37
60	1.00	0.39	0.39
65	0.90	0.39	0.41
75	0.80	0.39	0.44
90	0.66	0.39	0.48
100	0.60	0.39	0.50
150	0.40	0.39	0.62

Table 6.3: QT derived from different heart rates associated with constant QTc interval (0.39 sec)			
HR/min	R-R/sec	QT/sec	QTc/sec
50	1.20	0.43	0.39
55	1.10	0.41	0.39
60	1.00	0.39	0.39
65	0.90	0.37	0.39
75	0.80	0.35	0.39
90	0.66	0.32	0.39
100	0.60	0.30	0.39
150	0.40	0.25	0.39

square root of 1.0 second is still 1.0 second, the QT and QTc intervals will be constant.

2. With increasing heart rates (diminishing R-R intervals), the QTc interval is increased but measured QT is decreased.

3. With decreasing heart rates (increasing R-R intervals), the QTc interval is decreased but measured QT is increased.

4. The more the deviation of heart rate from 60 bpm (R-R interval of 1.0 sec), the greater will be the correction.

5. When heart rate is >60 bpm, QT interval is increased by correction to QTc; and the faster the heart rate, the greater is the correction.

6. When heart rate is < 60 bpm, the QT interval is shortened after correction to QTc; and slower the heart rate, the greater is the correction.

- *As a general rule, the QT interval does not exceed 0.39 sec with heart rates between 60 to 80 bpm.*
- *A useful rule of the thumb states that with normal heart rate of 60-100 bpm, the QT interval should not exceed half of R-R interval.*

The QTc derived from different heart rates associated with constant QT interval are depicted in Table 6.2 and QT derived from different heart rate with constant QTc interval are depicted in Table 6.3.

The causes of long and short QT (QTc) are given in Table 6.4.

Danger – It has dangerous consequences such as prolonged QT may lead to torsade de pointes (ventricular tachycardia).

QT Dispersion (QTd)

Recent studies have defined QT dispersion (QTd) as interlead QT variability on the surface electro-

Table 6.4: Causes of long and short QT or QTc
Long QTc
• Physiological – during sleep
• Congenital – Prolonged QT syndrome – The Jervell and Lange-Nielsen syndrome and Romano-Ward syndrome
• Acquired
- Hypocalcaemia
- Acute myocarditis
- Acute myocardial infarction
- Quinine, Quinidine and Procainamide effect
- Antidepressants (tricyclic and tetracyclics)
- Head injury with intracerebral bleed
- Hypothermia
- Idiopathic hypertrophic cardiomyopathy
- Advanced or complete heart block
- Ventricular tachycardia - Torsade de pointes
Short QTc
- Digitalis effect
- Hyperthermia
- Vagal stimulation
- Hypercalcaemia

NB: It is essential to measure QTc in patients on anti-arrhythmatic drugs (quinidine and procainamide) or on quinine therapy

cardiogram and it may reflect regional variations in myocardial recovery of excitability. The finding of a decreased QT dispersion in patients with heart diseases treated with class III agents (sotalol, amiodarone) further support the concept.

QTd is calculated on electrocardiograms where at least 9 leads show measurable QT interval. The QTd is the difference between the longest and shortest QT interval measured on the 12 lead surface ECG.

QTd = QT *maximum* – QT *minimum*
Corrected QTd (QT$_c$d) = QTc *maximum* – QTc *minimum*

The QT interval is measured from the beginning of QRS to the end of T wave (i.e. return to the TP baseline). If U waves are present, then QT interval is measured to the nadir of the curve between the T and the U waves. For calculation of QTd , 3 consecutive cycles are measured in each lead and the mean of these 3 cycles is taken as mean QTc of that lead. The QT may be corrected by Bazett's formula already discussed.

Clinical Conditions Associated with Wide QTd Interval

There are a large number of conditions associated with wide QTd interval, the pathogenesis of which is unclear (Table 6.5).

Table 6.5: Conditions associated with wide QTd
1. Congenital or acquired prolonged QT syndrome
2. Hypertrophic cardiomyopathy
3. Mitral valve prolapse
4. Coronary artery disease

The normal mean $QT_c d$ is 45 ± 15 ms

Clinical Significance

1. QTd is believed to be a measure of electrical inhomogenity in the heart that decreases an individual's threshold for ventricular arrhythmias, hence greater the QTd, greater is the chance to develop an arrhythmia.
2. Heart rate, reflex vagal activity and cardiac afterload physiologically alter the QT dispersion.
3. A significant QT dispersion was found both in patients with congenital and acquired long QT intervals, which is presumed to be the cause of Torsade-de-pointes in these conditions.
4. Certain antiarrhythmic drugs decrease the QT dispersion, hence, QT dispersion may be used to evaluate the efficacy of the drug.

A wide QT dispersion is a stimulus for arrhythmogenesis

The QU Interval

It is the interval between the beginning of the Q wave to the end of U wave provided U wave is inscribed; and it represents total ventricular depolarisation and repolarisation time including that of Purkinje fibres.

When the end of T wave is not well visualised or demarcated due to superimposition of a U wave, then QTU (QU) interval may be measured in place of QT interval. In hypokalaemia, U wave becomes prominent and QTU is prolonged while actual QT is within normal limit.

4. The P-P Interval (Fig. 6.27)

It is the interval between two successive P waves. It is measured from the beginning of first P wave to the beginning of next P wave (Fig. 6.27). The P-P interval will be regular in normal sinus rhythm and will be equal to R-R interval. However, when ventricular rhythm becomes irregular or when atrial and ventricular rates are regular but differ from each other, then P-P interval will be measured between any 2 consecutive beats to calculate the atrial rate.

5. The R-R Interval (Fig. 6.27)

It is the interval between two successive R waves. It is measured from the beginning of one R wave to the beginning of next R wave of QRS complexes. The R-R interval will be regular like P-P interval in regular sinus rhythm. The R-R interval is used to calculate the ventricular rate. The calculation of heart rate (ventricular rate) by R-R method has already been discussed. Slight variation in R-R interval may be normal due to respiratory effect–called *respiratory sinus arrhythmia*. Irregular R-R interval indicates irregular ventricular response or rhythm.

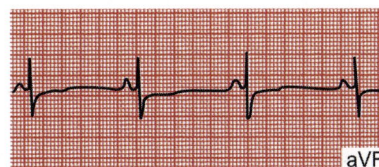

Fig. 6.27: The P-P interval. The electrocardiographic lead aVF shows normal P-P and R-R intervals

6. The JT Interval

It is the interval between the J point (the beginning of ST segment) to the end of T wave, indicates total ventricular repolarisation. In patients of bundle branch block, QT interval includes abnormally wide QRS complex, in such patients, JT interval gives accurate assessment of ventricular repolarisation time.

SECTION TWO

NORMAL SEGMENTS AND JUNCTIONS ON ECG

1. PR segment
2. ST segment
3. TP segment
4. R-S junction

1. The PR Segment

Usually in electrocardiography P-R interval is measured in reference to time and PR segment is measured in reference to distance. The PR segment is the distance from the end of P wave to the beginning of QRS complex. It serves as a baseline to evaluate depression of ST segment, hence, acts as reference baseline (Fig. 6.28) because it is isoelectric. A prominent Ta wave (atrial repolarisation wave) may depress the P-R segment in such way that it may mimic q wave of infarction. Prominent Ta waves are seen in conditions that cause atrial injury—atrial hypertrophy/enlargement, atrial infarction, pericarditis, etc.

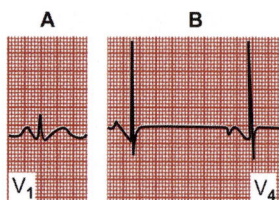

Fig. 6.28: A: The normal PR segment,
B: The depressed PR segment

2. The ST Segment

It is the distance from the end of S wave to the beginning to T wave. The point at which S wave joins the baseline is called 'J' point. Therefore, actually the portion of an ECG complex from the 'J' point to the onset of T wave is ST segment and is usually isoelectric. It may vary in shape and position with reference to baseline in certain disorders which will be discussed in appropriate sections.

The greater part of ventricular repolarisation is represented by ST segment. It leaves the baseline immediately after its origin from the end of QRS, and becomes isoelectric. The ST segment merges smoothly with the proximal limb of T wave, so, it is difficult to separate them (Fig. 6.29).

The elevation/depression of ST segment is decided with reference to baseline joining the termination of

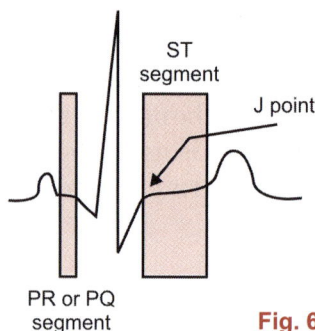

Fig. 6.29: The normal ST segment

T wave and the beginning of next P wave (T-P line or segment).

3. TP Segment

It is the portion of tracing between the end of T wave and the beginning of the next P wave. At normal heart rates, it is usually isoelectric and is used as baseline for determination of ST segment deviation. At rapid heart rate, it shortens and even P wave may come very near to T wave or may encroach the T wave, eliminating the isoelectric TP segment.

4. The R-S Junction

This is a point called 'J' point at which QRS ends with S wave returning to the baseline and ST segment starts. The 'J' point in electrocardiography is important in evaluation of initial ST segment deviation, i.e. elevation/depression (Fig. 6.28).

THE VOLTAGE MEASUREMENT

This is an important parameter of electrocardiographic interpretation. The voltage of an upright deflection is measured from the baseline to the top of deflection. The voltage of a negative deflection is measured from the lower portion of baseline to the bottom of the wave (Fig. 6.30). If the voltage of QRS

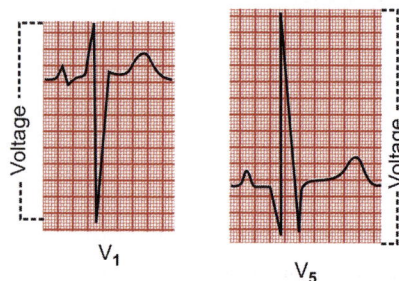

Fig. 6.30: The voltage measurement. The method of voltage measurement (diagram) includes both positive and negative deflections

complex does not exceed 5 mm in any standard leads (I, II, III, aVR, aVL, AVF) and 10 mm in the precordial leads (V_1 to V_6) it is considered as a low voltage graph. The voltage of QRS complex includes both positive and negative deflections. The voltage criteria is useful for diagnosis of left ventricular hypertrophy. The conditions associated with low voltage graph are listed under chronic obstructive pulmonary disease (Chapter 27).

THE ELECTROCARDIOGRAM IN INFANTS (FIG. 6.31)

In foetus, there is right ventricular dominance, therefore, at birth or during infancy, there is relative hypertrophy of the right ventricle. The ECG in an infant will resemble right ventricular hypertrophy in the adult. Thus, there will be right axis deviation with tall R waves in right precordial leads (V_1-V_2). However, an initial 'q' wave will never appear in V_1. Ventricular activation time in these leads is not prolonged. Within few days of birth, upright T waves may be seen in V_2-V_6, however, in V_1 it may be upright or inverted, after some time, T waves normally become inverted in leads V_1-V_3.

THE ELECTROCARDIOGRAM IN CHILDREN (FIG. 6.32)

The tall R wave and inverted T wave may persist in right precordial leads (V_1-V_2) for first few years of life. The tall R wave usually becomes smaller and smaller after 5 years of age and becomes smaller than S wave after 10 years of age. The inverted T waves in the right precordial leads frequently

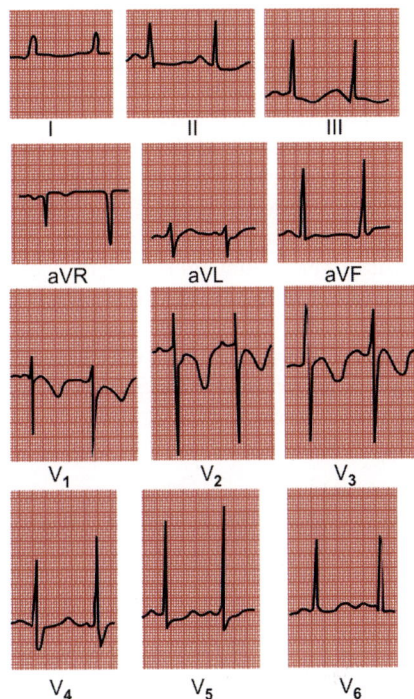

Fig. 6.32: The electrocardiogram from a child (6 years of age)

persists up to 2nd decade of life. This is called *juvenile pattern*. The frontal QRS axis gradually shifts to the left.

The normal electrocardiogram in adult (Fig. 6.33) is depicted for comparison. The r wave in V_1-V_2 is smaller than in children.

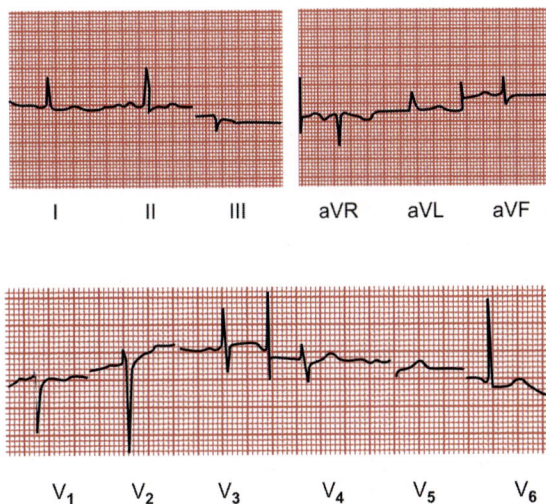

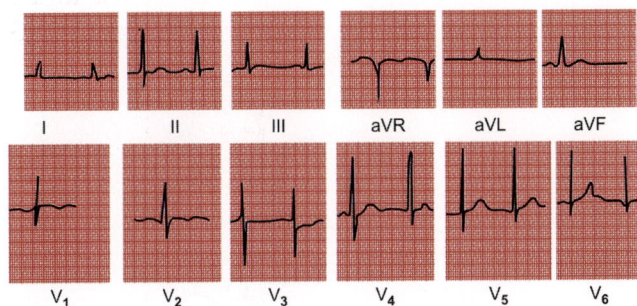

Fig. 6.31: The ECG taken from an infant shows right axis deviation with right ventricular dominance (R wave > S in V_1-V_2) with T wave inversion

Fig. 6.33: The normal electrocardiogram in an adult. Note rudimentary r wave in V_1-V_2 as compared to ECG of a child (Fig. 6.32) and an infant (Fig. 6.31)

Suggested Reading

1. Baett HC: An analysis of the time-relations of electro-cardiograms. *Heart* **7**:353, 1920.
2. Burgess MJ, Green LS, Miller K et al: The sequence of normal ventricular recovery. *Am Heart J* **84**:660, 1972.
3. Durrer D, VanDam RT, Freud GE et al: Total excitation of human heart. *Circulation* **41**:899, 1970.
4. Goldschlager N, Goldmann J (Eds): Principles of clinical electrocardiography, 13 edn, Prentice-Hall International Inc. 1989.
5. Lepeschkin E: Physiologic basis of U wave. In Schlant RC, Hurst JW (Eds): *Advances in Electrocardiography*. New York: Grune and Stratton Inc 1972.
6. Report of Committee on Electrocardiography, American Heart Association: Recommendations for standardisation of leads and of specification for instruments in electro-cardiography and vector–cardiography. *Circulation* **52**:11, 1975.
7. Scher AM: The sequence of ventricular activation. *Am J Cardiol* **14**: 287, 1964.
8. Surawicz B: The pathogenesis and clinical significance of primary T wave abnormalities. In Schant RC, Hurst JW (Eds): *Advances in Electrocardiography*. New York: Grune and Stratton Inc 1972.
9. VanDam RT, Durrer D: The T wave and ventricular repolarisation. *Am J Cardiol* **14**:294, 1964.
10. Watanabe V: Purkinje repolarisation as a possible cause of U wave in electrocardiogram. *Circulation* **51**:1030, 1975.

SECTIONTWO

7

Normal Electrocardiographic Variants in Adults

- ■ *General aspects of normal electrocardiographic variations*
- ■ *Conditions associated with recognisable electrocardiographic variants*

NORMAL ELECTROCARDIOGRAPHIC VARIANTS IN ADULTS—GENERAL ASPECTS

The electrocardiogram is a clinical test like any other test, helps in making the diagnosis and does not give the clinical diagnosis. It is interpreted in settings of clinical conditions like any other test, hence, is a subject of clinical variations. The arbitrary limits of normalcy are set in the 95th–98th percentile range for any given electrocardiographic finding, therefore, 2-5% of normal persons will have an abnormal ECG.

Certain recognised factors such as age, sex, body mass index, configuration of thoracic cage, position of the heart, race, heavy meals, variations in temperature, exercise, smoking, hyperventilation and position of electrodes on the chest, are known to cause variations in ECG. Therefore, ideally an ECG should be recorded when patient has at least rested for 15 minutes, should not have smoked 30 minutes before and should not have had a recent meal. The correct placement of electrodes is mandatory for normal electrocardiogram.

The electrocardiographic patterns which appear to be abnormal, yet occur in healthy individuals without any heart disease are termed as *'normal variants'*. In clinical practice, a large number of patients may consult the doctor for an abnormality on ECG done just as routine during health check up. A second group of patients include those who are referred to physicians for abnormal ECG which has been done routinely for pre-anaesthetic check up. Therefore, the physician after examining the patient, interprets the electrocardiogram, and many times, he/she may not find any obvious reason for the abnormality. In case of doubt, patient may be subjected to further diagnostic work-up. A physician should not give any diagnosis just on the basis of an abnormal ECG. The result of a specific test, i.e. ECG, although being outside the normal range, in itself, does not necessarily predict the disease in the subject being tested. According to Bayer's theorem, predictive value of the test depends on the prevalence of the disease in the population being tested, i.e. if prevalence is low, then predictive accuracy will also be low and vice versa.

Thus, an abnormal ECG in an asymptomatic individual does not always warrant diagnostic work-up. Some abnormal ECG patterns are known to occur in normal individuals that have been determined from studies of large groups of clinically normal individuals. Some normal variants are easily recognisable at a glance and have distinct patterns, have been designated by specific terms; others may be less specific and affect mainly the T wave (repolarisation phase). The important normal variants of P-QRS-T morphology are given in the box.

Normal Electrocardiographic Variants

1. **P wave variants:**
   - Abnormally tall P waves with normal duration.
   - Notching of P waves with normal duration.

2. **The QRS complex variants:**
   Abnormal Q wave of normal duration may appear in normal persons depending on the body built, heart position and thoracic cage abnormality and pneumothorax.

3. **Tall T waves:** Certain normal individuals record tall T wave in precordial leads due to anterior orientation of QRS vector on horizontal plane.

4. **High voltage in precordial leads:** Thin chested normal individuals and persons with large ventricular mass may exhibit high voltage on ECG.

5. **AV nodal or intraventricular conduction delay:** Certain vagotonic individuals develop notched QRS complexes, bundle branch block pattern and long P-R interval.

6. **Persistent juvenile pattern:** Certain black persons (Negroes) exhibit juvenile pattern up to 3rd decade of life.

7. **The early repolarisation syndrome:** It can occur in certain normal persons below 30 years of age.

8. **Nonspecific T wave variants (Figs 7.1 and 7.2):** Nonspecific T wave inversion may occur in those leads where the T waves are normally upright, for example, as a normal response to anxiety, fear, obesity (Fig. 7.2), apprehension, heavy meal, hyperventilation or as a orthostatic response. It can occur without any obvious reason.

9. **Early transition or counterclockwise rotation—A normal variant.** The early transition is normally seen in an infant or child due to right ventricular dominance but may be seen occasionally in an adult (Fig. 7.3). Sometimes, R wave may not progress from V_1-V_4 in an adult—a normal variant (Fig. 7.4).

10. **The ST segment variations:** The J point and ST segment may be elevated upto 2 mm in the precordial leads in normal persons,

occasionally, ST elevation occurs up to 4 mm. The ST elevation in normal person is concave upwards with upright T wave. The late inversion of T wave may occur in those leads with ST elevation, is also a normal phenomenon especially in black people.

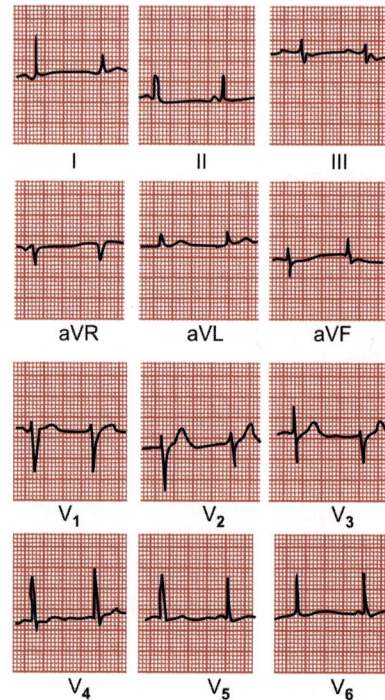

Fig. 7.1: Nonspecific ST-T changes—a normal variant. The electrocardiogram recorded from a healthy individual shows T inversion in lead III and minimal ST depression with T inversion in aVF. These changes are non-consequential in absence of an q wave or significant ST depression. The stress test performed in the patient was normal

CONDITIONS ASSOCIATED WITH WELL RECOGNISED ELECTROCARDIOGRAPHIC VARIANTS

Juvenile Pattern in Adults (Fig. 7.5)

The T wave inversion (normal in children) in precordial leads V_1 to V_3 or V_4 in a normal adult is called *persistent juvenile pattern*. This pattern may persist in black adults up to 3rd decade of life after which these changes may be considered as abnormal.

1. Hyperventilation and Anxiety States

Certain normal persons under the effect of anxiety or hyperventilation may exhibit prolongation of P- R

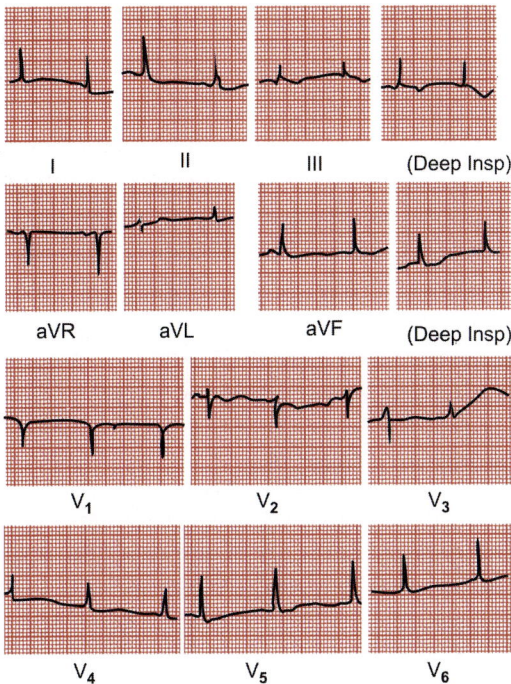

Fig. 7.2: The effect of obesity on ECG changes (Iatrogenic ECG heart disease). The electrocardiogram was recorded from a 35 yr obese female without symptoms of heart disease. There is downsloping of ST segment with inversion of T waves in leads II, III and aVF suggesting silent inferior wall ischaemia. She was subjected to stress electrocardiography and coronary angiography which were reported to be normal. There was no other cause to explain these ST-T changes except truncal obesity. These changes could be due to positional effect of the heart due to obesity. Misinterpretation of significance of ST-T wave abnormality is the most common cause of iatrogenic ECG heart disease. These changes being physiological may be considered as normal variant

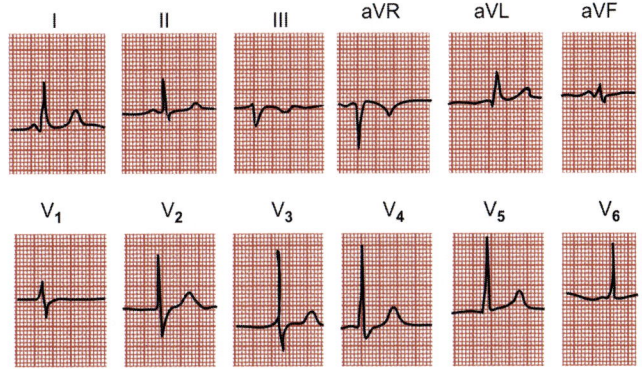

Fig. 7.3: Early transition or counterclockwise rotation—A normal variant. The electrocardiogram recorded from a 40 yrs female shows:
(i) There is early transition due to counterclockwise rotation shifting the transition zone rightwards, i.e. towards V_1
(ii) There is significant tall R wave in lead V_1 but is less than S wave which may be confused with posterior wall infarction, but absence of reciprocal ST depression in lead V_1-V_2, absence or decrease in voltage of R in V_5-V_6 and absence of associated changes of ischaemia either in the inferior or lateral leads rule out the possibility of posterior wall infarction

interval, sinus tachycardia, and ST segment depression with or without T wave inversion in inferior oriented leads (II, III and aVF) simulating myocardial ischaemia. These abnormalities have been documented to occur in persons with no obvious heart disease and with normal coronary angiograms (Fig. 7.6). These changes have been considered due to an imbalance of autonomic nervous system.

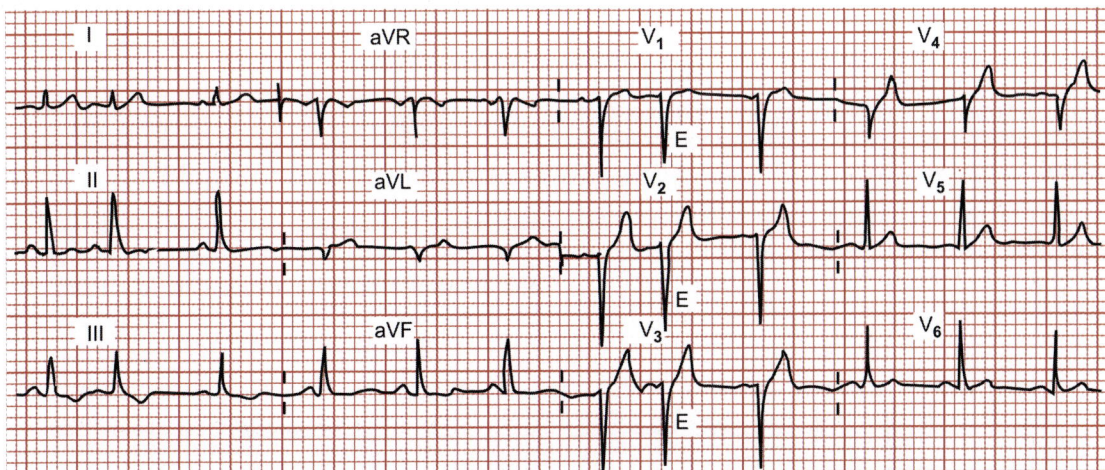

Fig. 7.4: *Nonprogression* of R wave from V_1-V_4 (a normal variant). The ECG shows small rudimentary r wave from V_1 to V_4 without any ST-T change. It was recorded from a healthy stout young man without any heart disease. Therefore rS pattern in V_1-V_4 can occur normally; should not be misinterpreted as an anteroseptal infarction. The T wave inversion is lead III is normal. There are atrial ectopics seen in leads V_1-V_3 labelled as E; are also of no consequence

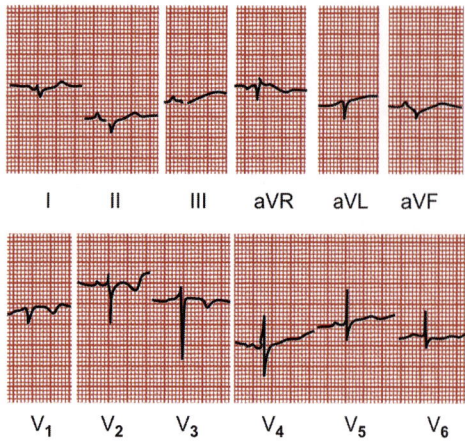

Fig. 7.5: Persistent juvenile pattern in an adult. The electro-cardiogram recorded from 20 yrs healthy female shows T wave inversion from V₁-V₃

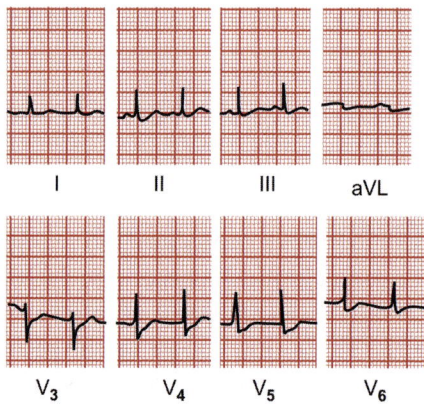

Fig. 7.6: Anxiety neurosis. The ECG recorded from a 24 yrs female during acute phase of anxiety shows:
(i) Sinus tachycardia (HR >100/min regular)
(ii) The J point and ST segment depression in leads II, III and precordial leads. All these changes appeared to be anxiety induced because they do not fit into any fixed coronary artery syndrome due to widespread distribution. This was confirmed when anxiolytics and small dose of propranolol brought these changes back to normal (ECG not shown)

Normalisation of these changes have been reported with drugs such as atropine, propranolol (β-blocker) and potassium.

2. *Effect of Heavy Carbohydrate Meal (Fig. 7.7)*

The ST segment depression or T wave inversion or both have been reported to occur following a heavy carbohydrate meal. This is considered due to a physiological response to carbohydrate meal. The high glucose metabolism may shift the potassium intracellularily and may result in these changes. These ECG changes can also occur pathologically in certain conditions, hence, must be interpreted carefully and should be declared as normal after ascertaining that there is no other cause to explain them.

3. *The Athlete's Heart (Fig. 7.8)*

The concept of '*Athletic heart syndrome*' refers to physiological adaptation of the heart to profound exercise in well conditioned persons. It is a well recognised variant. The ECG changes that occur commonly in athletes are given in the box. These changes most likely reflect an increased vagal tone and increased ventricular mass in conditioned athletes.

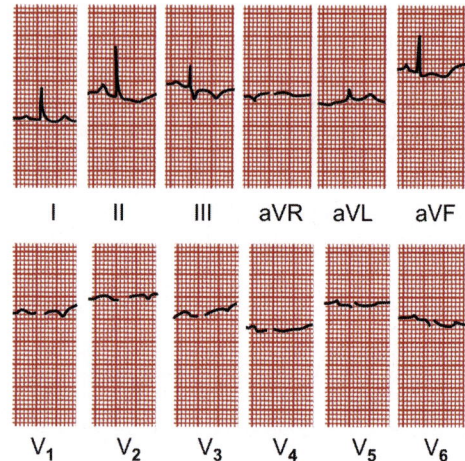

Fig. 7.7: The electrocardiographic changes after heavy carbohydrate meal. There is inversion of T wave in leads II, III and aVF which became normal after few hours

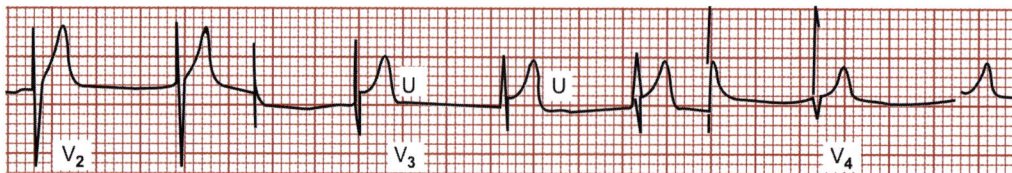

Fig. 7.8: The athlete heart. The ECG (leads V₂-V₄) was recorded from a young wrestler which shows sinus bradycardia (HR 43/min). There are tall T waves in mid-precordial leads. The P wave and P-R intervals are normal. There are prominent U waves following T waves best seen in V₂ and V₃

The electrocardiogram of an athlete

1. **Changes due to hypervagotonaemia**
   - Sinus bradycardia
   - Sinus arrhythmia.
   - Wenckebach second degree AV block
   - Wandering pacemaker

   These changes can be reverted to normal sinus rhythm with active exercise or by the administration of atropine or isoproterenol.

2. **Due to increased left ventricular mass**
   - Voltage criteria of LVH (i.e. $SV_1+RV_5 >35$ mm)
   - Increased amplitude of T waves
   - Presence of U waves
   - Increase in P-R and QRS intervals but not beyond upper limit of the normal
   - ST-T changes mimicing ischaemia

NB: It has also been reported that unsuspected hypertrophic cardiomyopathy is most common abnormality found at autopsy in young competitive athletes who die suddenly.

4. *Early Repolarisation Syndrome*
   (Figs 7.9A and B)

Normally, ventricular depolarisation is followed by repolarisation. The ST segment and T-U waves represent ventricular repolarisation on ECG. The endpoint of S wave (the point at which S wave returns to baseline) and beginning of ST segment is called 'J' point. The early repolarisation refers to an early onset of repolarisation in a portion of ventricular myocardium before the process of depolarisation is completed in other areas of the myocardium. It is a well recognised normal electrocardiographic variant. Early repolarisation is also known to occur in myocardial diseases such as cardiomyopathies, myocarditis, myocardial ischaemia, etc.

Grant and his associates in 1951 found a distinct notch or hook on the descending limb of QRS in the form of a wave called 'J' wave in mid-precordial leads (V_2-V_4) in certain individuals. They documented 'J' wave due to an early and rapid repolarisation. Later on, some workers found elevation of ST segment with concavity upwards, while others found abnormalities of T waves (tall symmetric upright T waves), tall R

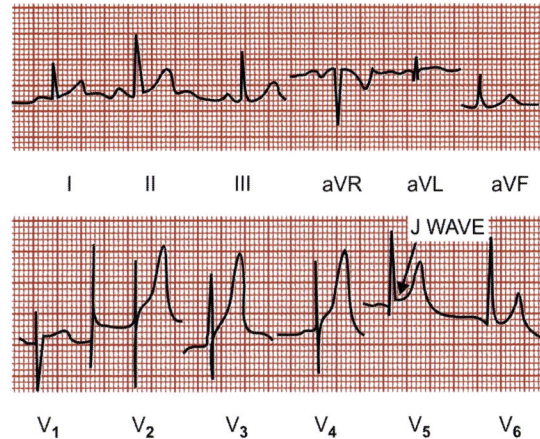

Fig. 7.9A: Early repolarisation syndrome. Note the following features:
   (i) Proment J waves (labelled as J) are seen in leads V_5-V_6
   (ii) ST segment elevation with concavity upwards seen in leads V_2-V_6
   (iii) Tall, peaked T waves more than R wave in leads V_2-V_4
   (iv) Early transition or counterclockwise rotation is reflected by shifting of transition zone rightwards between V_2-V_3 instead of normal (V_3-V_4)

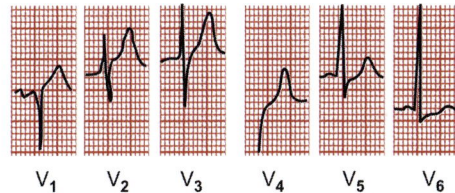

Fig. 7.9B: Early repolarisation syndrome. The electrocardiogram recorded from a normal healthy adult shows;
   (i) Early transition: The transition zone is shifted rightwards, lies in the lead V_2
   (ii) Elevation of ST segment with concavity upwards. The ST segment is minimally elevated in leads V_1-V_4, best seen in V_2-V_3 with concavity upwards
   (iii) Tall peaked symmetric upright T waves seen in leads V_1-V_6. These T waves are taller than normal. The T wave in V_1 is taller than V_6

waves and prominent U waves, a tendency to counterclockwise rotation or early transition, etc. in normal individuals. All these abnormalities now-a-days are included in electrocardiographic manifestations of a well defined *early repolarisation syndrome*. The term 'syndrome' is being retained for the purpose of these electrocardiographic normal variants. Therefore, ECG features of this syndrome include;

SECTION TWO

i) *Prominent 'J' waves*: The J or junctional wave is nothing but a distinct notch or hook on the descending limb of QRS and is separated from it. These J waves are best seen in leads V_2-V_4 but are uncommon in frontal plane leads. The prominent J waves indicate an early repolarisation. These J waves actually constitute an early part of the ST segment.

ii) *Elevation of ST segment with concavity upwards*: The ST segment elevation with concavity upwards along with tall, pointed upright T waves are seen in early repolarisation syndrome. The elevation of ST segment is variable (0.05 to 5 mm) but usually does not exceed 2 mm in precordial leads. This manifestation occurs in precordial leads (V_2-V_6) but best seen in mid-precordial leads V_3 or V_4.

iii) *Tall, peaked, symmetric upright T waves*: The T waves taller than normal are seen in precordial leads in this syndrome.

iv) *Inverted T waves*: Infrequently, inversion of T waves in leads V_5 and V_6 have been seen in early repolarisation syndrome. These should be considered due to early repolarisation syndrome when other features such as 'J' waves are present in these leads.

v) *Prominent 'q' waves and tall R waves in left precordial leads*: Prominent 'q' and a large or tall R wave simulating left ventricular diastolic overload may be seen in left precordial leads (V_5-V_6).

vi) *Prominent 'U' wave*: A prominent and easy identifiable U waves may be seen in mid-precordial leads. The 'U' wave is produced after T wave due to delayed repolarisation.

vii) *Early transition and counterclockwise rotation*: An early transition from characteristic 'rS' complexes of right ventricle to 'qR' complexes of left ventricle may occur during early repolarisation. A tendency to counterclockwise rotation leading to shifting of the transition zone from V_3 to V_2 may be seen in early repolarisation syndrome.

viii) *Sinus bradycardia or slow sinus rates*: Slow sinus rhythm or sinus bradycardia may occur in early repolarisation due to hypervagotonaemia.

Suggested Reading

1. Bachman S, Sparrow D, Smith KL: Effect of aging on the ECG. *Am J Cardiol* **48**:513, 1981.
2. Balady CJ, Cadiogam JB, Ryam TJ: Electrocardiogram of the athlete. An analysis of 289 professional football players. *Am J Cardiol* **53**: 1339, 1984.
3. Fenichel NN: A long term study of concave RS-T elevation. A normal variant of the electrocardiogram. *Angiology* **13**:360, 1962.
4. Goldschlager NC, Goldman KJ: Principles of electrocardiography. Appleton and Lange publication, 1975.
5. Grant R, Estes EH, Doyle JT: Special vector-electrocardiography. The clinical characteristics of ST and T vectors. *Circulation* **3**:182, 1951.
6. Kambara H, Phillips J: Long term evaluation of early repolarisation syndrome (normal variant) RS-T elevation. *Am J Cardiol* **38**:157, 1976.
7. Littman D: Persistence of Juvenile pattern in the precordial leads of healthy adult negroes. *Am Heart J* **32**:370, 1946.
8. Maron BJ, Isner JM, McKenna WJ: 26th Bethesda Conference: Recommendations for determining eligibility for competition in athletes with cadiovascular abnormalities. Task Force 3: Hypertrophic cardiomyopathy, myocarditis, and other myopericardial diseases and mitral valve prolapse. *J Am Coll Cardiol* **24**: 800, 1994.
9. Mirvis D: Evaluation of normal variations in ST segment pattern by body surface isopotential mapping: ST segment elevation in the absence of heart disease. *Am J Cardiol* **50**:122, 1982.
10. Ostrander LD Jr: Left axis deviation: Prevalence, associated conditions and prognosis: An epidemiologic study. *Ann Intern Med* **75**: 23, 1971.
11. Parisi AF, Beckmann CH, Lancaster MC: The spectrum of ST elevation in electrocardiogram of healthy adult men. *J Electrocardiol* **4**:137, 1971.
12. Surawicz B: Assessing abnormal ECG patterns in the absence of heart disease. *Cardiovas Med* **2**:269, 1977.
13. Wasserburger RH, Alt WJ: The normal RS-T segment elevation variant. *Am J Cardiol* **8**:184, 1961.
14. Zeppilli P et al: T wave abnormalities in top-ranking athletes. Effects of isoproterenol, atropine and physical exercise. *Am Heart J* **100**:213, 1980.

Chamber Hypertrophy or Enlargement

SECTION THREE

8

Atrial Hypertrophy/ Enlargement

- ■ *Anatomy and physiology of human heart*
- ■ *Chamber enlargement and the abnormalities of P wave*
- ■ *Atrial hypertrophy and enlargement–general aspects, causes, ECG criteria in reference to normal P wave characteristics*
- ■ *Left atrial hypertrophy or enlargement*
- ■ *Right atrial hypertrophy or enlargement*
- ■ *Biatrial hypertrophy or enlargement (combined right and left atrial hypertrophy)*
- ■ *Other P waves abnormalities – low atrial, left atrial pacemaker and coronary sinus rhythm, etc.*

ANATOMY AND ELECTROPHYSIOLOGY OF HUMAN HEART

The human heart is 4 chambered, i.e. 2 atria and 2 ventricles; the right atrium and right ventricle form the right side of the heart; while left atrium and left ventricle constitute its left side. The atria are thin walled than the ventricles. The left ventricle is the thickest of all the chambers (Fig. 8.1).

The electrophysiology and genesis of various complexes of electrocardiogram has already been discussed. For revision sake, P wave is the wave of atrial depolarisation and Ta or Pa wave is atrial repolarisation wave. The QRS complex indicates ventricular depolarisation and ST segment and T wave indicate ventricular repolarisation. The depolarisation is a continuous process, occurs first of all in both the atria synchronously followed by simultaneous depolarisation of both the ventricles.

CHAMBER ENLARGEMENT

Chamber enlargement may involve the atria or ventricles or both. It implies either enlargement or dilatation or hypertrophy. Dilatation implies an increase in the internal diameter of the cardiac chamber, occurs mostly due to volume overload. Actually, hypertrophy implies thickening of the walls of the chambers, usually occurs either due to pressure or systolic overload or both. Chamber enlargement whether due to dilatation or due to true hypertrophy is often called 'hypertrophy' in electrocardiographic terms. Although chamber enlargement is suggested by many ECG clues, it is actually impossible to

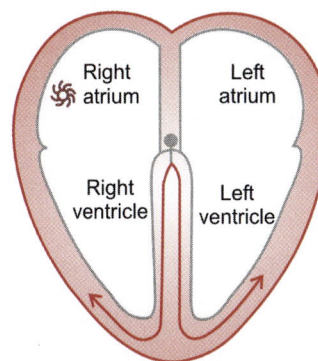

Fig. 8.1: Normal four chambered heart of humans (diagram).

differentiate the dilatation from hypertrophy on the basis of ECG alone. In such a situation, echocardiography forms an important diagnostic tool to differentiate between them.

Atrial chamber(s) enlargement/hypertrophy is reflected in abnormalities of P waves; while ventricular enlargement/hypertrophy is reflected in abnormalities of QRS.

The P Wave Abnormalities (Fig. 8.2)

The P wave abnormalities (Fig. 8.2) may manifest in height (tall P wave) or width or abnormal conduction (inverted P wave). Right atrial enlargement/hypertrophy increases the height of the P wave while left atrial enlargement widens the P waves (Fig 8.3). These P wave abnormalities are discussed below in relation to atrial hypertrophy.

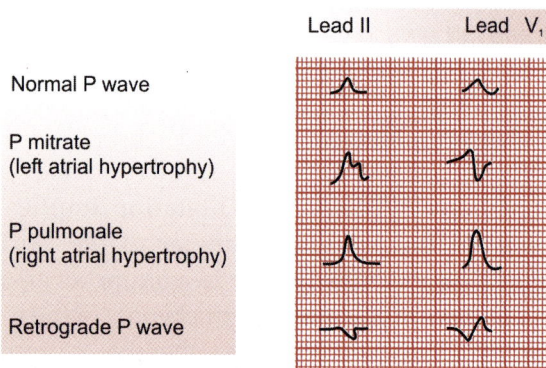

Fig. 8.2: Different shapes of P waves

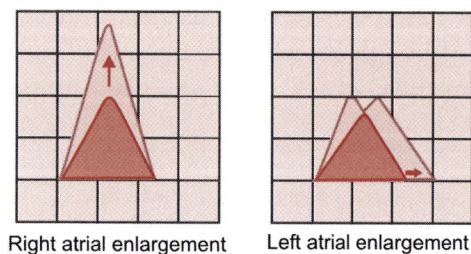

Fig. 8.3: The shape of P waves in atrial enlargement (diagram)

ATRIAL HYPERTROPHY AND ENLARGEMENT

As already stated above, atrial hypertrophy means an increase in the thickness of atrial muscle mass with or without increase in its internal diameter.

Hypertrophy later on may be followed by dilatation. For example, mitral stenosis produces left atrial hypertrophy initially followed by its enlargement in long standing cases; on the other hand, mitral regurgitation produces left ventricular and left atrial dilatation followed by slight increase or decrease of left atrial muscle mass depending on its response to volume overload and chronicity of the disease. In chronic cases of mitral regurgitation, left atrium may become giant with loss of atrial muscle mass.

Aetiology

The causes of atrial hypertrophy- right or left or both are briefly discussed below. There may be an isolated atrial hypertrophy or it may be associated with ventricular hypertrophy.

1. *Valvular heart disease*: Both the stenotic and regurgitant valvular lesions produce atrial hypertrophy by increasing workload on an atrium or atria which may either be in the form of pressure or volume overload. It is often associated with ventricular enlargement. For example, mitral stenosis first of all, produces left atrial hypertrophy followed by right ventricular hypertrophy (Fig. 8.4). Isolated right atrial hypertrophy may occur in tricuspid stenosis.

2. *Congenital heart disease*: Intra-atria shunt such as atrial septal defect produces right atrial hypertrophy due to volume overload (Fig. 8.4B).

3. *Atrial hypertrophy secondary to ventricular hypertrophy*: Atrial hypertrophy commonly occurs secondary to ventricular hypertrophy. Left atrial and left ventricular hypertrophy occur in mitral regurgitation, aortic valve disease and hypertensive cardiovascular disease (Fig. 8.4C).

4. *Pulmonary stenosis and pulmonary arterial hypertension*: Pulmonary stenosis is a congenital lesion. Pulmonary arterial hypertension develops due to variety of reasons and conditions. Irrespective of its cause, both the diseases are associated with pressure overload on right ventricle and consequently on right atrium leading to their enlargement. This type of chamber enlargement is seen in cor pulmonale and pulmonary stenosis (Fig. 8.4D).

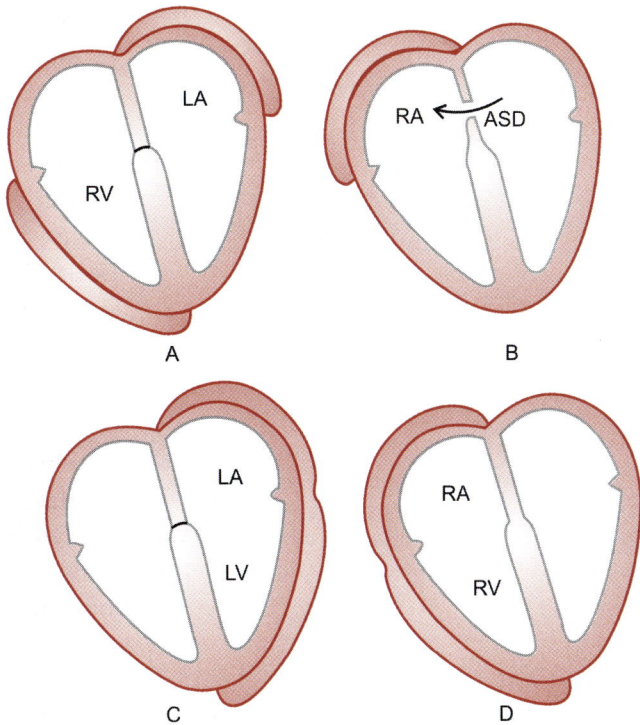

Figs 8.4A to D: Diagrammatic illustration of chamber(s) hypertrophy. **A:** Left atrial and right ventricular hypertrophy in mitral stenosis. **B:** Right atrial hypertrophy (shaded area) of atrial septal defect. **C:** Left atrial and ventricular hypertrophy (shaded area) due to aortic valve or hypertensive heart disease. **D:** Right atrial and right ventricular hypertrophy (shaded area) seen in cor pulmonale and pulmonary stenosis

The Electrocardiographic Criteria

The atrial hypertrophy and enlargement is electrocardiographically expressed as P wave abnormalities. It is difficult to distinguish atrial hypertrophy and atrial enlargement on ECG. For sake of revision, the normal characteristics of P wave are again summarised in the box.

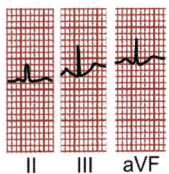

Fig. 8.5: The normal P waves. The electrocardiogram (leads I, II, III) shows normal characteristics of P waves. Both the height and width of P wave is < 2.5 mm

Characteristics of Normal P Wave (Fig. 8.5)

The normal P wave is best evaluated in terms of following parameters;

i. *Frontal plane P wave:* The P wave is best seen in lead II because frontal plane P wave axis is directed to the positive pole of that lead. The normal P wave is pyramidal in shape with rounded apex. The duration of P wave is 0.08 to 0.10 second normally but is never greater than 0.11 second. The normal maximum amplitude is 2.5 mm.

ii. *Normal P wave in lead V_1:* The P wave in this lead is usually studied because P wave is biphasic having an initial positivity and terminal negativity; the initial positive and terminal negative components are clearly defined and easily separated in this lead.
Explanation: The biphasic P wave in lead V_1 is because the SA node lies in right atrium, activates it first and right atrium being anterior to left atrium, the vector of right atrial activation is directed anteriorly and slightly to the left, i.e. towards lead V_1, hence, this lead records an initial positive deflection. Left atrial activation begins slightly later and overlaps the terminal activation of right atrium. Due to posterior position of left atrium, the left atrial vector is oriented posteriorly, hence, is away from the lead V_1, resulting in terminal negative deflection of P wave. Thus P wave in this lead is composite of deflections of both right and left atrial activation.

iii. *Frontal plane P wave axis* is directed to the region of + 45° clockwise to +60° or 65°. The P wave axis more than +70° indicates right axis deviation of P wave. P wave axis less than + 45° reflects left axis deviation of P wave.

Sinus tachycardia tends to deviate the frontal plane P wave axis minimally to the right for about 10 to 15°, for example if P wave axis is 45° at rest and becomes 55° during excercise, then P wave becomes taller in lead II as compared to P wave at rest in that lead.

SECTION THREE

LEFT ATRIAL HYPERTROPHY OR ENLARGEMENT

Causes

1. Mitral valve disease. Both isolated mitral stenosis and mitral regurgitation or both produce left atrial enlargement.
2. Systemic hypertension.
3. Associated with left ventricular hypertrophy in aortic valve disease or systemic hypertension.
4. Sometimes, acute pulmonary oedema due to myocardial infarction produces left atrial hypertrophy.
5. Cardiomyopathies.

In left atrial hypertrophy, there is increased thickness of left atrial walls and delayed conduction through them, therefore, the basic electrocardiographic effects are due to;

  (i) Prolongation and delay of the terminal or left atrial component of atrial activation
  (ii) Increased posterior deviation of left atrial vector
  (iii) Left axis deviation of frontal plane P vector.

The Electrocardiogram (Figs 8.6 and 8.7)

The evolution of electrocardiographic patterns of left atrial hypertrophy due to above mentioned mechanisms is reproduced below:

1. *Prolonged and delayed activation of left atrium.* Due to increased left atrial mass, there is prolonged and delayed activation of left atrium that follows right atrial activation, hence, total atrial activation process is virtually split into its two individual atrial activations (right and left), therefore, the P wave shows following characteristics (Fig. 8.6);

  i) Notched or double peaked (M shaped) broad P wave.
  ii) Duration of P wave is increased > 0.1 second (2.5 mm).
  iii) The duration of notch or distance between the two peaks of M shaped P wave is > 0.04 second.

These features are best seen on frontal plane leads depending on the P wave axis. If the P wave axis is directed to + 50° or + 55°, then morphology of P wave is best seen in lead II as the positive (+) pole of this lead lies at + 60° on the hexaxial system. However, if

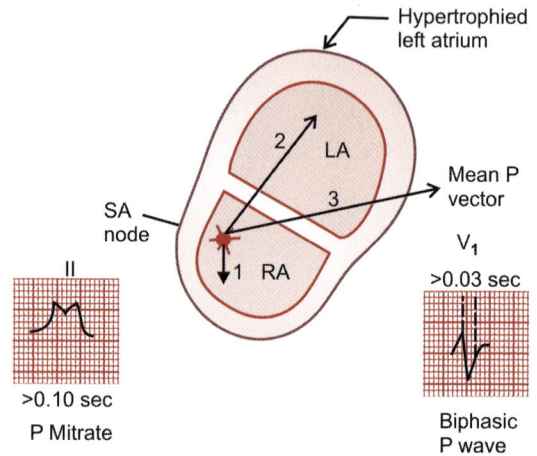

Fig. 8.6: Diagram illustrating the electrocardiographic effects of left atrial enlargement on the P waves in leads II and V_1. Arrow 1 → Right atrial vector, Arrow 2 → Left atrial vector, Arrow 3 → Mean P vector, RA = right atrium, LA = left atrium

there is left axis deviation of P wave (+ 45° clockwise to - 30°) then these features of P wave will appear in leads I, aVL and left precordial leads V_5 -V_6.

Left atrial enlargement produces a notched or bifid (double peaked – M shaped) P waves called - P mitrale, is characteristically seen in left atrial hypertrophy due to mitral stenosis – hence–its name. The first component or peak of this bifid P wave indicates right atrial activation and second peak is due to left atrial activation which is larger than the first. The duration of P is increased to > 0.11 second (>2.5 mm in width). The P wave is best seen in standard leads I, II, aVL or aVF depending on its axis.

2. *Posterior deviation of left atrial vector.* The P wave vector has two components – an initial right atrial vector directed anteriorly and terminal left atrial vector directed posteriorly. These two components are best demonstrated in a biphasic P wave of lead V_1 where initial upright deflection is due to right atrial vector and terminal negative deflection is due to left atrial vector. Due to left atrial hypertrophy, the left atrial vector gets directed more posteriorly (Fig. 8.8), hence, the negative deflection of biphasic P waves in lead V_1 becomes deep, delayed and widened. If this terminal negative component is > 1 mm deep and > 0.03 second in duration, it indicates left atrial hypertrophy.

Left atrial hypertrophy produces a deep and wide negative deflection of biphasic P wave in lead V_1.

3. *Left axis deviation of P wave axis.* In left atrial hypertrophy, there is left axis deviation of P wave on the frontal plane, i.e. it lies between + 45° counterclockwise to - 30°, hence the shape of P wave is best seen in leads I, II, aVL or aVF and V_5-V_6.

Left atrial hypertrophy produces left axis deviation of P wave (+ 45° counterclockwise to -30°)

Clinical Significance

1. Left atrial hypertrophy may be the only sign of left ventricular hypertrophy in the presence of left bundle branch block (LBBB).
2. Left atrial enlargement is frequent electrocardiographic manifestation of systemic hypertension and may be the earliest and only electrocardiographic sign.
3. Left atrial hypertrophy may also appear as a transient phenomenon in acute pulmonary oedema reflecting left atrial stress.
4. It is subsequent to haemodynamic alterations, hence, does not require any specific treatment except the treatment of the cause.

RIGHT ATRIAL HYPERTROPHY OR ENLARGEMENT (Fig. 8.8)

Right atrial hypertrophy produces an increase in its muscle mass or volume with slight delayed conduction through it which is reflected in the increased voltage of P wave. In addition, it produces a rotational effect which is reflected in QRS abnormalities.

The Electrocardiogram (Figs 8.9 to 8.11)

The ECG manifestations of right atrial hypertrophy can be divided into;
1. Direct
2. Indirect.

1. **Direct**: Right atrial hypertrophy / enlargement is reflected directly by one or more of the following manifestations;

i) *Increase in the height of P wave – P pulmonale* (Fig. 8.9) : Right atrial hypertrophy produces an increased amplitude of the P wave (> 2.5 mm) with a slight increase in its duration which usually does not exceed 0.11 second. The increase in amplitude results in a tall and peaked P wave, called *P pulmonale* – a characteristic feature seen in right atrial hypertrophy secondary to the disease of lung (cor pulmonale) – hence, its name. It is best seen in leads II, III and aVF since the frontal plane axis is directed toward the right, i.e. + 80° to + 90°, is aligned to the positive poles of the above mentioned leads. If P wave axis lies within normal limits or is around +60°, then tall P waves will be seen in lead II. Therefore, the leads reflecting the P wave abnormality depend on the P wave axis.

SECTION THREE

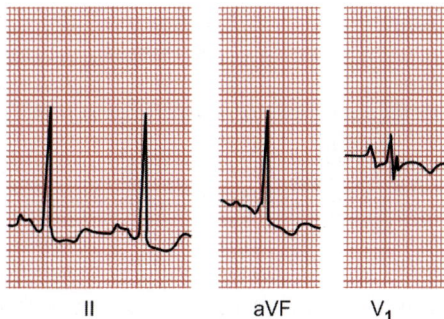

Fig. 8.7: The P-mitrale. The standard leads II and aVF show wide, notched P wave with width greater than 2.5 mm but height is normal. In lead V_1, P is biphasic with wide, prominent negative component

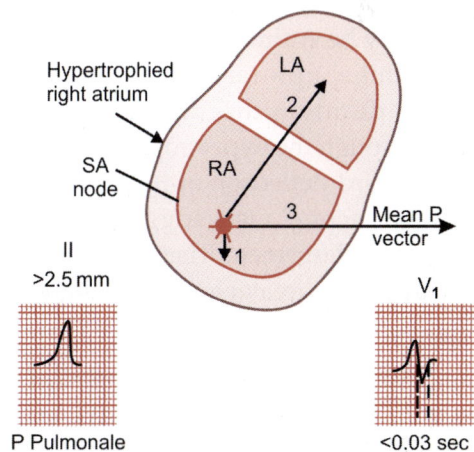

Fig. 8.8: Diagram illustrating the electrocardiographic effects of right atrial enlargement on the P wave in leads II and V_1. Arrow 1 → Right atrial vector, Arrow 2 → Left atrial vector, Arrow 3 → Mean P vector, RA = right atrium, LA = left atrium

Right atrial hypertrophy produces tall (> 2.5 mm) and peaked P waves in leads II, III and aVF. The duration of P wave is either normal or slightly increased but does not exceed upper limit of the normal, i.e. < 0.11 second.

ii) *Abnormalities of the P wave axis*

a) *Right P wave axis deviation.* In acquired heart diseases with right atrial enlargement / hypertrophy, there is a tendency to shift the P wave axis towards right, i.e. + 60° clockwise to + 90°, especially seen in cor pulmonale. The right axis deviation of P wave is the earliest and diagnostic manifestation of diffuse lung diseases producing cor pulmonale, hence, absence of such right axis deviation militates against its diagnosis.. When the tall and peaked P wave is associated with right axis deviation of P wave, it is called *P pulmonale,* a characteristic feature seen in right atrial hypertrophy secondary to lung diseases.

*Right atrial hypertrophy / enlargement produces right axis deviation of P wave (+ 60° clockwise to + 90°). The tall peaked P wave with right axis deviation is called **P-pulmonale.***

b) *Large dominant initial upright deflection of biphasic P wave in lead V_1:* In right atrial enlargement, the initial upright deflection of biphasic P wave in lead V_1 becomes taller and symmetrically pointed (Fig. 8.9). The initial upward deflection will exceed 1.5 mm and is greater than terminal negative deflection; at times, the P wave may be entirely positive. The right atrial component (initial upward deflection) may also be increased in duration due to slow and delayed conduction through the hypertrophied atrium. Thus, the initial upward deflection of the biphasic P wave in V_1 > 0.04 second also suggests right atrial hypertrophy or enlargement. These features of P wave in lead V_1 are due to greater and more aligned first or right atrial vector toward that lead (Fig. 8.8).

Exception: *Normal P wave axis or a potential left axis deviation of P wave:* The normal P wave axis (+ 40° clockwise to + 70°) is exceptionally seen in right atrial enlargement due to congenital heart disease such as pulmonary stenosis and tetralogy of Fallot. Occasionally, P wave axis may deviate from + 45° counterclockwise to 0°. Marked left axis deviation of

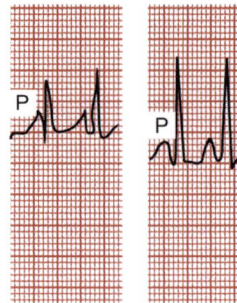

Fig. 8.9: The P-pulmonale. The leads (V_1 and V_2) show tall P waves (>2.5 mm) but width is normal. There is an evidence of right ventricular hypertrophy (a tall R wave and R:S >1 in V_1-V_2)

tall and peaked P wave may even be seen in Ebstein's anomaly, the mechanism of which is complex rather than simple right atrial hypertrophy. A tall peaked P wave with left axis deviation of P wave is called '*P-congenitale*' seen in congenital heart diseases – hence its name.

A tall peaked P wave with its left axis deviation is referred as P – congenitale, is seen in congenital heart diseases.

c) *Early terminal negative deflection of P wave in lead V_1:* The terminal negativity of biphasic P wave in V_1 is seen both in right as well as left atrial hypertrophy, hence, at times, it may be difficult to differentiate between them. In right atrial hypertrophy, the downslope of P wave (intrinsicoid deflection of P wave) is early and its negative deflection does not exceed 0.03 second in duration; while in left atrial hypertrophy the negative deflection is late, becomes wide and its duration is always longer than 0.03 second. When right atrial hypertrophy / enlargement manifests with an early and rapid inscription of negative component of biphasic P wave in lead V_1, then lead V_2 will also usually reflect tall and pointed P waves which may even be seen in all the precordial leads.

Right atrial enlargement / hypertrophy produces an early and rapid negative deflection of P wave in lead V_1 which is less than 0.03 second. In contrast to this, left atrial hypertrophy produces late and wide (> 0.03 second) negative deflection of P wave in V_1.

2) Indirect: Abnormalities of P wave reflect right atrial enlargement directly. It is becoming increasingly evident that diagnosis of right atrial hypertrophy or enlargement can frequently be made from the changes of QRS complex and, at times, with greater reliability than from the direct abnormalities of P wave. Two characteristic ECG manifestations of QRS complex suggest right atrial enlargement in the absence of direct evidences:

1. A 'qR' complex in lead V_1.
2. Diminution in height of QRS complex in lead V_1 with marked increase in its height in lead V_2.

1. A 'qR' complex in V_1: A 'qR' complex is lead V_1 indirectly reflect right atrial enlargement and such right atrial enlargement is usually seen due to tricuspid regurgitation. The tall R wave indicates associated right ventricular hypertrophy. The initial small 'q' is the result of anatomical shift of the heart consequent to right atrial enlargement. The genesis of 'qR' complex is thus due to an anatomical shift of hypertrophied right ventricle by an enlarged and dilated right atrium. Sodi-Pallares and his associates in 1952 postulated that lead V_1 reflects a small initial slur or even a notch on QRS, or on a tall R wave, but when 'qR' complex appears in lead V_1, then the lead V_2 under such circumstances reflects a tall R wave

with a small initial slur or notch and is produced due to rotation of heart by enlarged right atrium such that proximal high basal region of the interventricular septum becomes oriented to the lead V_1 (Figs 8.10 and 8.11).

2. Diminution in the height of QRS deflection in V_1 with a marked increase in QRS complex amplitude in lead V_2:

Tranchesi, J (1965) first of all, described a marked increase in QRS amplitude in the transition between lead V_1 and V_2 in some cases of right atrial enlargement, which later on was confirmed by echocardiography by Reeves and associates (1981). Thus, the QRS complex is strongly suggestive of right atrial enlargement if;

i) The magnitude of QRS is small in lead V_1.
ii) The QRS amplitude in lead V_2 is three times greater than in lead V_1. This manifestation has been attributed to large volume of blood in right atrium that lies between the ventricles and precordial electrode V_2.

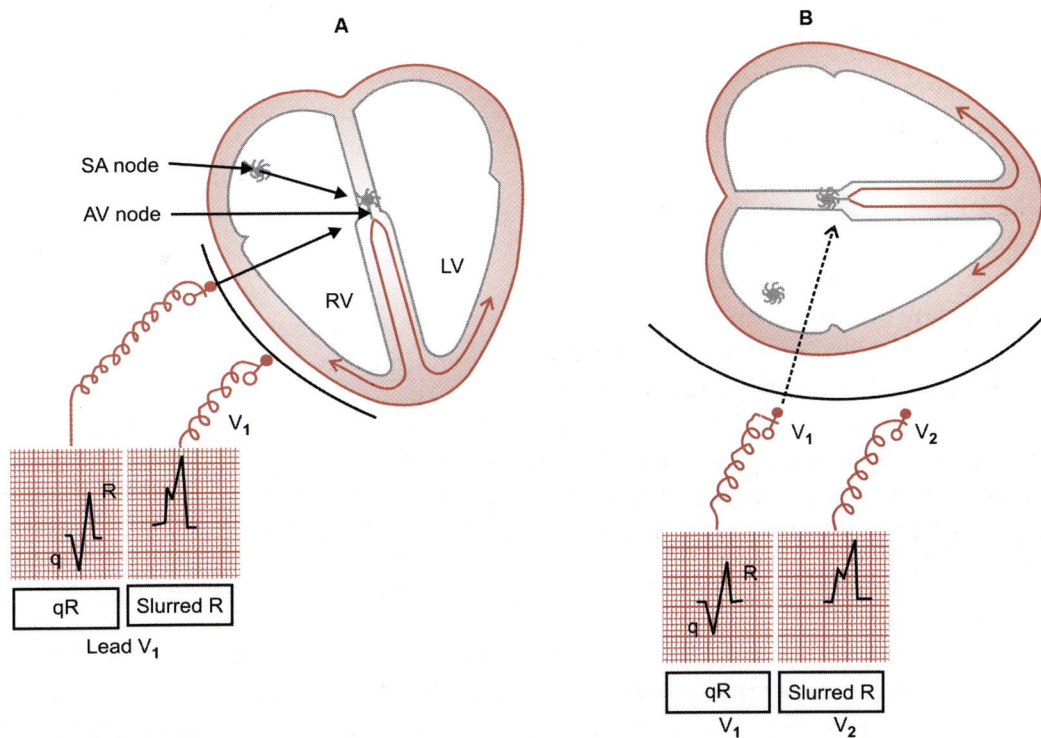

Fig. 8.10: Diagrammatic representation of indirect evidences of right atrial hypertrophy. **A:** The effect of right ventricular hypertrophy. **B:** The effect of right ventricular and right atrial hypertrophy on leads V_1 and V_2

SECTION THREE

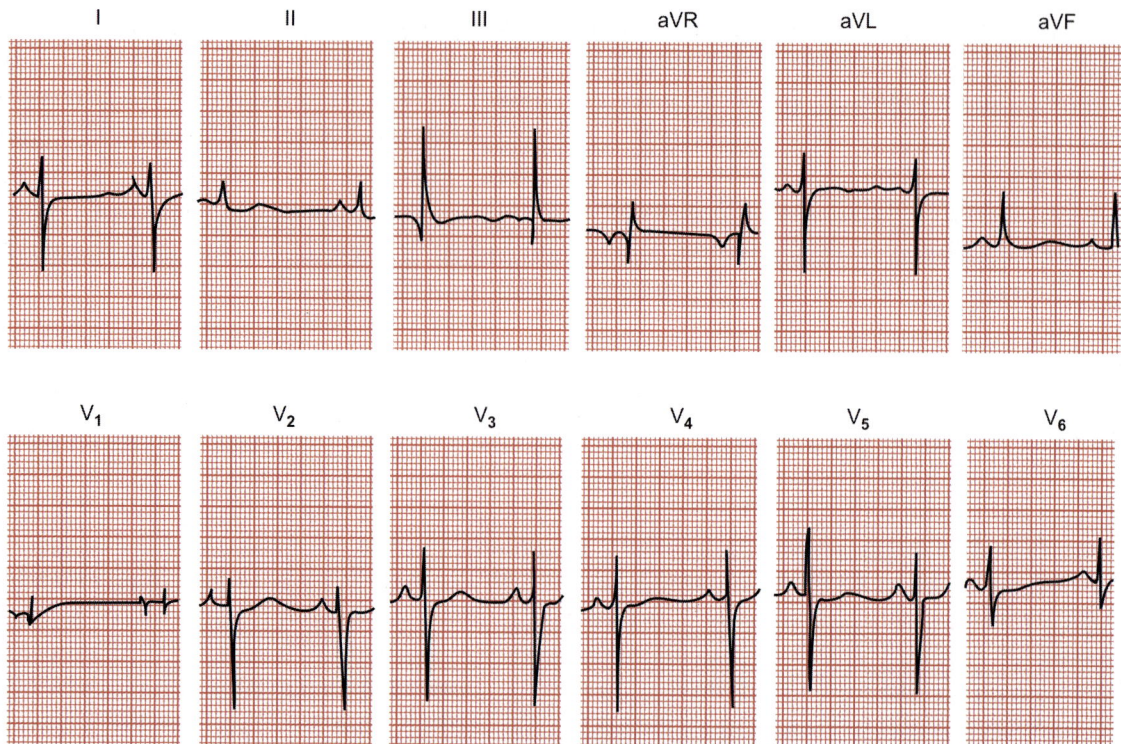

Fig. 8.11: The electrocardiogram showing right atrial and right ventricular hypertrophy. The frontal plane QRS axis is of +120° (right axis deviation). There is a qr pattern in lead V_1 with deep S wave in V_5 and V_6 and clockwise rotation; indicates right ventricular hypertrophy. The P wave amplitude of > 2.5 mm in lead I, II and precordial leads is compatible with right atrial hypertrophy. Right atrial and right ventricular hypertrophy is consistent with diagnosis of chronic cor pulmonále

SUMMARY OF RIGHT ATRIAL HYPERTROPHY

i) The frontal plane QRS axis is >110° (right axis deviation).

ii) Tall peaked P waves in leads II, III, aVF (P pulmonale) with biphasic P in lead V_1 where positive component is large indicates right atrial hypertrophy directly.

iii) There is a qR complex in lead V_1 with clockwise rotation, i.e. transition zone lies in V_6 with deep S wave in this lead. This is due to anatomical shift of right ventricle by hypertrophied right atrium. These findings with right axis deviation and associated right atrial hypertrophy suggest indirect right ventricular hypertrophy.

COMBINED RIGHT AND LEFT ATRIAL HYPERTROPHY (BIATRIAL HYPERTROPHY)

Aetiology

The important causes of both right and left atrial hypertrophy are:

1. Mitral stenosis with pulmonary hypertension.
2. Combined mitral and tricuspid stenosis.
3. Mitral stenosis in patients with COPD with secondary (functional) tricuspid regurgitation.
4. Atrial septal defect.
5. Lutembacher's syndrome (ASD with acquired rheumatic mitral stenosis).
6. Dilated cardiomyopathy with mitral and tricuspid regurgitation.

The Electrocardiogram (Figs 8.12 and 8.13)

In biatrial enlargement, both anterior and posterior forces of P wave vector are increased. The abnormality includes a prominent initial part of the P wave coupled with left axis of terminal portion of P wave and a biphasic P wave in V_1 and V_2. The ECG characteristics of biatrial enlargement include the presence of independent criteria for both left and right atrial enlargement as listed in the box. In biatrial hypertrophy, the P wave becomes taller usually more than 3 mm in height and also becomes wider (≥ 0.12 second), is characteristically seen in leads I, II and left precordial leads. The lead V_1 shows a biphasic P wave whose initial component is tall and terminal negative component is deep and wide.

ECG Characteristics of Biatrial Enlargement

- *Wide and notched P waves* (>0.10 sec) are seen in frontal (leads I, II) and left lateral precordial (V_5-V_6) leads. In addition, there is an increased amplitude of the P waves (> 2.5 mm).
  P-Tricuspidale : When P wave is notched or bifid, the initial upward component represents right atrial and second upward component represents left atrial activity. When initial component is taller than the terminal component (Fig. 8.12), it is called P-tricuspidale. It derives its name from tricuspid valve disease, because of its association with it. It is an electrocardiographic counterpart of–a bifid or notched P wave (P-mitral) of left atial hypertrophy where second upward component is taller than the first.
- *Tall and wide biphasic P wave:* The P wave in lead V_1 is biphasic, whose initial upward component is taller than normal and is peaked and, the terminal negative component is deep, wide and delayed (Fig. 8.12).

Other Abnormalities of P Waves

For convenience, the other abnormalities of P wave are discussed here in this chapter.

1. P wave of retrograde conduction: Retrograde activation of atria results from an impulse originating from the site low in atrium or from AV node. The frontal plane axis of P wave is directed to the region of - 80° to - 90° (left axis deviation of P wave). Consequent to this, the main electrical force of P wave is away from the leads II, III, aVF, i.e. towards their negative poles, thus, results in negative deflection of P waves in these leads. The negative P wave is written as P dash (P-) or (P'). The lead aVR faces the mean electrical force (positive pole of aVR faces P wave vector), hence, it records an upright P wave. The P' wave of retrograde atrial activation will be represented in lead V_1 by a tall, totally positive narrow and peaked deflection resembling P wave of right atrial activation from which it is easily differentiated. The characteristic features of retrograde conduction are again summarised in the box and explained with the help of diagram (Fig. 8.14, see Fig. 8.2 also).

P Wave Characteristics in Retrograde (ventriculoatrial) Conduction

- *Retrograde P wave (P')* Inverted P (P') in leads II, III, aVF.
- *Tall positive narrow peaked P wave* in lead V_1.
- *An upright P wave* in lead aVR.

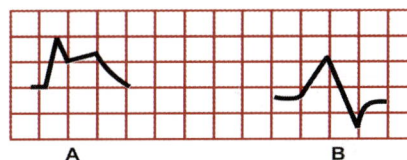

Fig. 8.12: The P waves of combined right and left atrial hypertrophy (graph paper tracing) **A:** P-tricuspidale. Note the initial component of P wave is taller than the second component. **B:** The biphasic P wave: Note the initial upright component is wider and taller than terminal negative component

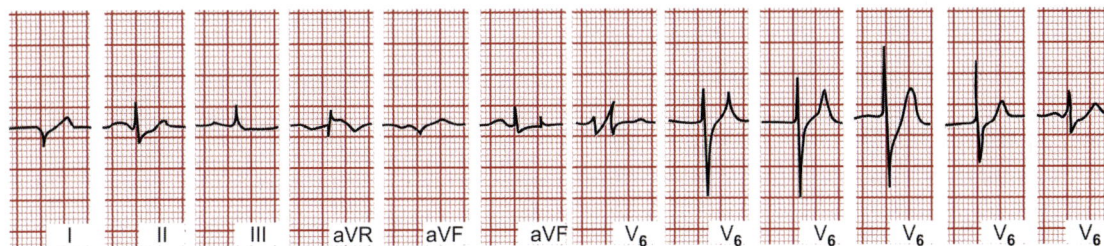

Fig. 8.13: Biatrial enlargement with right ventricular hypertrophy in mitral stenosis. The ECG shows:

i. *Biatrial hypertrophy:* Note the P mitrale (bifid, wide P wave > 2.5 mm) in leads II, III, and aVF. The lead V_1 shows biphasic P wave whose positive (initial) and negative (terminal) components are wide and accentuated. All these features suggest biatrial hypertrophy.

ii. *Right ventricular hypertrophy:* There is tall R wave in V_1 (R > S, R:S > 1) with clockwise rotation and persistence of prominent S wave in V_5-V_6

SECTIONTHREE

SECTIONTHREE

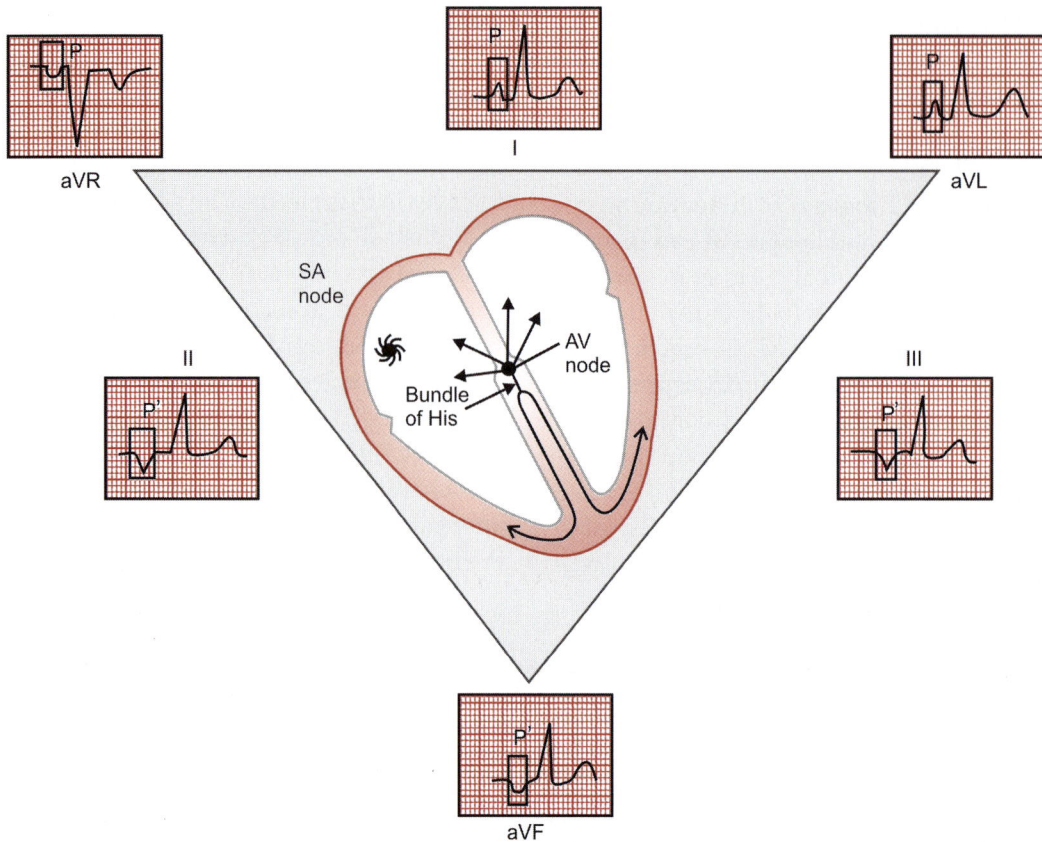

Fig. 8.14 Junctional rhythm with retrograde atrial activation producing inverted P waves (P′) in leads II, III and aVF, and upright P wave in aVR (diagrammatic illustration)

2. **P waves of low atrial rhythm**: The left atrial rhythm has more or less same pattern of inverted P (P′) waves in leads II, III and aVF due to retrograde activation of atria through the internodal conduction pathways. There may also be negative P waves in left precordial leads (V_4-V_6) due to shift of P wave axis away from these leads. The 'dome and dart' appearance (initial rounded dome-shaped upward deflection followed by terminal sharp spike) may be seen in lead V_1.

3. **Pseudo-P pulmonale**: The P pulmonale (tall P wave seen in leads II, III and aVF) in the absence of right atrial enlargement is termed as *'pseudo-P pulmonale'* is seen in left atrial hypertrophy due to a variety of disorders of left heart including coronary artery disease, and less often in the absence of left heart disease. It has been suggested that in the presence of left heart disease, pseudo-P pulmonale reflects an accentuation of left atrial component of P waves. The initial component of P wave representing right atrial depolarisation remains normal. The pseudo-P pulmonale due to severely damaged left atrium can be confirmed by the presence of deep, wide negative deflection of P wave in lead V_1. This finding is supported by the recent observations that left atrial stress or damage increases the right atrial vector and damage to the right atrium stimulates left atrial enlargement.

4. **Left atrial rhythm**: It is a disputed problem but term is still retained. The diagnostic criteria (Fig. 8.15) include (i) dome and dart appearance of P wave in lead V_1 or V_2 (ii) negative P waves in lead I and (iii) essential and most specific is a negative P wave in V_6. All these criteria have been deducted from victorial studies of P waves. This rhythm is seen in ASD (sinus venous defect) and can also be produced by right atrial pacing. The inverted P waves in II, III and aVF in sinus venosus type of ASD indicates left atrial ectopic pacemaker.

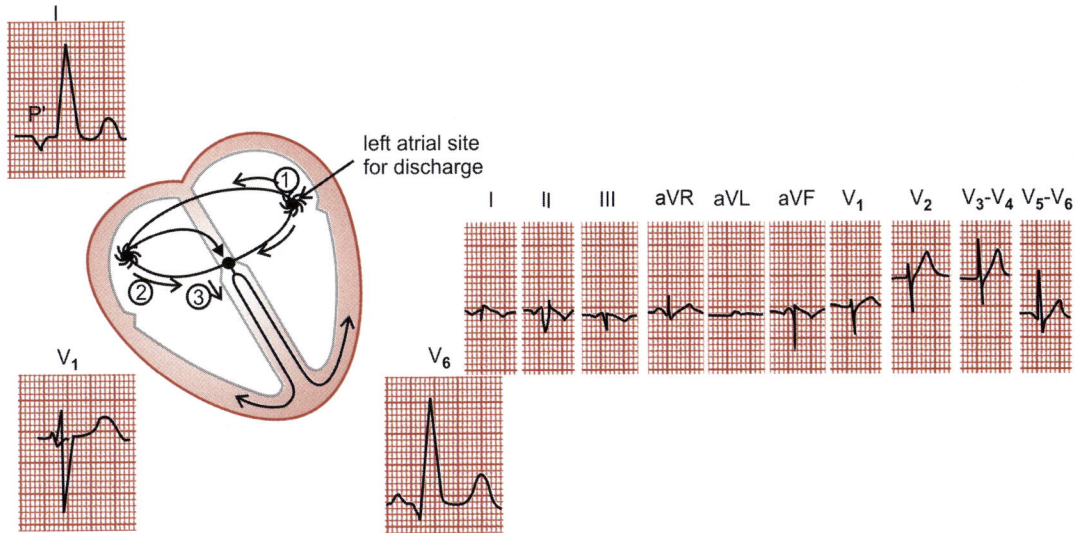

Fig. 8.15: Left atrial rhythm. **A:** Diagram. Due to shift of P wave axis to right (–90°), there is inverted P' waves in leads I and V$_5$-V$_6$ and superior orientation results in inverted P' in leads II, III and aVF and upright in aVR. There may be dome and dart appearance of P waves in leads V$_1$-V$_2$. **B:** The 12 lead surface ECG shows frontal plane P wave axis of -90° resulting in an inverted or negative P (P') wave in leads I, II, III and aVF with positive upward P in aVR. This type of rhythm can be produced by left atrial pacemaker. This type of rhythm has been described in atrial septal defect (sinus venosus type)

5. Left atrial pacemaker: If pacemaker lies in left atrium rather than right atrium then it will produce an inverted P (P') wave in lead I like dextrocardia. The ECG pattern will resemble dextrocardia.

Explanation

i) There is rapid retrograde passage of impulses from left atrium (site of rhythm) upwards through inter-nodal pathways (arrow 1).

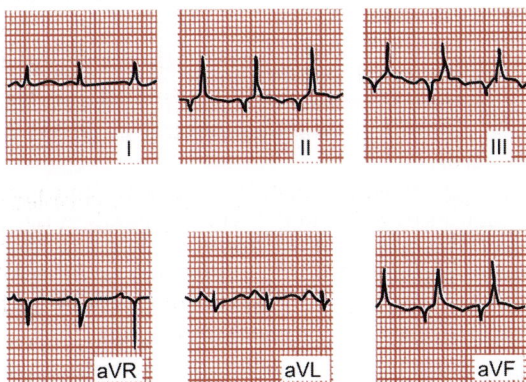

Fig. 8.16: Coronary sinus rhythm: The electrocardiogram showing inverted P (P') waves preceding normal QRS in leads II, III and aVF with upright P in aVR. It resembles a nodal rhythm. The ECG was recorded from a medical student without any evidence of heart disease. The rhythm disappeared next day

ii) Resultant depolarisation of atria is occurring normally as represented by arrow 2.
iii) Normal antegrade conduction of impulses occurs to AV node and bundle of His.

6. Coronary sinus rhythm: The coronary sinus lies in right atrium near the opening of inferior vena cava. It is placed low in right atrium. The coronary sinus rhythm will produce same pattern of P wave inversion (P') in leads II, III, aVF and upright P wave in aVR as described in junctional or nodal rhythm (Fig. 8.16).

REVIEW AT GLANCE

ATRIAL HYPERTROPHY OR ENLARGEMENT ON ECG

1. Right atrial hypertrophy and enlargement is reflected by tall large (>2.5 mm) P wave called P pulmonale in inferior leads (II, III, aVF) with increased upstroke of P wave in lead I. The initial upright deflection of biphasic P wave in lead V$_1$ becomes taller while its terminal negative deflection may be attenuated. The P wave width remains normal. These are direct evidences of right atrial hypertrophy.

SECTION THREE

Indirectly a 'qR' pattern in V_1 and diminished height of QRS in V_1 with increased height of QRS in V_2 also suggest right atrial hypertrophy if direct evidence is lacking.

2. Left atrial hypertrophy is diagnosed by wide and notched (M shape) P waves called 'P-mitrale' and there is deep negative component of biphasic P wave in lead V_1. P wave becomes wider than normal (> 0.1 second).

3. Combined left and right atrial hypertrophy is diagnosed by wide and notched P waves with an increase both in its height (>2.5 mm) and width (>0.10 sec). P mitrale or tricuspidale may be seen; if present then the initial component is larger and wider than terminal component. In biphasic P wave of V_1, the initial upward component is taller and wider than terminal component.

4. Inverted P waves (P´) in leads II, III and aVF with upright P wave in aVR occur in (i) junctional rhythm (ii) low atrial rhythm (iii) coronary sinus rhythm.

5. Left atrial rhythm on ECG produces pattern like dextrocardia.

Suggested Reading

1. Brody DA, Arzbaecher RC, Woolsey MD et al: The normal atrial electrocardiogram. Morphologic and quantiative variability in bipolar extremity leads. *Am Heart J* **74**:4, 1967.

2. Chou TC, Helm RA: The pseudo-P-pulmonale. *Circulation* **32**:96, 1965.

3. Cokkinos DV, Leachman RD, Zamalloa D et al: Influence of atrial mass on amplitude and duration of the P wave. *Chest* **61**: 336, 1972.

4. DiBianco R et al: Left atrial overload: A haemodynamic, electrocardiographic, echocardiographic and vector-cardiographic study. *Am Heart J* **98**:478, 1979.

5. Dines DE, Parkin TW: Some observations on P wave morphology in precordial lead V1 in patients with evaluated left atrial pressures and left atrial enlargement. *Proc Staff Meet, Mayo Clin* **34**: 401, 1959.

6. Gelb AF, Lyons HA, Fairster RD, et al: P-pulmonale in status asthmaticus. *J Allergy Clin Immuno* **64**: 18, 1979.

7. Goldreyer BN, Bigger JT: Ventriculoatrial conduction in man. *Circulation* **41**:935, 1970.

8. Gooch AS, Calatayud JB, Gorman PA et al: Leftward shift of the terminal P forces in ECG associated with left atrial enlargement. *Am Heart J* **71**: 727, 1966.

9. Ikeda K, Kubota I, Takahashi K et al: P wave changes in obstructive and restrictive lung diseases. *J Electrocardiol* **18**:233, 1985.

10. Josephson ME, Kastor JA, Moraganroth J: Electrocardiographic left atrial enlargement: Electrophysiologic, echocardiographic and haemodynamic correlates. *Am J Cardiol* **39**:967, 1977.

11. Kaplan JD, Evans GT, Foster E et al: Evaluation of electrocardiographic criteria for right atrial enlargement by quantitative two-dimensional echocardiography. *J Am Coll Cardiol* **23**:747, 1994.

12. Leatham A: The chest lead electrocardiogram in health. *Br Heart J* **12**:213, 1950.

13. Medano GA, De Micheli A, Osornio S: Interatrial conduction and STA in experimental atrial damage. *J Electrocardiol* **20**:357, 1987.

14. Minoswki M, Neill CA, Taussig HB: Left atrial ectopic rhythm in mirror image dextrocardia and in normally placed malformed hearts. Report of 12 cases with 'dome and dart P waves'. *Circulation* **27**:864, 1963.

15. Mirowski M: Left atrial rhythm: Diagnostic criteria and differentiation from nodal arrhythmias. *Am J Cardiol* **17**:203, 1966.

16. Morris JJ Jr, Estes EH Jr, Whalen RE et al: P wave analysis in valvular heart disease. *Circulation* **29**:242, 1964.

17. Piccolo E, Nava A, Furanello F, et al: Left atrial rhythm. Vectorcardiographic study and electrophysiologic critical evaluation. *Am Heart J* **80**:11, 1970.

18. Reeves WC, Hallahan W, Schwiter EJ et al: Two dimentional echocardiographic assessment of electrocardiographic criteria for right atrial enlargement. *Circulation* **64**:387, 1981.

19. Romhilt DW, Scott RC: Left atrial involvement in acute pulmonary oedema. *Am Heart J* **83**:328, 1972.

20. Rutenberg Hl, Soloff LA: Simulation of left atrial rhythm by right atrial pacing. *Am J Cardiol* **26**:427, 1970.

21. Saunders JL, Calatayud JB, Schultz KJ et al: Evaluation of ECG criteria for P wave abnormalities. *Am Heart J* **74**: 757, 1967.

22. Sodi-Pallares D, Bisteni A, Hermann GR: Some views on significance of qR and QR type complexes in right precordial leads in the absence of myocardial infarction. *Am Heart J* **43**:716, 1952.

23. Surawicz B: Electrocardiographic diagnosis of chamber enlargement. *J Am Coll Cardiol* **8**:714, 1986.

9

Ventricular Hypertrophy/ Enlargement

- General aspects – systolic and diastolic overload–ECG characteristics
- ECG changes in ventricular hypertrophy–mechanisms, criteria of hypertrophy and ventricular strain
- Left ventricular hypertrophy
- Right ventricular hypertrophy
- Biventricular hypertrophy

General Aspects

Ventricular hypertrophy is a pathophysiologic consequence of sufficient workload on the either ventricle. The load may be systolic or diastolic. Systolic overload is an expression of resistance to ventricular outflow or ventricular systolic contraction. In fact, ventricle hypertrophies as a compromise to augment ventricular contraction during systolic or pressure overload. The important causes of systolic overload are given in the Table 9.1.

The diastolic or volume overload is the expression of overfilling of the left ventricle in diastole, so that left ventricular compromise occurs during diastole. The some important causes of diastolic overload on left ventricle are given in the Table 9.1.

The type of ST-T changes which occur due to systolic or diastolic overloading of left ventricle are diagrammatically represented in Figure 9.1.

Mechanisms of ECG Changes in Ventricular Hypertrophy

The electrocardiographic pattern of ventricular hypertrophy depends on;

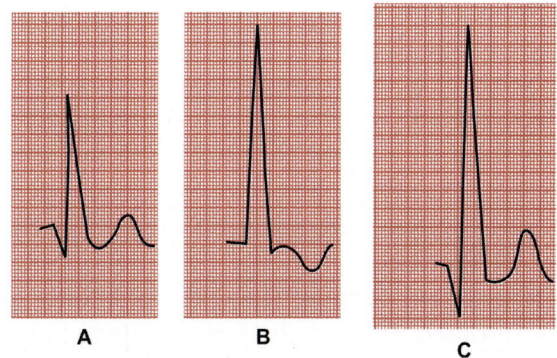

Fig. 9.1: Diagrammatic illustration of systolic and diastolic overload on left ventricle. **A:** Normal, **B:** Systolic overload, **C:** Diastolic overload

Table 9.1: Some important causes of systolic/diastolic overload on left ventricle	
Systolic	*Diastolic*
1. Aortic stenosis, i.e. valvular, supravalvular or subvalvular	1. Mitral regurgitation or incompetence
2. Coarctation of aorta	2. Aortic regurgitation or incompetence
3. Systemic hypertension	3. Moderate to large left to right shunt (PDA, VSD, etc.)
4. Hypertrophic cardiomyopathy	4. Beri-beri heart disease or other high cardiac output syndromes

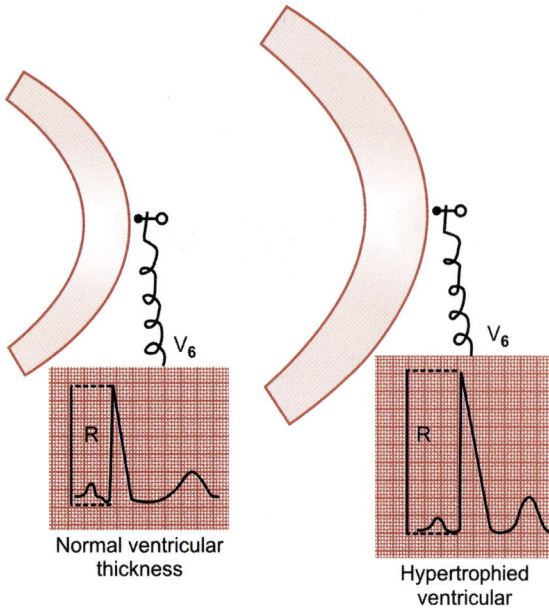

Fig. 9.2: Diagram illustrating height of R wave in normal and hypertrophied ventricle

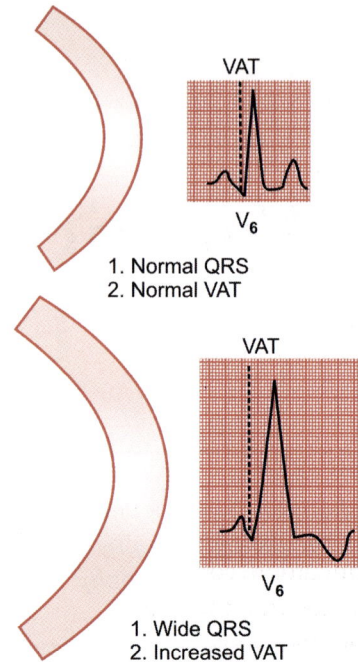

Fig. 9.3: Normal versus delayed conduction through hypertrophied ventricle

1. **Thickness of free wall of the ventricle**: More is the thickness of free wall of a ventricle, more will be the height of R wave in the leads representing that ventricle (i.e. V_5 and V_6 in left ventricular hypertrophy; V_1 and V_2 in right ventricular hypertrophy). The height of R wave of a hypertrophied ventricle produces corresponding deep S wave in leads representing nonhypertrophied ventricle. The mechanism of increased voltage is not well understood but is related to the altered geometric projection of electrical forces. This is not due to increase in the motor units or increase in muscle cells per unit. This is demonstrated with the help of diagram (Fig. 9.2).

2. **Delay in conduction**: The QRS originating from hypertrophied ventricle becomes widened due to delayed conduction through its thick muscle wall but does not exceed 0.12 second. Ventricular activation time is increased (Fig. 9.3).

3. **Endomyocardial changes**: The ST segment depression occurs in those leads which record the epicardial complexes of that ventricle (V_5-V_6 in left ventricular hypertrophy and V_1-V_2 in right ventricular hypertrophy). This is probably initially due to relative ischaemia and later on due to fibrosis of hypertrophied ventricle.

4. **Changes in repolarisation**: It is a general principle of electrocardiography that T wave electrical force or vector is directed away from the diseased or compromised ventricle. The T wave is inverted in ventricular hypertrophy and is seen in precordial leads representing that ventricle (Fig. 9.4). The T wave inversion is commonly seen in systolic than diastolic overload of a ventricle.

The ECG criteria of ventricular hypertrophy are briefly summarised in the box.

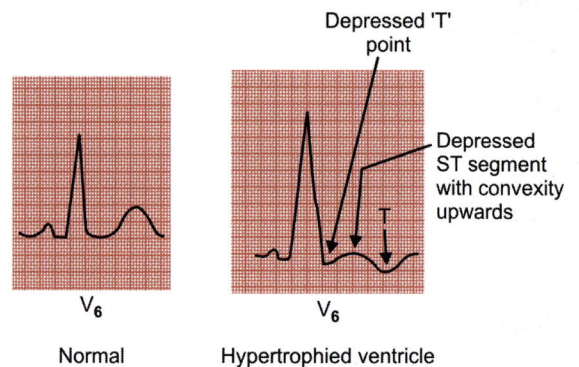

Fig. 9.4: Changes in repolarisation in hypertrophied ventricle

ECG Criteria for Ventricular Hypertrophy

- A tall R wave in leads representing the hypertrophied ventricle and a corresponding deep S wave in leads representing nonhypertrophied ventricle.
- Prolongation of QRS in leads representing the hypertrophied ventricle.
- Prolongation of VAT in leads representing the hypertrophied ventricle.
- Axis deviation and position of the heart depend on the ventricle hypertrophied, i.e right ventricular hypertrophy is mostly associated with right axis deviation, clockwise rotation and vertical heart position. Left ventricular hypertrophy mostly produces left axis deviation, counterclockwise rotation and horizontal heart position.
- ST segment depression or depression of 'J' point in leads representing the hypertrophied ventricle.
- T wave inversion in leads representing the hypertrophied ventricle.

  NB: For practical purposes, leads V_1-V_2 represent right and V_5-V_6 represent left ventricle on ECG.

Ventricular Strain

Ventricular strain in terms of electrocardiography means changes in the ST segment and T wave. The '*strain*' probably reflects the expression of relative ventricular ischaemia due to hypertrophied ventricle. Clinically, the term is used to describe more acute and probable reversible changes that affect the muscle of the ventricle.

As a rule of electrocardiography, the T wave forces shift away from the diseased or involved, hypertrophied or compromised ventricle resulting in T wave inversion in the leads representing the diseased or hypertrophied ventricle. These changes are interpreted as strain pattern or ischaemic pattern. There is no correlation between ECG and anatomical findings during ventricular strain.

An incomplete or complete bundle branch block may be the electrocardiographic pattern of clinical acute ventricular strain. For example, sudden appearance of incomplete or complete right bundle branch block pattern in a patient with acute pulmonary embolism suggests acute right ventricular strain.

LEFT VENTRICULAR HYPERTROPHY (LVH)

It refers to hypertrophy of free walls and apical regions of left ventricular as a compromise to systolic and diastolic overloading of left ventricle.

The causes of left ventricular hypertrophy (LVH) due to systolic and diastolic overload have already been discussed in the beginning.

The Electrocardiographic Criteria

The criteria mentioned under the heading of ventricular hypertrophy when applied to those leads which represent left ventricle will allow to build the ECG criteria for LVH. The specific leads in which the pattern will appear depend on the position of the heart which will be discussed subsequently.

Left Ventricular Hypertrophy Patterns

The two haemodynamic disturbances (systolic and diastolic) will be reflected electrocardiographically by the basic abnormal QRS voltage manifestations with minor differences between them. The differences are outlined in the Table 9.2.

A left ventricular hypertrophy on ECG can often be made when LVH is anatomically present. In fact, ECG diagnosis is made before any radiological evidence of LVH, hence, both do not have any correlation, but electrocardiography remains the valuable diagnostic tool in this field.

The ECG changes of LVH depends on the position of heart as already mentioned, because the leads which record the left ventricle epicardial complex also vary due to it, hence, these will be discussed separately with respect to different heart positions. Irrespective of heart position, the changes of LVH are briefly enumerated.

1. Abnormalities of QRS

a) *Increased amplitude of QRS deflection*: In left ventricular hypertrophy, the height of R wave in left oriented leads (V_5-V_6) increases beyond normal, i.e.

Table 9.2: The electrocardiographic manifestations in systolic and diastolic overload of left ventricle	
Systolic overload (Fig. 9.5)	*Diastolic overload (Fig. 9.6)*
• Attenuation of small 'q' wave in left oriented leads(V_5-V_6) • Ventricular activation time (VAT) is increased due to hypertrophied ventricle • ST segment shows strain pattern, i.e. depression with slight convexity upwards in V_5-V_6 • T waves inversion in V_5-V_6, I, aVL and upright in V_1, V_2 and aVR	• Initial q wave is increased in amplitude in V_5-V_6 • It remains usually normal • Minimally elevated ST segment in leads V_5-V_6 with concavity upwards. There may be slight elevation of 'J' point • Relatively tall symmetric upright T waves in left precordial leads (V_5-V_6). It is inverted in aVR

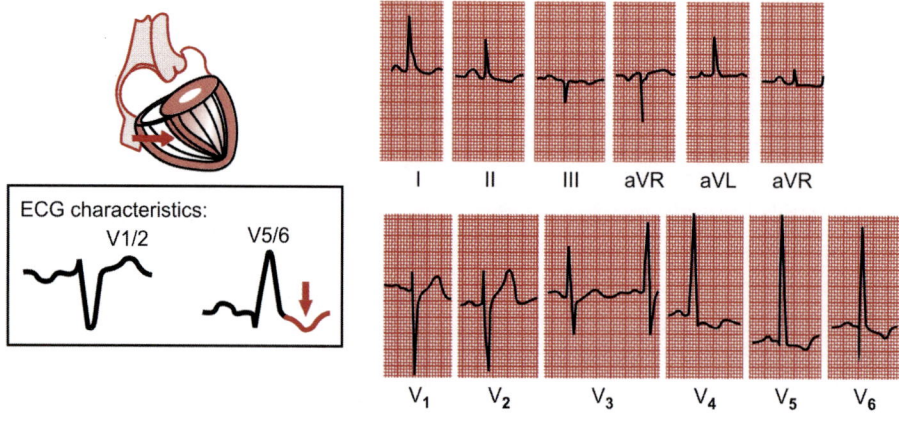

Fig. 9.5: Systolic overload

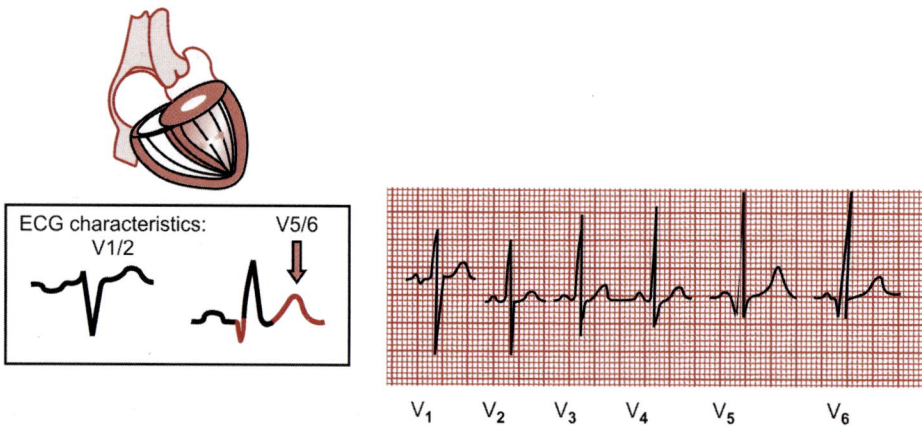

Fig. 9.6: Diastolic or volume overload. The electrocardiogram recorded from a patient with pure aortic regurgitation shows;
(i) Left ventricular hypertrophy. There is high voltage in precordial leads, i.e. R wave in V_6 > 26 mm. The voltage criteria of LVH is seen RV_5 + SV_1 > 35 mm
(ii) The QRS axis on frontal plane is normal
(iii) The q wave is prominently seen in V_5-V_6
(iv) The ST segment is isoelectric with upright T wave in precordial leads

> 26 mm due to increased bulk of the left ventricle. Corresponding to this large R wave, a deep S wave will appear in right oriented leads (V_1-V_2). The sum total of RV_5 + SV_1 is > 35 mm in adult over 35 years of age.

RV_5+SV_1 > 35 mm indicates LVH

Normally, R wave in lead V_5 is greater than R wave in V_6, but in left ventricular hypertrophy there occurs just reverse to normal, i.e. $RV_6 \geq RV_5$.

The voltage criteria and amplitude of R wave in standard leads (I, II, III, aVR, aVL and aVF) is discussed in left ventricular hypertrophy under different heart positions.

A new diagnostic criteria of "total QRS voltage" has been described in LVH; wherein the sum total of voltage of all the 12 leads is taken. Normally the total voltage of QRS is < 175 mm; if it exceeds this limit in an individual over 30 years of age, it suggests left ventricular hypertrophy.

The total voltage of QRS in all 12 leads > 175 mm suggests LVH

b) *Attenuation or absence of small initial q wave in lead V_4-V_6:* The normal small q wave of qRS complex in leads V_4-V_6 due to left to right septal activation may become attenuated or may even disappear in left ventricular hypertrophy. This happens either due to increased left ventricular pressure on the interventricular septum or development of incomplete bundle branch block. This phenomenon is seen in systolic overload of left ventricle while in contrast to it, the q wave becomes accentuated in diastolic overload of left ventricle.

The small q wave in leads V_4 – V_6 may either disappear or may even get accentuated depending on the type of overloading of the left ventricle.

c) *Increased ventricular activation time (VAT) or intrinsicoid deflection:* It is the time taken by the impulse to travel from endocardial to epicardial surface of the ventricle. Normally VAT of left ventricle is less than 0.05 second in leads V_4 –V_6. In left ventricular hypertrophy, it is increased beyond normal and may go upto 0.09 second due to increased thickness of the left ventricle.

VAT is > 0.05 second in left ventricular hypertrophy in leads V_4 –V_6.

d) *Increased duration of QRS :* The QRS interval indicates time taken for overall depolarisation of a ventricle including ventricular activation time. It is increased (> 0.10 second) in left ventricular hypertrophy due to increased muscle mass. It usually does not exceed 0.12 second.

The total QRS duration is increased in LVH

e) *Counterclockwise rotation :* In left ventricular hypertrophy, heart rotates counterclockwise on horizontal axis such that the transition zone which normally lies between $V_3 – V_4$, gets shifted rightwards (patient's right and reader's left) towards leads V_2 or V_1.

In LVH, there is counterclockwise rotation of the heart on horizontal axis resulting in shifting of the normal transition zone (V3 – V_4) towards right (V_2 or V_1)

f) *QRS axis:*

i) Frontal plane: The frontal plane QRS axis in early stages of left ventricular hypertrophy is normal, i.e. +55° to + 60°. This is due to symmetric hypertrophy of left ventricle which does not disturb the axis unless complicated.

With long standing left ventricular hypertrophy, the QRS axis tends to deviate towards left due to development of associated fibrosis which affects the anterior fascicle of left bundle leading to delayed conduction through it. Therefore, QRS may be deviated to the region of 0° in the beginning and to - 30° in the later stages. The left axis deviation of > 30° indicates associated left anterior fascicular block or hemiblock.

ii) Horizontal plane: The QRS axis on the horizontal plane is directed normally to the left but gets deviated somewhat posteriorly such that it lies between V_1 and V_6 axes, resulting in more or less equal amplitude of R wave in V_6 and S wave in lead V_1.

2. ST- T Changes

a) *ST segment depression in the leads representing left ventricle (V_5-V_6):* In left ventricular hypertrophy, the left ventricle is strained due to systolic overload, hence, there is relative ischaemia of left ventricle which results in minimal depression of ST segment with convexity upwards in left precordial leads. Corresponding to it, the ST segment in right precordial leads is minimally elevated with concavity upwards.

b) *The T wave changes:* According to general principle of electrocardiography, the T wave force or vector is directed away from the compromised left ventricle, hence, it gets directed to the right instead of being normal to the left. The T wave vector is in the region of ± 180° on frontal plane. As result of this change, the T wave will be inverted in left precordial leads (V_5-V_6) and standard leads (I and aVL); and T is upright in right precordial leads (V_1-V_2) and standard lead aVR. In contrast, the T wave remains upright in V_5-V_6 in left ventricular diastolic overload.

TV$_1$ taller than TV$_6$ syndrome: It is an early expression of rightward T wave deviation on horizontal plane, seen in left ventricular hypertrophy in which T wave remains upright in leads V_1-V_6. This is an infrequent change seen in left ventricular hypertrophy.

c) *Abnormalities of U wave:* The change in U wave is similar to T wave provided U wave are visible. The hypertrophied left ventricle results in inversion of U wave in left precordial leads (V_4-V_6). This is a sensitive sign of an impaired left ventricular function but is rarely seen. The genesis of inverted U wave is not clear but is commonly seen in left ventricular diastolic overload than systolic overload.

d) *Wide QRS-T angle:* In left ventricular hypertrophy, the frontal plane QRS axis is in the region of +0° and T wave axis in the region of ± 180° due to which there is maximum widening of frontal QRS – T angle (i.e.180°). Similarly, T wave axis on horizontal plane is directed away from lead V_6 and is directed towards lead V_1 due to rightward shift of axis. This change also widens QRS –T angle on horizontal plane.

Consequent to widening of QRS – T angle beyond +45° on frontal plane in early stages, the T wave in lead I in left ventricular hypertrophy will be of low amplitude while T wave in lead III will be tall and upright – called *"the T$_{III}$ taller than T$_I$ syndrome"*. With long standing hypertrophy of left ventricle, T wave axis is directed to the region of ± 180° due to which T wave will be maximally inverted in lead I; and lead aVF will record a small equiphasic QRS complex and a flat T wave since both QRS and T wave axes are ⊥ to it but opposite in direction.

e) *Associated left atrial enlargement:* The electrocardiographic features of left atrial hypertrophy (wide notched P wave in standard lead I and prominent and deep terminal negative deflection in lead V_1), if present, constitute a contributary evidence to left ventricular hypertrophy. This is a significant pointer to potential left ventricular hypertrophy in the presence of left bundle branch block.

The Electrocardiogram

Due to rotation of the heart on anteroposterior axis, two positions commonly evolve.
1. Horizontal heart position
2. Vertical heart position

The electrocardiogram in left ventricular hypertrophy based on the changes described above is discussed with respect to heart positions.

1. Left Ventricular Hypertrophy with Horizontal Heart

This is the most common position of the heart in left ventricular hypertrophy. The 12 leads electrocardiogram is as follows:

The Electrocardiogram (Figs 9.7 to 9.9)

1. *Standard leads (I, II, III)*: The frontal plane QRS axis is between 0° to -30°. More than -30° left axis deviation, indicates left anterior hemiblock rather than left ventricular hypertrophy. Due to this axis (0° to -30°), lead I records an R wave and lead III records a deep S wave. There is ST segment depression and T wave inversion in leads I and II. Therefore, voltage criteria for LVH on frontal leads is;

> *R wave in lead I > 15 mm*
> $R_I + S_{III} > 26 mm$ *(Fig. 9.7)*

2. *Unipolar leads (aVR, aVL, aVF)*: The frontal plane axis points towards positive pole of aVL, hence, a tall R wave with ST segment depression and T wave inversion will be visible in this lead. Therefore;

> *R wave in aVL >13 mm suggests LVH (Fig. 9.8)*

3. *Precordial leads (V_1-V_6)*: In the absence of rotation on the long or horizontal axis (clockwise or counterclockwise), left ventricular hypertrophy produces tall R waves with depressed ST segment and inverted T waves in leads V_4 to V_6, and corresponding deep S waves in right precordial leads V_1 to V_2. Therefore;

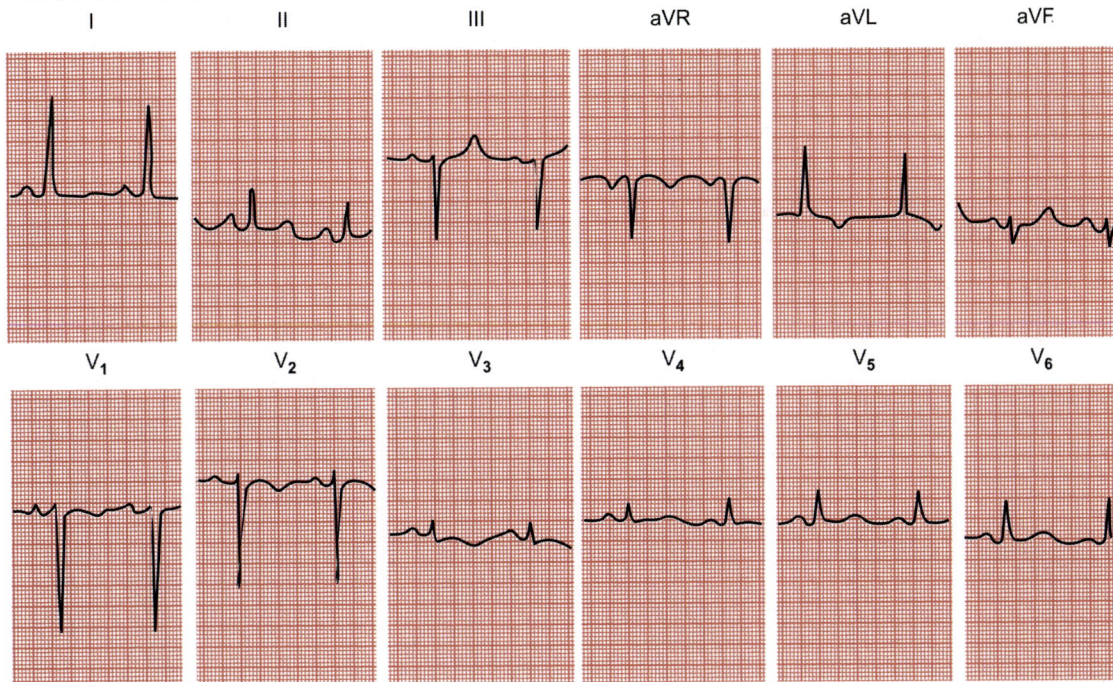

Fig. 9.7: Left ventricular hypertrophy with horizontal heart. The voltage criteria of LVH are met in standard leads. i.e. R wave in lead I > 15 mm and $R_I + S_{III}$ >26 mm. The ST segment is depressed and T is inverted in leads I and aVL. There is no evidence of LVH in precordial leads

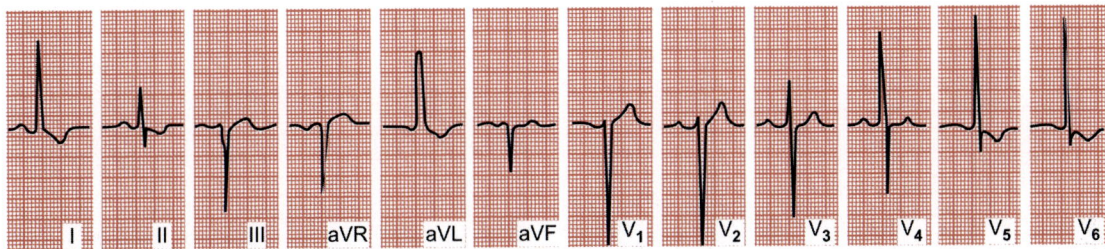

Fig. 9.8: Left ventricular hypertrophy with horizontal heart. Note the following ECG characteristics:
1. Tall R wave in V_5 and V_6 with deep S wave in V_1 and V_2, RV_5 or $RV_6 + SV_1$ = 52 mm
2. Tall R wave in aVL (19 mm). Normally R wave does not exceed 13 mm
3. Left axis deviation > -30°
4. ST segment depression and T wave inversion in lead I, II, aVL, V_5 and V_6
5. A small rS complex in aVF indicating QRS vector pointing toward negative pole of aVF and positive pole of aVL (RS complex) suggest horizontal heart

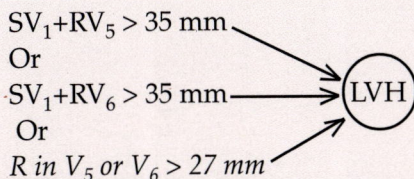

$SV_1 + RV_5$ > 35 mm
Or
$SV_1 + RV_6$ > 35 mm $\longrightarrow$ LVH
Or
R in V_5 or V_6 > 27 mm

NB: This voltage criteria as already stated is valid in persons > 35 years of age (Fig. 9.9) because certain other conditions can produce these voltage changes.

This voltage criteria suggests LVH in persons more than 35 years of age (Fig. 9.9). Other conditions such as fever, thyrotoxicosis, beriberi, and other high output states may also produce these changes. These changes frequently occur in young persons less than 35 years of age without any disease (Fig. 9.10).

SECTION THREE

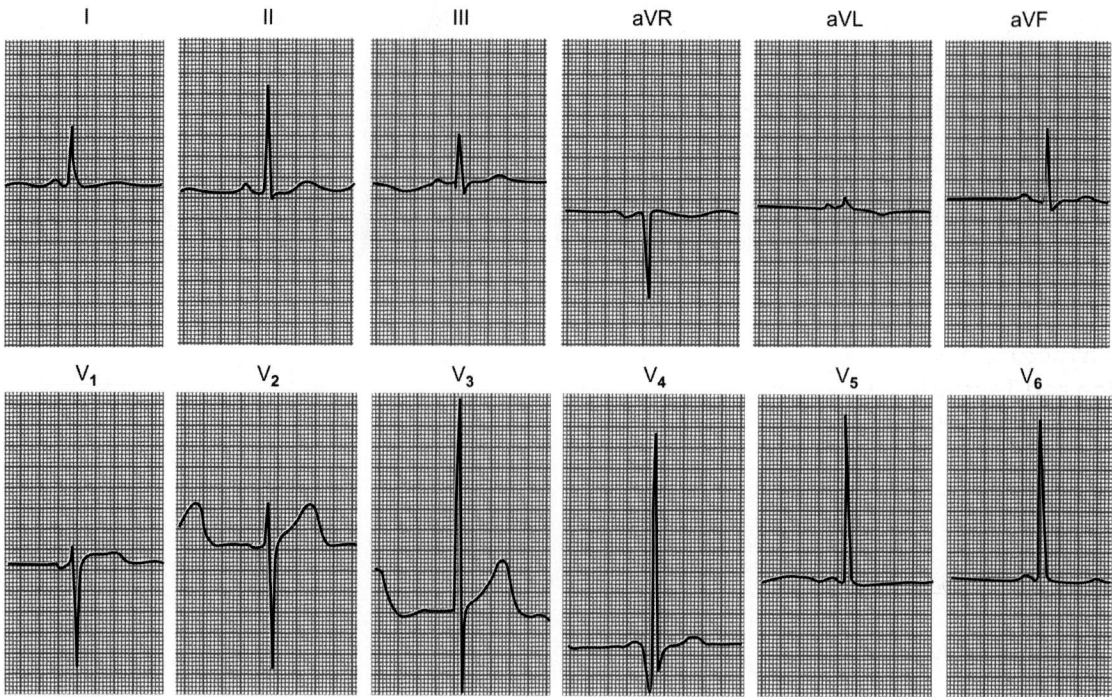

Fig. 9.9: Left ventricular hypertrophy. Note the following characteristic on ECG; (i) Right axis deviation, (ii) Intermediate heart position, (iii) $RV_5 + SV_1 = 43$ mm, (iv) T is flat or low amplitude in I, V_4-V_6 with inversion of T in aVL

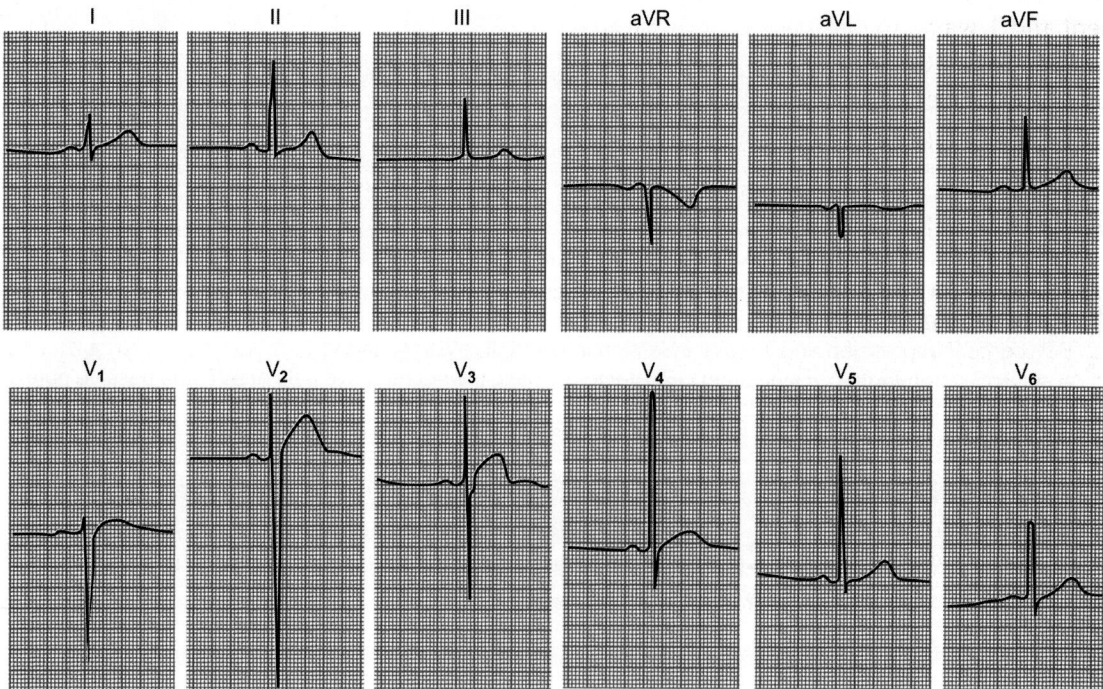

Fig. 9.10: High voltage graph in a normal boy of 18 years who came for medical check up. The total of $RV_5 + SV_1 = 40$ mm. It is normal according to his age

In addition to these above said voltage criteria, there will be ST segment depression and 'T' wave inversion in left precordial leads. The QRS interval may be more than 0.1 second and VAT may be greater than 0.05 second in left precordial leads (V_5-V_6).

4. *Vector analysis*: The magnitude of QRS vector is increased. There is slight change in its direction, i.e. it is oriented slightly superiorly and posteriorly. The ST and T vectors are opposite to QRS vector, i.e. away from the hypertrophied ventricle, hence, ST segment depression and T wave inversion occur in those leads which record left ventricular epicardial complexes (tall R waves). Due to an opposite direction of T wave vector to QRS vector, the QRS –T angle becomes widened.

QRS – T angle becomes widened (> +45°)

2. Left Ventricular Hypertrophy with Vertical Heart

The electrocardiogram (Fig. 9.11)

1. *Standard leads*: The frontal plane QRS is positive between +45° to +90°, therefore, tall R wave will be recorded in leads II and III with depression of segment and T wave inversion in the same leads.

2. *Extremities leads*: Since QRS vector is oriented towards aVF, hence, a tall R wave will appear in lead aVF with depression of ST segment and inversion of T wave in the same lead. Therefore;

R wave in aVF > 20 mm indicates LVH

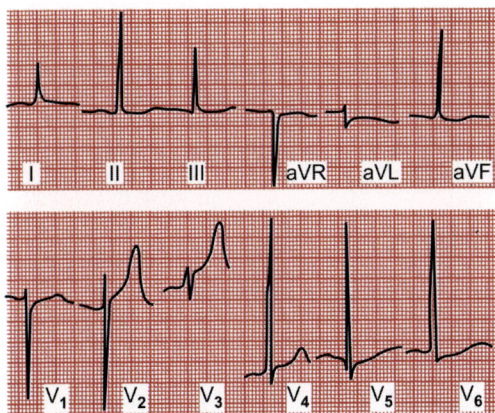

Fig. 9.11: Left ventricular hypertrophy with vertical heart

3. *Precordial leads*: In the absence of rotation on long axis, the pattern of precordial leads will be same as that seen in horizontal heart position.

Effect of Rotation on Left Ventricular Hypertrophy

The rotation on long axis may be:
1. Clockwise rotation
2. Counterclockwise rotation (common)

The counterclockwise rotation is common association with left ventricular hypertrophy; while in clockwise rotation heart can be vertical or horizontal.

1. *Clockwise rotation* (Fig. 9.12): The ECG pattern on clockwise rotation depends on the degree of rotation on the frontal plane. Marked clockwise rotation produces R wave in aVR.

The precordial leads show shift of transition zone towards left, i.e. towards V_5-V_6, so that a typical LVH pattern may not appear up to V_6, hence, leads V_7 to V_9 (from anterior to posterior axillary line) may be recorded to define left ventricular pattern.

2. *Counterclockwise rotation*: The ECG pattern in standard and extremity leads depends on the degree of rotation on anteroposterior axis.

The precordial leads show shift in the transition zone to the right, i.e. towards V_1, so that, left ventricular hypertrophy pattern may be seen in leads V_2 or V_3 or even V_1, in that case, V_{3R} lead will show right ventricular epicardial complex.

Left Ventricular Strain (Fig. 9.13)

The strain pattern means ST segment depression and T wave inversion in those leads which record left ventricular epicardial complex. There are no abnormalities of tall R wave or prolongation of QRS and VAT. The strain pattern arises due to relative ischaemia of left ventricle due to its hypertrophy. Some believe it as nonspecific ST-T change due to opposite QRS and T axes.

The differences in left ventricular hypertrophy with respect to systolic and diastolic overload are given in Table 9.2.

SECTIONTHREE

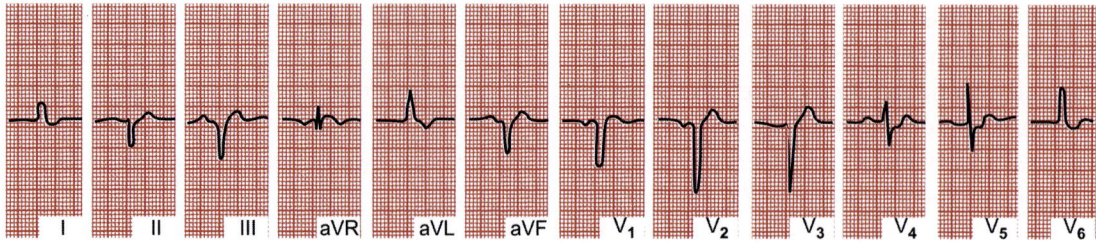

Fig. 9.12: Left ventricular hypertrophy with horizontal heart and clockwise rotation. The ECG shows; (i) Left axis deviation (> - 30°) and is superiorly oriented. (ii) Horizontal heart, (iii) Marked clockwise rotation (R wave in aVR and transition zone lies in V_5). (iv) The ST segment is depressed in leads I, aVL, V_4-V_6 but T is inverted in lead aVL

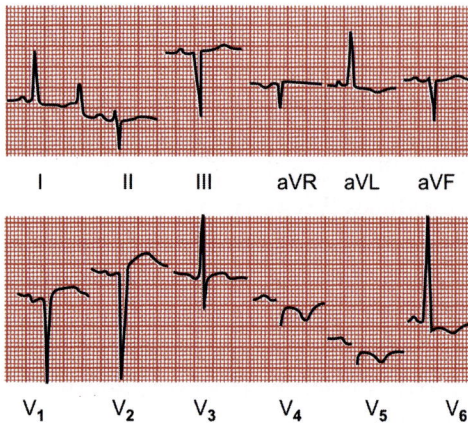

Fig. 9.13: Left ventricular hypertrophy with strain

REVIEW AT GLANCE

Left Ventricular Hypertrophy

1. *Voltage criteria*

> *R wave in V_5 or V_6 > 27 mm and RV_6 > RV_5*
> *R V_5 + SV_1 > 35 mm*

- *In horizontal heart:* There will be tall R wave in V_5, V_6, I and aVL associated with T wave inversion.
- *In vertical heart:* The T is upright in leads V_6 and V_1; and T wave is taller in V_1 than V_6 (TV_1 > TV_6).
- R in aVL (horizontal heart) > 13 mm
- R in aVF (vertical heart) > 20 mm
- R in lead I > 15 mm in horizontal heart position
- Total QRS voltage (in persons > 30 years with normal sized heart) of all 12 leads > 175 mm.

2. *Axis deviation:* There is left axis deviation (0° to - 30°) in most of the cases. Left axis deviation more than -30° is unusual, indicates associated left anterior fascicular block rather than LVH.

3. *QRS Interval:* It is prolonged in V_5-V_6 ($\geq$ 0.10 second).

4. *VAT:* It is increased to > 0.05 second in left sided leads.

5. *Counterclockwise rotation:* Due to this type of rotation, transition zone is shifted toward right, i.e. in leads V_1-V_2.

6. *Attenuation* of **initial q wave in V_5-V_6** in systolic and its accentuation in diastolic overload of left ventricle.

7. *ST-T change:* The ST segment is depressed with concavity upwards in the leads showing left ventricular hypertrophy pattern.

8. *The T wave:* It is inverted in V_5-V_6 in systolic overload, while it remains upright in diastolic overload of left ventricle.

9. *The wide QRS – T angle*

The scoring system proposed for left ventricular hypertrophy is given in the box.

The Romhilt and Estes point scoring system for LVH	
1. Increase in QRS voltage	- 3 points
2. ST-T changes	- 3 points (one point if patient is taking digitalis)
3. P wave indicative of left atrial enlargement	- 3 points
4. Left axis deviation	- 2 point
5. Increased VAT	- 1 point
6. Widened QRS	- 1 point

Note: At least five points are required to establish the diagnosis of LVH.

RIGHT VENTRICULAR HYPERTROPHY (RVH)

It refers to hypertrophy of the free walls of right ventricle leading to certain electrocardiographic criteria. Actually in RVH, there is hypertrophy of free walls of right ventricle associated with either paraseptal area or parabasal region or both of right ventricle.

Aetiology

The clinical conditions associated with right ventricular hypertrophy (RVH) are;
1. Pulmonary hypertension: It may be primary or secondary due to mitral valve disease especially mitral stenosis.
2. Chronic pulmonary disease and cor pulmonale. The chronic obstructive lung disease with pulmonary arterial hypertension leads to RVH.
3. Congenital heart diseases, i.e. pulmonary stenosis, tetralogy of Fallot, Eisenmenger's syndrome.
4. Associated with LVH. It may occur in association with left ventricular hypertrophy.
5. Right ventricular hypertrophic cardiomyopathy (rare).
6. Acute pulmonary thromboembolism.

7. Left to right shunt: Atrial septal and ventricular septal defects produce diastolic overload of right ventricle.

The Electrocardiographic Criteria

The electrocardiographic criteria discussed under ventricular hypertrophy when applied to leads recording the right ventricular epicardial complex give rise to ECG pattern of RVH.

Mechanisms

The ECG findings evolve due to following mechanisms (Fig. 9.14).
   i) The right ventricular hypertrophy results in generation of increased QRS forces due to increased muscle mass that are directed anteriorly and to the right.
  ii) Hypertrophy of right paraseptal region results in amplification of right paraseptal forces which are directed to the right and anteriorly.
 iii) Hypertrophy of parabasal area results in shifting of terminal forces of QRS superiorly and to the right.
  iv) Associated ST-T changes appear due to hypertrophied or compromised right ventricle.

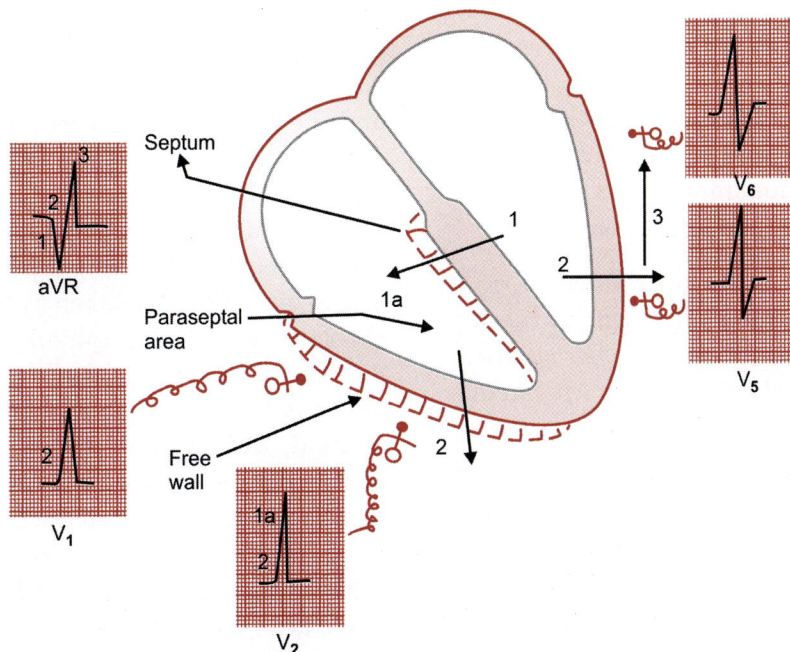

Fig. 9.14: The major sites of right ventricular hypertrophy (dotted lines) and their effects in different leads (diagram)

SECTIONTHREE

v) There may be changes of associated right atrial enlargement.

The Electrocardiographic Patterns

The electrocardiographic changes evolved due to above said mechanisms will be:

1. Abnormalities of QRS

a) *Right axis deviation*: It is the commonest, earliest and at times the only manifestation of right ventricular hypertrophy (RVH). The mean frontal plane QRS axis is deviated to the right, more commonly, in the right inferior quadrant, i.e. from $+90°$ clockwise to $+180°$ but mostly the right axis deviation is around $+120°$. This axis deviation reflects rightward direction of the electrical forces generated by the free walls of hypertrophied right ventricle.

When hypertrophy involves the parabasal region, the frontal plane axis deviates further to the right and in extreme cases, it may lie in right superior quadrant or "north–west zone". When this occurs, it will produce an intraventricular conduction defect resembling left anterior fascicular block. Such a combination of left anterior fascicular block with right ventricular hypertrophy may be seen in certain congenital heart diseases such as Fallot's tetralogy, Noonan's syndrome and persistent atrioventricular canal.

Isolated severe pulmonary stenosis with high right ventricular pressures usually has a frontal plane QRS axis in right inferior quadrant, and is uncommonly associated with right superior QRS axis.

Usually right axis deviation remains within right inferior quadrant in spite of high right ventricular pressure. The right axis in right superior quadrant indicates an additional defect such as left anterior hemiblock.

The only other condition that produces frontal plane QRS axis $> +140°$ is posterior fascicular block.

b) *Increased amplitude of R wave in right precordial leads (V_1-V_2)*: With dominance of right ventricle, the r wave of normal rS complex in right precordial leads increases in amplitude with respect to S wave in the same leads. This is probably due to combined effect of increased right paraseptal and right free wall ventricular forces (Fig. 9.14 vectors 1a and 2), but mainly is due to right ventricular free wall forces (Fig. 9.14 vector 2). Increasing height of r wave in lead V_1 in right ventricular hypertrophy will convert normal rS complex to RS, Rs, only R and qR complexes depending on whether right ventricular pressure exceeds (qR), is equal to (R or rR) or is lower (rsR' or RS) than the left ventricle.

In right ventricular hypertrophy the R wave is more than or equal to S wave ($R \geq S$), therefore $R : S \geq 1$.

c) *An initial slur on QRS complex in lead V_1*: At times, in right ventricular hypertrophy, an initial slur on dominant R wave may be seen which may simulate delta wave of pre-excitation syndrome.

Sometimes, the initial slur may take the form of a small positive deflection separate from dominant R wave producing rR pattern which may be mistaken for incomplete right bundle branch block. This pattern probably might be due to combined hypertrophy and dilatation of right ventricle as it is commonly seen in atrial septal defects.

This initial slur may take the form of a small Q wave resulting in qR complex in lead V_1. This is seen in marked right ventricular hypertrophy with right ventricle pressure exceeding the left ventricle and there may be associated tricuspid incompetence and right atrial hypertrophy. The dominant R of qR complex is inscribed by hypertrophied right ventricle and the initial q wave preceding R wave is due to rotational effect of associated right atrial hypertrophy (See Figs 8.10 and 8.11 on right atrial hypertrophy).

d) *Increased VAT*: The ventricular activation time (VAT) exceeds 0.03 second in right precordial leads. This is due to increased time taken by the impulses to travel through the hypertrophied right ventricle from endocardial to epicardial surface.

e) *A large S wave in left oriented leads*: The left oriented leads (I, aVL, V_5 and V_6) record a large S wave constituting Rs, RS or rS complexes. This is due to dominant right ventricular force generated by hypertrophied right ventricle which is directed towards lead V_1 and away from lead V_5 resulting in R wave in V_1 and corresponding deep S wave in leads V_5 and V_6. Therefore, an rS complex in V_6 wherein S wave is of greater magnitude than R wave (S > R) is highly suggestive of right ventricular hypertrophy.

f) *Clockwise rotation*: Due to right ventricular hypertrophy, a tall R wave with a deep S wave of more or less equal amplitude (RS complex) will appear in mid – precordial leads (V_3-V_4) due to clockwise rotation and these large equiphasic (RS) complexes may be shifted to leads V_5 and V_6 due to displacement of transition zone to the left (patient's left, reader's right). The large RS complexes in V_5-V_6 are due to increased right paraseptal forces (Fig. 9.14 – vector 1a). Occasionally, several precordial leads may reflect rS complexes.

g) *Increased QRS interval*: The QRS interval is increased (>0.10 second) in right precordial leads (V_1-V_2) but it usually does not exceed 0.12 second in any circumstance. If it increases further, then there may be associated right bundle branch block.

h) *The S_I, S_{II}, S_{III} syndrome*: This is an electrocardiographic expression of superior quadrantic QRS axis. Due to hypertrophy of parabasal area of right ventricle, the mean QRS forces get oriented superiorly and shift the QRS axis in right superior quadrant in the region of -150° (north-west zone, Read Chapter 15) on the frontal plane. This axis shift will produce a terminal S wave in all the three standard leads resulting in S_I, S_{II}, S_{III} syndrome. It must be remembered that, usually, the QRS axis does not shift in this region due to right ventricular hypertrophy, hence, if it occurs, the complicating factors such as left anterior hemiblock, atrial or ventricular septal defects or persistent atrioventricular canal or transposition of great vessels may be suspected.

2. The ST- T,U changes

The ST segment: In right ventricular hypertrophy, the right ventricle is strained due to increased pressure resulting in relative ischaemia of the ventricle leading to ST segment depression with convexity upwards in right precordial leads (V_1-V_2).

The T wave: According to principle of electrocardiography, the T wave axis on horizontal plane gets deviated away from the compromised ventricle, hence, in right ventricular hypertrophy, the T wave vector is directed away from the right, i.e. to the left and somewhat posteriorly resulting in inversion of T waves in the right precordial leads (V_1-V_2), which may even extend upto V_4. With marked clockwise rotation of the heart, the T wave inversion may be seen in most of the precordial leads.

The U wave: The U wave, if seen, also gets inverted in leads V_1 and V_2 and / or standard leads II, III and aVF. This may occur in both systolic and diastolic overload of right ventricle.

3. Associated right atrial hypertrophy

The electrocardiographic manifestations of right atrial hypertrophy (tall and peaked P waves in leads II, III and aVF) usually coexist with right ventricular hypertrophy irrespective of its cause. The P wave axis is directed to the right, i.e. +60° to +70°.

The electrocardiogram (Figs 9.15 to 9.17)

1. *Standard leads*:

i) Right axis deviation ($\geq 110°$) occurs in most of the cases. Some patients may not show abnormal axis deviation on frontal plane.

ii) Due to above said axis of the electrical forces, the leads II and III will register tall R waves and inverted T waves. This ECG pattern can also occur in LVH with vertical heart position, but the abnormal frontal plane axis will differentiate between the two.

2. *Extremities leads*: The pattern in extremities leads depends on the degree of rotation on the frontal plane. There is frequently clockwise rotation on horizontal axis due to which lead aVR will either record tall R wave as QR, qR, or R complex or may record pattern resembling leads II and III due to orientation of the frontal plane axis towards their positive poles and positive pole of aVR.

3. *The precordial leads*:

i) *Right ventricular precordial leads (V_1 and V_2):* They will record tall R waves. VAT is also increased in these leads. The QRS is also widened (> 0.10 second) in these leads but is always < 0.12 second. The ST segment is depressed and T waves are inverted in the above mentioned leads. Sometimes, these criteria may not be seen in leads V_1 or V_2 but may be seen in leads V_{3R} and V_{4R}, therefore, in cases of suspicion of RVH, these leads should be recorded.

ii) *An initial q wave preceding R wave or R wave with slur on its upstroke in right ventricular leads (V_1 or V_{3R}) may be seen.* This is due to delay in the activation of right ventricle resulting from its hypertrophy, suggests that right ventricular pressure exceeds (qR), is equal

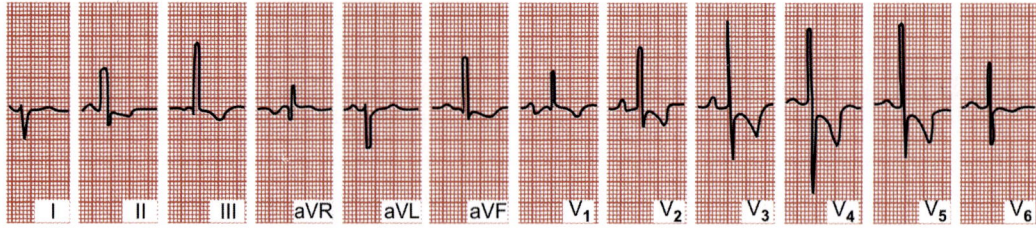

Fig. 9.15: Right ventricular hypertrophy. Note the following characteristics:
1. Large R wave in V_1 and deep S wave in V_5 and V_6. R:S in V_1 >1
2. Lead aVF resembles V_1 suggesting vertical heart
3. Right axis deviation
4. Clockwise rotation
5. Prominent P wave in leads II, aVF, V_1 - V_3 suggests of associated right atrial hypertrophy
6. There is qR pattern in V_1. This indicates concommitant right atrial hypertrophy indirectly

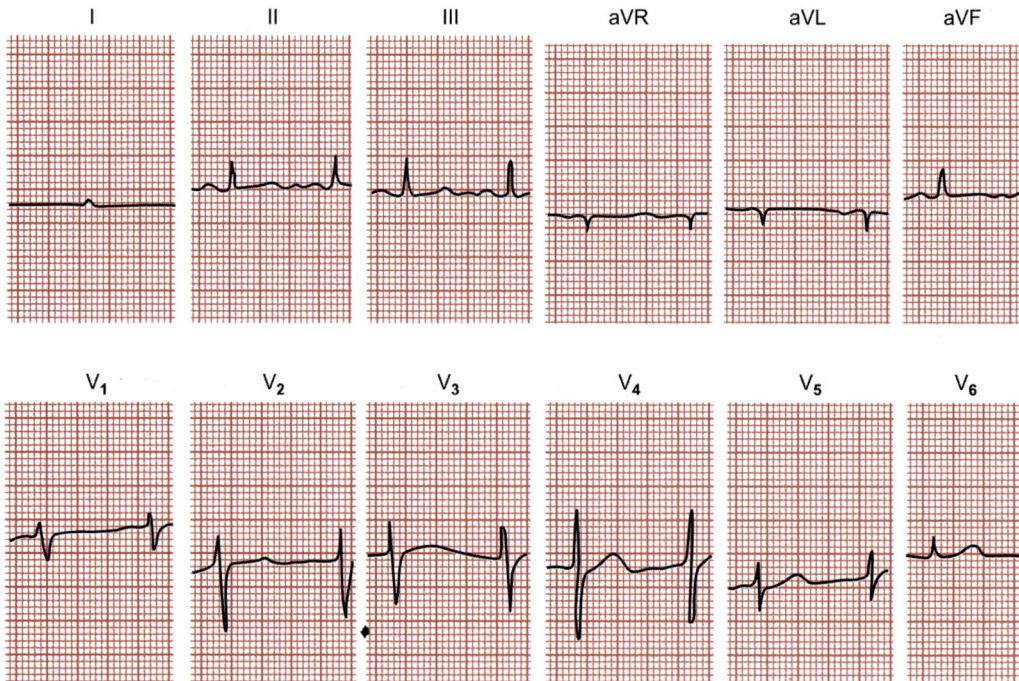

Fig. 9.16: Right ventricular and left atrial hypertrophy. The electrocardiogram shows:
(i) QRS axis is + 90°
(ii) P waves are broad (>2.5 mm) in leads II, III and aVF and there is right axis deviation of P waves
(iii) There are tall R waves in leads V_1 and V_2. The R wave in V_1 is more or less equal to S wave. There is clockwise rotation of the heart leading to persistence of deep S wave in V_5 and transition zone also lies in lead V_5
(iv) The VAT in leads V_1 and V_2 is increased
(v) The QRS duration in V_1 and V_2 is 0.10 sec
All these features suggest left atrial and right ventricular hypertrophy

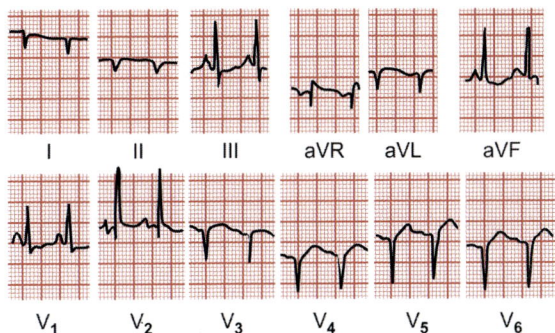

Leads: I, II, III, aVR, aVL, aVF

V₁, V₂, V₃, V₄, V₅, V₆

Fig. 9.17: Right atrial and right ventricular hypertrophy. The electrocardiogram shows:

(i) Mean QRS and P wave axes are markedly shifted to right.

(ii) Right atrial hypertrophy: Tall peaked P waves (>2.5 mm) are seen in leads III and aVF. The initial upward component of biphasic P is tall and peaked (>1.5 mm) in leads V_1-V_2

(iii) Marked right ventricular hypertrophy: The initial r wave in V_1 is absent resulting in Rs pattern (R > S or R:S >1). There is qR pattern in V_2; indicates marked right ventricular hypertrophy. The ST segment is isoelectric in V_1 and elevated in V_2 with T wave inversion, is consistent with RVH

(iv) Marked clockwise rotation. The rS pattern in leads V_4-V_6; the amplitude of R wave in V_6 is < 5 mm and shift of transition zone beyond V_6 indicates marked clockwise rotation

(v) A noticeable pronounced Ta wave is seen in leads III and aVF; indicates right atrial stress

to (R or rR) or is lower (rsR') than left ventricular pressure respectively. This pattern has been discussed in right atrial hypertrophy.

iii) *Shifting of transition zone to the left*, hence, RS or Rs complex will be seen upto V_5 and V_6 due to clockwise rotation of the heart.

iv) *Voltage criteria:* The height of R wave is increased in leads V_1 and V_2 due to RVH. Other causes which produce tall R wave in V_1 and V_2 include posterior wall infarction, right bundle branch block, myotonia, etc.

Voltage Criteria of RVH

- *Ratio of R and S in lead V_1 or $V_{3R} \geq 1$ (R:S ≥ 1)*
- Corresponding to tall R wave in V_1, there will be large S wave in V_5-V_6 due to clockwise rotation and hypertrophy of right parabasal segment and delayed spread of excitation through hypertrophied right ventricle.

4. *Vector analysis:* The mean QRS vector is oriented to right ($\geq$ +110°), anteriorly and either inferiorly (initial) and superiorly (later on).

REVIEW AT GLANCE

Right ventricular hypertrophy

- Right axis deviation – It is common (+110° or more).
- Vertical heart position – A common presentation.
- Clockwise rotation – A common manifestation leading to shift of transition zone to left, i.e. towards V_5 with qR pattern in aVR.
- A dominant R wave in right precordial leads (V_{3R}, V_1 and V_2)
- Voltage criteria:
  i) R/S ratio > 1 in V_1 or R > S in V_1
  ii) VAT in increased in right precordial leads (> 0.03 sec)
  iii) RS or Rs or rS complexes in left precordial leads (V_5-V_6)
  iv) Wide (> 0.10 second) QRS complexes in right precordial leads (V_1-V_2).

Diagnostic Clues

Direct – R/S ratio > 1 in lead V_1 is alone sufficient to diagnose RVH.

Indirect – Clockwise rotation with persistence of large S wave in V_5 and V_6 combined with right axis deviation >+ 110°

Right Ventricular Strain Pattern (Fig. 9.18)

Right ventricle is strained both in systolic and diastolic overload and produces ST depression and T wave inversion in right precordial leads. The ECG pattern does not form a criteria for differentiation between them. However, tall R waves with inverted T and U waves in right precordial leads (V_{3R}, V_1 and V_2) indicate systolic overload. In diastolic overload (volume overload) the pattern of incomplete or complete right bundle branch block (rsR') is common and may be seen up to V_3 or V_4. The U wave may or may not be inverted.

SECTION THREE

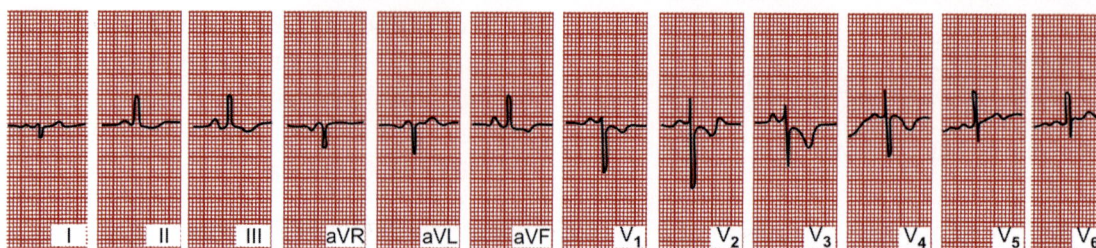

Fig. 9.18: Right ventricular hypertrophy with strain. The electrocardiogram shows right axis deviation, vertical heart, clockwise rotation and rS pattern with inverted T waves in leads V_1 to V_4. In such a situation, leads V_{3R} or V_{4R} may be recorded to get typical tall R wave equal to or more than S wave

BIVENTRICULAR (COMBINED RIGHT AND LEFT VENTRICLES) HYPERTROPHY

Sometimes, both ventricles of the heart are hypertrophied.

Aetiology

The clinical conditions associated with biventricular hypertrophy or enlargement include;
1. Dilated cardiomyopathy.
2. Congenital heart disease—Eisenmenger's syndrome, in which initial left to right shunt gets reversed due to development of right ventricular hypertrophy with pulmonary arterial hypertension.
3. Congestive heart failure due to valvular lesions or hypertension.
4. High cardiac output failure or states.

The Electrocardiographic Patterns

Mechanisms

In biventricular hypertrophy, the forces of left ventricular hypertrophy dominates over right ventricular forces, hence, characteristic pattern of LVH is usually seen in left precordial leads. Sometimes, if right ventricular hypertrophy also dominates and becomes equal to left ventricular hypertrophy, then the increased right ventricular forces cancel the left ventricular forces and a balanced state results, in such a situation, there are ECG changes of each ventricular hypertrophy in leads representing them, but transition zone remains at normal position (V_3 or V_4) and, also records both tall R wave and S waves which are equal indicating a balanced state of right

and left ventricular forces. Usually, increasing right ventricular forces cancel some of the left ventricular forces, in that situation, the voltage criteria of LVH may not be evident in leads V_5 or V_6, hence, other associated criteria may help in the diagnosis, for example, RVH associated with left axis deviation indicate biventricular hypertrophy provide there is no other cause for left axis deviation.

The electrocardiogram (Figs 9.19 and 9.20)

The criteria for biventricular hypertrophy on ECG include;
   i) *Left ventricular hypertrophy (LVH) associated with right axis deviation.* Voltage criteria of LVH are present. Instead of left axis deviation, there is a right axis deviation which may be the only evidence of right ventricular hypertrophy.
   ii) *Left ventricular hypertrophy with clockwise rotation of heart.* Voltage of criteria of LVH are present. Instead of counterclockwise rotation, there is clockwise rotation due to RVH leading to shifting of transition zone (RS) towards left (V_4 or V_5).
   iii) *Left ventricular hypertrophy associated with a tall R wave in lead V_1 or R/S ratio is more than I in that lead.* This means:
   • A tall R in left precordial leads (V_5-V_6).
   • A tall R in right precordial leads (V_1 or V_2 or V_{3R}).
   • A large equiphasic QRS (R=S) in mid-precordial leads (Katz – Wachtel phenomenon) indicates a balanced state of QRS forces in V_3-V_4 due to hypertrophy of both ventricles.
   • Right ventricular hypertrophy with left axis deviation provided there is no cause to explain the left axis deviation.

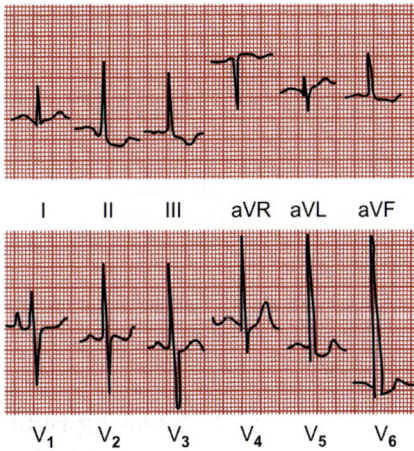

Fig. 9.19: Biatrial and biventricular hypertrophy. The electrocardiogram recorded from a patient with rheumatic heart disease with mitral senosis and mitral regurgitation shows the following characteristics:

(i) Right axis deviation of + 70°

(ii) Biatrial hypertrophy. P mitrale (M shaped) in leads II, III and aVF and bifid P waves where initial upright deflection is larger than terminal negative deflection

(iii) Left ventricular hypertrophy: There is tall R wave in V_6 (35 mm) and $RV_6 + SV_1 =$ 45 mm. There is ST segment depression in leads II, III, aVF, V_5-V_6. The T is inverted in leads aVL and III

(iv) Right ventricular hypertrophy. Tall R wave in V_1 and V_2. R is more or less equal to S wave in V_2 with inversion of T wave in V_1 and V_2. There is associated right atrial hypertrophy

(v) Katz-Wachtel phenomenon—R and S waves are tall and equal in V_3, also indicates biventricular hypertrophy

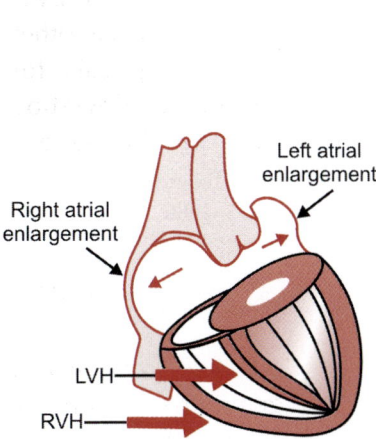

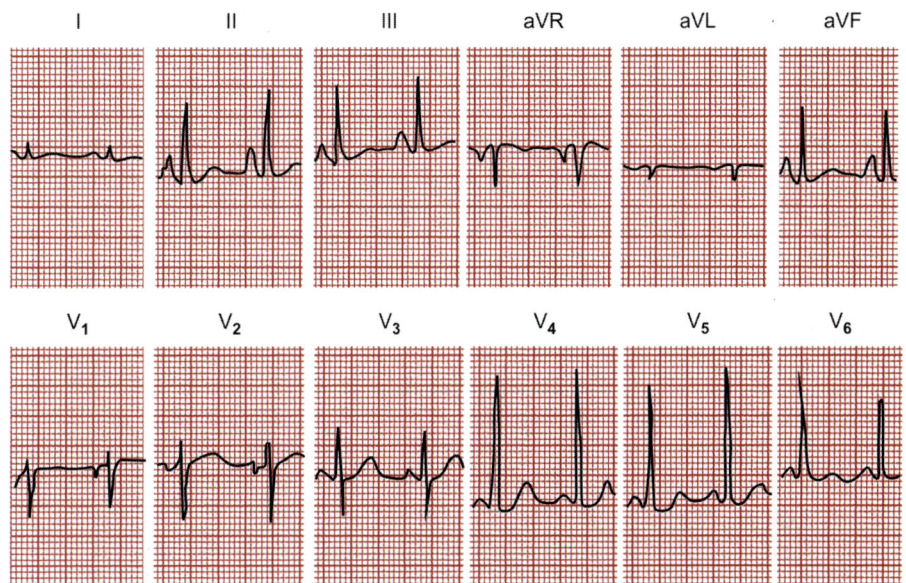

Fig. 9.20: Biatrial and biventricular hypertrophy. The ECG shows:

(i) Right axis deviation

(ii) Biatrial hypertrophy: The P waves are tall and wide (> 2.5 mm in height and width) in leads II, III and aVF. The P wave in lead V_1 is biphasic with accentuation of negative component.

(iii) Left ventricular hypertrophy. There are tall R waves in V_4-V_6; the R in V_5 is 26 mm. There is counterclockwise rotation with transition zone lies between V_2-V_3. There is associated ST depression in leads V_4-V_6 but T is upright

(iv) Right ventricular hypertrophy: It is evidenced by right axis deviation, significant R wave in V_1-V_2. All these features with right atrial hypertrophy suggest associated right ventricular hypertrophy.

Note: The voltage criteria of LVH and RVH are not evident clearly because of balance of forces due to hypertrophied both ventricles

iv) *When P wave indicating left atrial hypertrophy (wide M shaped P wave – P mitrale or tricuspidale) is associated with one of the followings;*

(i) *An R/S ratio in V_5 or V_6 = 1.*

(ii) *An S wave in V_5-V_6 is deep and > 7 mm*

(iii) *Right axis deviation > +90°*

Suggested Reading

1. –bid—Electrocardiography and vectorcardiography in heart disease, 2nd ed. E. Braunwald (Ed). Philadelphia, Saunders, 1984.

2. Carbrera CE, Monroy JR: Systolic and diastolic loading of heart. *Am Heart J* **43**:661, 1952.

SECTION THREE

3. Casale PN et al: Electrocardiographic deflection of left ventricular hypertrophy. Development and prospective validation of improved crtieria. *J Am Coll Cardiol* **6**:572, 1985.

4. Cooksey JD et al: Clinical vectorcardiography and electrocardiography, 2nd ed. Chicago, Year Book, 1977.

5. Fish C (Ed): Cardiovascular clinics, Vol 5, no. 3 Complex Electrocardiography I Philadephia, Davis, 1973.

6. Goldman MJ: Principles of clinical electrocardiography, 12th ed. Los Altos California, Lange Medical Publisher, 1986.

7. Griep AH: Pitfalls in electrocardiographic diagnosis of left ventricular hypertrophy. A correlative study of 200 autopsied patients. *Circulation* **20**:30, 1959.

8. Hoftman BF, Cranfied PF: Electrophysiology of the heart, New York: McGaw Hill, 1960.

9. Holt DH, Spodick DH: The RV6: RV5 ratio in left ventricular hypertrophy. *Am Heart J* **63**:65, 1962.

10. Kansal S, Roitman DI, Sheffield LT: A quantitative relationship of electrocardiographic criteria with echocardiographic left ventricular mass: A multivariate approach. *Clin Cardiol* **6**:456, 1983.

11. Loperfido F, Digaetano A, Santarelli et al: The evaluation of left and right ventricular hypertrophy in combined ventricular overload by electrocardiography: relation-ship with echocardiographic data. *J Electrocardiol* **15**:327, 1982.

12. Murphy ML, Thenabadu PN, De Soyza ND et al: Reevaluation of electrocardiographic criteria for left, right and combined cardiac ventricular hypertrophy. *Am J Cardiol* **53**:1140, 1984.

13. Parkash R: Echocardiographic diagnosis of right ventricular hypertrophy; Correlation with ECG and necropsy findings in 248 patients. *Cathet Cardiovas Diagn* **7**:170, 1981.

14. Piccolo E, Raviele A, Delise P et al: The role of left ventricular hypertrophy – An electrophysiologic study in man. *Circulation* **59**:1044, 1979.

15. Romhilt D, Estes EH Jr: A point-score system for ECG diagnosis of LVH. *Am Heart J* **75**:752, 1968.

16. Schamroth L, Schamroth CL, Sareli P et al: Electrocardio-graphic differentiation of the causes of left ventricular diastolic overload. *Chest* **85**:95, 1986.

17. Selzer A: The Bayer's theorem and clinical electrocardio-graphy. *Am Heart J* **101**:360, 1981.

18. Sokolow M, Lyon TP: The ventricular complex in LVH as obtained by unipolar, precordial and limb leads. *Am Heart J* **37**:161, 1949.

19. Surawicz B: Electrocardiographic diagnosis of chamber enlargement. *J Am Coll Cardiol* **8**:71, 1986.

SECTIONTHREE

Conduction Defects

SECTION FOUR

10

Intracardiac Conduction Defects

- *Classification of cardiac conduction defects*
- *The electrocardiographic manifestations of various conduction defects*
- *The graphic representation (ladder diagram) of intracardiac conduction defects*

An electrical impulse generated from the SA node, travels through the internodal bundles in the atria to AV node, then to the bundle of His, its branches (right or left) and Purkinje system of the ventricles. The abnormality in the conduction system may lie at various levels (Fig. 10.1). According to anatomical structures involved, they can be classified into many groups (Table 10.1).

Aetiopathogenesis

The primary disorders of conduction tissue are rare and are mostly due to congenital maldevelopment or heredofamilial in origin. The acquired disorders involving the conduction system are rather common and may be due to structural endomyocardial disease such as cardiomyopathy or there may be functional disturbance secondary to ischaemia, trauma, inflammation, tumour, etc. or it can be due to idiopathic fibrosis around the conduction tissue. The aetiology of individual conduction disorder is described in respective chapters.

The Electrocardiographic Manifestations

1. **SA node disturbance :** The disorders of SA node manifest as disturbance in impulse formation and its propagation through the atria, characterised electrocardiographically as intermittent sinus pauses or arrest and there may be sometimes, emergence of an escape rhythm from a subsidiary pacemaker. The SA node involvement may be temporary or functional and organic or structural warranting implantation of permanent pacemaker.

   Sinus pauses or sinoatrial blocks suggest sinus node dysfunction.

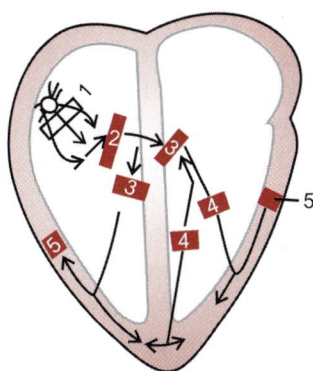

Fig. 10.1: Anatomical sites of intracardiac conduction defects. (Small squares represents the site of block) Site 1: Sinoatrial block, Site 2: AV block, Site 3: Bundle branch block, Site 4: Fascicular block, Site 5: Purkinje (peripheral) system block

2. **AV nodal conduction disturbances:** The conduction defects of AV node manifest as various grades of heart blocks producing either delay in the transmission of impulses leading to just prolongation

Table 10.1.: Classification of cardiac conduction defects

1. **Intra-atrial conduction defects**
   - First degree SA block
   - Second degree SA block
   - Third degree SA block
2. **Atrioventricular conduction defects**
   - First degree AV block
   - Second degree AV block
     - Mobitz type I (Wenckebach type)
     - Mobitz type II ; (fixed or variable)
   - Third degree or complete AV block
3. **Intraventricular conduction defects**
   A. *Bundle branch blocks*
      - Right bundle branch block (RBBB); complete and incomplete
      - Left bundle branch block (LBBB); complete and incomplete
      - Intermittent right or left bundle branch block.
   B. *Fascicular blocks or hemiblocks (peripheral left ventricular conduction defects)*
      - Left anterior hemiblock or fascicular block
      - Left posterior hemiblock or fascicular block
      - Left septal block
      - Peri-infarction block
   C. *Bilateral bundle branch blocks*
      i) Right bundle branch block with left anterior fascicular block.
      ii) Right bundle branch block with left posterior fascicular block.
      iii) Right or left bundle branch block with prolonged AV conduction, i.e. P–R interval > 0.20 second.
      iv) Trifascicular block.
      v) Alternating right and left bundle branch block.
4. **Indeterminate intraventricular conduction defects**

of P–R interval (first degree AV block) or blocking of some of the impulses while others get transmitted (second degree AV block) or there is complete barricade between atria and the ventricles (complete AV block) so that no impulse is conducted from either side.

AV nodal dysfunction manifests either in delay or block of some of the impulses or nontransmission of all sinus impulses to the ventricles.

3. **Bundle of His conduction disturbances:** They manifest similar to AV conduction disturbances but the site of involvement is defined by bundle of His electrocardiography.

4. **Conduction disturbances involving the bundle branch (es).** The bundle branch blocks produce specific electrocardiographic pattern in certain leads, i.e. left bundle branch block manifests in left precordial leads and standard leads while right bundle branch block manifests in right precordial

leads. The electrocardiographic pattern evolved is due to conduction of impulses first through the uninvolved bundle leading to activation of the ventricle supplied by it, then it passes through the involved bundle below the site of obstruction leading to delayed activation of the ventricle supplied by it thus completing the process of ventricular activation, resulting in prolongation of QRS interval on ECG. Therefore, the bundle branch block patterns are specific and easily identifiable electrocardiographic patterns. The bundle branch block may be complete or incomplete, both produce distinct ECG patterns. The bundle branch block is usually unilateral and rarely bilateral. Complete bilateral bundle branch block is not possible, therefore, in electrocardiography, bilateral bundle branch block means right bundle block with either one or both the fascicles of left bundle or a partial block of the left bundle. The bilateral bundle branch block invariably is intermittent, occasionally alternating and short-lived.

Bundle branch block patterns evolve due to delayed activation of the ventricle whose bundle is blocked resulting in wide QRS in leads representing that ventricle

5. **Conduction disturbance through the fascicle :** In electrocardiography, conduction system of the heart is considered trifascicular (right bundle branch, left anterior and left posterior fascicles), though some consider it to be quadrifascicular but the fourth or septal fascicle is not easily identifiable. All these fascicles fan out in the myocardium and meet with each other forming peripheral (Purkinje) system of conduction.

   The fascicular conduction block is mostly identified by an abnormal QRS axis deviation resulting in a specific ECG pattern. The left anterior fascicular block produces left axis deviation of QRS and ECG manifestations are consequent to it. Similarly, the posterior fascicular block results in abnormal right axis deviation and ECG pattern evolved is due to it. Therefore, abnormal axis deviation is a hallmark of fascicular block on ECG.

Abnormal left axis (> − 30°) or right axis deviation (> + 120°) suggests a fascicular block provided there is no other cause to explain the abnormal axis.

6. **Conduction disturbance involving Purkinje system (peripheral conduction defect):** The involvement of peripheral Purkinje system of conduction does not produce any specific pattern on ECG. It manifest as an indeterminate intraventricular conduction defect producing widening of QRS in certain leads which do not confirm to any specific bundle branch or fascicular block pattern. This type of intraventricular conduction defects in certain leads may be confused with myocarditis, but in such a situation, other electrocardiographic features of myocarditis help to differentiate between the two.

Peripheral (Purkinje) conduction defects result in widening of QRS in some or all leads which does not fit into any described bundle branch or fascicular block pattern.

BASIC CONCEPTS OF CONDUCTION

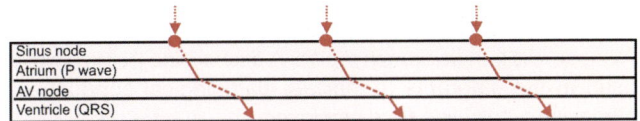

The conduction diagram represents a simplified projection of impulse conduction at the various anatomical levels of the heart on a time axis. Using typical ECG recordings a 1:1 correlation of the impulse components is made with the anatomical levels. The arrows are designed to help with recognition of the start of sinus rhythm and of the P wave. The passage of beat through atria, AV node and ventricle is represented by a relatively steep slope (↘)

A. Formation of Impulse in SA Node

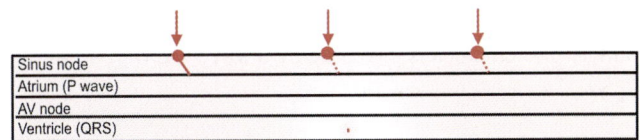

The formation of the electrical impulse in the sinus node is necessary to give rise to so-called sinus rhythm. Formation of an impulse in the sinus node is not conspicuous in the superficial ECG itself and can only be detected indirectly from atrial depolarisation (P wave).

   To better explain rhythm disorders in the region of the sinus node, impulse formation and conduction at the sinus node are represented schematically using a dot with line (in the ECG) and schematically in the diagrams by a line (↖).

B. Atrial Depolarisation with Formation of P Wave

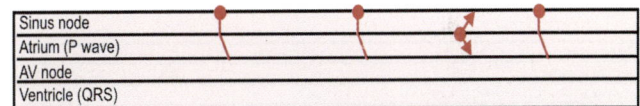

The first electrical activity conspicuous in sinus rhythm is depolarisation of the atria: a P wave occurs. The beginning of the P wave is indicated by a solid black dot and conduction in the diagrams by a solid line (\ ).

   In sinus rhythm the P wave has the largest positive deflection in lead II (the atrial vector runs parallel to lead II in sinus rhythm).

   The occurrence of supraventricular extrasystoles (SVES) is indicated by a dot with two arrows (⚡) and always occurs midway at atrial level.

C. Conduction through AV Node

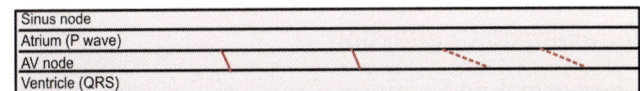

Following successful atrial depolarisation, the electrical impulse is further conducted via the AV node, the bundle of His and the bundle branches. The individual components of conduction,

SECTION FOUR

however, cannot be visualised in the superficial ECG. The time from the end of the P wave to formation of the QRS complex is equated with a simplified explanation of rhythm disorder in the AV node-His bundle branch region. A dashed line (\) is always used in the diagrams to indicate pathological conduction, otherwise a solid line (\) is employed.

D. Ventricular Depolarisation (QRS Complex)

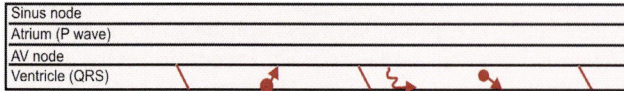

The depolarisation is represented by a QRS complex and is indicated by a solid line (\).

Ventricular ectopics are represented by a dot with a solid arrow (•↗).

Asynchronous ventricular excitation, for example due to bundle branch block is indicated by a wavy line with an arrow (ξ→).

E. Conduction Block

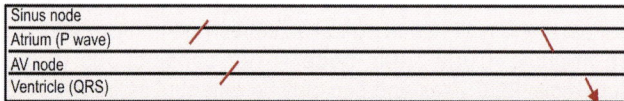

Blockade of conduction arises between the sinus node and the atrium or in the region of the AV node (between the atrium and the ventricle).

A complete conduction block is characterised by a red line; a single interruption of conduction is represented by a diagonal line (/) and a longer block by a horizontal line (—).

F. Re-entry Mechanism

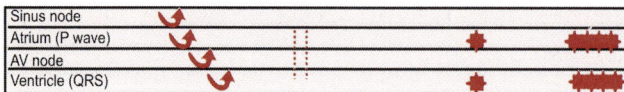

Re-entry mechanisms are indicated by (↻).

An accessory conduction pathway (e.g. a Kent fibre) is indicated by a double line (II).

The occurrence of supraventricular or ventricular ectopics is characterised by a star (✲).

With supraventricular non-entry tachycardia (e.g. atrial fibrillation) and ventricular non-reentry tachycardia a group of stars are seen (****).

The Graphic Representation of Intracardiac Conduction

The normal and abnormal intracardiac conduction may be conventionally represented by a ladder diagram. It is convenient and customary to draw a ladder diagram below the electrocardiogram showing a conduction disturbance. The "ladder" diagram is nothing but a graphic representation in which *ordinate* represents the anatomical sites of SA node, atria, AV node and ventricles; the *abscissa* represents the time (Fig. 10.2). The pathway of conduction at various levels is represented by a line which shows steep slope in case of rapid conduction and gradual slope in case of delayed or slow conduction. The interruption of conduction is represented by a small *bar* at the site of block. The site of origin of an impulse, is represented by a *'black dot'*.

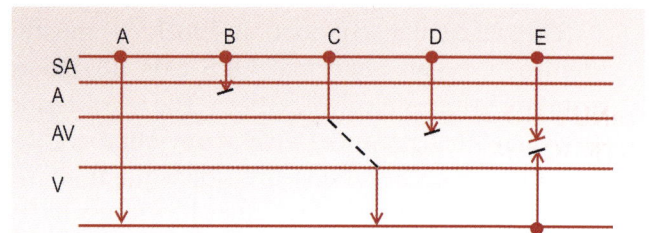

Fig. 10.2: Graphic representation of intracardiac conduction by a ladder diagram. The *ordinate* reflects the anatomical sites and *abscissa* reflects time.

A. *Normal conduction:* There is normal conduction of sinus impulse (black dot) arising from the SA node and passing relative quickly through the atria, AV node and ventricles and is represented by a relatively steep slope (↓).

B. *SA block:* The impulse arising from the SA node is immediately blocked just after its exit and at entry into atria (↴).

C. *Delayed AV nodal conduction:* The impulse arises from SA node and passes through the atria normally but is delayed in the AV node as represented by a gradual slope. The intraventricular conduction is normal. This type of conduction pattern represents first degree AV block (\). The dotted line indicate pathologic conduction.

D. *AV block:* The impulse arising from SA node and after passing through the atria normally, is blocked at AV node as represented by bar (↴).

E. *Complete AV block:* There is dissociation of sinus impulse from ventricular impulse (dual rhythm). The two impulses; one from SA node and other from ventricle arise and conduct antegradely from SA node and retrogradely from ventricle, collide and interfere at AV node. None of them is conducted either way.

11

Sinus Node Dysfunction

- Various disorders of sinus node
- Sinus pause or sinus arrest
- Various grades of SA blocks
- Sick sinus syndrome

SINUS NODE DYSFUNCTION AND STRUCTURAL NODAL DISEASE

Physiology of Sinus Node

The sinus node is a naturally occurring dominant cardiac pacemaker. It maintains normal heart rate due to its inherent property of impulse generation and has intrinsic discharge rate. It is controlled by autonomic nervous system, hence, can accelerate its rate during exercise and can slow it during rest and sleep. It has both types of innervation, i.e. sympathetic and parasympathetic. Increase in heart rate normally results from an increase in sympathetic tone acting via beta-adrenoreceptors and/or a decrease in parasympathetic tone acting via muscarinic receptors. Slowing of heart rate normally occurs due to opposite mechanisms, i.e. decrease in sympathetic tone and increase in parasympathetic tone.

Disorders of SA node

1. **Sinus arrest or sinoatrial arrest.** This is a disorder of impulse formation by SA node.
2. **Sinoatrial block**—A disorder in which sinus impulses are either delayed or blocked in the atria before they reach AV node.
   - First degree SA block
   - Second degree SA block
   - Third degree SA block

3. **Sick sinus syndrome**—A structural or functional nodal disorder expressed on ECG by varied electrocardiographic manifestations.

Sinoatrial or Sinus Arrest

A sinus pause entails the failure of the SA node to discharge its one or more impulses. Since sinus discharge *per se* produces ECG deflection (P–QRS–T), a sinus pause is manifested by absence of a P–QRS–T complex or complexes. Ordinarily, if a sinus pause occurs for a prolonged period, an AV junctional pacemaker takes over the control of ventricular activation. In case of depressed heart, even the escape rhythm may take origin from one of the ventricles. If there is uniform failure of all the pacemakers (SA node, AV node, bundle of His, ventricles); then cardiac asystole may result, which is an invariable phenomenon associated with sinus arrest in which impulse formation in SA node presumably ceases completely for a prolonged period. Therefore, sinus arrest is always intermittent. Sinus pause may follow an ectopic beat (atrial, nodal or ventricular) that is conducted retrogradely, discharges the SA node prematurely, and, as a consequence, results in a pause on ECG. The sinus pause following an ectopic is called compensatory pause.

Aetiology: Causes of sinus arrest are given in the box.

The sinus pause on ECG is not exact multiple of basic P-P interval

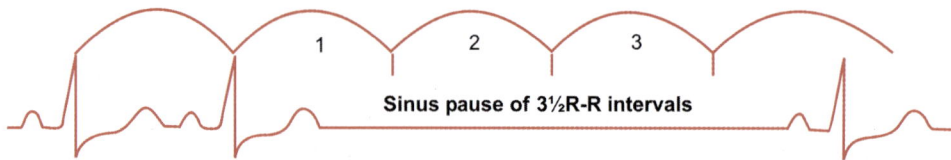

Sinus pause of 3½R-R intervals

Fig. 11.1: Diagrammatic illustration of ECG showing a sinus pause of 3½ R-R intervals. The basic underlying rhythm is sinus. Following two sinus beats there is a long pause due to failure of sinus discharge. The pause is not multiple of basic P-P or R-R interval

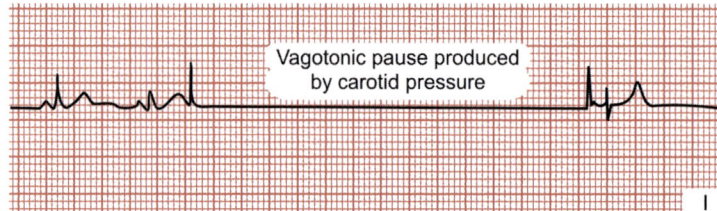

Vagotonic pause produced by carotid pressure

Fig. 11.2: Sinus pause. The electrocardiogram shows first two sinus complexes followed by a long pause produced by carotid massage, indicates atrial standstill (no P-QRS-T complex recorded) in a vagotonic individual due to failure of sinus discharge. This pause is not multiple of basic P-P or R-R interval (pause is 120 mm and P-P or R-R is 25 mm) and is more than normal sinus pause (≤ 3 sec) and shorter than the pause due to hypersensitive carotid reflex (> 5 sec)

Causes of sinus arrest

- Vagotonic individuals
- Digitalis administration
- Hypoxaemia
- Sick sinus syndrome
- Stroke
- Athletes
- Uraemia or acidosis
- Hypokalaemia
- A structural sinus disease

The Electrocardiogram in Sinus Pauses or Arrest (Figs 11.1 and 11.2)

1. The rhythm is irregular because an entire P–QRS–T complex is dropped intermittently and a pause is produced on ECG. As the impulse formation by the SA node fails, hence, atria are not depolarised producing an atrial standstill (no P wave) and subsequently ventricles are not activated (no QRS–T complex).
2. The P–P interval surrounding the pause is variable and is not multiple of basic P–P interval – a fact that distinguishes it from sinoatrial block where it is exactly multiple.
3. If more than one sinus cycle is dropped, the pause between sinus complexes can be lengthy. If pause

is long enough, then atrial, junctional, or ventricular escape beats may be observed.

SINOATRIAL BLOCKS (SA BLOCKS)

In SA block, impulse formation by the SA node is normal, but, however, it is blocked within sinoatrial junction, i.e. the junction between SA node and the surrounding atrial myocardium. As a result, a pause with no P–QRS–T complex is recorded. The SA blocks are called *'exit blocks'* because the impulse cannot exit from its pacemaker site. The SA block may occur at regular intervals, e.g. 2:1, 3:1 SA block or it may occur irregularly as an isolated phenomenon (rare). Following SA block, the subsequent beat may be a normal sinus beat, or an AV nodal or a ventricular escape beat.

Causes

The causes of sinoatrial exit blocks are given in the box.

SECTION FOUR

Causes of sinoatrial blocks

1. Excessive vagal stimulation
2. Acute myocarditis
3. Acute myocardial infarction (especially an inferior infarction)
4. Fibrosis involving the atrium
5. Drugs such as quinidine, procainamide

Types There are three types of SA blocks
A. First degree SA block
B. Second degree SA block
C. Third degree SA block

First degree SA block: It denotes a prolonged conduction time from the SA node to the surrounding atrial myocardium. It cannot be recorded on a standard 12 leads ECG, but requires invasive intracardiac recordings.

Second degree SA block: It denotes a regular intermittent failure of conduction of impulses from SA node to surrounding atrial myocardium. It is manifested on ECG as regular intermittent absence of P–QRS–T complex producing an interval which equals approximately twice or thrice or four times the normal P–P interval (Fig. 11.3). During type I (Wenckebach) second degree SA block, the P–P interval progressively shortens prior to the pause, and duration of the pause is less than 2 P–P intervals. Second degree SA block is akin to second degree AV block where P waves are formed but not regularly conducted. The main distinguishing features between the two are given in the Table 11.1.

Table 11.1: Distinguishing features between second degree SA and AV block	
Second degree SA block	*Second degree AV block*
• Neither the P wave nor QRS–T complex is recorded at the time of block.	• All P waves are recorded but blocked 'P' waves are not followed by QRS.
• Sudden acceleration of the heart occurs with effort or atropine.	• There is gradual acceleration of the heart with effort or atropine.

The Electrocardiogram in Second Degree SA Block (Fig. 11.4)

1. The P–P and R–R intervals are regular because the impulses are generated regularly by sinus node but they do not find exit into the atria, hence, entire P–QRS–T complexes are dropped for sometime producing a pause or an interval similar to sinus arrest.

2. The interval exactly equals two, three or four times the normal P–P interval in second degree SA block with 2:1, 3:1 or 4:1 conduction. During type I (Wenckebach) second degree SA block, the P–P interval progressively shortens prior to pause,

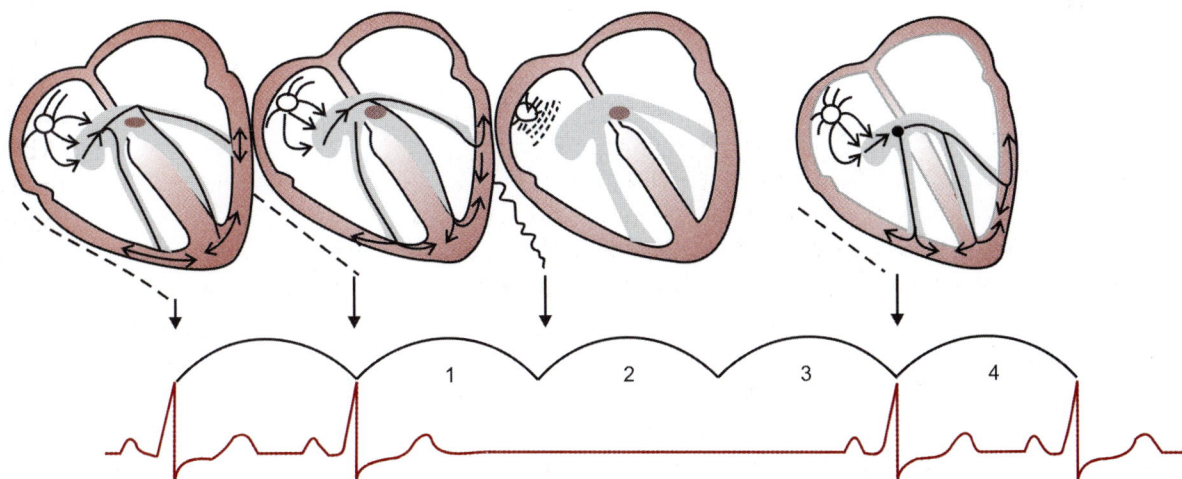

Fig. 11.3: Sinoatrial block of exactly 3 R–R intervals (diagram). The sinus impulse fails to depolarise the atria, so an entire P-QRS-T complex is dropped. The P-P or R-R interval surrounding the pause is exact multiple of underlying P-P (and R-R) interval

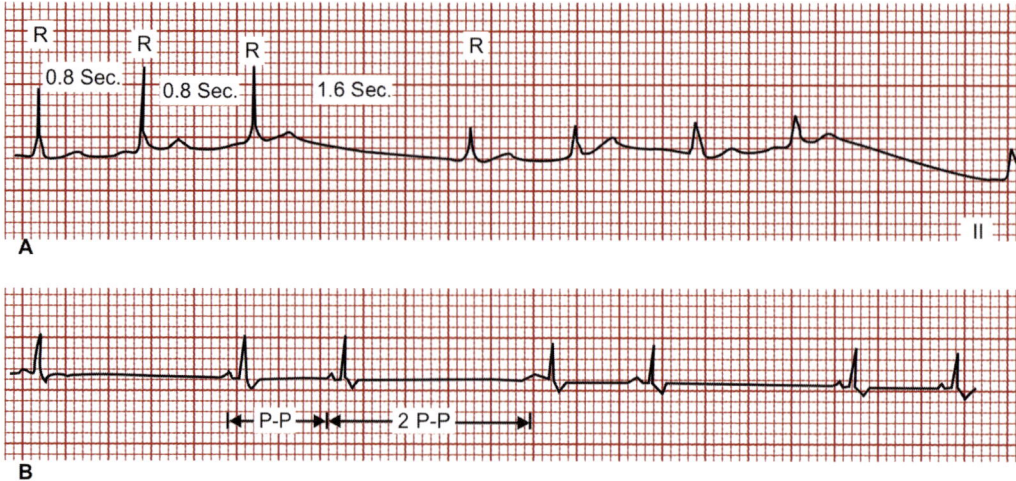

Fig. 11.4: Second degree SA block. **A:** The ECG (lead II) shows intermittent sinus arrest creating a pause which is exact twice of basic P-P or R-R interval. The QRS complex of sinus beat is wide and bizarre due to aberrant intraventricular conduction. **B:** The lead II shows normal sinus rhythm at a rate of 60/min. The P waves are distributed in bigeminal grouping of long and short intervals. The short intervals is 0.10 sec (P-P interval)alternates with long interval of 0.2 sec (2 x P-P interval). This indicates that after 2 successive P-QRS complexes, one P-QRS-T is dropped constituting 3:2 SA block

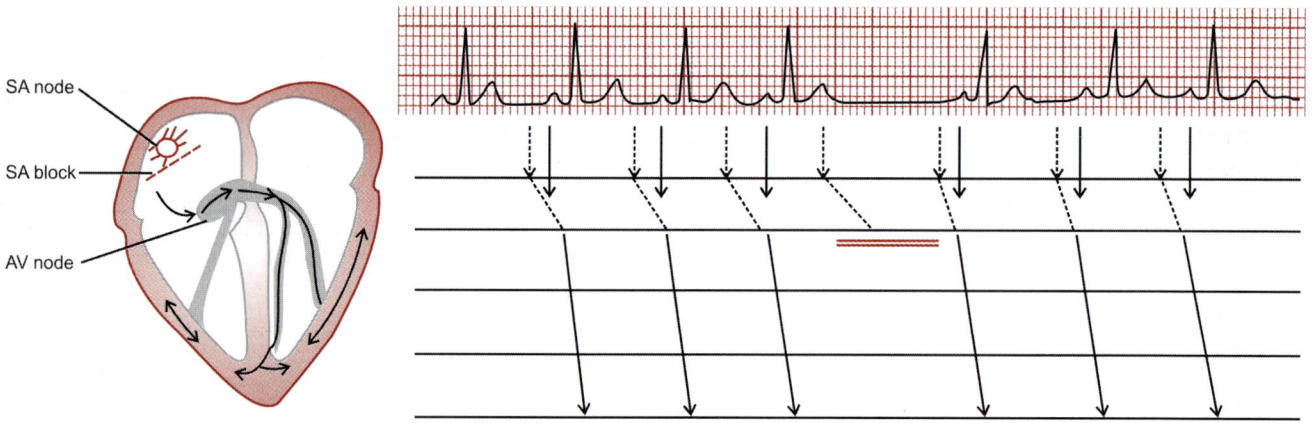

Fig. 11.5: Second degree SA block (Wenckebach type)

hence, the duration of pause is less than two P–P cycles resembling sinus pause (Fig. 11.5).

The pause due to sinoatrial block is exact multiple of the preceding normal P–P interval, –a fact that distinguishes it from the sinus pause due to sinus arrest.

Third degree SA block : Third degree or complete SA block, is characterised by complete lack of atrial activity (absent P waves) for sometime. On ECG, it will produce sinoatrial arrest in the form of a long atrial standstill. The ECG characteristics are given in the box.

ECG Characteristics of Third Degree SA Block

- Pause with no P wave
- Absence of several sinus P waves
- Length of pause > 2 × PP intervals

SICK SINUS (LAZY SINUS, UNSTABLE SINUS) SYNDROME–THE STRUCTURAL NODAL DISEASE

The term 'sick or lazy or sluggish sinus syndrome' was used to describe an inherent abnormality of SA node. Now, it has become abundantly clear that it is not only the SA node which is sick but also, the AV node and its appendages, and possibly other pacemaker centres as well. It has also become evident that it is a disorder not only of impulse conduction but also of impulse formation, therefore, double nodal disease would be an appropriate term for this syndrome. Now a days 'structural nodal disease' is well accepted term, since, it embraces disease of both SA and AV nodes and their appendages, and clearly separates diseases due to structural change from metabolic and pharmacological abnormalities.

The sick sinus syndrome is a useful clinical concept but it is not a specific ECG entity, hence, should not be used in the description of ECG. The sick sinus syndrome refers to a combination of symptoms (dizziness, confusion, fatigue, syncope and congestive heart failure) caused by sinus node dysfunction and its manifestations on ECG such as marked sinus bradycardia, SA blocks or sinus arrest, etc. It is very difficult to relate the symptoms of sick sinus syndrome on the basis of ECG findings. The clinical recognition of the multiple disorders that make up this syndrome is important because they can be treated effectively by a variety of permanent artificial pacemakers.

Aetiology: The causes of structural nodal disease include:

1. Acute myocardial infarction (e.g. inferior infarction)
2. Cardiomyopathies
3. Metastatic disease involving the heart
4. Primary muscular dystrophies
5. Amyloid heart disease
6. Tuberculosis involving the heart
7. Degenerative fibrotic disease of the atria.

Structural nodal disease occurs in 5–10% cases of acute myocardial infarction due to either involvement of left circumflex or right coronary artery, since either of these supplies the SA node. SA node dysfunction occurs in 5% cases with acute inferior myocardial infarction. Conversely it has been noted that when SA node dysfunction manifests in acute myocardial ischaemia or infarction, it is transient and resolves with recovery.

The Electrocardiographic Manifestations of Sick Sinus Syndrome

The following ECG features suggest sick sinus syndrome (SSS)–

1. **Sinus bradycardia**: The sinus bradycardia of less than 50–60 bpm in an adult may be due to structural nodal disease provided nonstructural causes, i.e. digitalis, beta-blockers, quinidine, procainamide, uraemia, obstructive jaundice, hypothyroidism, raised intracranial pressure, or vagotonaemia have already been excluded. The isolated bradycardia is more common due to nonstructural causes rather than sick sinus syndrome. Isolated bradycardia in sick sinus syndrome may be episodic or constant (Figs 11.6 and 11.7).

2. **Nonrespiratory sinus arrhythmia**: The sinus bradycardia when associated with nonrespiratory sinus arrhythmia suggests structural sinus node disease (Fig. 11.7).

3. **Inadequate tachycardia response to physiological and pharmacological means:** Normally, fever, pain, congestive heart failure produce

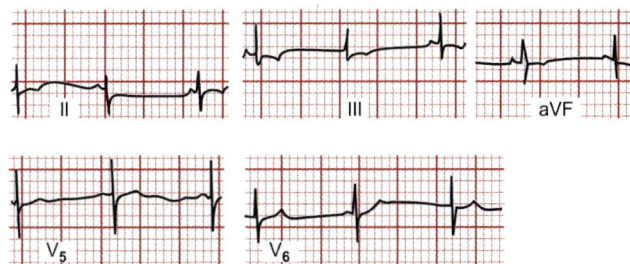

Fig. 11.6: Sinus bradycardia in a patient with inferior wall ischaemia. The electrocardiogram shows sinus bradycardia at a rate of 43/min and an inferior wall ischaemia (T wave inversion in leads II, III and aVF).

Note: Isolated sinus bradycardia is not common in structural nodal disease rather is more common in AV nodal dysfunction due to ischaemia especially inferior wall. This is transient phenomenon in inferior wall infarction due to transient ischaemia of AV node. When sinus bradycardia is associated with sinus arrhythmia, it indicates, sinus node dysfunction rather than AV nodal dysfunction

SECTION FOUR

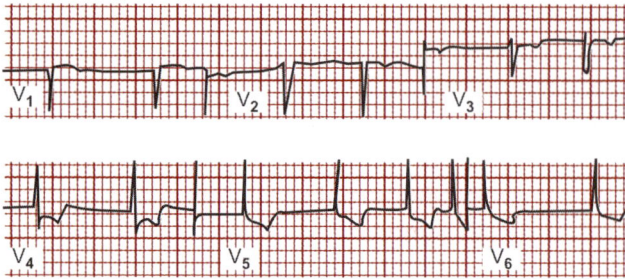

Fig. 11.7: Sinus node dysfunction. The electrocardiogram (V_1-V_4) recorded from a patient with coronary artery disease shows:

(i) Sinus bradycardia and sinus arrhythmia. The two beats shown in leads V_2-V_3 are sinus conducted (P wave precedes QRS) at a rate of 50 bpm and R-R interval is irregular (sinus arrhythmia)

(ii) Nodal escape beats/rhythm. The P wave are seen preceeding QRS in leads V_1-V_3 but are invisible in leads V_4-V_6 indicating emergence of nodal rhythm. The rhythm tries to accelerate at the end of V_5 (last three beats) but decelerates again in V_6

(iii) The coving ST segment in V_1-V_3 with T wave inversion and marked ST segment depression with T wave inversion in leads V_4-V_6 indicate acute coronary ischaemia

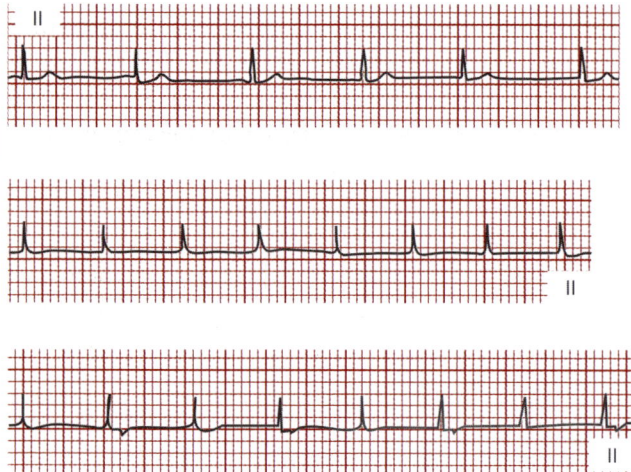

Fig. 11.8: Uncomplicated escape rhythm due to sick sinus syndrome. The ECG lead II shows;

(i) Upper strip: There is sinus bradycardia (HR < 60/min) with sinus arrhythmia (irregular R-R intervals)

(ii) Middle strip: The strip was taken from same patient at different time shows AV nodal rhythm at a rate of 60/min

(iii) Atropine response (lower strip): It was recorded after giving 1 mg IV atropine and ECG recorded immediately showed no response. The AV nodal rhythm persisted with alternate beat showing inverted P' wave indicating retrograde atrial activation

All these features on ECG suggest structural nodal disease.

sinus tachycardia which is an expected response. If adequate tachycardia response does not occur, then sinus node disease may be suspected. Similarly, if sinus node fails to accelerate its rate with exercise or after atropine administration, then diagnosis of sick sinus syndrome is most likely.

4. **Uncomplicated escape rhythm** : With marked SA node depression, a lower subsidiary pacemaker (AV node or ventricle) may take over the control of the rhythm of the heart producing an idionodal or an idioventricular rhythm. For example, an idionodal rhythm (an escape rhythm) at a rate of 45–60 bpm with antegrade conduction to ventricles and retrograde conduction to the atria (inverted P waves in leads II, III and aVF) indirectly suggests sick sinus syndrome (Figs. 11.8, 11.9).

5. **Sinus bradycardia associated with AV block** : When sinus bradycardia is associated with first, second or complete AV block, then sick sinus syndrome may be suspected as the underlying

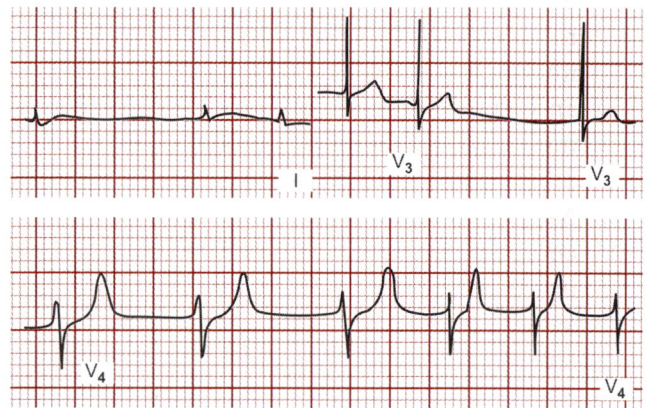

Fig. 11.9: Sinus pauses and nodal escape rhythm with its acceleration in sick sinus syndrome. The ECG shows:

(i) Lead I shows a sinus pause followed by a normal sinus beat (P-QRS-T)

(ii) Lead V_3 recorded from the same patient shows sinus conducted beats (Ist and 2nd) followed by a sinus pause and then a sinus conducted beat

(iii) As the ECG was being recorded, the lead V_4 starts showing nodal escape beats (first 3 beats) and then as sinus node did not pick up function, it was followed by accelerated nodal escape rhythm to maintain normal heart rate.

These are electrocardiographic manifestations of structural nodal disease (sick sinus syndrome)

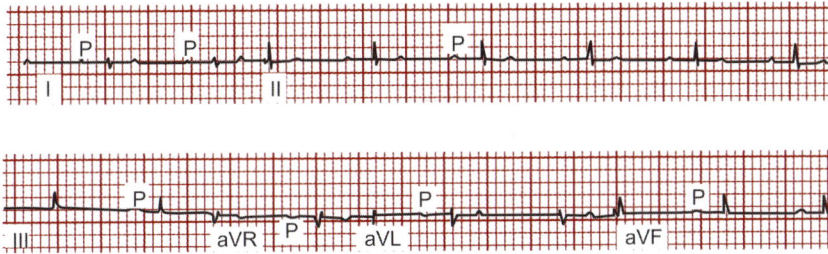

Fig. 11.10: Dual nodal disease (Sick Sinus Syndrome). The electrocardiogram (standard leads) show low voltage graph, wandering atrial pacemaker (variable shapes of P waves), sinus arrhythmia, slow atrial rate (< 60/min). All these features suggest sinus node dysfunction. The P-R interval is much prolonged (0.44 sec). There is second degree 2:1 AV block. The QRS complexes are widened and deformed (intraventricular conduction delay). Both these features suggest AV nodal dysfunction

cause. The AV block may manifest on ECG or may be revealed on atrial pacing. The AV block with sinus bradycardia occurs in two-third patients of sick sinus syndrome, called a *'double nodal disease'* (Fig. 11.10).

6. **Sinus bradycardia, sinoatrial arrest with escape rhythm:** Usually, the sinus bradycardia or sinoatrial arrest leads to an emergence of an escape rhythm, mostly an idionodal escape rhythm. If the electrocardiogram shows an interplay of sinus rhythm, sinoatrial arrest and an escape rhythm, then sick sinus syndrome must be suspected and should be explored by other sophisticated tests.

7. **Normal sinus rhythm or sinus bradycardia complicated by SA and AV blocks, and failure or delayed appearance of escape rhythm:** Various grades of SA blocks occur commonly in structural nodal disease but it is second degree SA block (type–II or type–I Wenckebach conduction) which is detected on electrocardiogram. The SA block may be associated with sinus bradycardia, normal sinus rhythm or may be associated with AV block. With marked SA node suppression, idionodal escape rhythm occurs and; if both SA node and AV node are involved then idioventricular rhythm will appear. The failure of an escape rhythm to appear after long sinus pauses in the presence of sinus bradycardia with suppression of SA node and AV node function (SA and AV blocks) indicates sick sinus syndrome.

The non-appearance or delayed appearance of an idionodal escape rhythm in the presence of marked SA suppression (bradycardia, sinus pauses or sinoatrial block) indicates sick sinus syndrome.

8. **Slow ventricular response in atrial fibrillation or atrial flutter:** In atrial fibrillation, digitalis or verapamil or betablockers are used to slow the rapid ventricular response. However, if ventricular response in atrial fibrillation or flutter is naturally slow (< 60 bpm) in the absence of drug treatment, then sick sinus syndrome may be suspected as its cause.

9. **Failure to resume sinus rhythm after cardioversion for atrial flutter or fibrillation:** Usually, after cardioversion for atrial flutter or fibrillation, the sinus rhythm is restored; the failure of or delayed restoration of sinus rhythm indicates structural nodal disease or sick sinus syndrome.

10. **Prolongation of return cycle following premature discharge of SA node pacemaker :** The atrial premature beat or retrogradely conducted AV nodal or ventricular ectopic beat tends to suppress SA node momentarily leading to the prolongation of return cycle, which normally is less than 25% of the basic sinus cycle length. If return sinus cycle is prolonged more than 25% of the basic sinus cycle length, it indicates structural nodal disease.

11. **Intra-atrial block and/or an atrial escape rhythm:** The deformed and wide P waves indicate atrial disease and may be an evidence

SECTION FOUR

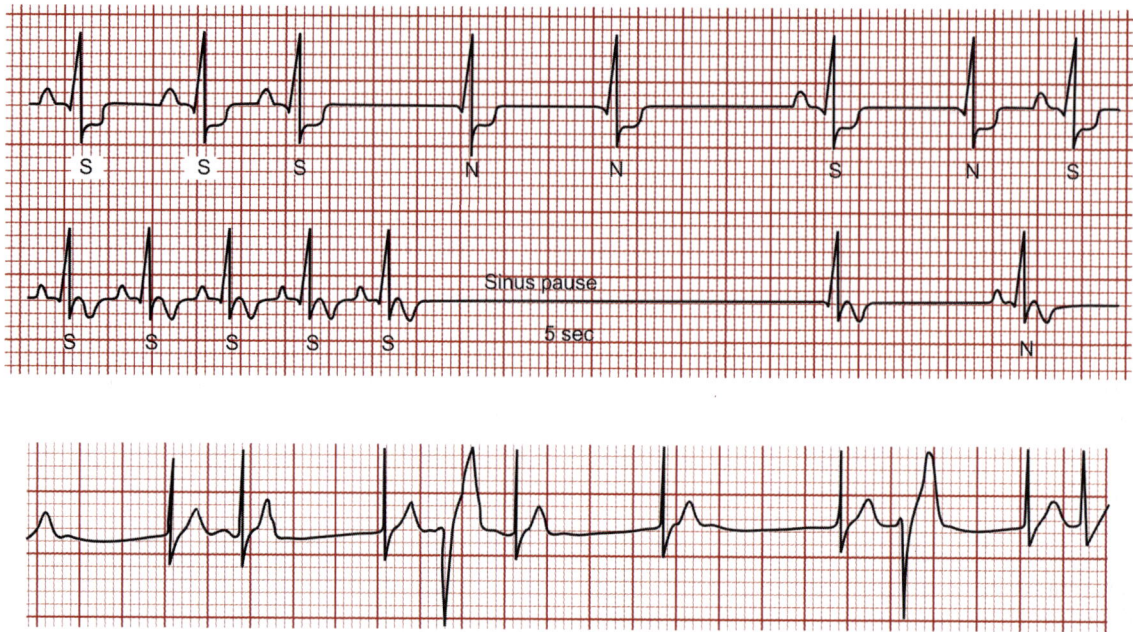

Figs 11.11A and B: Bradycardia—Tachycardia syndrome—a manifestation of sick sinus (A: Diagrammatic illustration)
Top strip: There is sinus bradycardia and sinus arrhythmia in the beginning (first three complexes) followed by junctional (nodal) escape beats (N) at irregular intervals)
In the bottom strip, there is paroxysmal atrial tachycardia followed by a long pause of almost 5 sec of asystole followed by resumption of nodal escape beats (N)
  All these features suggest sick sinus syndrome with varied manifestations including bradycardia and tachycardia syndrome.
B. The ECG (long strip) lead shows bradycardia and tachycardia (in the beginning and at the end) syndrome

of structural nodal disease. Changing shapes of P waves reflect atrial escape rhythm or wandering atrial pacemaker, may be secondary to sinus node suppression.

12. **The Bradycardia – Tachycardia syndrome** (Fig. 11.11): The bradycardia – tachycardia syndrome is characterised by periods of bradycardia and episodes of supraventricular tachycardia. The bradycardia may be due to sinus arrest or sinoatrial exit block, reflects sinus node dysfunction (sick sinus syndrome) associated with subsequent junctional or ventricular escape rhythms. The supraventricular tachycardia may be paroxysmal atrial tachycardia or atrial fibrillation or atrial flutter or AV nodal tachycardia, singly or in combinations. The tachyarrhythmic manifestations may ultimately become established as a chronic atrial fibrillation.

The diagnosis may be suspected when, following the termination of a paroxysm of atrial flutter, fibrillation or tachycardia, there is a short period

of exceptionally slow sinus bradycardia (25–35 bpm).

The bradycardia–tachycardia syndrome reflects depressed conduction with hyperexcitability, indicates diffuse disease of the conduction system, is not necessarily be associated with structural nodal disease.

The bradycardia–tachycardia syndrome is manifested on ECG as inappropriate (> 3 sec) pauses in sinus activity following spontaneous cessation of tachyarrhythmias (Fig. 11.11)

13. **Hemiblocks:** Aforementioned abnormal rhythms may be associated with hemiblocks (especially left anterior fascicular) in sick sinus syndrome.

Diagnosis

It is suspected clinically by symptoms, signs and electrocardiographic manifestations; the confirmation is done by provocative tests.

The diagnosis of sick sinus syndrome is suggested by symptomatic bradycardia which is not due to metabolic acidosis, hypothyroidism, uraemia or drug effect, e.g. digitalis, beta-blockers, calcium channel blockers and ECG shows an evidence of SA node suppression in the form of sinus arrest or SA block with escape rhythm or supraventricular tachyarrhythmias. Due to intermittent nature of the changes, it consequently becomes necessary to institute Holter's monitoring. This is further especially important in symptomatic patients to relate symptoms to certain physical acts or other events. The diagnostic clues to sick sinus syndrome on ECG are again summarised in the box.

Diagnostic clues to sick sinus syndrome

1. Sinus bradycardia alone or associated with one or more of the followings:
    1. Sinus arrhythmia
    2. SA block or sinoatrial arrest
    3. SA block or AV block or both
    4. With or without an escape rhythm
    5. Failure of appearance of escape rhythm after prolonged bradycardia.
2. Slow ventricular response in atrial flutter or fibrillation.
3. Failure to resume sinus rhythm after cardioversion for atrial flutter or fibrillation.
4. Prolongation of return cycle following a premature SA node discharge by an ectopic (atrial, nodal or ventricular).
5. Intra-atrial block and/or atrial escape rhythm or wandering atrial pacemaker.

Provocative Tests

1. *Physiological tests*: The simplest test is exercise. Normally, sinus rate accelerates with mild to moderate exercise, the failure of an increase in heart rate or inadequate tachycardia response to exercise points to the existence of structural nodal disease.

2. *Pharmacological tests:* The intravenous administration of 1–2 mg atropine will accelerate the heart rate beyond 90/ min. in case of vagotonaemia (Fig. 11.12) but will not accelerate it if structural nodal disease is suspected.

    Similarly, intravenous administration of 1–2 mg isoprenaline in a suitable vehicle may not accelerate the heart rate in structural nodal disease, but may accelerate the rate in autonomic dysfunction.

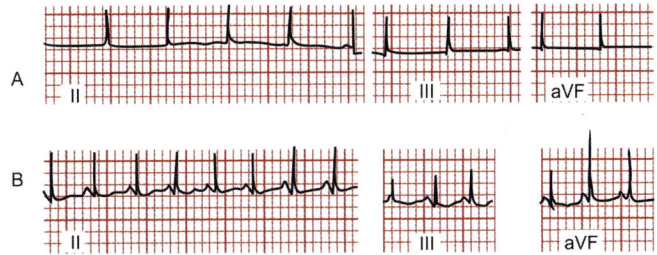

Fig. 11.12: Sinus bradycardia due to vagotonaemia. The ECG recorded from a 50 years male complaining of syncope and fatigue, shows:

A. There is sinus bradycardia (HR < 60 bpm). The P waves, P-R intervals and QRS complexes are normal (best seen in lead II).

B. After atropine: The ECG was repeated after atropine (1 mg) shows increase in heart rate (HR is 90/min) indicating vagotonaemia as the cause of bradycardia. Now the P waves, P-R intervals and QRS complexes are well seen and normal.

The pateint cannot be labelled as a case of sick sinus syndrome after atropine response. Further electrophysiological studies are needed in this case, i.e. sinus node recovery time and sinoatrial conduction time

Adenosine use has also been suggested as a noninvasive test of sinus node function.

3. *The electrophysiological tests:*
1. *Sinus node recovery time:* The sinus node recovery time is assessed following overdrive suppression by atrial pacing. A pacing rate of 120–140 bpm for 2–4 min is used in most cases; when atrial pacing is discontinued, a pause indicating sinus node recovery time occurs prior to restoration of spontaneous sinus rhythm. The rapid atrial pacing will momentarily suppress SA node so that resumption of normal sinus rhythm is delayed because sinus node recovers slowly following overdrive suppression. Therefore, time taken by the sinus node to recover following overdrive suppression forms the basis of this test. The interval between the last paced high atrial response and first sinus (spontaneous) response after termination of the pacing is measured to determine the sinus node recovery time. Because the sinus node recovery time is influenced by spontaneous sinus node cycle length, hence, the value is corrected by substracting the spontaneous sinus node cycle length (prior to pacing) from the sinus

node recovery time; thus corrected sinus node recovery time may be rewritten as :

> *"Sinus node recovery time (corrected) = Sinus node recovery time – Sinus cycle length before pacing (normal values of sinus node recovery time are < 525 msec.; prolonged values indicate structural nodal disease)."*

Direct recordings of sinus node electrocardiogram have documented that sinus node recovery time is also influenced by prolongation of sinoatrial conduction time, as well as changes in sinus node automaticity, especially in the first beat after cessation of pacing. After cessation of pacing, the first return sinus cycle can be normal, and can be followed by secondary pauses. Secondary pauses are more common in sinoatrial exit block–structural nodal disease. It is also important to evaluate AV nodal and His-Purkinje function in patients with sick sinus syndrome since both may exhibit impaired AV conduction.

2. *Sinoatrial conduction time:* Determination of the conduction time from the sinus node to the atrium allows for the differentiation of abnormalities of sinoatrial conduction from abnormalities of sinus impulse formation. The conduction time equals one half of the pause following termination of brief periods of pacing *minus* the sinus cycle length. Alternatively, it can be measured from direct sinus node electrocardiogram with extracellular electrodes placed in the region of sinus node and correlates well with sinoatrial conduction time measured indirectly in patients with normal sinus node function.

The sensitivity and specificity of both the tests, i.e. sinus node recovery time and sinoatrial conduction time is about 50 and 88% respectively. Thus, if they are abnormal, the likelihood of sinus node dysfunction is high, but, if they are normal, that does not exclude the possibility of structural nodal disease.

HYPERSENSITIVE CAROTID SINUS SYNDROME

The prevalence of carotid sinus hypersensitivity in an asymptomatic population is reported to be 5–25%, occurring primarily in older persons (> 60 years) and mainly in men. About 5–20% individuals with abnormal carotid sensitivity suffer from syncope called *"carotid sinus syncope"*. Attacks are precipitated by factors that exert pressure on carotid sinus, e.g. tight collar, shaving and sudden turning of head. Syncope occurs commonly in older individuals above 60 yrs. of age and the majority have coronary artery disease and/or hypertension. Other precipitating factors include; neck pathology such as enlarged lymph nodes, tissue scars, carotid body tumours, parotid, thyroid and, head and neck tumours. Possible association with digitalis, alpha–methyldopa and propranolol have been reported. Sinus node dysfunction and atrioventricular abnormalities may co-exist in carotid sinus hypersensitivity.

The Electrocardiographic Manifestations

The condition is recognised most frequently by ventricular asystole due to cessation of atrial activity from sinus arrest or SA exit block. AV block is observed less frequently. This condition has to be differentiated from sick sinus syndrome.

The condition is diagnosed by a sinus pause or pauses of > 3 seconds, occurring spontaneously or following unilateral carotid sinus massage, which is greater than the sinus pause that can occur normally (< 3.0 sec.). Atropine abolishes the sinus pause(s) due to hypersensitive carotid sinus syndrome.

Mechanism: It is due to either a high resting vagal tone, or excessive release of acetylcholine, or hyper–responsiveness of carotid sinus to acetylcholine, or baroreceptor hypersensitivity, or inadequate cholinesterase activity. This cardio-inhibitory carotid sinus reflex is abolished by atropine.

Suggested Reading

1. Asseman P, Berzin B, Desry D, et al: Postextrasystolic sinoatrial exit block in human sick sinus syndrome. Demonstration by direct recording of sinus node electrocardiograms. *Am Heart J* **122**: 1633,1991.

2. Benditt DG, Sakaguchi S, Goldstein MA, et al: Sinus node dysfunction: Pathology, clinical features, evaluation and treatment. In: Zipes DP, Jalife J (Eds): *Cardiac Electrophysiology: From Cell to Bedside*, 2nd ed, Philadelphia: WB Saunders Company 1994.

3. Brignole M, Oddone D, Cogorno S, et al: Long-term outcome in symptomatic carotid sinus hypersensitivity. *Am Heart J* **123**: 687, 1992.

4. DeMarneffe M, Gregoire JM, Waterschoot P, et al: The sinus node function: Normal and pathological. *Eur Heart J* **14**: 649, 1993.

5. Einks WR: The Lazy sinus syndrome. *Proc Roy Soc Med* **63**: 1307, 1970.

6. Ferrer MI: The sick sinus syndrome in atrial disease, *JAMA* **206**: 645, 1968.

7. Ibid: The sick sinus syndrome. *Circulation* **47**: 67, 1973.

8. Lown B: Electrical reversion of cardiac arrhythmias. *Br Heart J* **29**: 469,1967.

9. Mandel W, Hayakawa H, Danzig R, et al: Evaluation of sinoatrial node function in man by overdrive suppression. *Circulation* **44**: 59,1971.

10. Narula OS, Samet P, Javier RP: Significance of sinusnode recovery time. *Circulation* **45**:150, 1972.

11. Narula OS: Atrioventricular conduction defects in patients with sinus bradycardia. *Circulation* **43**:1096, 1971.

12. Rasmussen K: Chronic sinoatrial heart block. *Am Heart J* **8**: 38,1971.

13. Resh W, Feuer J and Wesley RC Jr.: Intravenous adenosine: A noninvasive diagnostic test for sick sinus syndrome. *PACE* **15**: 2068, 1992.

14. Rosen KM, Loeb HS, Sinno Z, et al: Cardiac conduction in patients. with symptomatic sinus node disease. *Circulation* **43**: 836, 1971.

15. Rubenstein JJ, et al: Clinical spectrum of the sick sinus syndrome. *Circulation* **46**: 5,1972

16. Schamroth L: Disorder of Cardiac Rhythm, 2nd edn, Oxford: Blackwell Scientific Publications, 1980.

17. Straberg B, Sagie A, Erdman S, et al: Carotid sinus hypersensitivity and carotid sinus syndrome. *Prog Cardiovasc Dis* **5**: 379,1989.

18. Wu DL, Yeh SL, Lin FC, et al: Sinus automaticity and sinoatrial conduction in severe symptomatic sick sinus syndrome. *J Am Coll Cardiol* **19**:355,1992.

19. Zipes DP: Specific arrhythmias–Diagnosis and treatment. In: Braunwald E (Ed): Heart Disease—A Textbook of Cardiovascular Medicine, 5th ed WB Saunders Company 1997.

SECTION FOUR

12

Atrioventricular (AV) Blocks

- Definition
- Classification
- Mechanisms of production
- Bundle of His electrocardiography
- First degree AV block
- Second degree AV Block
- High grade AV Block
- Complete AV Block
- Congenital versus acquired AV blocks

Definition

Atriovenricular block is a disturbance in conduction of sinus or atrial impulses through the specialised conducting system (AV node and bundle of His). It may be complete or incomplete.

Classification

I. **Incomplete AV block**
   A. First degree
   B. Second degree
      i. *Mobitz type I (Wenckebach type)*
      ii. *Mobitz type II (periodic or constant)*
II. **Complete AV block or third degree AV block**

INCOMPLETE AV BLOCKS

A. First Degree AV Block

Definition : Prolongation of P–R interval beyond 0.20 sec. constitutes first degree heart block at normal heart rate in an adult and beyond 0.18 sec in children. At heart rate of 60 bpm, P–R interval > 0.22 second suggests first degree AV block. The underlying rhythm in first degree AV block remains preserved.

Aetiology: Causes are;
1. Vagal stimulation or vagotonaemia.
2. Acute infectious diseases especially acute rheumatic fever.
3. Digitalis, beta-blockers, calcium channel blockers, class
   IC antiarrhythmic agents, etc.
4. Coronary artery disease.
5. Congenital heart diseases.
6. Hyperkalaemia.
7. Myocarditis.
8. Degeneration of conducting pathways associated with ageing.
9. Idiopathic.

Mechanisms: First degree AV block results either from a functional or pathological defect in AV node, bundle of His or bundle branches resulting in prolonged delay in the conduction of sinus impulses. Increased vagal tone delays conduction by producing a functional block. Digitalis produces AV block partly by vagal stimulation and partly by AV nodal delay. In first degree AV block, all the sinus impulses are conducted to the ventricles but the conductivity is consistently delayed resulting in the prolongation of P–R interval.

Site of block. His bundle electrocardiography is a clinical tool for classification of the mechanisms and site of first, second and third degree AV block.

Normally there is a slight delay of sinus impulses in AV node; further delay results in first degree AV block

His Bundle Electrocardiography

The technique of His bundle electrocardiography was introduced during late 1960s and early 1970s. This provides a great deal of informations regarding normal and abnormal conduction in humans.

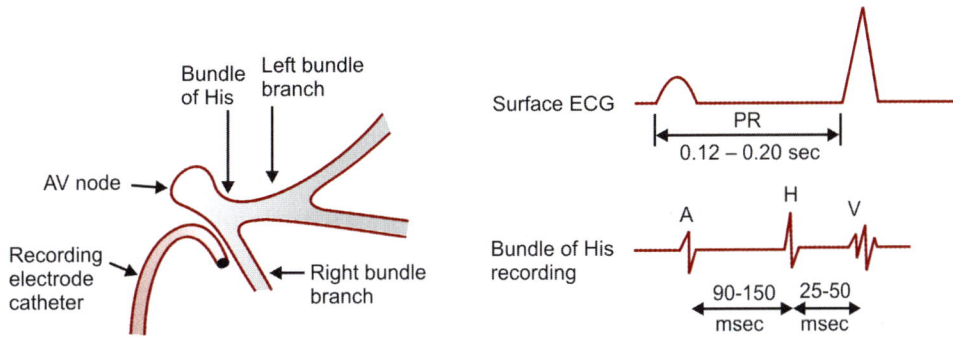

Fig. 12.1: Bundle of His electrocardiography (diagrammatic illustration). A multipolar electrode catheter is placed near to the bundle of His (as shown). The catheter records the electrical activity of low atrium, His bundle and right bundle branch, and ventricles. The surface electrocardiogram is shown for measurement of intervals. Atrial depolarisation begins with inscription of P wave on surface ECG. Since the catheter lies at low atrial level, therefore, the initial portion of atrial depolarisation (P–A interval) is not detected by it. It only records low atrial deflections (denoted by A), His spike (denoted by H) and ventricular deflections (denoted by V). The various intervals are calculated for site of block

The technique consists of placing a multipolar electrode catheter in the proximity of AV node–bundle of His in order to record electrical activity as it passes through these structures (Fig.12.1). Simultaneous ECG is usually recorded from one or more body surface leads. The electrical deflections recorded by this catheter are then related to events on the surface ECG. Several multipolar catheters can be placed in both the right and left atria and ventricle, as well as in coronary sinus in order to know the pattern of conduction of an impulse. In addition to defining of conduction pathway of impulse transmission, electrical pacing through the intracardiac electrodes used in His bundle electrocardiography, can be performed from different regions of the heart and one can study and map out the pattern of conduction of stimuli applied. Such 'mapping' of cardiac conduction is useful in diagnosis and management of certain arrhythmias and conduction system disorders. His bundle electrocardiography is also useful in evaluating the refractory period of cardiac tissue at different locations and, thus, has helped in evaluation of effects of cardiotonic and antiarrhythmic drugs. The uses of His bundle electrocardiography are summarised in the box.

Usefulness of His bundle electrocardiography
- To define the conduction pathway of an impulse transmission during normal or baseline cardiac rhythm in order to localise the site of AV block.
- To diagnose and to plan management of certain arrhythmias and conduction tissue disorders.
- To evaluate the effects of cardiotonic and antiarrhythmic drugs.

The bundle of His electrocardiography records three deflections, i.e. atrial (designated as A), His bundle (designated as H) and ventricular (designated as V). These recordings are now related to the P–R interval recorded by one or more leads on surface ECG. Depending on His bundle electrocardiography, the total P–R interval is divided into three intervals (Fig. 12.2).

1. **P–A interval:** This is the time interval between the beginning of P wave as recorded on surface ECG and A wave recorded by bundle of His electrode catheter from low atrium (designated as A). This interval is of no clinical significance unless conduction time from SA node is studied. It is 10–50 msec.

2. **A–H interval:** The time interval between low atrial (A) depolarisation to the bundle of His spike (H), is called A–H interval. Normal A–H interval is 90–150 msec.

3. **H–V interval :** The time interval between bundle of His spike (H) to the beginning of ventricular depolarisation (V) is called H–V interval. It is 25–50 msec normally.

Clinical significance: In first degree AV block (prolonged P–R interval), the site of block is deter-

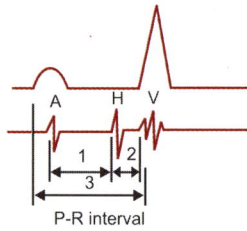

A. Normal AV conduction
1 = AH interval
2 = HV interval
3 = P-R interval

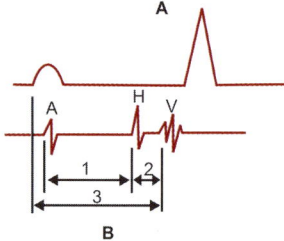

B. First degree AV block
1 = AH interval prolonged
2 = HV interval normal
3 = Total PR interval prolonged
  • The block is in AV node proximal to bundle of His

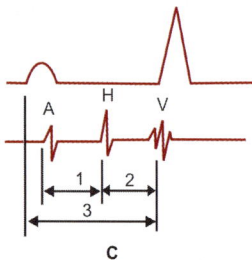

C. First degree AV block
1 = AH interval is normal
2 = HV interval is prolonged
3 = Total PR interval prolonged
  • Site of block is AV node distal to bundle of His

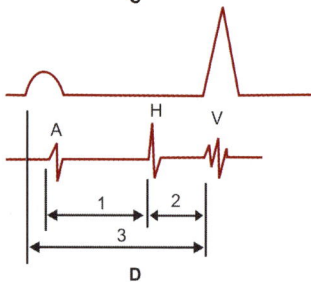

D. First degree AV block
1 = AH is prolonged
2 = HV is prolonged
3 = Total P-R is prolonged
  • Site of block is throughout the bundle of His

Fig. 12.2: Analysis of first degree AV block by bundle of His electrocardiography with reference to normal (diagrammatic illustration)

mined as given in the Table 12.1 and illustrated by diagram (Fig. 12.2).

The Electrocardiogram in First Degree AV Block (Figs 12.3 and 12.4)

1. The rhythm remains regular, i.e. P–P and R–R intervals remain constant. Atrial and ventricular rates are same and there is 1:1 conduction.
2. Every P wave is followed by a QRS complex. There is no dropped beat.
3. The P–R interval is consistently prolonged beyond upper limit of normal, i.e. 0.20 second at normal heart rate or > 0.22 sec at heart rate of 60/min. The P–R interval in first degree AV block may be prolonged upto 0.60 sec. In rare instances P–R interval of 0.70 to 0.80 seconds have been reported. The prolongation of P–R intervals indicates delay in conduction from SA node to AV node, bundle of His and its branches.
4. The QRS complex. It may be normal or wide resembling a bundle branch block pattern. A normal QRS indicates delay in the AV node, rarely within His bundle. The wide QRS indicates delay within AV node and/or His-Purkinje system. In this latter instance, His bundle electrocardiography is necessary to localise the site of conduction delay.

B. Second Degree AV Block

In this type of block, some of the sinus impulses are conducted to the ventricles, while others are blocked. Thus, second degree AV block manifests with regularly occurring P waves, some of which are not followed by QRS complex due to intermittent failure or interruption of AV conduction.

Aetiology: The causes of second degree AV block are:
1. Vagotonaemia.
2. Acute rheumatic carditis.

Table 12.1: Measurement of intervals and site of block	
Intervals	*Site of block*
1. Prolonged A–H interval and normal H–V interval.	Block is above the bundle of His (e.g. AV node)
2. Normal A–H interval and prolonged H–V interval.	Block is below the bundle of His
3. A combination of both, i.e. prolonged A–H and H–V intervals.	Block is present both proximal and distal to bundle of His, i.e. throughout AV node and His bundle

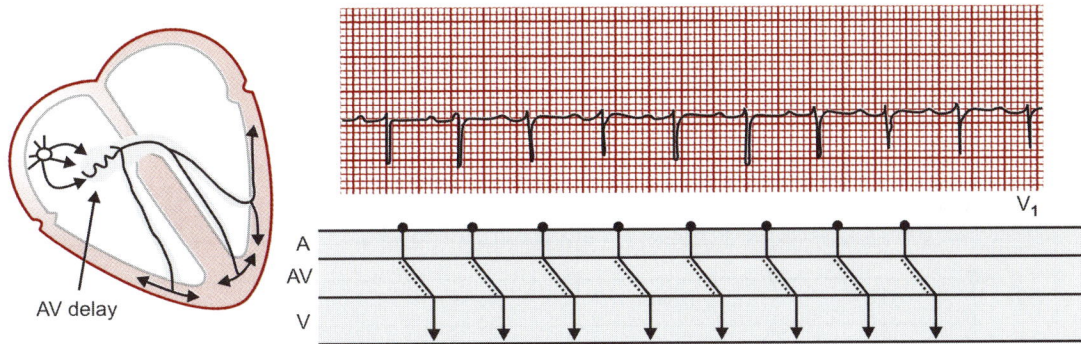

Fig. 12.3: First degree AV block. The electrocardiogram shows the following features;
 (i) The P-R interval of each conducted beat is fixed (0.28 sec) and is longer than normal
 (ii) P wave is of normal shape and occurs regularly
 (iii) R-R interval is constant. Heart rate is 84/min. QRS is normal
The ladder diagram below indicate the levels of AV conduction. The atrium (A), the AV node and the ventricles (V) with delay in AV conduction represented by steep slope in AV node

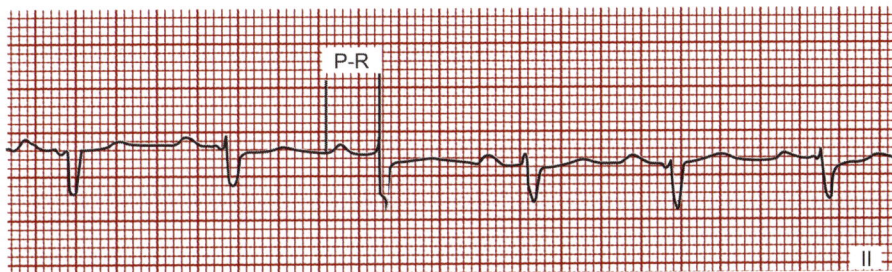

Fig. 12.4: First degree AV block with phasic aberrant intraventricular conduction. The ECG lead II shows P-R interval 0.28 sec. The QRS complexes are wide; indicating phasic aberrant intraventricular conduction

3. Acute diphtheric myocarditis
4. Coronary artery disease
   • Inferior wall infarction (AV nodal ischaemia)
   • Right ventricular infarction (AV nodal ischaemia)
   • Anterior wall myocardial infarction.
5. Digitalis toxicity – paroxysmal atrial tachycardia with varying degree of AV block (2:1, 3:2 etc) is a classical manifestation of digitalis toxicity.
6. *Physiological :* It may be physiological in certain situations such as atrial tachycardia, atrial flutter, atrial fibrillation, etc. This is protective mechanism to slow the heart rate. It can be a normal variant phenomenon (especially in athletes)
7. Aortic valve disease (syphilis).
8. Infiltrative heart disease.
9. Idiopathic fibrosis of conduction system (Lenegre's disease).
10. Calcification of mitral or aortic or both valves.

Types

i. *Mobitz type I (Wenckebach) AV block:* In this type of second degree AV block, one of the atrial impulse (P wave) fails to evoke a ventricular response in a cyclic fashion (group beating is present). The first atrial impulse of the cycle or group beating is with normal P–R interval. With each succeeding beat, P–R interval becomes progressively longer until one P wave (atrial impulse) is not followed by QRS complex (beat is dropped). A long diastolic pause results after each cycle and then the cycle is repeated (Fig. 12.5). Bundle of His electrocardiography has shown that block is proximal to bundle of His.

In Mobitz type I (Wenckebach) AV block, there is progressive lengthening of successive P–R intervals till one sinus P is blocked.

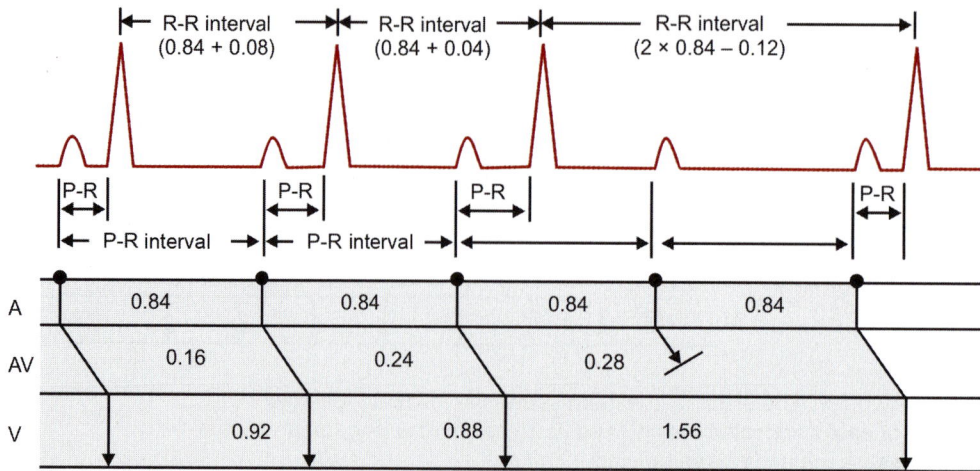

Fig. 12.5: A typical Wenckebach period (diagrammatic illustration)
There is 4:3 AV conduction during this period (4 P waves for 3 QRS complexes). The cycle length (P-P interval) is constant at 0.84 sec. There is progressive lengthening of P-R interval from 0.16 to 0.24 to 0.28 sec; thus the increment in P-R interval between the Ist and 2nd intervals is 0.08 sec and between 2nd and 3rd P-R intervals is 0.04 sec, indicating that increment in P-R interval is less with time. The P-R intervals equal the P-R interval plus the increment in P-R interval; thus successive R-R interval gets progressively shorter. The R-R interval encampassing the nonconducted P wave is twice the P-P interval minus total increament in all P-R intervals during the Wenckebach period.

Below is drawn the ladder diagram to show the conduction and nonconduction of P waves to ventricles. The various intervals are represented numerically in seconds.
A = Atria, AV = AV node, V = Ventricle

Conduction ratio or Wenckebach period: The second degree AV block is expressed in terms of an AV conduction ratio.

Definition: Conduction ratio is defined as ratio of number of P waves to number of QRS complexes in any one sequence. A *'sequence'* begins with the first conducted sinus beat following a pause created by 'dropped beat'; ends with and includes the P wave of blocked sinus beat. For example, in a sequence, there are 4 P waves (a P wave of sinus beat following the pause, next two P waves of other conducted beats and 4th P of blocked beat), out of which 3 have been conducted (P followed by QRS complex), then block is said to be 4:3. Similarly we can label 2nd degree AV block as 5:4, 6:5, 8:7 conduction, etc. The period of a group beating is called Wenckebach period in type I second degree AV block.

Conduction sequence in second degree AV block irrespective of its type begins with P wave of sinus conducted beat following the pause created

by blocked P; ends with and includes P wave of ensuing blocked beat

Mechanisms of Wenckebach period: The sinus rate is constant. Progressive prolongation of P–R interval occurs due to increasing conduction delay with each successive beat. However, the increment of conduction delay from one P–QRS complex to the next is not constant but is slightly less each time; resulting in shortening of R–R interval relative to preceding R–R interval. Finally, a P wave is not conducted. The R–R interval encompassing the blocked P wave is less than twice of the preceding R–R interval (Fig. 12.5).

The Electrocardiogram (Fig. 12.6)

1. The P–R interval of successive beats progressively lengthens in a cyclic manner until one P is blocked (not followed by QRS) following which the cycle repeats again
2. The R–R intervals are irregular due to dropped beats, causing the QRS complexes to appear in

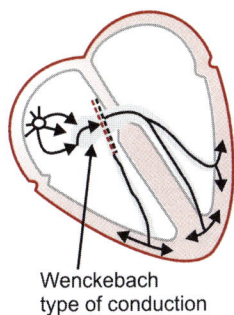

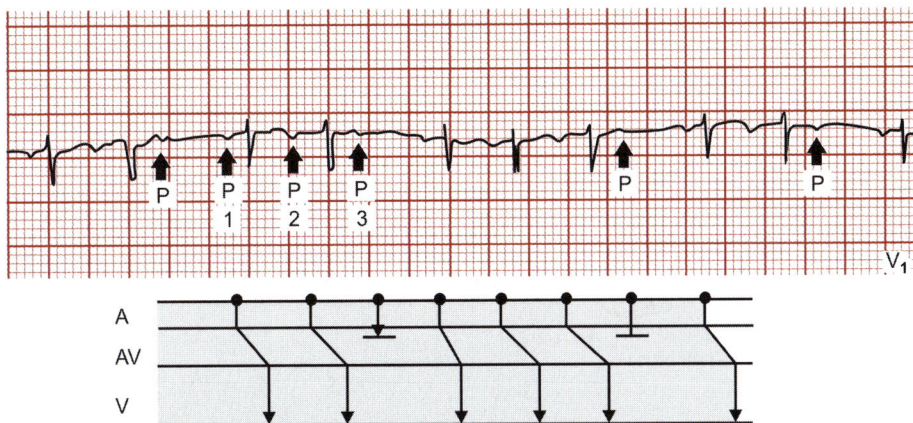

Fig. 12.6A: Mobitz type I (Wenckebach) second degree AV block with variable conduction (⋮⋮). Note the following characteristics on ECG (Lead V₁)
  (i) P wave is biphasic with prominent negative deflection
 (ii) Group beating is present. First P wave is conducted at P-R interval of 0.16 sec, Second P is conducted with P-R interval of 0.24 and third P (↑) is dropped. Therefore the conduction ratio of this group beating is 3:2. In this group beating all the P waves are shown by arrows (↑). In next group beating there are 4 P waves out of which 3 are conducted with progressive lengthening of P-R intervals and 4th P is blocked as shown by arrow (↑). The conduction ratio of this group beating is 4:3. Next group beat again consists of 3:2 conduction sequence
(iii) The P-R interval encompassing the blocked P is less than twice of preceding R-R interval.

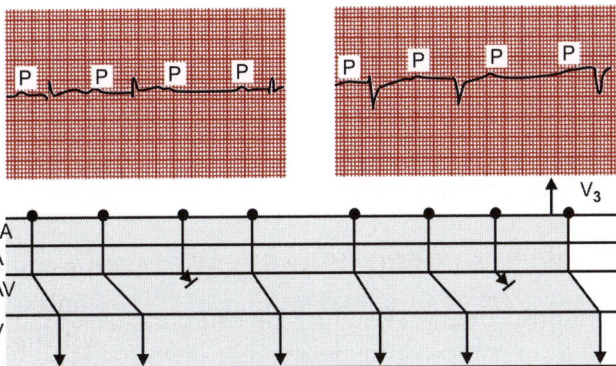

Fig. 12.6B: Mobitz type I (Wenckebach) AV block with 3:2 conduction. The leads II and V₃ are depicted. Note the followings;
  (i) First beat in both leads is conducted with P-R interval 0.28 sec and second is conducted with P-R interval of 0.40 sec and third beat in both leads is blocked indicating 3:2 Wenckebach conduction
     The ladder diagram drawn below indicates the origin and conduction of impulses.
     SA = Sinoatrial node, A = Atria, AV = Atrioventricular node, V = Ventricular

clusters. This phenomenon is called a group beating, is a hallmark of type I second degree AV block.
3. The group beating is present. The first P–R interval in a group of beats may be normal or prolonged. Subsequent P–R intervals lengthen gradually with smaller and smaller increments.
4. As the P–R intervals get longer, the R–R intervals get shorter.
5. The basic rhythm is sinus. The P–P intervals are constant. The QRS complexes are narrow unless intraventricular conduction is aberrant.
6. The conduction ratio may vary. AV conduction is mostly 1:1 with dropped QRS appearing intermittently. However, conduction ratio may be 3:2, 4:3 or greater.

ii. **Mobitz type II AV block:** In this type of block, P–R interval of all the conducted beats remains constant or fixed. There is no Wenckebach phenomenon. The associated QRS complexes are frequently abnormal. The heart rate is constant due to fixed block, i.e. 4:3, 3:2, 2:1, etc.

In Mobitz type II AV block, certain sinus beats are conducted and some are blocked in a variable or fixed fashion

The lesion in this type of block is distal to bundle of His, hence, QRS complexes often show a bundle branch block pattern (Fig. 12.9).

SECTION FOUR

SECTION FOUR

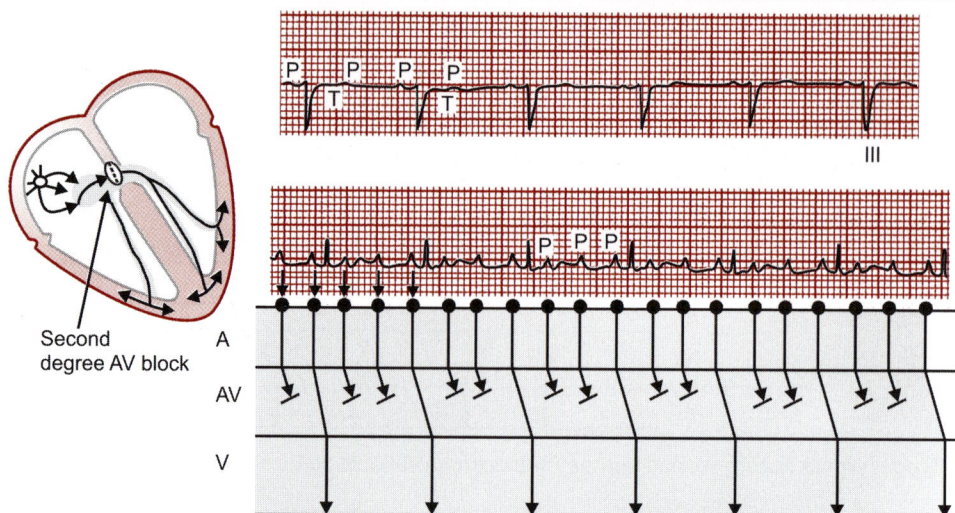

Fig. 12.7: Second degree (Mobitz type II) AV block (→)

   1.   Upper strip (lead III) shows the first sinus P conducted with normal P-R interval of 0.18 sec and next P is blocked. The cycle is repeated indicating Mobitz type II (2:1) AV block. The QRS complexes are wider than normal indicating aberrant intraventricular conduction of conducted impulses

   2.   Lower strip (lead III) shows atrial tachycardia with second degree AV block. Atrial rate is 150/min, regular indicating atrial tachycardia. The ventricular rate is just 50/min (one third of atrial rate). One sinus P wave is conducted with normal and fixed P-R interval and two successive P waves are blocked; and cycle is repeated indicating 3:1 second degree Mobitz type II AV block.

      Below ladder diagram shows the origin of impulses and their transmission at various levels.

      A = Atria, AV= AV node, V = Ventricle

The Electrocardiogram in Mobitz Type II AV Block (Fig. 12.7)

1. The P–R interval is constant and fixed. Although P–R interval of conducted beats may be normal or prolonged, but it does not vary because the site of block is below AV node,
2. The P–P intervals are constant and regular.
3. The R–R interval is variable because of the intermittent appearance of dropped beats. The P wave of the dropped beat appears on time, but no QRS follows.
4. The QRS complexes are wider than normal because of associated intraventricular conduction delay.
5. The conduction ratio may be fixed or variable. However, relatively fixed conduction ratio such as 2:1 (two P for every QRS), 3:1 or greater may be seen.

2:1 AV block (Mobitz type I versus Mobitz type II): Second degree of AV block with 2:1 conduction ratio could either be Mobitz type I (Wenckebach) or Mobitz type II since 2 consecutive P–R intervals are not recorded. The differentiation is difficult, however, certain points listed in the Table 12.2 may help to distinguish between them.

COMPLETE (THIRD DEGREE) AV BLOCK

The third degree AV block or complete heart block refers to complete or permanent obstruction to the conduction between atria and the ventricles, i.e. all the sinus or supraventricular impulses are blocked within the conducting system. Therefore, there are two independent pacemakers; one controlling the activation of the atria (usually sinus pacemaker) and the other controlling the ventricles–called a subsidiary pacemaker situated below the level of obstruction. The two rhythms (atrial and ventricular) are not only unrelated or independent; but are asynchronous also.

Definition

Complete AV block is said to be present when a fast supraventricular rhythm is completely dissociated from ventricular rhythm, the latter may be either a slow idionodal (< 45 bpm) or idioventricular

Table 12.2: Distinguishing features of two types of 2:1 second degree AV block

Mobitz type I (Wenckebach) 2:1 AV block (Fig. 12.8)	Mobitz type II AV block (Fig. 12.9) with 2:1 conduction
• The P–R interval of first conducted P wave is prolonged and the QRS complex is narrow and appears normal. • Carotid sinus massage, atropine or exercise will often unmask its nature by converting 2:1 to 3:2 in which progressive lengthening of P–R interval can be seen. • Bundle of His electrocardiography has shown the site of the block at AV node (intranodal) proximal to bundle of His.	• P–R interval of first conducted P wave is usually normal but, at times, may be prolonged and QRS complex is wide and bizarre (bundle branch block pattern). • All these maneuvers do not show any change in P–R interval. It is fixed 2:1 block. • Site of block is probably distal to bundle of His.

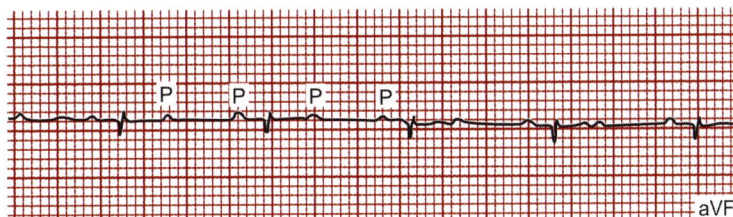

Fig. 12.8: Mobitz type 1 second degree AV block with 2:1 AV conduction
The characteristic features in lead aVF are:
1. Every alternate P wave is conducted (AV conduction ratio is 2:1).
2. The P-R interval of conducted P is lengthened (0.32 sec) and next P is blocked, it is called 2:1 Wenckebach type I second degree AV block.
3. The qRS complexes are normal. The q wave in aVF suggests an old inferior wall infarction.
Out of two P waves, one P is conducted regularly

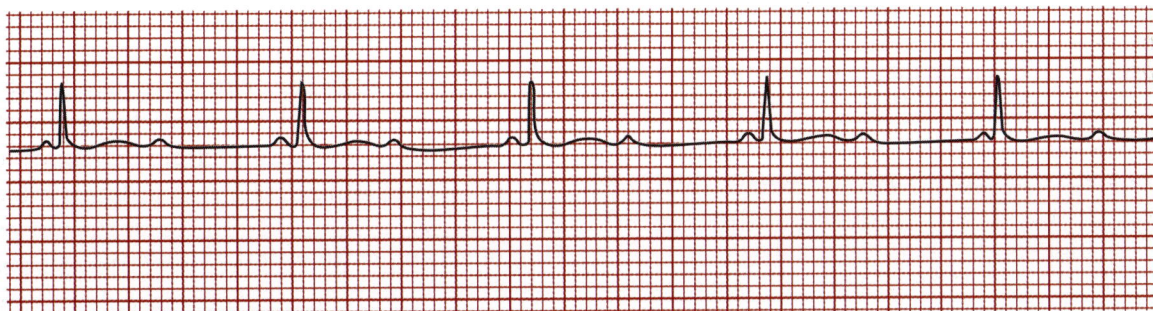

Fig. 12.9: Second degree (Mobitz type II) 2:1 AV block. The lead II shows first beat (P wave) conducted with normal P-R interval of 0.16 sec and the next P is blocked. The cycle is repeated regularly indicating second degree (Mobitz type II) AV block with 2:1 conduction. The P-R and R-R intervals are constant. The conducted QRS complexes are narrow indicating normal intraventricular conduction

(< 35 bpm) escape rhythm and long continuous recordings donot reveal any capture beat.

In complete AV block, there is a complete barrier to conduction of supraventricular impulses to the ventricles, hence, impulses originate from a subsidiary pacemaker cells of the ventricles to maintain the rhythm–called an idioventricular rhythm.

Aetiology: The causes of complete heart block include;
1. Drug toxicity (digoxin, beta-blockers, calcium channel blockers).

2. Excessive vagal tone (hypervagotonaemia).
3. Acute myocardial infarction, e.g. inferior wall, right ventricular or acute anterior extensive infarction. Complete heart block may be transient in myocardial infarction.
4. Age-related degeneration of the electrical conduction system.
5. Calcific stenosis of aortic or mitral or both valves.
6. Myocarditis and endocarditis.
7. Acute rheumatic carditis.
8. Intracardiac surgery.
9. Amyloid heart disease.
10. Myxomatous infiltration of conduction system in myxoedema can occasionally produce complete heart block.
11. Tumours, parasitic infestations, pyogenic and granulomatous infections. *Chagas'* disease is the commonest cause of AV block in Central and South America.
12. Congenital heart diseases, i.e. ostium primum type of ASD, ventricular septal defect, corrected transposition of great vessels, etc.

The Electrocardiogram

1. The P–P intervals are usually constant.
2. The R–R intervals are also constant.
3. *The atrial and ventricular rates are different;* atrial rate being faster than ventricular. The ventricular rate depends on the origin of the subsidiary pacemaker. If pacemaker is in the bundle of His or one of the bundle branches, the ventricular rate ranges between 40–60 beats/min. More distal is the subsidiary pacemaker, the slower is the ventricular rate, hence, it is slowest when pacemaker lies in the ventricles itself.
4. *No relationship between P and QRS:* The P waves 'march through' the QRS complexes, hence, some P waves may precede, some may merge with QRS and deform them, and others may follow QRS. There is complete dissociation between the P waves and the QRS complexes. No capture beat is seen.
5. *QRS configuration:* The configuration or morphology of QRS depends on the origin of the subsidiary pacemaker. If there are two subsidiary pacemakers, then there will be two different types of QRS complexes.

i. QRS complex is normal or near normal if the subsidiary pacemaker is situated in the AV node below the level of block or in the bundle of His (Fig. 12.10)
ii. If the subsidiary pacemaker lies in one of the bundle branches (Fig. 12.11); the QRS complexes will have pattern of a bundle branch block (right or left).
iii. If ectopic pacemaker is peripheral and situated in the ventricular myocardium or Purkinje fibres, then the activation of ventricles will be bizarre and QRS complexes will be abnormal being broad, notched or slurred (Fig. 12.12).
iv. In case of two or more subsidiary pacemakers, there will be competition between them for control of the ventricles, hence, one pacemaker will result in one form of QRS complexes followed by change of QRS complexes produced by the other pacemaker. The change or shift of pacemaker leads to Stokes–Adams syncopal attacks, which are not infrequent in complete heart block.

6. *Basic rhythm:* The basic underlying rhythm in complete heart block may be sinus or one of the supraventricular type (e.g. atrial tachycardia, atrial flutter, atrial fibrillation, etc.). In atrial fibrillation, regular R–R intervals indicate complete heart block. In atrial flutter, slow ventricular response indicates complete heart block. In complete heart block, atrial tachycardia may degenerate into atrial flutter (Fig. 12.13) or into atrial fibrillation.

Diagnosis and differential diagnosis: The complete heart block may be congenital or acquired. The differentiating features are summarised in the Table 12.3. The congenital complete AV block is common in children.

Clinical Significance of Second Degree AV Block and Complete AV Block

The second degree AV block may change to third degree, and in transition, may lead to *Stokes-Adams attacks*. They are infrequent in complete heart block *per se*.

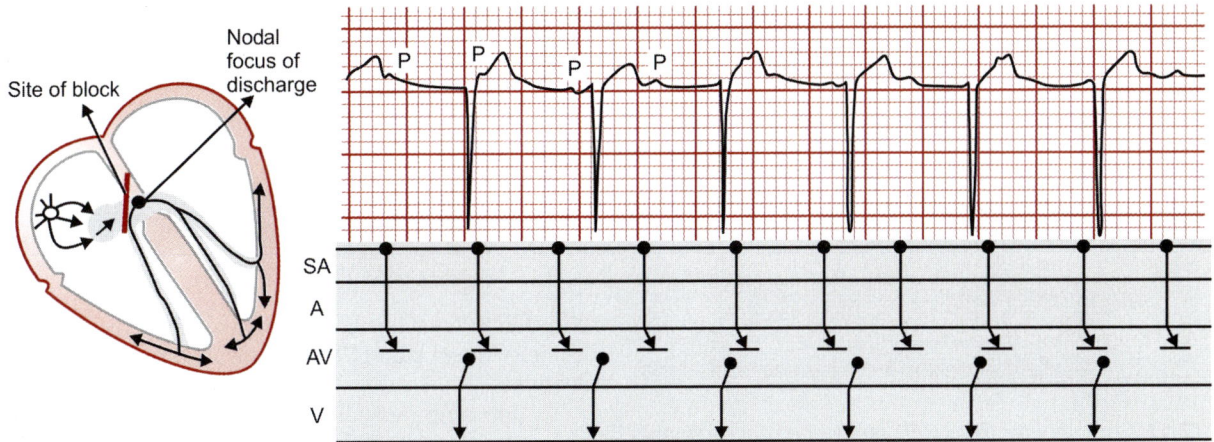

Fig. 12.10: Complete AV block with Idionodal escape rhythm. The ECG lead V_1 shows
 (i) The P-P intervals are constant
 (ii) R-R interval is constant. Ventricular rate is 54/min
 (iii) There is no relationship between P waves and QRS complexes
 (iv) Atrial rate is more than ventricular rate, hence, P waves and QRS complexes are independent
 (v) The QRS complex is not wide and bizarre, appears near to normal, hence, the subsidiary pacemaker lies in bundle of His or just below it.

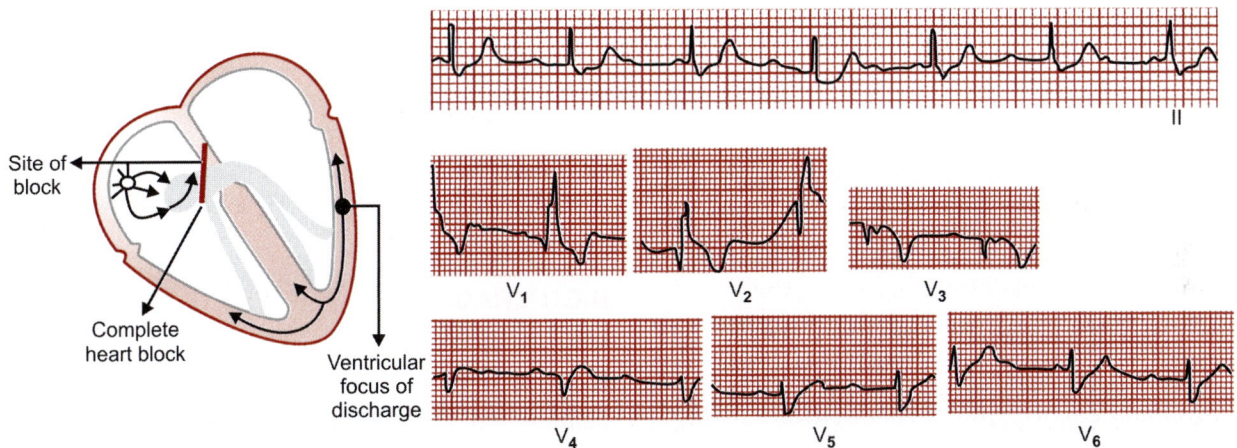

Fig. 12.11: Complete AV block in acute MI with idioventricular escape rhythm of RBBB pattern. The ECG shows:
 (i) The lead II shows complete AV block with atrial rate of 120/min regular (atrial tachycardia) and ventricular rate of 50/min regular. Some P waves are nicely seen while others are superimposed on the ST segment or T wave and deform them. The P wave are unrelated to QRS.
 (ii) Acute anterior MI. There is wide, deep Q waves in leads V_1-V_2 with QS pattern in V_3 and nonprogression of R wave from V_1-V_6. The ST segment is elevated in V_1-V_3 with deep wide symmetric T wave inversion. The lead V_4 shows ST elevation with flat T wave probably due to superimposition of P waves. The ST segment is depressed in V_5-V_6. The patient had raised CPK (MB)
 (iii) Idioventricular rhythm of RBBB type. The wide qR with slurred or notched R in V_1-V_2 with wide deep S in V_4-V_6 indicate RBBB pattern; idioventricular focus lies in left bundle branch producing RBBB pattern due to orientation of wave of excitation from left to the right and anteriorly

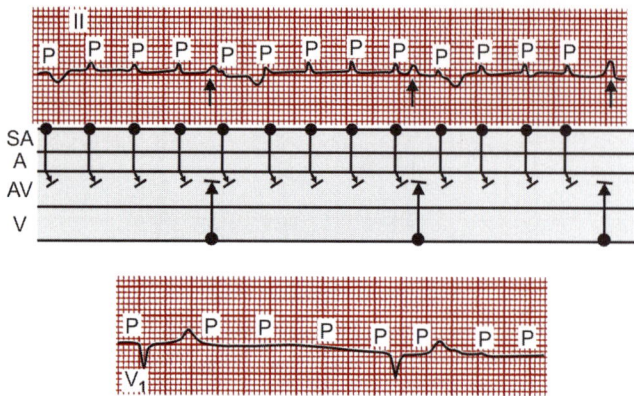

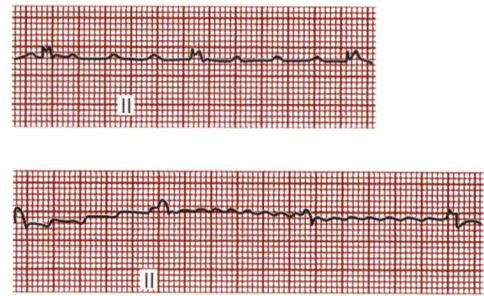

Fig. 12.12: Complete AV block with ventricular escape rhythm. The ventricular rate is 17/min approx. The ECG was recorded from a patient before developing cardiac arrest. The ladder diagram below lead II shows dual pacemaker (atria and ventricle) with their pathways of conduction. SA = Sinoatrial level, A = Atrial, AV = AV nodal, V = Ventricular level

Fig. 12.13: Atrial tachycardia degenerating into atrial flutter in complete heart block. The electrocardiogram shows following features:

1. Top strip (lead II). Atrial tachycardia in presence of complete heart block. The P waves are seen at a rate of 110/min and are regular but do not show any relation to QRS (independent atrial rhythm). Some of P waves distort QRS complexes. The QRS complexes are wide and occur at a rate of 30/min (idioventricular rhythm)
2. Bottom strip (lead II) from the same patient shows increase in atrial rate to >150/min, seen in the beginning of the strip which degenerated into atrial flutter evidenced by flutter (F) waves producing saw-toothed appearance of the baseline. The atrial rate is about 300/min, regular; the QRS complexes have same morphology as seen in the top strip and ventricular rate remains constant

Stokes-Adams Attacks

These are syncopal attacks occurring due to ventricular asystole or standstill and are frequently seen in third degree AV block under following situations ;

1. *During transition from second degree to third degree (complete) AV block.*

   This is due to some delay before a dormant or sluggish pacemaker is aroused.
2. When two or more subsidiary pacemakers compete with each other for the control of ventricles. The Stokes-Adams attacks occur during shift or change of pacemaker from one to another.
3. During paroxysms of ventricular flutter or fibrillation.

Pathognomonic sign of Stokes-Adams attack on ECG. Very large, broad, bizarre and inverted T waves called

'Giant' inverted T waves in leads V_2–V_4 str suggestive and virtually pathognomonic of a recent syncopal attack. This phenomenon is associated with prolongation of QT (QTc) interval. Giant T wave inversion and prolonged QTc are results of syncopal attacks.

HIGH GRADE AV BLOCK (Fig. 12.14)

High grade AV block may be defined as intermittent block of two or more consecutive supraventricular beats when supraventricular rate is very fast (140/min or less). In higher grade AV block, the AV

Table 12.3: Distinguishing features between congenital and acquired complete AV block	
Congenital complete AV block	*Acquired complete AV block*
• QRS complexes are frequently normal, but may be abnormal	• QRS complexes are frequently abnormal
• Heart rate is higher, i.e. ranges between 55–60 bpm	• Heart rate is slower i.e. between 20–40 bpm.
• The ventricular rate tends to increase slightly with emotion and exercise, thus, it is under some autonomic influence	• Heart rate or rhythm is stable and does not change under autonomic influence
• Syncopal attacks are rare	• Common
• It is permanent	• It may be transient such as in an infarction or may be permanent if there is fibrosis of the conduction tissue

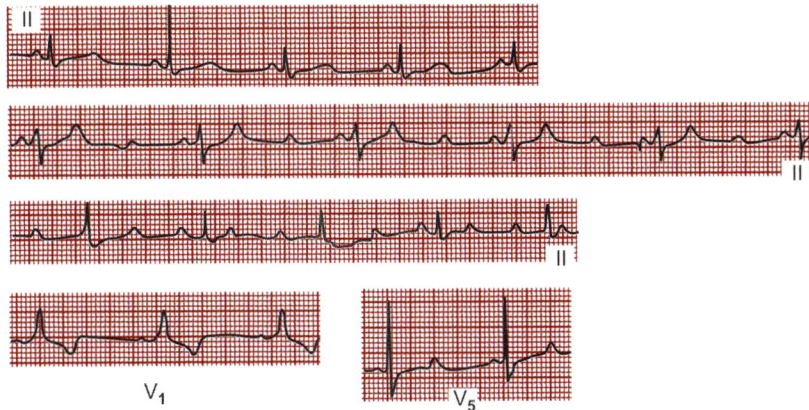

Fig. 12.14: High grade AV block progressing rapidly to complete AV block. The lead II (upper strip) shows P-R interval of conducted P waves of 0.16 sec, followed by blocked P wave that falls regularly on T wave and deforms it. Thus, there is second degree 2:1 AV block. The 2:1 AV block rapidly changes upto 3:1 in the next (second strip of lead II). The P-R interval of conducted P is 0.16 sec followed by blocked two consecutive P waves one of which falls again on the T wave and deforms it. The atrial rate is 114/min and ventricular rate of 38/min. The 3:1 AV block constitutes high grade AV block which rapidly progresses to complete AV block (third strip of lead II) with infranodal (focus below AV node) rhythm at a rate of 50/min. The QRS are normal but wider than sinus complexes. The tall R in V_1 indicates left to right ventricular excitation.

Table 12.4: Differences between high grade AV block and complete AV block

High degree AV block	Complete AV block
• Occasional conduction of supraventricular impulses to ventricles does occur.	• No sinus impulse is conducted to the ventricles, and the atria and the ventricles are depolarised independently of each other.
• Ventricular rate is fast.	• Ventricular rate is very slow.
• Escape rhythms are unusual and occur only when the ventricular rate slows down below the firing range of escape pacemaker due to changes in AV conduction ratio.	• There is always an idionodal or idioventricular escape rhythm; the morphology of QRS complexes and their rate will depend upon the origin of rhythm.

conduction ratio will be 3:1, 4:1, 5:2, etc. which means that occasional conduction of atrial impulses to ventricles does occur. In higher grade AV block, ventricular escape rhythm usually does not occur, but will occur if the ventricular rate slows below the inherent discharge rate of the ventricular pacemaker due to changes in the AV conduction ratio. (Fig. 12.14). The differences between high grade AV block and complete block are given in the Table 12.4.

Physiologic AV block. A physiological barrier to a fast supraventricular rhythm (atrial flutter or fibrillation) to reduce the ventricular rate, without which a chaos will occur in the ventricles, is called physiological AV block. In atrial flutter or fibrillation, atrial rate is fast (more than 300 bpm); and if all these atrial beats are conducted to the ventricles, the ventricular rate becomes very fast leading to a chaos in ventricular conduction, hence, a barrier at the AV node is must to reduce the ventricular response. This type of physiological or functional AV block is not a classified AV block, because it does not reflect a true inherent increase in refractoriness.

DIAGNOSING AV BLOCKS AT GLANCE

• *Guidelines:* Three ECG parameters are to be examined.

1. Look at P-R interval. Is it constant or changing?
2. Look at the number of P waves for each QRS complex. Is there one or more ?
3. Look at the R-R interval. Is it regular or irregular ?

Results and Conclusions

A. *If R–R interval is regular*, the block is probably either first degree or third degree.

- If conduction ratio is 1:1, i.e. every P wave is followed by QRS and P–R interval is prolonged beyond normal (> 0.20 sec.) and constant, then it is first degree AV block.
- If there is more than one P wave for every QRS complex, P–P and R–R intervals are constant, and there is no relationship between P wave and the QRS complex (P wave may precede, follow or merge with QRS), it indicates the third degree AV block.

B. *If R–R interval is irregular,* the block is probably second degree Mobitz type I (Wenckebach) or Mobitz type II.

- If P–R interval changes in a cyclic manner (P–R progressively lengthens till one P is blocked); it is second degree AV block—Mobitz type I (Wenckebach).
- If P–R interval stays the same, it is probably second degree AV block (Mobitz type II).
  NB: 'Second degree AV block associated with multiple dropped beats can exhibit either the fixed or variable conduction ratio (2:1, 3:2, 5:3, etc) so, the regularity of the R-R interval does not form diagnostic clue to Mobitz's 'second degree AV block'.

- If there are more than one P for every QRS, if P–R intervals are constant, a second degree AV block either with fixed or variable conduction is present.

Suggested Reading

1. Cahen, Doctor L, Pick A: The significance of AV block complicating acute myocardial infarction. *Am Heart J* **55**: 215, 1958.
2. Dhingra RC, et al. Incidence and sites of atrioventricular block in patients with chronic bifascicular block. *Circulation* **59**: 278,1979.
3. Dreifus LS, et al: Atrioventricular block. *Am J Cardiol* **28**: 371,1971.
4. Jacobson D, Schrire V: Giant T wave inversion. *Br Heart J* **28**: 768, 1966.
5. James TN: The morphology of human atrioventricular node, with remarks, pertinent to its electrophysiology. *Am Heart J* **62**: 756, 1961.
6. Kastor JA: Atrioventricular block (2 parts). *N Engl J Med* **292**: 462, 572, 1975.
7. Lenegre J: Contribution a l'etude des blocs de branche. Paris J. B. Balliere.
8. Lev M: Anatomical basis of AV block. *Am J Med* **37**: 742, 1964.
9. Mangiardi LM, et al: Bed side evaluation of atrioventricular block with narrow QRS complexes: Usefulness of carotid sinus massage and atropine administration. *Am J Cardiol* **49**: 1136, 1982.
10. Martin P: The influence of parasympathetic nervous system on AV conduction. *Circ Res* **41**: 593, 1977.
11. Narula OS, et al: Atrioventricular block: Localisation and classification by His bundle recordings. *Am J Med* **50**: 146, 1971.
12. Sherif N, et al: A typical Wenckebach periodicity simulating Mobitz type II AV block. *Br Heart J* **40**: 376,1978.
13. Strasberg MD, Amat–Y–Lean F, Dhingra RC, et al: Natural history of chronic second degree AV block. *Circulation* **63**: 1043, 1981.

13

Bundle Branch Blocks

- *Intraventricular conduction defects—definition and sites of block*
- *Bundle branch blocks—terminology, aetiology, electrocardiographic characteristics, significance and types (incomplete and complete)*
- *Right bundle branch block (complete and incomplete) – definition, causes, ECG patterns and their mechanisms, ventricular hypertrophy in presence of right bundle branch block, intermittent right bundle branch block*
- *Left bundle branch block (complete and incomplete) – causes, ECG patterns, left bundle branch block associated with fascicular blocks, ventricular hypertrophy with left bundle branch block*
- *Bilateral bundle branch block*
- *Nonspecific or indeterminate intraventricular conduction defect*

DISORDERS OF INTRAVENTRICULAR CONDUCTION

Definition—An abnormality of conduction through one or more divisions of the intraventricular conduction system distal to bundle of His is called *an intraventricular conduction defect*. The conduction defect may lie at different levels (Fig. 13.1). The sites of block include;

1. The right bundle branch (site 1)
2. The left bundle branch (site 2)
3. The left anterior fascicle (site 3)
4. The left posterior fascicle (site 4)
5. The septal fascicle from the left bundle and its ramifications that enter the myocardium (site 5)
6. At combinations of one site with the other (1+3, 1+4, 1+3+4, etc.)
7. The peripheral Purkinje fibres (site 6)

Aetiology : The causes of intraventricular conduction delay or block in adults are given in the Table 13.1.

BUNDLE BRANCH BLOCKS

A delay or block of conduction within a bundle (right or left) is termed as a *bundle branch block*. The bundle branch block is an electrocardiographic diagnosis

Table 13.1. Some important causes of intraventricular conduction delay in adults

1. Congenitally present in some normal individuals (right bundle branch block is common).
2. Lenegre's disease in which there is an idiopathic fibrosis of the conduction system.
3. Lev's disease (calcification of cardiac skeleton)
4. Cardiomyopathies
   a) Dilated
   b) Hypertrophic (concentric or asymmetric)
   c) Infiltrative
   - Tumours
   - Chagas' disease
   - Hypothyroidism or myxoedema
   - Cardiac amyloidosis
5. Ischaemic heart disease
   - Acute myocardial infarction
   - Post–myocardial infarction
   - Coronary atherosclerosis without myocardial infarction.
6. Aortic stenosis (left bundle branch block is common)
7. Infective endocarditis with formation of an abscess in conduction system.
8. High potassium levels.
9. Cardiac injury.
10. Massive pulmonary embolism, i.e. acute corpulmonale (transient right bundle branch is common).
11. Ventricular hypertrophy (conduction delay is common rather than complete bundle branch block pattern).
12. Myocarditis.

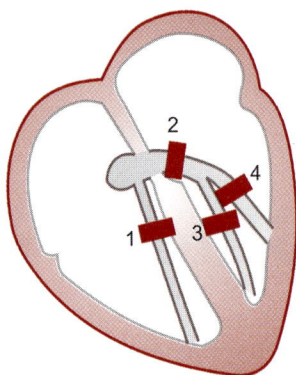

Fig. 13.1: Intraventricular conduction system and sites of conduction defects. The sites of block are represented by small boxes (diagram)

based on the specific ECG pattern that results from delayed conduction through the blocked bundle. It is not a clinical diagnosis; however, it can be suspected clinically on physical examination because;

1. Right bundle branch block (RBBB) produces a wide splitting of second heart sound.
2. left bundle branch block (LBBB), on the other hand, produces a paradoxical splitting of second heart sound.

Terminology Used

Intraventricular conduction delay is commonly referred to as 'block' which may be complete or incomplete depending on the conduction delay. Complete bundle branch block refers to an abnormal lengthening of QRS interval; while incomplete bundle branch block implies a conduction delay that does not result in abnormal prolongation of QRS interval. Neither of the term is accurate, hence, are best avoided and the term *"bundle branch block pattern"* is used, because the term *'block'* has no anatomical or electrophysiological counterpart and describes only a conduction pattern.

Mechanisms

The sinus impulse passes uninterruptedly upto the bundle of His and produces a normal P wave with normal P–R interval. Due to block in one of the bundle branches, the same impulse now passes through the unblocked bundle branch and activates the ventricular myocardium or ventricle supplied by it. The ventricular myocardium or the ventricle supplied by the blocked bundle branch is activated abnormally

by transmission of the same impulse through the interventricular septum to the blocked bundle branch beyond the site of block; and as well as transmission of the impulse from one ventricle to the other through the continuous Purkinje system. Therefore, an abnormal and delayed activation of the ventricle supplied by the blocked bundle branch results in QRS abnormalities and ST–T wave changes constituting *"a bundle branch block pattern"*.

Clinical Significance

Bundle branch block *per se* does not affect the prognosis. The prognosis depends on the underlying cause of it. The presence of left bundle branch block in acquired heart disease such as ischaemic heart disease is considered as an ominous sign. On the other hand, congenital right bundle branch block is inconsequential.

The left bundle branch block is always acquired. The right bundle branch is mostly congenital.

The Electrocardiographic Criteria

1. **Complete bundle branch block pattern**
   (Fig. 13.2A)
A. *QRS morphology and duration*
   i) *Abnormal QRS complex:* An abnormal QRS complex (ventricular depolarisation) results due to delayed and abnormal spread of excitation through the ventricle whose bundle is blocked. In bundle branch block, rsR' complex is recorded instead of QRS–a traditional term used in electrocardiography to represent the ventricular depolarisation. The abnormal QRS complex appears in the leads representing the ventricle whose bundle branch is blocked.
   ii) Prolongation of QRS interval to 0.12sec. or longer in leads recording the pattern of bundle branch block.
   iii) Ventricular activation time (VAT) is prolonged beyond normal in leads recording the bundle branch block pattern.
   iv) Axis deviation. The mean frontal plane QRS axis remains within –30° to +110°. Axis deviation beyond this limit indicates conduction delay through one of the fascicles in addition to bundle branch block.

B. *Associated ST–T changes*

iv) Depression of ST segment with convexity upwards and inversion of T waves occurs in leads that record the terminal abnormal R´ waves; on the other hand, leads showing terminal S wave deflection will record minimally elevated ST segment with concavity upwards and upright T wave.

2. **Incomplete bundle branch block pattern** (Fig. 13.2B).

Bundle branch block is said to be incomplete if QRS (rSR´) duration is less than 0.12 sec but more than 0.10 sec. VAT is prolonged but less than that seen in complete bundle branch block pattern . It is actually an arbitrary subclassification of complete bundle branch block.

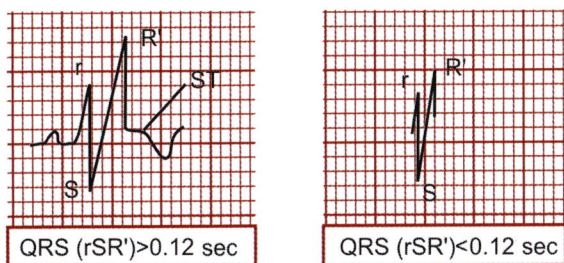

QRS (rSR')>0.12 sec   QRS (rSR')<0.12 sec

Fig. 13.2: A rSR' pattern in complete and incomplete bundle branch block (diagram)

A. Note rSR' is > 0.12 sec and VAT is increased, ST segment is slightly depressed with convexity upwards and T is inverted. These changes are characteristic of complete bundle branch block

B. Note rSR' is widened but not < 0.12 sec. VAT is slightly prolonged. T is inverted. This pattern indicates incomplete bundle branch block.

Note: Theoretically wide rSR' is a pattern of a bundle branch block irrespective of its type, but this pattern is seen only in RBBB. In left bundle branch block (LBBB) the small r and s are not seen being too small, hence, loss of q wave and wide slurred R is a characteristic feature

RIGHT BUNDLE BRANCH BLOCK PATTERN

The right bundle branch block is the result of a delay or complete interruption or block of conduction within the right bundle branch. A delay of conduction results in *incomplete bundle branch block*, while a complete interruption of conduction results in *complete bundle branch block*.

Complete Right Bundle Branch Block (RBBB) Pattern

Definition: A complete interruption or block of conduction of impulses through the right bundle branch is called, *'right bundle branch block pattern'*. It is an electrocardiographic finding and does not indicate a specific cardiac disease. It may be functional or organic. A functional RBBB pattern occurs commonly during phasic aberrant intraventricular conduction. It can be transient or may be permanent.

Causes: Some important causes of it are given in box.

Causes of Complete RBBB

1. *Congenital:* Right bundle branch block may be present in normal healthy persons as an isolated congenital abnormality in the absence of any heart disease. It is common in children (Fig. 13.4B).
2. *Acquired:* It is associated with congenital and acquired heart diseases.
   i. Coronary artery disease.
   ii. Cardiomyopathies
   iii. Hypertensive heart disease.
   iv. ASD or VSD
   v. Ebstein's anomaly
   vi. A manifestation of massive pulmonary embolism in some cases.
   vii. Phasic aberrant intraventricular conduction
   viii. Cardiac contusion
   ix. Idiopathic

NB: Consequently, the right bundle branch block must always be evaluated in the prospective of the associated clinical and electrocardiographic manifestations.

Mechanisms

A. The pathogenesis of abnormal QRS (rSR´) complex in right precordial leads (V₁–V₂)

A. The pathogenesis of abnormal QRS (rSR´) complex in right precordial leads (V_1–V_2)

The spread of excitation from SA node to AV node and through bundle of His occurs in normal fashion, hence, P waves are normal in shape and duration.

The septal activation in right bundle block occurs normally from left to the right. The steps of ventricular activation from the bundle of His onwards are as follows:

1. *The septal activation* from left to the right produces an initial prominent r wave in leads V_1 and V_2 and a small q wave in leads V_5 and V_6 due to orientation of septal vector towards right and anteriorly (Fig. 13.3, vector I)

2. *Normal left paraseptal and ventricular activation.* Normal left paraseptal activation occurs next, followed by the impulse spreading transversely from the endocardium to epicardium through the free wall of left ventricle (Fig. 13.3, vector 2). This free wall ventricular vector is directed to the left and left ventricular activation occurs first producing R wave in V_5 and V_6 with a corresponding S(s) wave in V_1 and V_2.

3. *Activation of the right ventricle is delayed and abnormal* due to blockage of its bundle. The slow and abnor-

mal depolarisation of right side of the intraventricular septum, right paraseptal region and free wall of right ventricle occurs by activation front that arises from the left side of the septum and jumps to the opposite side beyond the site of block in the right bundle branch, and then spreads transversely from endocardium to epicardium, is reflected electrocardiographically by large slowly inscribed vectors which are oriented anteriorly and to the right (vector 3 of Fig. 13.3) resulting in a large R' wave in V_1, hence, the complex in V_1 will be either rSR' or notched R or RR' wave (Fig. 13.3 vector 4). Due to this effect on V_1, a large slurred S wave in V_5 and V_6 is inscribed resulting in qRS pattern. All these events producing rSR' pattern in V_1 and qRS pattern in V_6 are summarised in the box.

	Electrocardiographic Deflections in V_1 and V_6 in Complete RBBB		
Vector	*Direction of vector*	*Lead V_1 (rSR')*	*Lead V_6 (qRS)*
1. Septal	Left to right	An initial r wave	An initial q wave
2. Left ventricular free wall	Left	A S wave follows r wave	A large R wave follows q wave
3. and 4. Right ventricular free wall	Right and anterior	A large R' wave	A large slurred S wave

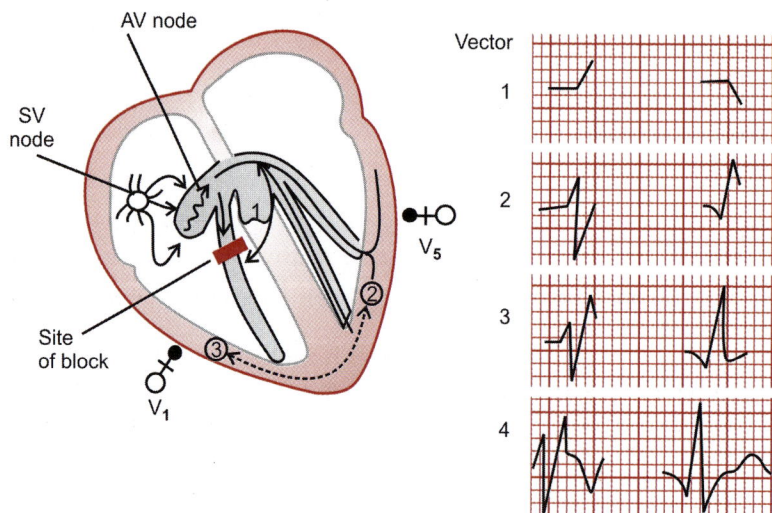

Fig. 13.3: Diagrammatic illustration of intraventricular conduction in RBBB (complete).
Vectors   1. Septal activation vector
            2. Activation of free wall of left ventricle
            3 & 4. Slow and abnormal depolarisation of the free walls of right ventricle due to orientation of terminal QRS vectors to the right and anteriorly.

For explanation, leads V_1 and V_5 are chosen for the diagram. The lead V_1 will record rSR′ or notched R wave and lead V_5 will record qRS pattern. If vector is oriented superiorly, it will record S wave in aVF; and if vector is inferiorly oriented, R wave will be recorded in aVF.

B. The associated ST–T changes

The ST segment and T wave changes in uncomplicated RBBB are usually secondary to abnormal intraventricular conduction rather than a primary change due to myocardial involvement, hence, are called the associated changes. The ST segment and T wave forces are opposite to terminal forces of ventricular depolarisation, i.e. terminal QRS deflections, hence, as the terminal deflection is an R′ wave in V_1 or V_2 – a diagnostic finding in complete RBBB, the ST segment is slightly depressed with convexity upwards and T is inverted. On the other hand, the terminal deflection is an S wave in leads V_5–V_6 in RBBB, the ST segment is slightly elevated with concavity upwards and T is upright.

> NOTE: Any deviation in the secondary ST–T changes as described above should be considered as a primary change due to myocardial involvement, in addition to complete RBBB. The presence of a q wave in leads V_1–V_2 (QR pattern) with ST elevation may indicate myocardial infarction, however, a qR pattern can occur in severe right ventricular hypertrophy but ST segment is depressed in these leads.

The Electrocardiogram (Fig. 13.4)

The electrocardiographic pattern of complete right bundle branch block is characterised by the followings:

1. A tall, wide and frequently notched R wave (RR′) or rSR′ complex instead of normal rS in the lead V_1 or V_1–V_2.
2. Consequent to the above change, a prominent, delayed and widened S wave (qRS complex) is seen in left precordial leads, i.e. V_5, V_6 and leads I and aVL.
3. The QRS duration is increased to more than 0.12 sec in the leads that record rSR′ complex (V_1–V_2).
4. VAT is increased in the leads with rSR′ complexes.
5. There is depression of ST segment with convexity upwards and inversion of T waves in leads that

records rSR′ complex (V_1 and V_2) and on the other hand, the leads with terminal S wave deflection (V_5 or V_6) will show slight ST elevation with concavity upwards and T is upright.

> *An rSR′ complex in lead V_1 or in both V_1 and V_2 invariably indicates right bundle branch block irrespective of its cause*

Incomplete Right Bundle Branch Block Pattern (Fig. 13.5)

Definition: A delay in conduction of impulses through the right bundle branch is called *'incomplete right bundle branch block pattern'*.

The electrocardiogram

The pattern of incomplete RBBB is similar to complete right bundle branch block with the following exceptions;

1. The QRS interval lies between 0.10 to 0.12 second.
2. The VAT in V_1 is slightly increased. There is rSR′ or rSr′ complex in V_1 (Fig. 13.5)

Now a days right intraventricular conduction delay is preferred term than incomplete bundle branch block because;

1. This pattern may be a variant of normal.
2. This pattern is frequently seen in right ventricular hypertrophy.
3. Some clinical conditions produce patterns of incomplete bundle branch block without involvement of the bundle. These are;
   1. Atrial septal defect
   2. Anomalous pulmonary venous drainage.
   3. Chronic obstructive pulmonary disease (COPD).
   4. Pulmonary embolism.

However, this term is still being retained in clinical textbooks of medicine, hence, described here.

Mechanism: In incomplete RBBB, the conduction through the right bundle branch is still possible but is delayed. A small delay in right bundle branch causes delay in the inscription of right paraseptal force or vector, which now occurs synchronously with the free wall forces. This will diminish the S wave in lead V_1–V_2 which is the earliest sign of incomplete RBBB. As the delay in right bundle branch increases, the activation of right ventricular free wall is delayed and occurs later than activation of free wall of left ventricle

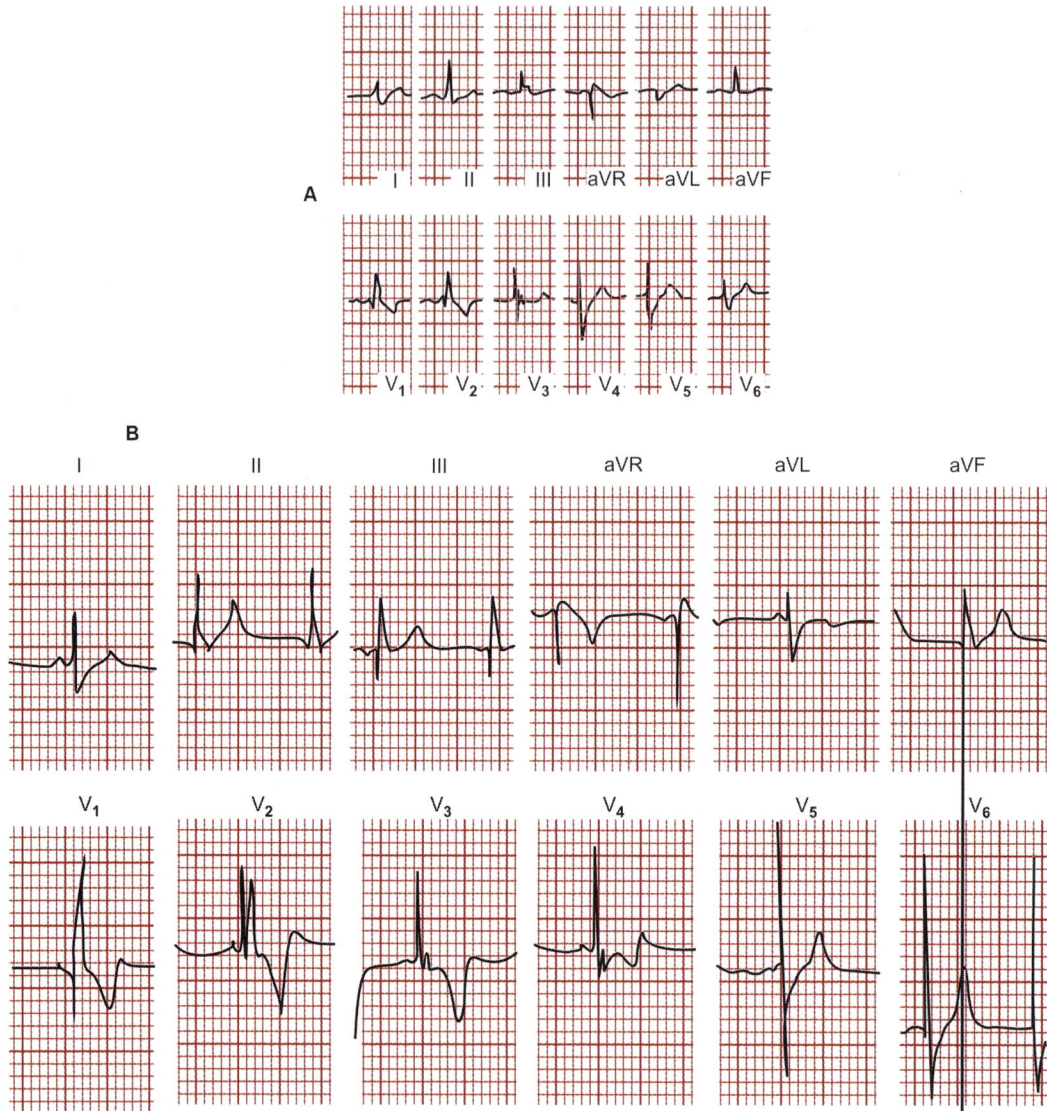

Fig 13.4: Right bundle branch block.

A. The ECG shows: (i) The mean frontal plane axis of +70°, (ii) The QRS interval is 0.12 sec, (iii) A wide, slurred rSR' pattern is prominently seen in V_1-V_2 with depressed ST segment and inverted T waves and (iv) Wide slurred S wave is seen in V_4-V_6 and lead I

B. Congenital right bundle branch block in a child. ECG from a five years child found to have wide variable split of 2nd heart sound shows congenital RBBB with high voltage and short P-R interval. The QRS duration is 0.12 sec. The broad late S wave in leads I, V_5 and V_6 and broad late R wave in aVF, V_1 and V_2 show that this conduction defect is due to RBBB. The frontal plane axis of +110° is compatible with RBBB as well as for his age, hence, is not much help in the diagnosis of RVH. The presence of marked right axis deviation, right atrial hypertrophy, and Q waves in V_1 and/or V_2 are much more helpful clues toward RVH in such a situation, but are absent in this case. The ST depression and T inversion in V_1-V_4 are compatible both for his age as well as for RBBB and are not due to RVH. This child has RBBB only. The P-R interval is short (0.09 sec) which is also compatible for his age

resulting in r' wave in right precordial leads (rSr' pattern). If delay is longer, then a large R' will be recorded (rsR' complex) in V_1 and V_2. The R wave is not widened. The duration of QRS remains between 0.10 to 0.12 sec. The VAT is also not increased much and even may be normal as conduction through the bundle is still possible.

The ST segment depression and T wave inversion in right precordial leads occurs secondary to bundle branch block as explained in complete RBBB.

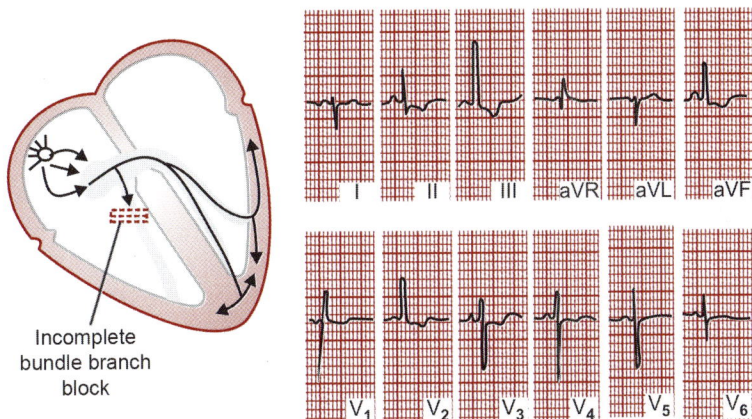

Fig. 13.5: Incomplete right bundle branch block. Right axis deviation of + 120° (aVR shows equiphasic complex and tallest R wave seen in lead III). The QRS interval is 0.10 sec. rSR' pattern in V_1 with tall R wave in V_2. This could be interpreted as right ventricular hypertrophy but this magnitude of right axis deviation with rSR' in V_1 and tall R' in V_2 favour incomplete bundle branch block

REVIEW AT A GLANCE

ECG Changes in Complete and Incomplete RBBB

- A tall R wave (rSR') or notched tall R wave (rR') in lead V_1 and V_2 and a deep, wide and prominent S wave in leads V_5, V_6 and standard leads 1 and a VL is seen in complete right bundle branch block. In incomplete bundle branch block, a wider rSr' or rSR' is common in V_1–V_2.
- QRS (rSR') duration is > 0.12 sec. in complete RBBB but it remains in between 0.10 to 0.12 sec. in incomplete RBBB.
- VAT is prolonged in V_1–V_2 (> 0.03 sec.) in complete RBBB but is normal in incomplete RBBB.

- ST segment is slightly depressed and T is inverted in V_1 and V_2, while ST is slightly elevated with concavity upwards in leads V_5–V_6 and T is upright in these leads. These changes are seen both in complete and incomplete RBBB.

RIGHT BUNDLE BRANCH BLOCK WITH LEFT VENTRICULAR HYPERTROPHY (Fig. 13.6)

In this situation, RBBB (rSR') pattern will be seen in right precordial leads (V_1 –V_2), in addition to, the pattern of left ventricular hypertrophy–a tall R wave with ST–T changes in leads I, aVL and V_4 through V_6. The position of the heart will be horizontal due to LVH resulting in an abnormal R wave in aVL. To

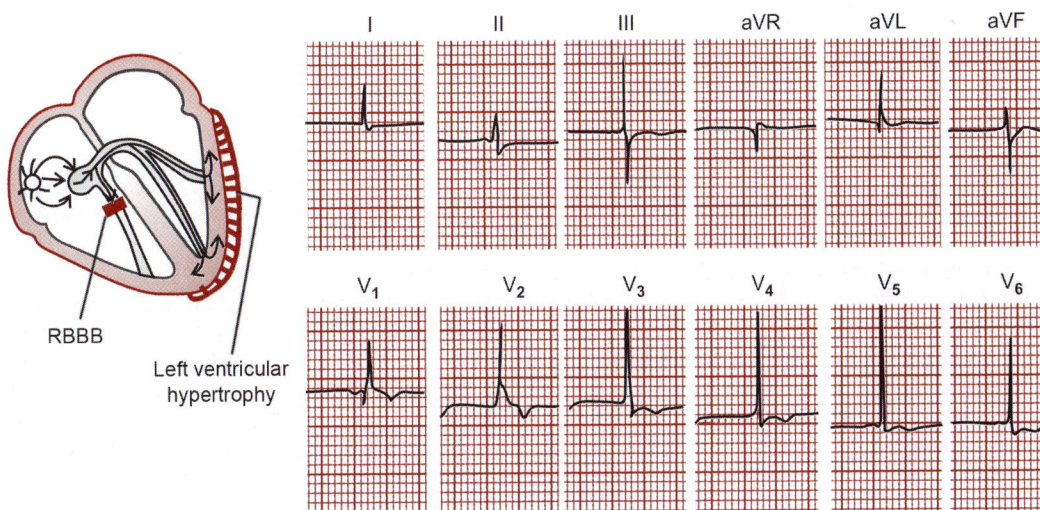

Fig. 13.6: Right bundle branch block with left ventricular hypertrophy. *Note* the following characteristics on ECG:
1. RBBB: It is indicated by a wide QRS with broad late S wave in leads I, V_5 and V_6; and there is rSR' pattern in V_1
2. Left ventricular hypertrophy: (i) There is mean QRS axis of -30° (left axis deviation). The heart is horizontal, (ii) The R wave in V_5 is 28 mm with ST-T change

Note: The RBBB distorts the depolarisation in such a manner to invalidate the voltage criteria for LVH, but still presence of high voltage in V_5, therefore, is stronger evidence of LVH

summarise, both RBBB and LVH will express on ECG independent of each other (Fig. 13.6).

INTERMITTENT RIGHT BUNDLE BRANCH BLOCK (Fig. 13.7)

When the pattern of right bundle branch block appears in between normal complexes, it is called *intermittent right bundle branch block* (Fig. 13.7). It may simulate a run of phasic aberrant intraventricular conduction of right bundle branch block type. The following points help in their differentiation.

1. The phasic aberrant conduction is rate–dependent, i.e. bradycardia or tachycardia may be the underlying mechanism. Change in heart rate may abolish aberrancy, but this is not a hard and fast rule. In contrast, the intermittent RBBB is rate–independent.

2. The initial deflection of QRS of aberrantly conducted beats is always similar to the beats conducted without aberration in the same lead but this does not occur in intermittent RBBB.

RIGHT BUNDLE BRANCH BLOCK WITH RIGHT VENTRICULAR HYPERTROPHY

Right ventricular hypertrophy affects the late and right bundle branch block affects the early as well as the late forces of activation of right ventricle, hence, co-existent of both supplement the late electrical effects of each other. Right ventricular hypertrophy itself can cause conduction delay in right ventricle, however, marked widening of QRS (> 0.12 sec) is not expected of right ventricular hypertrophy, hence, if present in leads V_1–V_2, indicates co-existing right bundle branch block. Similarly an abnormal right axis deviation $> + 90°$ cannot be expected from right bundle branch block, hence, if right axis deviation is $> + 110°$ in the presence of right bundle branch block, then co-existing either right ventricular hypertrophy or left posterior fascicular block may be suspected. In addition, QRS morphology in lead V_1 is either qR or pure R wave in right ventricular hypertrophy; and rSR′ morphology occurs in right bundle branch block, when both co-exist, then either rSR′ or rR′ complex is seen in V_1 while lead V_2 shows invariably rR′ complex. Finally, VAT over the right ventricle more than 0.06 second favours right bundle branch block than right ventricular hypertrophy. Therefore, a wide rR′ pattern in V_1 with increased VAT > 0.06 sec in presence of marked rightward frontal plane QRS axis suggest existence of both. The differentiating features between isolated right ventricular hypertrophy and RBBB are given in the Table 13.2.

Table 13.2: Differentiating features of right ventricular hypertrophy and right bundle branch block	
Right ventricular hypertrophy	*Right bundle branch block*
• QRS interval is < 0.12 sec.	• QRS interval is 0.12 sec. or more
• Only an R wave or qR complex or rR′ complex in V_1.	• rSR′ complex in lead V_1.
• VAT is between 0.03 to 0.05 second.	• VAT in right precordial leads (V_1 or V_2) is 0.06 second or more.

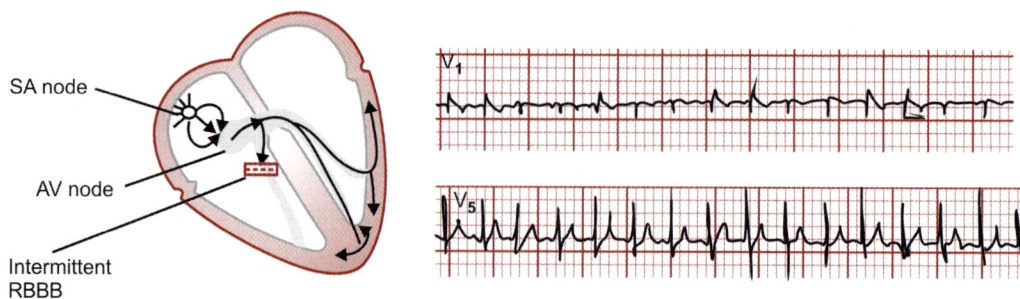

Fig. 13.7: Intermittent right bundle branch block. The electrocardiogram (lead V_1) shows sinus rhythm at a rate 100/min. In between sinus complexes, there are complexes with wide rSR′ pattern with associated T wave inversion which indicates intermittent RBBB pattern. These types of complexes can occur in phasic aberrant intraventricular conduction also (for differentiation, read the text)

The presence of complete RBBB pattern (rsR′ in V₁–V₂) with marked rightward axis shift > +110° suggest RBBB with RVH.

Right Bundle Branch Block with Persistent ST Segment Elevation (Brugada Syndrome)

Brugada syndrome was first reported 10 years ago, has now become a distinct clinical and electrocardiographic syndrome. It is now being diagnosed with increasing frequency in patients with acute ST segment elevation with incomplete or complete right bundle branch block pattern in right precordial leads (V_1-V_2) without any evidence of structural heart disease. It is one of the important causes of sudden death in South Asian males. The increased prevalence in South East Asia is attributed to genetic predisposition as a familial occurrence was noted to be present in approximately 50% of patients. The basic genetic defect is mutation in the gene one word SCN 5 A that encodes cardiac sodium channel. The result is loss of proper action potential dome in right ventricular epicardium but not in endocardium results in S segment elevation. This electrophysiological heterogeneity predisposes to development of ventricular fibrillation. The sodium channel blockers can reproduce the ECG phenomenon explaining the role of sodium channels in its pathogenesis.

Clinical Significance

It is associated with idiopathic ventricular fibrillation and sudden death.

Electrocardiogram (Fig. 13.8)

1. There is ST segment elevation with either convexity upwards (coved′) or concavity upwards ('saddle type') in right precordial leads (V_1-V_2).
2. There is complete or incomplete bundle branch block pattern in leads V_1-V_2.
3. These changes can lead to idiopathic ventricular fibrillation and some patients have absorted sudden death.

Diagnosis and Treatment

A patient with presumptive diagnosis of Brugada syndrome on ECG and a positive family history of sudden death should be referred for electrophysiological studies. During electrophysiological testing (EP testing), patients with Brugada syndrome will have inducible polymorphic VT during programmed electrical stimulation, may result in haemodynamic collapse requiring electrical cardioversion for termination. Electrophysiologists confirm the diagnosis by administering the class I antiarrhythmic (ajmaline, flecainide, procainamide) which will increase the elevation of ST segment in patients with Brugada syndrome.

Treatment is placement of an AICD (automatic intracardiac defibrillator) with 10 years survival almost in all patients. Antiarrhythmics, e.g. beta-blockers, amiodarone have not been found useful.

NORMAL rSr′ COMPLEXES IN V₁–A NORMAL VARIANT (Fig. 13.9)

A rSr′ complex in lead V_1 may be seen normally in 5% individuals of a population. The normal rSr′ comp-

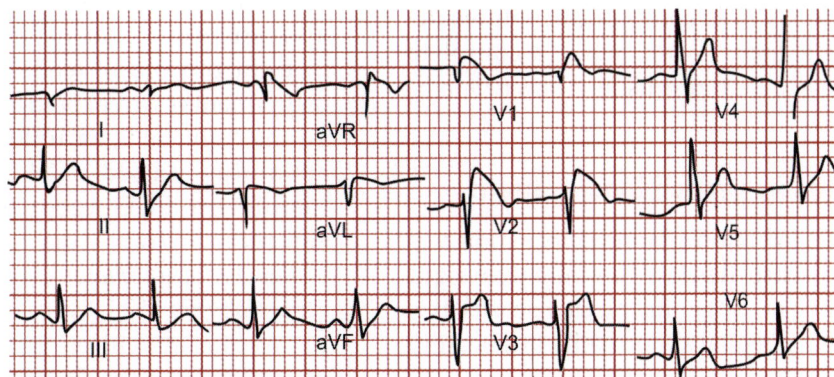

Fig. 13.8: Brugada syndrome. Note the followings
I. RBBB. There is right axis deviation with wide rSR' in V1-V3 with persistent of wide S wave in V_5-V_6.
II. ST segment elevation. There is ST segment elevation in leads V_1-V_3, i.e. leads showing RBBB pattern. The T is upright. The ST segment elevation is "saddle shape."

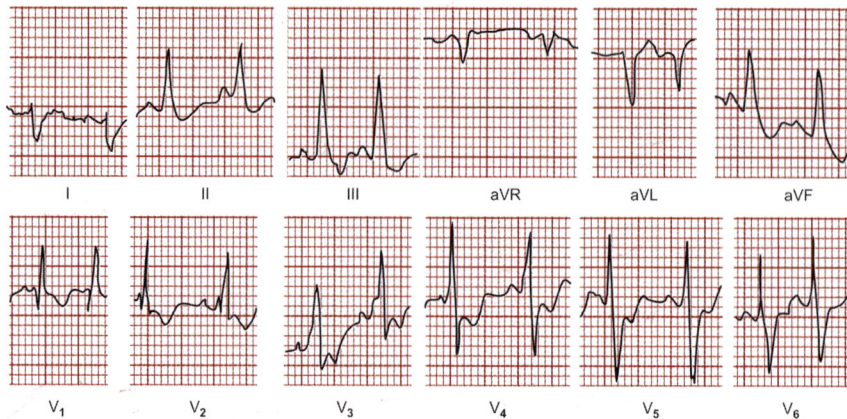

Fig. 13.9: Right bundle branch block with right ventricular hypertrophy. Note the followings:

   i. Right axis deviation > + 110°
  ii. Vertical heart and clockwise rotation
 iii. RBBB. There is rSR' in V_1-V_2 with tall RS complexes with deep S wave in V_4-V_6
 iv. RVH (right axis deviation > + 110° and tall RS complexes V_5-V_6) and the associated right atrial hypertrophy (tall peaked P waves).

SECTION FOUR

lex can resemble the rSr' complex of incomplete right bundle branch block in lead V_1. Sometimes, it is difficult to differentiate between them. The features that help to differentiate between the two are given in the box.

Differential diagnosis of rSr' complex in lead V_1	
Normal rSr' complex–a normal variant	Incomplete RBBB (rSr')
• r' wave in V_1 is narrow	r' wave in V_1 is wide.
• r' wave is small	r' (R') wave is large.

LEFT BUNDLE BRANCH BLOCK (LBBB) PATTERN

The left bundle branch block is the result of a delay or complete interruption or block of conduction within the left bundle branch. A delay of conduction results in *incomplete bundle branch block,* while a complete interruption of conduction results in *complete bundle branch block.*

Complete Left Bundle Branch Block Pattern

Causes: A complete left bundle branch block indicates an organic heart disease. It is less common than right bundle branch block in congenital heart diseases. It is rare as an isolated congenital abnormality in a healthy person. It can occur in:

1. Coronary artery disease
2. Cardiomyopathy
3. Aortic valve disease
4. Hypertensive heart disease
5. Sometimes, seen in phasic aberrant intraventricular conduction.

Mechanisms (Figs 13.10A and B)

The spread of excitation from SA node to AV node and bundle of His is normal, hence, there is no abnormality of P waves.

A: The QRS complex

The pattern of left ventricular activation and analysis of vectors due to LBBB are as under;

1. *Right to left septal activation :* Instead of normal left to right activation, the septum is activated from right to left (R → L). This results in a small right to left septal vector (Fig. 13.9 vector 1). This vector manifests as a small initial positive deflection (r wave) in left oriented leads V_6, I and aVL. This also results in a small negative deflection (q wave) in right precordial leads (V_1 and V_2). The first component (r wave) being very small in leads V_1–V_2 may not be seen unless sensitive recording apparatus is used. However, it is occasionally visible on ECG recorded by conventional electrocardiography machine.

2. *Delayed and anomalous left septal and paraseptal activation* (Fig. 13.10 vector 2). The left septal and paraseptal activation occurs in a delayed and anomalous manner. The right paraseptal activation proceeds normally. The right ventricular activation may occur slightly earlier due to blocked left bundle resulting in a small (r') wave in lead V_1

and a small S wave in lead V_5. Sometimes, because of relative thinness of right ventricle, this r' wave in V_1 and S wave in V_5 may not reach isoelectric line and may produce a notch on the S wave in V_1 and R wave in V_5. This ECG pattern is due to a vector of large magnitude (Fig. 13.10. vector 2) which is oriented to the left, posteriorly and superiorly.

3. *Delayed and anomalous activation of free left ventricular wall.* After left paraseptal activation due to jumping of the impulse from right to left beyond blocked left bundle, there occurs activation of left free ventricular wall in an anomalous manner and it is delayed. This activation results in a vector of large magnitude which is directed to the left, posteriorly and superiorly (Fig. 13.10 vector 3) which will be reflected by;

1. A tall R wave in left oriented leads (V_5,–V_6, aVL and lead I).
2. A deep S wave in right precordial leads (V_1–V_2).

B: *The associated ST–T changes*: In intraventricular conduction defect, the ST and T vectors get oriented opposite to QRS, hence, in LBBB, the left oriented leads I, aVL, V_5 and V_6 registering positive deflection of QRS, will have ST depression with convexity upwards and T is inverted. On the other hand, leads registering negative deflection (QS complex in V_1–V_2) will show minimally elevated ST segment with concavity upwards and T is upright.

Due to LBBB, there is neither an initial q wave nor a terminal S wave in the left oriented leads (V_5–V_6 and standard lead I).

The Electrocardiogram (Fig. 13.11)

The Precordial Leads (V_1–V_6)

1. ***QRS morphology and duration.*** The ECG pattern of LBBB is characterised by the followings:
   (i) A wide slurred R wave or RR', rsR' or RSR' complex is leads V_5 to V_6 and absent q waves in these leads. The S wave is slurred in right oriented leads (V_1–V_2) and an initial r wave in these leads also disappears resulting QS complex. The leads V_3 and V_4 show transition complex.
   (ii) QRS interval (rsR', slurred R or RSR') is more than 0.12 second in leads V_5–V_6.
   (iii) VAT is more than 0.09 second in V_5 to V_6.

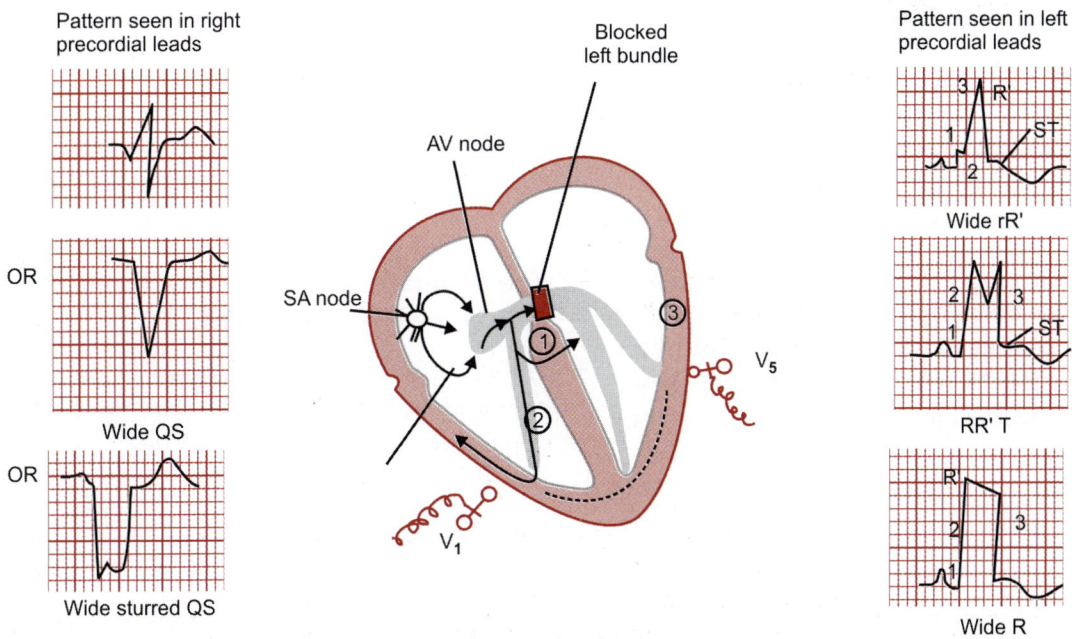

Fig. 13.10A: Diagrammatic illustration of complete LBBB patterns and various vectors
1. Right to left septal activation
2. Right ventricular and left paraseptal activation
3. Delayed and anomalous activation of free walls of left ventricle.

SECTION FOUR

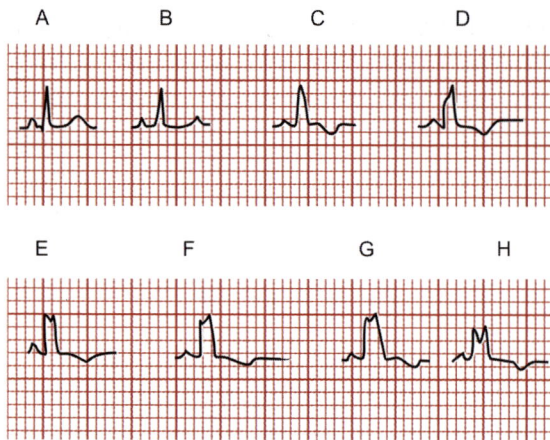

Fig. 13.10B: The electrocardiographic illustration (lead V_5) shows progression from normal intraventricular conduction through various phases of incomplete left bundle branch block to complete left bundle branch block

    A. The complex reflects normal intraventricular conduction. Note the presence of q wave with normal qRS pattern.

    B. It reflects earliest stage of incomplete left bundle branch block. The initial q wave has disappeared and a small initial slur is visible on the upstroke of R wave

C to D. The complexes reflect increase in amplitude of slur and there is progressive increase in width of QRS

E to F. They reflect the notch which is deep and wide with progressive increase in width of R wave

G to H. There is widening of QRS >0.12 sec with clearcut notch on the R wave producing its M-shaped pattern. This occurs in complete left bundle branch block.

    Complexes C to H reflect increasing ST segment T wave changes associated with both incomplete and complete left bundle branch block.

2. *The associated ST–T changes. The left oriented leads* $(V_5–V_6)$ show the minimal depression of the ST segment which has convexity upwards. The T wave is inverted in these leads. The right oriented leads $(V_1–V_2)$ show minimal elevation of ST segment with concavity upwards. The T wave is upright in these leads.

    These ST–T changes are secondary to bundle branch block itself. If there is any deviation in these changes, the primary myocardial disease may be suspected.

NOTE: The normal initial q wave in V_5– V_6 and r wave in leads V_1–V_2 disappear in left bundle branch block due to right to left septal activation. The presence of a q wave in V_5– V_6 in LBBB indicates associated myocardial infarction.

    The depression of ST segment in leads I, V_5–V_6 is secondary to LBBB; if there is an elevation of ST segment (reversal of normal pattern) myocardial

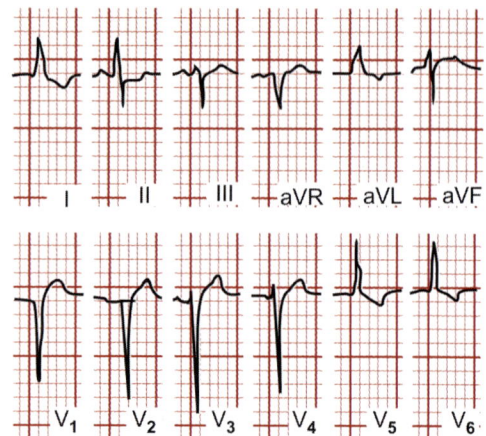

Fig. 13.11: Left bundle branch block (LBBB). The electro-cardiogram shows the following characteristics:

  (i) Mean frontal plane QRS axis is 0°

 (ii) The heart is horizontal

(iii) A wide slurred R wave is seen in lead I, aVL, V_5 and V_6 with ST segment depression and T wave inversion. Q wave is absent in these leads.

(iv) A deep wide S wave is seen in lead V_1 extending upto V_4 with upright T wave

 (v) QRS is widened (> 0.12 sec) in leads I, aVL, V_5 and V_6

(vi) VAT is prolonged in V_5-V_6 (>0.06 sec)

disease such as an infarction should be suspected and patient is investigated further to confirm it by serial cardiac enzymes and other sophisticated tests.

    The QS complexes in V_1-V_2 may, occasionally, extend upto V_3 should not be interperted as anteroseptal infarction in the presence of LBBB. These occur as a consequence of LBBB.

B. *The Standard and Extremities Leads (I, II, III, aVR, aVL and aVF)*

1. *The effect of position of the heart.* Extremities and standard leads reflect the different patterns depending on the position of heart which is as follows;

    A. *Horizontal heart:* The frontal plane QRS axis is 0° to –30°, therefore, lead I will have a wide slurred R wave with ST segment depression and T wave inversion. The QRS interval is more than 0.12 sec. The lead III records rs complex.

    The lead aVL will record a left ventricular epicardial complex (rSR´ or wide slurred R) with ST segment depression and T wave inversion, i.e. the QRS morphology seen in lead V_5.

The lead aVF will record right ventricular epicardial complex (qrs, QS or rS) with elevated or an isoelectric ST segment and upright T wave similar to lead V_1.

The precordial leads (V_4–V_6) will show a typical left ventricular epicardial complex (rSR′ or RsR′ or wide slurred M shaped RR′ complex). The VAT is prolonged to more than 0.09 sec. The ST segment is depressed and T is inverted. The right precordial leads (V_1 or V_2) will have right ventricular epicardial complex (qrs, QS, rS).

Vector analysis: The initial vector of QRS instead of being normal (L →R) is reversed (R→L), which explains the absence of a normal septal q wave is leads I and V_5–V_6. The abnormal and delayed activation of left ventricle due to delayed orientation of QRS to left and anteriorly leads to broad and slurred R wave in these leads. The ST–T vectors are oriented to right and anteriorly, hence, ST segment is depressed and T is inverted in these leads (V_5–V_6).

B. *Vertical heart:* Normal mean vertical plane axis leads to a wide slurred R wave in leads I, and II with ST segment depression and T wave inversion.

The lead aVF will show left ventricular epicardial complex (a wide, slurred R or rSR′ pattern).

The precordial leads will have same QRS morphologies as described in horizontal heart position.

Vector analysis: It remains same and constant as already discussed.

2. *The cavity complexes*
Right ventricular cavity complex. Since septal activation occurs from right to left (R → L), the right ventricular cavity will remain negative throughout the ventricular depolarisation, hence, will produce a wide QS deflection in aVR. The ST segment is elevated and T is upright in the same lead (aVR) due to a secondary change.

Left ventricular cavity complex. Since septal activation is from right to left, hence, left ventricular cavity becomes positive, an initial r wave is recorded in aVL. Left ventricular depolarisation proceeding from the endocardial to epicardial surface results in a large positive deflection as an R wave. Hence left ventricular epicardial complex seen in aVL is, therefore, rR or RSR′ or wide R wave.

Effect of Deep Respiration on LBBB

Deep inspiration and expiration by altering the position of heart can modify the ECG pattern especially in the extremities leads. The horizontal heart will become vertical during deep inspiration, hence, there will be shift from left ventricular epicardial complex to slight right ventricular epicardial complex in lead aVL. The same change will give rise to typical left ventricular epicardial complex in aVF.

Incomplete Left Bundle Branch Block Pattern

Incomplete left bundle branch block in electrocardiography means that conduction through the left bundle branch is not completely cut off, is still possible but is delayed. The electrocardiographic pattern that evolves in incomplete left bundle branch block depends on the degree of delay within the left bundle branch and its ramifications. The earliest and diagnostic ECG manifestation of incomplete LBBB is disappearance of q wave in left precordial leads and disappearance of the initial small r wave in right precordial leads (V_1–V_2) resulting in QS complex. Following this earliest change, progressively increasing delay within left bundle branch results in sequential changes in QRS morphology, i.e. first there is an initial slurring of R wave which progressively increases and ultimately produces a wide M-shaped or RsR′ or RR′ complex of left bundle branch block (Fig. 13.10B).

Mechanisms

In incomplete LBBB, there is delay in the formation and inscription of normal left sided septal vector. Due to this delay, right sided septal vector now has more time to develop so that it equals the magnitude of left sided septal vector. The two septal vectors being equal

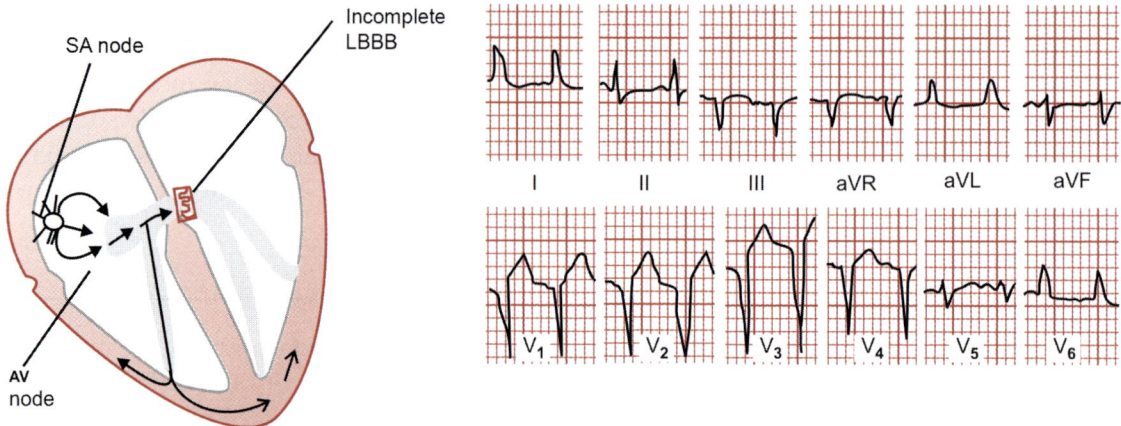

Fig. 13.12: Incomplete left bundle branch block (LBBB) pattern. The electrocardiogram shows; (i) There is loss of normal q wave in q wave containing leads (I, aVL, V₅-V₆), (ii) There is widening of R wave > 0.10 but < 0.12 sec in leads I, aVL and V₆, (iii) There is slur or notch on R wave of the above mentioned leads, (iv) There is QS pattern in leads V₁-V₃ and (v) There are associated ST-T changes in above mentioned leads indicating delayed intraventricular conduction through the left bundle branch

SECTION FOUR

and opposite, cancel or nullify each other, thereby resulting in disappearance of q waves in left sided leads and r wave in right sided leads. The pathogenesis of QRS is more or less similar to complete LBBB.

The Electrocardiogram (Fig. 13.12)

(i) The first and the earliest ECG manifestation of incomplete LBBB is loss of q wave in left sided leads (V_5–V_6, aVL and I) resulting in single tall R wave in these leads.

(ii) The small initial r wave in right precordial leads (V_1–V_2) disappears resulting in a QS complex.

(iii) With further increasing delay in conduction through the LBBB results in slurring and widening of R wave in left sided leads. The duration of QRS (duration of R wave) in incomplete LBBB remains within 0.10 to 0.12 sec. The VAT in these leads is also not much increased, remains within 0.06 to 0.09 sec.

(iv) The associated ST–T changes. These are similar to that seen in complete LBBB.

LEFT BUNDLE BRANCH WITH LEFT ANTERIOR FASCICULAR BLOCK (Fig. 13.13)

Both left bundle branch block and left anterior fascicular block shift the QRS axis leftwards. The left axis deviation in LBBB is usually in the range to 0° to –30°. The QRS forces in LBBB are oriented inferiorly and to the left, resulting in a wide R wave in leads I, V_5–V_6; while in anterior fascicular block, the QRS forces are oriented superiorly resulting in rS pattern in leads II, III and aVF. Therefore, when both LBBB and left anterior fascicular block are present, the early QRS forces become oriented inferiorly and late forces become oriented superiorly leading to left axis deviation of more than –30°.

LBBB pattern when associated with marked left axis deviation (> –30°) which is not expected from LBBB alone, indicates associated left anterior hemiblock.

LEFT BUNDLE BRANCH BLOCK WITH LEFT POSTERIOR FASCICULAR BLOCK (Fig. 13.14)

When left bundle branch block is associated with right axis deviation, then, it is either due to bilateral bundle branch block or due to a combination of left bundle branch with left posterior fascicular block. The electrocardiogram will show a typical pattern of LBBB but mean frontal plane QRS axis will be rightward due to left posterior fascicular block. The rightward axis deviation is due to delayed conduction through the posterior fascicle of left bundle branch, resulting in early forces being oriented anterosuperiorly through anterior fascicle and late forces being oriented infero–posteriorly.

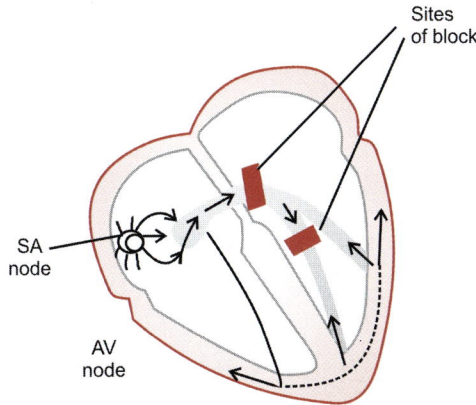

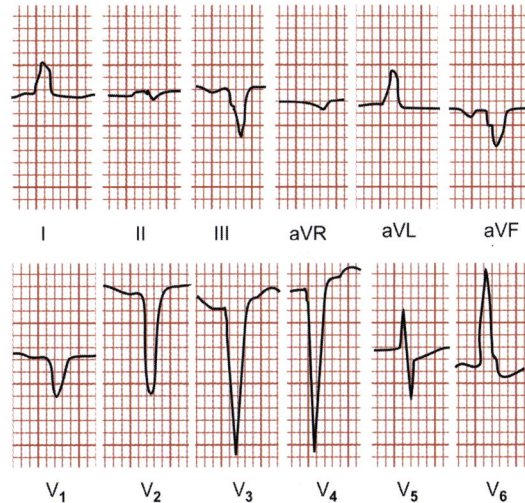

Fig. 13.13: Left bundle branch block with left anterior fascicular block. The leads I, aVL and V_5-V_6 indicate pattern of LBBB (wide R wave) and their is absence of normal q wave in V_5-V_6, and lead I. The dominant posterior vector is producing QS pattern in V_1-V_4 which is wide due to LBBB. The initial small r wave with deep wide slurred S wave in III and aVF with small r wave in II indicates superior axis to the left (> -30°), indicates additional conduction delay in left anterior fascicle of left bundle branch because one would not expect so much leftwards axis from LBBB alone

Note: The QS pattern from V_1-V_4 should not be confused with infarction unless ST-T evolutionary changes of infarction are present. In this case, this pattern is due to LBBB

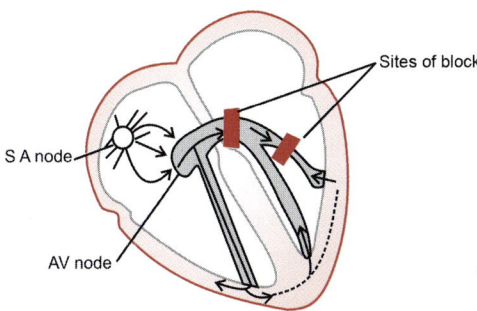

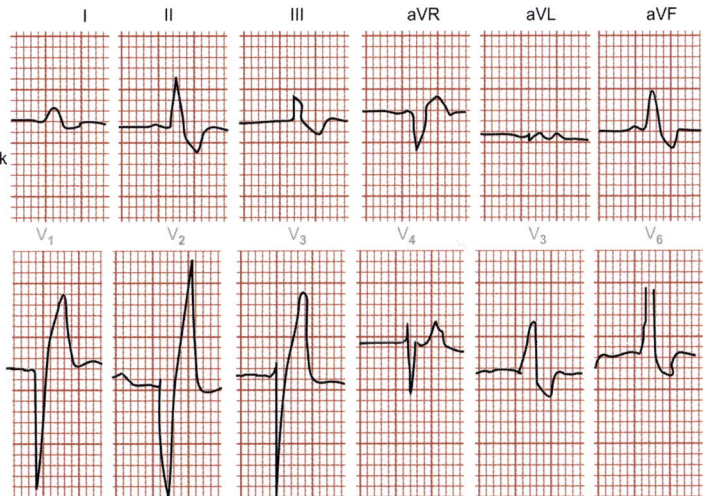

Fig. 13.14: LBBB with left posterior fascicular block. The ECG shows:
(i) *Left bundle branch block.* Loss of q wave, a wide (>0.12 sec) notched R wave (QRS) in leads I, aVL and V_5-V_6 with ST segment depression and T wave inversion indicate LBBB. Corresponding to these changes, there is QS pattern in lead V_1 and rS complex in leads V_2-V_3
(ii) *Left posterior fascicular block.* The mean frontal plane QRS axis even in the presence LBBB is +60° indicating early forces being directed through anterior fascicle and late forces through posterior fascicle towards infero-posterior direction. There is vertical heart position resulting in slurred R in leads I,II and aVF with ST segment depression and T wave inversion. All the features in the absence of other cause for right axis deviation and vertical heart position suggest associated left posterior fascicular block

LBBB pattern with right axis deviation suggests an associated left posterior fascicular block in the absence of other explainable cause.

LEFT BUNDLE BRANCH BLOCK WITH AV CONDUCTION DELAY: First degree AV block (Fig. 13.15) and other grades of AV block can occur

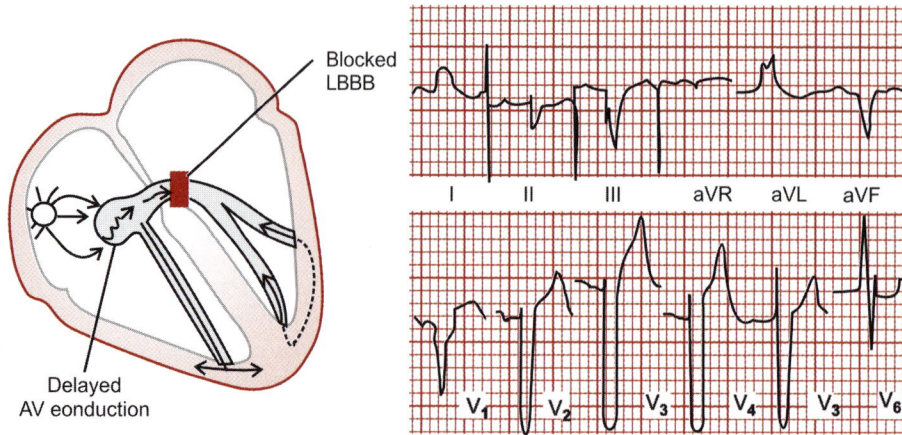

Fig. 13.15: Left bundle branch block with first degree AV block and abnormal left axis deviation: The electrocardiogram shows following characteristics:

1.   Left axis deviation of –60° (aVR shows small negative deflection and there is largest S wave in lead III than II and aVF)
2.   P-R interval is 0.24 sec (1° AV block)
3.   LBBB is evidenced by wide R wave in lead 1 and notched wide R wave in aVL and wide RsR' pattern in V_6. QRS is wide (>0.12 sec). VAT is prolonged; the heart is horizontal. A wide S wave is present in V_1-V_4

Note: A left axis deviation of –60° is not expected in LBBB, therefore possibility of associated left anterior hemiblock cannot be ruled out

concomittently with LBBB especially in hypertension and ischaemic heart disease.

INTERMITTENT LEFT BUNDLE BRANCH BLOCK:

When pattern of LBBB appears interspersed with sinus conducted complexes; it is called an intermittent LBBB. The left bundle branch block pattern can uncommonly be seen in aberrantly conducted supraventricular impulses (Fig. 13.16).

LEFT BUNDLE BRANCH BLOCK WITH LEFT VENTRICULAR HYPERTROPHY

Certain clinical conditions can produce a left bundle branch block in the presence of left ventricular hypertrophy. The differentiating features are given in the box. It is difficult to comment LVH in the presence of left bundle branch block.

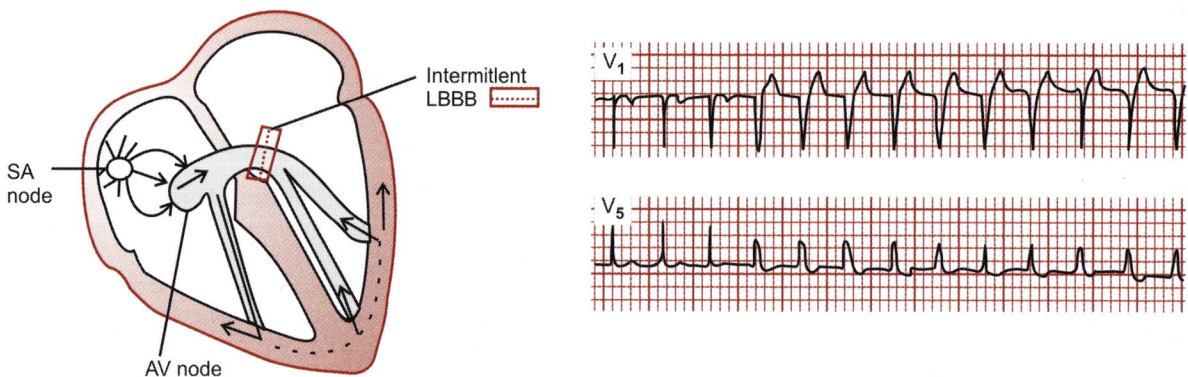

Fig. 13.16: Intermittent left bundle branch block (LBBB) pattern. The electrocardiographic leads V_1 and V_5 show first three beats as sinus conducted beats with normal QRS complexes followed by wide QRS (>0.12 sec) complexes which are upright in V_5 and downwards in V_1 indicate left bundle branch block pattern at a same rate as that of sinus conducted beats. These wide complexes are preceded by P wave and normal P-R interval. These complexes can be confused with aberrant intraventricular conduction but they are occurring at normal sinus rate, hence, this possibility is ruled out

Differentiating Points between LBBB and Left Ventricular Hypertrophy

Left bundle branch block (LBBB)	Left ventricular hypertrophy (LVH)
• Slurred R, RsR´ or M-shaped R wave in $V_5 - V_6$.	• A QRS pattern is seen in $V_5 - V_6$.
• Absence of q wave in leads I, $V_5 - V_6$ due to septal activation from right to left (R→L)	• q waves are present and may be deep due to normal septal activation from left to right (L→R)
• There is loss of initial r wave in $V_1 - V_2$ resulting in QS complex	• There is either rS complex or QS complex in leads $V_1 - V_2$.

REVIEW AT GLANCE

- ECG changes in complete and incomplete LBBB. Precordial leads V_1 and V_5 are best for diagnosis of LBBB.
- The leads V_5, V_6 and standard lead 1 show wide slurred R wave or RsR′ to RR′ complex with absent q wave. The initial small r wave in V_1 disappears. There is a slurring of S wave (if seen) in V_5–V_6 due to activation of *posterobasal* region.
- QRS interval is > 0.12 second resulting in QS pattern in V_1–V_2. In incomplete bundle branch block, QRS remains between 0.10 to 0.12 sec.
- VAT is > 0.09 second in complete LBBB. It is less increased in incomplete LBBB.
- ST segment depression with convexity upwards and T wave inversion occurs in leads I and V_5–V_6, while on the other hand, leads V_1–V_2 may show mild elevation of ST segment with concavity upwards and T is upright in these leads. This change is seen in both complete and incomplete LBBB.
- Horizontal heart position will reveal similar morphology of QRS in leads I, aVL and V_5–V_6. Vertical heart position will show similar morpologies of QRS in leads II, aVF and V_5–V_6.
- In LBBB (complete or incomplete), there is always an absence of q wave in leads I, V_5–V_6 due to septal activation from right to left. The presence of q wave in these leads suggests an associated myocardial infarction.

ALTERNATING RIGHT AND LEFT BUNDLE BRANCH BLOCK (INTERMITTENT BILATERAL BUNDLE BRANCH BLOCK)

Complete simultaneous block of both the bundles is not possible as it will lead to complete heart block, hence, bilateral bundle branch block will manifest intermittently, one at a time, alternating with the other. In this type of bilateral bundle branch block, the ECG will demonstrate a typical complete right or left bundle branch block at one time and within a few minutes or hours or days, it will show the opposite type of bundle branch block. The bilateral bundle branch block is transient, but is very ominous sign and predictive of complete heart block unless it is due to some reversible factor such as drug toxicity, myocardial ischaemia (Fig. 13.17) etc.

MASQUERADING BUNDLE BRANCH BLOCK

It is a rare form of bundle branch block. It is manifested electrocardiographically by pattern of RBBB with marked left axis deviation and absence of a significant S wave in leads I, aVL and V_6, hence, can be confused with bifascicular (RBBB with left anterior fascicular) block. In masquerading bundle branch block, there will be LBBB pattern in limb leads and right bundle branch block pattern in precordial leads. In contrast to bifascicular block, the masquerading BBB is usually associated with significant heart disease and is a bad prognostic indicator.

BUNDLE BRANCH BLOCK ALTERNANS

Bundle branch block alternans is a rare finding and manifests electrocardiographically as alternans of;
1. Alternate RBBB and LBBB without normal QRS complexes in between
2. Alternate RBBB and LBBB with normal of complexes in between intermittent bilateral bundle branch block)
3. Alternate complete and incomplete RBBB or LBBB.

NONSPECIFIC OR INDETERMINATE INTRAVENTRICULAR CONDUCTION DEFECT (FIG. 13.18)

The QRS complex may be abnormally prolonged without following the characteristic pattern of either

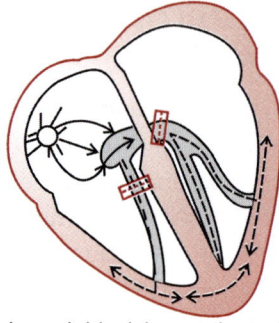

Fig. 13.17: Alternating bundle branch block in a patient with myocardial infarction. The electrocardiogram shows:

A. There is (i) right bundle branch block pattern (rSR' in V_1) with left axis deviation indicating bifascicular block (right bundle and left anterior fascicular block). (ii) Anteroseptal infarction: it is evident from wide, abnormal Q waves in leads V_2-V_4

B. The electrocardiogram recorded after several hours late shows: (i) Left bundle branch block pattern with lateral wall infarction (wide qR pattern in V_5-V_6 indicates lateral wall infarction with left bundle branch block). Now R wave is seen in leads V_1-V_4

    This tracing illustrates how lateral Q waves with LBBB may paradoxically reflect anteroseptal myocardial infarction

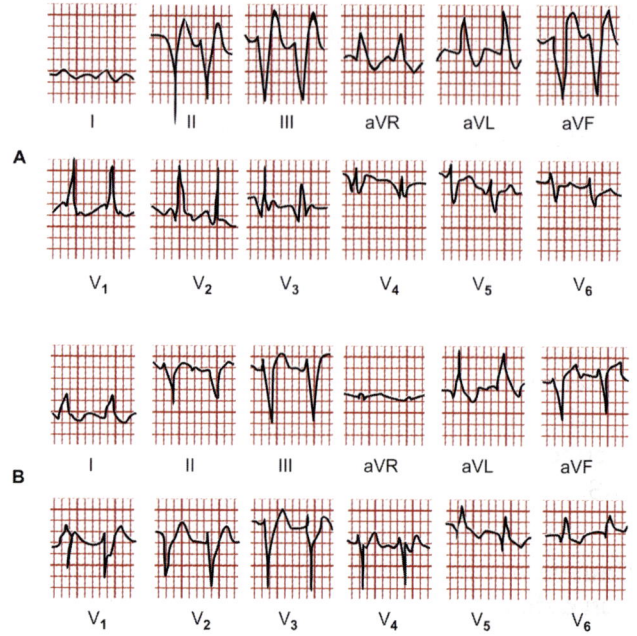

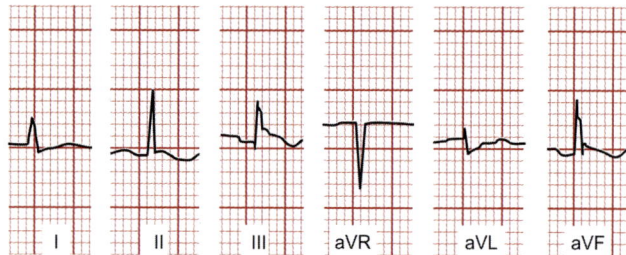

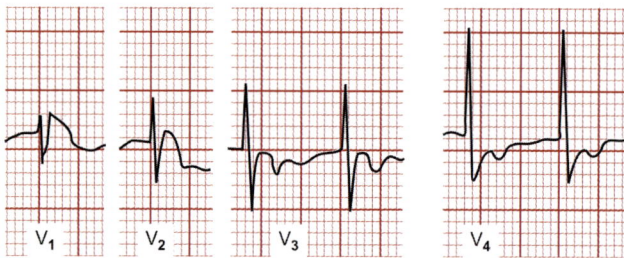

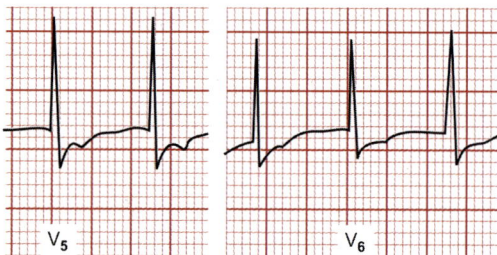

Fig. 13.18: Nonspecific intraventricular conduction delay or defect. The electrocardiogram shows:

(i)   Normal QRS axis

(ii) Wide QRS complexes in all the leads. In some complexes there is slurring of R waves (leads II, aVF) and S waves (aVL and aVR). There is rSr' pattern in V_1 and slurring of S wave; while there is RS pattern in V_2 with slurred S wave. This does not fit into pattern of RBBB.

(iii) There is q wave in lead I, III, V_5-V_6 with widening of QRS complexes. This does not suggest LBBB

(iv) There are diffuse widespread ST-T changes, i.e. ST depression with T wave inversion in leads I, II, aVL V_4-V_6. There is elevation of ST in lead V_1-V_2, III and aVF.

    All these features suggest widespread peripheral Purkinje system defect (nonspecific intraventricular conduction defect rahter than a specific bundle branch or bifascicular block

RBBB or LBBB. Such conduction delays are termed as *nonspecific intraventricular conduction defects*. These conduction delays resemble LBBB or RBBB with an abnormal left axis deviation–a combination suggesting bifascicular block. Presence of a normal Q wave in wide QRS complex supports the conduction delay in peripheral conduction system. The nonspecific intraventricular conduction delay can be due to many causes given in the box. An interesting form of right ventricular conduction delay has been obeserved in patients with arrhythmogenic right ventricular dysplasia, where delayed activation is inscribed as a sharp deflection after termination of QRS, i.e. during the ST segment or upstroke of T wave.

Causes of nonspecific intraventricular conduction defect

- Drugs
- Electrolyte disturbances
- Organic heart disease
- Arrhythmogenic right ventricular dysplasia

Suggested Reading

1. Brugada P, Brugada J: RBBB, persistent ST segment elevation and sudden cardiac death. A distinct clinical and ECG syndrome. A multicentric report. *J Am Coll Cardiology* **20**: 1391-96, 1992.
2. Dhingra RC, et al: Significance of chronic bifascicular block without apparent organic heart disease. *Circulation* **60**: 33,1979.
3. Fahr G: Some fundamental principles of electrocardiography. *Arch Intern Med* 27:126-30,1921.
4. Fisch C, Zipes DP, Mechtenry PH: Rate–dependant aberrency. *Circulation* **48**: 714,1973.
5. Flowers NC: Left bundle branch block: A continuously evolving concept. *J Am Coll Cardiol* **9**: 684, 1987.
6. Gold FL: From AHL; Alternating bundle branch block. *J Electrocard* **13**: 405, 1980.
7. Gussak I, Antezelevitcz C, Birregard P et al: "The Brugada syndrome." Clinical, electrophysiologic and genetic aspect. *J Am Coll Cardiol* **35**: 5-15, 1999.
8. Johnson RL, Averill H, Lamb LE: Electrocardiographic findings in 67, 375 asymptomatic individuals. Part VI: Right bundle branch block. *Am J Cardiol* **6**: 143,1960.
9. Massumi RA: Bradycardia-dependent RBBB. A critique and proposed criteria. *Circulation* 38:1066,1968.
10. McAnulty JH et al: Natural history of high risk bundle branch block. Final report of a prospective study. *N Engl J Med* **307**: 137,1982.
11. McAnulty JH, Rashimtoola SH: Bundle branch block. *Prog Cardiovasc Dis* **26**: 333,1984.
12. Moore EN, Hoffman BF, Patterson DF, et al: Electrocardiographic changes due to delayed activation of right ventricle. *Am Heart J* **68**: 347-61,1964.
13. Narula OS, Samet P: Right bundle branch block with normal left or right axis deviation. *Am J Med* 51:432,1971.
14. Richman JL, Wolff L: Left bundle branch block masquerading as right bundle branch block. *Am Heart J* **47**:383, 1954.
15. Rodriquez MI, Sodi–Pallares D: The mechanism of complete and incomplete bundle branch block. *Am Heart J* **44**: 715,1952.
16. Rosenbaum MB, Elizari MV, Lazzari JO, et al: The differential electrocardiographic manifestations of hemiblocks, bilateral bundle branch block and trifascicular blocks. In Advances in Electrocardiography, Eds, Schlant RC, Hurst JW. New York. Grune and Stratton 149-220, 1972.
17. Rosenbaum MB: Types of left bundle branch block and their clinical significance. *J Electrocardiol* **2**: 197, 1969.
18. Rosenbaum MB: Types of right bundle branch block and their clinical significance. *J Electrocardiol* **1**: 221, 1968.
19. Schamroth L, Myburgh DP, Schamroth CL: The early signs of right bundle branch block. *Chest* 87:180,1985.
20. Schneider JF, Thomas HE Jr, McNomara PM, et al: Clinical electrocardiographic study of newly acquired left bundle branch block : The Framingham study. *Am J Cardiol* **55**: 1332-8,1985.
21. Sodi–Pallares D, Medrano GA, Bisteni A et al: Deductive and polyparametric electrocardiography. Instituto Nacional de Cardiologia de Mexico.
22. Walston AH, Bioneau JP, Spach MS, et al : Relationship between ventricular depolarisation and QRS in right and left bundle branch block. *J Electrocardiol* **1**: 155, 1968.

14

The Fascicular Blocks or Hemiblocks

- Applied anatomy and physiology
- Left anterior fascicular block
- Left posterior fascicular block
- Left septal fascicular block

- Bifascicular block (right bundle branch block with either left anterior or left posterior fascicular block)
- Trifascicular block

FASCICULAR BLOCKS

Definition

A delay or interruption of conduction through one of the two major divisions or fascicles of left bundle is called a *'fascicular blocks or hemiblock'*. It, therefore, constitutes a peripheral left ventricular conduction defect.

Applied Anatomy and Physiology

The left bundle immediately after its origin divides into two major divisions or fascicles, i.e.

i) *Anterosuperior division or anterior fascicle* which arises distally and fans out as a broad band of fibres over the anterior and superior endocardial areas of the left ventricle. It is narrower than posterior division.

ii) *Posteroinferior division or posterior fascicle* which arises proximally and fans out over the posterior and inferior areas of the endocardium of the left ventricle.

The peripheral fibres of these two divisions arborise thereby forming a closed conduction network for rapid and synchronous conduction through both these divisions. This results in a normally directed QRS axis (– 30° to + 110°) in the frontal plane.

However, if one of the divisions is involved, then the conduction will proceed through the other uninvolved division, thus, altering the mean QRS vector. Since the spread of the conduction through the left bundle and Purkinje system is rapid, hence, QRS interval does not get prolonged in fascicular blocks or hemiblocks (Figs 14.1A to D).

QRS interval usually remains normal in fascicular blocks or hemiblocks

The left anterior fascicular block or left anterior hemiblock is commoner than left posterior fascicular block due to following reasons;

1. The anterior fascicle is long and thin; whereas posterior is short and thick

2. The posterior fascicle has dual blood supply; in contrast, the anterior fascicle has single source of blood supply.

3. The anterior fascicle is supplied by a septal branch of anterior descending artery which supplies the right bundle branch also. This is the reason for the frequent involvement of right bundle branch and left anterior fascicle in myocardial infarction–collectively called a bifascicular block.

4. The anterior fascicle is closer to the aortic valve, hence, is more likely to be involved in diseases involving the aortic valve.

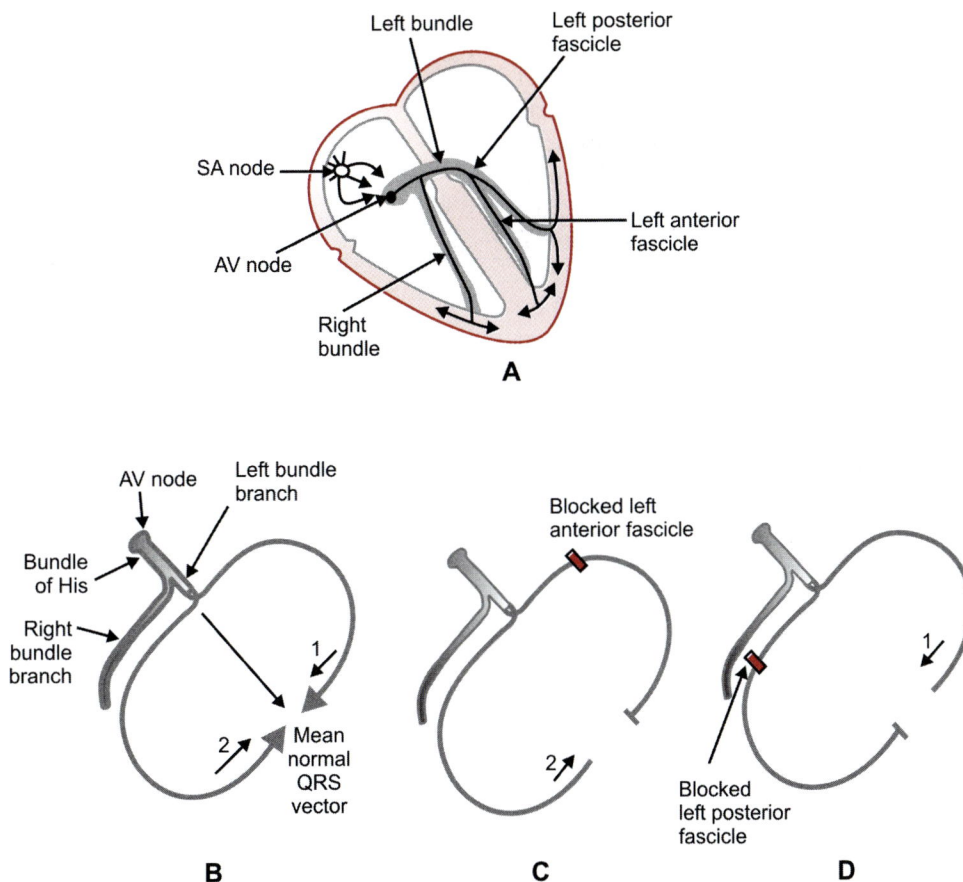

Figs 14.1A to D: Diagrammatic illustration;
A: Two divisions of left bundle and their anastomosis on endocardium.
B: The spread of conduction through both the fascicles and electrical forces (1 and 2) are directed opposite to each other.
C: The effects of block of anterior fascicle. The conduction proceeds through posterior fascicle.
D: The effects of block of posterior fascicle. It will result in conduction of impulses through anterior fascicle.

Left anterior fascicular block is commoner than left posterior fascicular block

Note: *For the purpose of electrocardiography, there are three fascicles in conduction system. The left bundle has two fascicles—anterior and posterior; whereas the right bundle itself acts as a third fascicle.*

THE LEFT ANTERIOR FASCICULAR BLOCK (LEFT ANTERIOR HEMIBLOCK)

Definition: A delay or block in conduction through the anterosuperior division (anterior fascicle) of left bundle branch is called *'left anterior fascicular block or left anterior hemiblock'.*

Aetiology: It may be due to following causes:
1. Coronary artery disease
2. Myocarditis or cardiomyopathies
3. Long standing systemic hypertension
4. Aortic valve disease (aortic stenosis or regurgitation)
5. Long standing congestive heart failure
6. Congenital heart disease, i.e. endocardial cushion defects
7. It may be transient due to myocardial infarction or may appear transiently during arrhythmias.

During arrhythmias and acute myocardial infarction, the left anterior fascicular block is transient.

SECTION FOUR

Mechanisms

The conduction from SA node to AV node, then to left main bundle branch before its division proceeds normally. Due to block or delay in left anterior fascicle, the conduction or excitation wave proceeds through the posterior fascicle, hence, posteroinferior surface of left ventricle is to be activated first. Thus, the initial QRS vector is directed inferiorly and to the right (Fig. 14.2. B–vector 1). This initial activation is followed by delayed activation of anterosuperior and anterolateral regions of left ventricular wall beyond the site of block of left anterior fascicle through interconnecting Purkinje system. This results in dominance of terminal QRS vector (Fig. 14.2. – vector 2) which is directed to the left and superiorly in the frontal plane leading to left axis deviation of > – 30°. It is directed somewhat posteriorly in the horizontal plane.

Due to difference in orientation of initial and terminal QRS vectors, the mean vector (Fig. 14.2. vector 3) remains to the left and superiorly. The various QRS vectors and their effects on different limb leads on hexaxial system are represented in the diagram (Fig. 14.2).

Vector 1: Initial QRS vector. It is directed to the right and inferiorly with the result that an initial R(r) wave will be recorded in inferior leads II, III and aVF, and q wave in leads I and aVL.

Vector 2: The terminal QRS vector. It is to the left due to which a R wave will be seen in lead I, and superiorly resulting in a deep S wave in leads II, III and aVF.

Vector 3: Mean frontal plane QRS axis: The mean frontal plane QRS vector is directed to the left resulting in

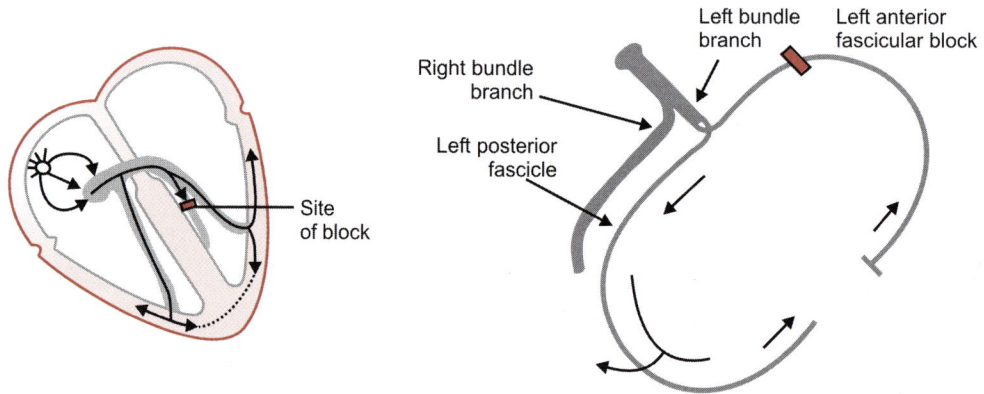

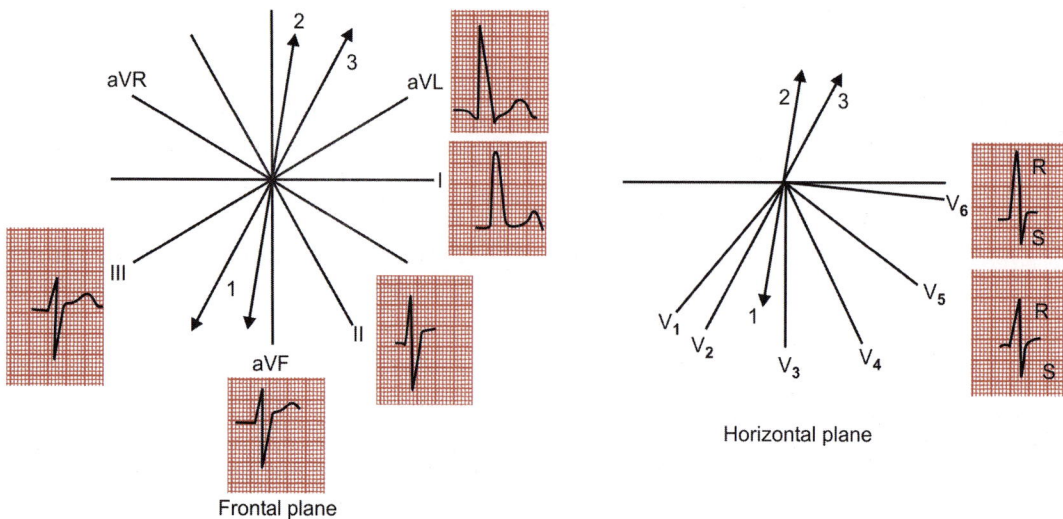

Fig. 14.2: The left anterior fascicular block; the mechanism of evolution of electrocardiographic patterns (diagram)

left axis deviation more than –30°. The precordial leads face the brunt of superior and left orientation of terminal QRS vector. This results in diminution or absence of small q waves in V_5-V_6 leading to RS complexes in V_5-V_6. The height of R wave is diminished due to superior orientation of axis. The QRS interval may be slightly prolonged but does not go beyond 0.11 second. The VAT is also slightly prolonged.

The Electrocardiogram (Fig. 14.3)

This evolves as follows:

1. *Left axis deviation is more than –30° (–30° counterclockwise to – 80°):* As left axis deviation is the hallmark of left anterior fascicular block, therefore, other causes of left axis deviation, e.g. inferior wall infarction, hypertrophic cardiomyopathy, hypertensive heart disease, Wolff-

Parkinson-White syndrome, etc. should be excluded before the label of left anterior fascicular block is applied.

2. *The rS complex in leads II, III and aVF:* The S wave is deeper in standard lead III than II. The QRS complex appears in leads I and aVL with prominent R wave in lead aVL than lead I. The q wave in these leads is either attenuated or absent. The lead aVR may reflect a late slurred r wave.

3. *The VAT* is increased due to delay in intrinsicoid deflection in leads oriented to high lateral or superior aspect of left bundle, i.e. aVL.

4. *The QRS change in precordial leads*
   i. There is usually no effect on QRS duration; in some cases, there may be slight prolongation, but it is always less than 0,11 second, best seen in lead aVL.

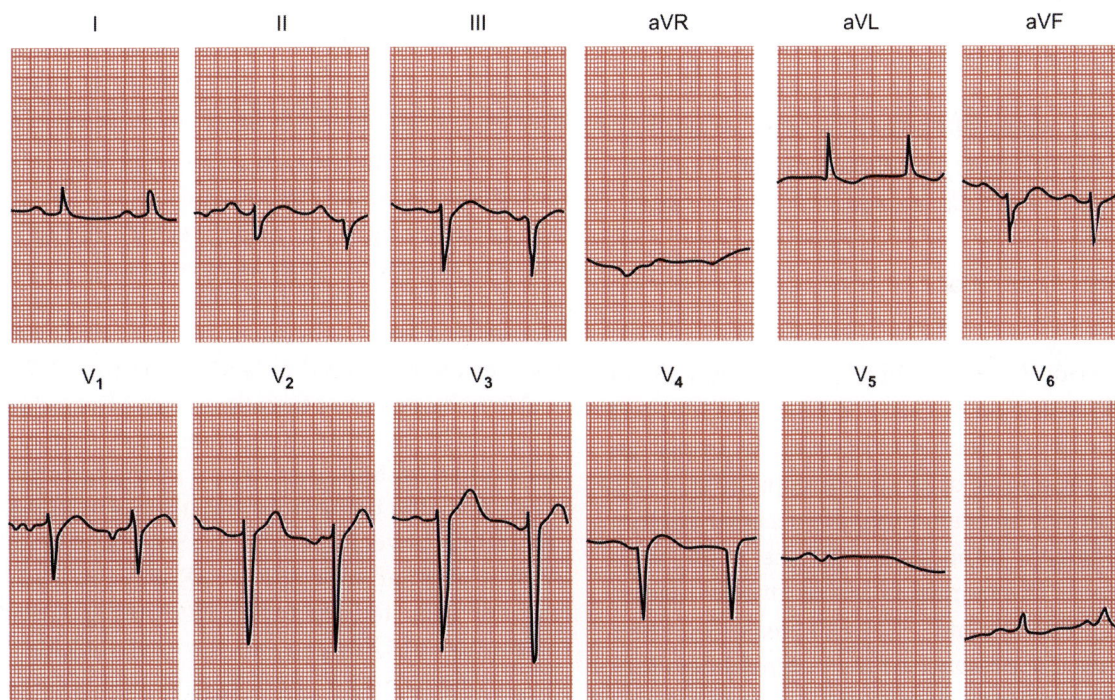

Fig. 14.3: Left anterior fascicular block or hemiblock (LAH). The electrocardiogram recorded from a patient with an old anterior wall myocardial infarction shows;
  (i) Left axis deviation of frontal plane QRS > –30°
  (ii) A rS pattern with deep wide S wave in leads; II, III and aVF, the S wave being deeper in lead III than II and aVF
  (iii) A qR pattern is seen in leads I and aVL
      All these features suggest left anterior fascicular block
  (iv) Features of an old myocardial infarction. There is QS pattern in V_4 with small truncated r wave in V_5-V_6 indicating peri-infarction block. In addition, there is nonprogression of R wave from V_1-V_6 and q waves of infarction not seen in V_5-V_6 due to left anterior fascicular block. There is ST segment depression and T wave inversion in leads I, aVL and V_6

ii. A tendency for the normal small initial q waves in left precordial leads (V_5-V_6) to disappear.

iii. Attenuation of R waves in left oriented precordial leads due to superiorly directed QRS vector. Due to this vector orientation, a deep S wave will be seen in precordial leads leading to RS pattern in leads V_5-V_6.

The normal QRS configuration of V_5-V_6 is changed to RS configuration in left anterior fascicular block.

5. **The ST and T changes:** The T wave vector deviates opposite to QRS as occurs usually in any type of intraventricular conduction block, the leads which register positive QRS complexes will register low to inverted T waves; whereas the leads with negative QRS complexes will register an upright T wave. This is called secondary ST-T changes due to intraventricular conduction defect. This is of no clinical significance. However, if there is deviation from the associated ST-T changes, myocardial involvement may be suspected.

In a fascicular block, ST-T change is opposite to QRS deflection, any deviation from this change constitutes a primary change and indicates myocardial involvement

Clinical Significance of Left Anterior Fascicular Block

1. Left anterior fascicular block, if detected as an isolated finding on ECG in the absence of an overt cardiac disease does not necessarily imply an adverse prognosis or does not constitute a risk factor. Long-term evaluations are necessary before the prognostic implications can be made with confidence. The manifestation of an isolated left axis deviation beyond – 30°, is, at least, a pointer to the possible presence or the potential development of a cardiac disease.

2. However, when LAH occurs in association with right bundle branch block (bifascicular block), it usually indicates an adverse prognosis and may lead to development of complete heart block. Further, if LAH occurs in association with left bundle branch block (a difficult situation to diagnose on ECG), the mortality and morbidity due to left bundle branch block itself is slightly accentuated.

LEFT ANTERIOR FASCICULAR OR HEMIBLOCK (LAH) BLOCK WITH LEFT VENTRICULAR HYPERTROPHY (Fig. 14.4)

Uncomplicated left anterior fascicular block rarely shifts the frontal plane QRS axis beyond – 60° leftwards (left axis deviation > – 60°). Higher grades of left anterior fascicular block will, merely, increase the amplitude and duration of QRS, i.e. the lead III may show deep S wave (> 15 mm). The left axis deviation more than – 60° and amplitude of S wave more than 15 mm in lead III indicate either high grade (both LBBB and LAH), or advanced left anterior fascicular block or there is an associated left ventricular hypertrophy with left anterior fascicular block.

LEFT POSTERIOR FASCICULAR BLOCK OR LEFT POSTERIOR HEMIBLOCK (LPH)

Definition : A delay or block of conduction through the posterior fascicle of left bundle is called' *left posterior fascicular block or left posterior hemiblock'*.

Mechanisms: Due to block in the left posterior fascicle, the activation wave spreads through the left anterior fascicle resulting in an initial vector oriented to the left and superiorly (Fig. 14.5. vector 1). Due to this initial vector orientation to the left, there appears a R(r) wave in lead I, and due to its superior orientation, q waves are registered in leads II, III and aVF.

Now the posterior fascicle is also activated beyond the site of block through the interconnecting network of Purkinje system, this results in the terminal QRS vector oriented to the right and inferiorly. Right-ward orientation of vector results in a S wave in lead I; and inferior orientation results in a R wave in leads II, III and aVF (Fig. 14.5 vector 2). Due to slight posterior orientation of QRS axis, all the anterior chest leads will register rS in V_1 and V_2 and Rs in V_5-V_6 with transition zone between V_3-V_4.

As usual with disturbances in intraventricular conduction, left posterior fascicular or hemiblock (LPH) is associated with secondary ST-T changes. As T wave vector deviates away from mean QRS vector, therefore, leads that register positive deflection of QRS will have ST segment depression with convexity upwards and low to inverted T waves (leads II, III

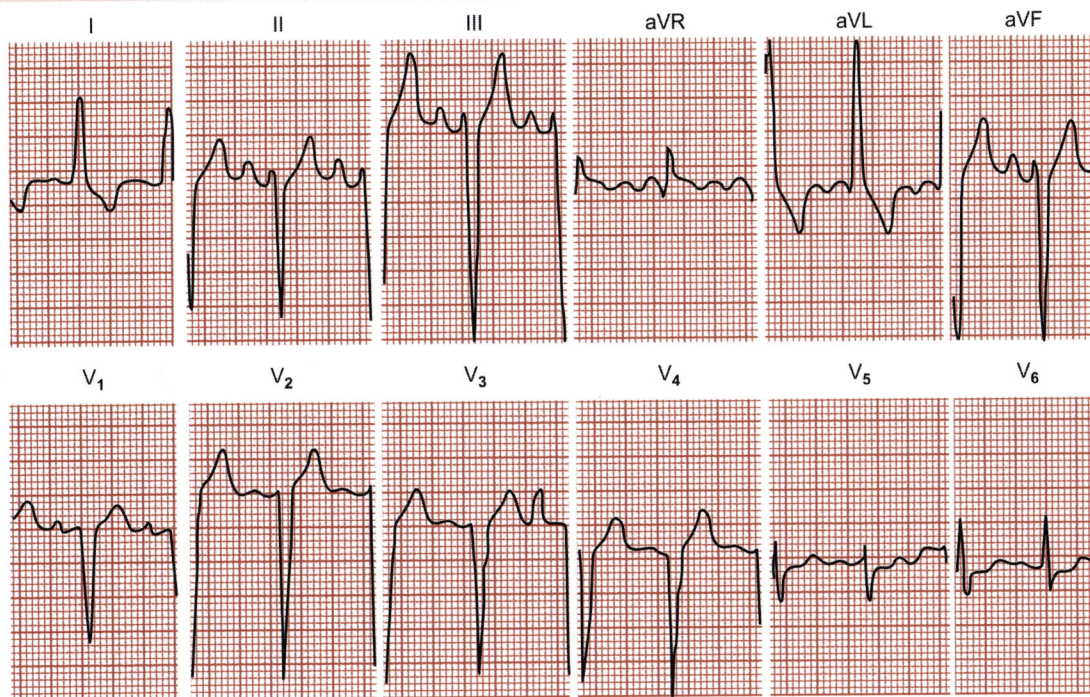

Fig. 14.4: Left anterior hemiblock associated with left ventricular hypertrophy. The ECG (recorded at half standardisation) shows:

1. *Left ventricular hypertrophy:* There is high voltage in standard leads. The index of Lewis (the net positive deflection in lead I plus the negative deflection in lead III) is 43 mm (well beyond the normal of 21 mm). The R wave in aVL is 23 mm (well beyond the normal of 13 mm). The lead V_5 and V_6 do not statisfy the voltage criteria due to superior axis of –60°. The QRS axis is oriented to the left and posteriorly (zone of transition seen in V_5) with loss of q wave in V_5-V_6 and poor progression of R wave in right precordial leads support LVH. The ST and T vectors are opposite to QRS; ST segment is depressed and T is inverted in lead I and aVL where R is tall.
2. *Left anterior hemiblock.* The extreme left axis of –60° is not expected due to LVH, hence indicate associated left anterior hemiblock.
3. The tall peaked P waves in II, III and aVF indicate associated right atrial hypertrophy

and aVF). The leads that register negative QRS deflection (leads I and aVL) will have upright T waves with minimal elevation of ST segment with concavity upwards.

The Electrocardiogram (Fig. 14.6)

1. Right axis deviation on frontal plane leads (+ 120° clockwise to + 180°), usually ≥ + 140°
2. A small r wave and a deep S wave (rS complex) is seen in leads I and aVL, and a small q wave and a tall R wave (qR or qRs complex) in leads II, III and aVF.
3. A rS complex is also seen in leads V_1-V_2 and Rs (tall R with small S wave) complexes are seen in leads V_5-V_6.
4. The duration of QRS complex is slightly prolonged but does not exceed 0.11 sec.

5. Low to inverted T waves in leads II, III and aVF; and upright T waves in lead I.

Note: As right axis deviation is the hallmark of left posterior fascicular block, therefore, other causes of right axis deviation, e.g. lateral wall myocardial infarction, obstructive lung disease, right ventricular hypertrophy, etc. should be excluded before the label of left posterior fascicular block is applied

Clinical Significance

The appearance of left posterior fascicular block during a myocardial infarction implies an extensive muscle damage and may lead to significant arrhythmias and heart failure.

Frontal plane

Horizontal plane

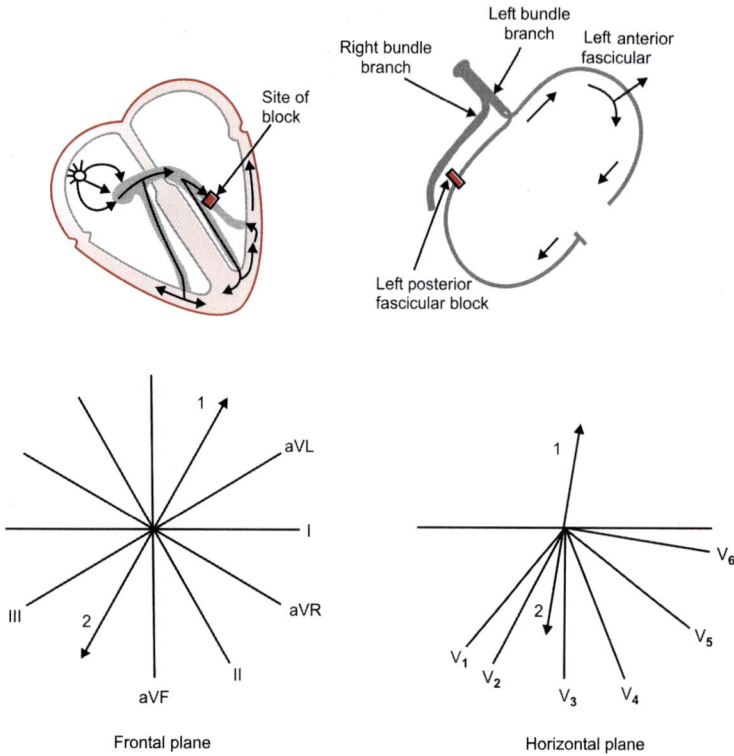

Fig. 14.5: Left posterior fascicular block (diagram). The mechanism of evolution of electrocardiographic patterns

(i) Vector 1. Initial QRS vector. It is directed to the left and superiorly due to which there will be initial r′ wave in leads I and aVL and a q wave in leads II, III and aVF

(ii) Vector 2. Terminal large QRS vector. It is directed to the right and inferiorly leading to a deep S wave in leads I and aVL (rS complex) and a large R in leads II, III and a VF (qR complex).

(iii) Mean frontal plane QRS vector, i.e. to the right and inferiorly >+110°

(iv) There will be rS complex in precordial leads (V_1-V_3) and RS pattern in leads V_4-V_6 due to the posterior orientation of mean QRS axis in horizontal plane

(v) Associated ST-T changes will be seen in leads II,III and aVF. This is due to the fact that ST-T vector is always opposite to mean QRS vector in any intraventricular conduction block

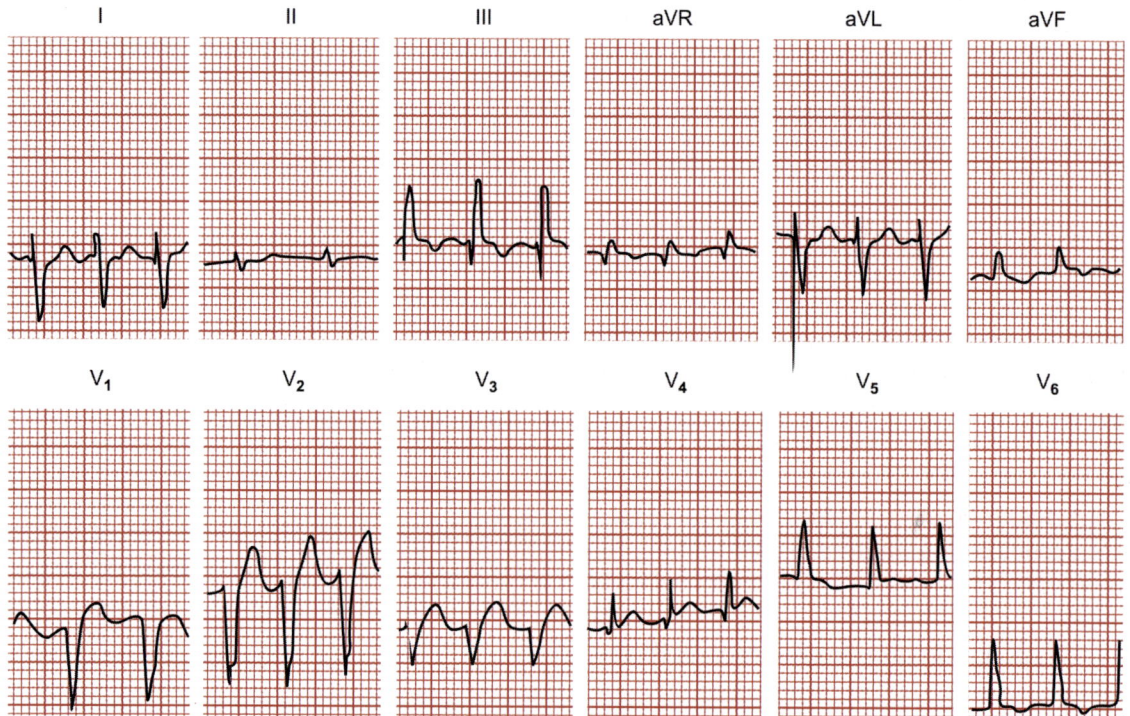

Fig. 14.6: Left posterior fascicular block. The electrocardiogram shows the following features with vector analysis shown in Fig. 14.5. (i) The mean frontal QRS axis is +135°, (ii) There is rS complex in leads I and aVL and qR complex in leads III and aVF, (iii) There is rS complex in leads V_1-V_3 with Rs in leads V_5-V_6 , (iv) There is associated change in ST segment and T waves. The T waves are inverted in leads III and aVF and upright in leads I and aVL

Note: There is neither any evidence of RBBB or RVH to explain extreme right axis duration, hence, these changes are due to left posterior fascicular block

LEFT SEPTAL FASCICULAR BLOCK

Some clinicians consider the intraventricular conduction system comprising of four fascicles and septal fascicle is considered as the third fascicle of left bundle, though, it is actually not. It arises by the septal fibres from the proximal portion of left bundle branch and supplies fibres to septum and leads to its activation from left to right (L→R) normally, resulting in an rS complex in right oriented (V_1 and V_2) leads and a qRs complex in left oriented V_5-V_6 leads with transition zone in V_3-V_4.

Interruption or block of septal fibres due to fibrosis, or septal infarction or due to any other cause will block the left to right activation of the septum resulting in loss of r wave in right oriented and q wave in left oriented leads. Therefore, as an isolated finding, there will be loss of q wave in leads I, V_5 and V_6, and QS pattern seen in leads V_1-V_2 and even in V_3, may simulate anteroseptal infarction.

The septal fibres donot constitute a separate fascicle because;

(i) Its isolated involvement is rare.

(ii) The origin of septal fibres and their orientation is variable.

(iii) Its electrocardiographic expression as loss of q wave in left oriented leads (I, aVL, V_5-V_6) forms a diagnostic criteria of left bundle branch block, hence, for purpose of electrocardiography, it is considered a part and parcel of left bundle branch.

(iv) The loss of q wave in leads I, V_5-V_6 may be a normal variant in 20% individuals. This does not disapprove the concept of left to right septal depolarisation but indicates that intraventricular septum is parallel to the frontal plane of the body. Even though, the septum is activated from left to right. The projection of this force will be oriented anteriorly rather than to the right resulting in loss of q waves in leads I, V_5 and V_6.

PERI-INFARCTION BLOCK

Peri-infarction block refers to a delay in conduction within the tissue surrounding the infarcted zone. This block is discussed in chapter on myocardial infarction.

REVIEW AT A GLANCE

A. Left anterior fascicular or hemiblock (LAH)

- Mean left QRS axis deviation is more than $-30°$.
- A rS complex in leads II, III and aVF. The S wave is deeper in lead III than lead II.
- A qR complex is present in leads I and aVL.
- A slight increase in QRS duration in these leads but less than 0.11 sec.
- VAT is slightly prolonged.
- ST segment depression and T wave inversion in leads registering positive QRS deflection. T wave is upright with slight elevation of ST segment in leads registering negative QRS deflection.
- Precordial leads will have RS complex with slurring of S wave in V_5–V_6.

B. Left posterior fascicular or left posterior hemiblock (LPH)

- Mean right QRS axis deviation (+ 120° clockwise to + 180°)
- Prominent S waves in leads I and aVL (rS complex), a tall R waves in leads II,III and aVF (qR or qRs complex); the R wave will be taller in lead III than II and may be slurred.
- Precordial leads show rS complex in V_1 and V_2 and Rs in V_5 and V_6 with transition zone in V_3 through V_4.
- The ST segment depression and T wave inversion appears as a secondary change in leads registering positive QRS deflection. T is upright in leads with negative QRS deflection.

C. Left septal block

- Loss of q wave in leads I, V_5 and V_6.
- QS pattern in leads V_1 to V_3 resembling anteroseptal infarction.

COMBINED FASCICULAR BLOCKS

In electrocardiography, the right bundle constitutes one fascicle and left bundle branch consists of two fascicles, i.e. left anterior and left posterior. Therefore, right bundle branch is invariably involved in bifascicular and trifascicular blocks. Bifascicular

SECTION FOUR

blocks are also called bilateral bundle branch blocks because one bundle is constituted by right bundle and other bundle is represented by one of the fascicles of left bundle. Complete bilateral bundle branch block is not possible, hence, conduction must occur through one of the fascicles of left bundle for ventricular activation.

BIFASCICULAR BLOCKS

The combination of right bundle bundle branch block with either left anterior or left posterior fascicular block constitute *bifascicular block.*

Combinations: Following combinations can occur;
1. Right bundle branch block (RBBB) *plus* left anterior fascicular block (LAH)
2. Right bundle branch block (RBBB) *plus* left posterior fascicular block (LPH)
3. Right bundle branch block (RBBB) *plus* AV conduction delay (prolonged P-R interval)
4. Right bundle branch block (RBBB) *plus* intermittent left bundle branch block (LBBB)

The last combination in fact indicates bilateral bundle branch block, hence, for purpose of electrocardiography, it is considered as a separate entity, hence, is discussed in Chapter 13.

Aetiology; The causes are;
1. Atherosclerotic heart disease.
2. Hypertensive heart disease.
3. Cardiomyopathies.
4. A complication of heart surgery.
5. Idiopathic fibrosis of mitral and aortic valve rings with subsequent calcification.
6. In association with myocardial infarction.

Clinical Significance

1. Right bundle branch block with left anterior fascicular block is the commonest bifascicular block. This type of block carries high risk of going into complete heart block.
2. When right bundle branch block is present in association with left anterior fascicular block in patients with myocardial infarction, the prognosis is bad because of two reasons;
   i. This type of bifascicular block indicates an extensive myocardial infarction.
   ii. There is risk of developing complete heart block in patients with myocardial infarction.

1. *Right bundle Branch Block with Left Anterior Fascicular Block (Figs 14.7A and B)*

This is the commonest type of bifascicular block. When right bundle branch block and left anterior fascicular block are present, then ventricular activation occurs through the midseptal fibres and left posterior fascicle. The ECG pattern will be a combination of:

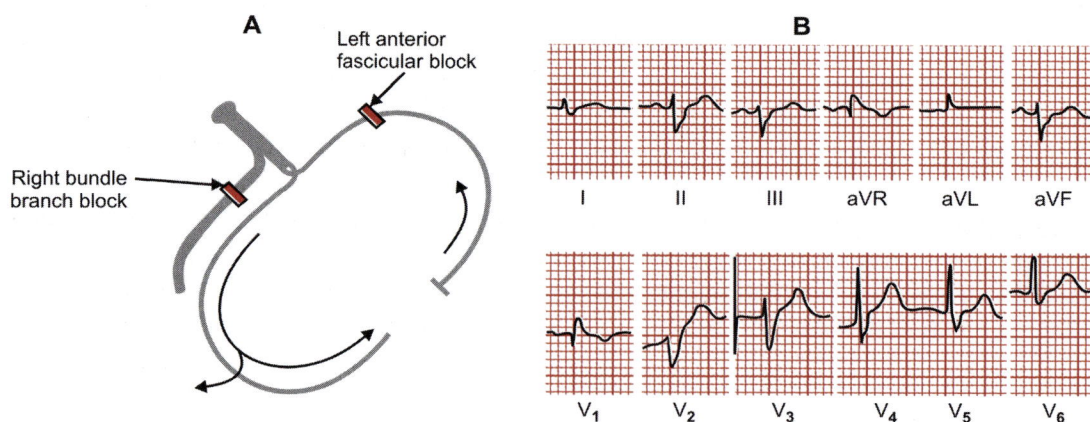

Fig. 14.7: Right bundle branch block with left anterior fascicular block (bifascicular block): **A:** Diagrammatic illustration of wave of excitation passing through the posterior fascicle leading to delayed terminal QRS forces to the right and anteriorly (shown by arrows). **B:** *The electrocardiogram:* Bifascicular block (RBBB plus left anterior fascicular block). Note the following characteristics on ECG: (i) Right bundle branch block: There is rSR' complex in lead V₁ with wide and deep S wave in V₅-V₆ and lead I, (ii) Left anterior fascicular block: The mean frontal QRS axis is superior and to the left beyond – 30° due to which there is rS complexes in leads II, III and aVF. The net negative deflection is towards the negative pole of lead III (–60°)

SECTION FOUR

i. *Right bundle branch block* – a wide R wave or rSR′ complex or R′ wave in leads V_1 and V_2 with a corresponding deep S wave in leads I, V_5 and V_6. This is due to delayed terminal QRS forces being oriented to the right and anteriorly.

ii. *Left anterior fascicular block* – It will be projected as abnormal left axis deviation > –30° on the frontal plane leads i.e. rS complex will be seen in leads II and III, where S wave will be deeper in lead III.

The pattern of RBBB with abnormal left axis deviation beyond – 30° invariably indicates a bifascicular block

2. Right Bundle Branch Block and Left Posterior Fascicular Block

Right bundle branch block with left posterior fascicular block is relatively uncommon. The ECG pattern of this disorder will be a combination of RBBB and left posterior fascicular block. The resultant vector of QRS is oriented inferiorly and to the right, and either slightly posteriorly or anteriorly due to right bundle branch block.

The Electrocardiogram (Figs 14.8A and B)
It consists of:

1. *Pattern of RBBB:* There is a wide R wave or rSR′ complex or R′ wave in V_1-V_2 with a wide slurred S wave in leads I, V_5, V_6.

2. *Abnormal right axis deviation (>+120°):* It produces taller R waves in lead III than R waves in lead II. This is due to left posterior fascicular block. Right bundle branch block alone shifts the axis towards right but not beyond +110°, hence, extreme right axis deviation > +120° occurs in the presence of left posterior fascicular block either alone or in combination with RBBB.

A combination of ECG pattern of right bundle branch block with abnormal right axis deviation beyond +120° indicates RBBB with left posterior fascicular block.

3. Right Bundle Branch Block (RBBB) with Prolonged AV Conduction

A prolonged P-R interval more than 0.20 second may be present in association with either right or left bundle branch block. The prolonged P-R interval could be due to delay in conduction through AV node (first degree AV block). In this instance, it would not indicate bifascicular block or bilateral bundle branch block. However, in most instances, bundle of His recordings have shown that the prolongation of P-R interval is due to delayed conduction distal to the bundle of His and therefore, it is an evidence of incomplete block in the opposite bundle, i.e. if right bundle branch is blocked, the prolonged P-R interval indicates delayed conduction through left bundle or its posterior fascicle. This fact is taken into consideration in the definition of trifascicular blocks which are discussed below.

The term bilateral bundle branch block be used rather than bifascicular block when alternating RBBB and LBBB are present in the same lead.

TRIFASCICULAR BLOCK (FIG. 14.9)

If all the three fascicles (right bundle branch, left anterior fascicle and left posterior fascicle) of intraventricular conduction system were completely blocked, it would be impossible to activate the ventricles by impulses from the supraventricular focus, and complete heart block with idioventricular rhythm would occur.

The term '*trifascicular block*' implies bilateral bundle branch block (right bundle branch and left anterior or posterior fascicle) with prolonged P-R interval due to; (i) delay in the intra-atrial conduction system or (ii) AV nodal delay or (iii) delay in His bundle conduction system. The normal P-R interval includes all the three above said components. Thus, P-R prolongation in the presence of bifascicular block does not always indicate a disease in the remaining fascicle of the intraventricular conduction system. In fact, there is 50% chance that AV nodal conduction delay is responsible for prolongation of P-R interval in patients with bifascicular block. Specialised technique (His bundle electrocardiography) is required to make the definite diagnosis of the location of the conduction delay.

His bundle recordings in trifascicular block have shown that the block in the conduction system lies distal to bundle of His, therefore, in the presence of right bundle branch block, the prolonged P-R interval

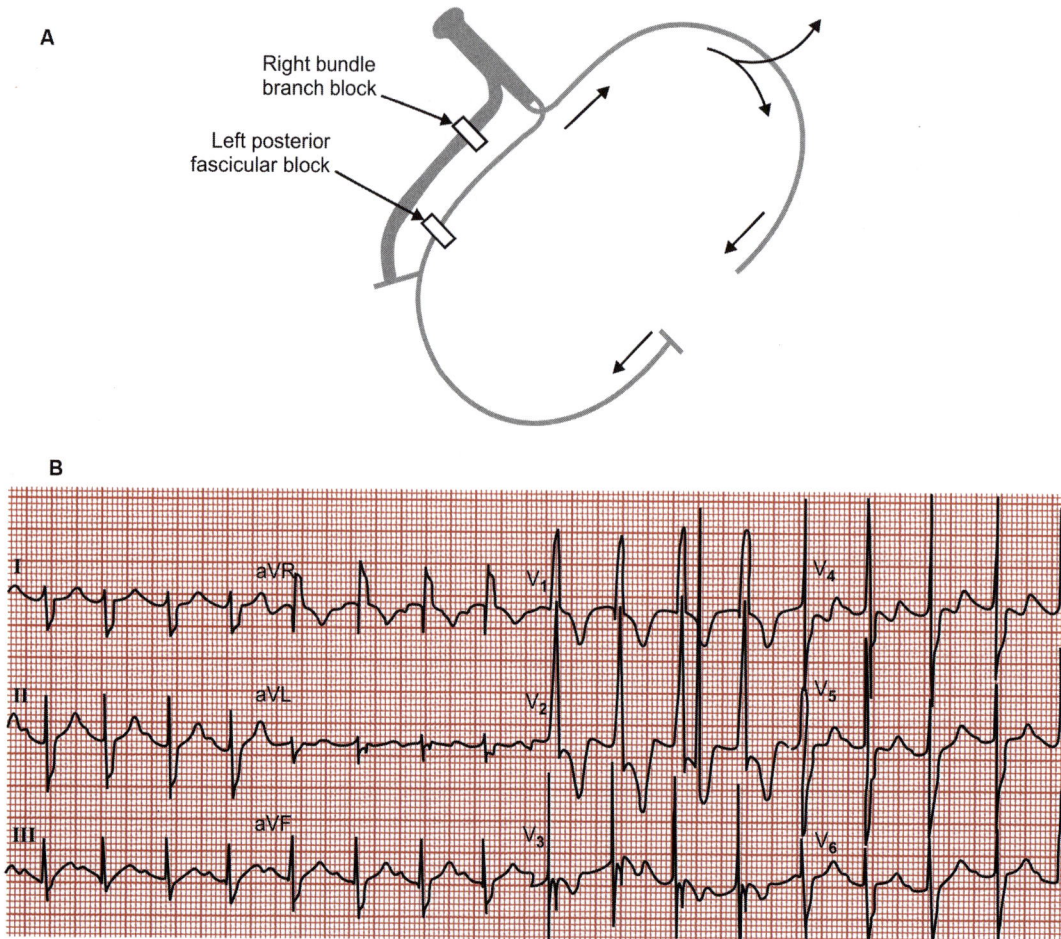

Figs 14.8A and B: Right bundle block with left posterior fascicular block.
A: Spread of excitation wave passing through the left anterior fascicle leading to terminal QRS vector oriented to the right, inferiorly and posteriorly or anteriorly (diagram).
B: Bifascicular block (RBBB plus left posterior fascicular block). The electrocardiogram was recorded from a patient who underwent surgery for ventricular septal defect (*courtesy* **Dr SS Lohchab, Head Cardiothoracic surgery**). The electrocardiogram shows: (i) *Right bundle branch block (RBBB) pattern:* There is a wide rSR' pattern in V_1-V_2 with T wave inversion. There is persistence of deep slurred S wave in V_5-V_6. (ii) *Left posterior fascicular block or hemiblock (LPH):* There is extreme right axis deviation >+ 140° of QRS on frontal plane. The right axis deviation of this magnitude can not occur with RBBB alone, indicates a delay in the left posterior fascicle in addition to RBBB

could be due to delay in conduction through the left bundle or through one of its fascicles, therefore, trifascicular block includes;
1. RBBB *plus* LAH (QRS axis > –30°) *plus* prolonged P-R interval > 0.20 sec, presumed to be due to delay of conduction through posterior fascicle. This is a commonest type.
2. RBBB *plus* LPH (right QRS deviation > + 120°) *plus* prolonged P-R interval > 0.20 sec presumed to be due to delay of conduction through anterior fascicle. This is uncommon type.

RBBB in presence of left axis deviation beyond – 30° and prolongation of P-R interval beyond normal indicate a trifascicular block of common type.

The AHA/ACC guidelines use the term 'trifascicular block' rather loosely. According to these guidelines, trifascicular block with 1:1 conduction include:
1. Alternating left bundle branch block with right bundle branch block
2. Fixed right bundle branch block plus alternating left anterior and left posterior hemiblock.

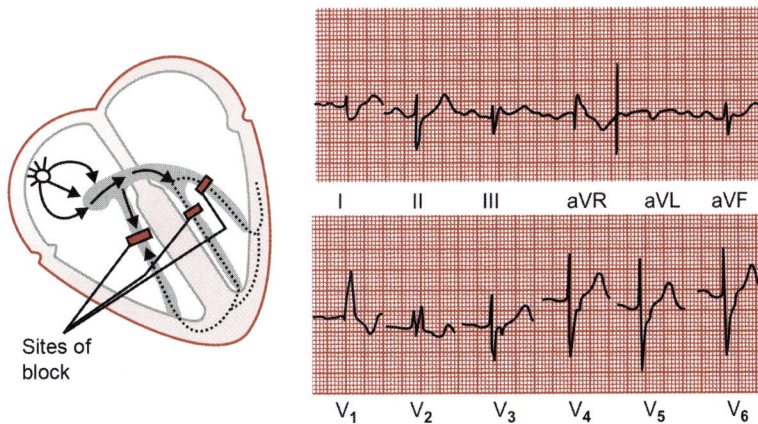

Fig. 14.9: Trifascicular block (left anterior and posterior fascicular plus RBBB)

A: Diagrammatic illustration of trifascicular block – left anterior and posterior fascicles plus right bundle branch. In this block both right and left bundle are not completely blocked. In fact, in the presence of left bundle branch block, there is still possible conduction through one of the fascicles mostly posterior fascicle which produces prolongation of P-R interval as shown by bundle of His electrocardiography.

B: The electrocardiogram showing trifascicular block (RBBB plus left anterior fascicular block and prolonged P-R interval).
Note: The following characteristics: (i) *Right bundle branch block:* There is rSR' complex in leads V_1 and V_2 with clockwise rotation and a deep, wide S wave in V_5-V_6 and lead I, (ii) *Left anterior fascicular block:* The mean frontal plane QRS axis is $-30°$ (left axis shift) and is oriented superiorly due to which there is rS complex in leads II, III and aVF. The S wave is deepest in lead II, (iii) *Left posterior fascicular block.* It is evidenced by prolongation of P–R interval which is 0.24 sec.

REVIEW AT GLANCE

Bifascicular or Bilateral Bundle Branch Block

A. Right bundle branch block (RBBB) with left anterior fascicular or hemiblock (LAH)
- Pattern of right bundle branch block (rSR' or rR' or slurred R) in V_1 and V_2 with wide S in leads I, V_5, V_6. This is due to terminal QRS orientation to the right and anteriorly.
- Left axis deviation is $> -30°$. This is due to initial QRS vector being oriented superiorly and to the left on frontal plane.

B. Right bundle branch block with left posterior fascicular block
- Typical features of RBBB as descussed above
- Right axis deviation $> +120°$.

C. Trifascicular block
1. *Right bundle branch block, left anterior fascicular block and AV conduction delay (commonest type)*
   - Pattern of RBBB as described above.
   - Left axis deviation $> -30°$.
   - Prolonged P–R interval > 0.20 sec.
2. *Right bundle branch block, left posterior fascicular block and AV conduction delay (uncommon type).*
   - Pattern of RBBB as described above.
   - Right axis deviation $> +120°$.
   - Prolonged PR interval > 0.20 sec.
3. *Right bundle branch block plus alternating left anterior and left posterior fascicular block*
   - Pattern of RBBB as described. It is fixed block.
   - Sometimes, left anterior fascicular block and, left posterior fascicular block alternates with RBBB.

Suggested Reading

1. Banchimol A, Desser KB, Barreto EC: Vectorcardiographic features of left anterior hemiblock combined with right bundle branch block. *J Electrocardiol* **4**: 322,1971.
2. Blondeau M: Complete left bundle branch block with marked left axis deviation of QRS. Clinical and anatomical study. *Adv Cardiol* **14**: 25, 1974.
3. DePasquale NP, Bruno MS: Natural history of combined right bundle branch block and left anterior hemiblock (bilateral bundle branch block). *Am J Med* **54**: 297, 1973.
4. Frink RJ, James TN: Normal blood supply to the human. His bundle and proximal bundle branches. *Circulation* **47**: 8,1973.
5. Ganbetta M, Childers RW: Rate-dependant right precordial Q waves: "Septal focal block". *AM J Cardiol* **32**: 196, 1973.

6. Kunstadt D, Punja M, Cagin N, et al: Bifascicular block: A clinical and electrophysiological study: *Am Heart J* 86: 173, 1973.

7. Lichstein E, Chadda KD, Gupta PK: Complete right bundle branch block with left axis deviation: Significance of vectorcardiographic morphology. *Am Heart J* **86**: 13,1973.

8. Lopas VM, Periera Mignel JM, doReiss DD, et al: Left posterior hemiblock: Clinical and vector cardiography study of 20 cases. *J Electrocardiol* **7**: 197, 1974.

9. Mangiola S: Intermittent left anterior hemiblock with Wenckebach phenomenon. *Am J Cardiol* **30**: 892,1972.

10. Rosenbaum MB, Elizari MV, Lazzari JO, et al: Intra-ventricular trifascicular blocks: The syndrome of right bundle branch block with intermittent left anterior and posterior hemiblock. *Am Heart J* **78**: 306, 1969.

11. Rosenbaum MB, Elizari MV, Lazzari JO, et al: The differential electrocardiographic manifestations of hemiblock, bilateral bundle branch block and trifascicular blocks. In Schlant RC and Hurst JW (Eds): *Advances in Electrocardiography*. New York: Grune and Stratton, 149–220, 1972.

12. Rosenbaum MB, Elizari MV, Lazzari JO: The hemiblock: New concept of intraventricular conduction based on human Anatomical, Physiological and Clinical studies (Olelsman, Fla: Tampa Tracings, 1970).

13. Scanlm PJ, Pryor R, Blount SG JR: Right bundle branch block associated with left superior or inferior intraventricular block, associated with acute myocardiol infarction. *Circulation* **42**: 1135, 1970.

14. Schweitzer P, Mellen HS, Rubendire M: Left posterior hemiblock. *J Electrocardiol* **4**: 204,1971.

15

The S$_I$, S$_{II}$, S$_{III}$ Syndrome

■ *Definition, mechanisms and aetiology*
■ *The electrocardiographic differentiation from left anterior fascicular block (hemiblock)*

Definition

It is an electrocardiographically expressed syndrome in which there are prominent S waves in leads I, II and III. To satisfy the definition of this syndrome, the S wave should be greater than R wave (R/S ratio < 1) in at least one of the three standard leads and the other two standard leads must register prominent S waves. However, *a small terminal s wave* in all the three standard leads which does not exceed the R wave in any lead, is not infrequent in normal electrocardiograms. This phenomenon of deep S waves in standard leads is, sometimes, referred to as the S$_I$, S$_{II}$,S$_{III}$ syndrome.

The presence of an S wave in all the standard leads (I, II and III) along with an S wave greater than R wave in any one of the three above mentioned leads constitute S$_I$, S$_{II}$, S$_{III}$ syndrome.

Mechanisms

Any condition which shifts the QRS vector superiorly and to the right, i.e. towards 'North–West zone or indeterminate axis' or "no man's land zone' (–90° counterclockwise to – 150°) will result in S$_I$, S$_{II}$, S$_{III}$ syndrome as follows.

1. Since the frontal plane QRS axis is to the right and superiorly, the mean QRS vector faces negative pole of lead II than negative poles of leads III and I (Fig. 15.1), hence, this lead will register deeper S wave than lead III and lead I. The QRS axis is aligned towards positive pole of lead aVR, hence, a R wave is recorded in this lead.

2. The extreme degree of right axis deviation will result in Qr or QR deflection in aVR and QS deflection in lead III. Therefore, S$_I$, S$_{II}$, S$_{III}$ pattern appears in the standard leads while remaining extremities leads (aVL, aVF) record rS deflections.

3. The terminal QRS vector is anteriorly oriented, so that, a positive deflection (r) wave will be seen in lead V$_1$. There may be clockwise rotation on long axis leading to RS pattern in precordial leads. The QRS duration is normal. There is ST segment depression in standard leads and aVF.

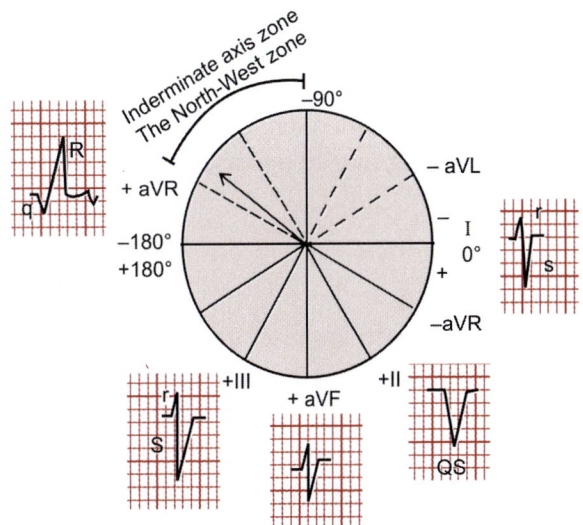

Fig. 15.1: The mean frontal plane QRS axis in S$_I$, S$_{II}$, S$_{III}$ syndrome (diagram)

Aetiology

The S_I, S_{II}, S_{III} syndrome may occur under following conditions;

1. *As a normal variant:* This may be a physiological phenomenon in young persons due to right ventricular dominance.

2. *As an expression of right ventricular hypertrophy:* The syndrome is commonly associated with right ventricular hypertrophy of congenital heart diseases, i.e. tetralogy of Fallot's, triology of Fallot's, pulmonary atresia, endocardial cushion defect or ventricular septal defect with pulmonary hypertension (Eisenmenger's syndrome) and in cases with complete transposition of great vessels.

   The S_I, S_{II}, S_{III} syndrome may also be associated with right ventricular hypertrophy of acquired heart disease, i.e. chronic cor pulmonale. When it occurs in cases of chronic cor pulmonale, then there will be both clinical and ECG evidences of right ventricular hypertrophy as well as P pulmonale of right atrial hypertrophy (Fig. 15.2). In chronic obstructive pulmonary disease, the amplitude of QRS will be markedly diminished.

3. *Anterior myocardial infarction:* This syndrome may be associated with anterior wall (apical) myocardial infarction and, once it appears, it remains permanent (Fig. 15.3).

4. *The straight back syndrome:* A pseudo-heart disease syndrome (straight back syndrome) in which there is straightening of upper dorsal spines due to loss of anterior concavity. It is a congenital osseous manifestation without any abnormality of heart. However, in extreme cases, cardiac displace-

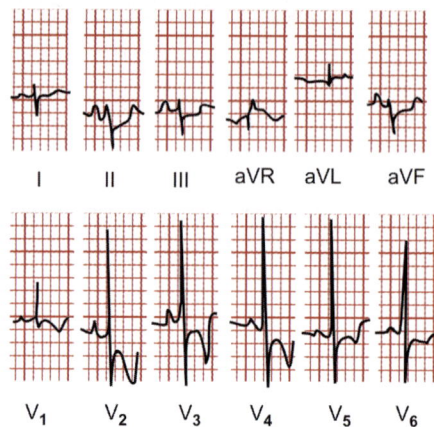

Fig. 15.2: S_I, S_{II}, S_{III} syndrome in chronic obstructive pulmonary disease with chronic cor pulmonale. The electrocardiogram shows the followings:

(i) *Right atrial hypertrophy.* The P wave axis is around + 85°, hence, P wave is taller in aVF than lead II. There is P-pulmonale-tall peaked P waves in leads II, III, aVF and all precordial leads

(ii) *Right ventricular hypertrophy with strain.* There is Rs complex in V_1 (R>S or R:S>1) through V_6 (deep S wave persists in V_5-V_6). There is marked clockwise rotation shifting the transition zone beyond V_6. The ST segment is depressed and T is inverted in leads V_1-V_6 and leads II, III and aVF indicating right ventricular strain and global ischaemia

(iii) *The S_I, S_{II}, S_{III} syndrome.* The QRS axis is shifted to North-West region and superiorly leading to S waves in leads I, II, III and S is deeper in lead II than lead III.

ment occurs and certain abnormalities appear which include;

   i. Left axis deviation.

   ii. S_I, S_{II}, S_{III} syndrome with rSr' in V_1.

The differences between S_I, S_{II}, S_{III} syndrome and left anterior hemiblock are given in the Table 15.1.

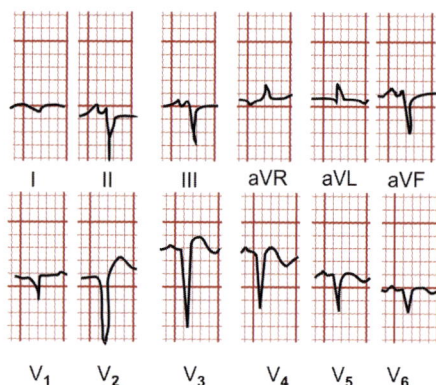

Fig. 15.3: The S_I, S_{II}, S_{III} syndrome associated with anterior wall myocardial infarction. Note the following characteristics on ECG:

(i) There is S wave in all standard leads (I, II and III). The QRS axis is oriented to North-West region along the negative pole of lead II as S wave is deeper in lead II than III, which indicates it around −140°. The QRS duration is normal

(ii) The anterior wall infarction. It is evident from QS pattern from lead V_1 through V_6 and there is ST segment elevation with convexity upwards in these leads

Table 15.1: Differentiating electrocardiographic features between S$_I$, S$_{II}$, S$_{III}$ syndrome and left anterior fascicular block or hemiblock	
S$_I$, S$_{II}$, S$_{III}$ syndrome	*Left anterior fascicular block or hemiblock*
• S wave is present in leads I, II and III.	• S wave is present in leads II, III and no S wave in lead I.
• S wave is deeper in lead II than III.	• S wave is deeper in lead III than lead II.
• QRS axis is markedly shifted to the right and superiorly facing the negative pole of lead II (–120°).	• QRS axis is shifted to the left facing the negative pole of lead III (> – 30°).

Suggested Reading

1. Delise P, Piccolo E, O'Este D, et al: Electrogenesis of S$_I$, S$_{II}$, S$_{III}$ electrocardiographic pattern. *J Electrocardiol* **23**: 23, 1990.

SECTION FOUR

Stress Electrocardiography

SECTION FIVE

16

Stress Electrocardiography

■ *Exercise electrocardiography; introduction, basis, indications, contraindications, safety and risks*
■ *Methods used and leads system employed*
■ *Sensitivity and specificity, ECG manifestations and adverse prognostic factors*
■ *Pharmacological methods–adenosine, dipyridamole, dobutamine*

EXERCISE ELECTROCARDIOGRAPHY

Introduction

Unfortunately, the diagnosis of ischaemic heart disease is often difficult to establish especially in those patients who are asymptomatic for the disease, and in those who have atypical chest pain associated with normal resting ECG. Early diagnosis is mandatory as it may benefit the patient by permitting him/her to adopt the surgical or medical therapy in time before permanent myocardial injury occurs. With this aim in mind, some forms of stress tests are used to detect or confirm the subclinical disease. These tests are performed only if control or resting ECG recorded just before commencing the test shows no acute abnormality.

Exercise electrocardiography is a noninvasive method to evaluate myocardial functions. It has become increasingly popular in early detection of ischaemic heart disease, for evaluating functional severity of ischaemic heart disease, for the effects of medical or surgical treatment and for rehabilitation of heart patients. It is hereby stressed that the electrocardiographic abnormalities observed during exercise are not *sine–quanon* for coronary artery disease and may be seen with other causes of myocardial ischaemia such as ventricular hypertrophy, anaemia; hypoxaemia, digitalis and diuretic therapy. These complicating factors must be excluded prior to exercise tests. A clinical evaluation including history, physical examination and a resting 12 lead ECG are pre-requisites for stress test. Exercise testing permits the physician to evaluate the patient by increasing workload that may result in reproduction of the patient's symptoms when they are secondary to myocardial ischaemia. Stress electrocardiography, in fact, is a noninvasive provocative test for myocardial ischaemia.

Since it is safe and simple noninvasive study; it can be repeated to assess the functional progress of the heart disease as well to test the efficacy of the therapy.

The Basis of Exercise Test

The sole aim of exercise test is based on the principle that exercise increases myocardial oxygen demand, which although adequate at rest, becomes inadequate during exercise. Consequently, the ECG manifestations which are normal or equivocal at rest, become abnormal and significant during exercise to diagnose ischaemic heart disease. Physiologically, the test evaluates the balance between O_2 demand and supply, therefore, ECG changes produced in response to exercise may provide conclusive evidence for the presence of myocardial ischaemia.

Indications of Exercise Tests

The exercise test is a simple, practical and cheap method of detecting ischaemic heart disease. It is emphasised that abnormal electrocardiogram on exercise is nothing but an electrical expression of myocardial ischaemia, and does not necessarily mean coronary artery disease as such. Certain other conditions and organic valvular lesions; for example aortic or mitral valve disease, may result in abnormal post-exercise ECG changes of myocardial ischaemia in the absence of coronary artery disease itself (False positive stress test). In these conditions, exercise can result in relative ischaemia with normal coronary arteries. Following are its indications.

1. To Evaluate the Coronary Artery Disease in Symptomatic Patients

A normal electrocardiogram does not exclude the likelihood of coronary artery disease in symptomatic patients, on the other hand, electrocardiographic changes developed in response to exercise may provide a confirmatory evidence in such patients. Therefore, the greatest diagnostic value of exercise test is in those patients; who either have an uncertain or equivocal evidence of ischaemic heart disease or have an atypical history of chest pain. It is useful in evaluation of the patients with post-myocardial angina, is also done as follow-up of patients who had a recent episode of infarction and in patients with known coronary artery disease.

It has been observed that majority of patients with occlusive coronary artery disease have a normal or near normal ECG at rest even though they may have long history of angina pectoris. Under these circumstances, exercise test is desirable for an objective confirmation of ischaemic heart disease.

2. For Screening of Asymptomatic Patients

The prevalence of ischaemic heart disease is also high in asymptomatic patients especially in those who are at high risk to develop it, such as patients with diabetes mellitus, familial hyperlipidaemia, myxoedema, etc. It has also been documented that coronary artery disease may be present in an apparent healthy and asymptomatic young men around 40 years of age. This too may be revealed by exercise test. This test has been documented as a screening procedure for the individuals who present themselves for a routine, often annual medical check up and/or applicants for life insurance. Secondly, it has been adopted as a screening procedure for men above 40 years who are in special occupations (pilots, firefighters, police personnel, drivers and rail road engineers), or who have two or more coronary risk factors or who plan to enter a vigorous exercise programme.

The exercise test can also form a baseline in patients with asymptomatic coronary artery disease for repeat evaluations in subsequent years.

3. Severity of Coronary Artery Disease

The abnormality of ST segment such as depression more than 2 mm on exercise test indicates a more severe disease than depression of 1 mm segment.

4. To Test Effectiveness of Treatment

A follow-up exercise test is done for this purpose, which may reflect the efficacy of treatment.
A. *Coronary artery bypass surgery:* The aim of exercise test is to document that expected improvement has been obtained after surgery and to evaluate patients with suspected incomplete coronary revascularisation and graft occlusion.
B. *Percutaneous transluminal coronary angioplasty (PTCA):* It is a useful parameter in evaluation of functional improvement after PTCA. It may be done 3-5 days after PTCA. Late testing during follow-up is useful to detect restenosis.

5. Evaluation of Symptoms

For evaluation of symptoms such as palpitation, dyspnoea, fatigue in patients with coronary artery disease, the exercise test is useful.

6. Arrhythmias Analysis

Exercise test is sometimes used in arrhythmias analysis in response to exercise such as ventricular ectopics to know whether they are abolished or aggravated by exercise.

7. Left Ventricular Functional Assessment

During rehabilitation of acute myocardial infarction, inducible ischaemia in this period reflects still viable and jeopardised myocardium. The decision to advise coronary angiography or revascularisation and balloon angioplasty depends on the outcome of these stress tests.

8. Prognosis in Coronary Artery Disease

The severity of ST changes and arrhythmias on exercise test indirectly are related to prognosis in ischaemic heart disease. The adverse prognostic factors on exercise test are discussed further in this chapter.

9. To Study Exercise Capacity in Valvular Heart Disease

Exercise testing is done to obtain exercise capacity in patients with valvular heart disease. This is useful guide in decision–making regarding cardiac catheterisation and surgery.

10. Evaluation of Congenital Heart Disease

Exercise test is useful in congenital mild aortic stenosis, and also in studying postoperative patients with tetralogy of Fallot and other complex defects. Severe or critical aortic stenosis is a contraindication for the test.

> *The most frequent indications for exercise or stress electrocardiography are; to aid in establishing the diagnosis of coronary artery disease, in determining functional capacity and in estimating prognosis.*

Safety and Risks of Exercise Testing

Exercise testing has an excellent safety record. In non–selected patients population, the mortality is 0.01% and morbidity is 0.05%. This risk is determined by the clinical characteristics of the patient subjected to this procedure. The risk is greater when the test is performed soon after an acute ischaemic episode. Symptom-related protocol is associated with more risk than low level protocol. Exercise testing can be performed safely in patients with compensated heart failure but risk is increased when test is performed in patients with life-threatening arrhythmias. After an uncomplicated acute myocardial infarction, it is wise to wait for one week before testing. The standard 12 lead ECG should be verified before the test for any acute or recent change. After an episode of unstable

angina, patient should be symptom-free (free of rest pain) at least 72 hours before testing. The contraindications of stress testing are given in the box.

Therefore it is pertinent that one must weigh the potential benefits of informations against the risks involved with an individual patient. The conditions associated with low risk are also summarised in the box.

Contraindications to stress testing

High risk individuals
- Unstable angina with recent chest pain.
- Uncontrolled cardiac arrhythmias (life-threatening).
- Severe congestive heart failure.
- Advanced atrioventricular blocks.
- Known severe coronary artery disease pattern, e.g. left main coronary artery stenosis.
- Impending or acute myocardial infarction.
- Critical aortic stenosis.
- Uncontrolled severe hypertension.
- Severe hypertrophic obstructive cardiomyopathy.
- Acute systemic illness.
- Ventricular aneurysm.
- Severe associated diseases such as pulmonary insufficiency, renal failure, uncontrolled diabetes or thyrotoxicosis, etc.

Low risk individuals
- Stable angina pectoris.
- Past history of supraventricular or ventricular arrhythmias.
- Conduction distrubances such as bundle branch blocks.
- Left to right shunts.
- Chronic stable valvular disease.
- Nonspecific ECG abnormalities of T wave or ST segment.
- Clinical or ECG evidence of ventricular hypertrophy.

The Standardised Methods for Exercise Testing

The exercise test must be performed in a standardised manner to permit comparison with other patient's data and evaluation of changes that occur with repeated testing. To obtain good results from exercise test, a competent physician, a willing well-informed and ambulatory patient, a standardised testing procedure and a suitable recording room are essential. An uncooperative patient will often '*under-achieve*' during an exercise test which may hamper the results or interpretations. Such uncooperative patients may be seeking disability compensation or may be using his apparent disabilities as a psychological crutch to obtain attention or reward. The physician must be alert for this type of patient who may purposely try to injure himself during an exercise test.

Methods

The standardised methods for exercise testing include;

  i) The Master's two steps exercise test (A submaximal exercise test).
  ii) Standardised protocols for treadmill exercise testing (multistage exercise testing).

The Master's Two Steps Exercise Test

Master and his associates standardised the technique according to age, sex and weight. Using these parameters, tables were constructed based on the return of BP and pulse rate to normal within 2 minutes. The exercise is performed on a special standardised two steps apparatus (wooden plateform) and the patient is required to do a certain number of ascents and descents in 12 minutes period over a device–two steps high with three steps; two of which are 9 inches above the floor and a top step is 18 inches high from the floor.

The validity of the test may be questioned because it is a submaximal test done to determine heart rate in response to exercise. It has been presumed that ECG changes following exercise parellel to the rise in pulse rate and BP. The sensitivity of exercise test as a predictor of the presence of significant coronary artery disease is directly proportional to the effort required by the exercise. In screening asymptomatic patients, the number of patients with positive response to the exercise test is increased by 15% when the end point of the exercise effort is increased from 85% of the age predicted maximal heart rate to minimal exercise effort. Provided its limitations as discussed, Master's two steps test has lost its significance due to availability of maximal stress test (bicycle ergometer or treadmill).

Master's two steps test is a submaximal test, not used nowadays

Bicycle Ergometer

Bicycle ergometer protocol involves incremental workload caliberated in Watts or Kiloponds (KPD)/meter/minute. One Watt is equivalent to 6 KPD/meter/min. Both mechanically braked and electronically braked bicycles may be used, the latter is preferred because it provides constant workload inspite of changes in pedalling rate but they are costlier. Most protocols begin at a workload of 25 Watts, and 25 Watts increments after every 2 minutes. Young patients may start with 50 Watts. Two types of protocol, i.e. ramp protocol and staged protocol can be employed. A ramp protocol differs from the staged protocols in that the patient starts at 3 minutes of unloaded pedaling at cycle speed of 60 rpm, workload is increased by a uniform amount each minute depending on the expected patient performance.

It is used when patient is unable to do treadmill exercise. It is method of exercise test during radio-nuclide ventriculography and for dynamic testing during cardiac catheterisation.

Treadmill Test (Fig. 16.1)

There are several protocols available, the choice of which depends on expected effort tolerance. Multistage treadmill exercise testing is a safe and a

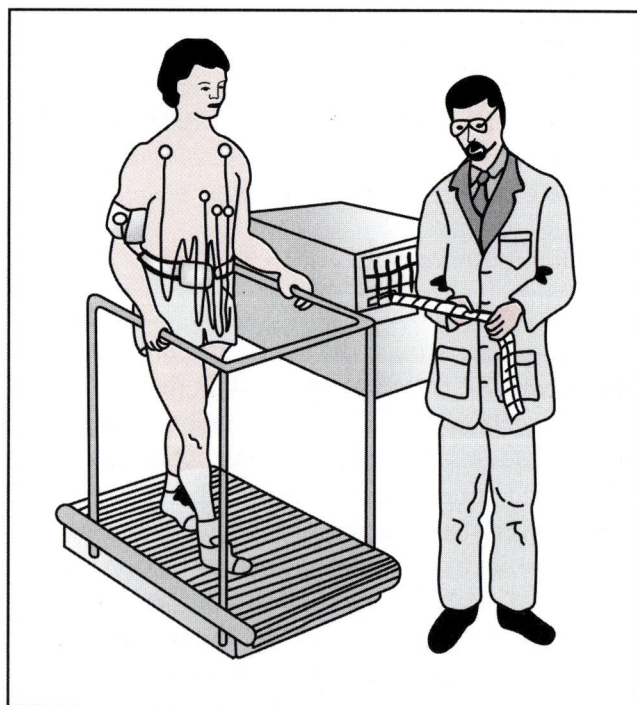

Fig. 16.1: Exercise treadmill test. The ECG and blood pressure are continuously recorded as the patient walks in place on treadmill. The inclination of slope and speed of the treadmill are gradually increased during the test

reliable method. Exercise performance on a treadmill is adjustable to three basic variables:

1. The speed of treadmill can be adjusted.
2. The grade and slope of treadmill can be varied.
3. The duration of exercise can be adjusted.

The amount of exercise prescribed may be maximal or submaximal. A maximal exercise test is individualised to a self-determined end point such as fatigue, chest pain of angina, dyspnoea, exhaustion–called '*symptom-limited testing*'. With submaximal exercise test, the amount of work load is predetermined to an arbitrary end-point, could be a predetermined target heart rate called '*heart rate-limited exercise testing*'.

Bruce Protocol

The most frequent protocol used for treadmill test is that devised by Bruce. This has a relatively higher initial workload with greater subsequent work increments. The subject starts at 1.7 MPH on a 10% incline and progresses to his/her maximum capacity at 3 minutes intervals.

With increasing speed and grade of incline of the treadmill (Table 16.1), depending on the exercise capacity of the individual, a total time may be as short as few seconds for a severely incapacitated class IV cardiac patients or as long as 21 minutes for the well trained long distance runner. The average time for ambulatory cardiac patient is 10-12 minutes, if each stage is spaced at 3 minutes interval.

Submaximal (heart rate limited) testing may also be performed by using Bruce's method of treadmill

Table 16.1: The Bruce protocol for treadmill testing

Stage (at 2 minutes interval)	Speed (MPH)	Grade %	Duration of exercise (minutes)	Approx O_2* cost
Rest	—	—	—	4
I	1.7	10	0-3	17
II	2.5	12	3-6	25
III	3.4	14	6-9	34
IV	4.2	16	9-12	44
V	5.0	18	12-15	56
VI	5.5	20	15-18	—
VII	6.0	22	18-21	—

* O_2 cost = Estimated O_2 consumption in ml of O_2/kg of body weight per minute.

Table 16.2: Age and maximal heart rates in normal males

Age (yrs)	Maximal heart rate (beats/min) Average	Range	85% maximal heart rate (beats/min)
20	204	184–215	174
25	200	180–210	170
30	197	180–210	168
35	194	180–202	165
40	191	180–200	163
45	189	178–204	161
50	182	162–194	155
55	179	174–195	153
60	177	164–192	151
65	173	—	148
70	169	—	144

Note: The numerical values are average values for age. Note the wide variation in heart rate. It is possible for a normal person of 50 years to have maximal heart rate of 194 and a 30 years young man to have maximum of only 180. The same limitations apply to 85% of predicted values.

speed and grade of incline (Table 16.2). The table shows the average heart rates at various ages at 85% and 100% maximal heart rate. The treadmill exercise is continued until the patient attains 85% of age predicted heart rate or until an indication for stopping the test develops.

Treadmill test is a commonly employed procedure by using Bruce protocol

By using Bruce protocol, one can compare a patient's data against a large body of collected data. The performa for modified Bruce protocol is given at the end of chapter.

The Naughton protocol This has low initial workload and small work increments in subsequent stages. It is used for patients with limited exercise tolerance such as patients after myocardial infarction or coronary artery bypass surgery or patients with congestive heart failure.

A protocol used for patients with limited exercise tolerance/capacity

The Cornell protocol. It is a modification of the Bruce protocol with smaller increments at 2 minutes stages, permitting a reliable estimate of ST/HR slope measurement, a parameter useful in diagnostic testing.

SECTION FIVE

Non-standardised Methods

With these methods, the amount of exercise given is according to the needs of the patients. The patient may be asked (i) to perform a few knee bends (ii) do a moderate degree of running on the spot or (iii) sit up a few minutes from supine position. The patient may be subjected to approximately amount of exertion which he/she knows will bring about an attack of angina pectoris. These are not used nowadays.

Preparation of the Patient

A detailed clinical examination and evaluation of resting 12 lead ECG must be done before treadmill test is ordered. The patient should be fasting for a least 2 hours before the test. If the purpose of the test is diagnostic, then every medicine being taken should be stopped; but when the purpose of the test is to evaluate functional capacity including response to treatment; then medication should be continued.

The conditions needed for successful performing of the test are listed in the box.

The Lead System Employed

1. *12 leads surface ECG:* This system is most frequently used for evaluation of ischaemic heart disease in which myocardial ischaemia may be detected in certain leads but not in others.

2. *Single bipolar lead system* – When single lead is monitored, then the most frequently used lead is CM_5 (Continuous monitoring lead V_5). However, it is infrequently used at present.

The patient is continuously monitored as he/she goes through various stages of exercise. Patient should be encourged so as to gain his/her confidence to enable him/her to perform a truely symptom-free exercise test.

A 12 lead surface ECG is employed for exercise electrocardiography

Post-test Evaluation

In post-exercise test, the sitting position is most frequently employed. Heart should be auscultated for any gallop sound, mitral regurgitation or pulmonary rales. Observations after exercise are continued for at least 6 minutes or longer till the exercise induced abnormalities have disappeared.

The Sensitivity and the Specificity of Exercise Testing

Since the accuracy of the interpretation of the exercise ECG for the disease being diagnosed depends on the

---

Pre-requisites for successful exercise test

- *Calm and quite atmosphere.*
- *Procedure to be fully explained to the patient so as to allay fear and anxiety. An informed written consent is required.*
- *No evidence of sinus tachycardia.*
- *No smoking at least 3 hours before testing.*
- *Test should not be performed within a week of cold or other infections.*
- *Test to be abandoned in case of chest discomfort, feeling of faintness or pallor.*
- *A sphygmomanometer cuff is wrapped around arm and a stethoscope diaphragm taped in position at point of apex beat.*
- *The exercise is performed according to standardised or non-standardised method.*
- *Physician presence is essential.*
- *Patient should wear comfortable shoes and loose-fitting clothes.*

- *Warm room (temperature between 18-22°C)*
- *Patient should be free of pain and congestive heart failure.*

- *Test should be performed before meals.*
- *Should stop vasodilators and beta-blockers for at least 3 to 5 half-lives of the drug and digitalis for 1-2 weeks before the test; if test is being done for diagnostic purpose.*
- *If angina is induced by cold and basal ECG being normal; the test is repeated with holding a piece of ice wrapped in gauze in each hand.*
- *The electrodes must be clean. The skin should be shaven propely for good electrode contact.*

Table 16.3: Prevalences of documented coronary artery disease on angiograms in patients undergoing stress tests for evaluation of chest pain

Description of chest pain	Age < 50 years		Age > 50 years	
	Men	Women	Men	Women
Nonspecific chest pain	10%	5%	20%	7%
Chest pain of probable cardiac origin	55%	30%	70%	35%
Chest pain of definite cardiac origin	85%	60%	95%	75%

prevalence of the disease (Table 16.3), careful clinical evaluation of the patient prior to exercise test is most important.

Techniques

A standard 12-leads ECG is recorded before the start of the test with the electrodes on distal extremities, a torso ECG (arm electrodes placed in torso position–upper limb electrodes below the clavicles and lower limb electrodes above the iliac crests) should be obtained in the supine position and in the sitting or standing position. Positional changes can bring out labile ST-T changes. Hyperventilation is not recommended before exercise, however, if a false positive test is suspected, then hyperventilation should be performed after the test and the tracing so obtained is compared with the maximum ST abnormalities observed. Now the patient is instructed how to perform the test, in case if symptoms (palpitation dyspnoea, pain chest, fatique) develop, he/she should raise an alarm. The heart rate, BP and ECG should be recorded at the end of each stage of exercise, immediately before, and immediately after stopping exercise, at the onset of an ischaemic response, and for each minute for at least 5-10 minutes in the recovery phase or until the ECG returns to the baseline pattern. Continuous ECG monitoring is done throughout the test since the limb leads are applied in torso position in exercising patient rather than upper and lower limbs. A torso ECG is recorded during exercise test to reduce motion artifact. The torso ECG results in right axis shift, increased voltage in the inferior leads and may produce a loss of inferior Q waves and development of new Q waves in lead aVL, thus, torso ECG can not be used to interpret a

diagnostic resting 12-leads ECG. The more proximal (cephalad) the leg electrodes, the greater is the degree of change and greater is the amplification of R wave potentiating exercise induced changes.

True positive ECG result: A patient with history of typical effort angina is likely to have underlying coronary artery disease, so, an exercise ECG suggesting myocardial ischaemia is likely to be positive, called true positive ECG result (an abnormal test result in an individual with disease).

False positive ECG result: In contrast to above, a patient with nonspecific chest pain not indicative of angina is unlikely to have coronary artery disease; so, an abnormal ECG on exercise, if present, is likely to represent false positive test result (an abnormal test result in an individual without disease). The causes of false positive ECG test are given in Table 16.4.

True negative ECG result: If an exercise ECG is normal in an individual without coronary artery disease; the test result is called true negative.

False negative ECG result: Patients with typical chest pain of angina who have a normal exercise ECG result but have coronary artery disease documented on angiogram, should be considered to have anatomical coronary disease which either is not associated with demonstrable myocardial ischaemia or does not produce ECG abnormalities for other physiological or technical reasons, are said to have false negative ECG result (normal test result in an individual with documented coronary artery disease). The causes of false negative ECG results are given in Table 16.5.

Table 16.4: Causes of false positive exercise ECGs

1. Hyperventilation
2. Abnormal depolarisation and repolarisation of left ventricle
   - LBBB
   - WPW conduction disturbance
3. Left ventricular hypertrophy (LVH)
4. Digitalis administration
5. Baseline abnormalities due to;
   - Nonspecific ST–T wave changes
   - Hypokalaemia
   - Positional ST–T changes
   - Mitral valve prolapse (MVP)
   - Vasoregulatory abnormalities

Definitions of terms in relation to some clinical tests

1. *Sensitivity of the test for the abnormality (%)* =

$$\dfrac{\text{No. of true positive results}}{\substack{\text{No. of patients with the abnormality}\\ \text{(True Positive + False Negative results)}}} \times 100$$

2. *Specificity of the test for the abnormality (%)* =

$$\dfrac{\text{No. of true negative results}}{\substack{\text{No. of patients without the abnormality}\\ \text{(True Negative + False Positive results)}}} \times 100$$

3. *Pre-test risk (probability of the abnormality in the patient undergoing test or prevalence of the abnormality)*

$$= \dfrac{\text{No. of patients in a given population having the abnormality}}{\text{All the patients in the given population}} \times 100$$

4. *Post-test risk (probability of the abnormality in the patient undergoing the test, who has a given test result)*

$$= \dfrac{\substack{\text{No. of patients with given pre-test risk and the}\\ \text{abnormality showing the given test result}}}{\text{All the patients with this test result}} \times 100$$

Or

$$= \dfrac{\text{Prevalence} \times \text{Sensitivity}}{(\text{Prevalence} \times \text{sensitivity}) + (1 - \text{prevalence})(1 - \text{specificity})}$$

Predictive value: percentage of patients with abnormal test who have the disease (CAD) =

$$\dfrac{\text{True positive results}}{\text{True positive + False positive results}} \times 100$$

Predictive value: percentage of patients with normal result out of normal test without disease (CAD)

$$= \dfrac{\text{True negative}}{\text{True negative + False negative}} \times 100$$

Test accuracy: percentage of true test result =

$$\dfrac{\text{True positive + True negative}}{\text{Total no of tests done}} \times 100$$

Likelihood ratio: (i) if test is abnormal = sensitivity (1–specificity)
(ii) if test is normal = specificity (1– sensitivity)

Table 16.5: Causes of false negative exercise ECGs

1. Angiographically documented lesions not able to produce functional myocardial ischaemia
2. Use of single monitoring ECG lead system
3. Postmyocardial infarction changes which obscures ischaemic ECG abnormalities

Table 16.6: Predictive accuracy of exercise ECG for the diagnosis of coronary artery disease

	Positive test		Negative test	
	Men	Women	Men	Women
Angina pectoris				
• Typical	100%	83%	55%	45%
• Probable	82%	45%	70%	71%
Non-cardiac chest pain	45%	0%	83%	97%

The definition of sensitivity or specificity, pre-test or post-test risk of any clinical test are given in the box. This applies to stress tests also.

For treadmill exercise testing, the mean test sensitivity based on meta-analysis of published reports is about 68% (sensitivity increases directly with increasing extent and severity of the ischaemia) and mean specificity of about 77% (Tables 16.3 and 16.6). The post-test risk of the disease will reflect the pretest risk for the disease together with the added information provided by the test itself.

End Points for Termination of Stress Test

Exercise tests are terminated when the patient develops symptoms and signs of myocardial ischaemia as given in the Table 16.7.

Electrocardiographic Manifestations of Stress Testing and their Interpretation

The exercise test is not a substitute for clinical diagnosis. It is just an aid to clinical diagnosis, hence,

Table 16.7: Indications for termination of stress tests

1. *Symptoms*
   - Anginal pain
   - Dizziness
   - Shortness of breath
   - Unsteady gait
2. *Signs*
   - Abnormal ST segment depression (≥ 3 mm) or elevation (≥1mm) in non–Q wave leads
   - Hypotension in the presence of pain and/or abnormal ECG
3. *Arrhythmias*
   - Ventricular tachycardia (3 or more VPCs in succession)
   - Multiform VPCs
   - Abrupt bradyarrhythmias
4. *Blood pressure abnormalities*
   - Systolic pressure > 250 mmHg
   - Hypotension (10 mm or more fall in systolic pressure below the basal value)
5. *Heart rate*
   - Decreasing heart rate

the proper evaluation of the exercise test is essential in context of clinical findings.

Two fundamental principles govern the interpretation of the exercise test;
1. Proper interpretation of ECG abnormalities on exercise testing.
2. Evaluation of these ECG abnormalities in terms of the associated circumstances, i. e.;
   i) The heart rate at which they appear
   ii) The exercise level at which they appear
   iii) The time course of their development
   iv) The clinical presentation

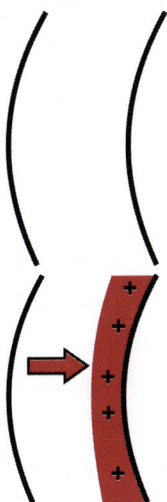

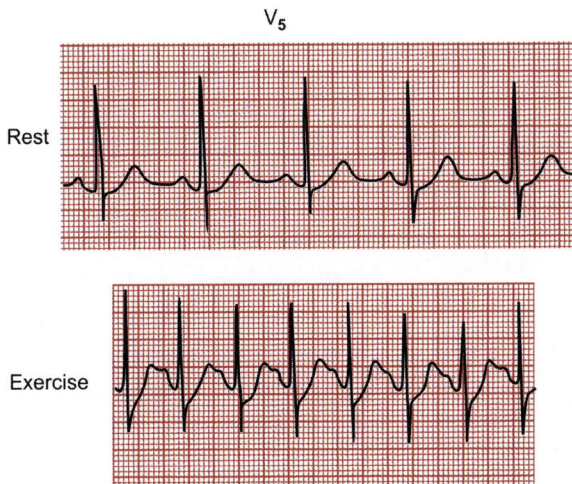

ECG Patterns and their Significance

1. **Normal exercise electrocardiogram** (Fig. 16.2)
When heart rate increases during exercise, certain predictable changes occur in normal ECG. The P-R, QRS and QT intervals shorten, the P wave becomes taller and atrial depolarisation wave (T_a wave) becomes prominent causing depression of PR segment. This results in depression of J point (junctional point between S wave and ST segment) for a short period of 0.04 sec. The normal ST segment with exercise is upsloping and slightly convex in form and returns to baseline within 0.04 to 0.06 sec after J point.

2. **Abnormal exercise electrocardiogram**
The quality of ST segment depression, shape and slope of the segment and time relationship of ST and T wave changes have emerged as most significant parameters of myocardial ischaemia. The abnormalities that can appear on ECG during exercise testing signifying myocardial ischaemia are ;

1. *The ST segment*
   - Depression of ST segment
   - Elevation of ST segment
2. *The T wave*
   - Inversion of T wave
   - Increased amplitude of upright T wave
3. *The U wave*
   - Exercise induced inversion of U wave
4. *The QRS complex*
   - A change in the amplitude of the R wave
   - A change in the magnitude of small initial Q wave

SECTION FIVE

V_5

Rest

Exercise

Fig. 16.2: Normal exercise response. The lead V_5 recorded at rest and during exercise shows the depression of J point 2 mm during exercise (-) with rapid upsloping ST segment. The ST segment is depressed about 1 mm for < 80 msec after J point. The ST segment slope is about > 3.0 mV/sec. This response is normal to exercise

5. *Conduction defects*
   - An intraventricular conduction defect such as a bundle branch block or a hemiblock.
6. *The Q-T interval*
   - Lengthening of QT_c on exercise.
7. *QX/QT ratio* (Fig. 16.3)
   - QX more than 50% of QT where X is the point at which ST segment meets isoelectric line.
8. *Cardiac rhythms*

   Exercise may affect the cardiac rhythm and may produce exercise induced arrhythmias.

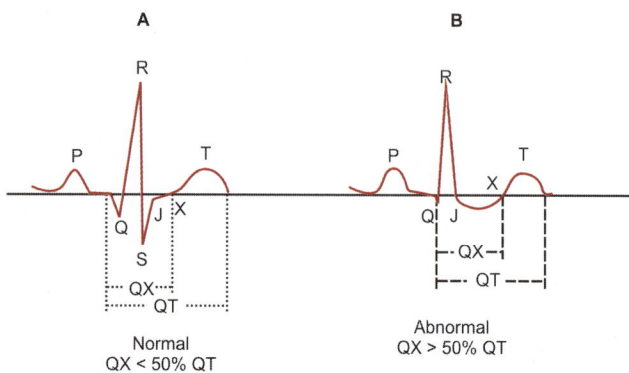

Fig. 16.3: QX /QT ratio. (A) Normal QX is less than 50% of QT interval (QX/QT ratio < 50%). (B) When QX is increased and becomes more than 50% of QT (QX/QT ratio > 50%) it indicates ischaemia

The concept of measuring the QX/QT was introduced as a method of evaluating ST segment depression in order to separate moderate J point changes from true ischaemic abnormalities (Fig. 16.3). At that time, it was assumed that ST depression due to ischaemia persists longer than that associated with tachycardia or changes in the ventricular gradient. It was proposed that a QX/QT ratio of 50% or more would be a reliable point of differentiation. Later on it was found that QX/QT ratio > 50% occurs in significant number of cases other than ischaemia and even in one study, it was reported upto 61%, therefore, it was considered as invalid in determining in presence of ischaemia, hence, is obsolete nowadays.

1. The ST Segment Changes

The J point, the ST segment and the ST slope are measured for any ST segment change (depression/elevation). The method of ST segment (non-computerised) measurement is demonstrated in Figure 16.4A and depression of J point, ST segment and its slope in Figure 16.4B. For submaximal tests, such as two step Master's test, a horizontal or downsloping of ST segment depression of 0.5 mm or more in any lead except aVR after exercise is an empirically established criteria for abnormality. In Bruce protocol, positive stress test is ST depression > 1 mm for 80 msec (Fig. 16.4C). For other submaximal tests, such as 85% of maximal predicted heart rate or for maximal tests, the followings are the parameters of abnormality for ST change (Fig. 16.5).

a) *Minor ST segment change:* The minor ST segment depression < 1.0 mm occasionally occurs in coronary artery disease (Fig. 16.5) but is not usually considered as positive response (Fig. 16.6).

b) *Upsloping ST segment:* The ST segment depression of 1.5 mm for 80 msec (0.08 sec) beyond the J point below the baseline constitutes a positive response.

c) *Horizontal ST segment:* When ST segment is horizontal or downsloping, 1.0 mm depression for 0.08 sec from the J point is considered as positive test and correlates well with the presence of ischaemic heart disease (Fig. 16.7).

d) *Rounded ST segment:* A rounded ST segment depression represents positive response; these patients with such configuration of ST segment are usually at high risk of future coronary events.

e) *Early onset and maximum ST depression during exercise:* In a significant number of cases, ST segment depression does not occur during or immediately after exercise but appears late in the recovery period (3-8 minutes). This is almost associated with normal coronary arteries. On the other hand, early onset, maximum depression of ST segment during exercise and its persistence into recovery phase constitutes an ischaemic response (Fig. 16.8).

f) *ST segment elevation* **(Fig. 16.9):** When ST segment elevation appears with exercise, it usually indicates either a ventricular akinetic or dyskinetic segment or a high grade lesion in the proximal left anterior descending coronary artery depending on whether it appears in a non-Q wave or a Q wave infarct lead.

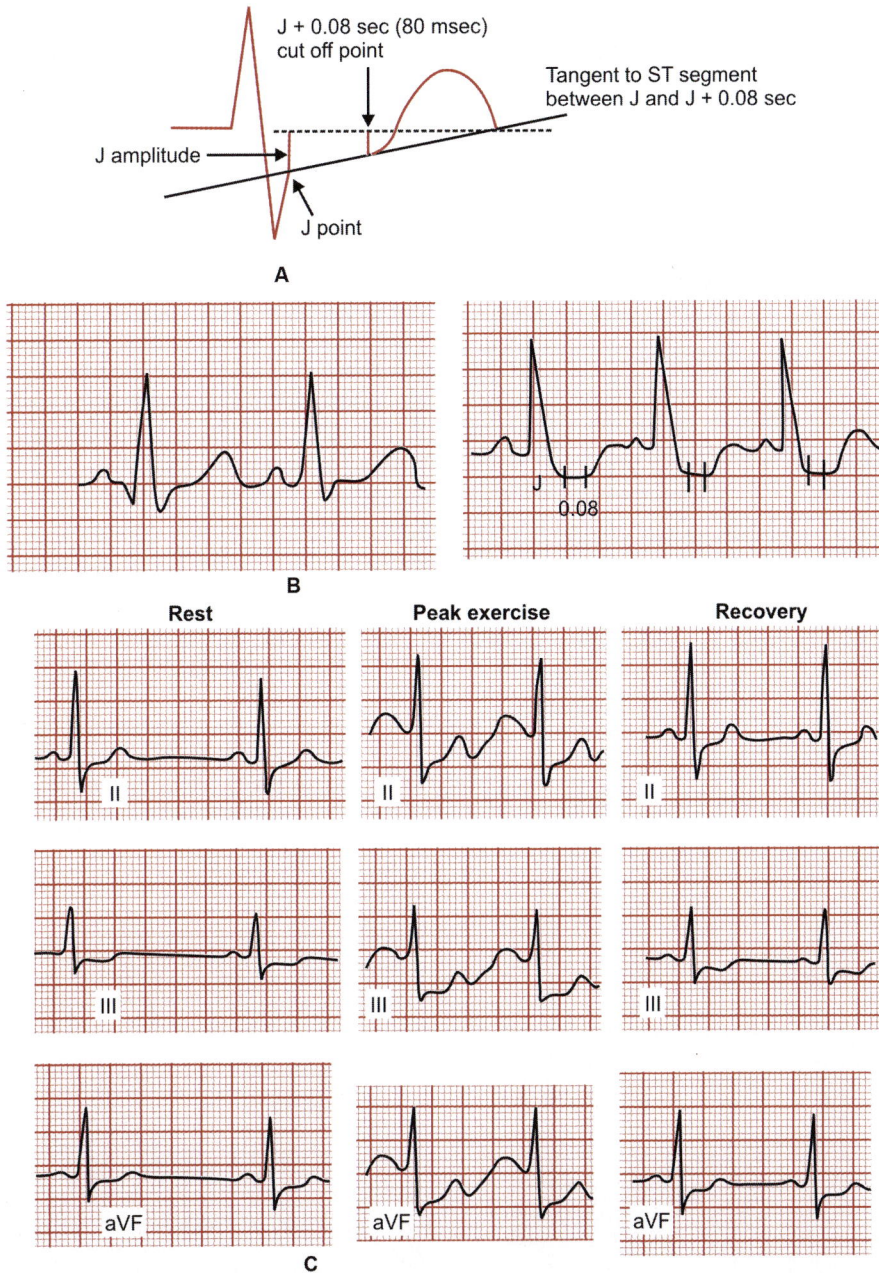

Fig. 16.4: The ST segment slope and ST segment area (diagram)

A: Method of measurement (noncomputerised)

B: Normal (rest) and abnormal ST segment during stress test (computerised measurement)

C: Positive stress test (Bruce protocol).

1. Normal ST segment and T wave recorded at rest
2. During exercise there is depression of the J point and ST segment by > 1 mm with horizontality for > 0.08 sec. The T wave is upright. The Changes persist in recovery phase.

Patients with Prinzmetal's angina–a variant angina due to coronary spasm, do not show ST change during exercise.

g) *ST intergral and slope:* ST segment integral is the area below the baseline subtended by ST segment. This area increases with increase in

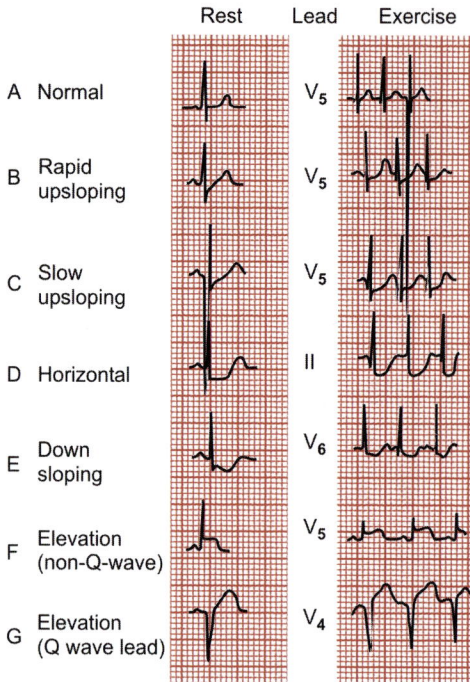

Fig. 16.5: The electrocardiographic illustration of various typical exercise patterns observed at rest and at peak exercise or stress. At least three average complexes with a stable baseline should meet the criteria for abnormality before the ECG is labelled as abnormal. The J point and ST segment slope at a fixed time point after J point to 80 msec of ST segment are analysed for any abnormality. The various patterns observed are;

A. Normal ST segment.

B. Rapid upsloping ST segment. This is a normal response to exercise. Depression of J point with rapid upsloping ST segment is common in old aged health persons.

C. *Slow upsloping ST segment depression:* It includes depression of J point, 80 msec ST depression of ≥ 0.15 mV and ST segment slope > 1.0 mV/sec. It demonstrates an ischaemic response in patients with documented coronary artery disease or those at high risk of coronary disease.

D. *Horizontal of ST segment depression:* It includes depression of J point and ST segment (80 msec from J point) of ≥ 0.1 mV and ST segment slope is within normal range (± 1.0 mV/sec). This form of ST segment constitutes classical criteria for myocardial ischaemia.

E. *Downsloping ST segment depression:* It includes depression of J point and ST segment (80 msec) of > 0.1 mV (mm) and ST segment slope is > 1.0 mV/sec. This is considered as an ischaemic response.

F. *ST segment elevation in a non-Q wave, noninfarct lead:* It includes elevation of J point and ST segment (60 msec) of ≥ 1.0 mV and indicates a severe degree of ischaemia.

G. *ST segment elevation in Q wave infarct lead:* It includes the same criteria as described above, but as it occurs in a Q wave lead, hence, indicates a severe wall motion abnormality rather than an ischaemic response.

Note: This is hand drawn noncomputerised electrographic expression.

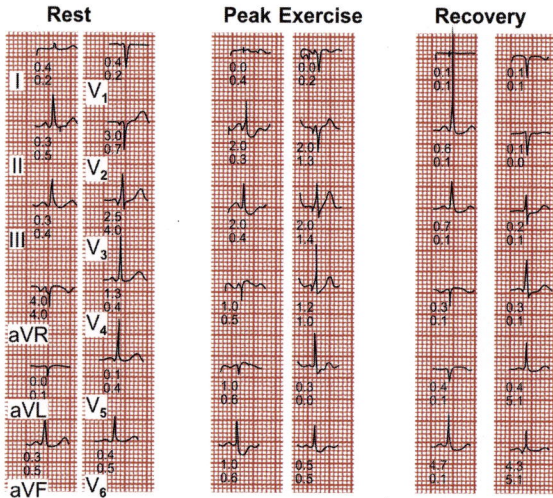

Fig. 16.6: Exercise electrocardiogram showing minor ST segment change (ST depression <1.0 mm) in leads V_4-V_6 during peak exercise and its normalisation during recovery period, occasionally, occurs in patients of ischaemic heart disease, but is not considered as positive response

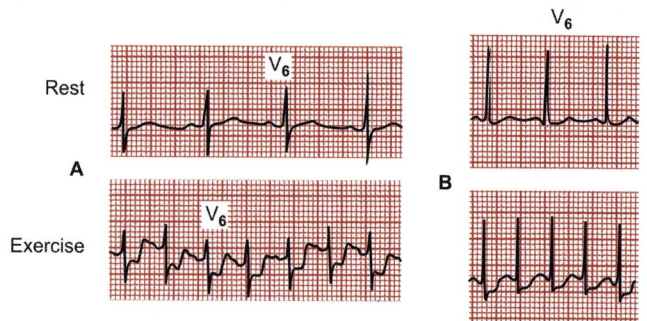

Fig. 16.7: Positive stress test. The electrocardiogram (lead V_6) shows:

A: There is downsloping ST segment depression of >1 mm along with J point, and stays for >80 msec during exercise

B: Depression of J point and horizontal ST depression > 1 mm that stay for > 0.8 sec (80 msec) after J point

ST segment depression. These are actually computer–derived measurements.

h) *ST/heart rate slope:* It has been claimed that calculation of ST/heart rate slope assists in separating individuals without significant coronary artery disease from those who have the disease. In patients with CAD, it may help in separating single vessel disease from multivessel disease. An ST/heart rate slope ≥ 2.4 mV/beat/min is considered as normal; and values ≥ 6 mV/beat/min are suggestive of triple vessel disease.

Lead II

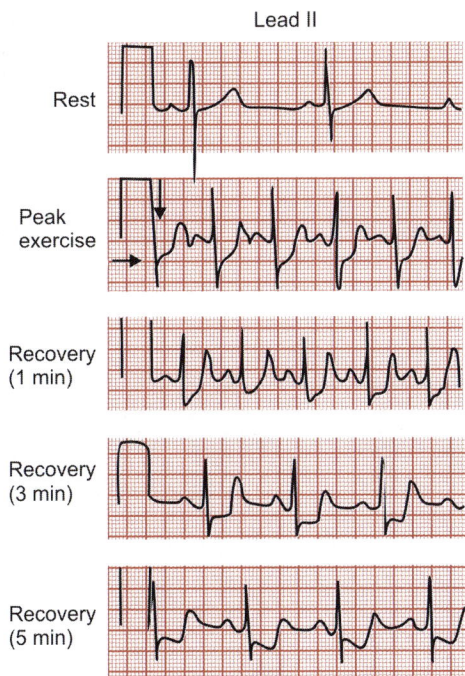

Lead V$_6$

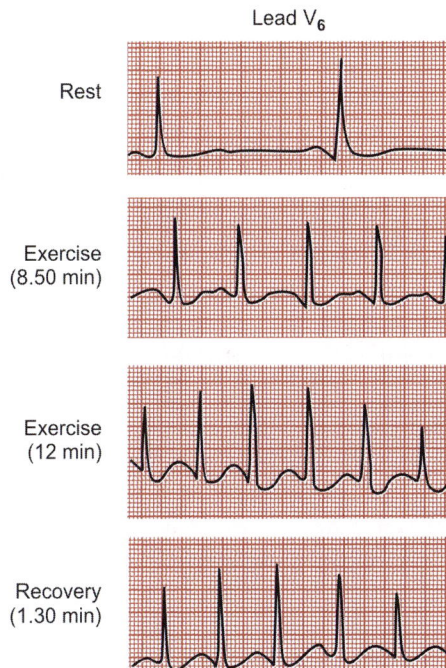

Fig. 16.8A: Bruce protocol (positive stress test). The stress ECG (lead II) shows:

(i) Depression of J point by 2.5 mm at peak exercise (J point should be at ↓ but is depressed as shown by →), ST segment depression of 80 msec (0.08 sec) by 1.6 mm with slow–upsloping ST segment

(ii) At 3 minutes of recovery phase: The ST segment depression with horizontality of initial 80 msec of ST segment is persisting, after which it becomes downsloping ST segment at 5 min of recovery phase.

Conclusion: Stress test is positive to provocative ischaemia

Fig. 16.8B: Positive stress test (Bruce protocol). The exercise electrocardiogram(lead V$_5$) shows an abnormal ST depression early in the test reaching 3 mm of horizontal (0.08 sec) ST depression at the end of excercise. This ischaemic change is persisting upto 1 min and 30 second into the recovery phase. Conclusion: This type of ST response (early onset, >3.0 mm ST depression of horizontal ST segment and its persistence during recovery) in consistent with severe ischaemic response to exercise

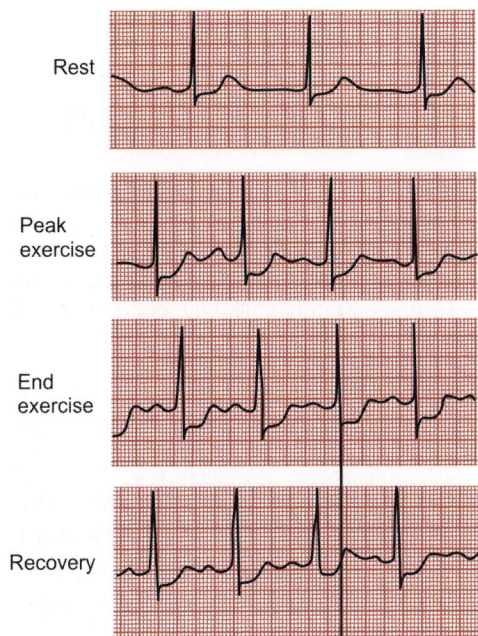

Fig. 16.8C: Bruce protocol (positive stress test). The rest ECG is normal. The stress electrocardiogram shows early ST segment depression with depression of J point, reaching 3 mm (0.3 mV) of horizontal ST depression at end of exercise. This ischaemic pattern persists into recovery phase. This type of ischaemic response, i.e. early onset, maximum depression of ST (3 mm) at end of exercise and persistence during recovery, is consistent with severe ischaemia.

Conclusion: The stress test is positive to provocative reversible ischaemia

SECTION FIVE

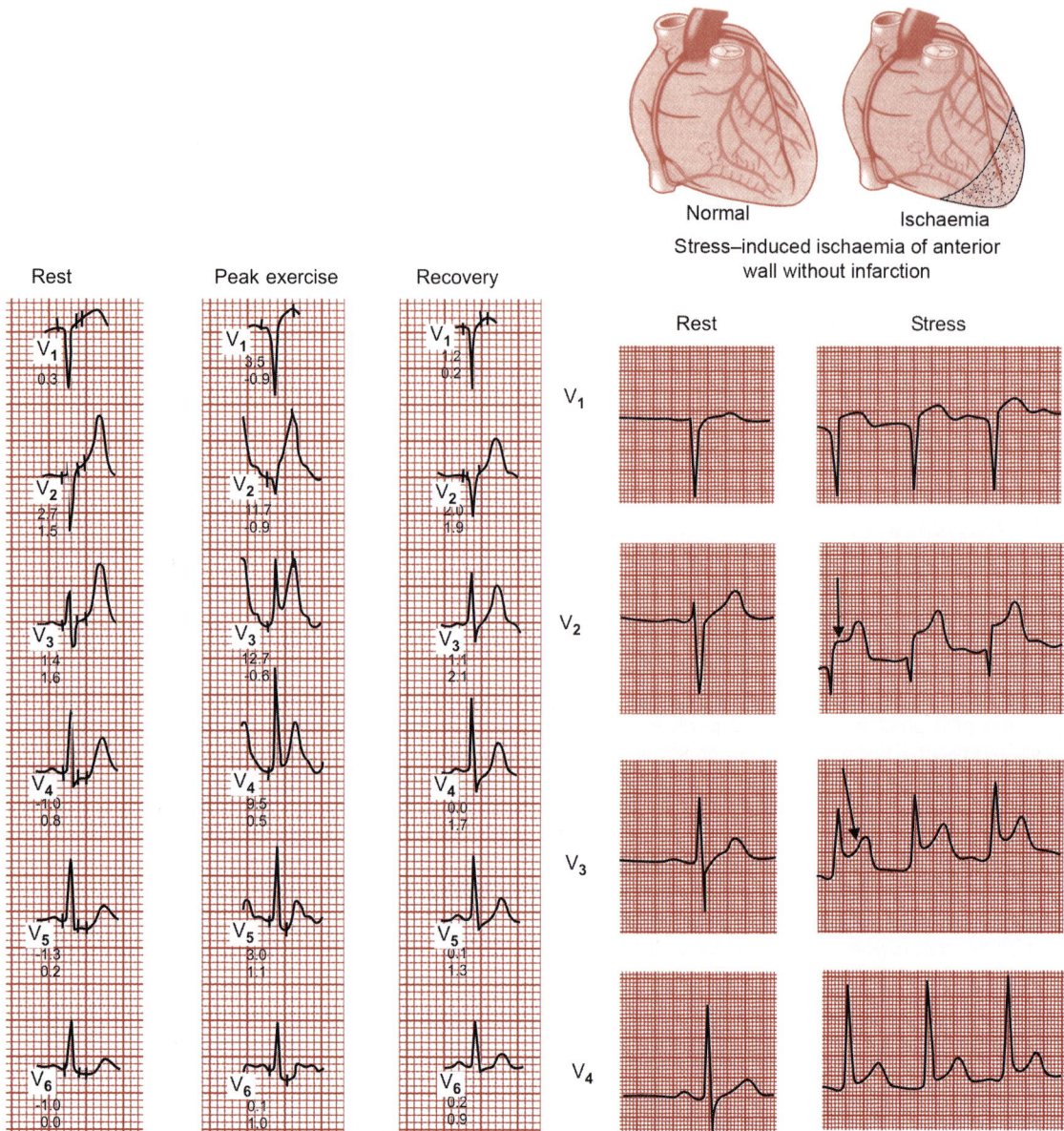

Normal   Ischaemia

Stress–induced ischaemia of anterior wall without infarction

Fig. 16.9: (A) Stress test (ST elevation of 3 mm in V_2-V_3 and 1 mm in V_4 with ST depression in V_5-V_6 during peak exercise.) (B) Bruce protocol (ST segment elevation during exercise). The resting ECG (precordial leads V_1-V_4 shown) is normal. The stress electrocardiogram recorded significant ST elevation (>4 mm) in leads V_2-V_3 ($\downarrow$) and lesser degree of ST elevation (>2 mm) in leads V_1 and V_4. The exercise test was terminated due to angina. This type of ECG response is usually associated with full thickness reversible myocardial ischaemia with significant intraluminal narrowing of coronary arteries. Rarely vasospasm may produce this type of response in the absence of intraluminal atherosclerotic narrowing

The elevation/depression of the J point, ST segment and ST slope are analysed for ischaemic response. The depression of J point (≥1 mm) with horizontal ST depression ≥ 1 mm for 0.08 sec from the J point in three successive beats constitutes a classic ischaemic response.

2. The T Wave Changes

- Tall T waves in lateral precordial leads after exercise are normal and are due to increased stroke volume.
- Isolated asymmetric T wave inversion during exercise is a nonspecific finding and is not considered

LBBB

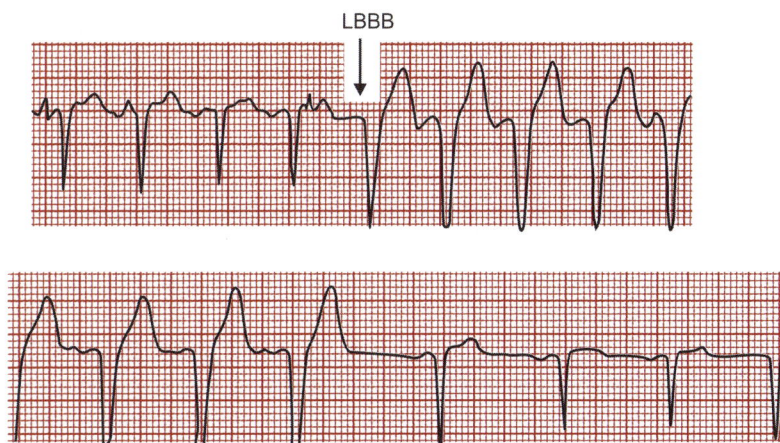

Fig. 16.10: Transient (rate dependant) left bundle branch block during stress electrocardiogram (Bruce protocol). The electrocardiogram (V_1) recorded from a patient of diabetes (controlled state) showed left bundle branch block which appeared during exercise at a heart rate of 136/min and disappeared during recovery (at 1.30 min) when heart rate slowed down, indicated rate dependant left bundle branch block (LBBB)

in the evaluation of ischaemia, but on the other hand, the evaluation of a downsloping T wave after exercise may suggest ischaemia under the following circumstances;

— Sharply pointed, symmetric T wave inversion.
— Inverted T wave of large amplitude.
— The associated ST segment tends to be iso-electric.
— The associated prolongation of Q-T interval.
— T wave changes appear at a relatively slow heart rate.

• Normalisation of T waves with exercise; such as flat or inverted T waves at rest becoming upright with exercise has been considered as a sign of ischaemia.

3. The U Wave Changes

Inversion of U wave after exercise is always indicative of presence of coronary insufficiency, in particular with high grade left anterior descending artery stenosis. This U wave change is commonly associated with ST change (depression/elevation).

4. The QRS Complex Changes

The exercise may induce the following changes.
1. *Tall R wave :* Normally, after exercise, R wave amplitude decreases, if on the contrary, amplitude of R wave increases, it indicates coronary insufficiency. False positive results are not infrequent, hence, this finding requires further confirmation with other ECG changes.

The R wave change combined with ST segment depression increases the specificity of the test.
2. *The q wave:* The normal qR or qRS complex in left precordial leads (V_5-V_6) increases in magnitude with exercise. The failure to do so, i.e. loss of septal q wave or a decrease in amplitude of qR suggests the presence of myocardial ischaemia.

The decrease in amplitude of q wave indicates multivessel disease with narrowing of left anterior descending artery. The changes in q wave are more reliable than those affecting the R wave in predicting coronary artery disease.

5. Intraventricular Conduction Changes

The development of left bundle branch block (LBBB) with exercise constitutes an abnormal response even if it occurs as an isolated phenomenon (Fig. 16.10).

Right bundle branch block (RBBB) development with exercise is of no consequence if it occurs as an isolated phenomenon, but if associated with other ECG changes of ischaemia, constitutes a corroborative evidence of the abnormality.

Occasionally left anterior hemiblock may occur with exercise leading to an abnormal left axis deviation. This is an abnormal response.

6. The Q-T Interval

The Q-T interval shortens with exercise normally. Lengthening of QT_c is an abnormal response. It is rarely used to diagnose ischaemia.

SECTION FIVE

7. Rhythm Disturbances (Exercise Induced Arrhythmias)

Sinus tachycardia is usual after exercise. Exercise has arrhythmogenic effect in patients with heart disease, may produce ventricular and supraventricular arrhythmias. The presence of multiform ventricular extrasystoles is diagnostic of cardiac disease and when they develop in response to exercise, they constitute a positive test.

The occurrence of ventricular arrhythmias during exercise is related to age as well as to the presence or absence of structural heart disease (Table 16.8). In asymptomatic individuals, the incidence of exercise induced arrhythmias increases with age, i.e. about 50% above the age of 50 years have these arrhythmias usually at rapid heart rate (>130 bpm). In patients with structural heart disease, these arrhythmias appear at lower heart rate (<130 bpm). The ventricular arrhythmias may be in the form of uniform or multiform VPCs, couplets or brusts of sustained or nonsustained tachycardia (monomorphic or polymorphic). Ventricular fibrillation is rare.

Sustained supraventricular tachyarrhythmias are seen in only about 1% of patients during exercise test. The usual rhythm is either atrial fibrillation or ectopic atrial tachycardia. Proxysmal supraventricular re–entrant tachycardia is unusual. These arrhythmias are usually self-terminating.

Exercise can normalise intraventricular conduction in patients with accessory AV conduction of WPW syndrome, due to both vagolysis and sympathetic overactivity induced by exercise.

Bradyarrhythmias are uncommonly seen with exercise due to high sympathetic tone. The overall incidence is about 1%. These are in the form of sinus bradycardia (reflex mechanism), sinus arrest and SA blocks due to rapid sinus rates with fatigue of the SA node. Similarly, AV blocks can occur if sinus rate is so high as to find His-Purkinje system refractory to conduction. AV blocks occurring during exercise usually result from conduction delay in His bundle or fascicular system or both. In such patients, pacing should be advised.

Rate–dependant intraventricular conduction delay occur infrequently (less than 1%). It is important to recognise them so as to avoid erroneous interpretation of the findings such as ventricular tachycardia or myocardial ischaemia or both.

The Post-extrasystolic T Wave Change (The Poor Man's Exercise Test)

Harold Levine and his associates have postulated the finding of post–extrasystolic T wave change in the tracing recorded at rest as a *'poor man's exercise test'*, since, it indicates an immediate evidence of an abnormality and obviates the need for a further more expensive stress test.

The abnormality consists of a T wave change in the first few sinus beats following an atrial or ventricular extrasystoles. The T wave usually becomes frankly inverted, at times, diminishes in amplitude. T wave inversion is not due to extrasystole *per se*, but is rather due to the pause which it produces. Inversion of U wave for one or two beats following an extrasystole carries the same significance as that of T wave.

The Significance of the Associated Phenomenon

1. Heart Rate

Heart rate is a parameter of workload on the heart. Thus, the heart rate at which abnormal ECG changes appear has an important bearing on their significance. If the abnormality appears at low heart rate (< 130 bpm), it is considered more significant as compared to when it appears at higher heart rate. The changes on ECG should be interpreted with caution because they may well constitute a false positive test or reflect only minimal myocardial ischaemia.

Table 16.8: Predisposing conditions for exercise induced arrhythmias
1. Normal subjects above the age of 50 years without structural heart disease
2. Coronary artery disease
3. Mitral valve prolapse
4. Cardiomyopathies of all types
5. Digitalis therapy
6. Long Q-T interval irrespective of its cause
7. Pulmonary disease
8. Congenital heart disease such as ASD or tetralogy of Fallot

In other words, a 1 mm ST segment depression which manifests at a rate of 110-115 bpm has more significance than a 1 mm ST segment depression which occurs at a heart rate of 170 bpm.

2. The Level of Exercise to Produce ECG Changes

The lower the exercise level at which the abnormal ECG changes appear; the more severe is the degree of coronary artery disease.

3. The Time Course of Abnormal ECG Changes

The more severe the myocardial ischaemia, the earlier is the onset of the abnormal ECG changes and the longer they tend to stay. Thus a moderate degree of myocardial ischaemia results in abnormal ECG changes during the first few minutes after exercise, and may persist for 8-10 minutes after exercise.

The abnormal ECG changes generally appear during exercise, reach a maximum at 3-6 minutes after exercise and persist for 10 minutes or longer after exercise. When resting ECG shows ST-T abnormalities, exercise results in the immediate exacerbation of ECG abnormalities, which persists for longer than 10 minutes and are more marked at 10 minutes than the tracing taken at rest.

Nonspecific Abnormalities and Exercise Test

Certain non-ischaemic and non-coronary causes (see the box) also produce abnormalities of the ST segment and T wave on the ECG taken at rest or may develop during exercise. These changes simulate morphologically with ischaemic ST-T changes. The non-ischaemic changes tend to vary during exercise and do not follow the time course characteristic of ischaemic changes. These nonspecific changes have a late onset and an early termination in contrast to ischaemic changes which tend to appear early and persist for longer period. Usually these nonspecific abnormalities present at rest, get normalised with exercise.

Cause of nonspecific ST-T changes	
• Anxiety	• Hyperventilation
• Mitral valve prolapse	• Athlete heart
• Neurocirculatory asthenia	• Atypical chest pain syndrome

Adverse Prognostic Factors on Exercise Testing

These include:
1. Duration of symptom–limiting exercise (<6 METs.)
2. Failure to increase systolic BP ≥ 120 mmHg, or a sustained decrease ≥ 10 mmHg, or below rest levels during progressive exercise.
3. ST segment depression ≥ 2 mm, downsloping ST segment starting at 6 METs involving ≥ 5 leads, persisting ≥ 5 minutes into recovery.
4. Exercise induced ST segment elevation (lead aVR excluded).
5. The development of multiform ventricular ectopics or reproducible sustained (>30 sec) or symptomatic ventricular tachycardia.
6. Angina pectoris during exercise.

Compilation of report: The data collected from analysis of exercise electrocardiography is compiled and interpreted as a report on the perform a given on the last page.

PHARMACOLOGICAL METHODS OF STRESS TESTING

Pharmacological stress testing is an alternative to exercise stress testing to identify the presence of ischaemia in those patients who are not able to perform exercise due to various reasons. Pharmacological stress testing is done in conjugation with electrocardiography, echocardiography and thallium (radionuclide) scanning. Chest pain, changes in BP or heart rate are parameters monitored.

Pharmacological stress testing does not require physical exertion by the patient, hence, is useful to evaluate the presence and degree of ischaemia in disabled patients. Pharmacological testing was developed in 1970. Many drugs or agents have been tried but most commonly used drugs in such testing nowadays are dipyridamole, adenosine and dobutamine. These drugs exert stress by increasing myocardial O_2 demand such as dobutamine (adrenergic–receptor agonist) or by inducing coronary vasodilation (adenosine, dipyridamole). Dobutamine produces haemodynamic stress similar to that produced by physical exercise, while adenosine and dipyridamole being vasodilators do not increase O_2 demand but produce disparity between areas supplied by normal coronary arteries and those supplied by diseased arteries because of differential ability of the arteries to dilate.

Pharmacological method of stressing is indicated in those who are not able to perform exercise due to varied reasons. Adenosine, dipyridamole and dobutamine are employed for this purpose

Pharmacological Agents and their Actions

1. *Adenosine:* Adenosine is a potent vasodilator of all vessels except renal. It is an endogenous coronary vasodilator in the presence of hypoxia. It has a rapid onset and short duration of action. Maximum response occurs after two minutes and lasts for 40 seconds after stopping infusion. Dose used is 0.14 mg/kg/min given as an infusion within 3-6 minutes. Hypotension and chest pain observed during infusion are reversed by stopping the infusion or by giving IV aminophylline. Though, in some centres, it is a preferred drug to dipyridamole in pharmacological stress testing but its use for this purpose has not been approved by FDA.

2. *Dipyridamole:* It increases the level of extracellular adenosine by blocking its reuptake by the endothelial cells. It is FDA approved drug and its half life in plasma is about 12 hours. Its vasodilator effect begins within 2-3 minutes after the start of infusion and peak effect occurs within 4 minutes. Recommended dose is 0.5 mg/kg given over a period of 4 minutes. Additional dose of 0.28 mg/kg after 5 minutes can be given for detecting wall motion abnormality on echocardiography.

Dipyridamole stress testing with thallium detection is equivalent to exercise stress with thallium detection for identifying ischaemia in patients with known disease diagnosed from symptoms or the occurrence of myocardial infarction or by angiography. Dipyridamole stress testing is also useful for detection of silent myocardial ischaemia. Sensitivity is 80-90%, with SPECT (Single Photo Emission Computed Tomography), the sensitivity is about 90% and overall being 97% in patients who had myocardial infarction and 89% in patients who had not previous myocardial infarction. With echocardiography, where the end point was development of wall motion abnormality, sensitivity of about 80% had been reported. Dipyridamole stress testing had demonstrated good results for detecting the effects of interventions, e.g. *'coronary artery bypass graft (CABG) or percutaneous transluminal coronary angioplasty (PTCA)'* on abnormalities in myocardial perfusion and wall motion. After PTCA, significantly more thallium was taken up in the regions of myocardium supplied by treated vessels than before PTCA. Similarly, after CABG, wall motion scores were significantly lower than before the surgery, Dipyridamole stress testing is especially useful in women in whom exercise test results are difficult to interpret because of nonspecific ST-T changes.

Major adverse effects include; fatal or nonfatal myocardial infarction, bronchospasm, coronary steal syndrome and ischaemic chest pain. Minor side effects also occur, Most of the effects occur during the infusion and disappear soon after it ends. Aminophylline should always be made available before dipyridamole stress testing.

3. *Dobutamine:* It is a β-adrenoreceptor agonist, hence, increases cardiac output and heart rate. Myocardial O_2 demand increases due to an increase in cardiac output. Dobutamine increases blood flow in normal coronary arteries and thus reduces perfusion pressure distal to coronary artery stenosis. The half-life is two minutes. The recommended dose for initial infusion is 5 µg/kg/min and is increased at 3-5 minutes intervals upto maximum dose of 40 µg/kg/min. End points in the test are attainment of maximum dose, achievement of target heart rate and development of segmental wall motion abnormalities detected on 2D echocardiography which is simultaneously performed. It has an advantage over dipyridamole and adenosine due to its flexibility in the infusion rate and resemblence to haemodynamic response to exercise.

Dobutamine is widely employed pharmacological method of stress testing

Clinical studies have addressed the use of dobutamine stress testing for evaluation of chest pain who have positive or incomplete exercise test results and patients after myocardial infarction before and after angioplasty. Dobutamine infusion offers an alternative diagnostic approach for patients who have contraindications to dipyridamole or adenosine infusion, such as those with bronchial asthma or chronic obstructive pulmonary disease, or for patients who are taking xanthine derivatives or who have consumed coffee. Dobutamine stress test, in fact, should be considered as a last resort in patients who cannot exercise, rather than a substitute for exercise. Sensitivity and specificity of the test for presence of ischaemic heart disease is 80-90%.

Adverse effects are less common and most patients are able to complete the test. Arrhythmias, chest pain, and fluctuations in BP may occur. If symptomatic ischaemia develops, nitroglycerine or beta-blockers may give rapid relief. Arrhythmias and haemodynamic instability warrant its discontinuation.

Proforma for Bruce Protocol (Modified) and Test Report

1. *Demographic data*

   Name   Test date

   Age   Medications

   Height   Doctor's reference

   Weight   Physician

   Sex   Technician

2. *Indications for the test*

3. *Exercise test*

Phase	Stage	Time of each stage	Duration of excessive (minutes)	Speed (MPH)	Grade (%)	HR (bpm)	BP (mmHg)	RPP	METs
Supine									
Standing									
Hyperventilation									
Exercise									
1.									
2.									
3.									
4.									
Peak exercise									
Recovery									

4. *Patient's clinical profile*
   - Coronary risk factor (s)   • Drug used
   - Resting ECG findings

5. *Exercise test results*
   - Protocol used ....
   - Reason for termination of the test
   - Haemodynamic data
     - a) Heart rate at rest ....   Peak ....
     - b) Blood pressure at rest.............   Peak ....
     - c) Per cent maximum achieved heart rate....... Maximum heart rate predicted....
     - d) Peak workload ....
     - e) Peak METS.............
     - f) Total duration of exercise in minutes.............

6. *Evidence for myocardial ischaemia*
   - Time of onset and offset of ischaemic ST segment deviation or angina.,
   - Maximum depth of ST segment deviation
   - Number of leads showing abnormal exercise change
   - Abnormal systolic blood pressure response

7. *Comments and conclusion*

Signature of the Physician

SECTION FIVE

Suggested Reading

1. Barlow JB, Pocock WA: Mitral valve prolapse, the Athlet's heart, Physical activity and sudden death. *Int J Sports Cardiol* **1**: 9, 1984.

2. Barlow JB: The false positive exercise ECG. Value of time course pattern in assessment of depressed ST segment and inverted T waves. *Am Heart J* **110**: 1328,1985.

3. Bogaty P, Dagenais GR, Cantin B, et al: Prognosis in patients with a strongly positive exercise electrocardiogram. *Am J Cardiol* **64**: 1284, 1989.

4. Borer JS, et al: Sensitivity, specificity and predictive accuracy of radionuclide cineangiography during exercise in patients with coronary artery disease. Comparison with exercise electrocardiography. *Circulation* **60**: 572,1979.

5. Bruce RA, Fisher LD, Pettinger M, et al: ST segment elevation with exercise: A marker for poor left ventricular function and poor prognosis. Coronary artery surgery study (CASS) confirmation of Seattle Heart Watch results. *Circulation* **77**: 897, 1988.

6. Bruce RA: Values and limitations of exercise electrocardiography. *Circulation* **50**: 1,1974.

7. Cahalin LP, Blessey RL, Kummer D et al: The safety of exercise testing performed independantly by physical therapists. *J Cardiopulm Rehabil* **7**: 269, 1987.

8. Chaitman BR, et al: The importance of clinical subsets in interpreting maximal treadmill exercise test results. The role of multilead ECG system. *Circulation* **50**: 560,1979.

9. Chaitman BR: Exercise stress testing–in Heart Disease—A textbook of Cardiovascular Medicine edited by Braunwald, 4th edn.Vol I WB Saunder Company, 1992.

10. Chaitman BR: The changing role of exercise electrocardiogram as a diagnostic and prognostic test for chronic ischaemic heart disease. *J Am Coll Cardiol* **8**: 1195, 1986.

11. Chung EK: Exercise electrocardiography. Practical approach. Baltimore, Williams and Willikins, 1979.

12. Ellestad MH: Stress testing, Principles and Practice. 2nd ed., Philadelphia; FA Davis, 1980.

13. Friesinger GC, et al: Exercise electrocardiography and vasoregularity abnormalities. *Am J Cardiol* **30**: 733, 1972.

14. Gerson MC, et al: Exercise induced U wave inversion as a marker of stenosis of the left anterior descending coronary artery. *Circulation* **60**: 1014, 1979.

15. Gianrossi R, Detrano R, Mulvihill D, et al: Exercise–induced ST depression in the diagnosis of coronary artery disease. A meta–analysis. *Circulation* **80**: 87, 1989.

16. Goldschlarger N, Selzer A, Cohn K: Treadmill stress tests as indicators of presence and severity of coronary artery disease. *Ann Int Med* **85**: 277, 1976.

17. Lachterman B, Lehmann KG, Detrano R, et al: Comparison of ST segment/heart rate index to standard ST criteria for analysis of exercise electrocardiogram. *Circulation* **82**: 44, 1990.

18. Lary D, Goldschlager N: Electrocardiographic changes during hyperperventilation resembling myocardial ischaemia in patients with normal coronary angiograms. *Am Heart J* **87**: 383,1974.

19. Lepschkin E, Surawic ZB: Characteristics of true positive and false positive results of electrocardiographic Master's two step exercise tests. *N Engl J Med* **258**: 511, 1958.

20. Lepschkin E: The U wave of electrocardiogram. *Med Conc Cardiovasc Dis* **389**:39, 1969.

21. Mark DB, Hlatky MA, Harrell FE et al: Exercise treadmill score for predicting prognosis in coronary artery disease. *Ann Intern Med* **106**: 793, 1987.

22. Martin JJ, Heng MK, Severin R, et al: Significance of T wave normalisation in the electrocardiograms during exercise stress test. *Am Heart J* **114**:1342, 1977.

23. Maseri A, Severi S, Denes M: 'Variant' angina: One aspect of a continuous spectrum of vasospastic myocardial ischaemia. Pathogenetic mechanisms, estimated incidence and clinical and coronary arteriographic findings in 138 patients. *Am J Cardiol* **42**: 1019, 1978.

24. Master AM, Friedman R, Dack S: The electrocardiogram after standard exercise as a functional test of the heart. *Am Heart J* **24**: 777, 1942.

25. McNeer JE, Margolis JR, Lee KL: The role of the exercise test in the evaluation of patients with ischaemic heart disease. *Circulation* **57**: 64, 1978.

26. Prinzemetal M, Kennamer R, Merliss R, et al: Angina pectoris; A variant form of angina pectoris. *Am J Med* **27**: 374, 1959.

27. Schlant RC, Blonqvist GC, Brandenberg RO et al: Guidelines for exercise testing: A report of the Joint American College of Cardiology—American Heart Association Task Force on Assessment of Cardiovascular procedures (subcomittee on exercise testing). *Circulation* **74**: (Supple III) 653a, 1986.

28. Sox HC Jr: Exercise testing in suspected coronary artery disease, DM **31**: 1, 1985.

29. Stuard RJ, Ellested MH: Natural survey of exercise stress testing facilities. *Chest* **77**: 94, 1980.

30. Weiner DA, Chaitman BR: Role of exercise testing in relationship to coronary artery bypass surgery and percutaneous transluminal angioplasty. *Cardiology* **73**: 242, 1986.

31. Yackee JM, Shrinder RM, Wasserman AG: Exercise induced ST segment depression and elevation in same patient. *Chest* **90**: 774, 1986.

PHARMACOLOGICAL METHODS OF STRESS TESTING

1. Eichorn EJ, Konstam MA, Salem DN et al: Dipyridamole thallium 201 imaging pre-and post-coronary angioplasty for assessment of regional myocardial ischaemia in humans. *Am Heart J* **117**: 1203, 1989.

2. Lavie CJ, Ventura HO, Murgo JO: Assessment of stable ischaemic heart disease, which tests are best for which patients? *Postgrad Med* **89**: 44, 1991.

3. Masini M, Picano E, Lattazi F et al: High dose dipyridamole echocardiography test in women, correlation with exercise electrocardiography test and coronary arteriography. *J Am Coll Cardiol* **12**: 682,1988.

4. Nesto RW, Watson FS, Kowalchuk CJ, et al: Silent myocardial ischaemia and infarction in diabetics with peripheral vascular disease; Assessment by dipyridamole thallium 201 scintigraphy. *Am Heart J* **120**: 1073, 1990.

5. Picano E, Lattanzl F, Masini M, et al : Usefulness of dipyridamole – Exercise echocardiography test for diagnosis of CAD. *Am J Cardiol* **62**: 67, 1988.

6. Pierard LA, Berthe C, Albert A et al: Haemodynamic alternations during ischaemia induced by dobutamine stress testing. *Eur Heart J* **10**: 783, 1989.

7. Ranhosky A, Kemphthorne–Rawson J: The safety of intravenous dipyridamole thallium myocardial perfusion imaging. *Circulation* **81**: 1205, 1990.

8. Russen J, Quillin J, Lopez A et al: Comparison of coronary vasodilation with dipyridamole and adenosine. *J Am Coll Cardiol* **18**: 485, 1991.

9. Zhu YY, Chung WS, Botvinick E, et al: Dipyridamole perfusion scintigraphy. The experience with its application in one hundred seventy patients with known or suspected unstable angina. *Am Heart J* **121**: 33, 1991.

Continuous Ambulatory Electrocardiographic Recording

SECTION SIX

17

Continuous Ambulatory Electrocardiographic Recording

- ■ *Continuous ambulatory electrocardiographic recording—Introduction, recording systems, duration of recording and lead system*
- ■ *Indications, analysis of Holter monitoring, its limitation and its superiority over exercise ECG*
- ■ *Methods of analysis of Holter monitoring*
- ■ *Artifacts and errors during Holter recording*

CONTINUOUS AMBULATORY (HOLTER) MONITORING

Continuous ambulatory electrocardiographic recording (Holter monitoring) is a method by which electrocardiogram is recorded for extended periods of time; the recording is analysed for rhythm, ST segment and T wave alterations. The main aim is to document and characterise the occurrences of random, spontaneous or activity induced cardiac disturbances or ST segment changes and to correlate the symptoms of the patients with these changes.

The Recording Systems

Technical advances in the past few years have provided numerous recording devices for ambulatory electrocardiography.

1. *Continuous Recorders*

The conventional Holter monitor which records the ECG channels on tape is a widely accepted method for continuous ambulatory recording. The tape recorder is battery-powered miniaturised device with very low tape speed (0.16 cm/sec) and is small enough to be suspended by a strap around the waist or over the shoulder to permit continuous data recording for 24 hours during normal daily activities of the patient. Most current recorders are equipped with an event recorder consisting of a button the patient pushes to note the time of symptoms. Activation of the event recorder marks the tape so that the patient's symptoms and recording can be interrelated during analysis. The patient also carries a diary in which he/she enters any symptom or symptoms experienced during the recording period, during activities, and the time at which symptoms appeared.

The lead systems on recorders vary from manufacturer to manufacturer. However, at least two leads should be recorded simultaneously either V_1 and V_5, or a bipolar limb or unipolar chest lead. Meticulous attention must be paid while placing the electrodes on the chest since poor electrode contact will produce technically inadequate recording.

2. *Event Recorders*

It is an alternative method of continuous electrocardiographic monitoring which records only abnormalities in rhythm or conduction, or records when the patient experiences symptoms. There are two basic types of event recorders. In the first, the rhythm is monitored continuously and only abnormalities in the rhythm and conduction are recorded. Operators select those parameters they wish the recorder to recognise as abnormal. Patients can activate the unit when they sense symptoms. Thus, an abnormal rhythm or an ECG synchronous with a symptom can be recorded spontaneously or in response to patient's activation.

In the second variety, rhythm is not monitored continuously but records are made when patient experiences symptoms. The patient can wear the recorder continuously, activating it when symptomatic. The recorded data are stored in the memory until the patient submits the information either directly or transtelephonically to an electrocardiographic receiver, where it is recorded.

Microcomputers (Digital Recording System)

The sophisticated microcomputers (all digital recording systems) amplify, digitise and store ECG in solid state memory. They have the potential to reproduce full-disclosure records and provide summaries of arrhythmias. The microcomputers sample the cardiac rhythm at real time, converts the analogue signals into a digital one, and analyse the data in terms of maximal and minimal rates, R-R interval, and changes in R-R intervals. Selected segments of ECG for brief periods, e.g. 6 to 10 second intervals can also be stored.

The record may be analysed by scanning the tape at high speed by writing it out directly or as in the case of microcomputers, by processing during recording, i.e. in the form of histograms covering the entire recording period, and a write out in real time of selected segments can be obtained. The microcomputers recording is similar to continuous tape recording except that actual ECG has not been recorded on tape.

Duration of Recording

A standard resting ECG records less than one minute of cardiac rhythm, detects ventricular premature beats in 8% of patients with known ischaemic heart disease; this frequency doubles if the recording period is extended to 12 hours. A 48 hr ECG recording time detects additional and more complex ventricular arrhythmias and supraventricular tachyarrhythmias,

and also displays the character and frequency of rhythm disturbances during sleep as well as during awake periods. Arrhythmias are often evanescent or may occur only rarely. In such patients, 24 hour Holter monitoring is unlikely to detect a rhythm disturbance. Even when the arrhythmias are frequent and revealed by 24 hours electrocardiographic monitoring, their marked variations in frequency and their complexity with variations occurring during and between days, need an extended period of monitoring.

The ideal duration of recording varies from patient to patient depending on the physician's goals. If the objective is to relate the symptoms with disturbance in the cardiac rhythm, then recording period must be extended sufficiently to include a symptomatic period, whether these intervals occur with a frequency of hours or days.

For screening purposes, 24 hours electrocardiographic tape recording (Holter monitoring) is optimal.

Lead System (Fig. 17.1)

The bipolar lead system needs 3 electrodes to record a single ECG lead, and 5 electrodes to record 2 leads simultaneously. Usually two leads (V_1 and V_5) are recorded during Holter monitoring. The placement of electrodes for these two monitor leads is as follows.

1. Two exploring electrodes are placed over the bone, one near the V_1 position (over the 4th or 5th rib just right to the sternum) and other at V_5 position (over the 5th rib at the midaxillary line).
2. Two indifferent electrodes are placed over the manubrium.
3. One ground electrode is placed over the 9th or 10th rib at the right midaxillary line.

This arrangement of bipolar lead system (Fig. 17.1) is termed as CM_1 or MCL_1 and CM_5 or MCL_5 respectively. This bipolar lead system thus is the same as used for bed side ECG monitoring in CCU and in telemetry.

The V_1 lead is especially useful in rhythm analysis since P waves are usually well seen in this lead. However, simultaneous recording of two ECG leads is preferred, whenever feasible, in order to avoid erroneous diagnosis based on low voltage signals or artifacts.

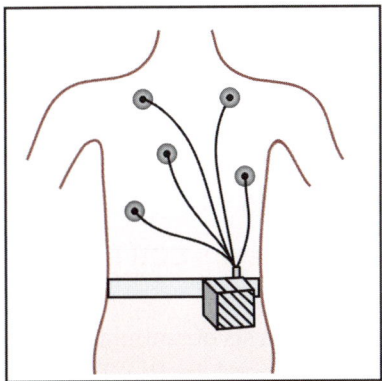

Fig. 17.1. Holter monitoring. Placement of electrodes on the body surface for continuous recording of ECG over a period of hours to days

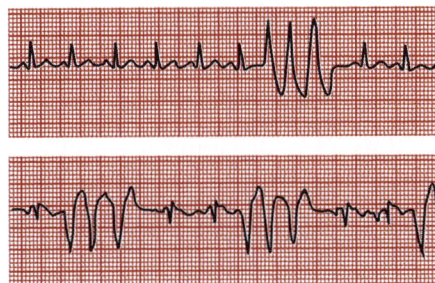

Fig. 17.2: Holter monitoring (24 hour record). The upper strip shows normal sinus rhythm with nonsustain VT. The lower strip shows self-terminating VT after every two sinus beats

Indications

1. Detection of an Arrhythmia (Fig. 17.2)

The widely accepted indication of continuous ambulatory ECG monitoring is to correlate cardiac arrhythmias with patient's symptoms, i.e. palpitation, syncope, dyspnoea, fatigue, etc. The recording may show symptomatic arrhythmia (brady or tachyarrhythmia) when patient experiences symptoms; or it may not show any arrhythmia during symptoms, in that situation, an arrhythmia is excluded as the cause of patient's symptoms. Sometimes, it may reveal asymptomatic arrhythmias about which the patient is not aware of. Therefore, if patient does not experience symptoms during the set period of recording, it is advisable to extend the recordings for longer durations. A majority of patients recovering from acute myocardial infarction exhibit ventricular arrhythmias within 6-24 hours of continuous ambulatory monitoring such as frequent ventricular premature beats, ventricular premature beats showing R on T phenomenon, ventricular tachycardia, etc. All these rhythm disturbances in patients with myocardial infarction increase the chances of sudden cardiac death.

There are certain cardiovascular conditions where single resting ECG may not reveal an arrhythmia, or potentially serious arrhythmias are likely to be missed, in such a situation, continuous ambulatory electrocardiography may expose them, for example, complex ventricular ectopy and dangerous arrhythmias in patients with hypertrophic cardiomyopathy, mitral valve prolapse, in patients with transient ischaemic cerebral attacks or unexplained syncope, in patients with sick sinus syndrome, bradycardia–tachycardia syndrome, the WPW syndrome or pacemaker malfunction.

Holter monitoring has also been found useful in evaluation of efficacy of antiarrhythmic therapy. A reduction in total number of premature ventricular complexes is the goal for antiarrhythmic therapy. The total number of premature ventricular complexes must be reduced by 80% as reported by various studies.

2. Assessment of Heart Rate Variability (R-R Interval Characteristics)

The ambulatory ECG is best suited to determine R-R intervals, i.e. heart rate variability, measured as the standard deviation of sinus cycle lengths. It is a measure of vagal input to the sinus node. It has now been recognised that beat to beat changes in heart rate or cycle lengths (R-R intervals) may contain useful informations for the diagnosis of certain conditions i.e. sleep apnoea, diabetic autonomic neuropathy, etc. Even in coronary heart desease, variability in R-R-intervals or cycle lengths after myocardial infarction form an independent prognostic indicator unrelated to ventricular arrhythmia or left ventricular function. Decreased heart rate variability correlates with an increased risk of sudden death.

Alteration in waveform morphology may be another clue to cardiac instability detectable by Holter monitoring.

SECTION SIX

3. Detection of Myocardial Ischaemia

Silent or painful episodes of myocardial ischaemia during day-time activities can be detected and documented by 24 hour Holter monitoring. Clinical studies have shown that transient ST segment depression is a sensitive and objective marker of reversible provocable myocardial ischaemia.

The prognostic significance of silent ischaemia during daily activity is similar to painful myocardial ischaemia during exercise. Therefore, the ambulatory ECG helps to identify a subgroup of patients with stable or unstable angina pectoris or postmyocardial infarction in whom ST-T wave alterations dictate guarded prognosis over the subsequent period of 1-12 months. These subgroups of patients are more likely to have severe angina, myocardial infarction or death. However, absence of such transient ECG changes on the other hand, does not guarantee a good prognosis.

Ambulatory ECG is also helpful in detecting the ST elevation in patients with Prinzmetal's variant angina (rest angina). Usually ST elevation does not occur during exercise in Prinzmetal's angina, hence, Holter monitoring is useful diagnostic parameter.

The Patient's Diary

The patient is instructed to maintain an activity diary during monitoring period so that clinical correlation could be made between electrocardiographic events (rhythm disturbance) with patient's symptoms. An event recorder on the recording system can be activated by the patient when symptoms occur. Some scanners automatically get activated by the event marker to write out the ECG in real time for later analysis by the physician.

Analysis of Ambulatory ECG Recording (Holter Monitoring)

A format to the analysis of ambulatory ECG recording is briefly summarised in the Table 17.1. Clinical correlation is required for all recorded events. The ECG recording is to be analysed for R–R intervals (Heart rate), rhythm and its disturbance, ST segment deviation and T wave changes.

Limitations of Ambulatory Electrocardiography in Evaluation of ST Segments and T Waves

The ambulatory ECG is an excellent tool for evaluation of rhythm disturbance during activity but for several reasons, both technical and physiological, it does not provide same degree of reliability in the interpretation of the pattern of ST segment and T wave as in detection of rhythm disturbance. Technical limitations include; unsatisfactory low frequency responses and the use of one lead system. Just as a single lead on standard ECG might not record ischaemic ST segment and T wave changes during myocardial ischaemia, so, a single lead system is inadequate here also for this purpose.

Table 17.1: Interpretation of ambulatory electrocardiographic recording

1. Determine the basic underlying cardiac rhythm and rate
2. Are premature beats present? If yes, then determine their origin, frequency and complexity.
3. Are sustained or nonsustained tachycardias present ? If yes, then;
   i. Determine its origin.
   ii. Determine its maximum and minimum duration.
   iii. Determine mode of onset and termination.
   iv. Is there any relationship with time of the day, heart rate, dose of medication or accompanying ST segment changes?
4. Are bradyarrhythmias present? if yes, then;
   What is its type (sinus, supraventricular, ventricular)? and what is its mechanism (slowing of SA node, sinus pauses, AV blocks, postextrasystolic pauses, post–tachycardia pauses)?
5. Is ST segment deviation present ? If yes, then;
   What is its type (downsloping depression, horizontal depression or elevation) ?
   Determine its frequency, minimum and maximum duration, any accompanying arrhythmia and its relationship with time of the day, heart rate and activity.
6. Is the patient has an implanted pacemaker? if yes, then;
   Are pacemaker functions (sensing, pacing) normal?

Note : Substantial variations of QRS-T morphology with body position can occur, therefore, prior to beginning of the ambulatory electrocardiographic recording, the electrocardiographic tracing should be performed with patient sitting, lying down and standing, in order to identify these positional changes upon play back of the tape.

Even more important than technical considerations are physiological limitations. For example, standing, eating, hyperventilation, anxiety, use of drugs, and any change in heart rate are all daily events that can result in ST segment depression and T wave inversion to mimic ischaemic changes. Striking ST segment elevation has been recorded during prolonged monitoring in patients without any evidence of organic heart disease. Despite these limitations, preliminary evaluation of ST-T change by the technique of prolonged electrocardiographic recording to detect ischaemic heart disease is indicated in some instances.

SUPERIORITY OF AMBULATORY ELECTROCARDIOGRAPHY OVER EXERCISE TESTING

1. Ambulatory electrocardiography proves superior to exercise testing in detecting Prinzmetal's variant angina (angina at rest accompanied by ST segment elevation). The ST elevation at rest in Prinzmetal's angina is not reproducible during exercise testing.
2. Ambulatory electrocardiography is an excellent method to correlate symptoms that occur during normal daily activities in a patients with an ECG evidence of ischaemia. On the other hand, stress used in exercise testing is not comparable with normal daily activities of the patient. In fact, stress testing does not correlate symptoms in time with ECG changes.
3. Ambulatory electrocardiography can be done in certain situations where exercise testing is not possible such as physical inability/disability.
4. Ambulatory ECG recording is also useful in patients where exercise testing gives negative results but symptoms are highly suggestive of myocardial ischaemia related to some other specific activities of the day.

Methods of Analysis of Ambulatory Electrocardiographic Recording

1. *Scanning techniques*: It includes technician–dependant analysis, in which a technician interprets the cardiac rhythm as it is played back at high speed on an oscilloscope. This scanning is coupled with human errors. To minimise the human error and to have accurate data, the tape can be analysed by semiautomated electronic analyser which quantitates the number of abnormalities it recognises. The accurary of this system depends on the system's ability to distinguish abnormal from normal.

2. *Computers analysis*: A computer can be interfaced with the scanner to quantitate the data even more accurately. The computers like electronic analysers are taught to recognise the patient's own QRS complex and then to recognise abnormal QRS complexes. The computers programme can provide summaries of the heart rates, frequency of premature beats (atrial or ventricular), coupling intervals, runs of tachycardia or other arrhythmias and variations in QRS, ST or T wave patterns during any period of time.

Scanning services are available and can generally give accurate analysis at less cost. An alternative method to scanning is the direct write out of the entire period. The electrocardiogram is compressed to reduce the amount of paper that the physician must examine.

Since microcomputers assess the ECG in real time as it is recorded and there is no need of technician or scanner when the results are written out. The physician evaluates the trend chart or any recorded rhythm strip.

Artifacts and Errors

Artifacts registered during ambulatory electrocardiographic recording may mimic every variety of supraventricular and ventricular brady or tachyarrhythmias and thus lead to an erroneous diagnosis.

Recording artifacts may result from incomplete tape erasure, tape drag within the apparatus, loose electrodes or mechanical stimulation of the electrode and battery depletion or failure.

Ventricular tachycardia is simulated by artifact produced by scratching of the electrode by the patient (Fig. 17.3). Incomplete tape erasure can result in the display of ECG tracing belonging to two different patients, confusing both the automatic scanner and the interpreter (Fig. 17.4). Tape drag due to failure of either the battery or the motor of the recorder, results

SECTION SIX

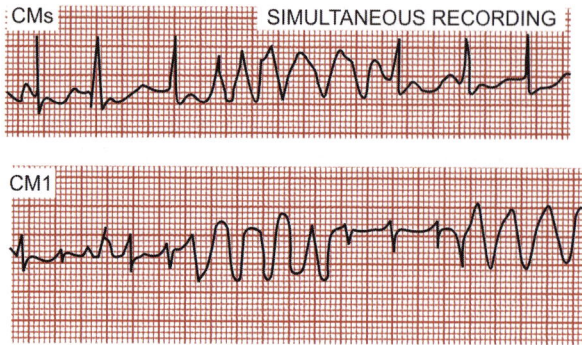

Fig. 17.3: Mechanical stimulation of electrodes mimicking ventricular tachycardia. The electrocardiogram (CM$_5$ and CM$_1$ leads) shows:

(i) Regular broad QRS complexes were repeatedly recorded in both monitor leads which maybe interpreted as non-sustained VT. However, the clue to the artifactual recording is the presence of normal QRS complexes marching through the ventricular tachycardia and the coupling, interval between first normal complex of CM$_1$, preceding tachycardia and the first normal complex of CM$_5$, preceding tachycardia; and the first normal complex following it is so short as to be unphysiological. Physiologically, the first QRS complex of VT must fall on the T wave of normal QRS complex and not before it.

(ii) The QRS complexes do not have smooth outlines. This patient admitted intense pruritis from the electrodes that led to scratching which explained the artifactual tracing

in slowing of the tape speed as the ECG is recorded. When played back, the heart rate will appear fast and may mimic tachycardia (Fig. 17.5). This can easily be diagnosed by the interpreter due to concomitant shortening of ECG intervals and complexes. Deceleration of tape due to sticking, slows the heart rate resembling bradycardia or AV block. The artifact is detected by wide spread out P waves, P–R intervals and QRS complexes (Fig. 17.6). Therefore, simultaneous recording of 2 ECG channels is extremely helpful in assessing recording artifacts.

Digital recording in solid state memory eliminates these various mechanical failures of tape recordings.

Suggested Reading

1. Berman Da, Rozanski AL, Knoebel SB: The detection of silent ischaemia: Cautions and precautions. *Circulation* **75**: 101, 1987.
2. Chung EK: Ambulatory Electrocardiography. Holter Monitor Electrocardiography New York: Springer-Verlag 1986.

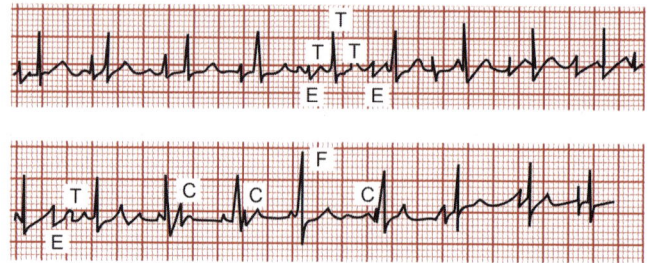

Fig. 17.4: Incomplete tape erasure. There are two independant ventricular rhythms, i.e. one with large QRS deflection is labelled as R and its P and T are also labelled and the other has small complex considered as ectopic is labelled as E with T labelled as T' (lower strip 2nd complex). This sequence appears as being due to superimposition of ECGs belonging to two different patients or it can be recorded in Siamese twins or piggyback heart transplant. Alternatively, the ectopic complex E may be misinterpreted as parasystolic rhythm because a fusion beat F is seen; but the very short coupling interval C and two dissociated cardiac rhythms preclude this possibility and indicates the artifact of tape erasure

Note: The ECG illustration is hand drawn.

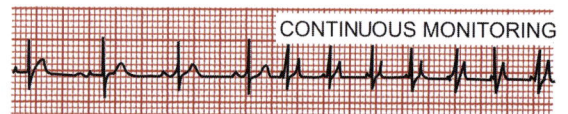

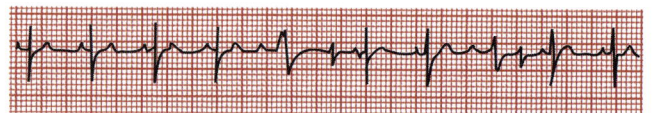

Fig. 17.5: Deceleration of tape due to battery failure resulting in fast rhythm resembling supraventricular tachycardia seen at the end of strip. When played back on recording paper at proper speed, the artifact was detected by shortening of all ECG intervals (PR, QRS, QT and RR) and duration of P wave
Note: The ECG illustration is hand drawn.

Fig. 17.6: Deceleration of tape during play back slows the heart rate resembling bradycardia or AV block. The artifact is detected by wide spread out P waves, P-R intervals and QRS complex. (5th and 9th complex of the strip)
Note: The ECG illustration is hand drawn.

3. Crawford MH, Mendoza CA, O'Rourke RA, et al: Limitations of continuous ambulatory electrocardiographic monitoring for detecting coronary artery disease. *Ann Intern Med* **89**:1, 1978.
4. Dreifus IS, Pennock R: Newer techniques in cardiac monitoring. *Heart Lung* **4**:568, 1975.
5. Fitzgerald JW, Spitz Al, Winkle RA, et al : Quantitation of ambulatory electrocardiogram. *Circulation* **56**: 178, 1977.
6. Gilson JS, Holter NJ, Glassock WR: Clinical observations using this electrocardiorecorder—AVSEP continuous electrocardiographic system. *Am J Cardiol* **14**: 204, 1964.

7. Golding B, Walf E, Tzivoni D, et al: Transient ST elevation detected by 24 hr. ECG monitoring during normal daily activity. *Am Heart J* **86**: 501, 1973.

8. Guidelines for ambulatory electrocardiography : A report of the American College of Cardiology/American Heart Association Task Force on Assessment of Diagnostic and Therapeutic Cardiovascular Procedures (Subcommittee on Ambulatory Electrocardiography). *J Am Coll Cardiol* **13**: 249, 1989.

9. Hinkle LE Jr, Meyer J, Stevens M, et al : Recording of ECG of active men. *Circulation* **36**: 752, 1967.

10. Holter NJ: New method for heart studies : Continuous electrocardiography of active subjects over long period is now practical. *Science* **13**: 1214, 1968.

11. Knoebel SB, Lovelace DE, Rasmusssen: Computer detection of premature ventricular complexes. A modified approach. *Am J Cardiol* 38: 440, 1976.

12. Krasnow AX, Bloomfield DK: Artifacts in portable electrocardiographic monitoring. *Am Heart J* **91**: 349, 1976.

13. Lopes MG, Runge P, Harrison DC, et al: Comparison of 24 hr versus 12 hours of ambulatory ECG monitoring. *Chest* **67**:269, 1975.

14. Malek J, Glushien A: To the Editors: Artifacts in portable ECG monitoring. *Ann Intern Med* **77**:1004,1972.

15. Morganroth J, Michelson EL, Horowitz LN, et al: Limitations of routine long-term ambulatory ECG monitoring to assess ventricular ectopic frequency. *Circulation* **58**: 408, 1978.

16. Sami M, Krermer H, Harrison DC et al: A new method for evaluating antiarrhythmic drug efficacy. *Circulation* **62**:1172, 1980.

17. Stern S, Trivoni D: Early detection of silent ischaemic heart disease by 24 hour ECG monitoring of active subjects. *Br Heart J* **36**: 48, 1974.

18. Winkle R: Curriculum in cardiology: Current status of ambulatory electrocardiography. *Am Heart J* **102**: 757, 1981.

19. Wold E, Tzivoni D, Stern S: Comparison of exercise test and 24 hr. ambulatory ECG monitoring in detection of ST-T changes. *Br Heart J* **36**: 90, 1974.

Coronary Artery Disease

SECTION SEVEN

18

Myocardial Ischaemia

- *Introduction, electrocardiographic manifestations and its pathogenesis*
- *Acute versus chronic ischaemia and their ECG manifestations*
- *Nonspecific ST-T changes*
- *Clinical and electrocardiographic correlation in angina pectoris*
- *Variant angina-Prinzmetal's angina and its electrocardiographic manifestations*
- *Asymptomatic electrocardiographic abnormalities*

MYOCARDIAL ISCHAEMIA

Myocardial ischaemia refers to the state of coronary blood flow that is inadequate to meet myocardial oxygen demands. By definition, it is a transient and reversible phenomenon, which clinically manifests as angina pectoris. The coronary blood flow may be sufficient at rest but becomes inadequate during exercise or stress or when there are additional factors which diminish the coronary blood flow such as coronary vasospasm. The ECG findings are limited to ST segment and T wave abnormalities, although transient 'q' waves may appear if ischaemia is of sufficient severity. As ECG manifestations are transient, therefore, a single ECG is never diagnostic of myocardial ischaemia. Similarly, fixed ECG changes in the form of ST-T wave abnormalities recorded weeks, months or years apart usually do not reflect myocardial ischaemia since ischaemia is a dynamic process not expected to remain constant or same over time. Therefore, diagnosis of myocardial ischaemia needs clinical and electrocardiographic evaluation during and after spontaneous angina, whether it occurs at rest or during exercise.

The ST-T changes must not be considered nonspecific and nondiagnostic unless or until myocardial ischaemia is ruled out. Many conditions unrelated to ischaemia can produce these ST-T changes such as electrolytes disturbance (hypokalaemia), left ventricular hypertrophy, drugs, myocarditis, and pericarditis, etc. A clinician must interpret electrocardiogram in the light of clinical findings.

The Electrocardiographic Manifestations

As myocardial ischaemia induces changes due to abnormal depolarisation and repolarisation, hence, they are mainly reflected as abnormalities of ST segment, the T wave, the U wave and QRS-T angle (Table 18.1).

Table 18.1: Electrocardiographic manifestations of myocardial ischaemia

1. *Abnormalities of ST segment*
   - Depression of ST segment
   - Elevation of ST segment
   - Alternation of ST segment (ST segment alternans)
2. *Abnormalities of T wave*
   - Low, flat, inverted T waves
   - Taller T waves in precordial leads (occasional)
3. *Abnormalities of U wave, if U wave is recorded*
   - Inversion of U waves
   - Low amplitude, biphasic U wave, etc.
4. *Abnormalities of QRS and QRS-T angle*
   - Transient q waves
   - Widening of QRS-T angle (>60°) in both frontal and horizontal planes

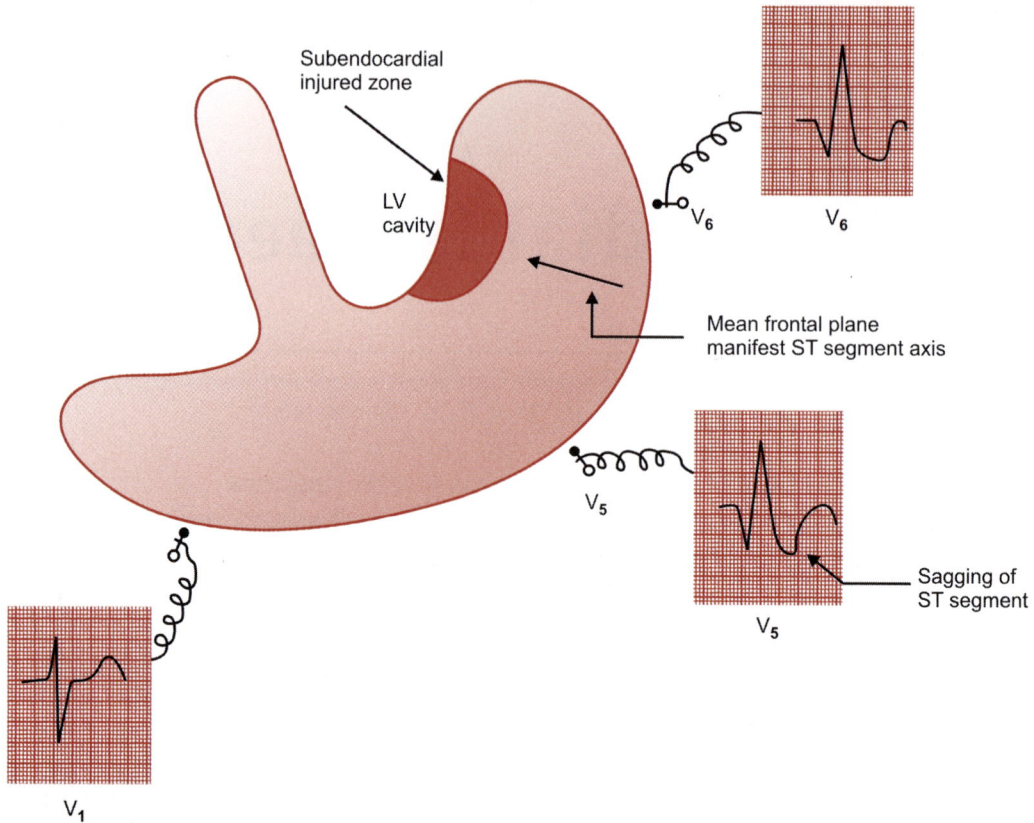

Fig. 18.1: Diagrammatic illustration of genesis of ST segment depression. Note a transient injury in subendocardial region shifts the mean ST segment manifest axis towards the injured surface (towards cavity) as represented by an arrow and away from the epicardial surface resulting in depression or sagging of the ST segment in leads V_5-V_6.

1. Abnormalities of ST Segment

A. *Depression of ST segment*: The ST segment depression is considered to reflect nontransmural myocardial or subendocardial ischaemia. The subendocardial portion of the heart is more prone to ischaemia because it bears most of the burden of systolic pressure developed by the ventricles that reduces that portion of blood supply which is derived from transmyocardial coronary artery perfusion pressure gradient, the portion of blood received through ventricular cavity remains, however, unaffected.

The ST segment depression is seen in left ventricular epicardial leads (V_4-V_6) and ST segment elevation (often not discernible) in leads facing the nonischaemic portion of the ventricular tissue (Fig. 18.1).

Pathogenesis : When ST segment is deviated above or below the baseline due to ischaemia, the mean frontal manifest ST segment axis is directed towards the surface of the injury. Thus, with injury to subendocardial portion of left ventricle, the mean manifest ST vector is directed towards the cavity of left ventricle and away from its epicardial surface, resulting in the depression of ST segment in left ventricular epicardial leads (V_5-V_6). This is represented diagrammatically in Figure 18.1.

Types and forms of ST segment depression (Figs 18.2A to H): The ST segment depression in the order of severity and forms are;

1. Horizontal ST segment depression
2. ST segment depression with upward sloping
3. Plane cove-plane ST segment depression (Fig. 18.3A)
4. Sagging ST segment depression
5. ST segment depression with downward sloping (Fig. 18.3B).

Table 18.2: Normal and abnormal ST segment characteristics

Type	Characteristics
A. *Normal ST segment* 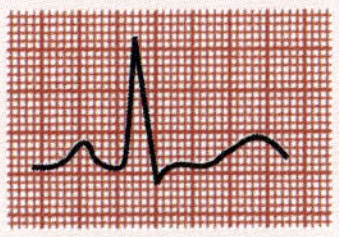 Normal P-QRS-TU complex	It leaves the baseline almost immediately after QRS, blends with the proximal limb of T wave. A very little part of ST segment is visible and is isoelectric.
B. *Junctional ST depression (physiological)* 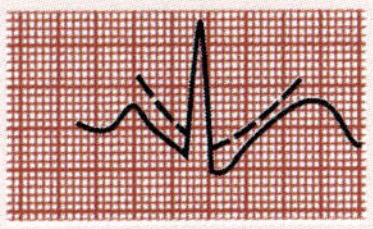 Junctional ST depression physiological	It may be physiological where distal limb of P wave, P-R segment, ST segment and proximal limb of T wave form a parabola and the horizontally depressed ST segment at the level of TP line is less than 0.08 second (two small squares) and it is not possible to separate T wave from ST segment.
C. *Junctional ST depression (pathological)* 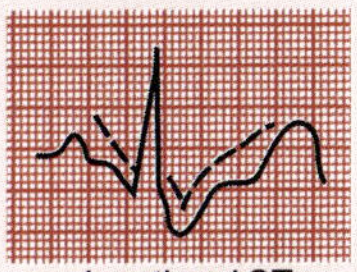 Junctional ST depression pathological	Pathological junctional ST depression does not form a parabola and depressed ST segment persists for more than 0.08 second below TP line and T wave is separated from ST segment by a distinct angle. It occurs in ischaemia.
D. *Horizontal depression of ST segment* 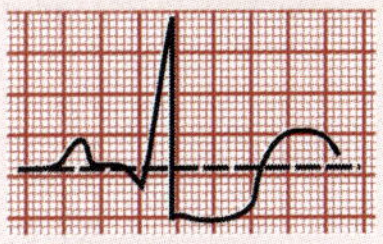 Horizontal depression. Note sharp angled ST-T junction	The ST segment depression remains horizontal for an appreciable time (i.e. 0.12 sec or 3 mm or longer). A sharp angle develops between ST segment and T wave, so, both can be identified and separated easily. The horizontality is in fact the earliest expression of ST depression, though ST segment does not go below the baseline, it may be viewed as depression of the distal part of the ST segment. It is the earliest change in myocardial ischaemia.
E. *Depressed ST with upward–sloping* 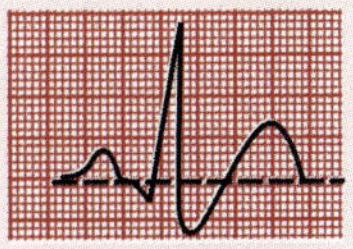 Depressed ST with upward slopping	There is junctional ST depression–proximal part of ST segment and its junction with QRS is depressed. It may be physiological (seen in normal persons) or pathological seen in myocardial ischaemia, therefore, differential diagnosis between them is essential.
F. *Plane ST segment depression* 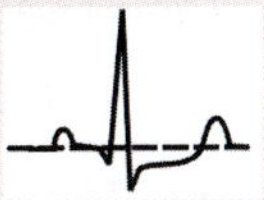 Plane ST depression with U wave inversion ('U')	ST segment is depressed in plane and horizontal or in coving manner. There is sharp angled ST-T junction. T wave can be separated easily from ST segment. This is seen mild to moderate myocardial ischaemia (Fig. 18.3A).

Table 18.2 contd...

Type	Characteristics
G. *Sagging ST segment* 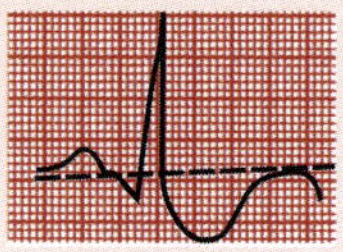 Sagging ST depression	The ST segment is sagged downwards and becomes cup-shaped. It is abnormal and indicates acute coronary insufficiency.
H. *ST segment depression with downsloping* 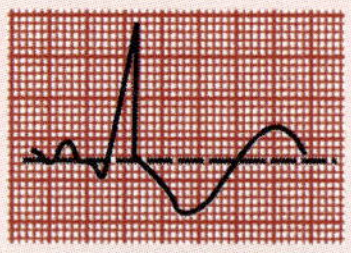 ST segment depression with downsloping	The ST segment is depressed below the isoelectric line at its origin and then it slopes further downwards. This indicates severe coronary insufficiency (Fig. 7.1.3B).

Figs 18.2A to H: Types and forms of ST segment depression (diagram)

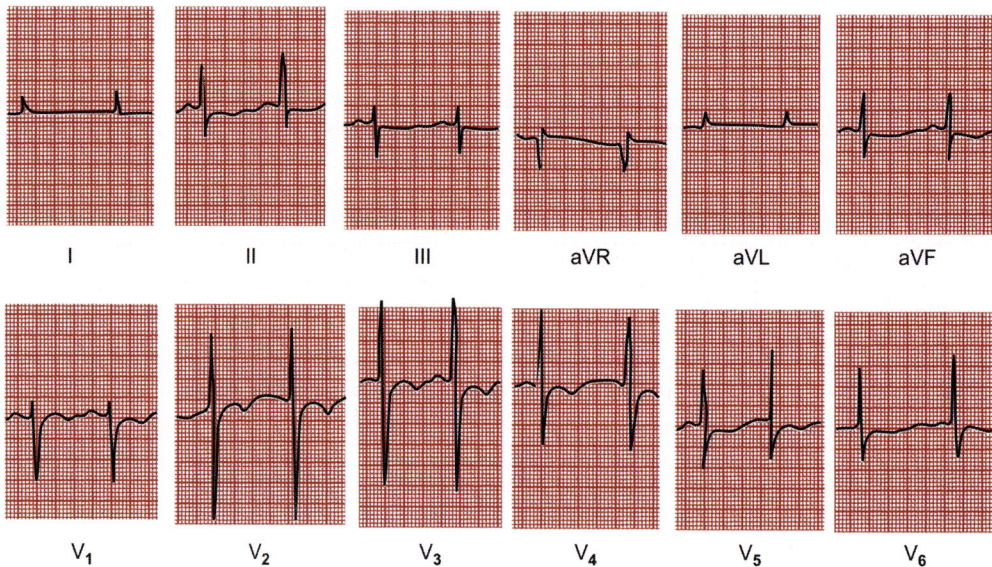

Fig. 18.3A: Acute coronary insufficiency (mild to moderate change). The electrocardiogram was recorded from a patient who complained of chest pain and palpitation. The ECG recorded shows features of acute global ischaemia involving anterior, inferior and lateral surface of the heart. Note the cove-plane ST segment depression in leads II, III, aVF and V_1-V_6. The ST segment is flat in lead I and aVL. The T wave is inverted in II, III, aVF and V_1-V_6 while it is flat in I and aVL

These changes are not sequential, may present in any of the above forms.

The characteristics of normal and abnormal ST segments are summarised (Table with Figs 18.2).

Clinical Significance of ST Segment Depression

1. The ST segment depression may manifest as a clinically silent phenomenon.

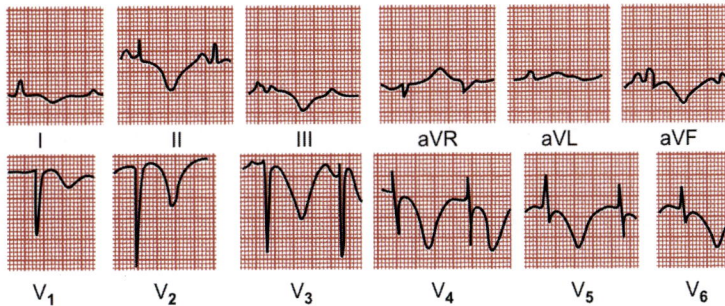

Fig. 18.3B: Acute coronary insufficiency (severe change). The ECG shows downsloping ST segment depression with deep and wide T wave inversion indicating severe coronary insufficiency

2. Transient ST depression is seen in classic form of angina pectoris (Heberden's angina).
3. The greater the ST segment depression in ischaemic heart disease, the worst is the prognosis.
4. The ST segment depression in a patient of angina during stress who had normal ST segment at rest, indicates positive stress test or provocable ischaemia, which is usually reversible.

B. *The ST segment elevation:* The ST segment elevation expresses transmural myocardial ischaemia, therefore, indicates more severe form of ischaemia than just ST segment depression. Transient, or reversible ST segment elevation, occurring at rest, is frequently observed in coronary vasospasm (Prinzmetal's angina). In Prinzmetal's angina, ST segment elevation occurs during acute episode of pain and may disappear with subsidence of pain. If ST segment elevation occurs during exercise, it may reflect critical narrowing of coronary arteries due to an organic lesion provided Q waves of previous myocardial infarction are not present. If Q waves are present, elevation of

Chief causes of ST segment elevation

- Prinzmetal's angina (rest angina, variant angina, vasospastic angina).
- Fixed narrowing of coronary arteries due to atherosclerosis–a chronic change.
- Acute myocardial infarction.
- Left ventricular aneurysm or tumour of left ventricle.
- Acute pericarditis.
- Impaired left ventricular function, wall motion abnormalities in a patient who had a previous myocardial infarction.
- Non-cardiac conditions, i.e. acute pancreatitis or cholecystitis, diaphragmatic pleurisy

ST segment during exercise reflects wall motion abnormality rather than ischaemia. The persistence of ST segment elevation after healing of an acute myocardial infaction indicates a weak ventricular scar or a ventricular aneurysm. The chief causes of ST segment elevation are given in the box.

Pathogenesis: Since mean manifest ST segment vector is directed to the surface of injury (Fig. 18.4), leads

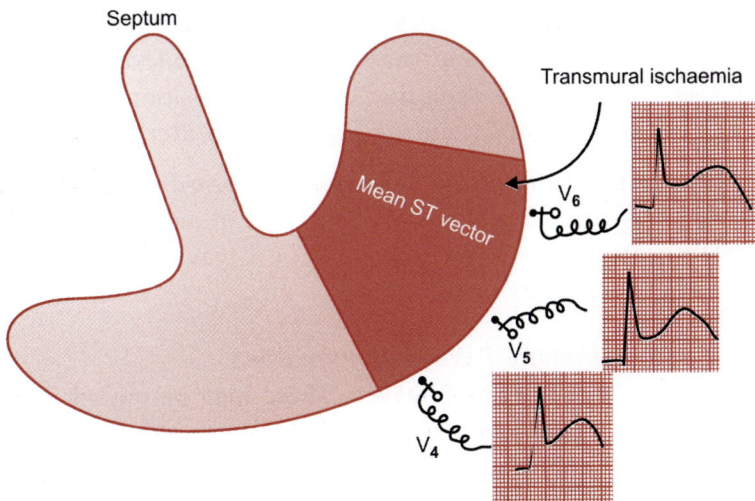

Fig. 18.4: Diagrammatic illustration of ST segment elevation in transmural ischaemia. Note, the mean manifest ST vector is going towards the epicardial surface, hence, the precordial leads (V$_4$-V$_6$ drawn) overlying the area of injury register ST segment elevation

SECTION SEVEN

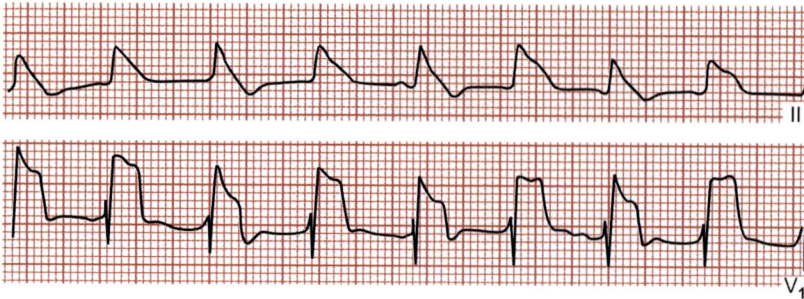

Fig. 18.5: The ST segment alternans in acute transmural ischaemia. The electrocardiogram was recorded from a patient with Prinzmetal angina (during episode of pain) shows ST-T alternation. The ST segment elevation alternates, i.e. 8-10 mm in one beat followed by 5-6 mm in next beat. The inverted T wave alternates with upright T wave. This type of ST-T alternans predisposes to ventricular arrhythmias

overlying the epicardial surface of injured myocardium reflect ST segment elevation. The ST segment elevation may be evident or confined to mid-precordial leads, anteriorly or inferiorly oriented leads depending on the part of injured myocardium. The ST segment elevation is more ominous than ST segment depression because it connotes a more severely injured ventricular myocardium.

C. *ST segment alternans:* Rarely, alternation in amplitude, duration and polarity of ST segment occurs in acute severe transmural ischaemia (Fig. 18.5). This may be accompanied by alternation in amplitude and duration of QRS complexes themselves. It is probably due to alternation in cellular action potential amplitudes and duration during ischaemia. The ST segment alternans though considered an insensitive marker but is highly specific for acute transmural ischaemia, and is even a predictor for the development of ischaemia-related ventricular arrhythmias.

Reciprocal change or additional ischaemia. The ST segment depression is often observed in leads opposite to those recording ST segment elevation. For example, anterior wall ischaemia may show reciprocal change in inferior (II, III and aVF) leads. This ST segment depression is considered either a reciprocal change due to diversion of electrical forces (mean ST segment manifest vector) away from these leads or may indicate an additional ischaemia in areas remote from those leads showing ST elevation (ischaemia at distance). A single ECG does not help to differentiate between them. However, on serial ECGs, if reciprocal change disappears with indicative change, then it does not indicate an additional ischaemia.

A reciprocal change is opposite to indicative change, observed either as ischaemia at distance or just as an electrical phenomenon in the leads placed at right angle or beyond to the leads showing an indicative change. First example, if anterior wall leads (V_1-V_6) show an indicative change (ST segment elevation), then inferior leads (II,III and aVF) will show a reciprocal change (ST segment depression).

PSEUDODEPRESSION AND PSEUDO-ELEVATION OF ST SEGMENT VS TRUE (ISCHAEMIC) ST DEPRESSION AND ELEVATION

For sake of convenience, distinguishing features are tabulated (Table 18.3). Some normal individuals show apparent ST depression or elevation at rest or duing exercise. This type of change is common during tachycardia or during anxiety and is attributed to the presence of T_a (prominent atrial repolarisation) wave.

In pseudodepression, the T_a wave continues through ventricular depolarisation, is inscribed after QRS complex and is evident on ST segment. In contrast, the true ST depression is indicated by depression of J point and horizontality of ST segment (Table 18.2). In pseudoelevation, due to superimposition of T_a on the P–R segment, the T-P line and ST segment, which normally maintain the isoelectricity, appear to be elevated (Fig. 18.7). In atrial flutter, this phenomenon of pseudoelevation and pseudodepression may also be seen due to superimposition of flutter waves on ST segment (Read atrial flutter).

II. *Abnormalities of T wave in myocardial ischaemia.* Normal T wave is asymmetrical in morphology, i.e. its two limbs are unequal. The T wave changes may be primary or secondary.

A. Primary T Wave Abnormalities
(i) Low, flat T waves: These may be recorded in necrosis-injury – ischaemia sequence of acute myocardial infarction. For example, in acute

Table 18.3. Distinction between pseudodepression and pseudoelevation of ST segment versus true ST depression and elevation

Pseudodepression (Fig. 18.6)	*True (ischaemic) depression (Fig. 18.6)*
• ST segment displays a continuous ascent with upward concavity. • Down sloping of PR segment due to T_a waves. T_a wave of atrial repolarisation may even continue through ventricular depolarisation and is still evident after QRS complex as pseudodepression of ST segment.	• 'J' point is depressed and ST segment is horizontal or downsloping. • No change in PR segment.
Pseudoelevation (Fig. 18.7)	**True elevation (Fig. 18.7)**
• Due to imposition of T_a on the PR, the TP line and the ST segment that represent the baseline and maintain isoelectricity appear elevated– called pseudoelevation of ST segment.	• The 'J' point and ST segment are elevated above the baseline and there is convex contour of ST segment with sagging of T wave upwards.

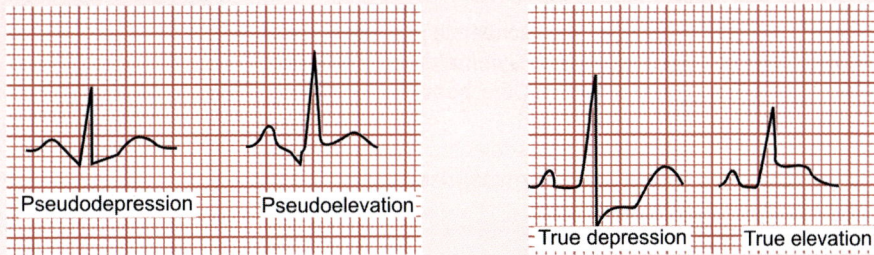

Fig. 18.6: Pseudoinfarction *vs* true depression and pseudoelevation *vs* true elevation

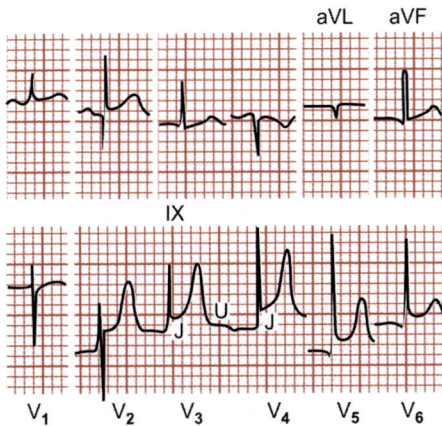

Fig. 18.7: Pseudoinfarction. The electrocardiogram showing pseudoinfarction which may be interpreted as true myocardial infarction. Note the following features:

i. There is pseudoelevation of ST segment and J point due to prominent Ta waves which brings down the P-R segment. When ST segment is measured from TP line, it is more or less isoelectric. The ST segment shows continuous ascent with concavity upwards. The T waves are tall and upright in precordial leads. A U wave (labelled) is seen in V_3

anteroseptal myocardial infarction, low to flat T waves may be seen in leads V_5-V_6 due to ischaemia of remote area (Fig. 18.8).

(ii) The T wave inversion (Fig. 18.9): Inversion of T wave may be seen in acute myocardial ischaemia such as acute coronary insufficiency or relative ischaemia during ventricular strain and during ventricular hypertrophy. Symmetrical inversion of T waves with sharp pointed apex is characteristic feature of subendocardial ischaemia or infarction. The T wave gets inverted during evolution of acute myocardial infarction and may persist thereafter for sometime or permanently.

(iii) Tall T waves : Occasionally, T wave may become taller (symmetric with pointed apex) in acute coronary insufficiency, but it is commonly seen after hyperacute myocardial infarction due to leakage of K^+ intracellularly or may be seen in true posterior wall infarction due to anterior orientation of T wave vector. Following exercise,

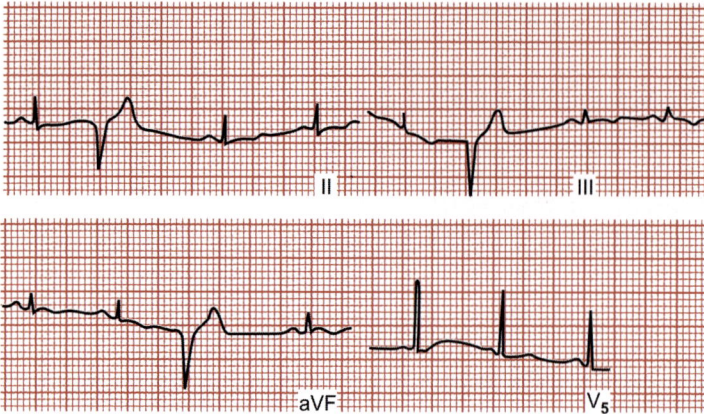

Fig. 18.8: Inferolateral ischaemia. The electrocardiogram shows coving ST segment with inversion of T waves in leads II, III and aVF indicating ischaemia of inferior wall. The low to flat T waves in V_5 indicates ischaemia seen in leads II, III and aVF further support inferolateral ischaemia

Fig. 18.9: Electrocardiogram illustration showing various forms of T wave inversion.
A. Asymmetric T wave inversion of ventricular strain: Note the depressed ST segment with convexity upward and is not isoelectric at any time. T is inverted asymmetrically but is blunt and deep.
B. Symmetrical inversion of T wave of subendocardial ischaemia or acute coronary insufficiency : Note the sharp pointed T wave with symmetric inversion (both limbs of T are equal). The ST segment embraces the baseline for a longer period.
C. Digitalis effect: The depressed ST segment is not isoelectric for any period. It shows a straight downward slope with a sharp terminal rise resembling the mirror image sign of correction or tick mark (✔)

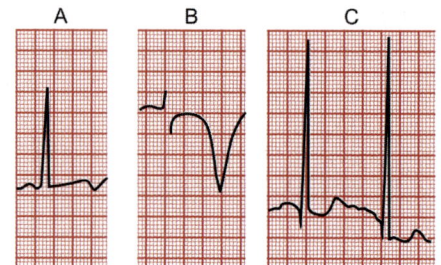

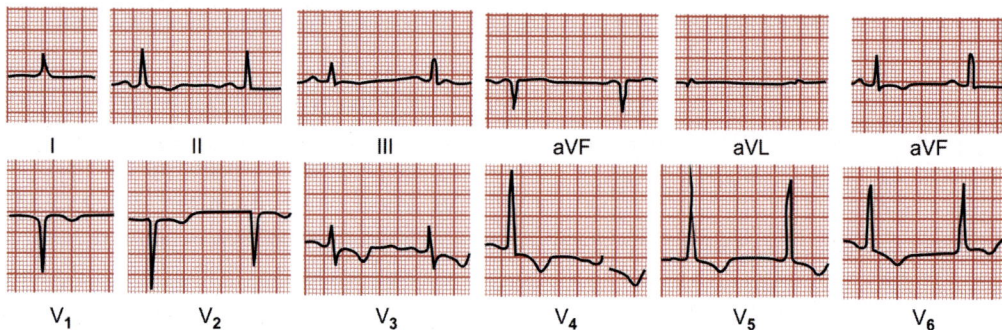

Fig. 18.10: Global T wave inversion recorded from an asymptomatic 30 years F who was referred to us for consultation regarding abnormal resting ECG with normal angiogram and stress test. The repeat ECG (depicted) shows T wave inversion in leads I, II, III, aVF and V_1-V_6 without any q wave or reduction in height of R wave or any significant ST change. The R wave progression in precordial leads is normal. The serum enzyme (CPK-MB) was normal. Persistence of these changes for a period of > 1 year with normal sophisticated test indicate them of no consequence

if the height of T wave increases more than the resting value, coronary ischaemia may be suspected (Fig. 18.10).

(iv) Global, diffuse symmetrical inversion of T wave is a nonspecific finding, most often seen in patients with myocardial ischaemia or infarction, cerebrovascular accidents, cardiac resuscitation, cardiomyopathy (hypertrophic nonobstructive), acute pulmonary embolism and rarely pheochromocytoma induced myocarditis. In small number of cases, it can occur without an evidence of organic heart disease especially in females.

B. Secondary T wave changes
These result from alteration of the timing or sequence of depolarisation or both, reflect an obligatory change in the order of repolarisation. For example in LBBB,

the left ventricular epicardial activation is delayed and prolonged because of slow conduction through ventricular myocardium. As a result of the above change, repolarisation begins in the subendocardium and an inverted T wave results in precordial leads due to orientation of T vector away from these leads. The change in the polarity of the QRS complex and T wave is identical but opposite in direction (i.e. if QRS is upright then T is inverted and if QRS is negative then T is upright). When LBBB is associated with upright T waves in left precordial leads, regional abnormalities due to myocardial disease may be suspected.

(i) Rate-dependant T wave changes (Fig. 18.11): These may be noted following a supraventricular or ventricular tachycardia. Abrupt change in cycle length may also produce T wave changes, seen following ventricular extrasystole (post-extrasystolic T wave change) or after an interpolated ventricular premature complex.

(ii) T wave alternans without QRS and P wave alternation: It is a rare abnormality and occurs due to alternans of phase 2 and 3 of the action potential of T wave without any change in the phase O. The T wave alternans may be seen during tachycardia or premature ventricular extrasystoles, advanced heart disease, severe electrolyte disturbance, following cardiac resuscitation, rarely with administration of amiodarone, acute pulmonary embolism and idiopathic long QT syndrome. When T wave alternans is associated with idiopathic prolongation of the QT interval, the risk is related to the prolonged QT interval rather than the T wave alternans.

(iii) Notched bifid T waves : These are common in the absence of heart disease especially in children, may be seen in congenital heart disease, the prolonged QT syndrome, central nervous system disorders, alcoholic cardiomyopathy, and following administration of drugs such as phenothiazines. The mechanism of bifid or notched T waves is not clear. It has been proposed that these may be caused by nonuniform repolarisation secondary to differential innervation of the anterior and posterior ventricular walls and, may reflect regional delay of repolarisation of the left ventricle in left ventricular disease.

(iv) Pseudonormalisation of T wave: The T wave may be abnormal (inverted) in a baseline ECG recorded from a patient with documented coronary artery disease, but during an episode of acute ischaemic pain, they may become either upright or less abnormal (e.g. lesser degree of inversion) in some ECG leads. This phenomenon is called *pseudonormalisation* of baseline abnormal T waves; and in the presence of acute cardiac pain, indicates myocardial ischaemia. However, since normalisation of T waves which are abnormal at baseline may occur in conditions other then ischaemia, needs clinical correlation.

C. The Abnormalities of U Wave

The U wave is a small positive deflection occurring just after the T wave and is best seen in leads showing the transition zone (V_3-V_4). It normally is in the same direction as the T wave. An inverted U wave is diagnostic of cardiac diseases, and when it develops after exercise, it invariably indicates ischaemia. Inversion of U wave may be seen in hypertension or hypertensive heart disease. Postectopic inversion of U wave can also occur.

D. The QRS-T Angle

The normal QRS-T angle usually does not exceed 40°, but does not go beyond 60° in any circumstance in the frontal plane. In myocardial ischaemia, QRS-T angle becomes widened in both the frontal and horizontal plane.

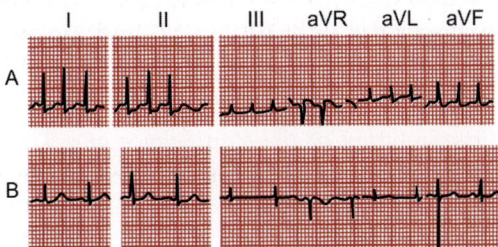

Fig. 18.11: Rate-dependant ST-T changes.
A. The electrocardiogram recorded from a patient with supraventricular tachycardia shows ST depression with low T waves during rapid heart rate
B. Disappearance of ST-T change with settling down of heart rate

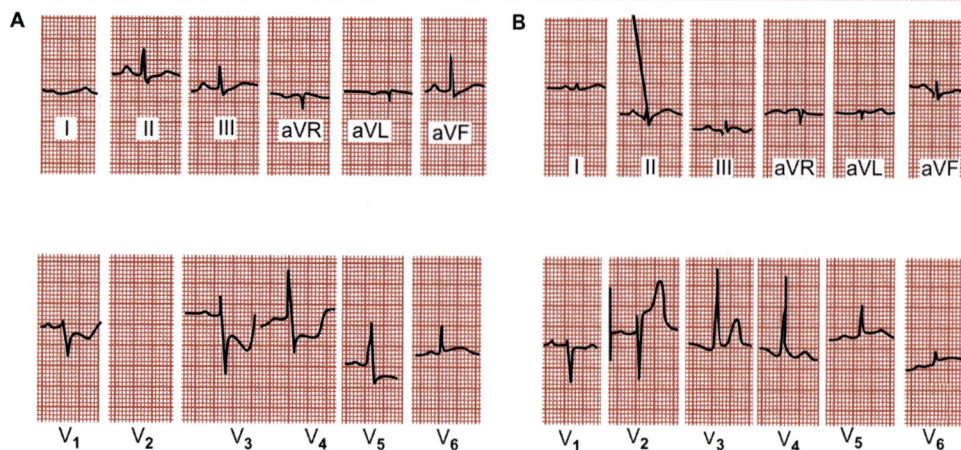

Fig. 18.12: Reversible ST segment depression in a patient with angina pectoris

A. The electrocardiogram recorded at the time of acute pain in emergency department shows acute depression of ST segment in leads V_1-V_4 indicating acute anteroseptal ischaemia

B. The electrocardiogram after admission with relief of pain showed reversal of these acute changes indicating provocable reversible ischaemia of angina pectoris

Pathogenesis: During ischaemia, the frontal plane T wave axis tends to deviate from the frontal plane QRS axis resulting in widening of the QRS-T angle. This manifests in positive QRS deflection and T wave inversion in lead I.

A widespread angle between the mean QRS and T wave axes is also evident in the precordial leads on horizontal plane. This wide angle results in taller T wave in V_1 than V_5-V_6 with QRS complex being dominantly upright in lead V_6. Further widening of the angle leads to inversion of T wave in lead V_6.

ACUTE VERSUS CHRONIC CHANGE

Acute depression of the entire ST segment below the baseline is transient, may occur spontaneously during an attack of angina pectoris (Fig. 18.12) or may be triggered by exercise. Such ST segment depression, however, may also become established and persists for long time (chronic change).

The common manifestation of chronic established ST segment abnormality is horizontality of ST segment without depression.

NONSPECIFIC ST SEGMENT AND T WAVE CHANGES

Although the ST segment and T wave represent different electrophysiological events and their respective changes may reflect different clinical conditions, but as per practice or convention the change in either one or both is referred to as ST-T changes; and frequently the abnormalities of both the ST segment and T wave frequently coexist.

Nondiagnostic ST segment and T wave changes (Fig. 18.13): These are most common ECG abnormalities and account for about 50% of the abnormal tracings recorded in a general hospital and 2.4% of all electrocardiograms. The T wave abnormality is most common because this wave is highly vulnerable to physiological, pharmacological and organic changes, hence, its isolated abnormality is least suggestive of any specific diagnosis.

Although an abnormal T wave suggests the presence of an abnormal, or, more appropriately an altered state of repolarisation, yet it can be recorded not infrequently in the absence of any disturbance. For example, T wave abnormality may occur as a reflection of physiological influence, e.g. following ingestion of cold water, heavy meal, in highly trained athletes or during an episode of paroxysmal supraventricular tachycardia (tachycardia induced ST-T change). For these reasons, T wave abnormality when occurs in isolation, must be interpreted with caution and always in the light of clinical and biochemical findings.

Misinterpretation of the significance of a T wave abnormality is the most common cause of "an iatrogenic ECG heart disease".

The specificity of purported 'classic ST-T- changes' such as those seen with LVH, digitalis intoxication and ischaemic heart disease, is relatively low. For example, T wave inversion seen as juvenile pattern can not be differentiated absolutely from the symmetrical T wave

Important causes of ST segment and T wave changes

1. *Physiological*
   - Positional
   - Temperature variation
   - Hyperventilation and anxiety state
   - High carbohydrate meal
   - Tachycardia induced
   - Neurogenic influences
2. *Drugs*
   - Digitalis
   - Psychotropic drugs (phenothiazines, tricyclics, lithium)
   - Antiarrhythmics
3. *Non-cardiac conditions*
   - Electrolyte disturbance
   - Cerebrovascular accidents
   - Infections
   - Acute abdominal disorders (Fig. 18.13B)
   - Shock
   - Anaemia
   - Endocrinal disorders
   - Pulmonary infarction
4. *Myocardial diseases*
   A. *Primary*
   - Myocarditis
   - Cardiomyopathies
   B. *Secondary*
   - Amyloidosis
   - Neoplasms
   - Connective tissue disorders
   - Haemochromatosis
   - Sarcoidosis
   - Neuromuscular disorders
   C. *Ischaemic heart disease*
   - Myocardial ischaemia
   - Myocardial infarction

inversion of myocardial ischaemia. The classic ST change of LVH, also may be due to ischaemic heart disease or digitalis effect. Similarly, marked ST segment depression due to ischaemia or subendocardial infarction may be simulated by the administration of digitalis in the presence of moderate or severe heart disease. However, when correlated with clinical and biochemical data, the ST-T changes assume a greater significance in terms of the predictive value.

Because of nonspecific and labile nature of ST segment and the T wave, they can occur in diverse disorders (see the box).

CLINICAL AND ELECTROCARDIOGRAPHIC CORRELATION IN ANGINA PECTORIS

Angina pectoris is purely a clinical syndrome of acute chest pain of a few minutes duration, relieved by rest or administration of sublingual nitrates. It is a transient disturbance, occurs when balance between O_2 demand and supply is disturbed. The most common cause of angina pectoris is coronary artery disease. The ECG is done for corroborative evidence. If changes of reversible ischaemia are present, it

strengthens the diagnosis of angina (Fig. 18.14A). In majority of cases, an ECG may not pick up the changes. In small number of cases, ECG changes may be seen during an episode of angina which is related to fixed effort (effort angina). The changes noticed during angina include ST segment depression and T wave inversion in leads V_5 and V_6. There is no specific ECG change diagnostic of angina pectoris. In some cases, ECG changes of ischaemia may be present in the absence of symptoms (*silent myocardial ischaemia changes*, Fig. 18.14B), which needs further evaluation because certain noncardiac disorders can bring about them.

The ECG changes brought on exercise or stress test and relieved by rest form a diagnostic clue to the syndrome of angina pectoris. Reproducibility of the critical level that precipitates angina, indicates angina due to an organic stenosis of a coronary artery (fixed luminal obstruction) and, no other factor such as vasospasm plays any role. The angina due to coronary vasospasm is a variant angina which mostly occurs at rest and is discussed below. The angina pectoris which occurs after a fixed effort and is reproducible is called '*Heberden's angina*' and ECG changes (ST

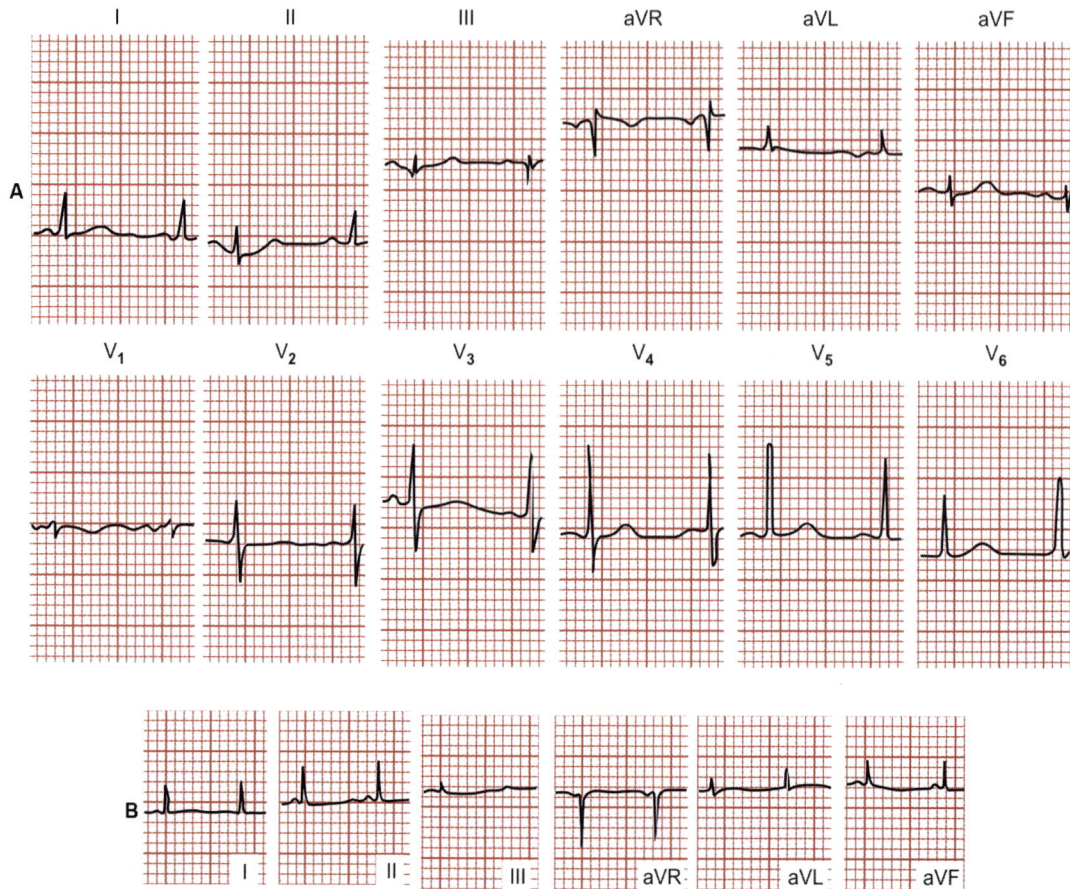

Fig. 18.13: Nonspecific ST -T changes. **A:** The ECG was recorded from a patient who was referred to us for physician check up. The mean QRS axis is +15°. There is no evidence of any chamber hypertrophy. The ST-T changes have posterior orientation, hence, are nonspecific in type. There is ST segment depression in leads II and III. T is in inverted in V_1 and flat in V_2. **B:** Acute cholecystitis. The ECG recorded from a patient (45 years F) shows ST depression and T wave inversion in leads II, III and aVF simulating inferior ischaemia

segment depression) appear during each time after a fixed effort.

VARIANT ANGINA (PRINZMETAL'S ANGINA) SYNDROME

In 1959 and 1960, Prinzmetal et al delineated a variant form of angina pectoris that differs from Heberden's classic angina pectoris in that the pain is frequently spontaneous, occurs at rest, and is unrelated to physical activity or emotion. The pain of Prinzmetal's angina lasts longer and may be severe than classic angina. Attacks tend to be cyclic, often occurring at a specific time of the day. It is not uncommonly encountered in clinical practice. It is, however, not usually preceded by a period of stable angina pectoris.

Electrocardiographically, it differs from effort or classic angina in that episodes of pain are accompanied by transient ST segment elevation in precordial and the standard leads as opposed to typical ST segment depression of classic angina if changes appear. In Prinzmetal's angina, ST segment elevation is an expression of acute transient transmural or dominantly epicardial injury. As the systolic current injury flows from the endocardial to epicardial surface and is oriented to the injured surface, hence, ST segment is elevated in leads overlying the injured surface. In contrast to this, in an effort angina, there is subendocardial injury and the current flows towards the injured surface, i.e. it flows from the epicardial to endocardial surface (e.g. away from the electrodes),

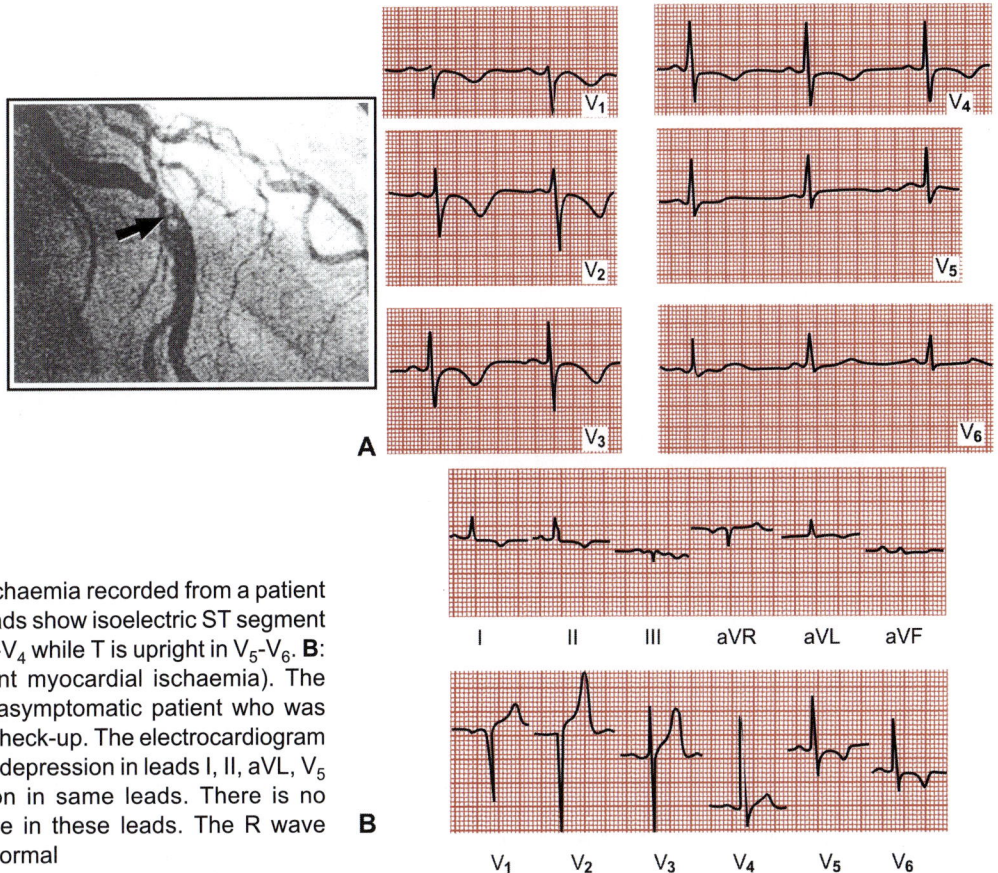

Fig. 18.14: A: Anteroseptal ischaemia recorded from a patient with angina. The precordial leads show isoelectric ST segment with T wave inversion from V_1-V_4 while T is upright in V_5-V_6. **B**: Anterolateral ischaemia (silent myocardial ischaemia). The ECG was recorded from an asymptomatic patient who was referred to us for anaesthetic check-up. The electrocardiogram shows horizontal ST segment depression in leads I, II, aVL, V_5 and V_6 with T wave inversion in same leads. There is no reduction in height of R wave in these leads. The R wave progression from V_1 to V_6 is normal

hence, ST segment depression is recorded in the leads overlying the injured surface.

The pathogenesis of Prinzmetal's angina has been explained by Maseri et al, who attributed it to be due to coronary artery spasm involving one of the coronary vessels in patients with normal angiograms. But, now, it has also been reported to occur in patients with angiocardiographically demonstrated focal lesions that affect the proximal segment of coronary arteries. It has been claimed that vasospasm occurs under autonomic influence.

The Electrocardiogram

The following electrocardiagraphic manifestations may be observed in Prinzmetal's angina.
  1. The ST segment change. The ST elevation is far more common than depression during an episode of pain and disappears with relief of pain.
  2. Abnormalities of T wave.
  3. The abnormalities of QRS complex.
  4. Inversion of U wave.
  5. Complex ventricular extrasystoles or arrhythmias.
  6. Varying degrees of conduction defects or AV blocks.

1. The Elevation of ST Segment
   (Figs 18.15 and 18.16)

Leads oriented to the injured surface register the elevation of ST segment usually of more than 4 mm but may be as high as 30-40 mm in amplitude. This is due to the fact that ST segment vector is always directed towards the surface of myocardial and epicardial injury (Fig. 18.15). The ST segment elevation manifests in leads V_2-V_6 due to involvement of usually epicardial surface of left ventricular apex and the adjacent anterior region. The mid-precordial regions of the heart being dominantly involved due to vasospasm, hence, ST segment elevation becomes more pronounced in leads V_2-V_4. If inferior region of

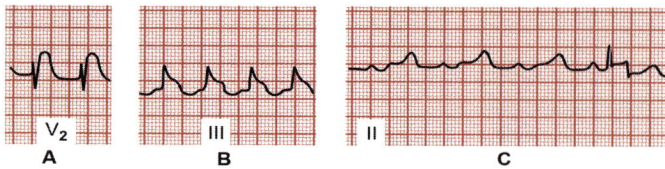

Fig. 18.15: Types of ST segment elevation. The electrocardiographic illustration shows:
A. Lead V_2 demonstrates ST segment elevation of hyperacute myocardial infarction
B. Lead III represents ST elevation seen in Prinzmetal's angina. The height of R wave is increased
C. Lead II demonstrates ST elevation seen in myopericardial disease. The ST is elevated with concavity upwards

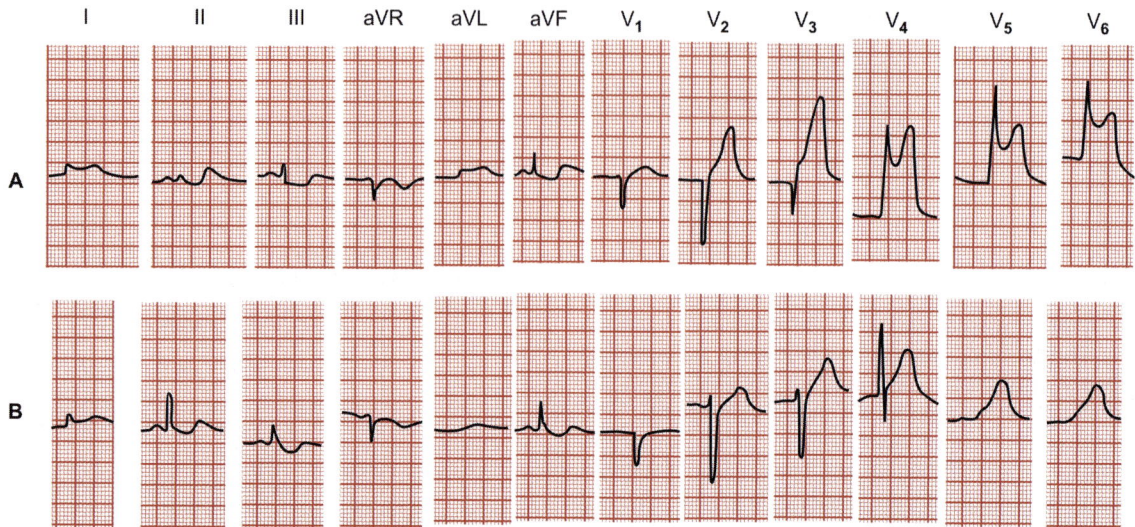

Fig. 18.16: Prinzmetal's angina (vasospastic angina). **A:** During acute pain, ECG (V_1-V_6) recorded shows acute ST elevation in precordial leads and leads I and aVL with T dragged upwards. Leads II, III and aVF depict reciprocal change (ST depression). **B:** These ECG changes reversed after 1 hour of cessation of pain which further confirmed the vasospastic nature of these changes

the heart is involved solely or dominantly, then standard leads II, III and aVF will register the elevation of ST segment.

The ST segment elevation is accompanied by a tall upright and widened T wave and the ST segment tends to have concavity upwards or upwards–sloping configuration similiar to slope elevation of ST segment seen in hyperacute phase of myocardial infarction (Fig. 18.16). In very severe cases, the tall R wave, the elevated ST segment and tall T wave may merge to form a monophasic complex, constitutes a potentially ominous sign as it may trigger complex ventricular arrhythmias.

Reciprocal ST segment depression may be seen in leads opposite to those recording ST segment elevation, i.e. inferior leads show ST depression if anterior leads show ST elevation and *vice versa*.

Hall mark of Prinzmetal's angina

Acute ST segment elevation (> 4 mm) in anterior or inferior leads during acute episode of cardiac pain that reverses after relief of pain.

Clinical Significance

I. Elevation of ST segment is due to coronary artery vasospasm, hence, occurs commonly in the absence of obstructive lesions of coronary artery and is commonly associated with normal angiograms (Fig. 18.17). In some cases, ST elevation has been shown to occur in angiographically demonstrated focal lesions that affect the proximal segment of coronary arteries.

II. The higher the ST elevation, the more severe is the coronary artery spasm or more severe is the

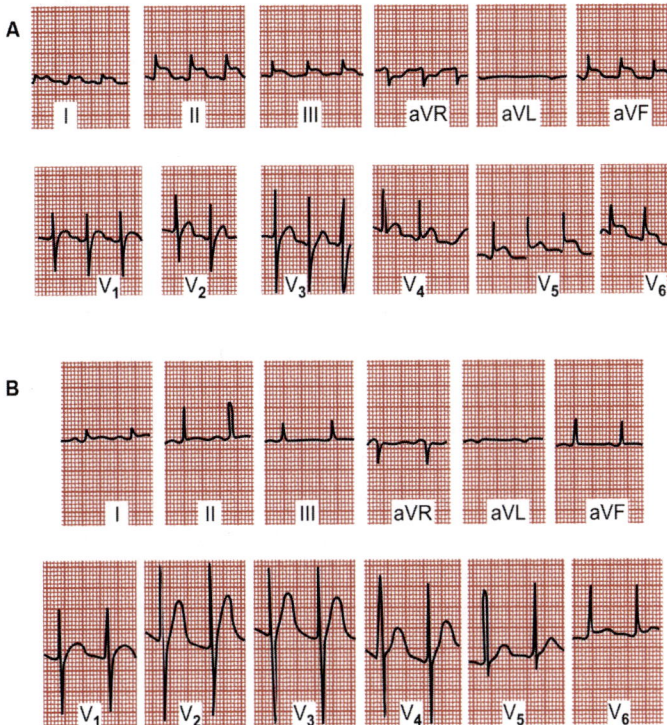

Fig. 18.17: Coronary vasospasm with normal coronary angiograms. The ECGs were recorded from a young boy of 18 years admitted with chest pain.
A. The ECG shows acute ST segment elevation >4 mm in lead I, II, III, aVF and V_5-V_6 with reciprocal ST depression in aVL and aVR. There is increase in height of R wave in leads showing ST elevation, and T is upright in these leads. The changes were thought due to coronary spasm under autonomic influence
B. After 1 hour, the ECG returned to normal. During hospital stay of 10 days, patient did not have any chest discomfort; and frequent ECGs subsequently recorded were normal. The echocardiogram done did not show any hypokinetic or akinetic segment. The coronary angiograms done at later stage outside was normal

coronary artery disease. The patients with triple vessels disease had been shown to have higher ST segment elevation than double vessels disease, who in turn, had higher ST elevation than those with single vessel disease.

III. The higher the ST segment elevation, the severer is the transmural ischaemia and higher is the incidence of complex ventricular arrhythmias.

IV. The coronary artery spasm may be variable and appear in different vessels at different times. The ST segment elevation may, for example, appear in precordial leads (V_2-V_6) during one attack and in the inferior leads (II,III and aVF) during another attack.

V. At times, ST segment elevation may be accompanied by T wave inversion, which may simulate the fully evolved phase of acute myocardial infarction.

VI. There may be ST elevation during one attack and ST segment depression in the same leads during another attack (Fig. 18.18). This is called alternation of ST segment change during different episodes.

VII. Some patients show ST segment depression during exercise which is followed by ST segment elevation during post-exercise period.

VIII. The ST segment elevation may occur spontaneously in patients with Prinzmetal's angina, but manifests with ST segment depression during exercise.

IX. The ST segment, sometimes, may appear as a primary change in complicating ventricular extrasystoles, i.e. the ST segment gets directed in the same direction as the main QRS deflection.

X. Selezer and co-workers reported that patients of Prinzmetal's angina with ST segment elevation in the inferior leads had normal coronary angiograms, ischaemia dependant AV blocks and bradycardia; while patient's who registered ST segment elevation in anterolateral leads, had coronary artery disease and ventricular tachycardia or fibrillation.

2. The Abnormalities of the T Wave

(i) The amplitude of T waves is usually increased and they also tend to become pointed and

SECTION SEVEN

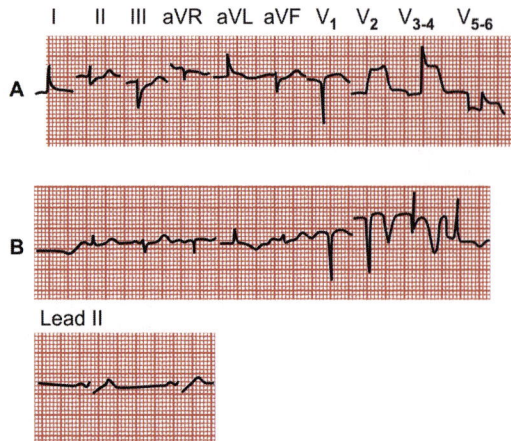

Fig. 18.18: Prinzmetal's angina. The electrocardiogram was recorded at rest. Two episodes of pain recorded different ECG patterns.

A. During first episode of pain: There is elevation of ST segment > 4 mm in leads I, aVL, V_2-V_6, marked elevation, i.e. 8-10 mm is seen in mid-precordial leads V_2-V_4. Reciprocal ST depression is seen in leads II, III and aVF. The height of R wave is increased along with VAT in leads V_4-V_6. The T is upright, and dragged up with ST segment. These changes disappeared within few minutes after nitroglycerin drip and with relief of pain.

B. Second episode occurred next day which showed deep symmetrical inversion of T wave in those leads which registered ST elevation during first episode. QS pattern was seen in leads V_1-V_2, RS pattern seen in V_3-V_4 and normal tall R wave in V_5-V_6. Nitroglycerin drip again relieved the pain and ECG changes reversed. The lower strip (lead II) shows bradycardia recorded during one episode of pain

widened like that of hyperacute phase of myocardial infarction. At times, in severe cases, the tall R wave, elevated ST segment and upright T wave form a monophasic complex.

(ii) Less frequently, T wave inversion may occur, if this occurs, then, it simulates the fully evolved phase of acute myocardial infarction.

3. Inversion of the U Wave

The U wave, if present, may show inversion and is best seen in mid-precordial leads during acute phase of vasospasm. This presentation is like that of inversion of U wave in myocardial infarction, if present, is diagnostic sign of ischaemia.

4. The Abnormalities of the QRS Complex

(i) *Increased height of the R wave in leads showing ST segment elevation:* In some patients, the height of the R wave becomes increased (> 10% increase over the pre-episode value or normal value) in leads that reflect an upright R wave and show marked ST segment elevation. This increase in height of R wave is mainly due to increase in terminal part (0.04 sec) of QRS complex.

There may be a slight increase in duration of QRS complex and increase in ventricular activation time (VAT) due to acute injury block.

Nicholas et al have shown that arrhythmias occur frequently during Prinzmetal's angina and correlates well with the degree of ST segment elevation and percentage increase in R wave.

(ii) *A dimination in the depth of S wave:* The increased amplitude of R wave seen in Prinzmetal's angina is associated with diminished depth of S wave in the leads showing RS complex, thus, RS complex changes to Rs complex. This is due to increased orientation of QRS vector towards injured surface of myocardium.

5. Complex Ventricular Arrhythmias (Fig. 18.19)

Complex ventricular extrasystoles (multifocal, showing R on T phenomenon, bigeminy or couplets, etc), ventricular tachycardia and fibrillation can occur during an acute severe episode of Prinzmetal's angina showing marked ST elevation (> 4 mm) and increased amplitude of R wave.

6. Atrioventricular Block and Intraventricular Conduction Defects

The following atrioventricular blocks and conduction defects have been reported during Prinzmetal's angina.

1. Sinus bradycardia.
2. Transient second degree and complete AV block. These AV blocks are commonly seen when inferior oriented leads are involved during vasospasm.
3. Transient left axis deviation due to involvement of left anterior fascicle during vasospasm.
4. Transient right or left bundle branch block.
5. Transient bifascicular block (right bundle branch block with left anterior hemiblock).

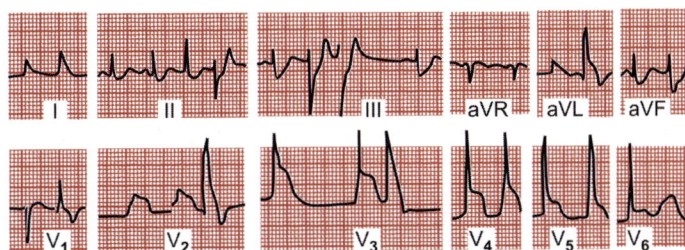

Fig. 18.19: Complex ventricular arrhythmias in Prinzmetal's angina. The electrocardiogram recorded during an episode of acute chest pain at rest in a young patient shows:
  i. Marked ST elevation in anterior leads (I, aVL, V_2-V_6). The T wave is upright and dragged up with elevated ST segment
 ii. Reciprocal ST depression with concave upward slope is seen in leads II, III and aVF
iii. Complex ventricular extrasystoles are seen. They are seen as a couplet in lead III, bigeminy type in leads aVL, V_1 and V_6, and as an isolated VPCs in leads II and V_3. These ectopics have same degree of ST elevation or depression. The major positive deflection of VPCs in V_1 and negative deflection in V_6 localises the site of origin from left ventricle

ASYMPTOMATIC ELECTROCARDIOGRAPHIC ABNORMALITIES

Asymptomatic ECG abnormalities have diagnostic significance – major abnormal Q waves indicate silent myocardial infarction and is a common cause for coronary artery disease (CAD) prevalence. Similarly, asymptomatic ST segment and T wave abnormalities may be indicative of CAD, but are most of the time interpreted as nonspecific findings especially in females. The prognostic significance of axis deviations (left or right), RBBB and asymptomatic ventricular arrhythmias is not clear, but, however, adverse prognosis of LVH, LBBB and complete heart block is well known. These abnormalities being silent and detected accidentally pose a problem for fitness of the patient for general anaesthesia. Previous record may be summoned, if any. The patient must be assessed by other means (stress ECG, echocardiography and myocardial scanning) to declare him/her fit. The prevalence of ECG changes in asymptomatic individuals are presented in the box.

Prevalence of ECG abnormalities among asymptomatic population

1. *Q wave:* An age-related increase in the prevalence and higher prevalence in males suggest pathological significance of these Q waves.
2. *Nonspecific ST segment depression and T wave inversion:* There is no set pattern and these changes do not *conform* to any specific coronary artery syndrome.
       These ECG changes may be totally asymptomatic in younger age groups but are more often associated with CAD in older individuals.
3. *Left ventricular hypertrophy:* In Framingham study, An ECG evidence of LVH was 2.9% in males and 1.5% in females. The Framingham cohort showed that persons with LVH on ECG have a higher chances of developing hypertension as well as adverse cardiac events at 10 years of its development.
4. *Right bundle branch block:* There is high prevalence of RBBB and asymptomatic atrioventricular conduction defects. The presence of incomplete RBBB may not have an adverse prognostic significance; the presence of first degree AV block (P-R interval > 0.20 sec) has a natural history of adverse outcome with progression to complete AV block. Presence of Mobitz type I and complete heart block in asymptomatic individuals suggest adverse prognosis.
5. *Other ECG changes are:*
    a) Axis deviations (right or left)
    b) R-wave changes
    c) Intraventricular conduction defects – more common in females than males.
    d) Ventricular arrhythmias, i.e. ectopics occur with equal frequency in males and females.
    Note : LVH on ECG is very specific for diagnosis of left ventricular mass and indicates adverse long-term outcome.

SECTION SEVEN

Suggested Reading

1. Bateman TM et al: Transient pathologic waves during acute ischaemic events: An electrocardiographic correlate of stunned but viable myocardium. *Am Heart J* **106**: 102, 1986.

2. Deanfield JE, Ribeiro P, Oakley K, et al: Analysis of ST segment changes is normal subjects *Am J Cardiol* **54**: 321;1981.

3. Demedina EOR, Haver RNW: Clinical utility of the ECG in patients with cardiac arrhythmias. In: Zipes D, Jalife J (Eds): Cardiac Electrophysiology from cell to beside. Philadelphia. WB Saunders Company **798**: 86; 1990.

4. Friedberg CK and Zager A: Nonspecific ST and T wave changes. *Circulation* **23**: 655, 1961.

5. Goldschlager N and Goldman MS: Principles of Clinical Electrocardiography 13th edition, Appleton and Lange Publication, 1989.

6. Kannel WB, Abbott RD: Incidence and prognosis of unrecognised myocardial infarction. An update on the Framingham study. *N Engl J Med* **311**: 1144; 1984.

7. Kannel WB, Gordon T, Qffutt D: Left ventricular hypertrophy by ECG. Prevalence, incidence and mortality in Framingham study. *Ann Intern Med* **71**: 89-96, 1969.

8. Levy D, Labib SB, Anderson KM et al: Determinants of sensitivity and specificity of electrocardiographic criteria of left ventricular hypertrophy. *Circulation* **81**: 815, 1990.

9. Maseri A, L'Abbate A, Chierchia S: Significance of spasm in pathogenesis of ischaemic heart disese. *Am J Cardiol* **44**: 788, 1979.

10. Maseri A, L'Abbate A, Desola A: Coronary vasospasm in angina pectoris. *Lancet* **i**: 713, 1977.

11. Maseri A, Mimmo R, Chierchia S et al: Coronary artery spasm as a cause of acute myocardial ischaemia in man. *Chest* **68**: 625, 1975.

12. Mckeigue PM, Ferrie JE, Pierpoint T et al: Association of early onset coronary heart disease in South Asian man with glucose intolerance and hyperinsulinaemia. *Circulation* **87**: 152;1993.

13. Ortega—Carnicer J, Payloss J: Transient right bundle branch block and left anterior hemiblock in Prinzmetal's angina. *J Electrocardiol* **16**: 419, 1983.

14. Parmley WW: Prevalence and clinical significance of silent myocardial ischaemia. *Circulation* **88**: 68;1989.

15. Pipapierto SE, Niess GS, Paine TD et al: Transient ECG changes in patients with unstable angina relation to coronary artery anatomy. *Am J Cardiol* **46**: 28, 1985.

16. Prinzmetal M, Kennamer R, Merliss R, et al: Angina Pectoris. I. A variant form of angina pectoris. *Am J Med* **27**: 374, 1954.

17. Rose G, Blacburn H: Cardiovascular Survey Methods (2nd Ed) Geneva WHO, 1982.

18. Rutherford JD, Braunwald E: Chronic ischaemic heart disease. In Braunwald E (Ed): *Heart disease–A Textbook of Cardiovascular Medicine* (4th edn), Philadelphia: WB Saunders Company, 1292, 1992.

19. Schmaroth L, Schmaroth C: *An Introduction to Electrocardiography* (7th edn): Blackwell Science, 1990.

SECTION SEVEN

19

Myocardial Infarction

- General aspects, ECG characteristics and the mechanism of pathogenesis of hyperacute infarction, evolution of acute myocardial infarction and effects of thrombolysis on ECG changes
- Chronic established or an old myocardial infarction
- Subtle or atypical changes of infarction
- Localisation of infarction–left and right ventricular infarction along with their ECG characteristics, infarction at combined sites (multiple infarctions) and, ventricular aneurysm and its ECG characteristics
- ECG changes and their relation to localisation of coronary artery occlusion
- Myocardial infarction with conduction and rhythm disturbances

MYOCARDIAL INFARCTION

Myocardial infarction is a designated term used to describe the necrosis of heart muscle secondary to deficient blood supply over a critical length of time or sudden complete occlusion of a coronary artery. Clinical myocardial infarction occurs primarily as a complication of coronary artery disease, i.e. thrombotic or embolic occlusion, or spasm in an artery and can be considered as the end stage of ischaemia-injury-necrosis sequence. Most infarctions are situated in the left ventricular free wall and interventricular septum, anteroseptal and inferior regions of the heart. Therefore, left ventricle is involved in virtually all instances of myocardial infarction. Isolated infarction of right ventricle is rare; however, if occurs, is usually associated with an inferior or inferolateral infarction. Atrial infarctions, though rare, are also not recognised on ECG easily.

A single ECG recorded during an acute myocardial infarction may be normal, may show nonspecific ST-T wave changes only, or may reflect transmural ischaemia and loss of ventricular forces; serial ECGs and clinical correlation are necessary for correct diagnosis.

Recently, it has been observed that terms previously used such as transmural and nontransmural infarctions depending on the presence and absence of Q wave respectively are no longer tenable. Autopsy findings have confirmed that patients diagnosed as having transmural infarction with presence of large Q waves on ECG, did not have necrosis of whole thickness of myocardium (endocardium to epicardium). Conversely, patients with infarctions showing no Q waves on ECG have been found to have necrosis of whole thickness of myocardium. Due to lack of this specificity, the myocardial infarction, nowadays, is described as 'Q wave' and 'non-Q wave' infarction.

The infarction process is evolved through three stages or phases, which can be recognised electro-cardiographically as (i) The hyperacute phase, (ii) The fully evolved phase, and (iii) The chronic established phase. The infarcted region consists of three zones, i.e. central zone of necrosis surrounded by a zone of injury and subsequently there is an outer zone of ischaemia and all of them behave differently on ECG. Since an electrode placed on the chest subtends a relatively large area, may include all the three zones and may reflect their ECG changes (Fig. 19.1),

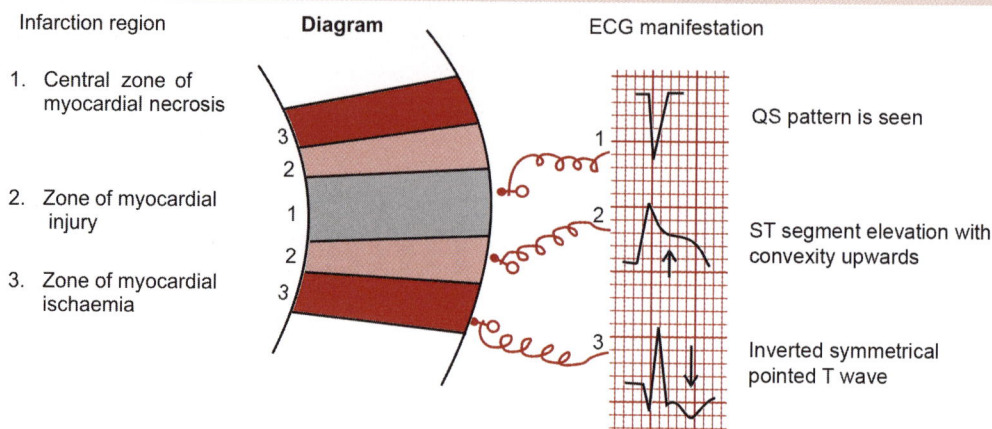

Fig. 19.1: ECG manifestations of various zones of infarcted region

otherwise, all the three zone may be detected separately in different leads.

The Electrocardiographic Characteristics

Mechanisms of Electrocardiographic Patterns

The electrocardiographic abnormalities seen in myocardial infarction are due to ischaemia-injury-necrosis sequence and include :

1. The QRS abnormalities
2. The ST segment changes
3. The T wave changes
4. The U wave changes

1. The QRS Complex Abnormalities and Their Pathogenesis

Since infarcted tissue is electrically silent, i.e. incapable of generating electrical potentials and is inexcitable; manifests electrocardiographically by QRS negativity and/or loss of QRS positivity in a lead overlying the infarcted region. Thus, ECG complexes may show one or more of the following characteristics of QRS;

   i. A QS complex
   ii. A Qr or QR complex
   iii. The loss of R wave height

(i) A QS complex: A QS complex is totally negative QRS, represents a complete loss of positivity, is evident most commonly in leads overlying the area of myocardial infarction. It represents zone of necrosis. *Pathogenesis:* The myocardial necrotic tissue being electrically negative, cannot be depolarised or activated, therefore, if it involves practically the full

thickness of myocardium (transmural), an electrical hole or a window becomes evident in the ventricular wall. An electrode overlying this hole or window will record the electrical activity of distant healthy muscle sensing through this hole. It is not due to transmission of negative electrical potential of left ventricular cavity, a concept previously held, has not been found valid when applied to body surface potentials. Nowadays, the mechanism that holds true is as follows;

"An electrode overlying the necrotic region of the left ventricle will first sense and reflect the resultant vector of septal depolarisation which is from left to right (Fig. 19.2 vector I), hence, being directed away from the electrode will result in a negative deflection (q wave). The electrode will then sense distant depolarisation of the free wall of the right ventricle, and since, this vector (Fig. 19.2 vector 2) is also directed away from the electrode will result in a further negative deflection. The negative deflections produced by these two vectors (1 and 2) result in total negative deflection of QRS producing QS complex."

From the above discussion, it has become abundantly clear that QRS negativity, thus, is the expression of QRS forces or vectors which are directed away from the electrode oriented to the infarcted region. Now it can be deduced that vectorial principle governing the electrocardiographic expression of myocardial necrosis states that "QRS vectors are directed away from the necrotic or infarcted myocardium."

The electrical forces during myocardial infarction are directed away from the infarcted area leading to QS complex in the leads overlying that area.

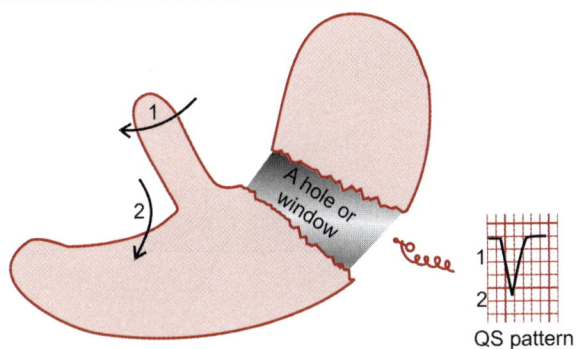

Fig. 19.2: Diagrammatic illustration of QRS vectors (1 and 2) resulting in negative deflections in an electrode oriented to the "electrical hole" produced by infarcted area of myocardium

The above principle is also applicable to any electrically silent region of the myocardial tissue, i.e. a large compact region of fibrosis or a ventricular aneurysm.

(ii) *The Qr or QR complex:* A QR complex consists of a deep, wide abnormal Q wave followed by a small ensuing r wave or R wave. The r or R wave indicates the terminal positivity; actually represents the depolarisation of the remaining viable (electrically excitable) myocardial tissue in the infarcted ventricular free wall (Fig. 19.3).

Pathogenesis: The significant loss of initial QRS forces will result in a pathological Q wave followed by late activation of viable myocardial tissue that will result in inscription of an r wave, the magnitude of which depends on the viable myocardium.

Pathological Q waves and its genesis : The most common diagnostic abnormality of myocardial infarction on ECG is wide (> 0.04 sec) and deep (> 25% of R wave in same lead) q waves or QS complexes. Small nonpathologic Q waves that do not meet the above mentioned criteria for width and height are seen in normal individuals in leads I, aVL, V_4 to V_6. The q waves in these leads indicate normal depolarisation of interventricular septum from left to right. The difference between normal and abnormal q waves are given in the box.

The Q waves

Normal
- A normal 'q' wave is < 0.03 sec (<1 mm) in width and does not exceed 25% of the R wave in the same lead.

Abnormal
- A wide 'q' wave (> 0.04 sec) that exceeds 25% of the R wave in same lead is abnormal.

Exceptions
1. The Q waves of 0.04 sec in duration and 25% of R wave can be seen in lead III normally in persons having mean frontal plane QRS axis between 0° to + 30 °, hence, is of no consequence. This axis will not produce Q wave in aVF, hence, diagnosis of infarction should not made only on the basis of Q waves in lead III only.
2. In vertical heart position with mean frontal plane axis ranging between +60° to +90°, Q

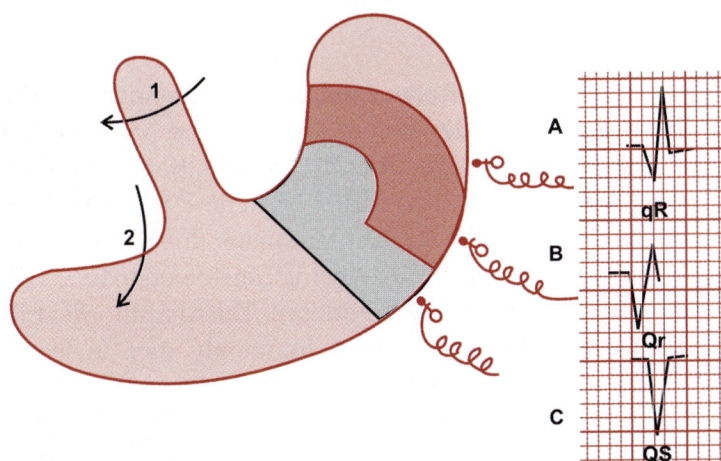

Fig. 19.3: Diagrammatic illustration of
A: Normal endocardial to epicardial QRS activation of an involved region.
B: Diminished QRS activation following a pathological Q wave.
C: The absent QRS activation associated with transmural necrosis.

SECTION SEVEN

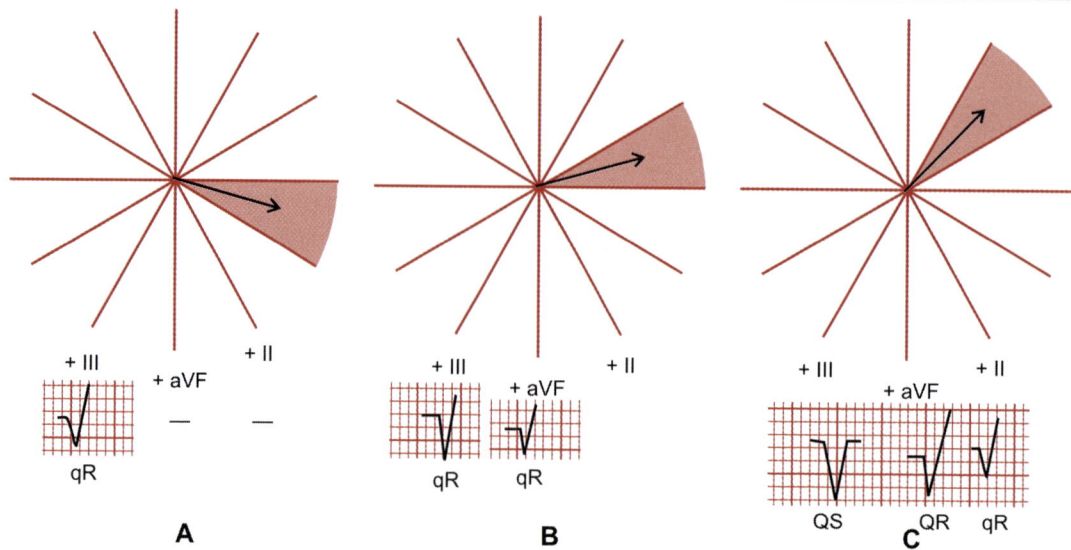

Fig. 19.4: Axis deviation and development of Q waves in leads II, III and aVF (Diagram)
A. Normal axis—small insignificant normal q wave in lead III only
B. Left axis deviation—q wave is seen in leads III and aVF only
C. Marked left axis deviation: QS pattern is seen in lead III, QR in lead aVF and qR in lead II

waves of more than 0.04 sec and more than 25% of R wave will appear in lead aVL. It is of no consequence if this is localised to this lead only.

3. A small insignificant 'q' wave (but not QR or QS complex) may be present in lead V_2 While any wide q wave in this lead is often an abnormal finding, and may indicate conditions other than myocardial infarction such as LBBB, left anterior hemiblock, left ventricular hypertrophy or chronic obstructive pulmonary disease, is thus, not helpful in establishing the diagnosis of myocardial infarction unless or until Q waves and evolutionally changes of ST segment and T wave are present in the adjacent leads.

4. Effect of axis deviation on the development of q waves in leads II, III and aVF (Fig. 19.4). Left axis deviation can produce q wave in leads III and aVF only which is narrow but marked left axis deviation can produce q waves in all inferior leads.

The genesis of Q wave is ascribed to the redirection of electrical forces as a result of loss of electrical forces from the infarcted area. When a myocardial infarction of significant size occurs, there is a change of direction of initial mean forces away from the infarction resulting in 'q' wave (or Qr or QS complex) in leads overlying the infarcted zone (Fig. 19.5).

A small infarction in which only a small amount of tissue is lost, may be insufficient to alter the mean QRS forces, so, a 'q' wave is not produced but it may merely reduce the magnitude of the normal mean force, resulting in a reduction of R wave height in leads overlying the infarcted area. It may be recalled that attenuation of R wave across the precordium may be an indicator of myocardial infarction provided other confirmatory ECG changes (ST-T changes) are also present.

iii) *The loss of R wave amplitude* : Attenuation of R wave amplitude without an associated pathological Q wave is a frequent ECG manifestation of a small nontransmural myocardial infarction. It tends to be neglected as a diagnostic parameter due to obsession of pathological Q waves being considered to be a sole important diagnostic evidence. The diminution of R wave amplitude is most commonly seen in leads oriented to the periphery of infarction, i.e. lead V_6. Normally R wave becomes progressively taller and taller as one goes through the leads V_1 to V_6.

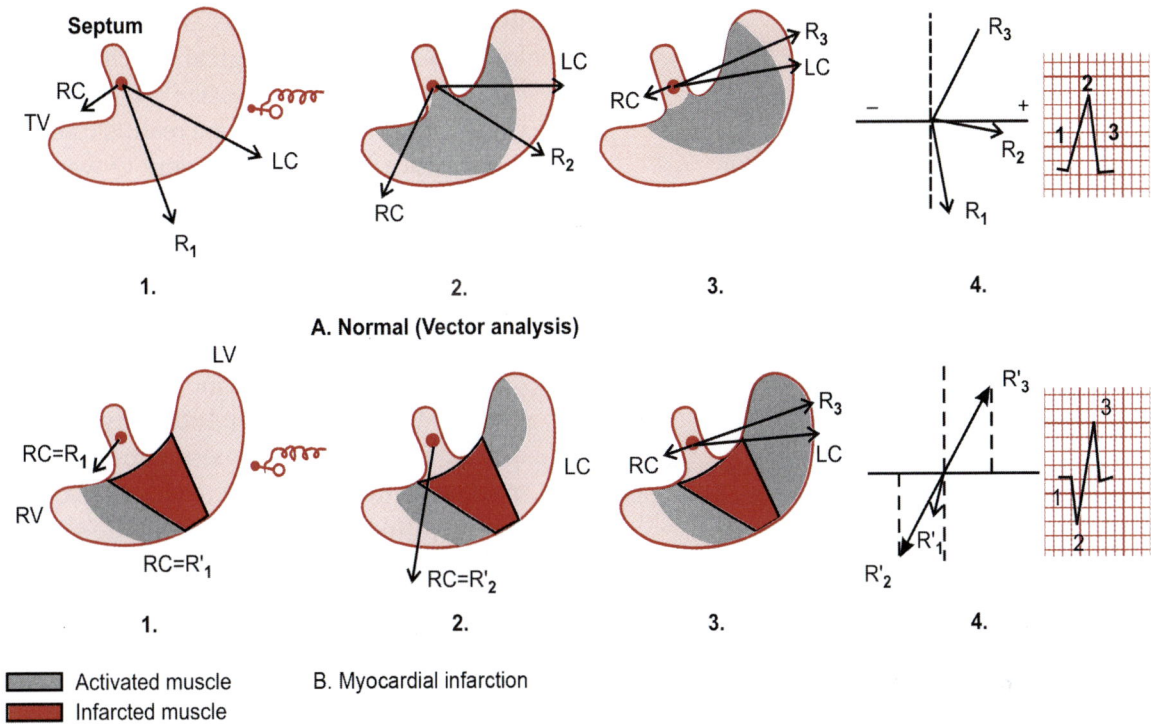

Fig. 19.5: Genesis of diagnostic Q waves and related QRS abnormalities in myocardial infarction. The activated wave-front in each ventricle, their component vectors representing electrical forces generated by them and resultant vectors of these two components are depicted as they exist at three different stages in the activation process. In **A(4)**, the three instantaneous vectors have been projected on the axis of derivation of transverse lead and the values obtained have been used to construct the ventricular complex recored by that lead. In **B**, myocardial infarction (Solid black) is represented, the electrically inert infarcted muscle fails to produce component vector LC in stages 1 and 2 of activation process, consequently right ventricle component vectors (RC) are unopposed and are equivalent to the resultant vectors R_1 and R_2; but R_3 is unchanged. In **B(4)**, all the three vectors produced during myocardial infarction have been employed to depict the genesis of Q wave or QR complex on transverse lead in contrast to R wave in **A(4)**

Progressive diminution of R wave or nonprogression of R wave may indicate myocardial infarction.

The height of R wave depends on the magnitude of QRS forces directed towards the electrodes overlying the infarcted area. A rind of subendocardial necrosis causes loss of QRS forces which try to balance or nullify the QRS forces produced by the viable myocardium. If loss of forces is of greater magnitude to overwhelm the QRS forces, a q wave or QR complex will be produced. Total loss of QRS forces result in QS complex. If loss of forces is not sufficient, then it will not produce Q wave but these forces may be sufficient to reduce the net QRS vectors resulting in decreased

amplitude of R wave (Fig. 19.6). In other words, R wave is produced by depolarisation of remaining viable myocardium encircling the infarcted region.

Pathogenesis: The mechanism of diminished 'R' wave amplitude is governed by the same principle as discussed above in transmural infarction. The QRS vectors (Fig. 19.6) directed towards electrode overlying the infarcted region are diminished in magnitude by a subendocardial or subepicardial rind of necrosis. This attenuated QRS vectors are still sufficient to nullify or balance the QRS vectors which are directed away from the infarction. The pathological Q waves do not appear as the net vector

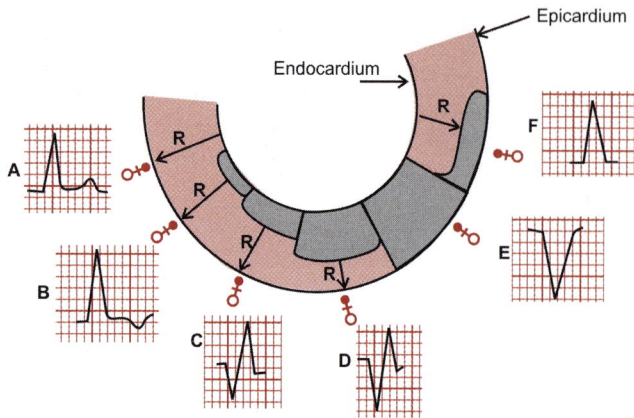

Fig. 19.6: The genesis of Q waves, QR complex or QS complex and reduced height of R wave in acute myocardial infarction (diagram).

A. Normal endocardial to epicardial activation producing normal R wave

B. *Minimal subendocardial necrosis* insufficient to produce q wave but may result in slight reduction in height of R wave. This type of infarction is non-Q wave characterised by T wave inversion only

C. *Significant subendocardial necrosis* leading to pathological Q wave and reduced height of R wave (QR complex)

D. *Nontransmural (not involving the whole thickness) infarct* resulting in significant reduction of muscle mass leading to an increase in depth of Q wave and reduction in height of R wave (Qr complex)

E. *Transmural necrosis* with total loss of QRS forces resulting in QS complex

F. *Subepicardial necrosis* leading to significant loss of QRS forces resulting in diminished R wave with no Q wave, indicates net QRS forces produced by viable myocardium responsible for variable height of R wave

though of less magnitude is deflected by the viable myocardium towards the electrode, hence, R wave of less amplitude is registered.

> *Presence of Q waves in infarction indicates a significant size of infarcted myocardial tissue; while reduction in the height of only R wave in leads overlying the area signifies a small infarcted area.*

Noninfarction Q Waves

While the vast majority of abnormal Q waves are due to myocardial infarction, a significant number are due to other causes :

Noninfarction Q waves may be transient or permanent. Transient Q waves have been experimentally documented in animals and observed in humans during ischaemic episode, are explained by transient loss of electrophysiological function – a condition called "*myocardial concussion'*. Q waves have been observed in shock and pancreatitis due to metabolic disturbance. Similarly transient Q waves have been noted during cardiac surgery, and are ascribed to transient ischaemia, hypoxia, coronary spasm, localised metabolic and electrolyte disturbance and possible hypothermia. Rarely a transient Q wave may appear due to tachycardia.

The largest group of noninfarction Q waves in myocardial diseases include, myocarditis, AIDS, cardiac amyloidosis, progressive muscular dystrophy, myotonia atrophica, Friedreich's ataxia, scleroderma, cardiac tumour, postpartum cardiomyopathy, idiopathic cardiomyopathy, sarcoidosis, coronary embolism and anomalous coronary artery. Noninfarction Q waves are common in hypertrophic cardiomyopathy and may simulate anterior or inferior myocardial infarction, are probably due to increased septal mass or abnormal septal depolarisation because of abnormal architecture of the septum, apical myocardium, or both.

Abnormal Q waves have been observed in COPD with or without cor pulmonale, pulmonary embolism and pneumothorax. In COPD, the ECG finding of QS complex in precordial leads frequently simulate anterior myocardial infarction. The mechanism responsible for the QS complex in COPD is clockwise rotation and downward displacement of the diaphragm and of the heart. As a result, the electrodes are located superior to the initial QRS vector; when this vector is directed inferiorly, a QS pattern results. By placing the electrode one space lower, it is often possible to record an R wave and thus provide strong evidence against myocardial infarction. Occasionally, in COPD, the Q waves may simulate inferior myocardial infarction. The positional origin of the anterior or inferior q waves in COPD may be suspected when the Q wave is accompanied by other ECG changes such as right atrial or ventricular hypertrophy. However, since both COPD and myocardial infarction may coexist in a patient, hence, at times, the differential diagnosis may be difficult or impossible.

Abnormal Q waves especially in lead III and rarely in lead aVF with an S wave in lead I can be recorded in acute cor pulmonale due to pulmonary embolism (S_I, Q_{III}, T_{III} syndrome). Clockwise rotation with superior orientation of the initial vector is most likely responsible for the Q waves in lead III. A q wave in lead II is rarely recorded. Occasionally, acute pulmonary embolism may simulate anterior myocardial infarction.

Spontaneous pneumothorax on the left side may result in a pattern simulating anterior myocardial infarction with occasional absence or decreased R wave in all the precordial leads (low voltage graph).

In LBBB, the initial vector of QRS is directed from the right to the left and is either superiorly or inferiorly. When the inferiorly directed forces dominate, a QR complex may be recorded in precordial leads simulating an anterior myocardial infarction. If the initial vector is oriented to the left and superiorly, a QS complex may be registered in inferior leads (II,III, aVF) suggesting inferior myocardial infarction. The vector analysis is mandatory to differentiate between infarction Q wave and noninfarction Q wave in LBBB.

With left anterior fascicular (divisional) block, the transition zone is shifted to the left and an initial Q wave may appear in right precordial leads. Loss of forces normally contributed by left anterior division results in a vector directed inferiorly, posteriorly and to the right. Consequently right precordial leads may register a qrS complex suggestive of an anteroseptal infarction. By placement of electrode one interspace lower, an rS complex can be recorded attesting to the positional nature of Q wave.

Noninfarction Q waves are frequent in WPW syndrome. In type B WPW syndrome, the initial forces are directed from right to left, hence, a QS complex may be registered in the right precordial leads, and may be mistaken for anteroseptal or anterior myocardial infarction. Rarely, pre-excitation of the left lateral wall with vector oriented anteriorly and to the right, simulates lateral wall infarction. Most often, however, WPW syndrome simulates inferior wall infarction. The Q waves recorded in leads II, III and aVF are due to superior orientation of the initial vector and may be seen with either type A or type B WPW syndrome (read Chapter on pre-excitation).

In left ventricular hypertrophy (LVH), failure to record an R (r) wave in leads V_1 to V_4 may simulate an anteroseptal infarction (Read Chapter in LVH). Similarly, a reciprocal elevation of the ST segment in these leads due to LVH may contribute to misdiagnosis of myocardial infarction. The exact mechanism of the initial negative deflection of QRS is not clear, but it may be related to posterior rotation or inferior orientation of the initial vector.

> *Noninfarction Q waves are seen in a variety of conditions, therefore, for diagnosis of infarction, the ST segment and T wave changes must be present. Vector analysis is helpful in differentiating the Q wave of infarction from the Q wave produced by other conditions.*

2. The ST Segment Changes

The indicative change: The ST segment elevation with coving/convexity upwards is first characteristic electrocardiographic manifestation of acute myocardial infarction. This ST segment change is called *indicative change* because it indicates the presence of an infarcted area. Thus, if the injury is dominantly epicardial involving the left ventricle, the ST segment is deviated towards the injured epicardial surface leading to raised ST segment in lead V_6. Conversely, a lead oriented towards the uninjured surface (e.g. lead aVR, Fig. 19.7A) will reflect a depressed ST segment called a *reciprocal change*. With a dominant subendocardial injury reverse will happen, i.e. lead aVR which is oriented to injured surface will reflect elevation of ST segment and lead V_6 which is oriented to uninjured surface will reflect depressed ST segment (Fig. 19.7B).

The reciprocal change: The depressed ST segment in leads vertical/opposite to the leads associated with acute myocardial infarction is called a *reciprocal change*. Leads that are placed approximately 90° to 180° from the area of infarction show reciprocal ST depression. This change is analogous to those described for injury currents in the isolated muscle strip. Significance of reciprocal change is not well recognised or appreciated because whether it represents an electrocardiographic phenomenon opposite to infarcted area or actually indicates the coexistent ischaemia in a vascular bed remote from the infarction, i.e. *'ischaemia at a distance'* is disputable, since, it is likely that remote ST

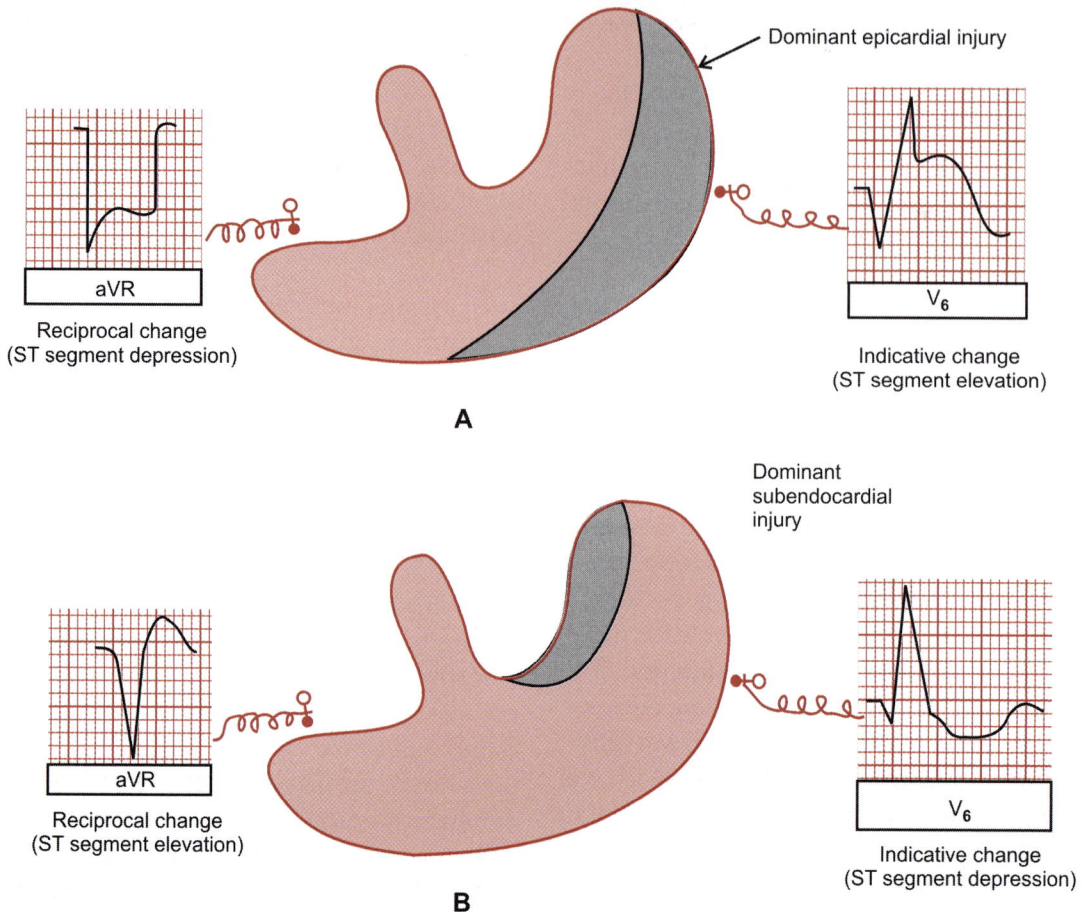

Fig. 19.7: Diagrammatic representation of indicative and reciprocal changes during dominantly epicardial **(A)** and dominantly subendocardial, **(B)** injury

depression could be due to either, thus, it is advised that reciprocal ST segment depression and ischaemia remote from the infarcted area (ischaemia at distance) must be evaluated further by independent means such as perfusion scintigraphy, because completely dead muscle is electrically inert or silent, hence, the occurrence of ST change in leads oriented to epicardial surface indicates the presence of some viable endocardial tissue (endocardial sparing) early in course of infarction.

The ST segment elevation with convexity upwards in leads overlying the infarcted area points out the indicative change; while the ST segment depression in leads placed perpendicular (⊥) to or beyond to the infarcted area, indicates a reciprocal change.

Pathogenesis: The changes of ST segment can be explained on the basis of injury current of rest and injury current of activity. Recent studies on transmural action potentials and epicardial electrocardiogram recorded simultaneously from the surface of the ventricles have shown:

1. During ischaemia, there is depression of ST segment on surface electrocardiogram (E-gram) due to decrease in the resting membrane potentials.

2. During ischaemia, there is decrease in action potentials duration, amplitude and rate of change of voltage producing ST segment elevation on surface electrocardiogram. There is prolongation of activation time over the involved tissue. The reduction in action potentials can render it incapable of propagating an impulse, and complete inability to stimulate the tissue may occur. These

changes may be transient or permanent depending on the duration of ischaemia.

Explanation on the Basis of the Electrophysiology of Normal and Excited Cardiac Cell

The membrane action potential recording of depolarisation and repolarisation as wave forms have already been discussed in Chapter 3.

For sake of convenience, they are again reproduced in relation to injury current of rest and injury current of activation. A healthy resting membrane of cardiac cell has positive charge over the surface and negative charge in the interior of the cell. The membrane is said to be polarised when the number of positive charges over the surface are equal to number of negative charges inside the cell (Fig. 19.8A).

The stimulated cell and injured cell behave in a similar manner during depolarisation and repolarisation. Therefore, when the cell is stimulated or injured, there is reversal of polarity due to flow of positive ions from outside to inside, and negative ions from inside to outside and when this process is completed, the membrane is said to be *depolarised* (Fig. 19.8B). During recovery, reverse happens and polarity of membrane is re-established due to return of positive charge again on outside surface and negative charge inside the cell. This state is called *repolarisation* which is analogous to resting cell. A series of cells normally having positive charge on the surface in the resting state, the dipole is not created, hence, no charge flows across them (Fig. 19.8C).

The dipole means two charges (positive and negative) are equal and opposite in direction, are placed next to each other on the surface of excited tissue and currents flows as explained below.

Injury Current of Rest and Activation

Injured or ischaemic muscle is electrically negative in contrast to normal or nonischaemic cell, resulting in the flow of currrent from ischaemic to normal cells, an opposite current flows in the rest of the heart. Depending on whether the ischaemia is transmural or nontransmural, current flows are established from endocardium to epicardium in which epicardial electrodes show QRS and ST changes that are reciprocal to endocardial events. The T wave alterations reflect differences in repolarisation of ischaemic and normal myocardium. If repolarisation of ischaemic tissue is prolonged than nonischaemic tissue, the T wave becomes negative, whereas it will be positive if repolarisation in ischaemic cells does not outlast that in nonischaemic cells.

Injured myocardium is reflected by a raised ST segment in leads facing the injured surface and by a depressed ST segment in leads facing the uninjured surface (reciprocal change). This occurs as follows:

Two phenomena—systole and diastolic currents of injury explain the ST segment displacement. Local reduction or loss of resting potential in the injured area results in *diastolic current of injuries;* while an unopposed current flowing from injured area during isoelectric ST segment results in *systolic current of injury.* Both these phenomena cannot be differentiated on conventional ECG recoding.

The concept of *diastolic current of injury* proposes that localised area of ischaemia/infarct is associated with flow of current from the healthy (nonischaemic

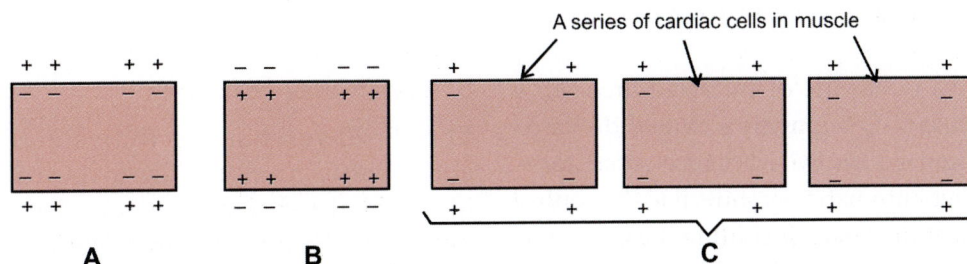

Fig. 19.8: Diagrammatic representation. **A:** A polarised or resting cell. **B:** A depolarised or activated cell. **C:** Repolarised cardiac muscle shown as a series of cells. No current flows as all have positive charge on surface. No dipole is created

At rest

After depolarisaion

Baseline

Normal baseline

Upward shift of baseline as injured area
repolarised early and rapidly

A. Systolic current of injury

At rest

After depolarisaion

Baseline

Injury
deflection

Downward shift of baseline
as injured area repolarised

Depressed baseline, as all areas
are uniformly depolarised

B. Diastolic current of injury

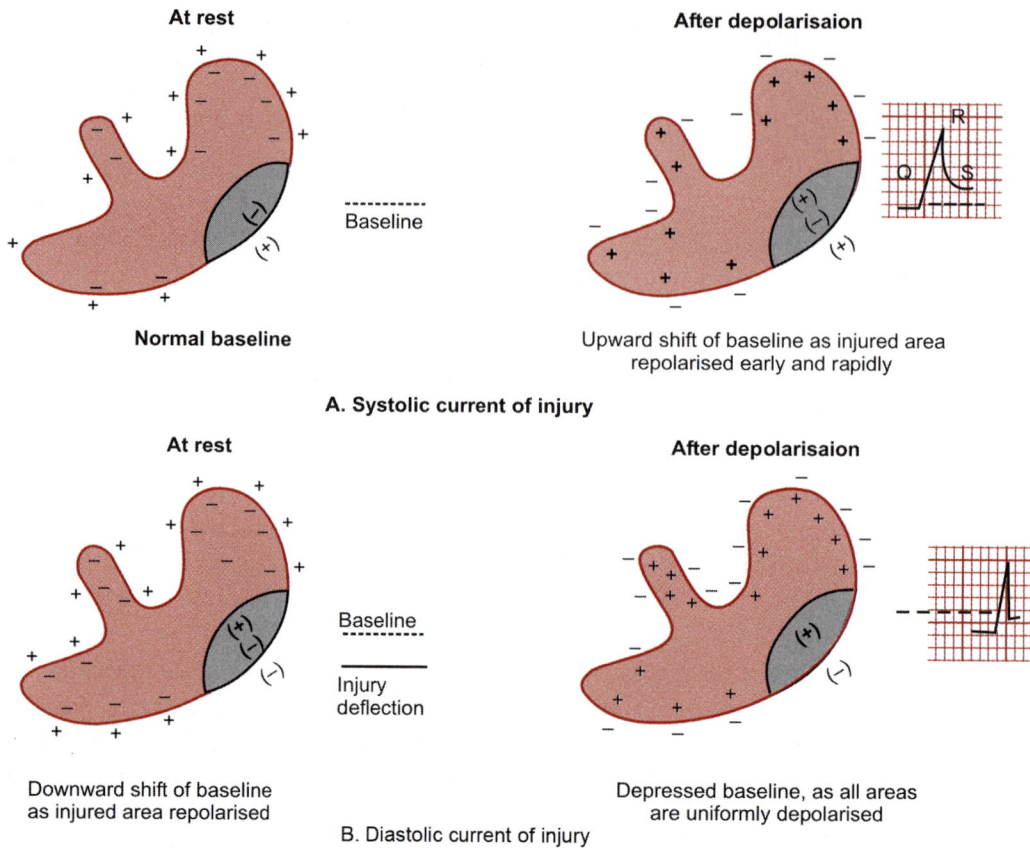

Fig. 19.9: Diagrammatic illustration of systolic and diastolic currents of injury

A: *Systolic current of injury (upper row). At rest,* the infarcted area (shaded) being electrically silent is identical to the normal myocardium, hence, there is no dipole and no current flows. As a result, there is no shift of the baseline. *During repolarisation* the infarcted area (shaded) has repolarised early and is positive relative to the rest of the depolarised heart, a current flows between infarcted area and adjacent healthy area as dipole is created. As a result, the baseline is shifted upwards (positive) and the ECG records an elevated ST segment. Similarly, if the infarcted area fails to depolarise with rest of the heart, then also it would be positive relative to rest of the heart and a positive ST segment would be recorded. This latter mechanism also may be operative.

B: *Diastolic current of injury (lower row).* The infarcted area (shaded) is depolarised at rest, thus, is negative relative to the rest of healthy myocardium, hence, the baseline is drifted downwards (negative). This drift is not recognised as it gets automatically corrected by the capacitor-coupled amplifier of the ECG. However, when the depolarisation of both infarcted as well as healthy myocardium is completed, the potentials of injured and healthy myocardium become identical and ST segment although isoelectric, is elevated with respect to depressed baseline; so that an elevated ST segment is recorded.

Both the mechanisms contribute to current of injury; but systolic current dominates.

adjacent area) to ischaemic or infarcted area. As a result the baseline (T-Q segment) is drifted dowards but is not recognised on ECG because capacitor—coupled amplifier automatically shifts it to the control level. When the entire heart (including the ischaemic or infarcted area) is depolarised, the ST segment is elevated with respect to the depressed baseline and is recorded on ECG (Fig. 19.9).

3. The 'T' Wave Changes

The T wave changes indicate repolarisation abnormality produced by myocardial infarction. Myocardial ischaemia leads to deep, symmetrical inversion of pointed T waves. The inverted 'T' waves, as such, are nonspecific and may be associated with other pathological states such as left ventricular overload, but deep and symmetrical inversion is

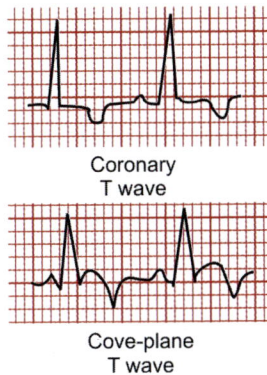

Fig. 19.10: Types of T wave abnormalities on ECG in acute myocardial infarction/ischaemia

usually indicative of myocardial ischaemia or infarction.

The vector analysis reveals that 'the T wave vector' is directed away from the region of myocardial ischaemia, hence, there is T wave inversion.

Deep symmetric inversion of T wave accompanying ST segment change indicates myocardial infarction.

The inverted T wave may have an isoelectric ST segment but shows an upward convexity–called 'coronary' T wave' (Fig. 19.10A) or it may have an elevated ST segment and an upward convexity–called 'cove-plane' T wave' (Fig. 19.10B).

A clinically important sequence of T wave change is *pseudonormalisation* of T wave, i.e. the T wave becomes upright, looking like normal, during an episode of ischaemia or infarction in the patient with pre-existing T wave inversion. Old ECGs must be compared to current ECGs in order to correctly diagnose– or rule out-ischaemia or infarction.

4. The U Wave Changes

An abnormal U wave (inverted or biphasic) is a frequent marker of ischaemic heart disease. Transient or permanent negative or biphasic U waves are seen in about 30% patients with chronic angina pectoris. It is recorded in leads I, II and V_4-V_6. Appearance of negative U wave during excercise indicates ischaemia, is considered to be specific of left anterior coronary artery disease. The negative U wave accompanying unstable angina or infarction frequency indicates multivessel disease with a severe lesion in anterior descending coronary artery. A negative U wave is seen in 10-60% patients with anterior infarction and in upto

30% patients with inferior wall infarction. Appearance of an negative U wave may precede other ECG changes of infarction by several hours. The presence of a negative U wave in setting of an infarction indicates an extensive infarction involving the apex and indicates poor left ventricular function.

HYPERACUTE MYOCARDIAL INFARCTION

Definition: The phase of first few hours of the onset of acute myocardial infarction before it gets fully evolved is called *"hyperacute phase"*. Although it is an appropriate term to be used but has not received much attention in the electrocardiographic literature, and is indeed, frequently ignored or not recognised probably because presence of Q wave is considered as an absolute diagnostic sign of an infarction.

The Electrocardiogram (Figs 19.11 and 19.12)

The hyperacute phase of myocardial infarction is characterised by the five characteristic features present in those leads that face the infarcted surface (Figs 19.11 and 19.12). These are:

1. Increased ventricular activation time or intrinsicoid deflection.
2. Increased amplitude of 'R' wave.
3. Slope elevation of ST segment.
4. Tall and wide T waves.
5. Absent Q waves.

1. *Increased ventricular activation time (VAT):* It is the time taken by the excitation wave to travel from endocardium to epicardium. It is also called an intrinsicoid deflection, is measured by the interval between beginning of QRS complex to the top of R wave of that complex. This is prolonged beyond 0.05 sec and may even reach upto 0.06 sec. This is illustrated in the Figure 19.13.

2. *Increased height of 'R' wave:* The taller 'R' wave than normal, at times, is seen in hyperacute phase of myocardial infarction particularly in inferior wall infarction where leads II, III and aVF represent this change (Fig. 19.13).

Pathogenesis: The increased VAT and tall 'R' wave are due to acute injury block (delayed conduction). The actually injured myocardial tissue is not yet necrosed, is still able to conduct impulses but at a

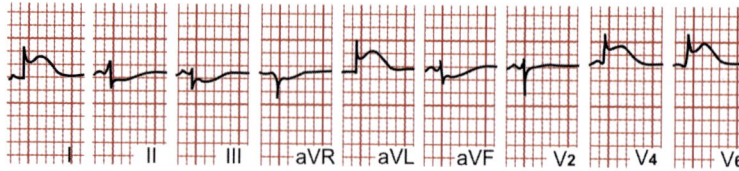

Fig. 19.11: Hyperacute anterolateral myocardial infarction. The electrocardiogram shows:
i. There is slope elevation of ST segment in leads I, aVL and V_4-V_6 with upright and widened T waves and increased height of R waves in the same leads
ii. The VAT is increased in leads showing ST elevation
iii. There is reciprocal depression of ST segment in leads II, III and aVF

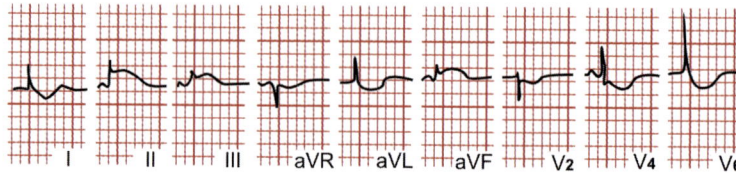

Fig. 19.12: Hyperacute inferior wall myocardial infarction. The electrocardiogram shows:
i. Elevation of ST segment with tall R and upright T waves in leads II, III and aVF
ii. The VAT is markedly prolonged in leads II, III and aVF
iii. Reciprocal change (ST depression) is seen in leads I, aVL and V_1-V_6

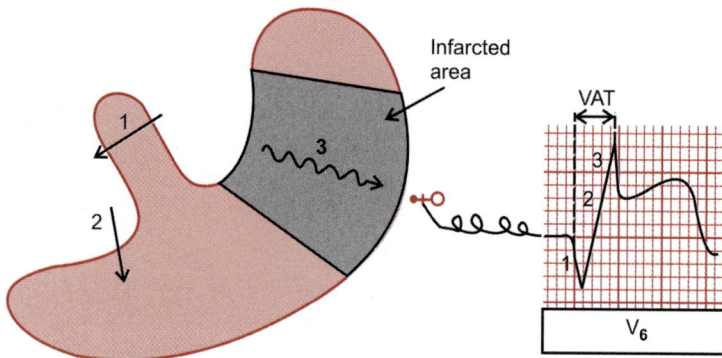

Fig. 19.13: Diagram illustrating the prolongation of ventricular activation time due to delay in intrinsicoid deflection as a result of acute injury or myocardial infarction (only lead V_6 is shown)

slower rate. As shown in the Figure 19.13, the vector 3, which represents the later part of excitation process remains unopposed by distal activation of right ventricular free wall, and is consequently increased in magnitude leading to a tall 'R' wave.

3. *Slope elevation of ST segment:* This means the ST segment first becomes straight and then becomes elevated resulting in slope elevation of ST segment. This is one of the most observable and characteristic change on ECG in hyperacute phase of myocardial infarction (Figs 19.11 and 19.12).

4. *The tall and wide 'T' wave:* The 'T' wave becomes tall and wide. The 'T' wave, at times, becomes taller than associated R wave of the same complex. Very tall and widened 'T' waves in precordial leads, may occasionally, be dominant characteristic feature of hyperacute phase of myocardial infarction. The tall and wide 'T' waves represent hyper-repolarisation of muscle cells due to leakage of K^+ from inside to outside the cells.

5. *Absent Q wave:* The Q waves take some time (few hours) to appear in myocardial infarction. Therefore, in hyperacute myocardial infarction, they are not seen, but appears later on serial ECG and then persist throughout evolution of myocardial infarction, and even in a healed old infarction.

SECTION SEVEN

Note: Prinzmetal's angina may produce identical presentation on ECG, but it resolves within 20-30 minutes following cessation of chest pain.

Clinical Significance

1. This phase is clinically important and significant because it is during this phase that the complications or primary ventricular arrhythmias such as ventricular fibrillation is likely to occur.
2. It is an indication for intensive coronary care monitoring.
3. The greater the elevation of ST segment and the taller the T wave, the more potentially critical is the situation.
4. During this phase of infarction, thrombolytic therapy is highly effective and successful.

THE EVOLUTION OF ACUTE MYOCARDIAL INFARCTION

In experimentally produced myocardial infarction, there appears, in sequence, the changes of subendocardial, myocardial and subepicardial ischaemia, subepicardial injury and, finally, myocardial infarction. However, the initial stage consisting of subendocardial ischaemia may be transient and probably occurs only during the first few minutes of an infarct in the form of tall, wide T waves called 'hyperacute phase of acute myocardial infarction' as discussed already. Generally, the ECG abnormality first seen is ST segment elevation due to subepicardial injury. At the same time or slightly later, there is diminution of the height of R wave. Thereafter follows the appearance of abnormal Q waves because of muscle necrosis. The presence of Q waves, ST segment elevation and beginning of T wave inversion indicate *fully evolved infarction*. The T wave inversion immediately follows as the ST segment returns towards the baseline, indicates the change in ventricular repolarisation and this change persists even after the ST segment has become isoelectric suggesting established phase of infarction. These changes are diagrammatically represented and discussed in the box. The sequence of these changes is sufficiently reliable for the approximate age of the infarct to be deduced (Fig. 19.14). Successful thrombolysis aborts the evolutionary changes of infarction in a significant number of patients, may not be seen in thrombolysed patients.

The fully evolved phase of acute myocardial infarction. An idealised representation of acute myocardial infarction is depicted in Figure 19.15A. The infarcted region consists of three zones – a central necrotic core surrounded by a zone of injury, which in turn, is surrounded by a zone of ischaemia. The electrocardiogram (Fig. 19.15B) explains the different zones of necrosis-injury-ischaemia sequence in different leads;

(i) Myocardial necrosis on ECG is represented by QS complex.

(ii) Myocardial injury is represented by an elevated and coved/convexed upward ST segment.

(iii) The myocardial ischaemia is reflected as deep, symmetric, pointed inversion of T waves.

A conventional electrode does not reflect or pinpoint the changes occurring inside the heart itself. It is actually situated on the chest some distance away from the heart, therefore, subtends a relatively large area including the zones of necrosis, injury and ischaemia. Such an electrode may reflect changes of all the three basic zones. Therefore, some leads may show all the three characteristic changes of fully evolved infarction; while other adjacent leads may show changes of either injury or ischaemia or both.

The reciprocal ST segment depression also evolves simultaneously with ST segment elevation, is seen in leads representing the uninjured surface, i.e. in inferior leads (II, III and aVF) in anterior wall infarcton; and in precordial leads (V_1-V_6) in inferior wall infarction. These changes also resolve simultaneously with infarction changes.

In subendocardial infarction, there is usually neither Q wave nor ST elevation but symmetrical T waves inversion develops. The ECG changes are best seen in the leads which face the infarcted area. They are fully discussed under the heading of subendocardial infarction.

The development and evolution of ST segment, Q wave and T wave changes following acute myocardial infarction are depicted in Figures 19.16 and 19.17A to C and the relationship of these change to time is shown in Figure 19.18.

Diagram		Duration	ECG complex
1.		Normal	Pre-infarct complex
2.	*The early change*	Few minutes to few hours	ST segment elevation appears in diagnostic leads. The T wave is often obscured by ST segment elevation. The height of R wave is reduced. The superimposition of ST elevation on the pattern of an old infarction usually signifies a fresh infarction in the region of previous involvement. This stage lasts for few hours.
3.	*Later change*	Few hours to few days	Abnormal Q waves or QS complexes make their appearance. Ordinarily Q wave develops while ST segment is still elevated. With the onset of infarction, the normal R wave may either be replaced by a QS complex or may become smaller, in that case, it is usually preceded by a abnormal Q wave (QR complex).
4.	*Late pattern*	Few days to few weeks	Deep, symmetrical inversion of T wave appears soon as the ST segment returns to the baseline. This stage indicates transmural ischaemia which has already been present through previous stages –2 and 3 but was masked by strong current of injury.
5.	*Very late pattern (chronic change)*	After several weeks to several months	After several weeks (beyond 6 weeks), the ST segment returns to the baseline but abnormal Q waves and inverted T waves persist. These changes may persist for months or years, in that case, they are called *changes of an old infarction*. Once ST elevation disappears after an infarction, it is very difficult to date the infarction on the basis of ECG.

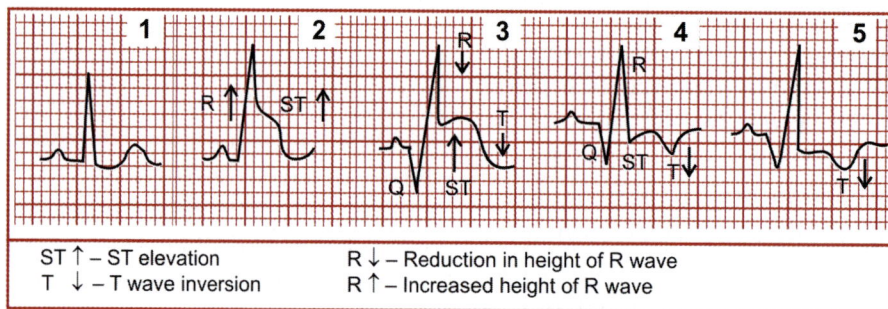

ST ↑ – ST elevation   R ↓ – Reduction in height of R wave
T ↓ – T wave inversion   R ↑ – Increased height of R wave

Fig. 19.14: The serial electrocardiographic changes during evolution of myocardial infarction. A single complex is drawn to represent the change

Note : *During acute chest pain due to infarction, the ECG changes do not appear simultaneously but take some time to appear, therefore, ECG taken immediately may be normal but a subsequent ECG taken few hours later may show changes. Hence, serial ECGs must be recorded before a patient is declared not having an infarction. Since the Q wave and inverted T wave of acute phase of myocardial infarction may persist, sometimes, for long period or indefinitely constituting an old infarction, therefore, in a patient with an episode of angina superimposed on an old acute myocardial infarction will be a difficult situation to diagnose on the basis of single record. Therefore, ask the history of an old infarction and summon the old ECG record if possible. In such a situation, other parameters such as raised cardiac enzymes and troponins may help.*

SUBTLE, ATYPICAL OR NONSPECIFIC PATTERN OF INFARCTION

Atypical or nonspecific characteristics of an early infarction are seen in 40-50% cases in first ECG. These includes a normal ECG, subtle ST-T changes, an isolated T wave abnormality, transient normalisation of ST segment, T wave or QRS complex. Similarly involvement of electrically 'silent areas' and/or masking effect of conduction defects may cause confusion. Awareness and recognition of early non-diagnostic atypical abnormalies will improve the diagnostic sensitivity of ECG.

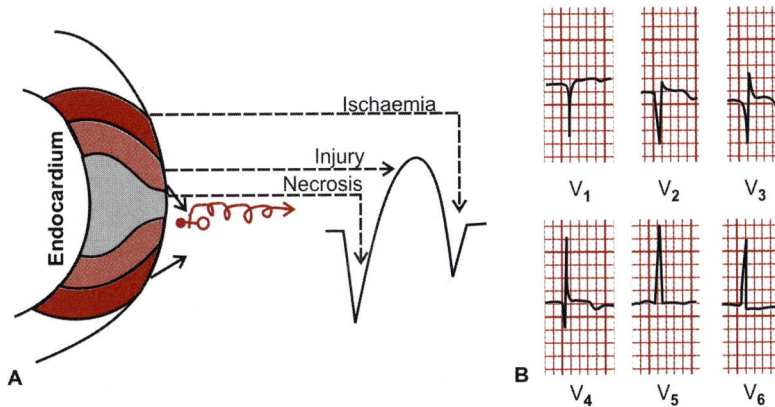

Fig. 19.15: Necrosis-injury-ischaemia sequence during fully evolved acute myocardial infarction
A. Diagrammatic illustration of an infarct which is pyramidal in shape with broad base towards endocardium. In the diagram, there is hypothetical rind of endocardial sparing. A lead placed over the infarcted area may represent any part or all the parts of necrosis-injury-ischaemia sequence depending on its placement and area subtended by it. A hypothetical lead showing all the three parts of this sequence is drawn
B. Myocardial infarction. The electrocardiogram (V_1-V_6) showing electrocardiographic changes of necrosis—injury—ischaemia sequence
   i. Myocardial necrosis is represented by QS complex in lead V_1
   ii. Myocardial injury surrounding necrosis is reveals by qR complex in lead V_2-V_4 with elevate and coved or convex upward ST segment
   iii. Myocardial ischaemic zone which lies away from necrosis zone is revealed by inverted T waves in leads V_5-V_6 without elevation of the ST segment
Note: It is difficult to point out zone of necrosis-injury-ischaemia on ECG because these changes can be pin-pointed only by placing the electrodes directly on the heart. Secondly one electrode may overlie an area of necrosis *cum* injury or necrosis *cum* injury *cum* ischaemia, hence such a lead will show either two or all the three changes i.e. Q wave, ST elevation and T wave inversion. Therefore, the changes shown in ECG are arbitrary and may not be real one due to superimposition of one change over the other

Although ECG changes can be documented immediately after infarction but, sometimes, such changes may be delayed. A normal initial ECG (Figs 19.19 and 19.20) in a patient with myocardial infarction may be due to (i) absence of ischaemia at the time of initial tracing, (ii) a delay in evolution of characteristic pattern, (iii) an initially small infarct that produces diagnostic ECG changes after extension, (iv) transient normalisation of the ECG in the course of evolution of acute myocardial and/or (v) an infarction of electrocardiographic silent areas of myocardium.

Subtle or atypical or nonspecific changes or normal ECGs are not uncommon during early phase of acute infarction. Subsequent or serial ECGs may demonstrate evolutionary changes (Q wave, ST elevation and T wave change)

The evolution of characteristic ST segment elevation along with appearance of Q wave and T wave inversion is highly specific for acute myocardial infarction. In the first ECG, the sensitivity and specificity of ST change alone, especially when marked, is high. With passage of time (4-12 hours), however, evolving changes in the ST segment must be demonstrated, to differentiate infarction from other conditions such as early repolarisation syndrome, pericarditis, ventricular aneurysm and a cardiac tumour which also produce similar ST segment elevation but it is usually a persistent change. Transient hyperkalaemia and Prinzmetal's angina may cause transient ST elevation simulating acute myocardial infarction. Although, subtle, minor ST segment elevation can be easily overlooked but it is a relatively common isolated early finding. Sometimes, the evolution of infarction may be delayed and changes may not appear within 24 hours, but persistence of cardiac pain indicates *"Infarct-in-evolution"*. In such cases, the ECG changes may be delayed beyond 24 hours of cardiac pain (Fig. 19.21).

SECTION SEVEN

A

I   II   III   aVR   aVL   aVF

V₁   V₂   V₃   V₄   V₅   V₆

B

I   II   III   aVR   aVL   aVF

V₁   V₂   V₃   V₄   V₅   V₆

C

I   II   III   aVR   aVL   aVF

V₁   V₂   V₃   V₄   V₅   V₆

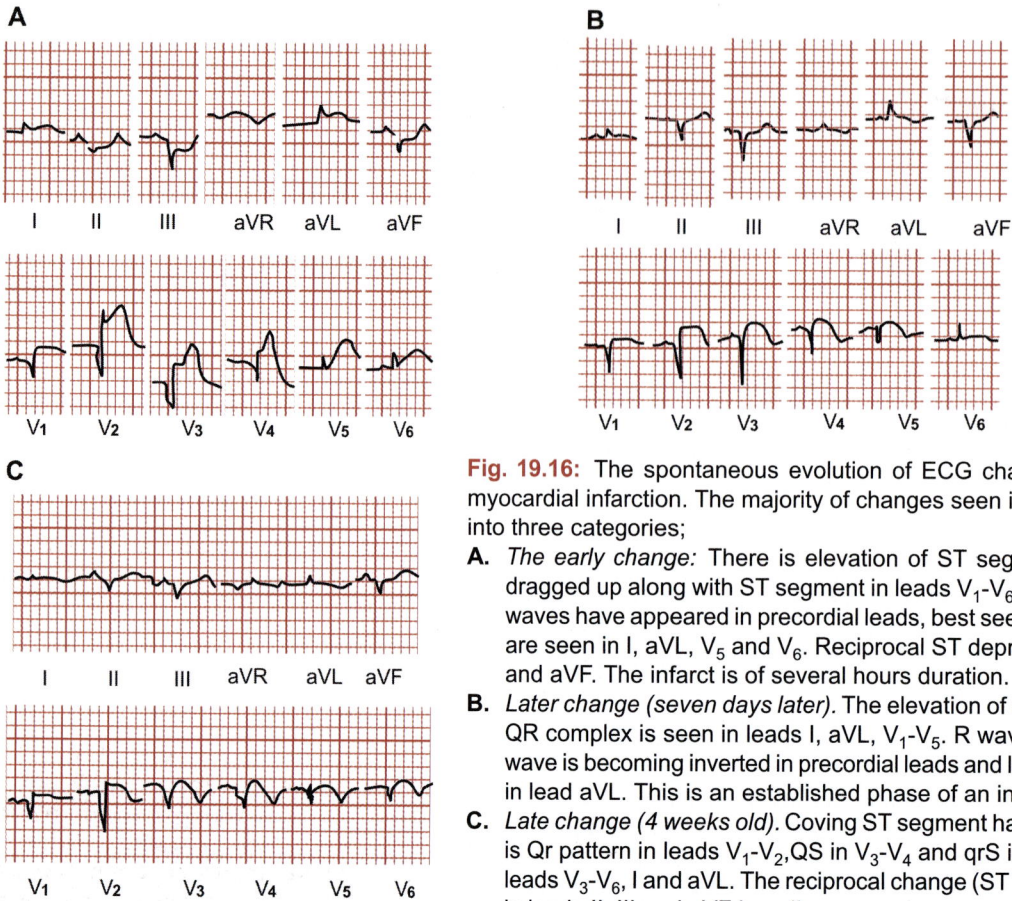

Fig. 19.16: The spontaneous evolution of ECG changes during acute anterior myocardial infarction. The majority of changes seen in clinical practice mostly fall into three categories;

A. *The early change:* There is elevation of ST segment with wide tall T wave dragged up along with ST segment in leads V_1-V_6 and leads I and aVL. The Q waves have appeared in precordial leads, best seen from V_1-V_4. Small q waves are seen in I, aVL, V_5 and V_6. Reciprocal ST depression is seen in leads II, III and aVF. The infarct is of several hours duration.

B. *Later change (seven days later).* The elevation of ST segment has decreased. QR complex is seen in leads I, aVL, V_1-V_5. R wave height is reduced in V_6. T wave is becoming inverted in precordial leads and lead I. It has become inverted in lead aVL. This is an established phase of an infarction.

C. *Late change (4 weeks old).* Coving ST segment has become isoelectric. There is Qr pattern in leads V_1-V_2, QS in V_3-V_4 and qrS in V_5-V_6. The T is inverted in leads V_3-V_6, I and aVL. The reciprocal change (ST depression) previously seen in leads II, III and aVF has disappeared.

Note: There is left axis deviation > −30°, i.e. wide rS pattern is seen in leads II, III and aVF. The T wave is upright in these leads. This could be due to left anterior hemiblock

Fig. 19.17: The evolution of acute inferior wall infarction. The electrocardiogram shows evidence of:

A. *Early change or recent infarction.* The q waves are seen in leads II and aVF with QS pattern in III with slope elevation of ST segment and T inversion in the same leads. Reciprocal ST depression is seen in leads I, aVL, V_1-V_6 . All these changes suggest recent or fresh acute inferior infarction.

B. *Later changes.* The ST segment elevation is reduced. The qr pattern appeared in leads II and aVF. QS pattern is present in lead III. Symmetric T wave inversion is seen in leads II, III, aVF. Reciprocal change disappeared.

C. *Late or old changes.* The ST segment has become isoelectric in the above said leads. The T waves have become upright in leads II, III and aVF. These changes, i.e. abnormal q wave may persist and will indicate an old infarction.

Note: The hyperacute phase of this infarction is usually not recorded because patient usually comes after few hours of infarction

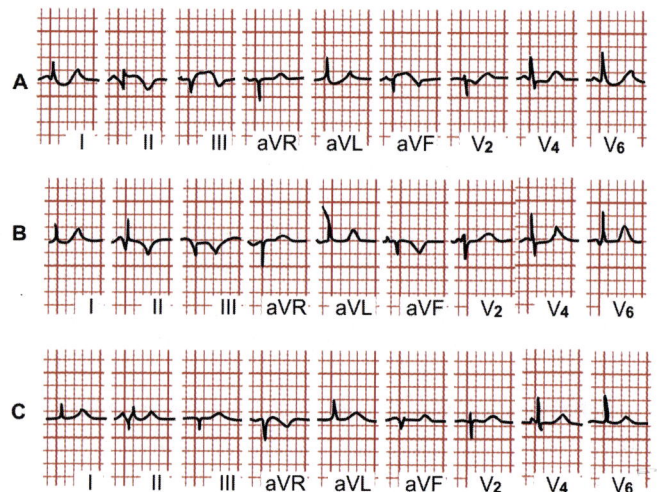

A   I   II   III   aVR   aVL   aVF   V₂   V₄   V₆

B   I   II   III   aVR   aVL   aVF   V₂   V₄   V₆

C   I   II   III   aVR   aVL   aVF   V₂   V₄   V₆

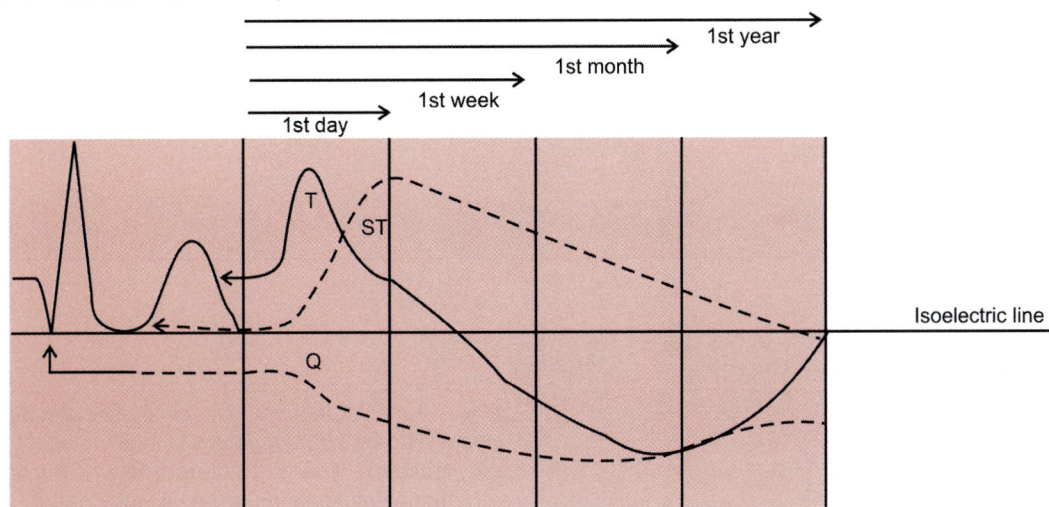

Fig. 19.18: Development and evolution of ST segment, Q wave and T wave changes accompanying myocardial infarction, as related to time of onset of infarction (diagram). The more a curve rises above the isoelectric line, the taller is the T or greater is ST segment elevation, while the greater the descent of the curve below the isoelectric line, the deeper is the Q wave or inverted T wave

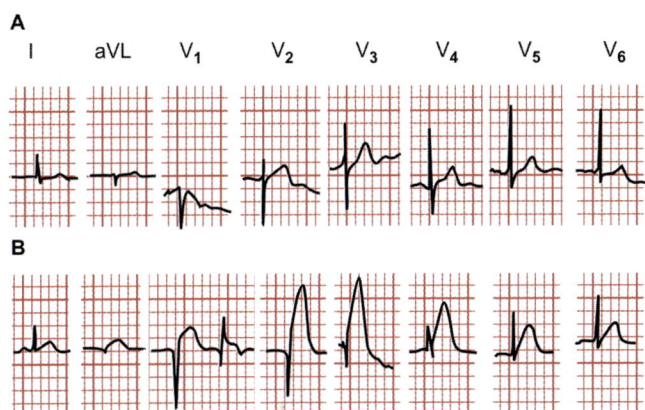

Fig. 19.19: Acute anterior myocardial infarction following an initial normal electrocardiogram. The initial electrocardiogram **A:** taken from a patient who had severe acute chest pain with diaphoresis was essentially normal. The electrocardiogram, **B:** taken after 6 hrs revealed changes of Q-wave acute myocardial infarction (abnormal Q waves, reduction in height of R wave, marked ST segment elevation with lifted T waves). A VPC is seen in lead V_1

Occasionally, the initial ECG in a patient of suspected of myocardial infarction may be normal, the reasons are mentioned in text (read the text) and subsequent serial ECG may reveal it as in this patient

---

Conditions associated with ST segment elevation other than acute myocardial infarction

- Early repolarisation syndrome
- Myopericarditis
- Ventricular aneurysm
- Prinzmetal's angina
- Hyperkalaemia
- A cardiac tumour

Note: The ST segment elevation in these conditions is persistent rather than transient seen in acute myocardial infarction and Prinzmetal's angina

---

The ST segment depression usually reflect subendocardial ischaemia or infarction (read subendocardial infarction), or a reciprocal change secondary to an infarction at a remote (opposite) site as already discussed, but recently it has been observed that the ST segment depression in anterior chest leads V_1-V_6 in patients with inferior wall infarction may indicate ischaemia secondary to obstruction of anterior descending coronary artery rather than just a reciprocal change. This observation needs further classfication and documentation.

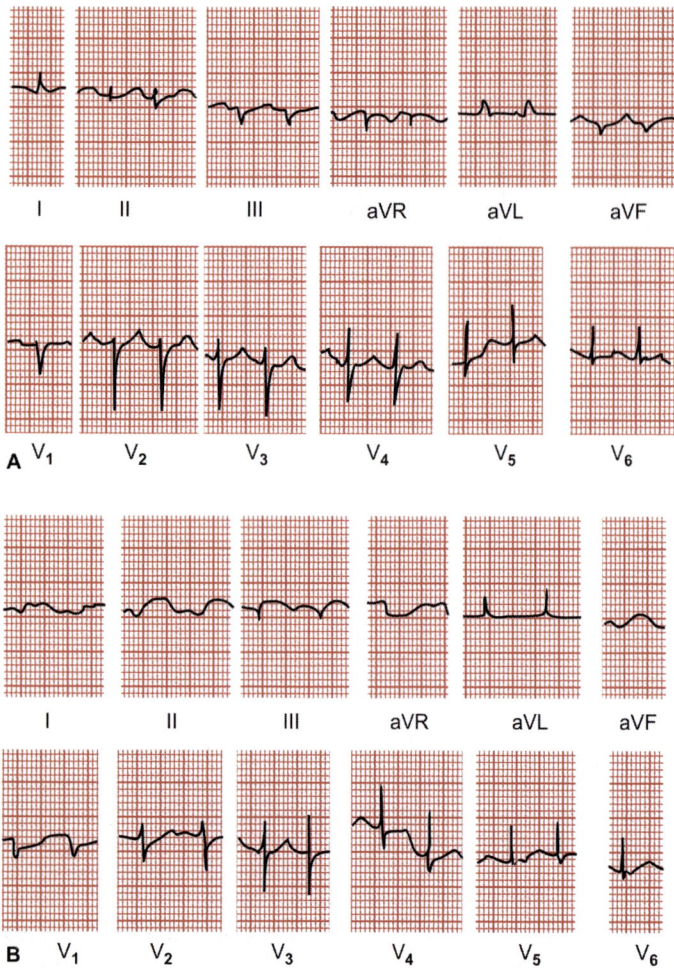

Fig. 19.20: Inferior wall infarction. The electrocardiograms were recorded from a patient with acute chest pain.

A. Normal. The initial electrocardiogram recorded immediately after chest pain was normal.

B. The electrocardiogram recorded subsequently after few hours showed inferior wall infarction (hyperacute) evidence by ST segment elevation with dragged upward T waves in leads II, III and aVF. The ST segment is convex without any q wave in leads II and aVF.

The initial ECG may be normal in 10% patients of acute myocardial infarction. Serial tracings increase the sensitivity to 95%. A single ECG may never be diagnostic. Serial ECGs may be recorded frequently during first few hours before a patient is labelled not to have the infarction. A normal initial ECG in this patient with subsequent acute myocardial infarction may be due to absence of ischaemia at the time of initial tracing, or a delay in evolution of characteristic pattern or may be an initial small infarct that produced diagnostic ECG changes after extension subsequently

Minor or atypical ST depression instead of an elevation is a common early finding of acute myocardial infarction, especially non= U-Q wave infarction, should not be just ignored but should be evaluated in the light of other clinical and laboratory findings.

Tall, peaked T waves are occasionally seen in coronary occlusion in humans and reflect subendocardial ischaemia (Fig. 19.22). More often, initially, the T waves are isoelectric, negative or biphasic in myocardial infarction. Subtle or nonspecific T wave abnormalities are often the earliest recorded sign of an infarction on ECG but their value is limited because of poor correlation. In about one fourth of patients with myocardial infarction, a T wave abnormality may be the earliest sign (Fig. 19.23).

ST alternans is seen in limb leads and anterior precordial leads in patients with myocardial

infarction, but is not specific of it as other conditions may also produce it as already discussed.

An abnormal QRS complex, ST segment and T wave may normalise transiently during evolution of acute myocardial infarction. This may be due to reversible ischaemia or injury or conduction defects, but is also frequently observed in normal evolution of acute myocardial infarction. Presence of an upright T wave longer than 48 hours after infarction or an early reversal of inverted T wave to upright T wave is indicative of post-infarction pericarditis and suggests the presence of a transmural infarction.

A premature ventricular complex (VPC) with a qR or QR complex without any other evidence of myocardial infarction on ECG suggests the presence of myocardial infarction and abnormal ventricular premature complex is presumed to be originating from it. This finding may prove particularly useful

| I | II | III | aVR | aVL | aVF | V$_1$ | V$_2$ | V$_3$ | V$_4$ | V$_5$ | V$_6$ |

Day 0

Day 1

Day 2

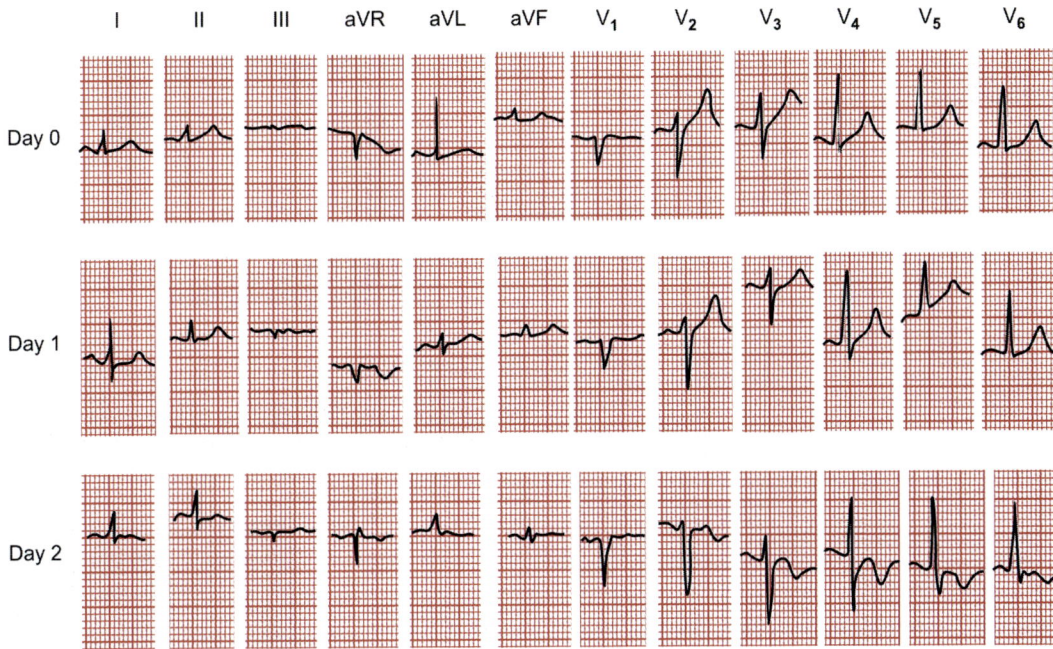

Fig. 19.21: Infarct-in evolution. The patient (50 yrs M) presented with acute cardiac pain with perspiration and palpitation. The ECGs recorded at different intervals shows:

1. *Day 0 (At the time of admission)* The ECG taken was normal. The patient was observed for 24 hours in emergency and casualty department and was discharged after relief of pain and was labelled as angina pectoris.

2. *Day 1 (Next day)* Patient again landed in casualty and emergency department with same symptoms. The ECG taken was again normal. As the patient had same episode of angina one day before and today also, we became suspicious that patient might be having repeated episodes of angina and ECG changes might not be appearing due to the fact that either it is transient or occurring in an electrical inert area or patient is passing through the stage of infarct-in evolution. The patient was hospitalised for observation and for recurrent angina.

3. *Day 2 (48 hours later)* The patient did not have cardiac pain. The ECG done routinely showed acute subendocardial infarction with coving ST segment and deep symmetric T inversion from V$_1$-V$_6$ and aVL. The cardiac enzymes were elevated. The ECG demonstrates the fact that sometimes ECG changes may be delayed beyond 48 hours in patients who are suspected of infarction on clinical grounds

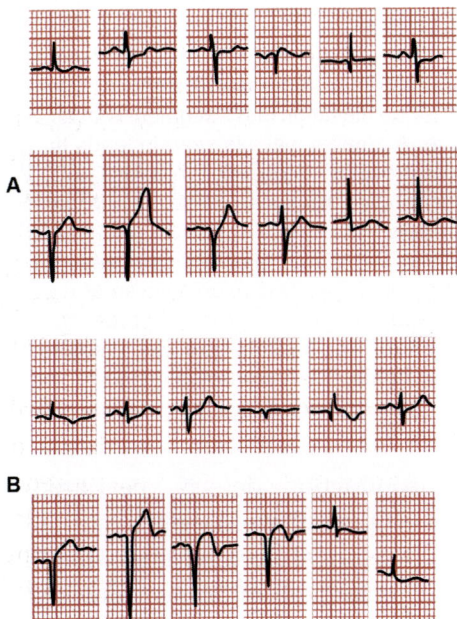

A

B

Fig. 19.22: Tall-peaked T wave preceding an episode of infarction. The electrocardiogram shows;

A: Tall, upright T waves in leads V$_1$ to V$_4$ recorded during early acute myocardial infarction. These are thought to reflect subendocardial ischaemia (leakage of K$^+$ extracellularly)

B: Anteroseptal myocardial infarction was recorded within few hours of previous (A) ECG. There is elevation of ST segment (V$_1$-V$_4$) with biphasic T wave in V$_1$ to V$_2$ and inversion of T in V$_3$ to V$_4$

SECTION SEVEN

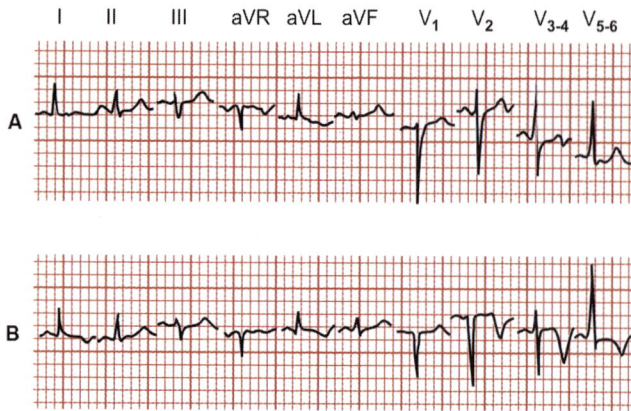

Fig. 19.23: Anterior wall infarction following subtle nonspecific T wave changes. The ECG recorded immediately after chest pain. **A:** showed flat T in lead I, inverted in aVL and biphasic T in V_3-V_4. The electrocardiogram recorded after 6 hr. **B:** showed frank inversion of T wave in leads I, aVL, V_2-V_6 which is deep and symmetric and is neither associated with ST elevation nor a q wave. The R wave height in precordial leads is slightly reduced. This indicated subendocardial (non Q-wave) infarction which was corroborated by raised cardiac enzymes and presistence of these changes on serial ECGs

when myocardial infarction is masked on ECG either by LBBB or by WPW syndrome. A recent study, however, has questioned its validity in the diagnosis of an infarction in the absence of other ECG changes of myocardial infarction.

The Serial ECGs and its Significance during Myocardial Infarction

1. A single initial ECG may be normal in about 10% patients even in the presence of myocardial infarction or may be abnormal but not diagnostic of an infarction in about 40% patients, hence, serial ECGs are must to prove or disprove the presence of an infarction.

2. Serial ECGs substantiate the evolution of changes of ST segment, Q wave and T wave during an infarction, hence, help to differentiate it from other conditions simulating myocardial infarction.

3. The intraventricular conduction defects (LBBB, a fascicular block, etc.) may initially obscure the pattern of an infarction, where repeat or serial ECGs may reveal it later on.

4. Serial ECGs help to determine the age of infarction in relation to time.

5. Serial ECGs help to record the other complications occurring during the course of infarction, such as

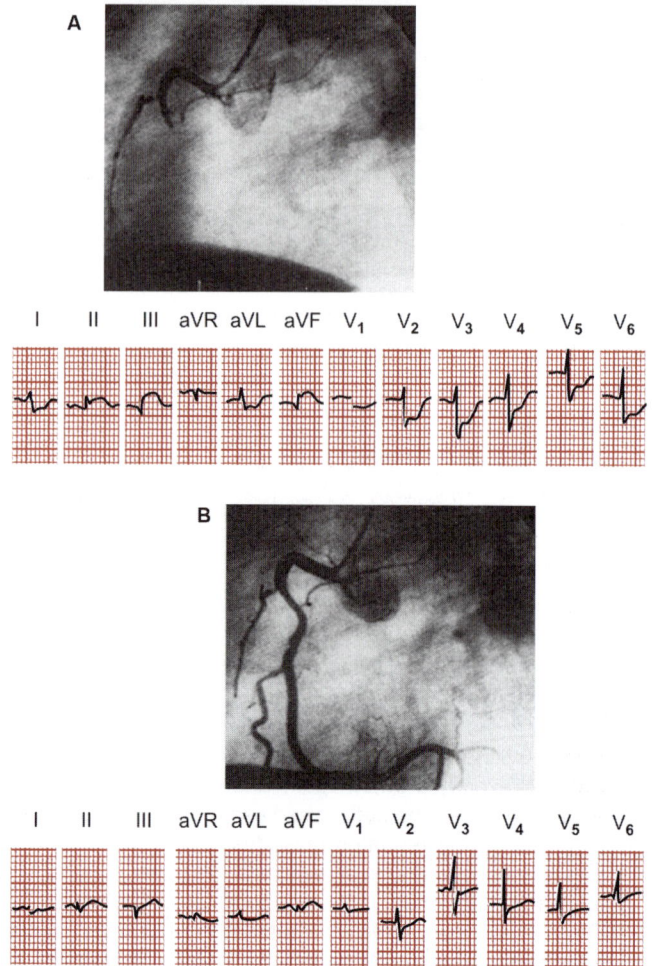

Fig. 19.24: The resolution of inferior wall infarction following thrombolysis. The electrocardiogram taken before **A:** and after, **B:** thrombolysis shows complete resolution of ST elevation (100%) after thrombolysis;

A: Before thrombolysis: There are hyperacute changes in leads II, III and aVF, i.e. increased height of R wave, prolonged VAT, slope elevation of ST segment with tall and widened T wave. A small q wave is seen in leads III and aVF. There is reciprocal ST depression in leads I, aVL, V_1-V_6. The coronary angiogram shows complete occlusion of right coronary artery.

B: After thrombolysis: There is more or less complete resolution of ST segment and T wave change but a small q wave is persisting in leads III and aVF. The reciprocal change has also disappeared. The thrombolysis was attempted in a private nursing home. The coronary angiogram shows appearance of right coronary artery following successful thrombolytic therapy.

arrhythmias, conduction defects, pericarditis, reinfarction, multiple infarctions, etc.

6. Persistence of ST segment elevation after 3 months of myocardial infarction indicates ventricular aneurysm.

7. Infarctions at combined sites, occurring concomitantly or at different intervals, need serial ECGs recording for correct evaluation.

Resolution of ST Segment Elevation on ECG Following Thrombolysis

Rapid resolution of ST segment elevation following successful thrombolysis has been reported in many studies but the usefulness of this change in identifying infarct artery patency status remains controversial. The resolution of ST segment elevation as predictive of successful reperfusion in acute myocardial infarction is highly variable in terms of sensitivity and specificity. An abrupt ST-T changes (> 2 mm resolution in ST elevation or depression and > 3 mm reduction in T wave height) has been used as an indicator of patency of an occluded artery. A stable ST segment within 100 minutes after completing successful thrombolysis on Holter monitoring was found to be 89% sensitive and 82% specific for detection of reperfusion. Similarly, 50% reduction in ST elevation in the leads showing maximal elevation was 67% specific and 93% sensitive for infarct artery patency. It has also been shown that quantification of the ST elevation in all electrocardiographic leads during acute coronary occlusion correlates well with both development of new wall motion abnormalities and final AMI size in non-perfused patients, thus, reduction of ≥ 20% in the sum total of ST elevation in all affected electrocardiographic leads, theoretically, proves superior to the single lead or few leads or on Holter lead analysis and has consistent 88% sensitivity and 80% specificity, which means the improvement in ST segment resolution still may not occur in about 20% cases. Recently, a prospective study, has demonstrated that complete (> 70%) ST resolution was associated with a patency (TIMI 2 or 3 flow) rate of 94%. Patients with partial resolution (30 to 70%) or no (< 30%) ST resolution has significantly lower rates of patency (72% and 68% respectively). The electrocardiograms before and after successful thrombolysis with relief of pain and complex resolution of ST elevation is depicted in Figure 19.24.

A significant reduction with partial resolution in sum total of ST deviation in eleven leads is depicted in Figure 19.25.

Electrocardiographic changes following successful thrombolysis

- Complete resolution or significant reduction of ST segment elevation
- Early T wave inversion
- Reperfusion arrhythmias–accelerated nodal or idioventricular rhythm, VPCs, transient sinus bradycardia, nonsustained VT, etc. are common. They usually do not require treatment because of transient and benign nature.

THE CHRONIC ESTABLISHED CHANGES

Following the fully evolved phase of myocardial infarction, there is spontaneous resolution of ECG changes. The elevated ST segment returns to the baseline and becomes progressively isoelectric. The inverted T waves gradually regain its positivity. Even the R wave may regain some of its lost positivity. It is clear that acuteness of myocardial infarction is diagnosed primarily by the changes of ST segment elevation and T waves inversion.

Old Infarction

The diagnosis of an old myocardial infarction on ECG is not only difficult but even impossible without documentation of acute episode on ECG, hence, serial records of ECGs or an old ECG may be summoned for this purpose. The diagnosis of an old infarction is based on the presence of pathological Q waves and T wave changes either alone or in combination (Fig. 19.26). Although abnormal Q waves may be present in nontransmural infarction and absent in transmural (full thickness) infarction, yet, the sensitivity and specificity of ECG for diagnosis of myocardial infarction depends on presence of abnormal Q waves. The specificity of abnormal Q wave is high and sensitivity is too low.

Since spontaneous healing of myocardial infarction takes 4-6 weeks, therefore, persistence of abnormal Q waves, normal ST segment and inverted T waves beyond this period indicate old changes. For confirmation, either serial ECGs must demonstrate evolutionary changes of an infarction or old record may be summoned to document an episode of previous acute infarction.

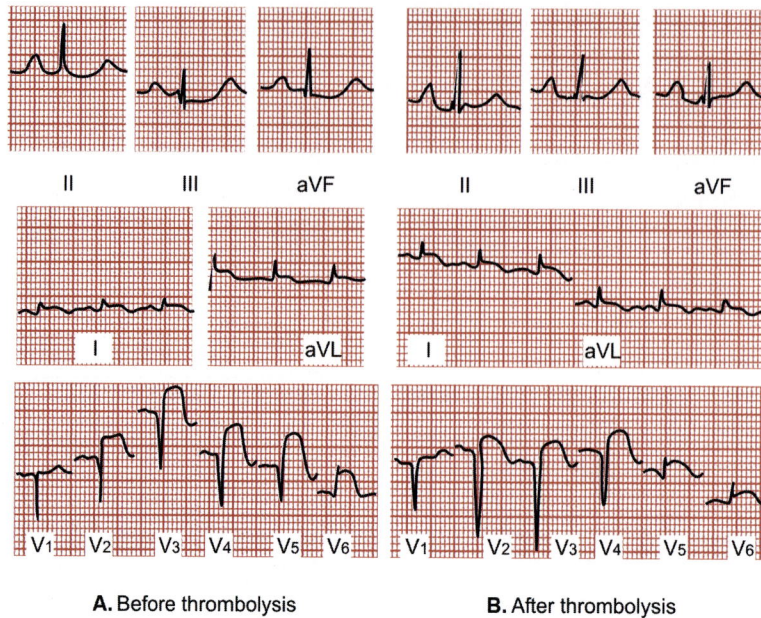

| II | III | aVF | | II | III | aVF |

| I | aVL | | I | aVL |

| V1 | V2 | V3 | V4 | V5 | V6 | | V1 | V2 | V3 | V4 | V5 | V6 |

A. Before thrombolysis   **B.** After thrombolysis

Fig. 19.25: The resolution of ST segement deviation after thrombolysis in acute anterior myocardial infarction. Resolution of ST segment 45% of total ST segment deviation in all leads except AVR after thrombolysis is considered significant (Partial resolution—TIMI grade 1-2 flow)

ST segment elevation in various leads				Reciprocal ST segment depression			
Before thrombolysis		After thrombolysis		Before thrombolysis		After thrombolysis	
Lead I =	2 mm	Lead I =	2 mm	Lead II = −1 mm		Lead II =	0
aVL =	3 mm	aVL =	2 mm	III = −2 mm		III =	0
V1 =	1 mm	V1 =	1 mm	aVF = −1 mm		aVF =	0
V2 =	5 mm	V2 =	3 mm	The leads are not shown			
V3 =	7 mm	V3 =	5 mm				
V4 =	8 mm	V4 =	6 mm	Total = −4 mm		Total =	0
V5 =	8 mm	V5 =	3 mm				
V6 =	6 mm	V6 =	2 mm				
Total =	40 mm	Total =	24 mm				

Net total ST deviation before thrombolysis = 40 + 4 = 44 mm   Net total ST deviation after thrombolysis = 24−0 = 24 mm

$$\text{Resolution of ST segment \%} = \frac{44-24}{44} = \frac{20}{11} \times 100 = \frac{500}{11} = 45\%$$

Within 6 to 12 months after an acute myocardial infarction, about 30% of the tracings although abnormal but are not diagnostic of an infarction by virtual absence of Q waves. Similarly by the end of 10 years or later, it has been observed that 6-10% electrocardiograms have reverted to normal. Regression of Q wave is common in small infarctions especially of anterior wall than at other sites. Still a large number of patients continue to demonstrate chronic established ECG changes for rest of their lives, particularly if they evolve Q waves.

Nowadays, in the era of thrombolysis, neither the evolutionary changes nor the old changes of infarction are seen frequently except in those cases where the thrombolysis has either failed or it was not attempted.

The Significance of Q Wave in Lead III

The causes of Q wave in lead III are given in the box. A Q wave in standard lead III is suggestive of an old inferior infarction, when following criteria are met with ;

1. The duration of the Q wave must be at least 0.04 sec (one small square in width).

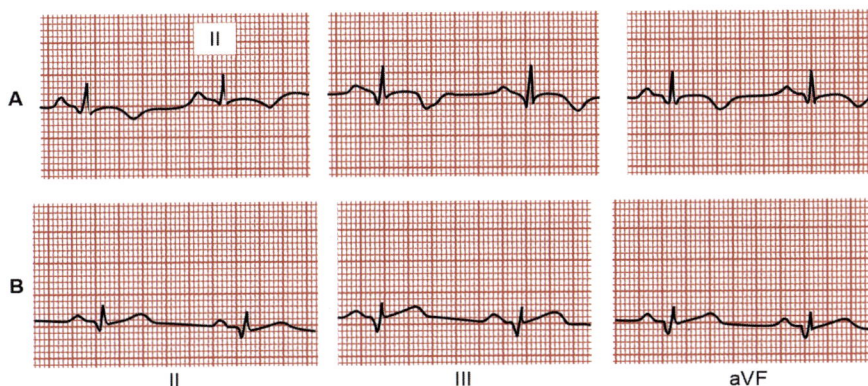

Fig. 19.26: Old inferior wall infarction. The electrocardiogram. **A:** taken at 6 weeks of infarction show;

   i. Presence of q wave in leads II, III and aVF
   ii. Isoelectric ST segment in above mentioned leads
   iii. Symmetric T wave inversion in leads II,III and aVF

All these features suggest presence of an old (chronic phase) inferior wall infarction. **B:** ECG taken at 2 years shows persistence of Q wave with normal ST segment and upright T waves

2. A Q wave of at least 0.02 sec in duration, i.e. half small square in width, must be present in aVF.
3. A 'q' or Q wave of any duration must be present in standard lead II.
4. The Q wave in lead III must be 25% of the R wave provided R wave is more than 5 mm in this lead.
5. The P wave in lead III must be upright. This is necessary to exclude some forms of AV block with retrograde conduction which produces inverted P (P)' waves simulating q waves in lead III.

Causes of Q wave in lead III

1. *Normal:* It may be normally present in this lead, but frequently disappears on deep inspiration. This should be a routine practice while recording standard lead III.
2. *Old inferior myocardial infarction :* The characteristics of abnormal Q wave have already been discussed.
3. *Acute pulmonary embolism* (Read the text in Chapter 27)
4. *Left posterior hemiblock* (Read the text in Chapter 14)
   NB : • *A negative delta wave in WPW syndrome may simulate a pathogical Q wave (Read Chapter 22)*
   • Marked left axis deviation more than – 70° will result in dominantly negative deflection in standard lead II, III and aVF which may, at times, mimic pathological Q waves.

Persistent ST Elevation (Read Ventricular Aneurysm Towards the End of Chapter)

The infarction usually heals by the end of 4 weeks and is replaced by a scar within 4-6 weeks. The ST segment by that time comes to baseline in majority of patients. In few cases, it may take longer time to resolve. However, persistence of ST segment elevation beyond 3 months following infarction suggests ventricular aneurysm or a fibrotic scar that bulges during ventricular contractions. Therefore, persistence of ST segment elevation over this time must be supported by serial ECGs done at different times, otherwise, it is difficult to decide whether ST segment elevation indicates a fresh infarction or a ventricular aneurysm. In case of history of a previous infarction where old ECG record is not available, in such a situation, serial cardiac enzymes, echocardiography, scintigraphy may aid to differentiate between them.

Persistent ST segment elevation beyond 3 months of myocardial infarction usually indicates either a weak fibrotic scar or a ventricular aneurysm.

LOCALISATION OF MYOCARDIAL INFARCTION BY ELECTROCARDIOGRAPHIC PATTERNS

The anatomical site of an infarction can be localised by the infarction pattern observed in specific leads but the functional extent of the infarction is not possible from the ECG. The site of infarction and the leads reflecting the infarction pattern are depicted in the box. Accuracy of such localisation is influenced

SECTION SEVEN

Localisation of myocardial infarction by ECG

Site of infarct	ECG leads showing infarction pattern
1. Left ventricle	
A. Anterior wall	
• Anteroseptal	V_1-V_3, sometimes, may involve V_4 also.
• Anterolateral	I, aVL and V_4-V_6
• Anteroapical	V_1-V_6
• Apical	V_5-V_6
• Extensive anterior	I, aVL, V_1-V_6
• High anterior	1 and aVL. ECG recorded one space higher up ($3V_2$-V_5) may show evidence of an infarction.
B. Inferior wall	II, III and aVF
• Inferoposterior	II, III, aVF and V_1-V_2
• Inferoposterolateral	II, III, aVF, V_1-V_2 and V_5-V_6.
• *Inferolateral*	II, III, aVF and V_5-V_6.
C. Posterior wall	*Mirror image changes of infarction are seen in right precordial leads*
• True posterior	V_{3R}, V_1-V_2.
• Posterolateral	V_1, 1 and V_5-V_6
2. Right ventricle	$V_{3R\text{-}6\,R}$ and V_1 or V_2 or both.

by the distance of an electrode from the heart which varies considerably among individuals. The area subtended by a given electrode also varies with anteroposterior diameter of chest and, is greater in persons with increased diameter. For example the same sized anterior infarct would be recorded in more leads in a person with normal AP diameter than in a person with increased AP diameter.

1. INFARCTION OF LEFT VENTRICLE

A. Anterior Left Ventricular Infarction

Anterior wall myocardial infarction involving the left ventricle is best reflected in the precordial leads (V_1-V_6). If lateral wall is also picked up by infarction, then leads I and aVL will also reflect the changes. The characteristic findings in the evaluation of a Q wave anterior wall myocardial infarction along with the orientation of infarction vector and other instantaneous vectors are depicted in the Table 19.1. The direction of ST vector in anterior wall infarction will be just opposite to the infarction vector as dipicted in Table 19.2. The reciprocal ST segment depression in anterior wall infarction is seen in leads II, III and aVF (inferior oriented leads).

B. Inferior Wall Infarction (Figs 19.31A and B)

The inferior surface of heart overlies the diaphragm, the infarction involving the inferior wall surface will be projected in leads II, III, aVF—called *inferior surface oriented leads*. The characteristic findings of Q wave infarction, infarction vector and other instantaneous vectors have already been presented in the Table 19.1.

The Q wave, ST segment elevation and T wave inversion limited to leads II, III and aVF indicated inferior wall infarction.

At times, the elevation of ST segment in leads II, III and aVF may produce reciprocal changes in leads I, aVL and precordial leads in the form of ST depression and low upright T wave. Later on, when

Table 19.1 : The relationship among the electrical site of infarction, direction of infarction vector, the VA vectors affected and the QRS changes in different leads

Site of infarction	Direction of infarction vector	Instantaneous VA vectors affected	Resulting QRS abnormalities in different leads
Anteroseptal	Left, posterior	0.01 sec septal and 0.02 sec apicoanterior VA vectors	QS patterns or abnormal Q waves in leads V_1-V_3 or V_4.
Anterior	Posterior	0.02 and 0.04 sec left ventricular VA vectors.	QS patterns or abnormal Q waves in leads V_2-V_4.
Anterolateral	Right, posterior	0.02 and 0.04 sec VA vectors	Abnormal Q waves in leads I, aVL, V_5 and V_6.
Extensive anterior	Right, posterior	0.01 to 0.06 sec VA vectors	Abnormal Q waves in leads I, aVL, V_1-V_6.
Inferior (diaphragmatic)	Superior	0.02 and 0.04 sec VA vectors.	Abnormal Q waves in leads II, III and aVF.
Posterolateral	Right, anterior	0.02 and 0.04 sec VA vectors.	Abnormally tall and/or wide R in lead V_1 and abnormal Q waves in leads I and V_6.
Strict posterior	Anterior	0.04 and 0.06 or 0.08 sec VA vectors	Low, vibratory RR or rsR' or R pattern in leads V_{3R} and V_1.

Table 19.2: The ST segment elevation depending on direction of ST vector in acute myocardial infarction

Effective electrical site of injury/ischaemia	Direction of ST vector	Leads showing ST elevation
• Anteroseptal	Right, anterior	V_1-V_3 or V_4 (Figs 19.27 A and B)
• Anteroapical or anterior	Anterior and slightly to left	V_1-V_6
• Anterolateral	Left, anterior	I, aVL, V_4-V_6 (Fig. 19.28)
• Extensive anterior	Anterior, or left and anterior	I, aVL, V_1-V_6 (Fig. 19.29)
• High anterior	Anterior and left	I, aVL (ECG to be recorded one space higher, i.e. 3rd space ($3V_{2-5}$) for infarction (Fig. 19.30).

T wave becomes inverted in inferior leads, the T wave in leads I, aVL will also become tall due to resolution of reciprocal changes.

C. Inferolateral Infarction (Fig. 19.32)

The infarction pattern (Q wave, elevated ST segment and T wave changes) is limited to inferior wall (leads II,III and aVF) and lateral wall (V_5-V_6) of left ventricle.

D. Posterior Wall Myocardial Infarction (Figs 19.33 and 19.34)

There is no conventional electrode which is oriented directly to the posterior wall of the heart. This is not feasible also because of interposition of too much of

tissue (muscles and bone) between an electrode and the posterior wall of the heart, with the result, there will be marked attenuation of deflections recorded on surface ECG. Therefore, infarction of the posterior wall is diagnosed by the *'inverse or mirror image changes'* which will be reflected by the electrodes oriented in the same plane to the uninjured anterior myocardial wall (Fig. 19.33). As we know, the changes of a fully evolved infarction are; a QS complex, elevated ST segment and inverted T wave in the leads overlying the injured myocardial wall, hence, inverse will be reflected in the anterior chest leads (V_1-V_3) representing the uninjured surface opposite to posterior wall. The inverse or mirror image changes in leads V_1-V_3 (Fig. 19.33) will be;

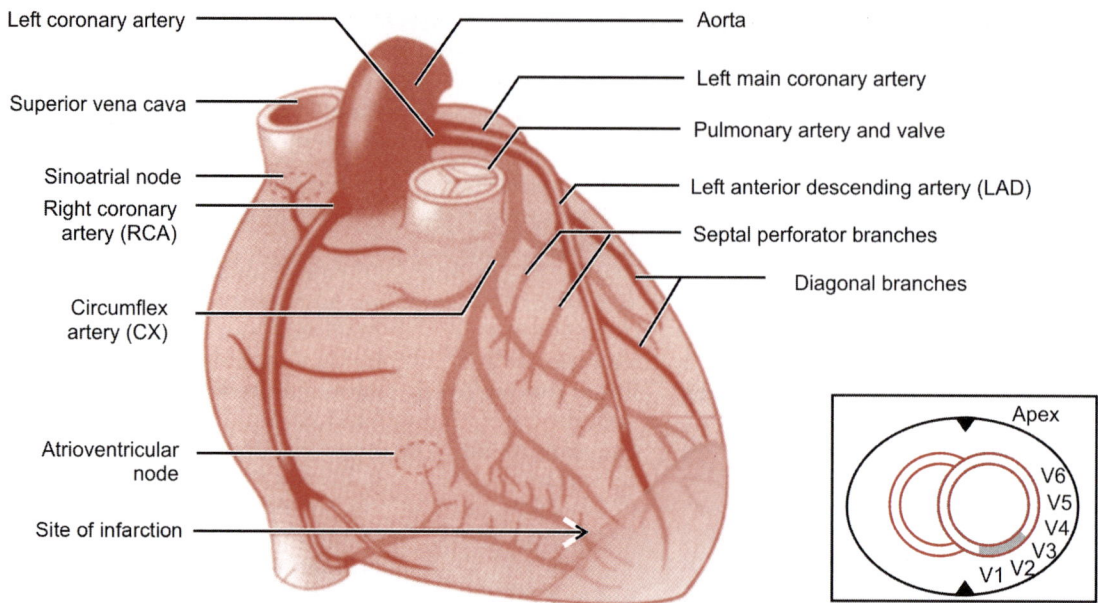

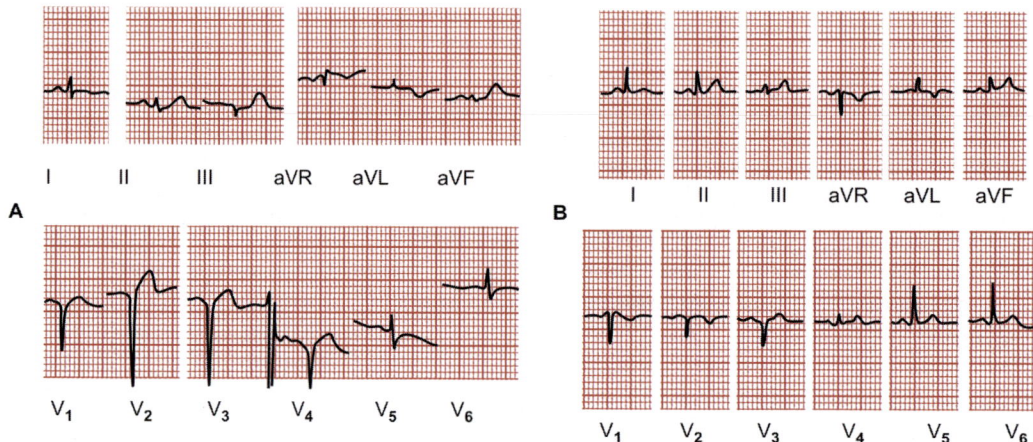

Fig. 19.27: Anteroseptal infarction. **A:** Recent anteroseptal infarction with lateral wall ischaemia. The ECG shows QS pattern in leads V₁-V₄ with elevated ST segment and T is dragged upwards. The T is inverted in leads I and aVL with isoelectric ST segment. Reciprocal ST segment depression is visible in leads II, III and aVF. **B:** Old anteroseptal infarction with QS pattern in V₁-V₃ with reduced height of R wave in V₄. The T is inverted in leads V₁-V₂ and aVL. The ST segment is isoelectric in V₁-V₃ and aVL. The inverted T wave seen in aVL is an additional finding, may indicate high lateral ischaemia

(i) The tall and wide R wave which is mirror image change of QS complex.

(ii) The depressed concave upward ST segment is recorded which is theoretically mirror image change of coved and elevated ST segment.

(iii) The upright, widened and usually tall or relatively tall T waves : This is a diagnostic change of posterior wall infarction and it is stressed that diagnosis should not be entertained without this change. This is mirror image change of inverted, deep and symmetric T wave.

The tall R wave in leads V₁ or V₂ with ST segment depression and tall or relatively tall upright T wave suggest true posterior wall myocardial infarction.

All these changes are due to anterior orientation of infarction vector as shown in the Table 19.1. The tall, widened and upright T wave may take a long time to resolve and may occasionally be present permanently.

An isolated true posterior wall myocardial infarction is unusual. Posterior wall infarction is

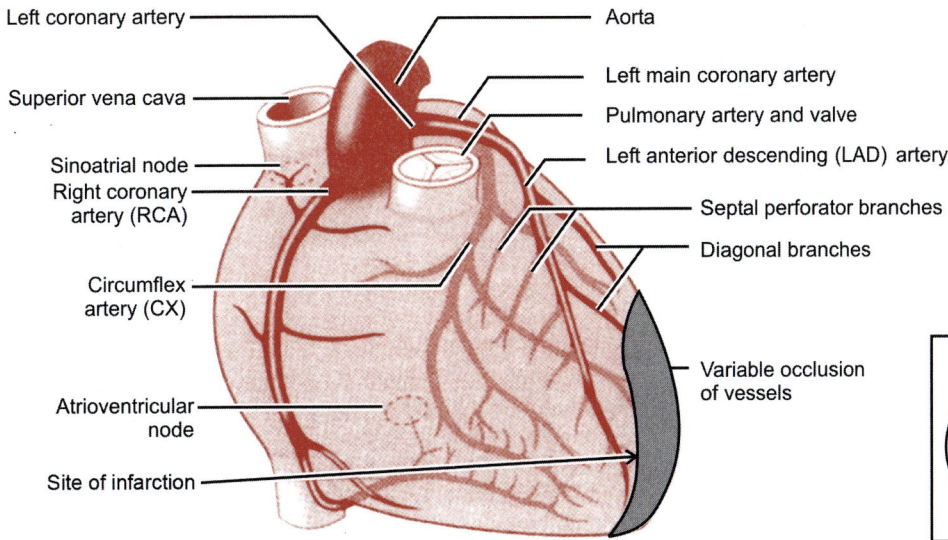

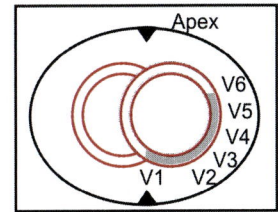

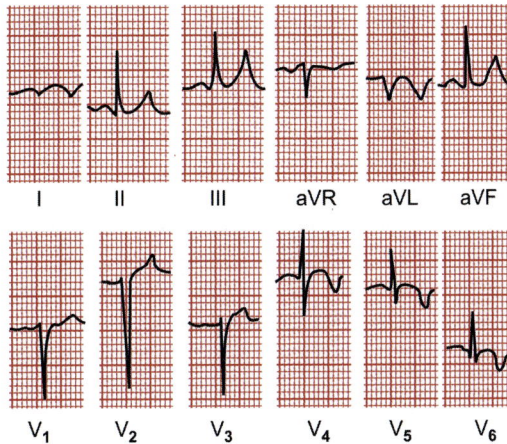

Fig. 19.28: Anterolateral infarction. The ECG shows Qr pattern in lead I and QS in lead aVL. There is coving ST segment with T inversion in leads I, aVL and V_4-V_6. The infarct is few days old

almost accompanied either by inferior (Fig. 19.34) or lateral wall infarction or both. In such a situation, the ECG changes of posterior wall infarction are added to the changes of inferior or lateral wall infarction.

E. Inferoposterolateral Myocardial Infarction (Figs 19.35 and 19.36)

The pattern of infarction will be recorded in anterior, inferior and lateral leads as given in the box.

F. Nontransmural Myocardial Infarction (Fig. 19.37)

For many years, ECG has been used to differentiate the transmural from nontransmural infarction on the basis of Q waves; but now it has been proved that it is not correct. It had been considered that subendocardial portion of the myocardium was electrically 'silent' and that depolarisation in this area would not be associated with an abnormal Q wave. However, correlations of ECG patterns with autopsy findings now have established the unreliability of ECG in an accurate differential anatomic diagnosis. Although many transmural infarctions are manifested by Q waves on ECG, a significant number is still not. Conversely, many anatomic nontransmural infarctions will demonstrate Q waves. When Q waves are not present, the electrocardiographic diagnosis of acute myocardial infarction depends on evolutionary changes on serial records and clinical correlation.

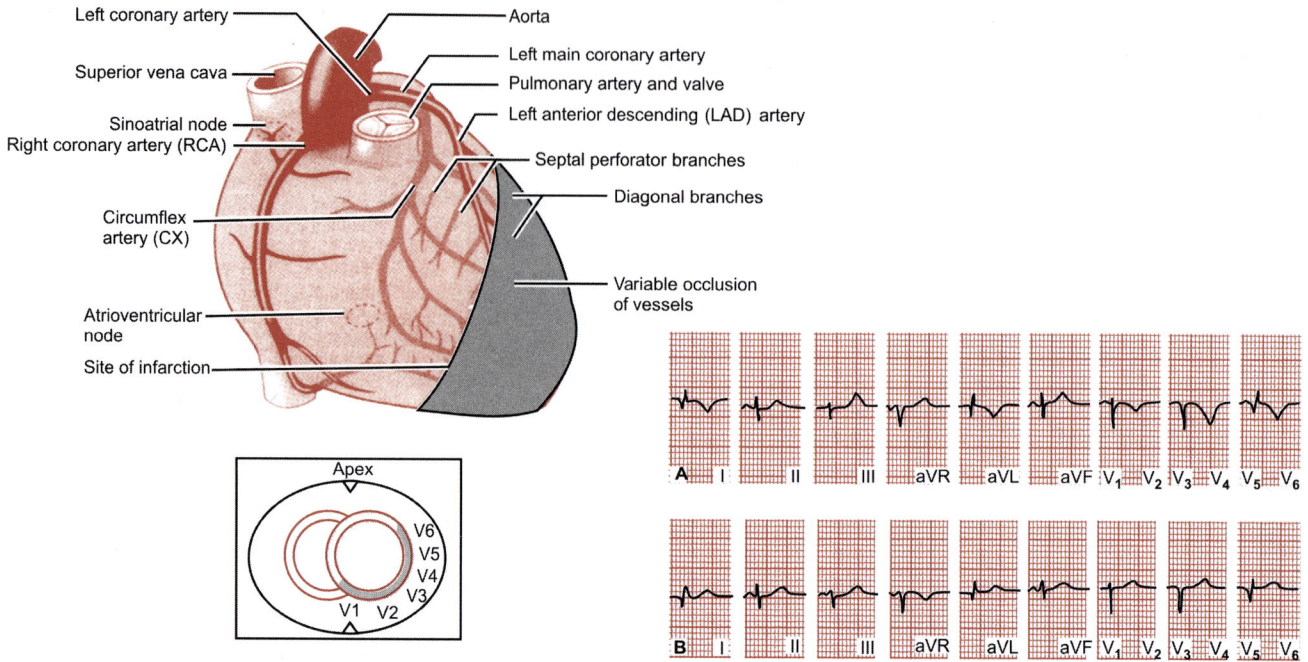

Figs 19.29A and B: Anterior wall infarction (extensive). The electrocardiogram.
A: Recent, **B:** Old. The electrocardiogram shows;

1. Recent infarction. It is evident by q waves in leads I, aVL, V_5-V_6 with QS pattern in V_3-V_4. ST segment is elevated wtih convexity upwards in I, aVL, V_5-V_6. Isoelectric in V_1-V_4. The T is inverted in I, aVL, V_1-V_6

2. Old (chronic) changes: The electrocardiograms taken after 6 months shows q wave in leads I, aVL, V_5-V_6 with QS in leads V_3-V_4 ST segment has become isoelectric in I, aVL, V_1-V_6 . The inverted T waves have become upright, i.e. regained their positivity

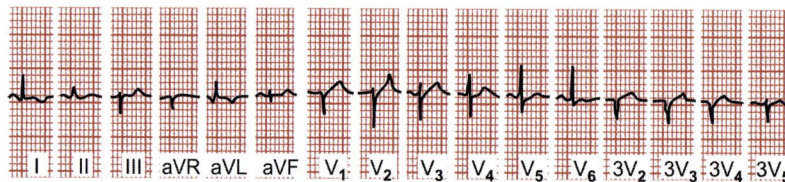

Fig. 19.30: High anterior myocardial infarction. The initial electrocardiogram recorded shows q wave, ST segment elevation and T waver inversion in leads I and aVL only. The precordial leads recorded at normal 4th space did not reveal any abnormality. The precordial leads (V_1-V_5) recorded at 3rd space ($3V_2$-$3V_5$) showed QS pattern in $3V_2$-$3V_4$ with upright T waves. Lead $3V_5$ showed small r wave (rS pattern). All these feature suggest high anterior infarction missed on conventional precordial leads, was reflected in high lateral leads (I and aVL)

Therefore, the importance of Q waves lie in the diagnosis of myocardial infarction and not in the differentiation between transmural and nontransmural infarction. The differential diagnosis of non-Q wave infarction from myocardial ischaemia likewise depends on the serial demonstration of evoluationary changes in the former and reversibility of changes to normal in the latter. For this purpose, a single ECG is insufficient for correct diagnosis (Fig. 19.37).

Nowadays infarction on ECG are designated as 'Q wave' and 'non-Q wave' rather than 'transmural' or nontransmural'.

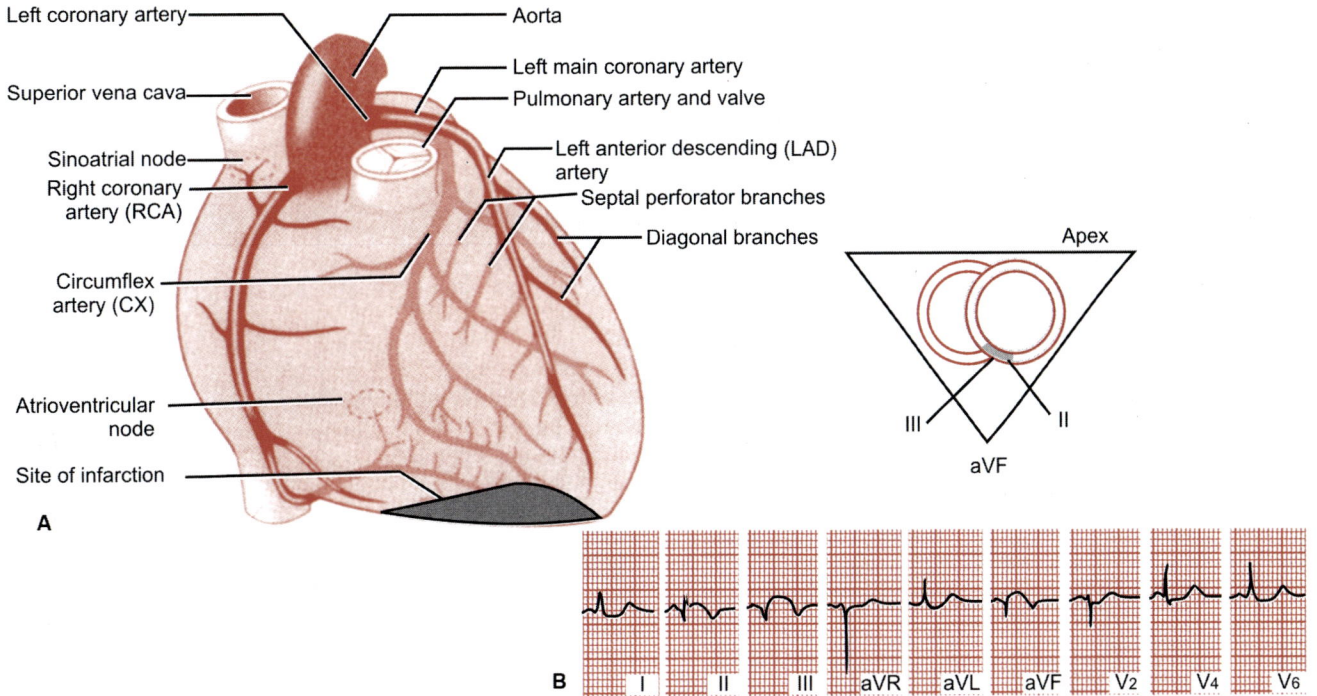

A

B | I | II | III | aVR | aVL | aVF | V₂ | V₄ | V₆

Fig. 19.31: Inferior wall infarction. **A:** Diagram showing site of infarction. **B:** The ECG shows fresh infarction. The presence of significant Q waves, ST elevation and T wave inversion in leads II, III and aVF with reciprocal ST segment depression in leads I, aVL and V₂-V₆ (anterior chest leads) indicate the fully evolved acute inferior wall infarction

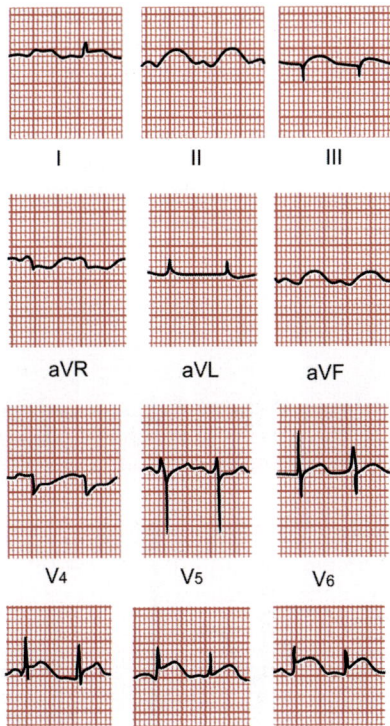

Fig. 19.32: Hyperacute inferolateral myocardial infarction. The electrocardiogram shows:

   i. *Inferior wall infarction.* There is elevation of ST segment (> 4 mm) in leads II, III, and aVF

   ii. *Lateral wall infarction.* There is ST segment elevation (>4 mm) in lateral leads (V₄-V₆) and lead I

The elevation of ST segment without appearance of q wave and T wave changes indicate it to be hyperacute

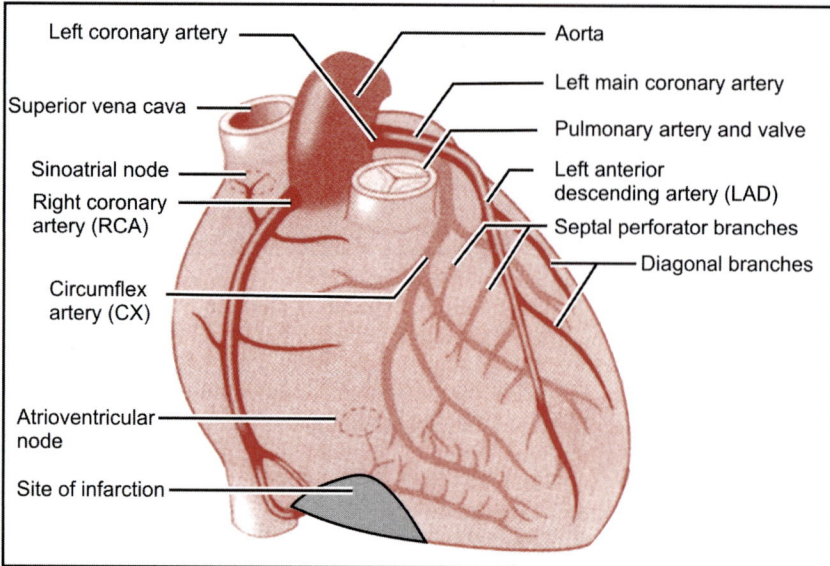

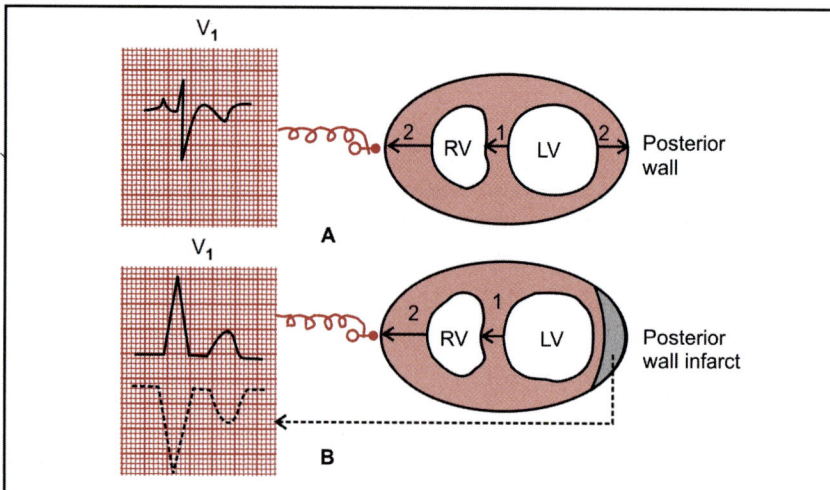

Fig. 19.33: Diagram showing **A:** Normal ventricular depolarisation and, **B:** Ventricular depolarisation during true posterior wall infarction. Note the tall, wide R wave with depressed concave upward ST segment and tall T wave (mirror image change of V_1) shown below in dotted lines. This change would have been picked up by the lead placed directly over the injured surface

Fig. 19.34: Posterior wall infarction/ischaemia. The ECG shows tall prominent R wave in right precordial leads with ST segment depression. These changes occur in posterior wall ischaemia/infarction but may occur in:

i. Anteroseptal subendocardial ischaemia or infarction
ii. Right ventricular hypertrophy
iii. Normal variant with early transition

The marked decrease in voltage in lateral precordial leads rule out normal variant with counterclockwise rotation or early transition. The upright T wave in right precordial leads with normal axis rules and right ventricular hypertrophy or strain. The ST segment depression in V_1-V_3 does not appear to be a primary change due to subendocardial ischaemia in the absence of T wave inversion but appears as a reciprocal ST segment change produced by posterior wall myocardial injury/ischaemia. Therefore the findings are suggestive of posterior wall infarction rather than subendocardial ischaemia of right ventricle

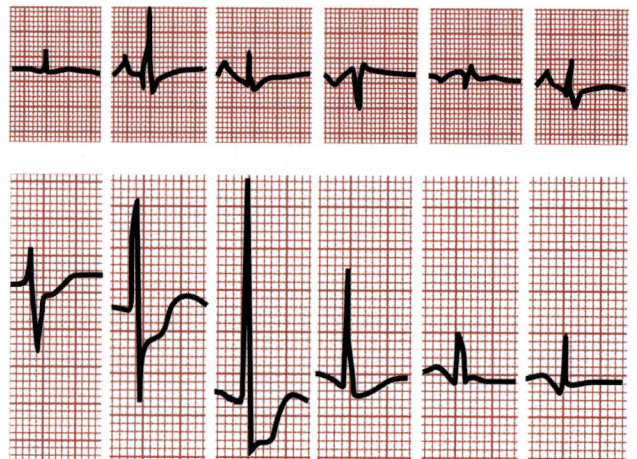

ECG changes of inferoposterolateral infarction

- Inferior infarction   Leads II, III, aVF   Abnormal Q waves, ST elevation and T waves inversion.
- Posterior infarction   Leads V_1-V_2 Tall R waves with upright T waves.
- Lateral wall infarction   Leads V_5-V_6 Abnormal Q waves and inverted T waves.

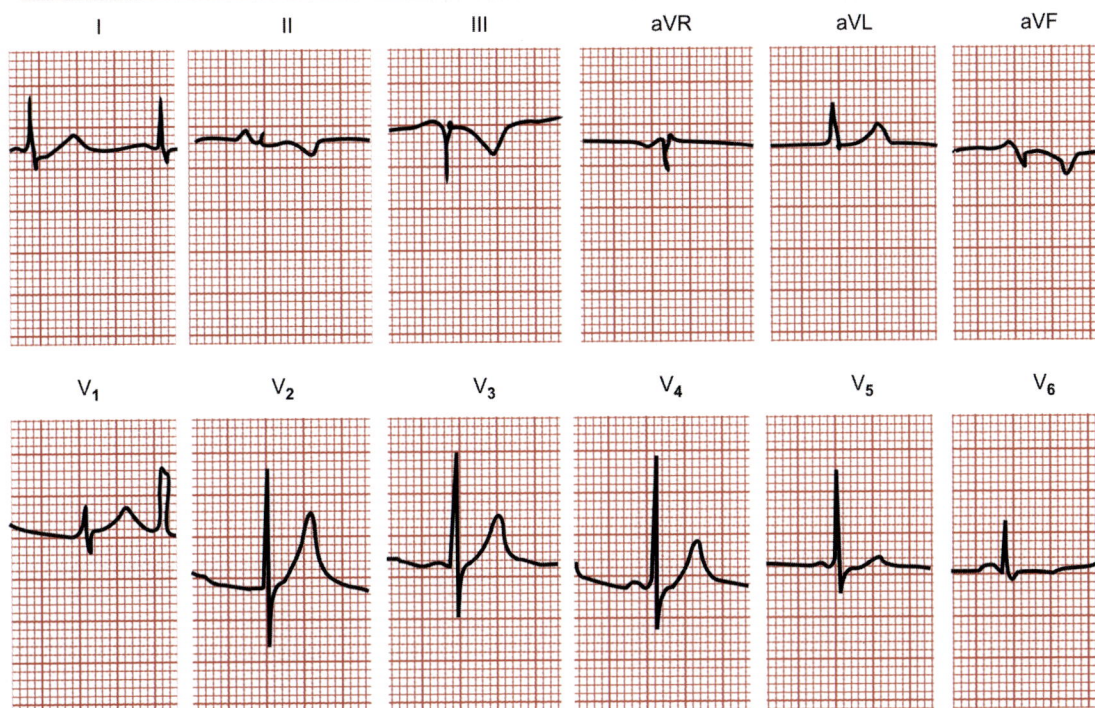

Fig. 19.35: Old inferior wall infarction with true posterior wall infarction. Note the following characteristics on ECG:
1. *Old inferior wall infarction.* There is q wave in leads II, III and aVF with T wave inversion and coving ST segment.
2. *True posterior infarction.* The R wave is taller and broader than S wave in V_1 and there is 19 mm tall R wave in V_2. Both these changes are due to anterior displacement of QRS due to loss of posterior left ventricular forces. There is relatively tall, peaked T wave in V_1 and especially in V_2. All these findings support true posterior infarction which is further supported by associated inferior myocardial infarction.

The Q waves in the ECG signify abnormal electrical activity but are not synonymous with irreversible myocardial damage. Non-Q wave infarction, conventionally called a subendocardial infarction, but in fact it is more than that because true pathological subendocardial anterior myocardial infarction, as recognised at autopsy is seen with ST segment depression and/or T wave inversion only about 50% of the time. Angiographic studies performed in anterior myocardial infarction without ST segment elevation show a higher incidence of subtotal occlusion of the culprit vessel and higher collateral flow to the infarcted zone.

The clinico-pathologic spectrum of non-Q wave acute myocardial infarction lies midway between unstable angina and acute myocardial infarction (see the box). Electrocardiographically, it is submyocardial infarction where loss of electrical forces from the infarcted area are not sufficient to produce Q wave, but the ST vector is either directed towards the epicardial surface producing ST elevation or is directed towards ventricular cavity leading to ST depression resembling subendocardial infarction (see the box).

Since changes in ST segment and T wave are quite nonspecific and may occur in variety of cardiac (stable

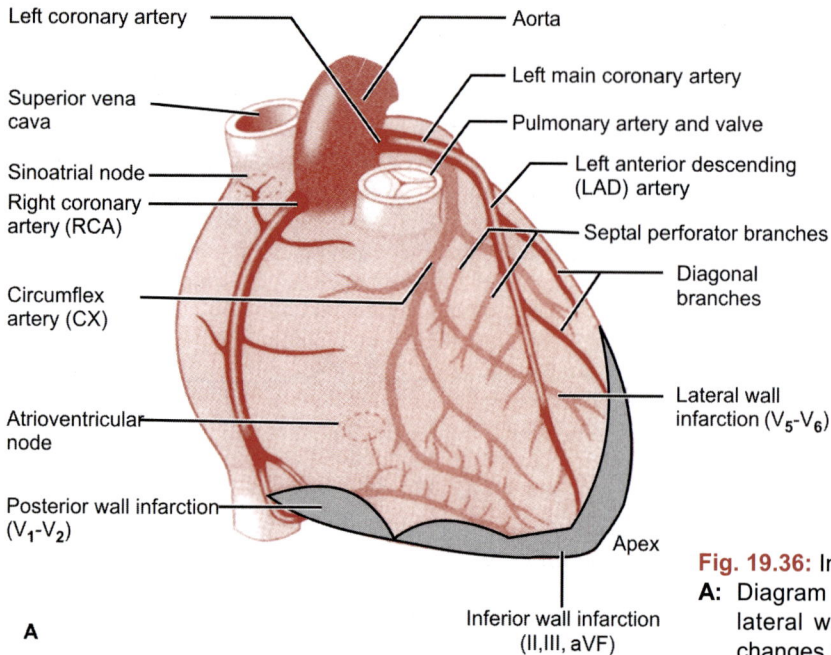

A

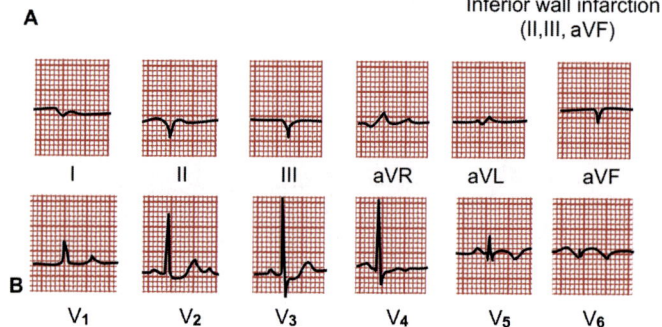

I   II   III   aVR   aVL   aVF

B   V₁   V₂   V₃   V₄   V₅   V₆

Fig. 19.36: Inferoposterolateral infarction.

A: Diagram showing infarction of inferior, posterior and lateral walls of left ventricle and the leads with the changes reflected in them

B: The 12 lead surface ECG shows

  i. *Inferior wall infarction:* The QS complexes and inverted T waves in leads II, III and aVF suggest an old inferior wall infarction.

  ii. *Posterior wall infarction:* The tall R waves and upright T wave in leads V_1-V_3 indicate posterior infarction

  iii. *Lateral wall infarction:* The presence of q wave and coving, ST segment with inversion of T wave in leads V_4-V_6 suggest recent lateral wall infarction

and unstable angina) and noncardiac conditions (ventricular hypertrophy, pericarditis, myocarditis, electrolyte and metabolic disturbance, early repolarisation syndrome or drugs induced, etc.), the distinction of non-Q wave infarction rests on the persistence of ST-T changes, while all other conditions described above produce transient changes. Therefore, a single ECG is never diagnostic of non-Q wave infarction. Serial ECGs must be done to show persistence of ST-T changes and non-evolution of Q waves.

The diagnosis of non-Q wave infarction is made when a patient presents with acute cardiac pain and there is biochemical evidence of myocardial necrosis (raised CPK-MB, cardiac troponin T or I) but ECG shows ST-T changes of myocardial ischaemia/infarction without pathological Q waves. In the final analysis, the diagnosis of non-Q wave infarction rests on the combination of clinical findings and elevation of serum cardiac enzymes and troponins rather than on the ECGs.

It has been observed that patients with non-Q wave infarction have a pattern of myocardial (transmural) necrosis that is less confluent and is more concentrated in the inner third of the ventricular wall because restoration of blood flow through collaterals, prevents the wavefront of necrosis from extending to the thickness of ventricular wall.

Clinical Significance

1. A crude categorisation of patients into Q wave and non-Q wave infarction based on the ECG is useful; Q wave AMI are usually associated with greater ventricular damage, a greater tendency to infarct's expansion and remodelling, and a higher mortality rate.

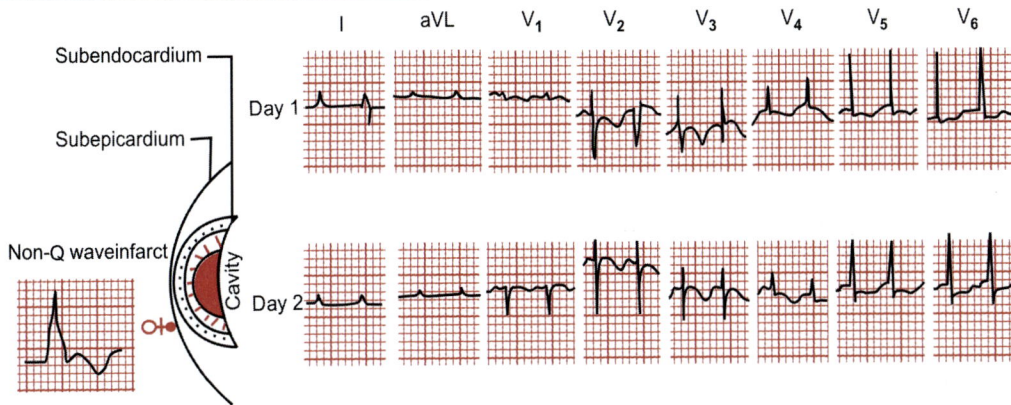

Fig. 19.37: Non Q-wave anterior wall infarction. Serial electrocardiograms were taken from a patient who had chest pain.
Day 1: The electrocardiogram taken at admission during pain reveals coving ST segment with T wave inversion in leads I, aVL, V_4-V_6 suggesting anterior wall infarction. Cardiac enzymes (CPK-MB) were raised. Serial electrocardiograms and continuous monitoring during day 1 did not reveal any deviation from the ECG taken at admission
Day 2: The ECG taken next day showed the same pattern. The Q wave did not appear.
NB: The ECG findings taken serially suggest non-Q wave anterior wall infarction.

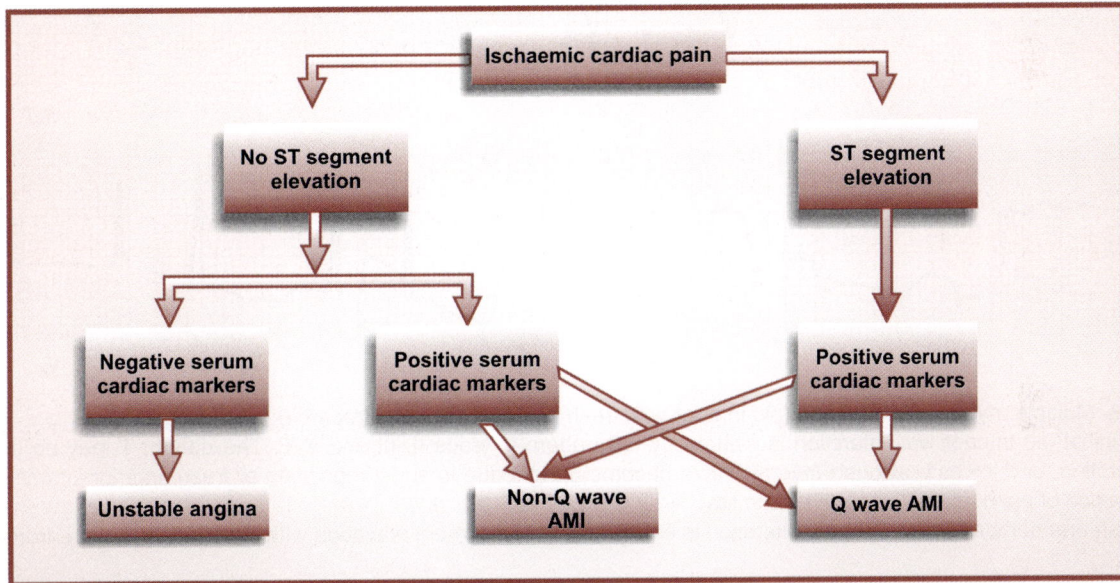

Note: Patient with ischaemic cardiac pain may or may not have ST segment elevation. The majority of the patients with ST segment elevation ultimately develop Q wave anterior myocardial infarction (AMI); while a minority may not develop it at all (non-Q wave AMI). On the other spectrum, the patients who have no ST elevation, a majority are diagnosed as unstable angina or non-Q wave AMI depending on the absence and presence of cardiac markers respectively. A minority of such patients may ultimately develop a Q wave AMI.

2. Nevertheless, non-Q wave AMI a distinct clinical entity, is increasing in frequency probably owing to a combination of factors including widespread use of anti-ischaemic therapy in the population (e.g. aspirin), increasing age of population and more sensitive assays for serum markers.

3. Mostly it is due to subtotal occlusion of the culprit vessel.

4. Following thrombolysis, the classification of infarcts into Q wave and non-Q wave should be deferred for the period of convalescence because of the tendency of Q waves to appear and regress after first 24 hours.

SECTION SEVEN

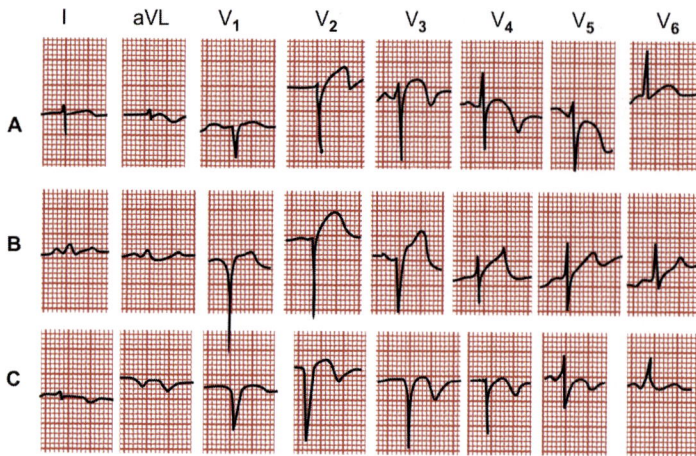

Fig. 19.38: Multiple myocardial ischaemia/infarction in same territory (anterior wall). The ECG recorded at different times during chest pain shows:

A. *During first episode.* The ST segment elevation with T wave inversion from V_1-V_6 and leads I and aVL indicates acute myocardial infarction.

B. *Second episode* of pain resulted in normalisation of T waves. The T wave inverted in (A) became upright from (I, aVL, V_1-V_6). The ST segment is just elevated in V_2 only.

C. *Third episode* of pain again recorded inversion of T waves in the same leads as in (A) i.e. I, aVL, V_1-V_6

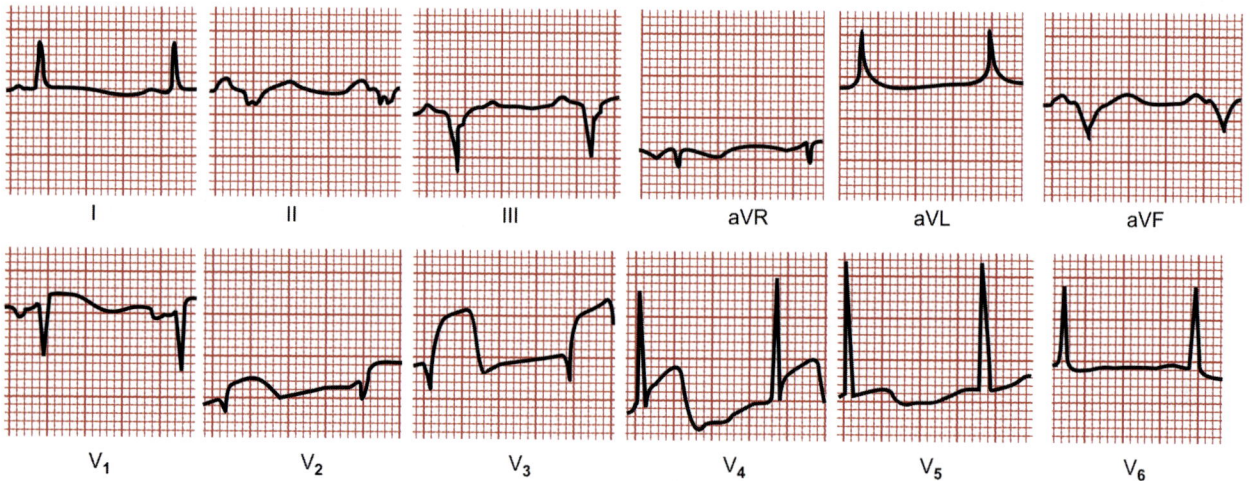

Fig. 19.39: Multiple myocardial infarction (old inferior with fresh anterior). The electrocardiogram shows;
  i. An initial old inferior wall infarction is evident by QS pattern in leads II, III and aVF. The upright T may be due to old infarction, or if it was previously inverted have become upright due to superimposition of fresh anterior infarction. In the absence of previous ECG it is difficult to say.
  ii. Fresh anterior wall (antero-septal) infarction is evident from ST segment elevation with dragged up T wave from V_1-V_4

Infarction at Combined Locations or Multiple Infarctions (Figs 19.38 to 19.40)

A myocardial infarction frequently involves several different areas of the left ventricle concomitantly, or an acute myocardial infarct may occur in a previously infarcted ventricle either in a proximate or a remote area. In most instances, each of the component of a combined infarct produces changes individually recognisable on the ECG because infarction in one region of the left ventricle ordinarily does not interfere with the diagnostic changes produced by infarction of another region. Perhaps, the major exception to this rule but a rare one is combined infarctions of anterior and posterior walls of the left ventricle. In such a situation, serial ECGs, if followed, will help. The initial ECG will show typical evolutionary changes of QRS, ST segment and T wave abnormality of an infarction at one site, say, for example, in anterior wall infarction in leads V_1-V_6; after sometimes, subsequent changes of posterior wall infarction in leads V_1-V_3 will appear, due to which the previously deflected QS complex or abnormally low R waves due to anterior infarction will now change into R waves of relatively normal

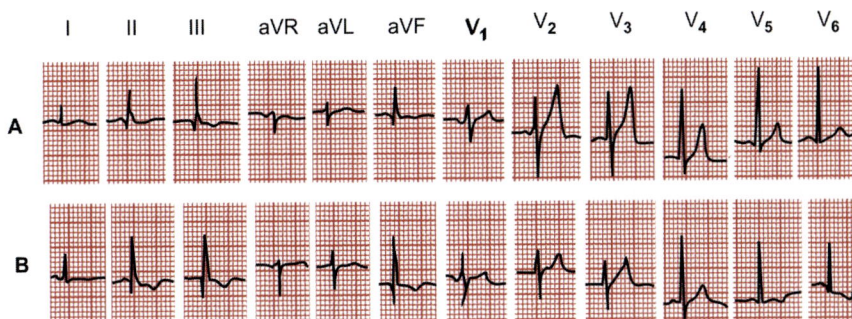

Fig. 19.40: Multiple infarction (Two episodes of infarction).

A: The electrocardiogram recorded 4-5 months back after recovery from first episode showed q wave, minimally elevated ST segment and inverted T waves in leads II, III and aVF indicating an old inferior wall infarction. There were tall peaked T waves in precordial leads which were dismissed as due to early repolarisation.

B: The electrocardiogram recorded during second episode of pain shows lateral wall infarction (q wave, convex coving ST segment and inverted T waves in V_5-V_6 only). The changes of old inferior wall infarction are still persistent. This type of multiple infarction is not common because inferolateral infarction in more common in one episode than to occur in two different episodes.

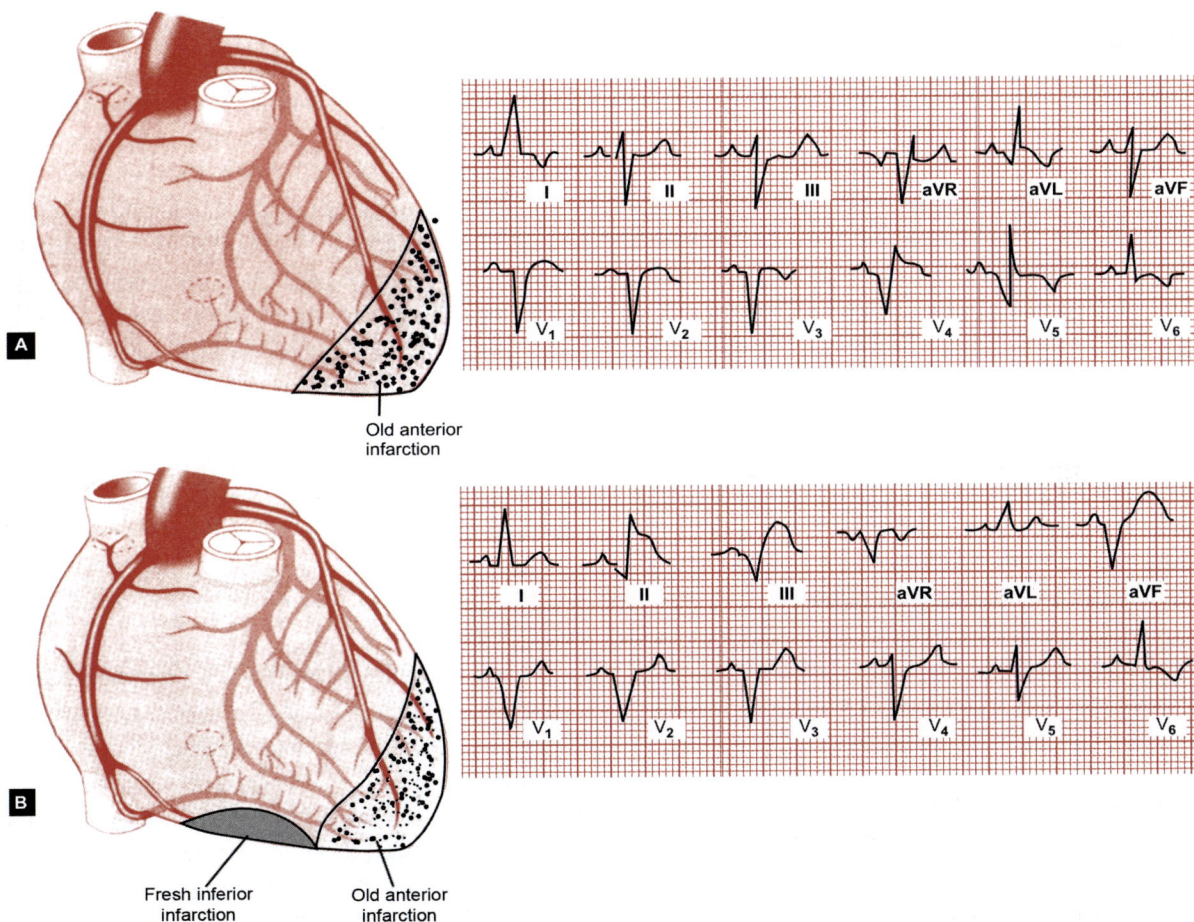

Fig. 19.41: Diagrammatic illustration of ECG showing multiple myocardial infarctions (an inferior wall infarction superimposed on an old anterior infarction. **A:** Initial old anterior infarction evidenced by QS pattern in V_1-V_5. The T waves are inverted in leads I, aVL and V_3-V_6. This pattern is stable infarction pattern. **B:** If patient develops inferior wall infarction in next episode then pattern will be as shown. A broad Q, raised ST segment in lead II, QS pattern with elevated ST in III and QS pattern with elevated ST and inverted T in aVF. As a result of superimposition of inferior wall infarction over anterior wall, the T waves that were previously inverted in precordial leads due to anterior infarction have now become upright in leads I, aVL and V_3-V_6

size and a normal precordial QRS transition results, since both are diagonally opposite to each other. In addition, now there will be ST segment depression in precordial leads, and the inverted T waves of previous anterior infarction will either become low upright or less inverted. These serial ECGs interpret the superimposition of posterior infarction on anterior infarction. If such a patient survives, the ECG recorded at some future date conceivably may not show an evidence of either infarction, since the electrical effects of one would counterbalance or nullify the effects of other. Here, vector theory will be valid to diagnose previous infarction.

> *The infarctions of anterior and posterior walls of left ventricle need serial ECGs for diagnosis. Changes of infarction of one surface (ST segment elevation and inverted T waves) will become reversed (ST depression and upright T wave) during infarction of opposite surface.*

If the ECG changes show an old initial infarction (i.e. Q waves and T wave inversion) of one region or surface, a second infarct of the same region or opposite surface will produce a pattern as would be expected with initial infarction, however, second infarction does not change the abnormal Q wave of previous infarction. The ST segment elevation expected due to second infarction will cause ST segment depression in the area of initial infarction. The inverted T waves expected as a result of second infarct will cause the previously inverted T waves of initial infarction to become upright by reversing its polarity.

> *Second infarction in the same area does not alter the Q wave of previous infarction but inverted T waves of previous infarction become upright.*

When a fresh infarction of a region or a surface gets superimposed on the old infarction of another region, it may mask the changes of old infarction which are likely to be missed or ignored especially non-Q wave infarction, if previous record is either not summoned or not available. However, if Q waves are present due to infarction, then situation is different because Q waves are not altered by second infarction.

This is illustrated with an example (Fig. 19.41), say a patient had an old anterior wall infarction with persistence of Q waves and inverted T waves in leads I, aVL, V_1-V_5, gets second episode of fresh infarction involving the inferior wall, now evolutionaly changes of inferior infarction (Q waves, ST elevation and T inverted in inferior leads) will cause ST depression; and inverted T waves of previous infarction become upright in leads I, aVL, V_1-V_4, hence, changes of an old inferior wall are masked by superimposed fresh anterior wall infarction.

Value of Electrocardiography in Localising the Site of Coronary Artery Occlusion

Coronary angiography is the gold standard to localise the site of coronary artery obstruction. However, attempts have been made to localise the site of coronary occlusion depending on the site of infarction. Electrocardiographically, anterior myocardial infarction is basically classified into anteroseptal, anterolateral and apical. Most studies have shown poor correlation between the ECG findings and the extent of myocardial involvement determined on autopsy. Recently important correlations have been made regarding the site of occlusion of a coronary artery and site of infarction on ECG with high degree of sensitivity, specificity and predictive value (Table 19.3).

Further, certain electrocardiographic predictors of left anterior descending artery occlusion have been highlighted with high degree of specificity and sensitivity (Table 19.4).

Comments

1. ST segment elevation in aVR, complete RBBB, ST ↑ in V_1 (> 2.5 mm) and ST ↓ in V_5 are some predictors of left anterior descending artery occlusion proximal to SI.
2. Abnormal Q waves in V_4-V_6 are indicative of occlusion distal to SI.
3. Q waves in aVL suggest proximal occlusion (proximal to DI) while ST ↓ in the same lead suggests distal occlusion.
4. ST depression > 1 mm in inferior leads (II,III, aVF) suggests occlusion before SI/DI whereas absence of these changes predict distal occlusion.

Table 19.3: Correlation of myocardial infection with side of occlusion of a coronary artery

ECG evidence of infarction	Site of coronary occlusion	Sensitivity (%)	Specificity (%)	Predictive value (%)
1. Anterior infarction	Left coronary	90	95	96
2. Inferior infarction	(i) Right coronary	56	97	80
	(ii) Right or left circumflex	53	98	94
3. Strict posterior or posterolateral infarction	(i) Left circumflex artery	24	98	75
	(ii) Right or left circumflex	53	98	94

Table 19.4: Electrocardiographic predictors of left anterior descending occlusion site in anterior myocardial infarction

Site of occlusion	ECG findings
1. Proximal to first septal perforator (SI)	1. ST $\uparrow$ (V$_1$) > 2.5 mm • Complete RBBB • ST $\uparrow$ aVR • ST $\downarrow$ V$_5$

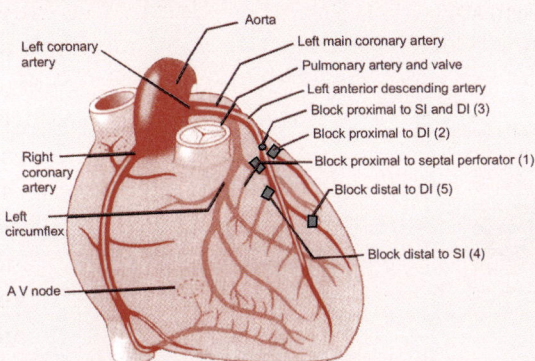

Aorta
Left coronary artery
Left main coronary artery
Pulmonary artery and valve
Left anterior descending artery
Block proximal to SI and DI (3)
Block proximal to DI (2)
Right coronary artery
Block proximal to septal perforator (1)
Block distal to DI (5)
Left circumflex
Block distal to SI (4)
A V node

2. Proximal to first diagonal branch (DI)	2. Q waves in aVL
3. Proximal to SI/DI	3. ST $\downarrow$ in inferior leads > 1 mm
4. Distal to SI	4. Q waves in V$_4$-V$_6$
5. Distal to DI	5. ST $\downarrow$ aVL

ST $\uparrow$ = ST elevation ST $\downarrow$ = ST depression

SECTION SEVEN

Clinical Significance

It is pertinent to define the site of occlusion of left anterior descending artery in the setting of acute myocardial infarction because proximal occlusion needs a more aggressive approach to revascularisation to prevent (i) extensive myocardial damage, (ii) development of sub-AV nodal conduction disturbance and (iii) occurrence of life-threatening arrhythmias.

Inferior Wall Infarction and Site of Coronary Artery Occlusion

Inferior wall infarction can result from occlusion of either right coronary artery (RCA) or left circumflex (LCX) artery. Anatomically, right coronary artery

supplies posterobasal and diaphragmatic segments of the left ventricle; while left circumflex (LCX) coronary artery supplies inferolateral and postero-lateral areas of the left ventricle. A good correlation with high degree of sensitivity, specificity and predictive value have been established between certain electrocardiographic findings in leads representing the areas supplied by right coronary and left circumflex arteries (Table 19.5).

Comments

1. The ST segment elevation ($\uparrow$) in lead III higher than lead II indicates right coronary artery occlusion. The area infarcted is localised to posterobasal and

Table 19.5. Electrocardiographic finding and its relation to the culprit vessel

Culprit vessel	ECG findings	Sensitivity (%)	Specificity (%)	Predictive value (%)
1. Right coronary artery (Fig.19.42)	• ST ↑ in III > II	99	100	99
	• ST ↓ in lead I	95	96	88
	• T wave upright in V_{4R}	89	100	92
2. Left circumflex (LCX) artery (Fig. 19.43)	• ST ↑ in II > III	93	100	98
	• ST ↑ in lead I	50	100	87
	• T is normally inverted in lead V_{4R}	79	100	94

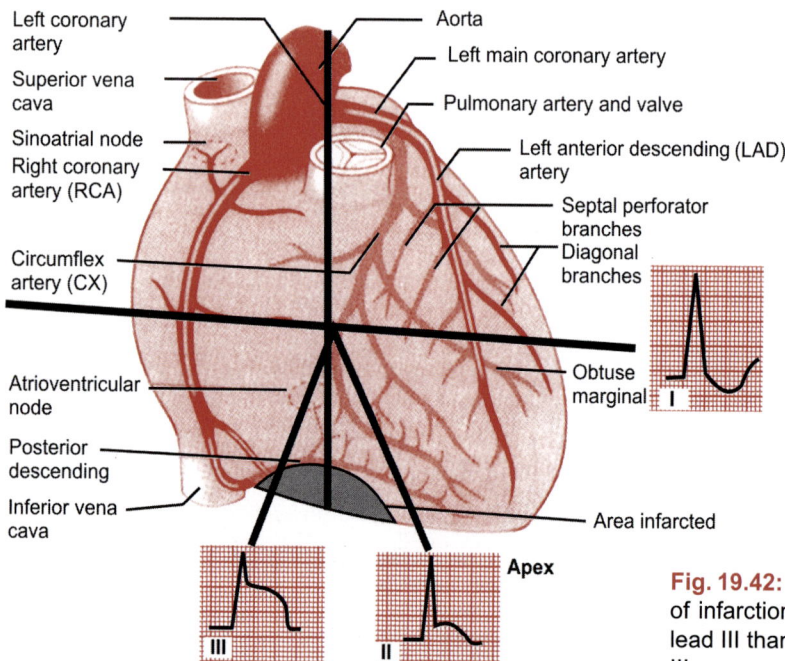

Left coronary artery
Superior vena cava
Sinoatrial node
Right coronary artery (RCA)
Circumflex artery (CX)
Atrioventricular node
Posterior descending
Inferior vena cava

Aorta
Left main coronary artery
Pulmonary artery and valve
Left anterior descending (LAD) artery
Septal perforator branches
Diagonal branches
Obtuse marginal
Area infarcted

I

III   II   Apex

Fig. 19.42: Right coronary artery occlusion with predicted area of infarction. The maximum ST segment elevation occurs in lead III than lead II due to orientation of ST axis towards lead III

diaphragmatic segments of left ventricle which is electrocardiographically represented by lead III (Fig. 19.42). This will produce ST depression (↓) in lead I as a reciprocal change, as lead I is placed > 90° away from the infarcted area. The upright T wave in V_{4R} is due to change in its polarity in right sided leads which if previously inverted becomes upright due to right coronary artery occlusion.

2. The ST segment elevation in lead II higher than lead III indicates left circumflex occlusion because the area infarcted due to occlusion of this artery is localised to inferolateral and posterolateral areas of left ventricle which are electrocardiographically represented by lead II (Fig. 19.43). The ST segment vector is oriented towards lead II, hence, produces marked ST elevation in this lead and lead I. The T wave is inverted in V_{4R} as usual as normal.

Differential Electrocardiographic Diagnosis of Myocardial Infarction

The conditions that mimic or simulate myocardial infarction on ECG are briefly discussed below.

1. Normal Individuals

The criteria for diagnosis of acute myocardial infarction rests on the presence of abnormal Q waves, e.g. wave duration > 0.04 sec and Q wave

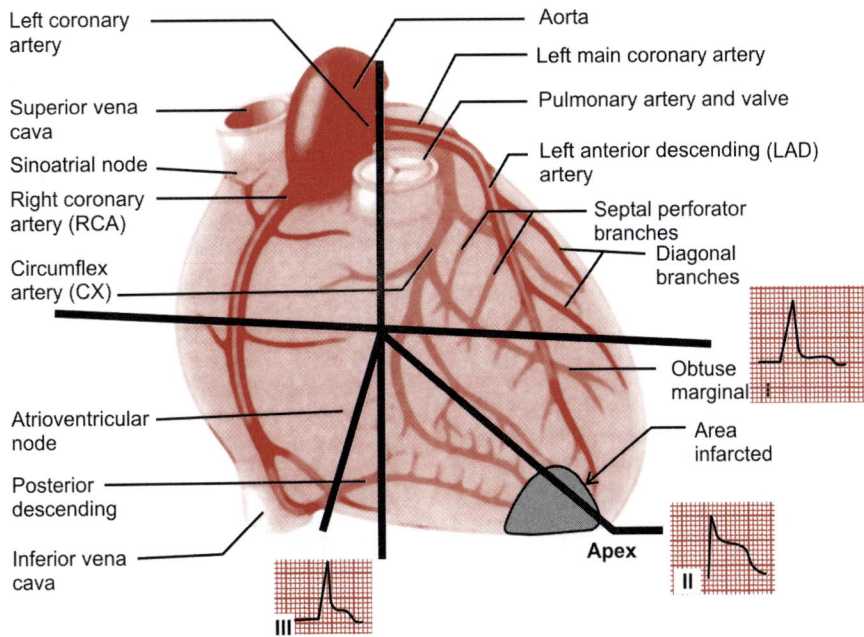

Fig. 19.43: Left circumflex artery occlusion with predicted area of infarction. The ST segment vector being oriented to lead II produces maximum ST elevation in lead II (ST↑ II>III)

should either be equal or exceeds 25% of the R wave in the same lead except in lead III. It has been observed that a large number of normal individuals may satisfy this criteria in lead III. Even lead III may show normal T wave inversion. It is advised to record lead III after deep inspiration and expiration as a means of identifying the inconsistency of Q wave in this lead. Majority of the individuals show either disappearance of Q wave or a small insignificant Q wave during deep inspiration. Therefore, sensitivity and specificity of Q wave in lead III alone in diagnosis of myocardial infarction is unknown. Never make the diagnosis of infarction only on the basis of lead III if it is not associated with other criteria of myocardial infarction (Fig. 19.44).

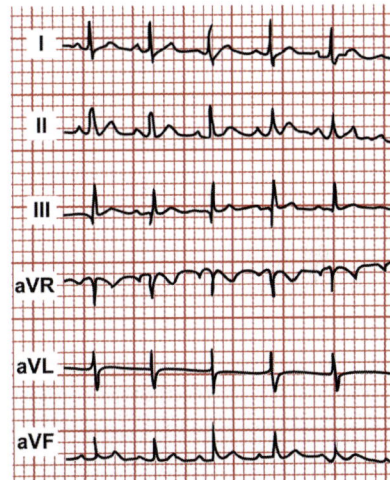

Fig. 19.44: Normal individual with Q waves in lead III

2. Left Ventricular Hypertrophy (LVH)

In left ventricular hypertrophy, QRS forces are directed *leftwards*, inferiorly and posteriorly, hence, QS complexes may be observed in leads V_1-V_2 and even in V_3 and V_4. In addition, ST segment depression in leads I, aVL and V_5-V_6 and ST segment elevation in V_1-V_3 due to left ventricular hypertrophy may mimic myocardial infarction (Read Chapter on LVH).

3. Hypertrophic Cardiomyopathy

In patients with marked septal hypertrophy, abnormal Q waves may be seen in several ECG leads. This is due to an abnormal and delayed depolarisation of interventricular septum from left to right. The abnormal Q waves in different leads may simulate anterior, inferior, lateral wall myocardial infarction. Coronary arteriography and autopsy data have proved the absence of myocardial infarction in such patients depicting abnormal Q waves. For details read Chapter on Hypertrophic Cardiomyopathy.

4. Chronic Cor Pulmonale (Chronic Obstructive Pulmonary Disease with Right Ventricular Hypertrophy)

Due to hyperinflation of the lungs in chronic obstructive pulmonary disease (COPD), there is marked reduction or total absence of anterior QRS forces resulting in small r waves or QS complexes in precordial leads V_1-V_4. If right ventricular hypertrophy is associated with chronic obstructive lung disease, a condition called *cor pulmonale*, the T waves may be inverted in these leads. Both these changes mimic ECG changes of acute anteroseptal myocardial infarction (Fig. 19.45).

For reasons that are not clear, pulmonary emphysema results in shift of QRS axis *leftwards* and superiorly. This leftward axis deviation should not be confused with left anterior hemiblock since there is no involvement of intraventricular conduction. In addition, abnormal Q waves, QS deflections may be recorded in leads I and aVF mimicking lateral or inferior wall infarction. These ECG findings in the presence of lung disease should not be interpreted as myocardial infarction unless or until there is clinical correlation.

Infarction in a patient with *cor pulmonale* otherwise is not uncommon. When it occurs, it becomes difficult to diagnosis because some of the features of infarction may be masked. However, changes of infarction limited to a territory (anterolateral, inferior wall, etc) suggest concomitant infarction which must be interpreted in the light of history, cardiac enzymes and other sophisticated investigations (Fig. 19.46).

5. Left Anterior Hemiblock

In the presence of left anterior hemiblock, the inferoposterior surface of the heart is depolarised in advance through left posterior fascicle than the anterosuperior surface. The initial inferoposterior forces will produce q wave in leads 1 and aVL which does not indicate infarction but occurs as a result of anterior fascicular block perse. In addition, small but

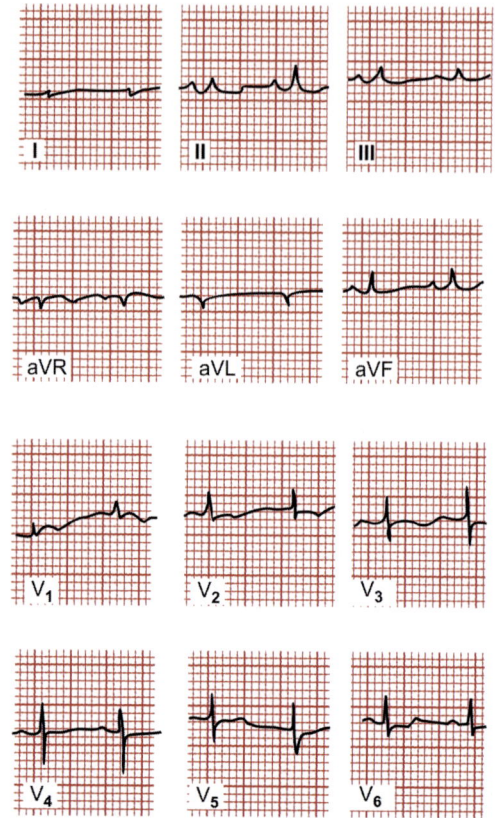

Fig. 19.45: The ST-T changes due to chronic obstructive pulmonary disease simulating anterior as well as inferior wall infarction. The ECG shows;

i. The ST segment depression with biphasic T wave in leads II, III and aVF. These changes mimic inferior wall ischaemia

ii. Coving ST segment with T wave inversion from V_1-V_3. These changes mimic anteroseptal infarction

The presence of low voltage graph, P pulmonale in leads II, III, aVF (right atrial hypertrophy) and right ventricular hypertrophy (tall R wave in V_1-V_2, clockwise rotation, large S waves in V_5-V_6), suggest chronic obstructive pulmonary disease with cor pulmonale. The changes in right precordial leads V_1-V_3 are due to right ventricular hypertrophy. The ST changes in leads II, III, aVF, I and V_5-V_6 are due to generalised hypoxaemia of COPD

not wide Q waves may be seen in leads V_1-V_2 as a result of loss of normal depolarisation sequence of anterior portion of interventricular septum (Read Chapter 14 on fascicular blocks).

RIGHT VENTRICULAR INFARCTION

Isolated right ventricular myocardial infarction was a rarely recognised entity till last decade. Numerous

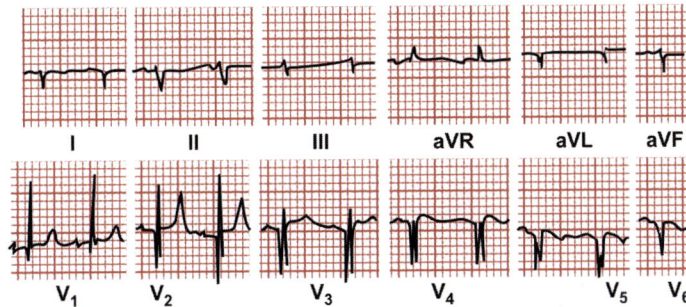

Fig. 19.46: Probable anterior wall infarction in a patient with cor pulmonale. The electrocardiogram was recorded from a 60 yrs male having cor pulmonate for the last 4 yrs, who was admitted with acute chest pain. The electrocardiographic findings include;

i. Low amplitude of QRS deflections in standard and limb leads. The QRS axis is in right superior quadrant producing S_I, S_{II}, S_{III} syndrome and R wave in aVR. Biphasic P wave is seen in lead V_1 with initial upright peaked component indicating right atrial hypertrophy which is further corroborated by peaked P wave in V_2 and V_3. The qR pattern in V_1 and qRS pattern in V_2 indicate right ventricular hypertrophy. All these features suggest COPD with right atrial and ventricular hypertrophy.

ii. Evidence of acute myocardial infarction. The presence of large significant q wave extending from V_1-V_4 with wide and slurred QS pattern in V_5-V_6 with convexity upwards and associated T wave inversion indicate lateral wall infarction with peri-infarction block. It may be possible that upright T wave in leads V_1-V_3 could be due to the fact that inverted T wave of concommitant right ventricular hypertrophy have become upright due to anterior wall infarction while Q waves of infarction is persisting. The diagnosis of infarction was confirmed by raised cardiac enzyme and by echocardiography.

NB: The ECG in COPD may simulate anterior wall infarction, in that case, there will be rS complexes in V_5-V_6 and not wide and slurred QS complexes. The T wave would be upright but could be inverted due to hypoxaemia, in that situation, it will be seen in all precordial leads and most of standard and limb leads.

The clinical history, electrocardiographic findings with raised cardiac enzymes and echocardiography confirmed the diagnosis of associated myocardial infarction which is otherwise common in a patient with COPD.

studies conducted during last decade or so have shown that it is not rare but is encountered infrequently, can be diagnosed on surface ECG. The reasons for its less occurrence has been, i.e. (i) smaller mass of right ventricle (ii) lower tension in right ventricular cavity and (iii) there is richer collateral circulation of right ventricle. It has been estimated that 30-35% cases of right ventricular infarction occurs in conjunction with inferior left ventricular myocardial infarction.

The Electrocardiographic Pattern (Fig. 19.47)

Various studies in recent past have documented changes affecting repolarisation; mainly ST segment and to some extent the T wave. The changes are:

1. *ST segment elevation in leads V_1 and/or V_{4R} (Extreme right precordial leads).* Right ventricular infarction should be strongly suspected, if in the setting of an acute inferior wall infarction (ST-T changes in leads II, III and aVF), there is ST segment elevation of 1 mm or more in leads V_1 and/or V_{4R-6R}. The V_{4R} lead is considered most

sensitive for this change. An ST segment elevation in V_{4R} than lead V_1 or V_2 offers the highest specificity and efficacy in the diagnosis of right ventricular infarction. Although Q waves and ST elevation may appear in leads V_1-V_3, their specificity is too low to be useful in diagnosis of right ventricular infarction.

2. *Failure of reciprocal ST depression in leads V_1-V_2.* If ST depression of appreciable depth in leads V_1-V_2 does not occur in patients with inferior wall infarction, it is indicative of right ventricular infarction. Lewis and his associates in an interesting study on inferior wall infarction found that ST segment depression in lead V_2 was 50% of the magnitude of ST elevation in lead aVF. They postulated that insignificant depression of ST segment in leads V_1-V_2 in the event of inferior wall infarction indicates associated right ventricular injury.

Mechanism : The principle of electrocardiography states that ST segment deviates towards the surface of myocardial injury, hence, the anterior upward

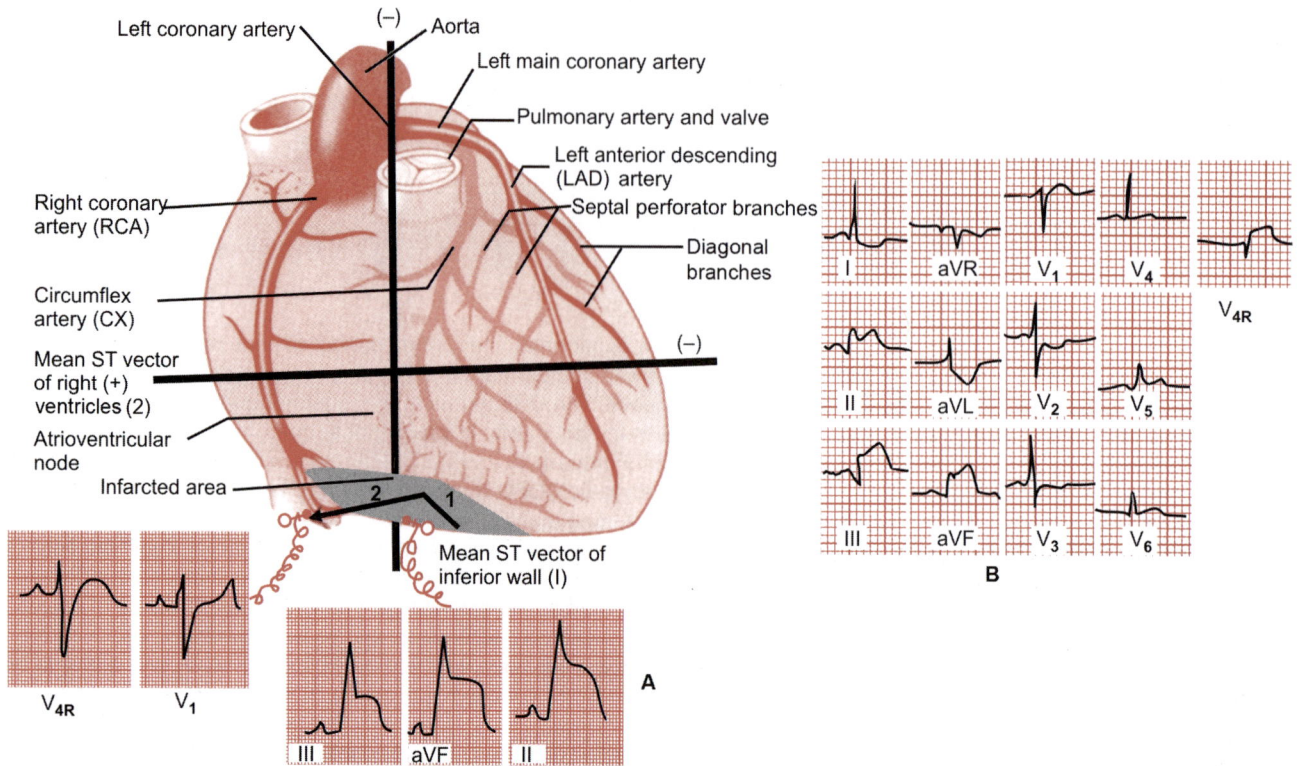

Figs 19.47A and B: Inferior wall infarction combined with right ventricular infarction.

A: Diagrammatic illustration shows the ST segment elevation in leads II, III and aVF due to inferior wall infarction due to alignment of mean infarction vector towards these leads. As a result of the above mentioned changes, one would expect reciprocal change in lead V_1 in the form of ST segment depression. Either failure of reciprocal changes in V_1 or elevation of ST segment in V_4R or V_3R indicates associated right ventricular infarction (as shown in figure)

B: The electrocardiogram shows characteristic of inferior wall and right ventricular infarction

   i. *The Inferior wall infarction* is evidenced by q wave, ST elevation with dragged T waves in leads II, III and aVF. Reciprocal ST depression is seen in leads I, aVL, and V_2-V_3. V_1 does not show reciprocal change

   ii. *Right ventricular infarction* was suspected due to nonappearance of ST depression in V_1 (reciprocal change) and even ST elevation was recorded in it. Therefore, lead V_4R was recorded which clearly revealed ST elevation more than 1 mm which confirmed associated right ventricular infarct. The ST elevation in V_1 and ST depression in V_2 (discordant pattern) is highly suggestive change of right ventricular infarction

ST segment deviated force towards right ventricular surface in right ventricular *infarct* would thus tends to nullify or counteract any other force which would tend to depress the ST segment in right precordial leads, for example, mean ST force of inferior wall infarction (Fig. 19.45). In other words, inferior wall infarct tends to depress ST segment in right precordial leads as a reciprocal change, hence, reciprocal change will not be allowed to occur in these leads if there is an associated right ventricular infarction.

3. *The ST segment elevation in lead V_1 with ST depression in lead V_2* (A discordant pattern). This discordant relationship also indicates the presence

of a right ventricular infarct (Fig. 19.47B). It has been suggested that simultaneous ST segment elevation in lead V_1 and depression in V_2 is an important and specific sign for right ventricular infarction.

4. *Lewis and his associates* have reported hyperacute phase of right ventricular infarction. This manifests primarily with slope elevation of ST segment only in lead V_4R or lead V_1. Now it has been estimated that sensitivity and specificity of ST elevation in lead V_4R alone is between 82-100% and 68-77% respectively.

The diagnostic clues of right ventricular infarction are summarised in the box.

Diagnostic Clues to Right Ventricular Infarction

- A diagnosis of right *ventricular infarction* should only be entertained if there is concomitant ECG evidence of an inferior or an inferoposterior myocardial infarction.
- The ECG changes of both inferior wall as well as right ventricular infarction will be as follows;
  - **(i) Changes of acute inferior wall infarction,** i.e. decreased amplitude of R wave, increased ventricular activation time, slope elevation of the ST segment with dragged up T waves and abnormal Q waves in leads II, III and aVF.
  - **(ii) Changes of right ventricular infarction,** i.e. slope elevation of ST segment (≥ 1 mm) and relatively increased amplitude of T wave in lead V_{4R} and V_1.

NB: In the presence of inferior wall infarction, the reciprocal ST depression in V_1 if is less than 50% of ST elevation in aVF in the absence of other evidence, suggests right ventricular infarction in addition.

SUBENDOCARDIAL INFARCTION (FIG. 19.48)

Anterior subendocardial infarction produces a ST and T vector directed towards the cavity of left ventricle, i.e. away from left ventricular leads, therefore, there is ST segment depression and T wave inversion in the left precordial leads especially in the midprecordial region. The diagnosis of subendocardial infarction on ECG is not as definite or clearcut as that of transmural or even epicardial infarction. Therefore, diagnosis should be entertained when;

I. The ECG presents ST segment depression and deep symmetric T wave inversion in mid and lateral precordial leads as well as standard leads I and II.

II. There is clinical and biochemical evidences of an acute myocardial infarction.

III. These abnormal changes persist for several days.

Since the ST segment changes persist for several days, subendocardial infarction are usually indistinguishable from changes of chronic coronary insufficiency, hence, the presence or absence of alterations

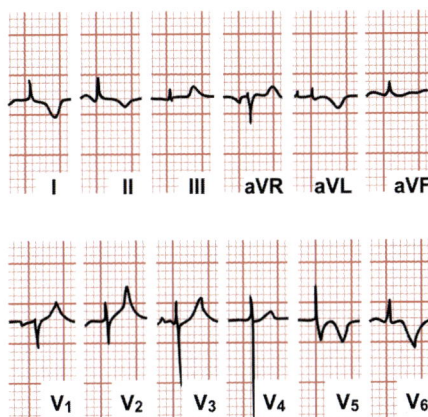

Fig. 19.48: Anterolateral subendocardial infarction. The electrocardiogram recorded from a patient with cardiac chest pain shows:
  i. Wide, deep inverted T wave in leads I, II, aVL, V_5 and V_6
  ii. There is no Q wave
  iii. ST segment is depressed with convexity upwards in leads I, aVL and V_5-V_6

Persistent changes subsequently confirmed the infarction. However, these changes must be confirmed by other tests (enzymes, echocardiogram, scanning) because these types of symmetrical inversion of T waves may be seen in cerebrovascular accidents and other noncardiac conditions

in QRS configuration assumes critical diagnostic significance. The association of QRS changes particularly abnormal Q waves indicate coronary insufficiency rather than subendocardial infarction, a fact that has been proved experimentally in dogs by Prinzmetal and his co-workers. They further concluded that pure subendocardial infarction does not alter the QRS complex in precordial leads, an opinion which is widely accepted nowadays. The diagnostic clues to subendocardial infarction are summarised in the box.

Diagnostic ECG clues to subendocardial infarction

- ST segment depression with deep symmetric T waves inversion in precordial or inferior leads or both.
- No change/alteration in morphology of QRS in these leads.
- Absence of Q wave in these leads.

INTERVENTRICULAR SEPTAL INFARCTION

Septal infarction occurs frequently in combination with infarction of left ventricular free wall, but rarely, septum may be the sole site of infarction. Septal infarction characterised by abnormal Q wave should be suspected; if any of the following abnormalities appear on the ECG.

(i) QS deflections in leads V_1-V_4 or the absence of an R wave in any of the leads V_2, V_3 or V_4 if an adjacent leads to the right show an initial positivity.

(ii) The presence of Q waves in leads V_5 and V_6 when there is complete left bundle branch block, or Q waves in leads V_1 and V_2 when there is complete right bundle branch block.

ATRIAL INFARCTION

Atrial infarction is rarely recognised because there is no distinct clinical presentation and the ECG manifestations are also inconspicuous and difficult to evaluate. Atrial infarction produces ECG changes by affecting atrial repolarisation represented by P-R segment which extends from the end of P wave to the beginning of QRS. Atrial infarction may further be corroborated by other features such as abnormalities of P waves, abnormalities of atrial rhythm and sinoatrial block or first degree AV block. The ECG features are summarised in the box. Atrial infarction is common in the setting of acute inferior wall infarction.

ECG Features of Atrial Infarction

In clinical setting of acute inferior myocardial infarction, the features suggesting atrial infarction are;

(i) P-R segment is usually minimally displaced in a direction opposite to that of P wave. It tends to be slightly depressed in leads II, III and aVF where P waves are upright and best seen.

(ii) P-R segment even may be elevated minimally in atrial infarction in the same direction as that of P wave, best seen in aVF.

(iii) Occasionally, a sharp angle between the P wave and P-R segment due to abnormal, horizontal depression of the P-R segment suggests an atrial infarction.

(iv) Corroborrative evidences such as abnormalities of P wave (wide, notched or slurred), abnormalities of atrial rhythm (atrial ectopics, atrial tachycardia, atrial flutter), sinus bradycardia, and sinoatrial or first degree AV block help to substantiate the diagnosis of an atrial infarct.

Sensitivity and Specificity of ECG in Diagnosing Myocardial Infarction

The ECG lacks sensitivity in making the diagnosis of acute myocardial infarction due to increased number of cases with false negative results. False positive cases are also a big handicap. The sensitivity and specificity of ECG with correlation to autopsy findings are given in the Table 19.6.

MYOCARDIAL INFARCTION WITH CONDUCTION DISTURBANCE

Failure of conduction may develop at four different levels in the conduction system of the heart; the SA node, the atrioventricular (AV) node, the bundle of His, and the more peripheral portions of the conduction system. If block occurs in AV node, the escape rhythm usually originates from the AV junction, i.e. lower part of AV node or bundle of His, and the QRS complexes are of usually normal duration. When the block occurs distal to AV node; the escape rhythm originates from one of the ventricles and the configuration of QRS is abnormal and its duration is prolonged. Disturbances of conduction may occur in a bundle branch or in one or two peripheral branches (fascicles) of conduction system and their recognition is of utmost importance so as to identify the patients at risk of developing complete AV block. When block occurs in any two of the three fascicles, *bifascicular block* is said to exist; complete AV block often develops in such patients. Thus, patients who have a combination of right bundle branch block and either left anterior or left posterior hemiblock or patients with bilateral bundle branch block are particularly at high risk of progression to complete heart block. These conduction disturbances adversely affect the mortality rates in patients with myocardial infarction. The conduction disturbances are more common with inferior wall than anterior wall infarction (Figs 19.49A to C and 19.50). The presence

Table 19.6: Sensitivity and specificity of ECG in diagnosing myocardial infarction

Causes of false negative cases
(Infarct is present but ECG does not show diagnostic changes)
- Second infarction
- Left ventricular hypertrophy
- Lateral and posterior wall infarction
- WPW syndrome.
- Nonspecific ST-T changes in absence of Q wave.

Causes of false positive cases
(Infarction absent but ECG shows diagnostic changes)
1. *A Q wave present but infarction changes absent*
   - Left ventricular hypertrophy
   - WPW syndrome
   - Chronic obstructive pulmonary disease
   - Fascicular blocks
   - Infiltrative heart disease
2. *Q waves are absent, ST changes present but infarction is absent*
   - Right ventricular hypertrophy
   - Drugs and electrolytes disturbance
   - Secondary ST-T changes in presence of bundle branch block
   - Chronic obstructive pulmonary disease
   - Acute pulmonary embolism
   - Hyperventilation
   - Myocarditis.

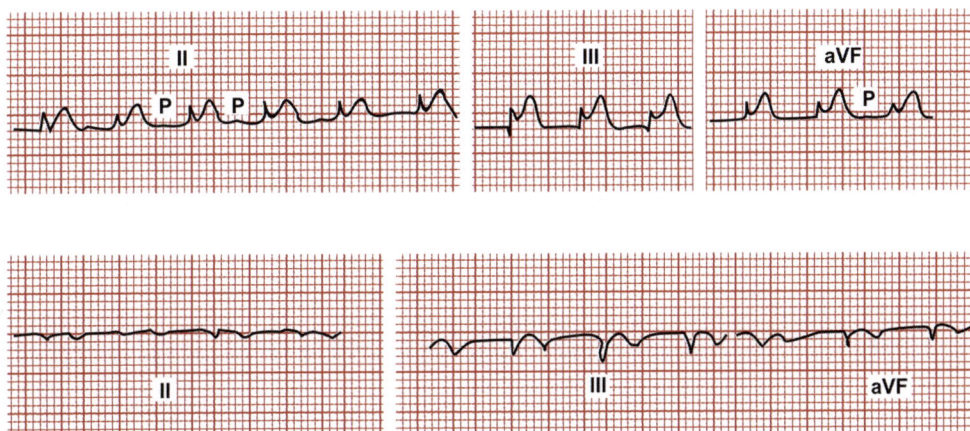

Fig. 19.49A: Inferior wall infarction with first degree AV block. The ECG (leads II, III and aVF) shows;
  i. *Inferior wall infarction;* There is ST segment elevation with T dragged upwards in leads II, III and aVF
  ii. *First degree AV block;* P-R interval is prolonged to 0.24 sec
      Lower strip: Following recovery, there is resolution of ST segment with inversion of T waves. The first degree AV block has disappeared. The P-R interval is 0.16 sec

of conduction disturbances in an anterior wall infarction usually indicates massive infarction.

Myocardial Infarction with Bundle Branch Blocks

Since septal activation occurs during 0.02 sec of QRS interval, and activation of all except the basal portions of left ventricle takes place between 0.02-0.04 second

of QRS interval, therefore, myocardial infarction produces abnormalities of the first 0.04 second of QRS deflection in the form of abnormal Q waves or changes in the R waves. In general, right bundle branch block (RBBB) does not obscure the pattern of myocardial infarction because initial activation of left ventricle follows a normal pattern and first 0.04 second of QRS is relatively unaffected by RBBB. The left bundle

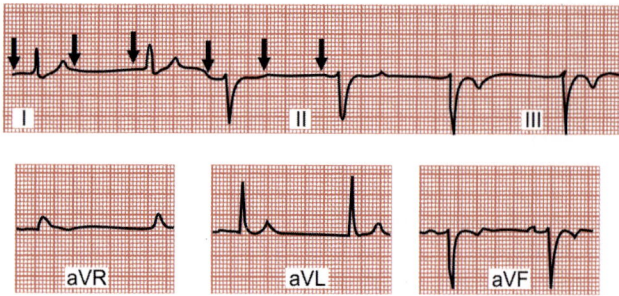

Fig. 19.49B: Second degree AV block. The ECG (standard leads) shows:
   i. *Second degree (2:1) AV block.* Every alternate P is conducted with fixed P-R interval.
   ii. *Inferior wall ischaemia*/infarction is suggested by coving ST segment in leads III and aVF with T wave inversion.
   iii. *Left anterior hemiblock* is suggested by left axis deviation >-30° and rS pattern in leads II, III and aVF.

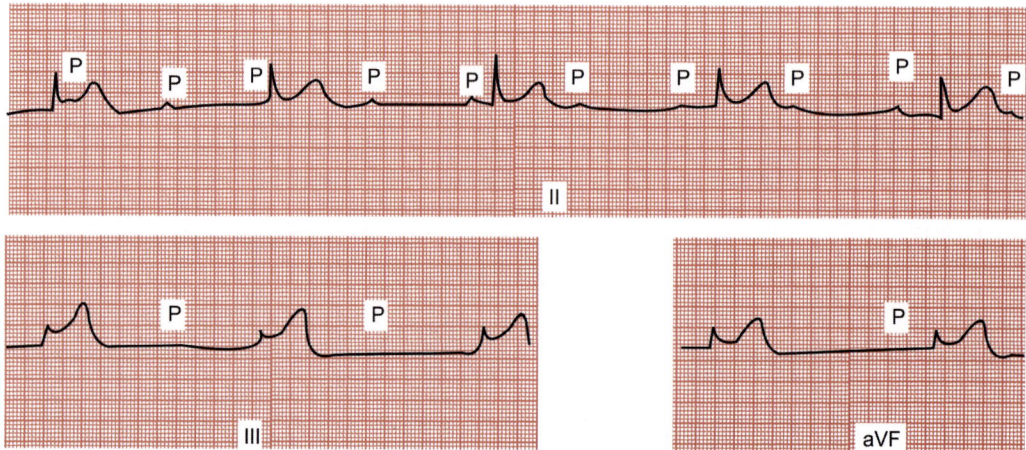

Fig. 19.49C: Complete heart block. Note the following characteristics on ECG (leads II, III and aVF);
   i. *Inferior wall infarction;* There is ST segment elevation in leads II, III and aVF The T is wide, upright and lifted with ST segment.
   ii. *Complete heart block.* The atrial rate is 75 bpm and is regular. The ventricular rate is 33 bpm and is also regular. The P waves are unrelated to QRS. The QRS complexes are wide indicating idioventricular rhythm

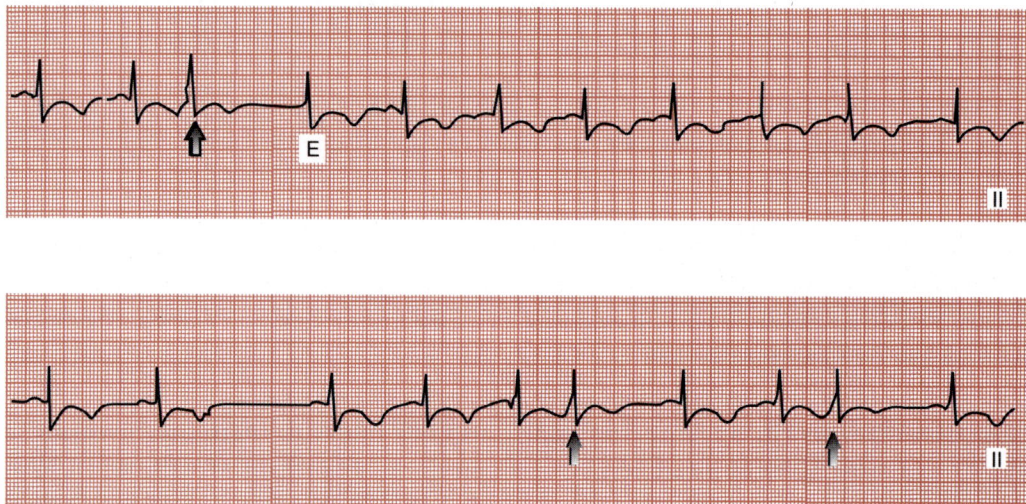

Fig. 19.50: Sinus node dysfunction in a patient with inferior wall infarction . The long rhythm strip (lead II) shows:
   i. *Sinus arrhythmia* (nonrespiratory). The P-R interval is variable
   ii. *Sinus pause.* The lower strip shows a sinus pause following a sinus beat indicating sinus arrest (no atrial activity or P wave visible between two sinus beats)
   iii. *Multiple intermittent AV nodal ectopics* (QRS complex not preceded by P wave) are seen. There is compensatory pause following each of them. Some of them are indicated by arrows. There is one nodal escape beat (E) seen following a nodal ectopic in upper strip
   iv. *Inferior wall infarction.* The ST segment elevation with T wave inversion in lead II suggest an inferior wall infarction

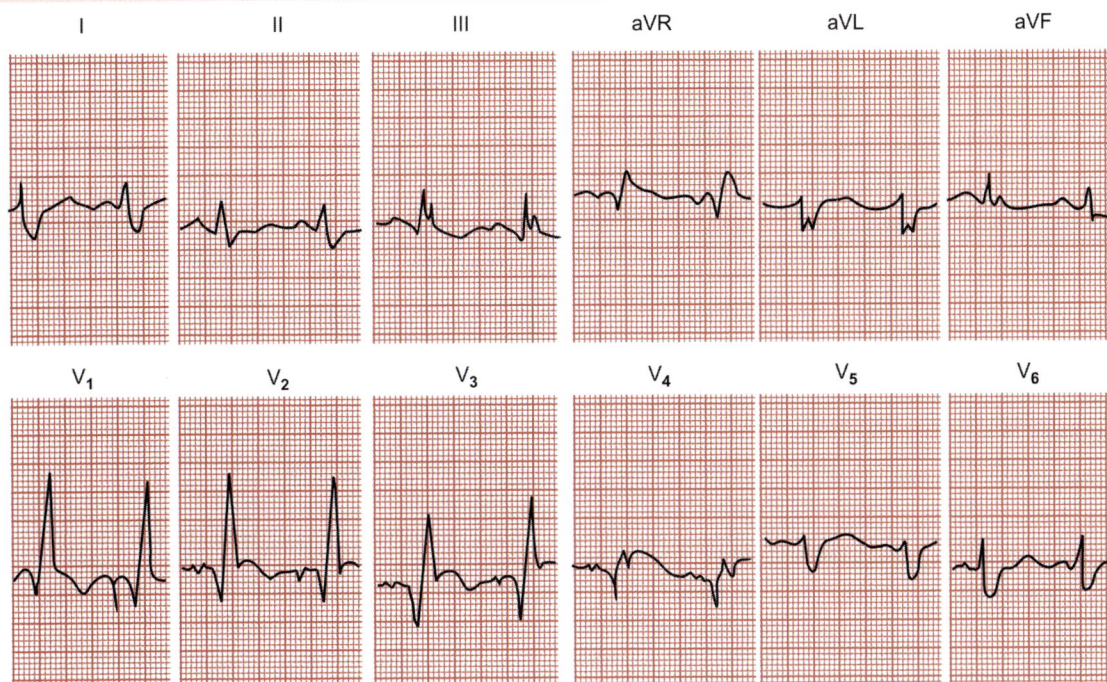

I   II   III   aVR   aVL   aVF

V_1 V_2 V_3 V_4 V_5 V_6

Fig. 19.51: Acute anterior myocardial infarction with right bundle branch block (RBBB). The qR pattern in V_1-V_4 with associated ST segment elevation and T wave inversion strongly support the diagnosis of acute myocardial infarction (anteroseptal). There is typical right bundle branch block pattern (wide qRS in V_1 with broad late S wave in I, V_5 and V_6). The initial r wave of RBBB in V_1 and V_2 has been replaced by wide deep q wave of infarction. Broad notched P wave are present in leads II, III and aVF, and bifid P waves with wide negative component in V_1-V_3 could be pseudo-P pulmonale due to left atrial enlargement

branch block, on the other hand, obscures the pattern of myocardial infarction by affecting the initial 0.04 second vector of QRS, hence, expected abnormal Q waves may not be inscribed.

1. Right Bundle Branch Block with Myocardial Infarction (Fig. 19.51)

As features of right bundle branch block (RBBB) are not blocked or disturbed by concomitant myocardial infarction, therefore, both express individually and can be easily recognised on ECG. Since most infarctions involving the left ventricle disturb the initial portion of QRS and RBBB disturbs the terminal portion of QRS, hence, both express on ECG individually. The ECG pattern that evolves in such a combination of RBBB and myocardial infarction will be as follows:

1. In extensive anterior myocardial infarction involving the interventricular septum as well, the initial r wave of rSR' complex of RBBB will disappear in right precordial leads resulting in QR or qR pattern. The disappearance of r wave and appearance of QR pattern in right precordial leads is due to septal infarction (Fig. 19.51).

2. The occurrence of RBBB in inferior wall infarction, the ECG pattern of RBBB (rSR') will appear in right precordial leads and changes of infarction (Q waves, elevated ST segment and inverted T waves) will appear in inferior oriented leads (II, III, and aVF). Right bundle branch block is common in inferior wall infarction because in most cases right bundle is supplied by right coronary artery which also supplies the inferior wall of left ventricle (Fig. 19.51).

3. The occurrence of RBBB in posterior wall myocardial infarction produces alteration in QRS complexes in right precordial leads. Instead of rSR' complex, either an abnormally tall, wide R wave or rR' complex will be inscribed in the right precordial leads (Fig. 19.51). This is due to the fact that RBBB alters late forces of ventricular depolarisation and posterior wall infarction alters

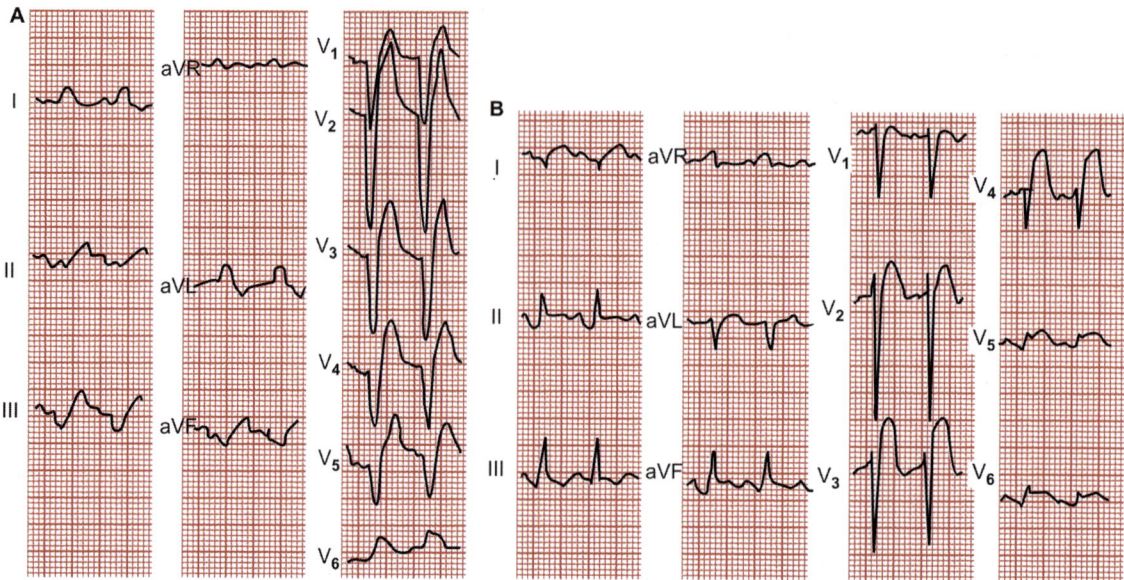

Fig. 19.52: Transient and reversible left bundle branch block in acute anterior myocardial infarction.

A: *During acute chest pain before thrombolysis.* The ECG shows non-Q wave infarction with evolutionary changes of ST elevation in precordial leads with dragged upwards T wave in V_1-V_6. There is non-progression of R wave from V_1-V_6 and slurring of S wave. The left bundle branch is characterised by wide QRS in leads I, aVL and V_6 with left axis deviation and ST depression and T inversion in I and aVL.

B: *Disappearance of pain after thrombolysis.* The ECG shows disappearance of left bundle branch block with fully evolved myocardial infarction characterised by q waves in V_5-V_6 with ST elevation in I, V_1-V_6 with convexity upwards and tendency towards inversion of T waves. All these features suggest that LBBB may mask the evidence of Q wave infarction and its disappearance reveals an Q wave infarction

the initial forces. Both the initial forces (due to myocardial infarction) and late forces (due to RBBB) are oriented anteriorly, hence, the pattern of tall, wide R or rR' appears in leads V_1 or V_2. A similar pattern may also be seen in patients of right ventricular hypertrophy with intraventricular conduction delay. It may also be present in RBBB alone. Therfore, confirmation of myocardial infarction must be sought with the help of other parameters.

2. Left Bundle Branch Block (LBBB) with Myocardial Infarction (Fig. 19.52)

Unlike RBBB, the left bundle branch block (LBBB) makes it quite difficult, often impossible to detect myocardial infarction, particularly if the infarction is an old one. In the acute stages of infarction, since changes of fresh infarction (ST segment elevation and T wave inversion) make their appearance even in the presence of LBBB, hence, problem becomes less formidable and can be diagnosed easily (Fig. 19.52).

Several attempts have seen made in the past to define the diagnostic ECG criteria for myocardial infarction in the presence of a left bundle branch block but have proven unsuccessful when correlated with autopsy findings. Left bundle branch block (LBBB) alone produces a wide QRS complex with ST depression and T wave changes in left precordial (V_5-V_6) and standard leads (I and aVL) and the normal 'q' wave is conspicuous by its absence in these leads. On the other hand, acute myocardial infarction is characterised by presence of abnormal q waves (> 0.04 sec and 25% of the R wave in the same lead), elevated ST segment and inverted T waves. When both occurs concomitantly, then following ECG findings are helpful in making the diagnosis with 90-100% accuracy:

(i) A Q wave in at least two leads representing acute anterior myocardial infarction (leads I, aVL, V_5 or V_6).

(ii) Nonprogression of R wave or R wave regression from V_1 to V_4.

(iii) Notching of the upstroke of S wave in at least two leads (V_3, V_4 or V_5).

(iv) Primary ST-T changes (ST elevation) in two or more adjacent leads. Evolutionary changes of ST segment elevation and T wave inversion on serial ECG recording suggests acute infarction.

Presence of Q wave in leads I, aVL, V_5 or V_6 in the presence of LBBB pattern indicates associated anterior myocardial infarction. The specificity and sensitivity increases if primary ST-T changes are associated with q waves.

The presence of q waves in inferior leads (II, III and aVF) and anterior leads (I, aVL, V_5-V_6) with pattern of LBBB indicates associated inferior wall and anterior wall infarction respectively.

Difficulty arises in diagnosis of acute myocardial infarction, when Q waves do not evolve during the course of acute infarction (non-Q wave infarction). In such a situation, the evolutionary changes of ST elevation, T wave inversion and regression of R wave in precordial leads with notching of S wave become diagnostic criteria, such an infarction must be corroborated by sophisticated investigations such as CPK (MB), echocardiography and myocardial scanning, etc. The development of LBBB in a patient with prior infarction obsures the ECG pattern of infarction which can no longer be detected. Similarly, myocardial ischaemia may also be not detected easily on ECG unless sophisticated means are employed to detect them.

Acute myocardial infarction in the presence of intermittent left bundle block is diagnosed by ECG changes of infarction during normal intraventricular conduction. Otherwise also, acute changes are recognisable in the presence of LBBB.

Clinical Significance

1. Conduction disturbances in acute infarction are limited to involvement of Purkinje system (peri–infarction block) or fascicles of left bundle (fascicular blocks). These conduction disturbances are common in inferior than anterior infarction.

2. The LBBB, on the other hand, is uncommon in anterior infarction; and if it occurs, indicates a massive infarction and constitutes a bad prognostic sign.

3. Conduction disturbances in acute infarction are mostly transient and reversible.

3. Fascicular Blocks

Fascicular block can occur transiently during the course of an acute myocardial infarction or can result from an old infarction. The conduction abnormalities produced by the fascicular block, on one hand, may mask the evidence of an infarction and, on other hand, the infarction may complicate the diagnosis of fascicular block. Sometimes, vectorcardiographic findings have suggested the diagnosis of fascicular block in presence of myocardial infarction.

Fascicular blocks in the presence of myocardial infarction result in changes of infarction in addition to abnormal *leftward* or *rightward* axis deviation. Left anterior fascicular block leads to left axis deviation (Fig. 19.53), therefore, it is difficult to recognise the existence of anterior fascicular block in presence of an old inferior wall infarction as both produce left axis deviation. In the above mentioned situation, the pattern of R wave due to anterior fascicular block in inferior leads (R in II > aVF > III) is reversed namely R in III > II.

The left anterior fascicular block in association with left bundle branch block is usually not defined on the basis of ECG, because changes produced by anterior fascicular block are masked by left bundle branch block, but abnormal left axis > – 60° suggests the existence of both because neither of them produce so much left axis deviation.

Abnormal right axis deviation (>+120°) in presence of myocardial infarction indicate left posterior fascicular block provided there is no evidence of either RBBB or right ventricular hypertrophy (Fig. 19.54).

The abnormal left axis deviation (> – 30°) or right axis deviation(> + 120°) in presence of myocardial infarction indicates left anterior or left posterior fascicular block respectively, provided other causes of abnormal axis deviation have been ruled out.

SECTION SEVEN

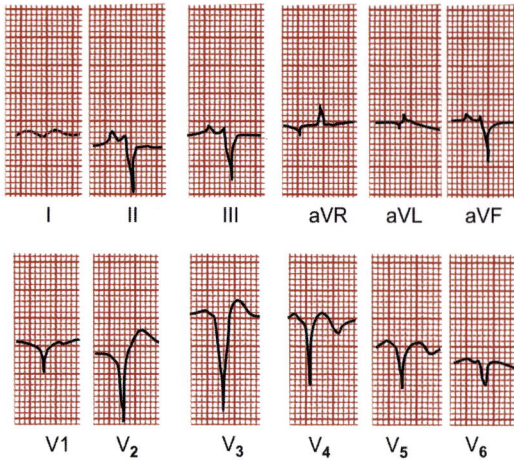

Fig. 19.53: Acute anterior myocardial infarction with left anterior hemiblock. The ECG shows;
  i. Acute myocardial infarction is evident by QS pattern from V_1-V_6 and lead I, and qR pattern in lead aVL with marked ST elevation with convexity upwards
  ii. There is marked left axis deviation > -30° (rS complexes in leads II, III and aVF).

Bifascicular block (right bundle branch block *plus* left anterior or posterior fascicular block) complicating myocardial infarction will result in changes of right bundle branch block, changes of myocardial infarction with abnormal leftward (Fig. 19.55) or rightward QRS axis shift. *Infarction Q waves* already present may be masked by the fascicular conduction delay.

Peri-infarction Block (Figs 19.56 and 19.57)

Conduction delay that is limited to the area surrounding the infarcted region is called *'peri-infarction block'*. In peri–infarction block, there is involvement of fibres of distant Purkinje system surrounding the infarcted area. The identifying features of peri-infarction block on ECG are:
  i) The QRS complexes that show an infarction pattern will appear to be more prolonged (0.11 to 0.12 sec) than the QRS complexes recorded

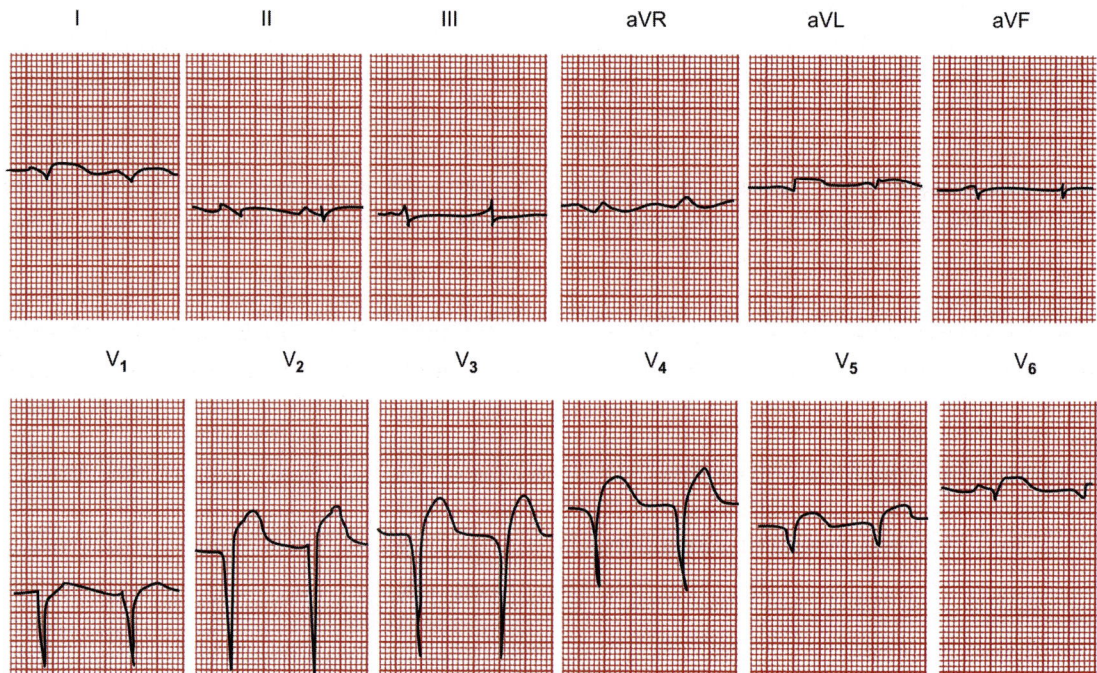

Fig. 19.54: Extensive anterior wall infarction with left posterior fascicular block. Note there is rightward shift of QRS axis between +150° to + 180° (The North-West zone), small R and deep S waves are present in V_1 and V_2, and QS complexes are seen in the remaining precordial leads. Inspection of lead I and aVL shows that in this case, the right axis deviation is due to anterior wall infarction and not due to RVH as in the latter RS complexes will be seen rather than QS deflections. The marked ST elevation in leads I, V_2-V_6 further supports the diagnosis of extensive anterior myocardial infarction (acute). Ordinarily, the Q wave of anterolateral component of an extensive anterior wall infarction is not so large a portion of the QRS that it results in right axis, but sometimes, it happens as in this case, if there is associated posterior fascicular block

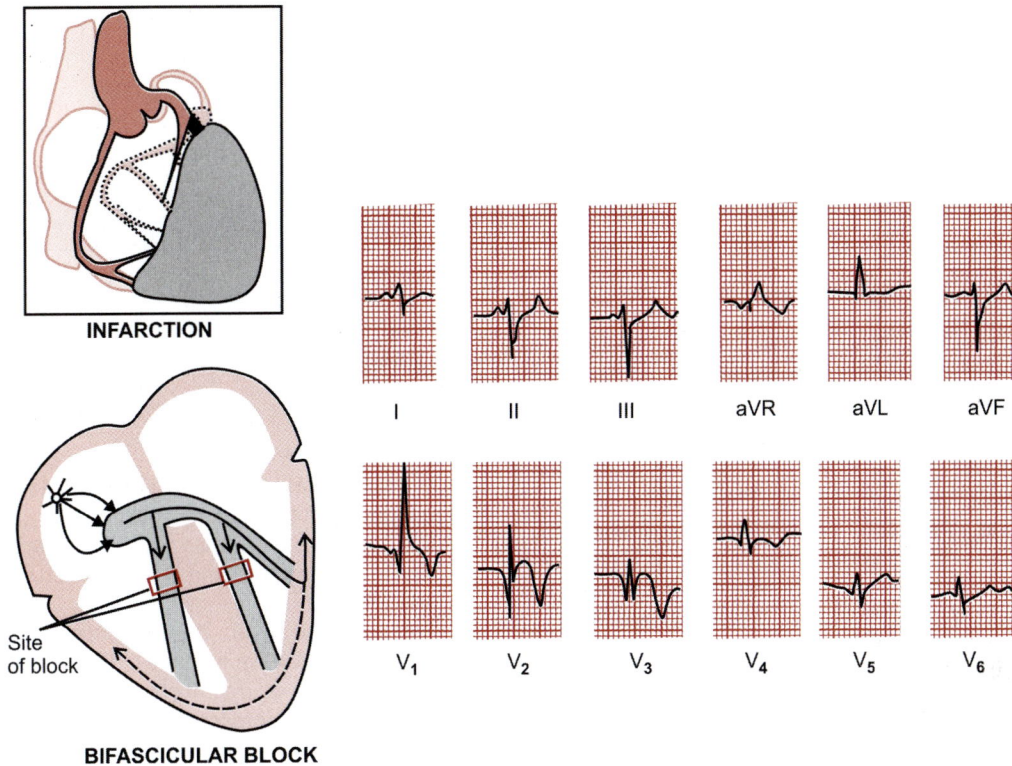

INFARCTION

Site
of block

BIFASCICULAR BLOCK

Fig. 19.55: The electrocardiogram shows bifascicular block in acute myocardial infarction. Note the followings;
   i. *RBBB* is evidenced by rSR' in V_1 with ST-T changes and persistence of S wave in V_5-V_6
   ii. *Left anterior fascicular block* is evident by left axis deviation > –30° with rS pattern in leads II and III. QRS duration in these leads is 0.11 sec
   iii. *Acute anteroseptal myocardial infarction*. There is q wave in leads aVL, and V_2-V_4 with elevation of ST segment in V_2-V_4 and T wave inversion in leads aVL and V_2-V_4. There is regression of r wave from V_1-V_4

from the area remote from infarction. Notching of these complexes may also be seen.

ii) Ventricular activation time is prolonged in precordial leads overlying the infarcted portion of left ventricle, while, it will be normal in leads overlying the univolved portion of the ventricles.

iii) There is an evidence of myocardial infarction on ECG.

The QRS complexes in peri-infarction block are widened and slurred due to delayed conduction in the leads showing infarction pattern, while they are normal in the leads recorded remote from the infarction.

All these changes in presence of normal QRS axis suggest peri-infarction block rather than fascicular block.

Peri–infarction block should not be interpreted as fascicular blocks. Fascicular blocks will produce axis deviation, whereas in peri–infarction block, the frontal plane QRS axis is not altered and the QRS duration in the leads that show Q waves is prolonged.

4. Rhythm Disturbance (Figs 19.58A to D)

The electrical disturbance in the heart (arrhythmia) is most common and dreadful complication of acute myocardial infarction. Ventricular fibrillation is most common cause of arrhythmic death in acute myocardial infarction, although ventricular premature beats and ventricular tachycardia may precede an episode of ventricular fibrillation, the latter often occurs without any warning arrhythmia. All types of arrhythmias arising from atria, AV node, bundle of His, ventricles have been described to occur during

SECTION SEVEN

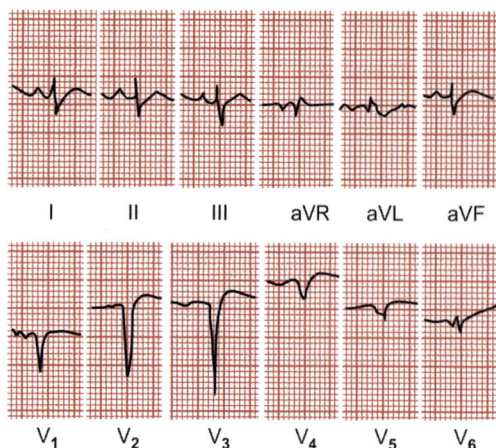

Fig. 19.56: Peri-infarction block (anterior myocardial infarction with intraventricular conduction delay). The ECG shows;
   i. Anterior wall infarction is present due to presence of q wave in lead aVL, QS pattern in V_1-V_5 with qrs in lead V_6
   ii. The QRS in leads V_4-V_6 is prolonged (>0.12 sec) with respect to V_1-V_2
   iii. The QS complex in leads V_4-V_6 is wide and notched due to peri-infarction block
   iv. Normal QRS axis on frontal plane.

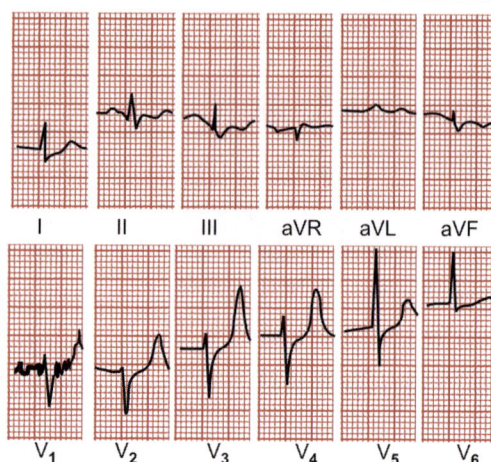

Fig. 19.57: Peri-infarction block in inferior wall infarction. The electrocardiogram shows;
   i. *Old infarction of inferior wall:* There are q waves with coving ST segment and T wave inversion in leads II, III and aVF.
   ii. *Peri-infarction block:* The presence of wide, deep QRS with slurred S wave in leads II, III and aVF
   iii. *The QRS axis on frontal plane is normal.*
The presence of left anterior hemiblock is ruled out due to tall R wave than S wave in II, III and aVF, hence, all these changes suggests intraventricular conduction delay in peripheral Purkinje system surrounding the infarcted area

acute setting, during clinical course and in follow-up cases of acute myocardial infarction. The ventricular arrhythmias are far more common than atrial; and anterior myocardial infarction is its leading cause. The conduction disturbances are common with inferior wall infarction.

Out of ventricular arrhythmias, ventricular ectopics (monomorphic, polymorphic, ectopics with R on T phenomenon), slow or accelerated idioventricular rhythm (AIVR), ventricular tachycardia are common. The ventricular bigeminy is rare in acute episode of myocardial infarction (Fig. 19.60). Similarly, all types of supraventricular (atrial and nodal)

arrhythmias are known to occur in acute myocardial infarction; atrial fibrillation being an uncommon.

The enhanced automaticity, triggered acitivty, re-entry and prolonged QT dispersion are proposed mechanism for pathogenesis of arrhythmias in infarction.

QT Dispersion and Arrhythmias in Coronary Artery Disease

Day and his colleagues first proposed that interlead variability of QT intervals in 12 leads electro-

Fig. 19.58A: An interpolated ventricular premature complex (VPC) and a nodal ectopic. The electrocardiogram (V_3) shows:
   i. Myocardial ischaemia is evident by ST depression and symmetric T wave inversion indicating subendocardial ischaemia/infarction
   ii. An interpolated VPC: The second beat with wide QRS and no visible P wave is a VPC which is sandwitched between two sinus complexes indicating it to be an interpolated beat
   iii. AV nodal premature complex (labelled as E). The 7th complex with narrow QRS and no visible P wave, followed by a compensatory pause is an AV nodal ectopic

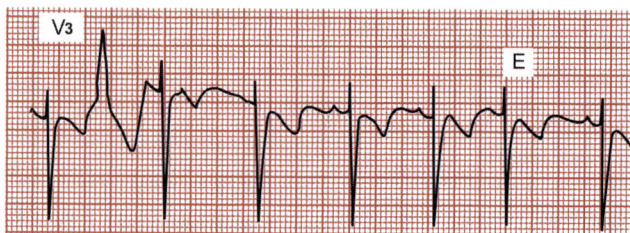

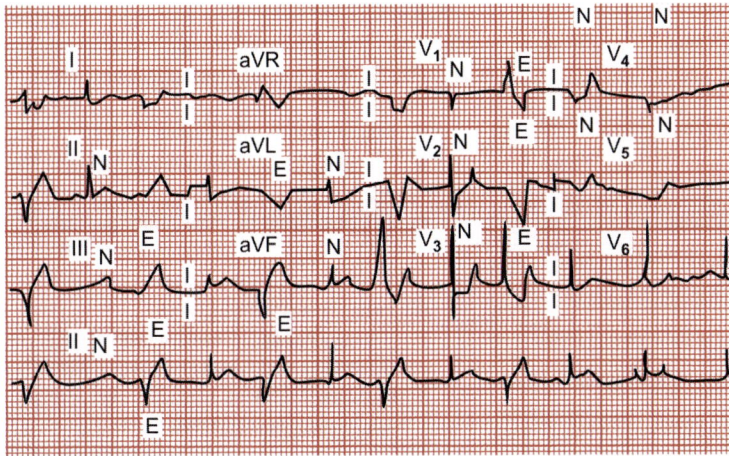

Fig. 19.58B: Ventricular bigeminy in acute inferior wall infarction with acute anterior wall ischaemia. The ECG shows;
   i. *Acute inferior wall infarction.* The ST elevation with dragged up T waves in leads II,III, aVF (best seen in III and aVF) indicates inferior wall infarction. The normal complexes showing ST elevation are labelled as 'N'.
   ii. *Additional anterior wall ischaemia.* The marked ST segment depression with horizontality and low upright T waves of normal complexes (N) in leads I, aVL and V_1-V_6 indicate additional ischaemia of anterior wall rather than just a reciprocal change due to inferior wall infarction. A reciprocal change in inferior wall infarction will not be so wide spread and does not produce so much deep ST depression and T waves are tall and upright.
   iii. *Ventricular bigeminy:* The ventricular premature complex—VPC (wide QRS with no preceding P wave-labelled as (E) alternate with normal complex (N) in most of the leads. The long lead II below highlights bigeminal pattern of VPCs
NB: The VPCs in lead V_1 have wide qR pattern indicating them to be of left ventricular origin; further strengthen an additional ischaemia of anterior wall of left ventricle

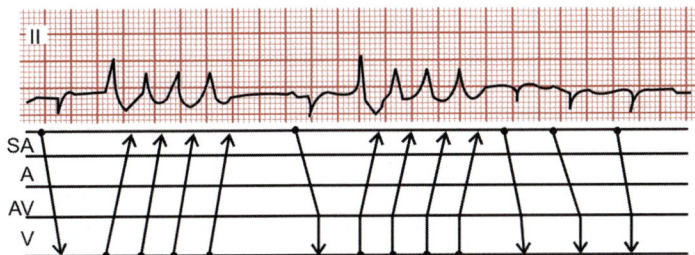

Fig. 19.58C: Repetitive short episodes (two in numbers) of a polymorphic ventricular tachycardia at a rate of 167/min repeatedly interrupt the normal sinus rhythm. These episodes are self-terminating. The long rhythm strip (lead I) was recorded from a patient with extensive old anterior wall infarction. The QS pattern in lead I with minimal ST elevation and flat to low inverted T waves suggest anterior wall infarction. There is first degree AV block (P-R interval 0.24 sec)

SECTION SEVEN

cardiogram called, *QT dispersion*, reflects dispersion of ventricular recovery time, thus, provide a convenient tool for clinical studies. The QT dispersion has been associated with susceptibility to malignant ventricular arrhythmias in long QT syndrome, hypertrophic cardiomyopathy, mitral valve prolapse, and patients operated on for tetralogy of Fallot.

In coronary artery disease, increased QT dispersion has been associated with ventricular fibrillation in acute myocardial infarction, however, its role has not been established in detecting patients who present with ventricular fibrillation not associated with acute myocardial infarction.

Nowadays, experimental and clinical studies have provided strong evidence for pathological mechanism

of dispersion of ventricular recovery time for genesis of ventricular fibrillation in acute myocardial infarction.

VENTRICULAR ANEURYSM (Figs 19.59 to 19.61 A and B)

Following an acute myocardial infarction, the elevated ST segment on the ECG ordinarily returns to the isoelectric line within several days to several weeks or months after the onset of acute episode. However, in a small number of patients, the ST segment remains elevated for many years or indefinitely and are usually associated with prominent Q waves or QS complexes. Most of these patients are found to have sustained

A

B

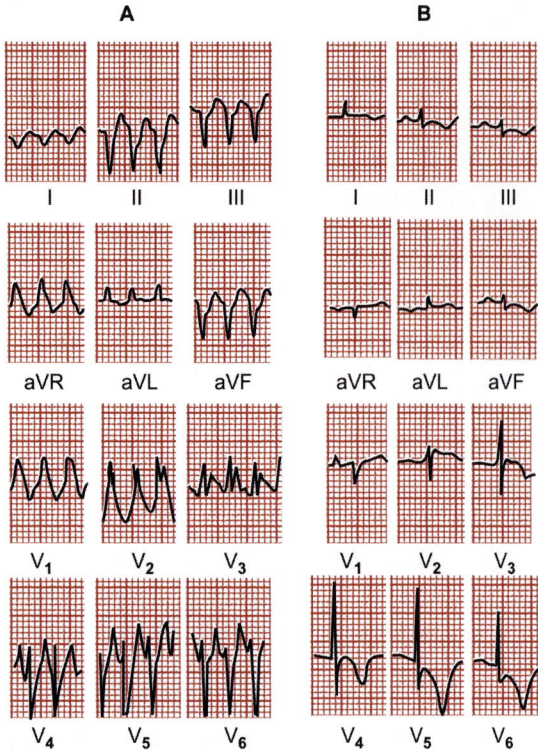

I   II   III

aVR   aVL   aVF

V_1 V_2 V_3

V_4 V_5 V_6

Fig. 18.58D: Wide QRS tachycardia with right bundle branch block pattern. The ECG was recorded from a patient with acute chest pain and palpitation

A: The ECG taken at admission shows:
   i. Superior axis of QRS with S_I, S_{II}, S_{III} syndrome
   ii. Heart rate > 200 bpm
   iii. Wide QRS complexes > 0.14 sec in majority of the leads especially V_4-V_6 with rS pattern
   iv. Right bundle branch block pattern (RR' in V_1-V_2 with wide rS in V_5-V_6)
   v. Nonconcordant pattern

All these features suggest;
1. Ventricular tachycardia with RBBB pattern
2. Supraventricular tachycardia with aberration
3. Left fascicular re-entrant tachycardia
4. Tachycardia in a patient with pre-existing right bundle branch block

B: After cardioversion, the ECG recorded shows a normal sinus rhythm with features of:
   i. Inferior wall infarction. There is coving ST segment with inversion of T waves in leads II, III and aVF. These changes suggest old inferior wall infarction.
   ii. Fresh anterior wall infarction. There is ST segment elevation in leads V_2-V_3 with dragged up T waves and there is depression of ST segment with inversion of T waves in V_5-V_6. These suggest anteroseptal infarction with subendocardial ischaemia of apical region of left ventricle.

In veiw of above features the tachycardia appears to be PSVT with aberrant conduction (right bundle branch pattern in V_1-V_6) rather than ventricular tachycardia or reciprocating tachycardia (pre-excitation syndrome). The pre-existing bundle branch block is ruled out because after reversion, bundle branch block pattern was not seen.

The rS pattern in leads V_4-V_6 virtually rules out VT unless or until pre-existing RBBB is present

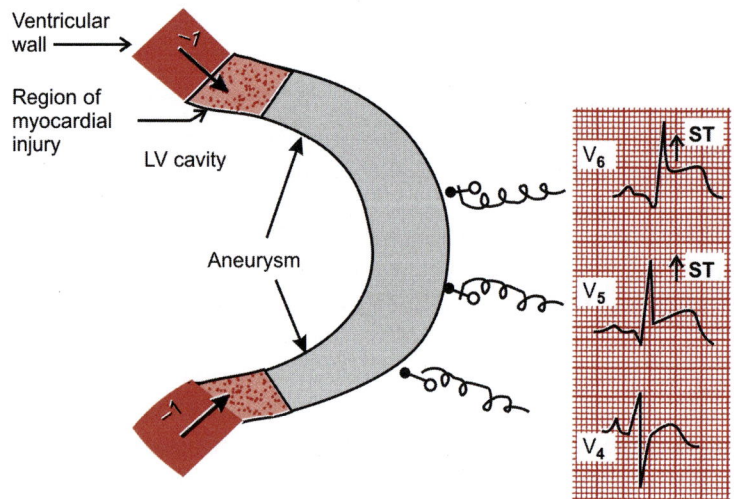

Fig. 19.59: Diagram showing mechanisms by which injury vector I is produced by ventricular aneurysm. The systolic expansion of thin, scarred fibrotic wall of the left ventricle exerts traction on the heart muscle around the periphery of an aneurysm. This, in turn, leads to appearance of the currents of injury at the end of electrical systole, can be represented by injury vectors as shown above. The vectors (I) project positive voltages on the overlying leads during early electrical diastole and so ECG registers elevated ST segment as shown in leads V_4-V_6 in left ventricular aneurysm

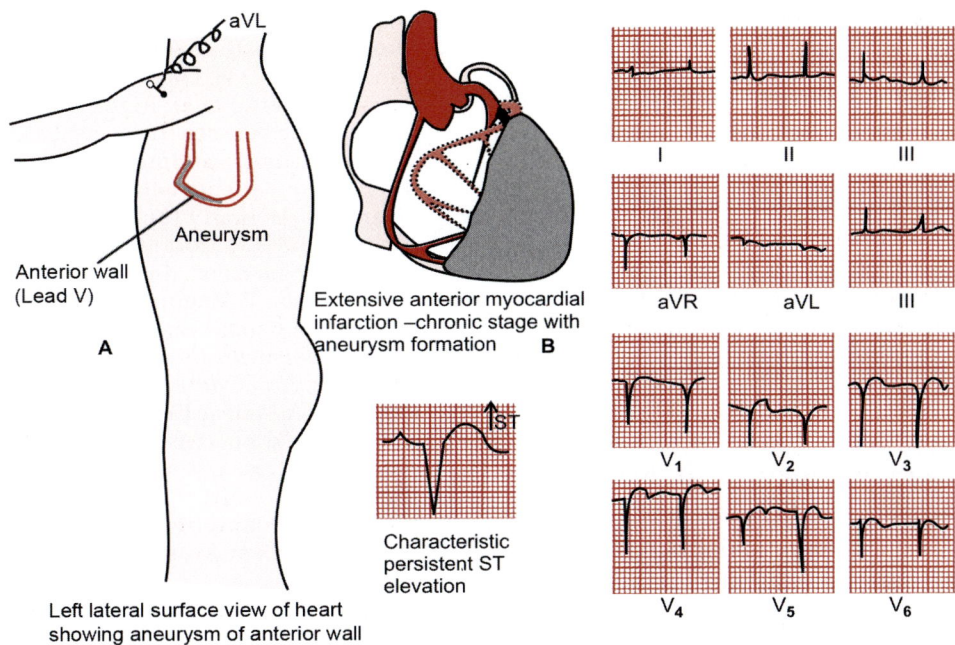

Fig. 19.60: Ventricular aneurysm. **A:** Diagrammatic illustration of aneurysm involving anterior wall. **B:** Ventricular aneurysm following acute extensive anterior myocardial infarction. The electrocardiogram recorded 6 months after the episode of acute infarction, shows persistent ST segment elevation in preordial leads (V$_1$-V$_6$). These changes could will be interpreted as acute myocardial infarction if the history of patient and duration of chest pain is not known. Other causes of persistent ST segment elevation include a weak fibrotic scar of left ventricle or metastatic tumour of left ventricle (rare)

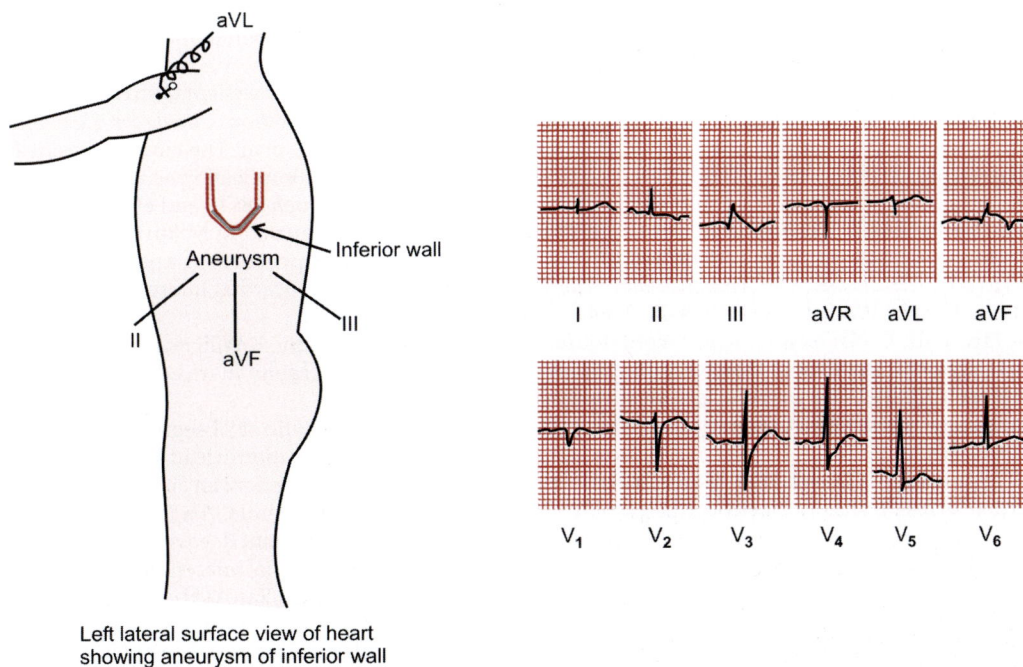

Fig. 19.61: Ventricular aneurysm. **A:** Diagrammatic illustration of aneurysm involving inferior wall. **B:** The electrocardiogram taken 1 year after infarction still shows ST segment elevation with T wave inversion in leads II, III and aVF simulating recent infarction. The aneurysm was proved on echocardiography with a thrombus

massive infarction previously. In many, but not all of these patients (approx. 50%), a ventricular aneurysm can be demonstrated. Conversely, some patients with ventricular aneurysm do not display persistent ST segment elevation. The mechanism responsible for the persistent injury vector accompanying ventricular aneurysm is not definitely established.

Ventricular aneurysm is suspected when there is persistent elevation of ST segment on ECG in a patient with an old and healed infarction, i.e. 3 months or longer.

Aneurysm is a pathologic term, however, it describes the morphological character of fibrotic or scarred muscle. Functionally aneurysmal tissue is either akinetic (loss of motion) or dyskinetic (paradoxical buldging motion during ventricular systole). The most common ECG abnormality characteristic of an aneurysm is persistent ST segment elevation in precordial leads overlying the area of aneurysm; are due to setting up of injury currents at both the ends of aneurysm during systole which project positive voltages in overlying leads, so, ECG registers ST elevation (Fig. 19.59). The electrocardiograms recorded from patients with ventricular aneursym following an old anterior and an inferior infarction are depicted in Figures 19.60 and 19.61.

Suggested Reading

1. Alpert JS, Braunward E: Pathological and clinical manifestations of acute myocardial infarction. In Braunwald E (Ed) *'Heart disease'. A textbook of Cardiovascular Medicine*, Philadelphia: WB Saunders, 1268–74, 1984.
2. Andersen HR, Falk E, Nielsen D: Right Ventricular infarction. Diagnostic accuracy of electrocardiographic right chest leads V3R to V7R investigated prospectively in 43 consecutive fatal cases from a Coronary Care Unit. *Brit Heart J* **62**: 328, 1989.
3. Ascher EK, Stauffer JE, Gaasch WH: Coronary artery spasm, cardiac arrest, transient electrocardiographic Q waves and stunned myocardium in cocaine–associated acute MI. *Am J Cardiol* **61**: 939, 1988.
4. Babbitt DG, Binkley PF, Schaal SF: Clinical significance of terminal QRS abnormalities in the setting of inferior myocardial infarction. *J Electrocardiol* **24**: 85,1991.
5. Bateman TM et al: Transient pathological Q waves during acute ischaemic events; an electrocardiographic correlate of stunned but viable myocardium. *Am Heart J* **106**: 1421, 1983.
6. Braunwald E, Kloner RA: The stunned myocardium: Prolonged postischaemic ventricular dysfunction. *Circulation* **66**: 1146, 1982.
7. Candell–Riera J et al: Right ventricular infarction. Relationship between ST segment elevation in V$_{4R}$ and haemodynamic, scintigraphic and echocardiographic findings in patients with acute inferior myocardial infarction. *Am Heart J* **101**: 281, 1981.
8. Chou T et al: Electrocardiographic diagnosis of right ventricular infarction. *Am J Med* **70**: 1175, 1981.
9. Clemmenson P, Magnus Ohman E, Sevilla DC, et al: Changes in standard electrocardiographic ST elevation predictive of successful reperfusion in an acute myocardial infarction. *Am J Cardiol* **66**:1407, 1990.
10. deLemes JA, Antman EM, Gingliano RP, et al: ST–segment resolution and infarct related artery patency and flow after thrombolytic therapy. *Am J Cardiol* **85**: 299, 2000.
11. DePasquale NP, Burch GE, Phillips JH: Electrocardiographic alterations associated with electrically silent areas of myocardium. *Am Heart J* **68**: 697,1964.
12. Edmunds JJ, Gibbons RJ, Bresnahan JF, et al: Significance of anterior ST depression in inferior wall infarction. *Am J Cardiol* **73**: 143, 1994.
13. Flowers NC, Horan LG, Wyids AC et al: Relation of peri–infarction block to ventricular late potentials in patients with inferior wall myocardial infarction. *Am J Cardiol* **66**: 658,1990.
14. Hands ME, Cook EF, Stone PH et al: Electrocardiographic diagnosis of myocardial infarction in presence of complete bundle branch block. *Am Heart J* **116**: 23, 1988.
15. Hands ME et al: Electrocardiographic diagnosis of myocardial infarction in the presence of LBBB. *Am Heart J* **116**: 23, 1988.
16. Hasset MA et al: Transient QRS changes simulating acute myocardial infarction. *Circulation* **62**: 975, 1980.
17. Hinduman MC et al: The clinical significance of bundle branch block complicating acute myocardial infarction (2 parts). *Circulation* **58**: 79 and 699, 1978.
18. Kataoka H, Kanzaki K, Mikuriva Y: Massive ST segment elevation in precordial and inferior leads in right ventricular myocardial infarction. *J Electrocardiol* **21**: 115, 1988.
19. Levine HD, Young E, William RA: Electrocardiography and vectorcardiography in myocardial infarction. *Circulation* **45**: 457, 1972.
20. Lew AS et al: Ratio of ST segment depression in lead V2 to ST segment elevation in lead aVF in evolving inferior acute myocardial infarction; an aid to early recognition of right ventricular ischaemia. *Am J Cardiol* **57**: 1047, 1986.
21. Madias JE: The Giant R waves' ECG pattern of hyperacute phase of myocardial infarction. *J Electrocardiol* **26**: 77, 1993.
22. Mak KH, Chia BL, Tan ATH et al: Simultaneous ST segment elevation in lead V$_1$ and depression in lead V$_2$. A discordant ECG pattern indicating right ventricular infarction. *J Electrocardiol* **27**: 203, 1994.
23. Oreto G, Saporito F, Donato G et al: The 'inverse' R wave progression in inferior leads in the presence of left anterior hemiblock. A Clinical Study. *J Electrocardiol* **24**: 277,1991.

24. Pelliccia F, Clantrocca C, Cristotani R et al: Electro-cardiographic findings in patients with hypertrophic cardiomyopathy. *J Electrocardiol* **23**: 213, 1990.

25. Ready GV, Schmroth L: The electrocardiology of right ventricular infarction. *Chest* **90**: 756, 1986.

26. Savage RM et al: Correlation of postmortum anatomic findings with ECG changes in patients with myocardial infarction. Retrospective study of patients with typical anterior and posterior infarcts. *Circulation* **55**: 279, 1977.

27. Scheiman MM, Abbott JA: Clinical significance of transmural versus of nontransmural ECG changes in patients with acute myocardial infarction. *Am J Med* **55**: 602, 1973.

28. Shugoll GI: Transient QRS changes simulating myocardial infarction–associated with shock and metabolic stress. *Am Heart J* **74**: 402, 1967.

29. Tamura A, Katooka H, Mikuriya: Electrocardiographic findings in a patient with pure septal infarction. *Brit Heart J* **65**: 166, 1991.

30. Toutouzas P et al: The electrocardiogram and vector-cardiogram in the diagnosis of old inferior myocardial infarction. *J Electrocardiography* **6**: 319, 1973.

31. Wackers FJ et al: Assessment of the value of electro-cardiographic signs for myocardial infarction in LBBB in: Wellens HJJ, Kulbertus HE (Eds), What's new in Electrocardiography Martinus Ni jhoff, 1981.

Congenital and Heredofamilial Disorders

SECTION EIGHT

20

Congenital Heart Disease

- *Congenital pulmonary stenosis—haemodynamic alterations and electrocardiographic features*
- *Primary pulmonary hypertension—the electrocardiogram*
- *Atrial septal defects—types, haemodynamic alterations and ECG features*
- *Atrial septal defect with pulmonary arterial hypertension—the Eisenmenger's syndrome—the electrocardiogram*
- *Common atrium—the electrocardiogram*
- *Ventricular septal defects—haemodynamic alterations, Eisenmenger's complex and ECG features*
- *Malposition of the heart—dextrocardia—the electrocardiogram*
- *Patent ductus arteriosus—haemodynamic alterations, electrocardiographic features*
- *Patent ductus arteriosus with pulmonary arterial hypertension—the Eisenmenger's syndrome—the electrocardiogram*
- *Complete transposition of great vessels—haemodynamic alterations and electrocardiographic features.*
- *Tetralogy of Fallot and its variants (Triology and Pentalogy)—haemodynamic alterations and electrocardiographic features*
- *Ebstein's anomaly—the electrocardiogram*
- *Persistent truncus arteriosus—haemodynamic alterations and electrocardiographic features*
- *Tricuspid atresia—the electrocardiogram*
- *Congenital aortic stenosis (bicuspid aortic valve)—the electrocardiogram*

SECTION EIGHT

CONGENITAL PULMONARY STENOSIS WITH INTACT SEPTUM

Obstruction to right ventricular outflow is common due to pulmonary stenosis which may occur at supra-valvular, valvular and infundibular or subvalvular levels, or may occur at combination of these sites.

Haemodynamic Alterations

With isolated pulmonary stenosis with intact inter-ventricular septum, there is pure obstruction to the flow of blood from right ventricle to pulmonary artery leading to pressure overload on the right ventricle which first hypertrophies and then enlarges. As there

is no safety valve to release this pressure, hence, it mounts to high levels depending on the severity of stenosis. The right ventricular enlargement is followed by right atrial enlargement.

The Electrocardiogram (Fig. 20.1)

A. In adults: The electrocardiographic changes occur due to:

1. Right ventricular hypertrophy/enlargement.
2. Clockwise rotation on horizontal plane due to hypertrophied right ventricle.
3. Right atrial hypertrophy/enlargement

The ECG findings in different grades of pulmonary stenosis in an adult are tabulated (Table 20.1).

Table 20.1: The electrocardiogram in different grades of pulmonary stenosis

Severity	QRS axis	ECG patterns
Mild or subin-fundibular	+ 40° to +60° (normal axis)	• **P wave:** Sharp pointed/peaked P waves < 2.5 mm in leads II and V_1. • **QRS:** Tall R waves in lead V_1 or V_2 which do not exceed the S waves in the same lead, thus, there will be RS pattern in V_1 and QRS in V_5-V_6. • **T wave:** T wave inversion is limited to right precordial leads (V_1 or V_2)
Moderate	+100° to + 120° (right axis deviation)	• **P wave:** Sharp pointed tall P waves > 2.5 mm in height in leads II and V_1. • **QRS:** Tall R waves in leads V_1-V_3 which exceeds S waves in these leads, hence, R:S is > 1. There is a clockwise rotation of the heart with shifting of transition zone to the left (patient's left, reader's right). • **T wave:** T wave inversion in V_1-V_2 that proceeds towards left precordial leads to V_4-V_5 due to shifting of transition zone as a result of clockwise rotation.
Severe	+120° to + 150° or more (marked right axis deviation)	• **P wave:** Tall, giant P waves (≥ 5 mm) may be seen in leads II and V_1. • **QRS:** R wave in lead V_1 is frequently tall > 20 mm in height and R: S ratio is more than I. The S wave is small or even may disappear in V_1 or V_2. There is RS pattern from V_2-V_6. This is due to marked clockwise rotation. A QR pattern in V_1 indicates severe stenosis. • **T wave:** T wave inversion is deep, symmetric and extends upto lead V_6, may be associated with ST depression with convexity upwards. The QRS - T angle is widened and T wave inversion appears in leads II, III and AVF due to shift to T wave axis to the left.

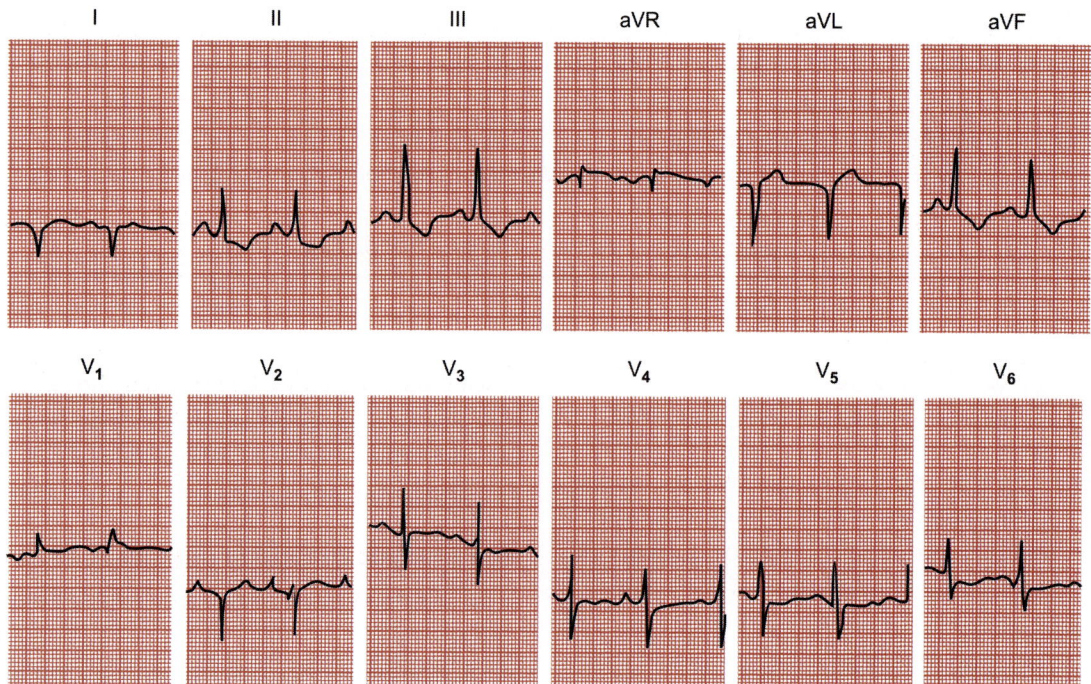

Fig. 20.1: Congenital pulmonary stenosis with intact interventricular septum. The electrocardiogram shows; (i) The frontal plane QRS axis is rightward to +110°, (ii) There is clockwise rotation of the heart, (iii) *Right ventricular hypertrophy.* A qR pattern with large R wave is seen in leads V_1-V_2 with prominent S wave in V_5 with sagging ST segment in V_5-V_6, (iv) *Right atrial hypertrophy.* The P waves are peaked and tall > 2.5 mm in leads II, III and aVF suggest associated right atrial hypertrophy, and (v) The ST segment is depressed and T wave is inverted in leads II, III, and aVF

B. *In infants and children* The children and infants generally generate more voltage in lead V_1 than the adults with similar pressure gradients. In assessing R wave height, it should be remembered that after infancy, R wave height in lead V_1 is usually 8.0 mm normally and even in younger children it never goes beyond 10.0 mm. The voltage of R wave greater than normal values suggest right ventricular hypertrophy in children.

In normal neonates, upright T waves in right precordial leads become inverted by the time the infant becomes 4 days of age. It is noteworthy that in infants and children with mild pulmonary stenosis, upright T wave in right precordial leads V_1-V_2 (a change reverse to normal) indicates right ventricular hypertrophy when associated with tall R wave in these leads (Fig. 20.2).

In neonates with pinpoint pulmonary stenosis and a small right ventricular cavity, the ECG findings are similar to pulmonary atresia with intact interventricular septum and resembles adult progression of R waves in precordial leads (V_1-V_6); and the QRS axis on frontal plane is virtually normal. Normal axis in pulmonary stenosis is exceptional. In addition to normal right axis deviation, depending on the severity of stenosis, extreme degree of right axis deviation has been observed in pulmonary valve dysplasia. Left axis deviation has been reported in infants with pulmonary artery stenosis and the rubella syndrome.

PRIMARY PULMONARY HYPERTENSION

Primary pulmonary hypertension is defined as an intrinsic, idiopathic obstructive disease of the small pulmonary arteries and arterioles and, is histologically reflected by plexiform lesions. The secondary pulmonary hypertension due to a variety of causes is far more common than primary.

Haemodynamic Alterations

The haemodynamic consequences of pulmonary hypertension (primary or secondary) are reflected by an increased resistance to blood flow through the pulmonary microvasculature. The pulmonary arterial pressure not only is elevated but also rises to levels well above the systemic pressure. As a result of this physiological consequence, the right ventricle first

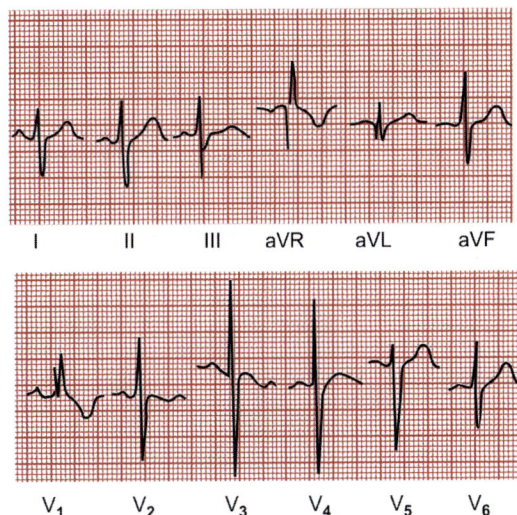

Fig. 20.2: Pulmonary stenosis with intact septum. The ECG recorded from a 10-year-old girl shows;

i. Right axis deviation. There is qR pattern in aVR
ii. *Right ventricular hypertrophy.* A wide slurred R wave (M shaped) in V_1 and tall R> 10 mm in V_2-V_3 with ST segment depression and T wave inversion indicates extreme degree of right ventricular hypertrophy with strain. There is persistence of large S wave in V_4-V_6 indicating marked clockwise rotation (transition zone lies in V_5)
iii. *Right atrial hypertrophy.* The peaked P wave in leads II, III and monophasic P with peaking in V_1-V_2 indicates associated right atrial hypertrophy

hypertrophies due to systolic or pressure overload, and then subsequently fails. There may be an associated right atrial hypertrophy in severe cases.

The Electrocardiogram

The electrocardiographic findings vary depending on the magnitude of hypertension and its related consequences. In early or mild cases, the ECG may be normal. Sinus rhythm is the rule, but late in the course, atrial arrhythmias (atrial fibrillation) may occur. The following ECG manifestations of right atrial or right ventricular hypertrophy may appear in advanced disease.

i) *Right atrial hypertrophy:* P wave is either normal or may show P pulmonale.
ii) *Right ventricular hypertrophy:* The frontal plane QRS axis is shifted to the right or may be normal. In late course of the disease, right precordial leads (V_1-V_2) exhibit tall monophasic R wave

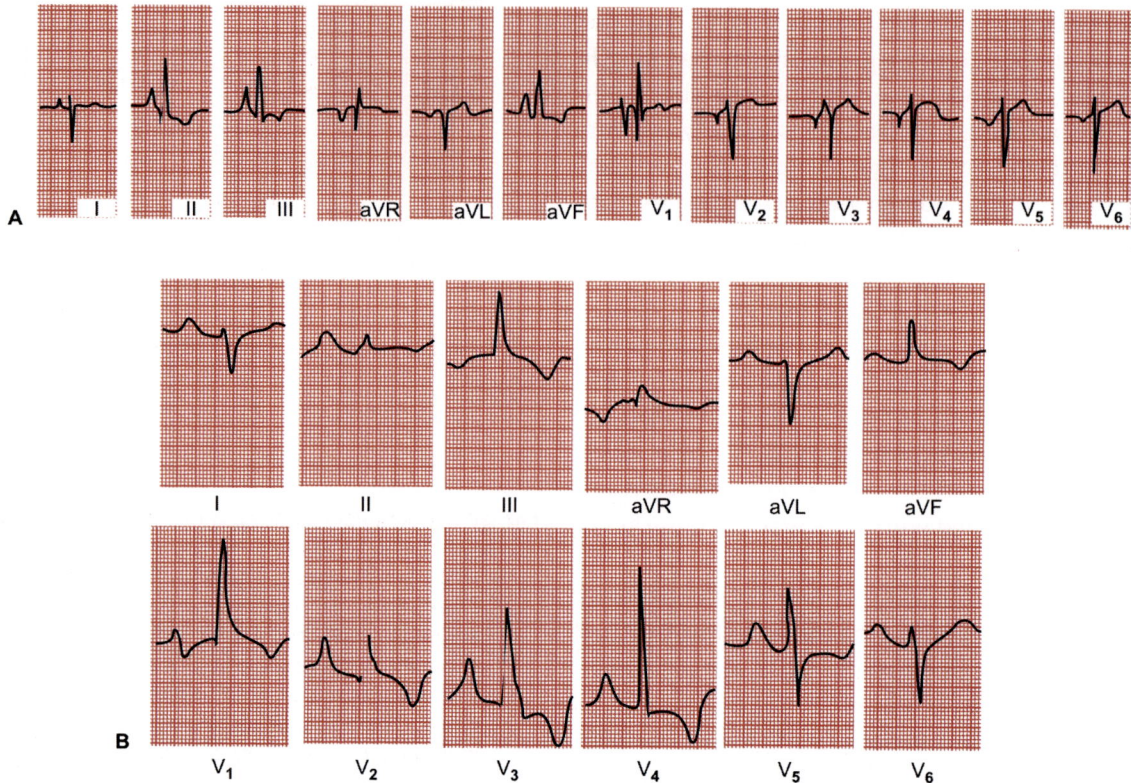

Fig. 20.3: Primary pulmonary hypertension.

A: The ECG shows (i) right axis deviation, (ii) *Biatrial atrial hypertrophy.* There are tall P waves (>2.5 mm) in leads II, III and aVF but the P wave in V_1 is biphasic and negative component is large indicating biatrial hypertrophy. (iii) *Right ventricular hypertrophy.* Tall R wave in V_1 (R > S) and rS pattern persisting through the precordial leads (upto V_6). There is clockwise rotation and transition zone lies beyound V_6

B: The electrocardiogram recorded from 30 yrs female reveals; (i) Right axis deviation of about +120°. (ii) Vertical heart position (iii) Clockwise rotation. The tall R wave extends upto V_6 with small S, therefore, the transition zone lies somewhere beyond V_6. (iv) *Right atrial hypertrophy.* Peaked but not tall P waves in leads I, II and aVF, and monophasic peaked P waves in V_1 and V_4 indicate right atrial hypertrophy in presence of RVH. (v) *Right Ventricular Hypertrophy.* Very tall R wave without S wave in V_1 – V_4 and persistence of large S wave in V_5-V_6 and associated ST segment depression with inverted T waves in right precordial leads indicate right ventricular hypertrophy.

(R>S) with ST segment depression and symmetric T wave inversion. Deep S wave will appear in left precordial leads V_5-V_6 (Fig. 20.3).

iii) The P-R and QRS durations may be normal or slightly prolonged.

ATRIAL SEPTAL DEFECT (ASD)

It is a clinically recognised acyanotic congenital heart disease in adults and is more common in females than males. Cyanosis develops when shunt gets reversed (R→L), a condition called *Eisenmenger's syndrome.*

Types of Defects

A. *SINUS VENOSUS TYPE:* The defect of this type occurs high in the septum near the entry of superior vena cava and is associated with anomalous connections of pulmonary veins from the right lung to the junction of superior vena cava and right atrium.

B. *OSTIUM SECUNDUM TYPE:* It is a midseptal defect and involves fossa ovalis. An ostium secundum defect may be associated with pulmonary stenosis, the both being present in triology of Fallot and pentalogy of Fallot.

Lutembacher's syndrome: The term is applied to a rare combination of ASD and mitral stenosis. The mitral stenosis in this combination is usually of rheumatic origin. Atrial fibrillation is more common with this combination than its occurrence in isolated ASD.

C. *Patent foramen ovale*: Anatomical obliteration of foramen ovale follows its functional closure soon after birth. Failure of closure results in probe patency of foramen which is a normal variant. Thus, there is no haemodynamic shunt or electrocardiographic abnormalities.

D. *Ostium primum type*: It occurs commonly in patients with Down's syndrome where other more common endocardial cushion defects are characteristically seen. The defect occurs due to developmental arrest at the time of fusion of septum primum with endocardial cushion. Therefore, as a result of this, there is not only an interatrial communication but there may be other abnormalities that are associated with primitive common atrioventricular canal development.

The various anomalies may be:
1. Cleft anterior leaflet of mitral valve. This leads to mitral regurgitation.
2. Cleft septal leaflet of tricuspid valve. This leads to tricuspid regurgitation.
3. Maldevelopment of anterior superior division of left bundle branch. This leads to left hemiblock. This is the cause of left axis deviation—a characteristic of septum primum defect.
4. There may be high membranous VSD.
5. Persistent atrioventricular canal (an ostium primum defect associated with VSD). This leads to shunting of blood from (a) left atrium to right atrium, (b) left ventricle to right atrium, (c) right ventricle to left atrium and (d) left ventricle to right ventricle.

The term endocardial cushion defect is used when ostium primum defect is associated with any of the above mentioned anomalies.

Haemodynamic Alterations

Ostium Secundum Type of ASD

The left atrial pressure usually is higher by 3-5 mm Hg than right atrium, hence, shunts the blood to right atrium (L →R). This results in;
  a. Overloading of right atrium.
  b. Overloading of right ventricle.
  c. Pulmonary plethora due to increased blood flow to the lungs.

Thus, the haemodynamic events are just limited to right side of the heart. Due to these haemodynamic alterations, there will be dilatation and hypertrophy of right atrium, dilatation of right ventricle (volume overload) and hypertrophy of crista supraventricularis (e.g. a crescent shaped muscular ridge over outflow tract of right ventricle). The greater the degree of volume overload of right ventricle, the greater is the hypertrophy of *crista supraventricularis*. The volume overload of right ventricle is followed by hypertrophy of its free walls.

Ostium Primum Type of ASD

This permits a left to right (L→R) shunt at atrial level. The other haemodynamic alterations depend on the associated anomalies (e.g. cleft mitral valve produces mitral regurgitation and left ventricular overload, the cleft septal leaf of tricuspid valve produces tricuspid regurgitation and, there may be an associated VSD).

The Electrocardiogram

The Ostium Secundum Defect
(Figs 20.4 and 20.5)

A. *The P wave abnormalities* The P wave are frequently normal or may reflect biatrial enlargement. The P waves are peaked and widened in leads II and aVF as mean frontal plane P wave axis lies in the region of +40° to +60°. If P waves are widened but not peaked, indicates left atrial enlargement commonly seen in patients with a small ASD. In biatrial enlargement, P waves increase in amplitude as well as in width, a common finding in large ASD. In lead V_1, biatrial enlargement is reflected in an increase in positive and negative components of biphasic P wave and both the components are sharp and peaked.

B. *The QRS abnormalities*
  (i) *Axis:* Frontal plane QRS axis is directed rightwards and inferiorly, the most common being in the region of +90° to + 120°.
  (ii) *Duration:* The QRS duration is usually normal, but may be slightly prolonged upto 0.11 sec and does not exceed 0.12 sec in any circumstance. This is due to right ventricular dilatation. Complete bundle branch block pattern (QRS > 0.12 sec) is rare.

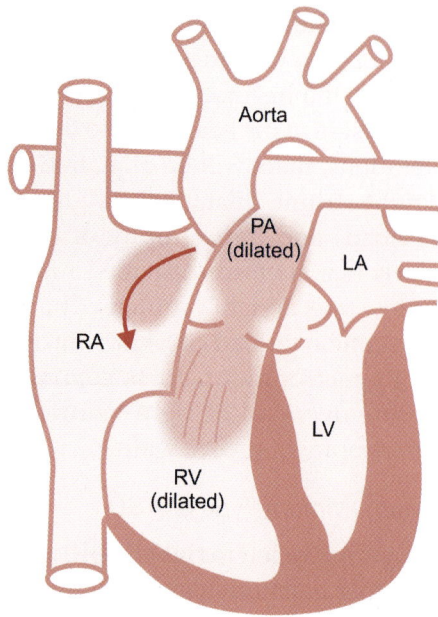

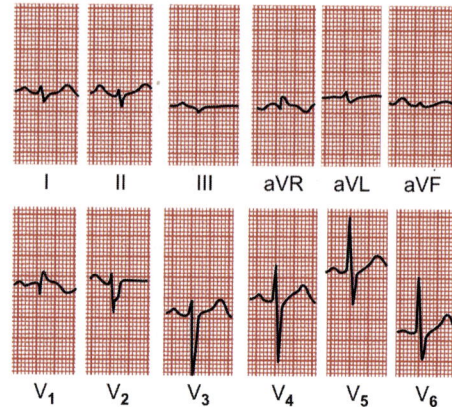

Fig. 20.4: Atrial septal defect (ostium secundum). The electrocardiogram recorded from a 30 yrs female shows;
  i. P wave axis is around +60°. The P wave is tall, wide and peaked in leads II and aVF and biphasic in V_1 with wide initial upright deflection. Indicating biatrial hypertrophy.
  ii. There is rSR' pattern in V_1 which is not wide, indicates incomplete right bundle branch block.

(iii) *QRS pattern:* In lead V_1 or right precordial leads, the QRS pattern is triphasic, commonly rSr' but may be rSR' or rsR' (Figs 20.4 to 20.6) which resembles the pattern of incomplete right bundle branch block (QRS < 0.12 sec). In this rSr' pattern, the secondary r' wave is due to depolarisation of outflow tract of right ventricle which becomes disproportionately thick and is last to be depolarised. The rSr' pattern in lead V_1 changes sequentially to an rsR' or an rR and ultimately to a tall monophasic R wave which, sometimes, is preceded by a q wave, indicates development of pulmonary arterial hypertension (Read Eisenmenger's syndrome).

In lead V_5 or left precordial leads, the R wave amplitude is diminished with slurred widened S wave. The q wave in these leads become prominent due to left ventricular diastolic overload. Therefore, pattern commonly evolved is qRs in left precordial leads.

C. *Clockwise rotation on horizontal plane* The clockwise rotation shifts the transition zone slightly leftwards to V_5-V_6. Therefore, there will be R wave in aVR, and rSR' pattern in lead V_1 may persist upto V_3-V_4.

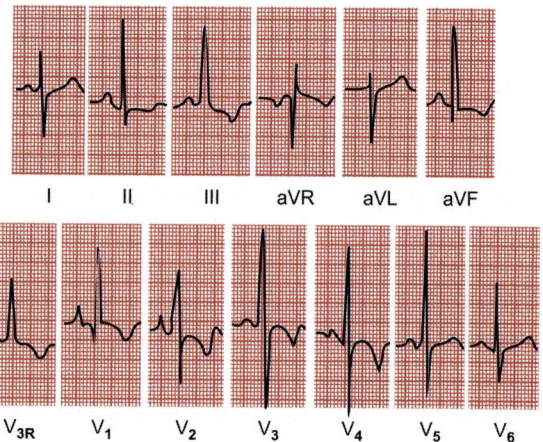

Fig. 20.5: Atrial septal defect (ostium secundum) in a 6-yr-old child. The electrocardiogram shows:
  i. Tall peaked P waves in leads II, III and aVF indicate inferior, and tall P wave>2.5 mm in lead V_1-V_3 indicate anterior orientation of P wave axis due to right atrial hypertrophy
  ii. Incomplete right bundle branch block. These is rSR' pattern in lead V_1 (R' is tall due to his age) with qRS pattern in leads II, III and aVF. The QRS duration is 0.10 sec

D. *The T wave abnormality* The T wave usually remains upright prior to development of pulmonary hypertension, when it develops, then the T waves are deeply inverted in right and midprecordial leads.

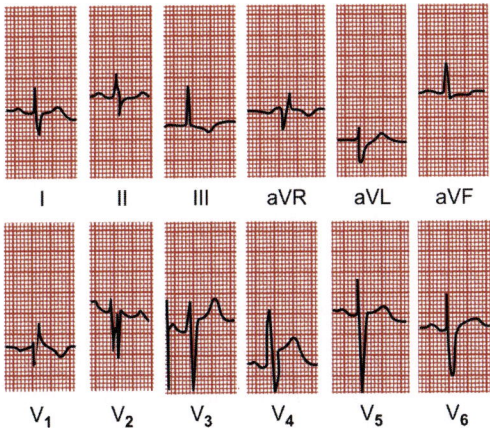

Fig. 20.6: Incomplete right bundle branch block pattern in ASD. The ECG shows:
  i. The P wave is slightly wider in leads I, II and aVF and negative component of biphasic P wave is accentuated suggesting left atrial enlargement.
  ii. Incomplete RBBB pattern. There is rSR' pattern in lead V_1 which does not exceed 0.12 sec in duration. There is associated deep wide slurred S wave in V_5-V_6. The T wave is inverted in V_1.
All these features suggest mild ASD with ostium secundum defect which was confirmed on Doppler study

E. *Rhythm and conduction disturbance* A large ASD may commonly be associated with atrial fibrillation, and less commonly with flutter or supraventricular tachycardia. The ASD is a common congenital anomaly associated with atrial fibrillation. Prolongation of P-R interval may be observed in all types of ASD specifically in ostium primum defect; is due to the prolonged internodal conduction time as a result of both increased size of the right atrium and increased distance between SA and AV node produced by the defect.

ECG clues to ASD in lead V_1
- The rSr' pattern is common in a small ASD
- The rsR' or rSR' pattern is common in a large ASD
- The change of rSr' or rSR' to monophasic R, or qR complex/pattern indicates development of pulmonary arterial hypertension—the Eisenmenger's syndrome.
Note: The Katz-Wachtel phenomenon—large equiphasic QRS complexes in the mid-precordial leads is rare in ASD.

Ostium Primum Defect (Fig. 20.7)

A. *The P wave abnormalities* The P wave changes are similar to ostium secundum defect due to left to right shunt and similar haemodynamic alterations. The P-R interval prolongation occurs approximately in 50% patients with endocardial cushion defect.

B. *The QRS abnormalities*
  (i) *Axis* There is 'left axis deviation' of QRS on frontal plane. Therefore, if there are other characteristics of ASD (secundum defect) present, then combination of left axis deviation points to the defect of primum type or common atrioventricular canal. The left axis is in region of 0° counterclockwise to –90°. The left axis deviation is due to congenital alterations in the excitation pathways resulting in delayed activation of anterosuperior portion through left anterior fascicle due to its large length in endocardial cushion defect.
  (ii) *Duration:* QRS duration remains either normal or < 0.11 second.

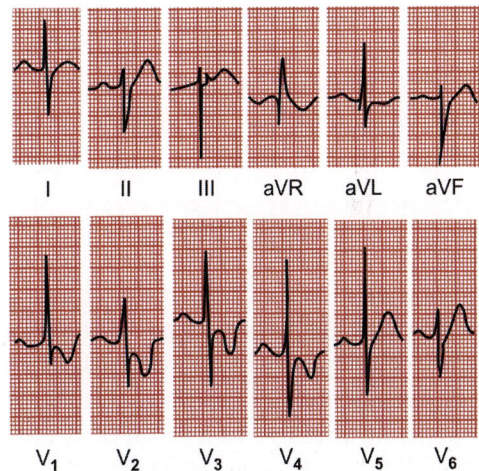

Fig. 20.7: Endocardial cushion defect (ostium primum defect with mitral regurgitation). The ECG recorded from 5-year-old male child shows;
  i. Prolonged P-R interval 0.22 sec.
  ii. Left axis deviation (rS pattern in leads II, III and aVF) with counterclockwise rotation
  iii. Right ventricular hypertrophy. There is tall R wave disproportionate to his age in leads V_1-V_2 with deep S wave in V_5-V_6
  iv. Left ventricular leads shows good voltage of R wave in V_5 indicating left ventricular overload

SECTION EIGHT

(iii) *QRS pattern:*
- Right precordial leads (V_1-V_2): It is same rSr' or rSR' pattern as seen in secundum defect.
- Left precordial leads (V_5-V_6): When ostium primum defect is complicated by mitral incompetence (cleft mitral valve), then left precordial leads V_5-V_6 will show tall or relatively tall R wave with QRS pattern. The q wave is prominent in these leads due to left ventricular overload.

C. *The T wave abnormalities* The T waves are also tall and symmetrically upright with concave upwards ST segment.

Common Atrioventricular Canal (Fig. 20.8)

The ECG changes in common atrioventricular canal are similar to ostium primum defect but left axis deviation is more marked. Frontal plane QRS axis occurs in left superior quadrant. The electrocardiogram may manifest with rsR' complex in V_1 as well as features of biventricular hypertrophy as a result of left ventricular volume overload.

Sinus Venosus Defect

The ECG abnormality include left axis deviation of P wave (Fig. 20.9). The P waves are inverted in III and aVF due to ectopic pacemaker. Rest the ECG findings are of ostium secundum defect type.

ATRIAL SEPTAL DEFECT WITH REVERSED SHUNT–THE EISENMENGER'S SYNDROME

The pulmonary arterial hypertension is a complication of atrial septal defect and is more common with ostium primum defect and a large ostium secundum defect. With development of pulmonary hypertension, there is an increase in right atrial pressure due to rising right ventricular pressure as a result of systolic overload. When right ventricular and right atrial pressures are very high, then there may be reversal of shunt, a condition called *Eisenmenger's syndrome.* Cyanosis appears in this condition due to right to left (R→L) shunt.

The Electrocardiogram

Ostium Secundum Defect with Pulmonary Hypertension (Fig. 20.10)

(i) There is a marked right axis deviation of QRS (+120° or more)

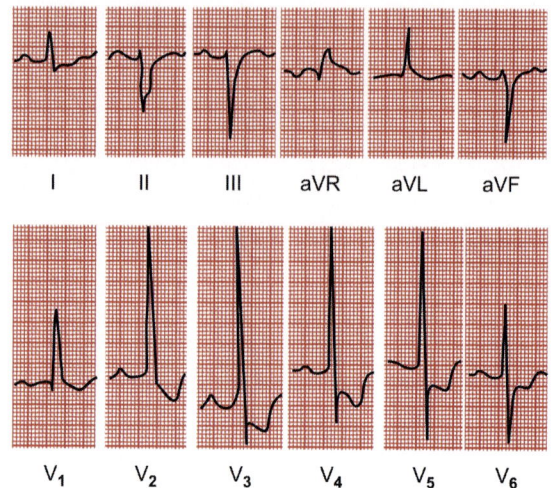

Fig. 20.8: Common atrioventricular canal with complete atrioventricular valve. The electrocardiogram of young adult male shows:
 i. *P-R interval* is 0.20 sec
 ii. *Left axis deviation* of QRS on frontal plane. The S wave in leads II, III and aVF is slurred and notched
 iii. *Right atrial hypertrophy.* There are peaked P waves in right precordial leads V_1-V_3
 iv. *Right ventricular hypertrophy.* The tall monophasic R in lead V_2 with qR pattern in lead V_1 and deep wide S wave in V_5-V_6 indicate right ventricular hypertrophy. There is also slurred R in aVR (qR Complex)
 v. *Evidence of biventricular hypertrophy:* The RVH with left axis deviation suggests biventricular hypertrophy. In addition, good voltage of R in V_5 (>27 mm) suggest associated LVH.

(ii) The P wave amplitude increases and P wave axis is shifted rightwards from +40° or + 60° to +80° or + 90°. The P waves are now tall in leads II, III and aVF.

(iii) There is a tall R wave in lead V_1 with diminution of S wave. Later on, S wave may eventually disappear producing only tall R wave.

(iv) There is diminution of R wave in leads V_5-V_6 with concomitant increase in S wave in these leads. The R: S ratio remains frequently less than I in these leads. An initial q wave in V_5-V_6 may also disappear.

Ostium Primum Defect with Pulmonary Hypertension

The ostium primum defect with pulmonary hypertension is frequently associated with biventricular hypertrophy due to left and right ventricular diastolic overload. The ECG changes include:

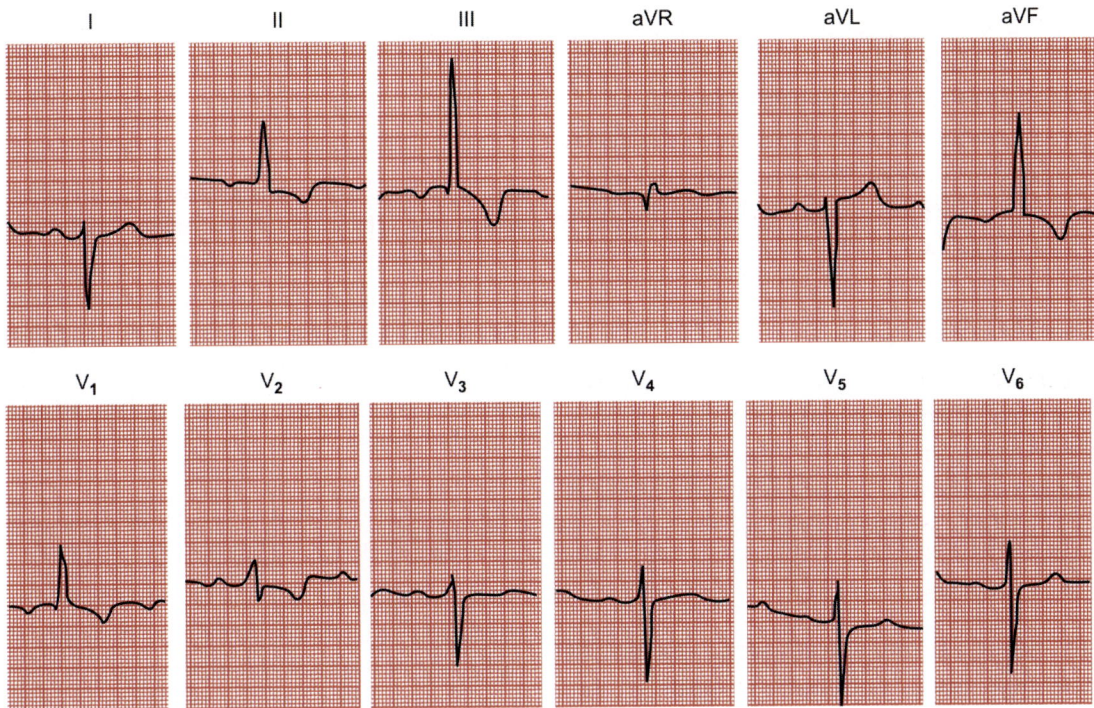

Fig. 20.9: Atrial septal defect (sinus venosus type) with pulmonary hypertension. The electrocardiogram shows:
   i. Superior and posterior axis of P waves (P is inverted in leads II, III, aVF and V_1)
  ii. Right axis deviation of QRS
 iii. P-R interval is prolonged (0.24 sec)
  iv. Right ventricular hypertrophy (R wave in V_1 is greater than S wave and there is persistence of S wave in V_5-V_6 with clockwise rotation)

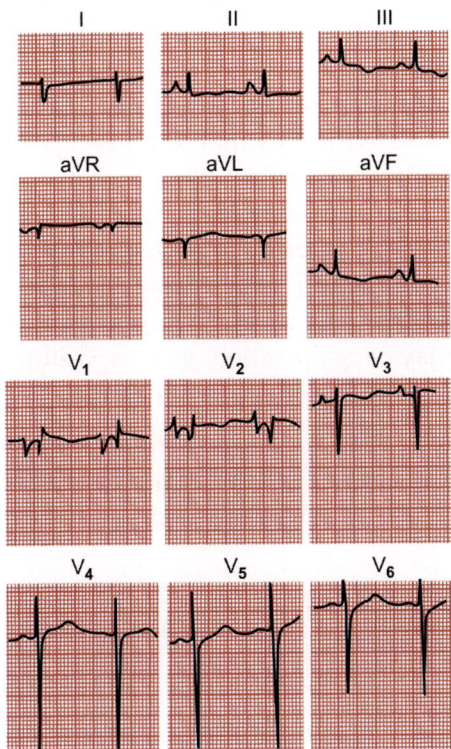

Fig. 20.10: Atrial septal defect (ostium secundum) with pulmonary hypertension. The electrocardiogram recorded from a 19 yrs female shows;
   i. Right axis of P wave is + 70°
  ii. Right axis deviation of QRS (+ 105°) on frontal plane
 iii. Marked clockwise rotation on horizontal plane producing rS pattern upto V_6 indicating transition zone is shifted beyond V_6
  iv. *Biatrial hypertrophy.* The P waves are tall, wide and peaked in leads II, III and aVF. In lead V_2, P wave is biphasic, the initial upwards component is tall and peaked, the terminal negative component is deep and wide. In lead V_1, the terminal negative deflection of biphasic P is deep and wide. The P is upright and peaked in lead V_3.
   v. *Right ventricular overload hypertrophy.* There is qR pattern in lead V_1 and V_2 with upward convex ST segment and inversion of T waves. A small initial q wave is seen in V_3 and T is inverted. There is diminution of R wave amplitude in leads V_5-V_6 and R:S is less than 1, i.e. rS pattern is seen from V_4-V_6.

All these features suggest gross right ventricular hypertrophy. A qR pattern in right precordial leads suggest increased right ventricular and right atrial pressure due to pulmonary hypertension

(i) A tall R wave will appear both in right precordial leads (V_1-V_2) and left precordial leads (V_5-V_6). Transition zone remains in lead V_3 or V_4.

(ii) T wave inversion occurs in right precordial leads due to right ventricular pressure overload while they remain upright in V_5 -V_6 due to diastolic left ventricular overload.

COMMON ATRIUM

It is a rare variety of interatrial septal disorder characterised by virtual absence of atrial septum, i.e. only vestigial remnants are present. Absence of atrial septum implies deficiency of septum at both the sinus venosus and ostium primum locations.

The Electrocardiogram

1. Due to sinus venosus atrial septal defect of superior vena caval type, there is tendency for leftward deviation of P wave axis.
2. Due to defect in septum primum location, there is left axis deviation of QRS complexes with counter-clockwise rotation.
3. Right ventricular volume overload: The precordial leads show features of right ventricular volume overload, i.e. tall R waves in V_1-V_2; the amplitude of the R wave is greater than in the ostium secundum atrial septal defect.

VENTRICULAR SEPTAL DEFECT (VSD)

This is a acyanotic heart disease with left to right shunt (L→R) at ventricular level; cyanosis appears when shunt gets reversed, i.e. right to left (R→L), a condition called Eisenmenger's complex which is similar to Eisenmenger's syndrome that occurs due to reversal of shunt in other conditions. In VSD, the defect may be in the membranous or muscular or both parts of the interventricular septum. Rarely, the complete interventricular septum may be absent, thereby constituting the congenital anomaly of a single ventricle. The clinical presentations of VSD are variable from asymptomatic disease without haemodynamic alterations (*maladie de Roger*) to symptomatic disease with moderate to large shunts producing pulmonary plethora and haemodynamic disturbances.

The Haemodynamic Alterations and the Electrocardiogram

The electrocardiographic manifestations depend on the haemodynamic alterations which, in turn, depend on the magnitude of the shunt and peripheral vascular resistance. They are given in the Table 20.2. When a small defect in the membranous septum takes the form of a congenital septal aneurysm, then there is an increased incidence of rhythm and conduction disturbances especially atrial fibrillation, paroxysmal atrial tachycardia, junctional rhythm, atrial flutter and complete heart block.

MALPOSITION AND MALFORMATION OF THE HEART

Anomalous position of the heart refers to those conditions in which cardiac apex is situated in the right side of the chest (dextrocardia), or in the midline (mesocardia). Sometimes, the heart is situated in the normal position on the left side but there is situs inversus-an abnormal position of the viscera (*isolated levocardia*). Mirror image dextrocardia is usually observed in patients with *situs inversus*; a condition which is commonly observed in patients whose hearts are otherwise normal except dextroposition. Associated cardiac anomalies are the rule in isolated dextrocardia without situs inversus. When heart occupies normal position but there is situs inversus only (isolated levocardia), the heart is usually seriously malformed. When situs inversus is indeterminate, there is an associated asplenia, or polysplenia with multiple cardiac anomalies; such as septal defects and, systemic and peripheral venous abnormalities. When asplenia is present with malposition of heart, there may be malposition or transposition of great vessels and double outlet right ventricle.

The Katz-Wachtel phenomenon (equiphasic large QRS defections in V_3–V_4) is seen in moderately large VSD with high pulmonary vascular resistance

DEXTROCARDIA (TRUE OR MIRROR IMAGE VERSUS TECHNICAL)

True Dextrocardia

It is a congenital abnormality in which there is complete transposition of both ventricles and atria. The

Table 20.2: Magnitude of defect and shunt, haemodynamic alterations and electrocardiographic findings

Defect	Magnitude of shunt	Haemodynamic alterations	Electrocardiographic findings Figs 20.11 to 20.14
i. An isolated small membranous defect	A) A small left to right shunt with normal pulmonary vascular resistance (maladie de Roger)	As there is a small left to right shunt, (Fig. 20.11) there is no haemodynamic alterations. There is little or no hypertrophy or enlargement of cardiac chambers	The electrocardiogram is normal
	B) Moderate left to right shunt with slight rise in pulmonary vascular resistance	i) Due to moderate left to right shunt, there is left ventricular diastolic overload and left atrial enlargement	(i) P waves may be normal or widened in leads II and I. There will be widening of terminal negative part of biphasic P wave in V_1. (ii) Prominent, deep but narrow Q waves of qR complexes in V_5-V_6. These prominent Q waves can be seen in leads II, III and aVF. (iii) Tall R waves in V_5-V_6. (iv) Slight elevated ST segment with concavity upwards. (v) T waves are upright and increased in amplitude
		(ii) If shunt is moderately large, then in addition to diastolic overloading of left ventricle, there will be right ventricular systolic overload	(i) In addition to above features, there will be features of right ventricular systolic overload, i.e. tall R wave in V_1 with an initial slur or notch or there may be qR complex with tall R wave indicating high right ventricular pressure (ii) T waves may be upright or inverted
	C. Large left to right shunt with high pulmonary vascular resistance	Large left to right shunt with high pulmonary vascular resistance leads to combined biventricular and biatrial enlargement	(i) Biatrial enlargement—Tall as well as widened P waves in leads II, III and aVF (ii) Right axis deviation beyond +120° (iii) Biventricular hypertrophy/enlargement. There is large amplitude of equiphasic QRS (RS pattern) in midprecordial leads V_3-V_4 called - The *Katz-Wachtel phenomenon*. In addition, there are large R waves in V_4 and qR (both waves prominent) in V_5-V_6 indicating biventricular hypertrophy/enlargement. (Fig. 20.12.) (iv) T wave may be inverted in lead V_1 **Note:** Infants may occasionally show right axis deviation with pure right ventricular hypertrophy. Even, then large equiphasic complexes are generally seen in one or more leads.

Contd..

SECTION EIGHT

Contd..

Defect	Magnitude of shunt	Haemodynamic alterations	Electrocardiographic findings (Figs 20.11 to 20.14)
	D. Reversal of shunt (R→L) due to high pulmonary vascular resistance; a condition called *Eisenmenger's complex*	Biventricular and biatrial hypertrophy. Right ventricular pressure is higher than the left ventricle.	(i) Signs of biventricular hypertrophy as discussed above (ii) Tall R waves or qR pattern with tall R in V_1 indicates right ventricular dominance (Fig. 20.13) (iii) Extreme right axis deviation. (iv) Marked clockwise rotation with shifting of transition zone to V_5 (v) Symmetrical inversion of T waves in V_1-V_3.
2. *Membranous defect with prolapse of aortic valve*	Due to prolapse of aortic valve in membranous part of defect, aortic regurgitation results	There is dual (systolic and diastolic) overloading of left ventricle. Due to superimposition of aortic regurgitation, there will left ventricular hypertrophy out of proportion than that produced by isolated VSD. Even features of VSD may be masked by aortic regurgitation.	(i) There will be tall R waves in V_5-V_6 with deep S wave in V_1-V_2. Voltage criteria of LVH, i.e. $RV_5 + SV_1 > 35$ mm may be present (Fig. 20.14). (ii) P-R interval is usually prolonged (iii) Counterclockwise rotation leads to shift of transition zone towards right, i.e. V_1.

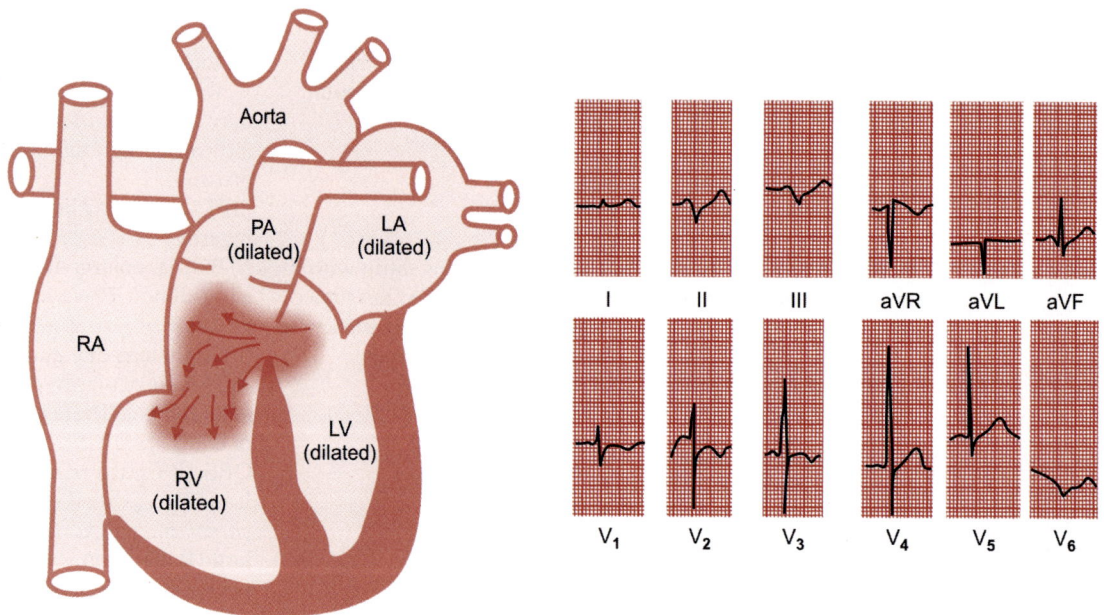

Fig. 20.11: Ventricular septal defect (maladie de Roger) in a child. The electrocardiogram is normal according to his age. Tall R wave in V_1-V_2 with large equiphasic complex in V_3-V_4 are normal to his age. The T wave inversion from V_1-V_3 shows juvenile pattern

aortic knob and the apex of the left ventricle are seen on the right side on chest X-ray. Electrically, there is reversal of polarity of limb lead I axis. The SA node present in the right atrium occupies the left upper part of the heart, hence, P wave vector is oriented to right and inferiorly instead of normal left, resulting in inverted P (P') waves in lead I and upright P waves in aVF. The mean QRS vector is directed to the right, inferiorly and posteriorly. The ECG in dextrocardia gets altered in following fashion, i.e. lead I is reversed, leads II and III exchange their positions, leads aVR and aVL also exchange their positions and only lead

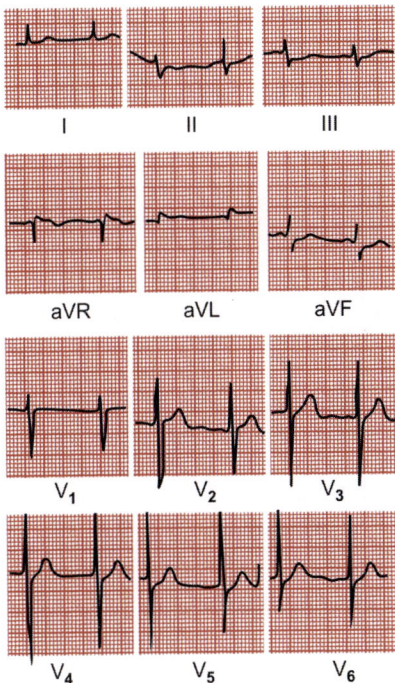

Fig. 20.12: Ventricular septal defect (moderate shunt) in a 18 yrs girl. The electrocardiogram shows biventricular volume overload—The Katz-Wachtel phenomenon. The large amplitude equiphasic QRS deflections in mid-precordial leads (V_2-V_4) indicate right as well as left ventricular volume overload due to balance of electrical forces from both the ventricles. The P waves are normal. QRS axis is normal.

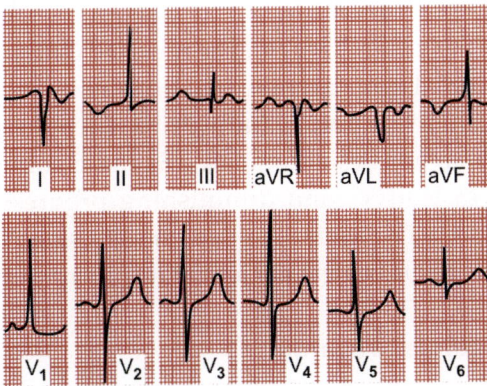

Fig. 20.13: Ventricular septal defect with right to left shunt (*Eisenmenger's complex*). The ECG recorded shows:
  i. Normal P waves
  ii. Right axis deviation of QRS
  iii. *Right ventricular hypertrophy*: There is a tall monophasic R wave in lead V_1 with persistence of S wave in V_5-V_6
  iv. The Q waves in left precordial leads are absent
  v. There is still good voltage of R wave in V_5-V_6.
  All these features suggest right ventricular pressure overload. The features of left ventricle volume overload have disappeared probably due to reversal of shunt at an early age

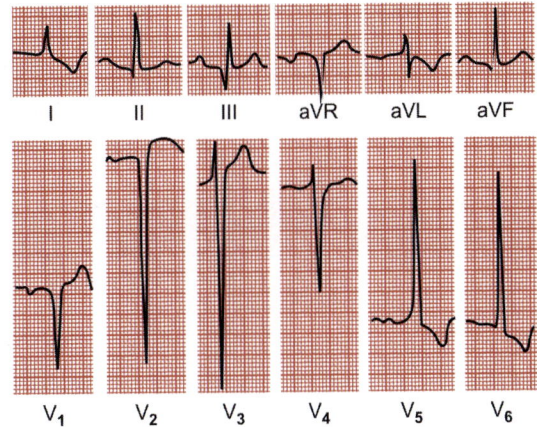

Fig. 20.14: Ventricular septal defect with aortic regurgitation. The electrocardiogram recorded from a 19 yr adult male shows features of aortic regurgitation rather than VSD in the form of:
  i. Left ventricular hypertrophy: There are tall R waves (>27 mm) in leads V_5-V_6 and RV_5+SV_1 is > 35 mm. There is concomitant QS pattern in leads V_1-V_2
  ii. P-R interval is prolonged (0.22 sec)
  iii. Clockwise rotation with shifting of transition zone towards left between V_4-V_5. Heart position is vertical.
All these ECG features are suggestive of aortic regurgitation, though VSD was present in this patient which did not express electrocardiographically as right ventricular volume overload due to dominant aortic regurgitation, but clockwise rotation vertical heart and rS pattern in V_3-V_4 suggest that there is right ventricular dominance which is counterbalancing the forces of LVH but is not expressed by direct voltage criteria in V_1-V_2.

aVF remains constant and normal. All precordial leads (V_1-V_6) record right ventricular epicardial complex (rS pattern), hence, ECG has to be recorded on right 4th intercostal space to get left ventricular epicardial complex (Fig. 20.15A). The polarity of different leads in true dextrocardia with respect to normal are depicted in the box.

Electrode	Leads	
	Normal	*True dextrocardia*
RA→LA	I	– 1 (Reversed, hence, P, QRS and T are inverted in this lead)
RA →LL	II	III Note: The leads II and III have exchanged
LA →LL	III	II their positions with respect to normal
	aVL	aVL these are also reversed in
	aVR	aVR their polarity with respect to normal
	aVF	aVF this is only lead which is constant

SECTION EIGHT

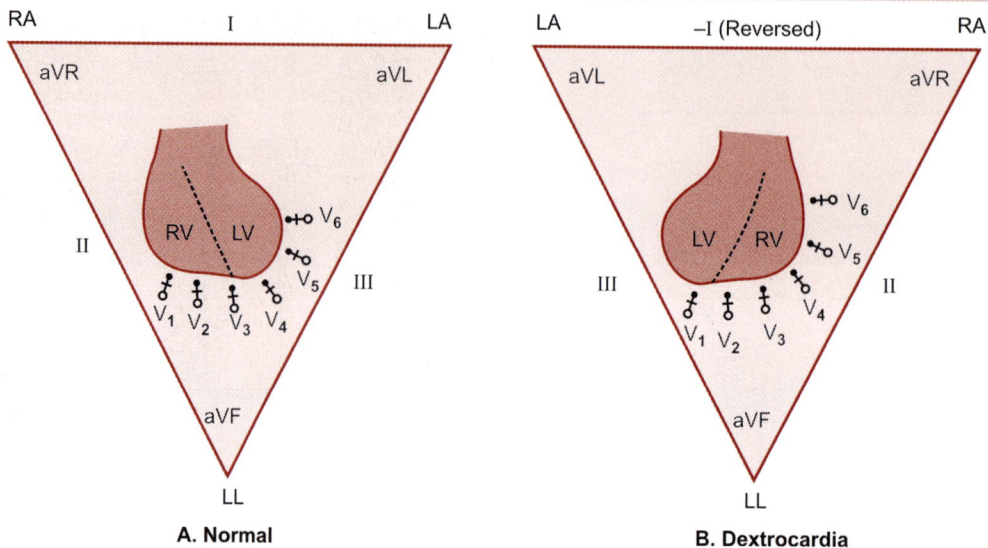

Fig. 20.15: Polarity of different leads. **A:** normal, **B:** True dextrocardia

Precordial (V$_1$-V$_6$)	Right ventricular epicardial complex (rS) in leads V$_1$ and V$_2$. Left ventricular epicardial complex qRS in leads V$_5$–V$_6$	All the precordial leads taken on left side (V$_1$-V$_6$) record right ventricular epicardial and back of the heart (rS) complexes Special leads V$_{3R-6R}$ which are similar to V$_3$-V$_6$ and occupy similar position on right side of the chest will now record left ventricular epicardial (qR) complex. If the ECG is recorded on the right side in a fashion similar to normal, then lead V$_1$ becomes lead V$_2$ and *vice versa*; the leads V$_3$-V$_6$ become V$_{3R}$, V$_{4R}$, V$_{5R}$ and V$_{6R}$ which will now record left ventricular epicardial qR complex.

The Electrocardiogram (Fig. 20.16B)

Because of reversed polarity of different leads, the ECG complexes will have different configurations. For recording the left ventricular complexes, repeat the ECG on right side in a fashion similar to left side (Fig. 20.16 A). The leads V$_{3R-6R}$ will record qR complex and confirm the position of left ventricle on the right side of the chest (Fig. 20.16 B).

I. Standard leads In mirror image dextrocardia, the P wave, QRS and T wave axes are directed to the right and inferiorly, hence, P waves will be inverted in lead I, upright in inferior oriented leads (II, III and aVF) and upright or equiphasic in aVR. Likewise, the QRS complexes will also be dominantly upright in leads II, III, aVF and aVR and, dominantly negative in leads I and aVL.

II. Precordial leads There will be reversed QRS pattern in precordial leads as compared to normal (Fig. 20.16 B versus C). The lead V$_1$ through V$_6$ will reflect right ventricular epicardial complex (rS); the rS complexes tallest in lead V$_1$ and diminishing progressively towards V$_6$. The leads recorded on right side (V$_{3R-6R}$) will reflect left ventricular epicardial complex.

Technical Dextrocardia

This occurs due to inadvertent interchange of right and left arm electrodes. This will produce dextrocardia in limb leads (standard and unipolar) but the precordial leads (V$_1$-V$_6$) remain normal. Therefore, the ECG pattern in unipolar and standard limb leads is similar to that seen in true dextrocardia. The only difference on ECG between technical dextrocardia and true dextrocardia is that the precordial leads remain normal in former but are reversed in the latter. The

B

C

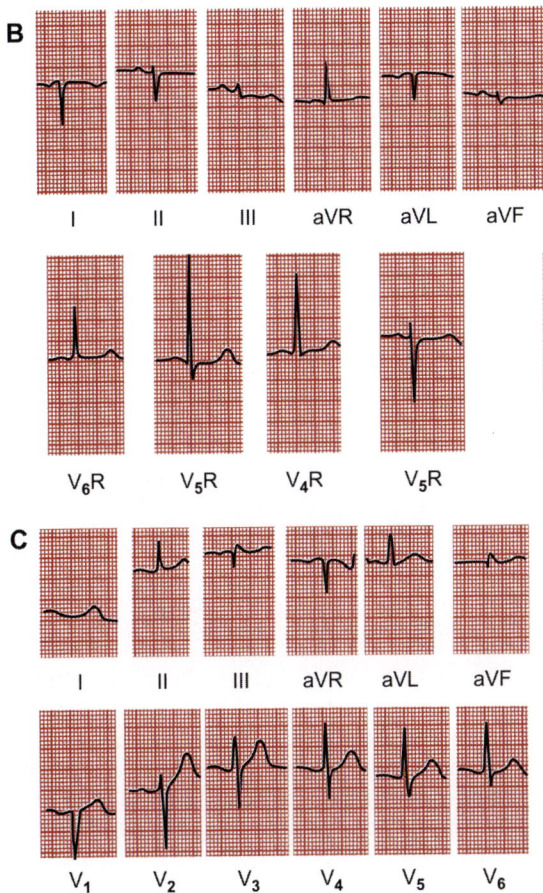

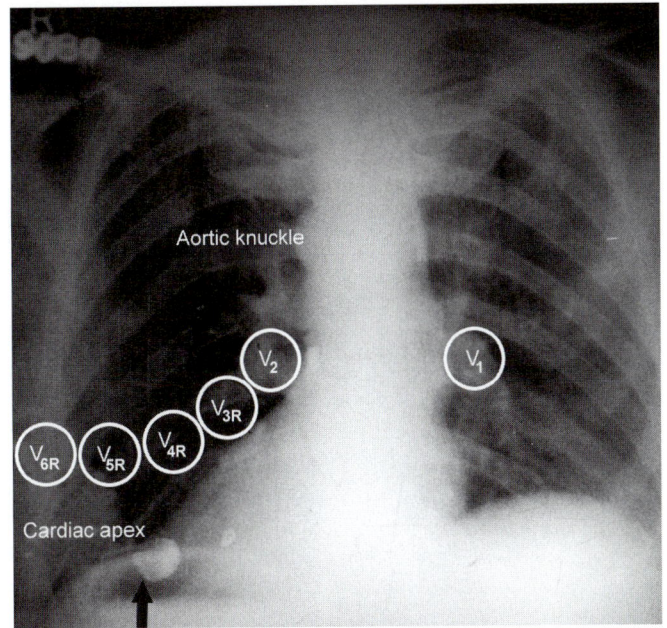

Figs 20.16 A to C: True (mirror image) dextrocardia. (A) X-ray Chest-PA view shows the placement of chest leads. (B) The electrocardiogram recorded normally from a patient with true dextrocardia shows: (i) Inverted P-QRS-T complex in lead I, (ii) Leads II and III have exchanged their positions, (iii) Lead aVR records all positive (P, QRS, T) complexes of aVL; and aVL recorded are negative (P, QRS, T) complexes of lead aVR, (iv) Precordial leads (V$_1$-V$_6$) record right ventricular epicardial complex (rS), (v) The leads V$_{3R-6R}$ recorded on 4th space right side show normal qRS complex of left ventricle.

All these features confirm the position of left ventricle on right side of the chest. (C) The normal electrocardiogram is displaced for comparison of complexes in different leads when left ventricle is at its normal position on left side.

ECG in technical dextrocardia is given in the Figure 20.17. Correct placement of electrodes will result in normal graph.

The Electrocardiogram (Fig. 20.17)

1. *Standard leads* In technical dextrocardia, the polarity of the leads and P, QRS and T waves axes are similar to mirror image dextrocardia, hence, ECG pattern will be similar to mirror image dextrocardia.

2. *Precordial leads* In contrast to mirror image dextrocardia, the precordial leads show normal P-QRS-T pattern. For comparison, ECG recorded after correction of arm electrodes is shown as Figure 20.17C.

PATENT DUCTUS ARTERIOSUS (PDA)

The ductus arteriosus is a vessel which connects the pulmonary trunk and the aorta distal to the origin of

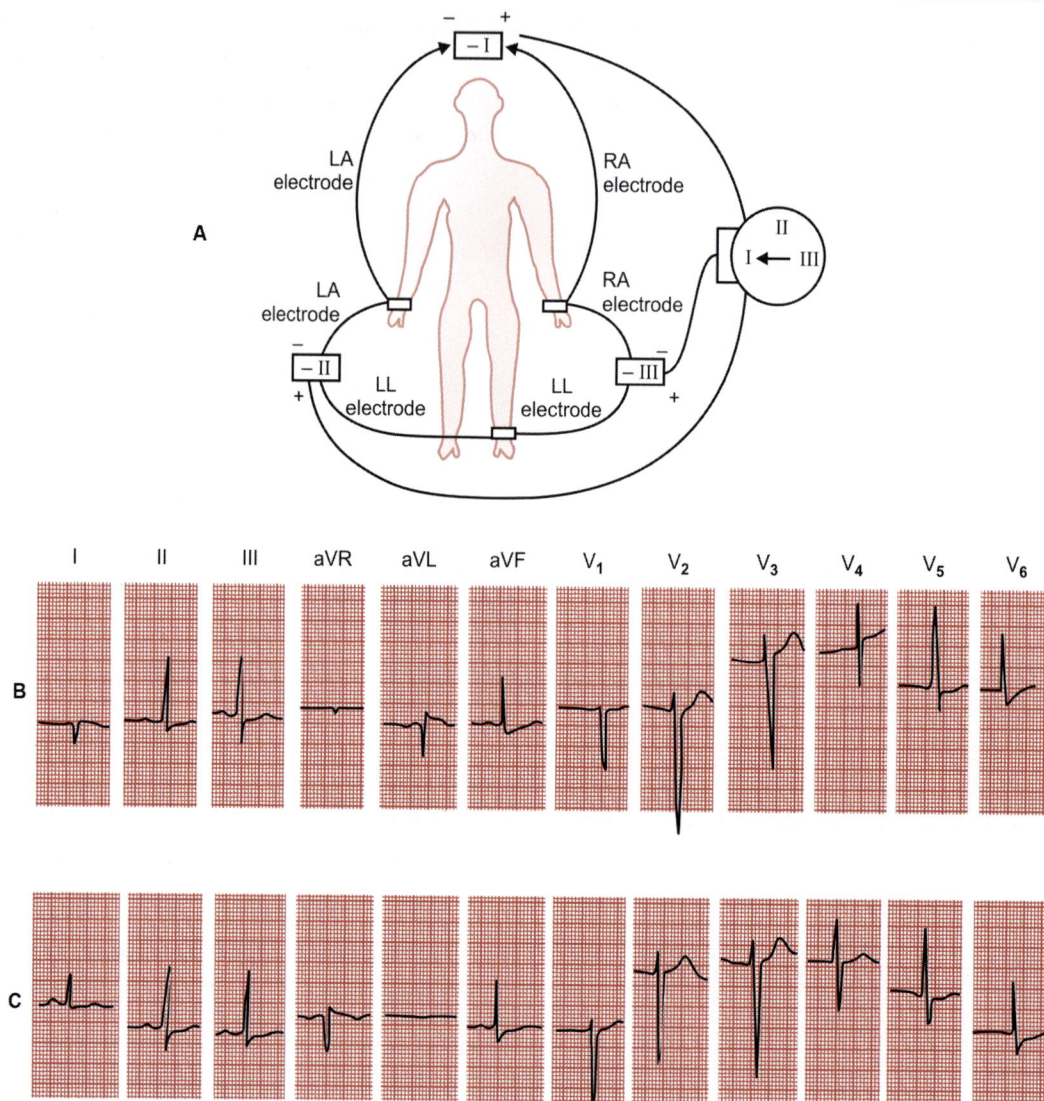

Figs 20.17A to C: Technical dextrocardia. **(A)** Interchange of arm electrode. **(B)** The electrocardiogram shows negative P, QRS and T waves in lead I. The lead II and III exchanged their positions with respect to normal depicted in **(C)**. The lead aVR records positive P, QRS and T wave of lead aVL which records negative P-QRS-T complex (cavitary pattern of aVR). All the precordial leads (V_1-V_6) are normal and show normal progression of R wave. All these features suggest technical rather than true dextrocardia. **(C)** The ECG recorded after correction of arms electrode is perfectly normal

left subclavian artery. Normally it gets closed immediately after birth due to sudden rise in arterial oxygen tension after cry of the child. Persistent patency of the ductus after birth is relatively common, occurring more frequently in females, in the offsprings of mothers whose pregnancies are complicated by rubella infection. It is also common in premature infants and children born at high altitudes.

HAEMODYNAMIC ALTERATIONS

The ductus communication leads to left to right shunt (L→R), hence, is a acyanotic heart disease. The haemodynamic alterations depend on the pressure in systemic (aorta) and pulmonary vessels and, cross-sectional area and length of the ductus. Most commonly, pulmonary vascular resistance being normal throughout the cardiac cycle (systole and diastole), the gradient persists between aorta and pulmonary artery throughout the cardiac cycle which causes a continuous 'machinery murmur'. The haemodynamic abnormality is reflected by left ventricular and left atrial enlargement due to volume (diastolic) overload. In large left to right shunt, there is an elevation of pulmonary vascular pressure which will result in right ventricular hypertrophy in addition to left; if the pulmonary arterial pressure exceeds aortic pressure, then shunt gets reversed (R→L), a condition called *Eisenmenger's syndrome*.

The Electrocardiogram (Figs 20.18 to 20.20)

The electrocardiogram is normal when the duct is small. Variations depend on the degree and duration of volume overload on the left side of the heart and pressure overload on the right ventricle. In patent ductus arteriosus with moderate left to right shunt, sinus rhythm is the rule, but occasionally atrial fibrillation has been reported in older children with large shunts. The bifid, prolonged left atrial P waves are sometimes seen in one or more standard and/or in left precordial leads. The P wave in lead V_1 may be biphasic with a deep broad negative component. The QRS axis in frontal plane is normal, i.e. deviated downwards and to the left. Occasionally, in an infant, there may be right axis deviation, and rarely, there may be left axis deviation. In patients with PDA and the rubella syndrome, the QRS axis may have superior orientation pointing upwards and either to the right or to the left. In neonates with PDA and respiratory distress syndrome, there is dominance of right ventricle.

Left ventricular volume overload in PDA with moderate shunt in an adult is reflected on ECG by a tall R wave in left precordial leads (V_5-V_6) and deep S wave in right precordial leads (V_1-V_2) and; the T waves remain tall and peaked. The q wave in V_5-V_6 becomes prominent (Fig. 20.18). If left ventricular hypertrophy/enlargement becomes marked, then ST segment is depressed but upright T wave persists. The voltage criteria of LVH ($RV_5 + SV_1 > 35$ mm) with left axis deviation and counterclockwise rotation may be seen.

A large left to right shunt with pulmonary hypertension results in biatrial and biventricular hypertrophy on ECG. Large equiphasic RS complexes

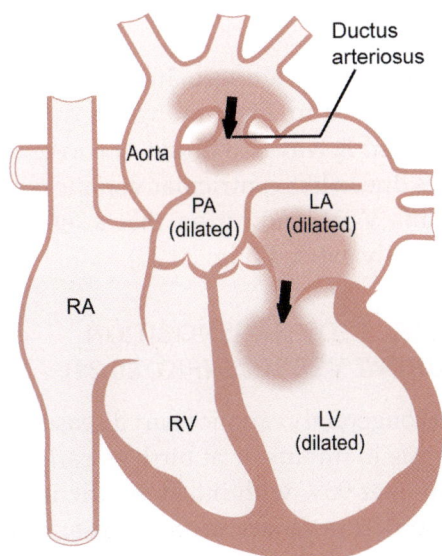

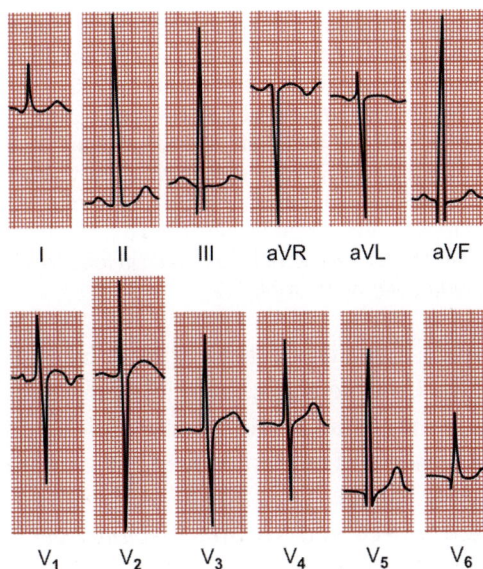

Fig. 20.18: Patent ductus arteriosus. The electrocardiogram from 18-yr-old male shows;
  i. The QRS axis is normal downwards and to the left
  ii. There is horizontal heart position with deep q wave and tall R in leads II, III and aVF. The q waves in V_5-V_6 are accentuated.
  iii. *Left ventricular volume overload.* It is evident from deep S wave in V_1 with tall R in V_5. $RV_5 + SV_1$ is > 35 mm. There are q waves in leads V_5-V_6 with upright T wave
  iv. *Evidence of biventricular hypertrophy.* There are large R and S waves in midprecordial leads (V_2-V_4) which are recorded on half standardisation except V_2

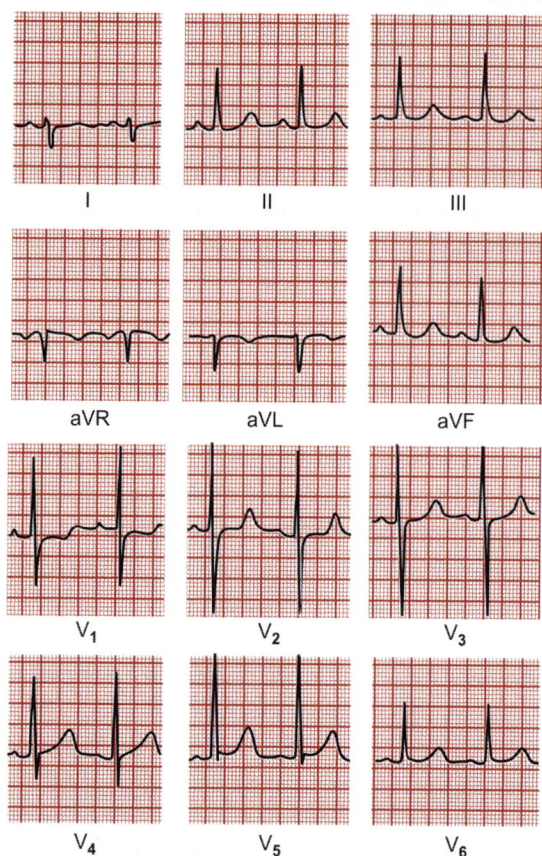

Fig. 20.19: Patent ductus arteriosus with pulmonary hypertension. The electrocardiogram recorded from 18 years female shows right axis deviation with biventricular hypertrophy. The *right ventricular hypertrophy* is evidenced by R:S >1 in lead V_1 (R>S wave) and both waves are tall. The lead V_5 shows high voltage complex (R>26 mm) with a small S wave and absent q wave. There is no S wave in lead V_6. The voltage criteric for LVH is still fulfilled, i.e. $RV_5 + SV_1 = 39$ mm. All these features suggest LVH. Large R and S wave deflections of equal amplitude (equiphasic complexes) seen in lead V_2-V_3 also indicate *biventricular hypertrophy*

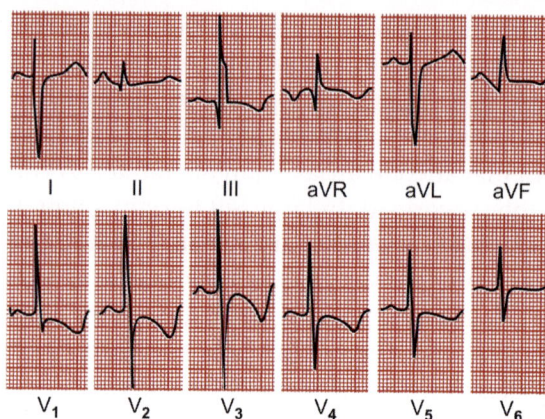

Fig. 20.20: Patent ductus arteriosus with reversed shunt (*Eisenmenger's syndrome*). The electrocardiogram recorded from a 30-yr-old male shows;

  i. The QRS axis is directed to the right (> +110°) and anteriorly

  ii. *Right atrial hypertrophy.* Peaked, tall P waves in leads II, and V_1-V_2

  iii. *Right ventricular hypertrophy.* The monophasic R wave in lead V_1 with clockwise rotation and shifting of transition zone towards left and persistence of deep S wave in V_5-V_6 suggest RVH. The ST segment is depressed and T wave is inverted from V_1-V_5

  iv. In spite of right ventricular hypertrophy, there is good voltage of R wave in V_5-V_6 indicating that there was a previous left to right shunt

can be present in most, if not, then at least in mid-precordial leads. In some cases, large RS complexes are confined to right and mid-precordial leads whereas tall R waves and moderate deep S waves are seen in V_5-V_6 (Fig. 20.19).

In PDA with reversed shunt (*Eisenmenger's syndrome*), peaked narrow P waves are seen in leads II, III and V_1. The P wave in V_1 may be biphasic with peaked initial upward component. The QRS axis now shows right axis deviation. The ECG criteria of right ventricular hypertrophy (tall R waves in V_1 and deep S waves in V_5-V_6 with inversion of T waves in right

precordial leads) are seen. In spite of right ventricular hypertrophy in Eisenmenger's syndrome, fairly developed R waves without Q wave, and upright T waves due to left ventricular volume overload persist in leads V_5-V_6 indicating that a left to right shunt previously existed (Fig. 20.20).

CORRECTED TRANSPOSITION OF GREAT VESSELS (FIG. 20.21)

It is a congenital cyanotic heart disease, manifests with cyanosis in infants or at birth as early as first day of life in over 90% with intact ventricular septum. The transposition (*trans* means cross; *position* means placement) means that aorta arises from the right ventricle (morphologic RV) and pulmonary artery arises from left ventricle (morphologic LV) but their relationship is changed in which aorta becomes anterior to pulmonary artery. This anomaly results in two parallel and separate circulations, therefore, some communication between the two must exist after birth to sustain life. Atrial, ventricular septal defects and patent ductus arteriosus are associated communications (Fig. 20.21A). Transposition is more common in males, occurs commonly in offsprings of diabetic mothers. It is a leading cause of death during infancy.

Haemodynamic Alterations

The ventricles are transposed or inverted, as a result, the left sided ventricle (morphologic LV) has the structure of right ventricle, i.e. it is thin-walled and has a tricuspid valve. The right sided ventricle (morphologic RV) has the structure of left ventricle, i.e. it is thick-walled and has a mitral valve. The dominant right ventricle forms the apex. The aorta arises from right ventricle (venous ventricle) and pulmonary artery arises from thick left ventricle (arterial ventricle).

The Electrocardiogram (Figs 20.21B and 20.22)

Due to transposition of ventricles and not of atria, the conduction of impulses from SA node to AV node is normal, but ventricular depolarisation is reversed, i.e. septal activation occurs from right to left and

dominant free wall depolarisation occurs from left to right. As a consequence of above said arrangement, the right oriented leads will register qR pattern (normal left ventricular epicardial complex) and left oriented leads will have rS or RS pattern (normal right ventricular complex). An initial q wave will thus be absent in leads I and left precordial leads (Figs 20.21 and 20.22). Since the right sided ventricle (left ventricle) is electrically dominant in this anomaly, hence, mean frontal plane QRS axis will be oriented to the right and inferiorly. Similarly, the T wave axis will also be oriented like QRS.

In horizontal plane, T wave vector is oriented to right and anteriorly, hence, T waves will be upright in all precordial leads (V_1-V_6) but it will be taller in lead V_1 than V_6. At times, the T wave may be inverted in V_6. Pure right ventricular hypertrophy is commonest in complete transposition of great vessels. Biventricular hypertrophy is a good evidence of VSD with volume overload of left ventricle with low pulmonary vascular resistance.

Tall, peaked right atrial P waves are common, not only because the right atrium is attached to a systemic right ventricle but also because of additive effects of

SECTION EIGHT

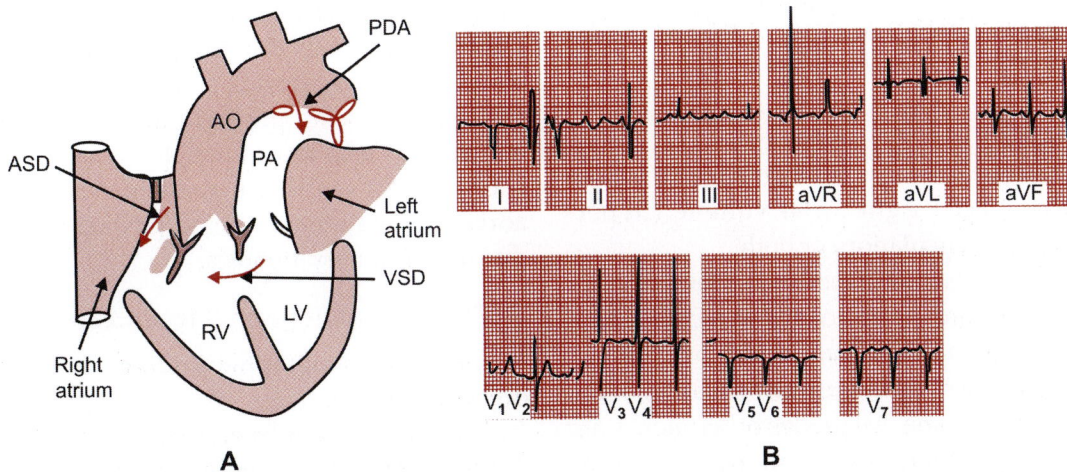

Fig. 20.21: Corrected transposition of great vessels.
A: Diagrammatic illustration of corrected transposition of great vessels. Aorta arises from right sided ventricle (morphologic RV) and is situated to the right and anterior to pulmonary artery (PA) which arises from left sided ventricle (morphologic LV). The great vessels run parallel to each other and do not cross. Three types of communications join the systemic and pulmonary circulation (i), ASD—atrial septal defect, (ii) VSD—ventricular septal defect, (iii) PDA—patent ductus arteriosus
B: The ECG taken from a 2-year-old child with corrected transposition of great vessels associated with VSD shows biventricular hypertrophy. The leads V_1, V_3, V_5 are recorded at half voltage

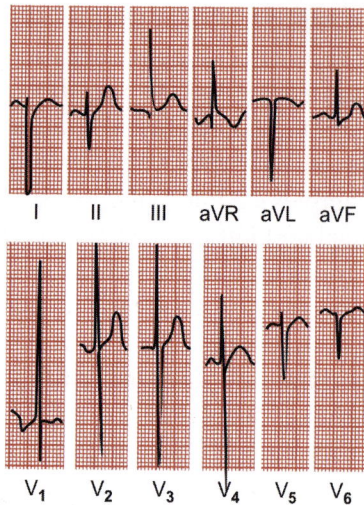

Fig. 20.22: The electrocardiogram from a 13-year-old boy with corrected transposition of great vessels with ASD shows:

   i. Left atrial bifid P waves in leads I, II and biphasic P wave with deep terminal negative deflection in lead V_1

   ii. Right axis deviation (+140°)

   iii. Inversion of depolarisation. The right oriented lead V_1 records left ventricular epicardial complex (qRS); while left oriented leads V_5-V_6 record right ventricular epicardial complex (rS) indicating reversal of depolarisation pattern. The transition zone (RS) is seen in lead V_2. There is regression of R wave from V_1-V_6 due to reversed depolarisation. Leads I and aVL also record rS pattern (right epicardial pattern).

   iv. The T is upright in all precordial leads. The T wave is taller in leads V_1-V_4 than leads V_5-V_6. The frontal plane T axis is +60° (The T is taller in lead II than III and aVF)

increased right atrial mean pressure (congestive heart failure) or increased right atrial volume (hyper-volaemic systemic circulation) or both.

Rhythm and conduction disturbance: Sinus rhythm is the rule with rare exceptions. Corrected transposition, rarely, may be associated with paroxysmal supraventricular tachycardia, atrial fibrillation or the pre-excitation syndrome. All grades of AV blocks are common. AV dissociation from idionodal or idioventricular tachycardia may occur because bundle of His in this anomaly is elongated and there is inversion of the conduction system which is subjected to greater pressure of the left ventricle. The manifestation of an AV block in association with a cyanotic congenital heart disease in an infant or a child should immediately arouse the suspicion of congenitally corrected transposition of great vessels.

THE TETRALOGY OF FALLOT

It is a cyanotic heart disease having four following components:

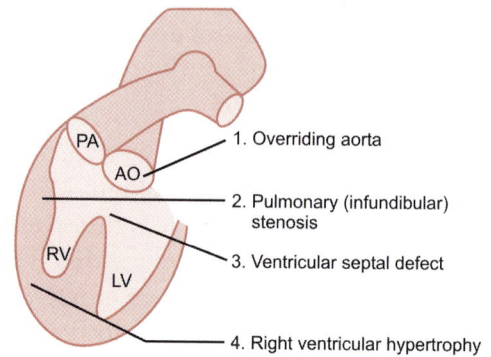

Haemodynamic Alterations

The pulmonary stenosis which is frequently infundibular and present since birth, obstructs the flow of blood from right ventricle to pulmonary artery leading to right ventricular hypertrophy. The right ventricular pressure is high and may even be equal to left ventricle. In tetralogy of Fallot, the right ventricular and left ventricular pressures remain more or less equal and both push their blood into over-rided aorta at the level of ventricular septal defect. This is the reason that VSD in tetralogy of Fallot does not produce murmur because of no pressure gradient. Central cyanosis is due to mixing of unoxygenated blood from right ventricle and oxygenated blood from left ventricle being pushed into aorta. Actually, the left atrium and left ventricle remain underfilled because right ventricle mainly pushes the blood into aorta and less amount being pushed into the lungs due to pulmonary stenosis.

The Electrocardiogram (Fig. 20.23)

The electrocardiographic findings in this anomaly occur due to:

1. Right ventricular hypertrophy
2. Right atrial hypertrophy
3. Clockwise rotation of heart on horizontal axis.

The genesis of electrocardiographic findings is similar to an isolated pulmonary stenosis with a slight difference, in the sense, that right ventricular and right atrial hypertrophy are marked in pulmonary stenosis than that in tetralogy of Fallot, because in the latter, there is an outlet to release pressure of right ventricle at level of VSD, which usually does not exceed left

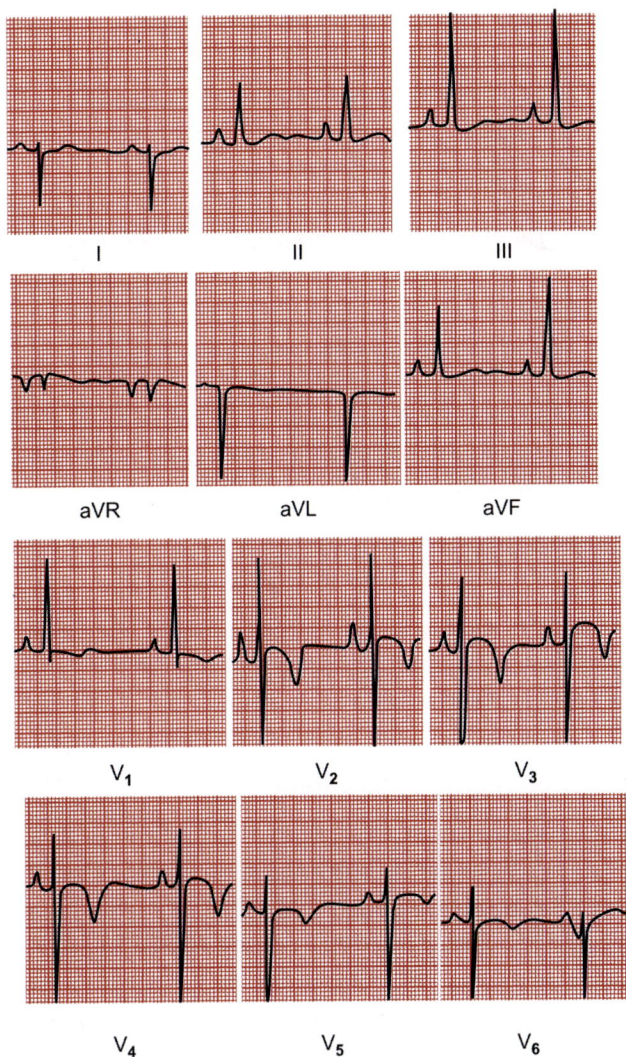

Fig. 20.23: Fallot tetralogy: The electrocardiogram shows:
  i. *Right axis deviation* > 110°. R wave is taller in lead III than aVF
  ii. *Clockwise rotation.* There is rS pattern in all precordial leads indicating shifting of transition zone beyond V_6.
  iii. *Right atrial hypertrophy.* Tall, peaked P waves are seen in all standard leads except aVL indicating marked right axis deviation of P wave (P in III > P in aVF > P in II). Tall, peaked P waves (tallest in V_2-V_4) are seen in all precordial leads
  iv. *Right ventricular hypertrophy:* Tall R wave in V_1 (R > S or R:S > 1) with persistence of S wave in V_5-V_6 (rS pattern) indicate RVH. Transition zone (R = S) lies between V_2-V_3 where both R and S are tall; indicate balancing of large right and left ventricular forces

ventricular pressure, hence, ECG findings frequently remain more or less confined to right precordial leads; whereas in an isolated or pure pulmonary stenosis, they frequently extend to the left precordial leads. The electrocardiographic findings include:

1. *Frontal plane QRS axis:* The QRS axis in the frontal plane is important because it is typically the axis of the normal newborn, i.e. downwards and to the right. This is because the functional requirements of right ventricle in Fallot's tetralogy are virtually identical before and immediately after birth and the sequence of ventricular activation is normal. For these reasons, the tracing is occasionally normal according to the age. As the neonates mature the QRS axis does not deviate to the left of vertical, therefore, depolarisation is clockwise with an rS pattern in lead I and prominent R wave in leads II and III. The QRS duration is normal. In adults, however, QRS prolongation of right bundle branch type may be seen due to defect in conduction in peripheral tissue. The QRS axis in adults is usually to the right and inferiorly in the region of + 90° counterclockwise to + 150° resulting in deep S wave in lead I and tall R wave in lead III. At times QRS axis is directed to North-West region producing S_I, S_{II}, S_{III} pattern.

Frontal plane QRS axis is downwards and to the right in the region of + 90º clockwise to + 150º

2. *Clockwise rotation on horizontal plane:* There is shifting of normal transition zone from V_3-V_4 leftwards to V_5-V_6. This will produce change of Rs to rS complex in leads V_2-V_6, in that situation, the lead V_6 will reflect rS complex and lead aVR shows a qR or QR pattern. Counterclockwise depolarisation with left axis deviation arouses suspicion of Fallot's tetralogy with endocardial cushion defects.

There is clockwise rotation on horizontal plane leading to shifting to transition zone leftwards

3. *Pattern of right ventricular hypertrophy:* The right ventricular hypertrophy pattern will be visible in lead V_1. The lead V_1 shows a tall R wave which may show a slur or notch or may be entirely positive. Very high pressures of right ventricle producing a qR pattern in lead V_1 is uncommon in tetralogy of Fallot as compared to pure pulmonary stenosis. The T waves are usually inverted in right precordial leads.

A characteristic feature of mild to moderate enlargement of right ventricle which is common to tetralogy of Fallot, is manifested by a sudden

SECTION EIGHT

change of amplitude of R wave from V_1 to V_2, i.e. lead V_1 shows a large R wave with inverted T wave, whereas the lead V_2 usually show diminished R wave (RS or rS pattern) with associated upright T wave. This sudden change of R wave from V_1 to V_2 indicates mild systolic overloading of right ventricle. When, uncommonly, right ventricular pressures are high with right to left shunt, the pattern of V_1 (R or slurred R) may extend through leads V_1 to V_3 and even may extend to V_6 if left ventricle is underfilled, and there is associated inversion of T wave in these leads. The Q waves are conspicuously absent. The presence and depth of Q waves and the amplitude of R wave in leads V_5-V_6 are sensitive signs of the magnitude of pulmonary blood flow and left ventricular filling.

A relatively balanced shunt produces small q waves and well-developed R waves in leads V_5-V_6. A left to right or a bidirectional shunt is associated with deeper left precordial Q waves and well-developed R waves in V_5-V_6.

The T wave axis in frontal plane is normal. T waves in leads V_1-V_2 are upright or inverted with equal frequency. Deep inverted T waves in right precordial leads seen in pulmonary stenosis are uncommon because usually right ventricular pressure does not exceed the left ventricular pressure in Fallot's tetralogy.

A sudden change in amplitude of R wave (a tall R wave with a slur or notch or entirely monophasic) in lead V_1 to V_2 (Rs or rS complex) is characteristic of tetralogy of Fallot.

4. **Right atrial hypertrophy:** The P wave reflects the atrial events. The P wave may be peaked in standard lead II and there is an increase in its amplitude but it may or may not exceed 2.5 mm. The 'P' pulmonale may uncommonly be seen but the duration of P wave is normal or short because of underfilled and relatively small left atrium. The right atrial enlargement in lead V_1 is reflected by accentuation of initial upright component of P wave which becomes peaked and exceeds the negative terminal component if P is biphasic in V_1. If P is positive in V_1, the peaking of P wave will be evident. The peaked P waves, sometimes, may also be seen in leads V_2-V_6.

The frontal plane P wave axis is usually in the region of +40° to +60° (downwards and to the left). The 'P' pulmonale is uncommon.

The P wave is frequently peaked rather than P pulmonale in standard leads but its duration and amplitude remain within normal limits. P wave axis is downwards and to the left.

5. **Right bundle branch block pattern:** In spite of presence of VSD, RBBB pattern does not occur in tetralogy of Fallot.

PENTALOGY OF FALLOT

It consists of all the four components of tetralogy. In addition, there is an atrial septal defect in the form of patent foramen ovale.

Haemodynamic Alterations

Due to presence of ASD (ostium secundum defect) in association with tetralogy of Fallot, there is shunting of blood from right atrium to left atrium (R→L) and, from right ventricle to left ventricle or into over-rided aorta through VSD, therefore, left atrium and left ventricle get overburdened. Thus, in the pentalogy of Fallot, there is enlargement of all the chambers of the heart.

The Electrocardiogram

The ECG findings will be of right atrial enlargement (tall peaked P waves—P pulmonale in leads II, III and aVF), right ventricular hypertrophy and minimal signs of left ventricular hypertrophy. Therefore, the leads V_5 and V_6 will have good height of R wave with small S wave due to left ventricular hypertrophy. There will be no or slight shift of transition zone to the left due to balancing of electrical forces between the two hypertrophied ventricles.

In case, right ventricular hypertrophy overwhelms left ventricle, which usually it does, then R wave in lead V_1 will be taller than S wave (R:S >1) with inverted T waves.

TRIOLOGY OF FALLOT

It consists of:
1. Pulmonary stenosis
2. Right ventricular hypertrophy
3. Atrial septal defect in the form of patent foramen ovale (commonest), or ostium secundum defect (uncommon), or ostium primum defect (rarest).

Haemodynamic Alterations

Due to presence of pulmonary stenosis, there is hypertrophy and enlargement of right ventricle and subsequently of right atrium (pressure overload). The increase in right atrial pressure results in shunting of unoxygenated blood to left atrium through patent foramen ovale or interatrial septal defect leading to cyanosis. Therefore, as there is no outlet to release the right ventricular pressure due to intact interventricular septum, the pressure in right ventricle rises further and may reach to high levels similar to an isolated pulmonary stenosis.

As a result of shunting of blood from right atrium to left atrium (R→L shunt), there will be volume overloading of left atrium, which, subsequently leads to volume overloading of left ventricle.

The Electrocardiogram

Basically, the electrocardiographic abnormalities arise due to:
1. Right atrial enlargement.
2. Right ventricular hypertrophy
3. Left atrial enlargement due to volume overload.
4. Possible left ventricular enlargement.

The ECG patterns consist of:
1. *Biatrial enlargement*: The P waves are increased both in height and width in leads II, III and aVF. In lead V_1, there will be prominence of both positive (right atrial enlargement) and negative components (left atrial enlargement) of P waves; if P wave is biphasic. If P wave is positive, then it will be of increased amplitude (> 2.5 mm), peaked and wide. In other chest leads, P wave will show the same characteristics as in V_1.
2. *Right ventricular or biventricular hypertrophy:* There will be increase in height of the R wave in lead V_1 with small S wave and inverted T wave due to right ventricular hypertrophy. The left ventricular volume overload may be reflected by qRS complex in V_5-V_6 with good voltage of R wave. The transition zone may remain within normal range, in that situation, both the R and S waves will have high voltage in leads V_3-V_4 due to balance of forces between two hypertrophied or overloaded ventricles.
3. *Right axis deviation on frontal plane:* In nut shell, the ECG diagnosis of triology of Fallot is suspected when there is right axis deviation, biatrial and right ventricular hypertrophy. The P waves are tall and widened. The widening of P wave is due to left atrial hypertrophy or overloading.

EBSTEIN'S ANOMALY

It is a rare congenital defect wherein tricuspid valve is malformed and is displaced downwards into right ventricular cavity resulting in hypoplastic right ventricle. As a result of this defect, a part of right ventricle gets incorporated into right atrium which becomes large, voluminous and hyperplastic; a condition called *'atrialisation of right ventricle'*. The functional part of right ventricle is reduced and consists of mainly an outflow region, a small apical part and an infundibulum. The cusps of tricuspid valve are fused with a narrow and deformed orifice. Chorda tendinea are short and poorly developed. One-third cases are acyanotic; while two-third cases have a patent foramen ovale or an atrial septal defect through which right to left shunt occurs leading to central cyanosis.

The right atrium is voluminous and accommodates a large amount of blood. The tricuspid valve being deformed and displaced into right ventricle, shows some degree of functional tricuspid regurgitation or stenosis or both. The tricuspid regurgitation is common in Ebstein's anomaly and forms a clinical diagnostic clue.

The Electrocardiogram (Fig. 20.24)

The electrocardiographic manifestations though bizarre but are distinct.

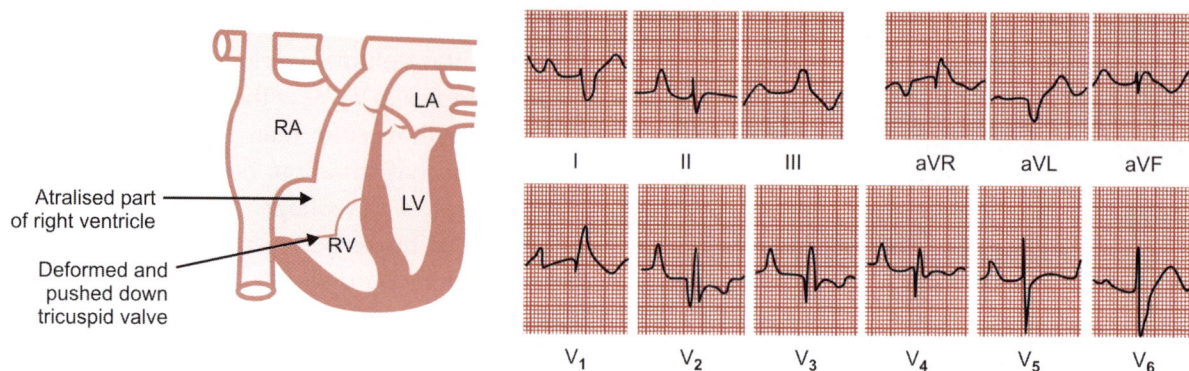

Fig. 20.24: Ebstein anomaly. The ECG recorded from 18-yr-old boy shows;
  i. *First degree AV block.* The P-R interval is 0.28 sec.
  ii. *Right bundle branch block (RBBB).* There is wide (>0.12 sec) rsR' pattern in leads V_1-V_4 with coving ST segment and inverted T waves. There is wide deep S wave in V_6
  iii. *Right atrial hypertrophy:* There is tall peaked P waves in leads II, III, aVF, V_2-V_5
      NB: Tall P waves (Himalyan P waves) along with conduction detects are highly suggestive of Ebstein anomaly

The P Wave Abnormalities

Due to abnormally large right atrium, P waves are bizarre, i.e. tall and widened with ragged limbs. Both P wave amplitude and duration are increased, distinctly seen in lead II. All the precordial leads may reflect tall upright P waves. The P waves are frequently taller than QRS in right precordial leads especially V_1. The frontal plane P wave axis lies in the region of +60° clockwise to +70°.

First Degree AV Block

The P-R interval is frequently prolonged, may be 0.20 sec or even more. This is seen in one-third cases. The increased P-R interval and increased width of P wave are due to prolonged conduction through the large right atrium.

The QRS Abnormalities

There is generalised low amplitude of QRS complexes in all the leads which may vary from 5 mm to 10 mm. The QRS duration is increased to 0.12 sec or longer. The QRS complexes may have pattern of right bundle branch block or may have bizarre intraventricular conduction delay.

Prominent initial Q or q wave is not unusual in right precordial leads (V_1-V_3) and, at times, in all the precordial leads. The prominent Q wave in right precordial leads forms an important characteristic of Ebstein's anomaly because large atrium pushes the right ventricle anteriorly and left ventricular posteriorly.

The mean frontal plane QRS axis is directed to right and inferiorly (+60 clockwise to +120° or more). Left axis deviation is a feature of associated pre-excitation.

Accelerated Conduction

At times or intermittently, pre-excitation due to right lateral kent bundle (type B-WPW syndrome) may be seen (5-25% cases), in which QRS complexes are dominantly negative in right precordial leads (V_1-V_3). Ebstein's anomaly is the only congenital cardiac malformation consistently associated with pre-excitation, commonly via right bypass tract, i.e. type B WPW pattern. Sometimes, during accelerated conduction a delta wave and normal P-R interval are present.

The T Wave Changes

The T wave changes are nonspecific. Frontal plane T wave axis has same orientation to that of QRS. The T wave is usually shallow in V_1, positive in V_2 and V_3. The left precordial leads may have upright or inverted T waves.

Arrhythmias

Tachyarrhythmias are frequent in Ebstein's anomaly. They even form one of the important electrocardiographic feature of this anomaly. Atrial and ventricular ectopics (extrasystoles) are common. Paroxysmal atrial or re-entrant supraventricular tachycardia or wide QRS reciprocal tachycardia via bypass tract may be present in 25% cases. Atrial fibrillation and atrial flutter are not uncommon.

PERSISTENT TRUNCUS ARTERIOSUS

Normally, truncus arteriosus is divided completely into aorta and pulmonary artery by a septum. Failure of this septum to develop results in persistence of a large single vessel (persistent truncus arteriosus) which leaves the heart and conveys blood to the systemic, pulmonary and coronary circulations. Incomplete division of truncus arteriosus results in aorto-pulmonary window. Persistent truncus arteriosus is a rare congenital anomaly and is always associated with VSD. At times, there may be single ventricle due to the absence of interventricular septum.

Haemodynamic Alterations

Since both the ventricles pump their blood into a common truncus arteriosus which has systemic vascular resistance, hence, both ventricles work against this resistance, therefore, there is hypetrophy of both the ventricles, more so, of right ventricle. There is an associated VSD which also equalises the pressures between both the ventricles. Since pulmonary vascular resistance being normal, the lungs are overflooded from the right ventricle, which return their blood to left atrium and left ventricle, thus, left ventricle is overburdened and hypertrophies. Thus, due to high pressure in the right ventricle, the right atrium in sequence gets hypertrophied.

The Electrocardiogram (Fig. 20.25)

The 12-leads ECG reflects volume overload of the left side of the heart and pressure overload of the right side. Sinus rhythm is the rule. P-R interval is usually normal. The P waves may be normal in infancy, but as the time passes, abnormalities of P wave, i.e. tall, peaked right atrial P waves appear in one or more leads and often there may be notched or bifid left atrial P waves.

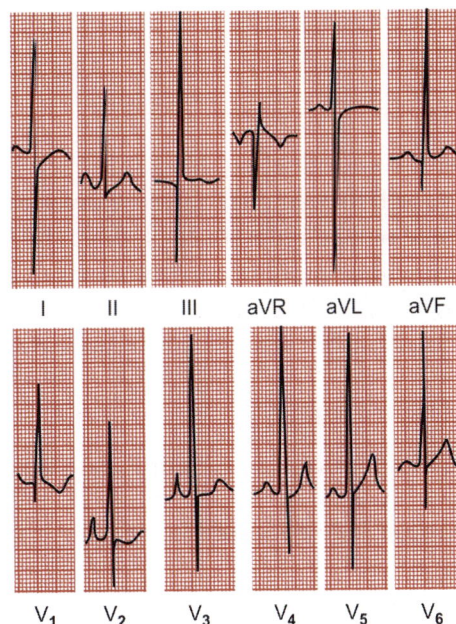

Fig. 20.25: Persistent truncus arteriosus. The electrocardiogram of < 1-yr-old girl shows:
  i. Right atrial hypertrophy. There are peaked right atrial P waves in leads II, aVF and V_2-V_4
  ii. Normal QRS axis
  iii. Left ventricular hypertrophy. Tall R waves and prominent peaked tall T waves in V_5-V_6 and tall R waves in leads III and aVF
  iv. Right ventricular hypertrophy. There is qR pattern in lead V_1 with inverted T wave and there is deep S wave in leads V_4-V_6

The frontal plane QRS axis is normal or inferior and slightly to the right. A rightward shift is more likely when pulmonary blood flow is reduced; and a leftward shift is more likely when pulmonary blood flow is increased, but marked deviation of axis either to left or right is uncommon. Due to clockwise depolarisation, Q wave may be found in leads II, III and aVF.

Precordial leads depict either left or biventricular hypertrophy. Pure right ventricular hypertrophy occurs in adult survivors with high pulmonary vascular resistance. When pulmonary blood flow is abundant, the features of volume overload of left ventricle (q waves in V_5-V_6 with tall R waves and upright T waves) appear. Right precordial leads(V_1-V_2) continue to exhibit tall R waves with deep S waves. In addition to features described above, the biventricular hypertrophy is reflected by equiphasic complexes (RS complexes) in midprecordial leads (V_3-V_4).

AORTO-PULMONARY COMMUNICATION (WINDOW)

Haemodynamic Alterations

Since there is shunting of blood from aorta (high pressure vessel) to pulmonary artery (lower pressure vessel), there will be pulmonary plethora. If shunt is large, there will be rapid rise in pulmonary vascular resistance, which will result in right ventricular systolic overload and left ventricular diastolic overload.

The Electrocardiogram

The ECG characteristics are similar to VSD and include:
1. Left ventricular hypertrophy due to diastolic overload.
2. Right ventricular hypertrophy due to systolic overload. Therefore, there will be features of biventricular hypertrophy.
3. Left atrial enlargement due to diastolic overload.

TRICUSPID ATRESIA

It is a congenital cyanotic heart disease in which the tricuspid valve is malformed or absent or hypoplastic and imperforate (atretic). The right ventricle is hypoplastic and an interatrial communication (patent foramen ovale) exists between right and left atrium. The left side of the heart is normal with normal mitral valve. In about 90% cases, the great vessels / arteries are normally related and there is an associated VSD to regulate the flow of blood from left ventricle to the pulmonary circulation.

Haemodynamic Alterations

Through an atrial septal defect, the left atrium receives the entire systemic venous return in addition to its normal venous return from the lungs directly. The mixed blood now flows into left ventricle which is overloaded and is only pumping chamber for systemic and pulmonary circulation. In the 90% cases, the great arteries being normally related, the blood flows from left ventricle to right through VSD and subsequently through pulmonary arteries to the lungs. A few additional anatomical and physiological alterations may also coexist in small number of cases.

The Electrocardiogram (Fig. 20.26)

The electrocardiogram will show features of right atrial or biatrial enlargement along with volume overloading of left ventricle:
1. ***Right atrial or biatrial enlargement:*** Tall, peaked right atrial P waves are almost always present

ASD: Atrial septal defect
VSD: Ventricular septal defect

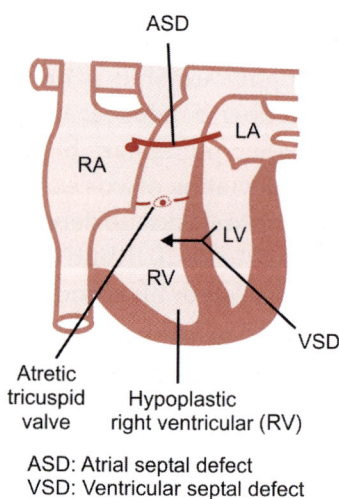

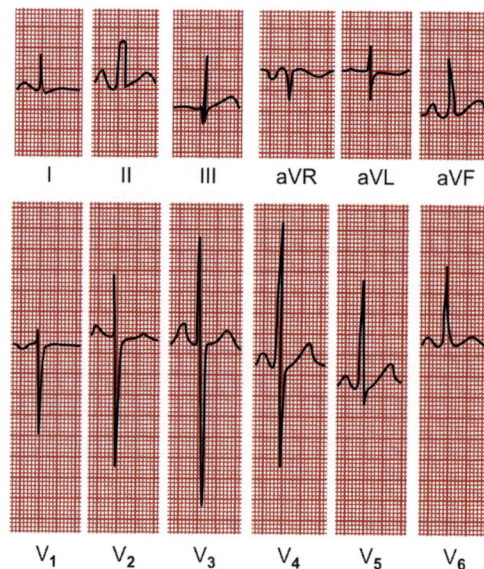

Fig. 20.26: Tricuspid atresia. The electrocardiogram recorded from a 3-yr-old boy with tricuspid atresia, complete transposition of great vessels and a large VSD shows:
   i. The QRS axis normal
   ii. Biatrial hypertrophy. There are tall peaked P waves in leads II, III, aVF and V_2-V_3 with biphasic P in V_1 where negative component is deep and prominent
   iii. There is progression of R wave from V_1-V_6 as occurs in adults, i.e. height of R wave increases as we proceed from lead V_1 towards V_6
   iv. Left ventricular overolad. The large S wave (rS complex in V_1-V_2) with good large R wave in V_5-V_6 where S in V_1 > R in V_6 indicate left ventricular overload.

especially in inferior limb leads and right precordial leads. The P waves are sometimes biphasic with initial positive component taller than negative in leads V_1 or V_{3R} but positive and peaked in V_2-V_3. Bifid or notched P waves (tall as well as wide) may also be seen and signify a large left atrial volume overload due to increased pulmonary blood flow.

2. *Left ventricular volume overload:* An abnormal leftwards QRS axis with counterclockwise rotation is characteristic feature of tricuspid atresia with normal great vessels and a small VSD. This is due to large left ventricular and absence of right ventricular forces in precordial leads resulting in rS pattern in V_1 and V_2 with large R waves in V_5-V_6. The left ventricle overload on ECG in adult survivors is reflected by q waves in V_5-V_6 with tall R waves. The ST segment is isoelectric but gets depressed with inversion of T waves in case of left ventricular hypertrophy.

The diagnosis of tricuspid atresia on ECG is suggested by the association of right atrial enlargement with left axis deviation and/or left ventricular hypertrophy.

CONGENITAL AORTIC STENOSIS

Valvular aortic stenosis is relatively rare congenital cardiovascular defect, while on the other hand, bicuspid aortic valve which is not necessary stenosed is the most common congenital malformation of the heart. It is more common in males and goes undetected during early life. Patients seeks medical help when either it becomes stenosed or becomes the site of infective endocarditis, otherwise, it may go undetected throughout life. Patent ductus arteriosus and coarctation of aorta are common associated lesions.

Haemodynamic Alterations

Haemodynamically significant obstruction causes concentric hypertrophy of the left ventricular wall and dilatation of ascending aorta.

The Electrocardiogram (Fig. 20.27)

It may be normal or may show signs of left ventricular systolic overload of left ventricle (read chapter on ventricular hypertrophy).

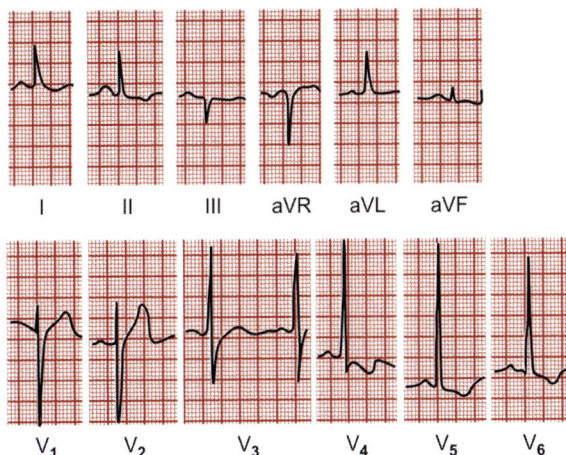

Fig. 20.27: Congenital aortic stenosis. The electrocardiogram was recorded from a 20 yr male with congenital aortic stenosis with gradient of 40 mm across the valve. Note the following features;
  i. Left axis deviation of mean frontal QRS.
  ii. Left ventricular hypertrophy. The precordial leads show criteria of LVH;
    a. The R wave in V_5 or V_6 > 27 mm
    b. $SV_1 + RV_5$ > 35 mm
  iii. There is associated ST segment depression and T wave inversion in leads V_4-V_6, I and II

Suggested Reading

1. Bharati S, Rosen K, Steinfield L et al: Anatomical substrate for pre-excitation in corrected transposition of great vessels. *Circulation* **62**: 831, 1980.
2. Char F, Adam P, Anderson RC: Electrocardiographic findings in 100 cases of verified ventricular septol defect. *Am J Dis Child* **97**: 48, 1959.
3. Davach F, Lucas RV Jr, Moller JH: The electrocardiogram and vectorcardiogram in tricuspid atresia. Correlation with pathological anatomy. *Am J Cardiol* **25**: 18, 1970.
4. Friedman WF: Congenital heart disease in infancy and childhood. "In Braunwald Heart Disease" Textbook of Cardiovascular Medicine. WB Saunders Company, 5th ed **2**: 1997.
5. Friedman WF: Congenital heart disease. In *Harrison's Principles of Internal Medicine* (14th International Edition). McGraw Hill Book Company, 1997.
6. Perloff JK: Congenital heart disease in adults. "In Braunwald—*Heart Disease Textbook of Cardiovascular Medicine* (5th ed), WB Saunders Company **2**: 1997
7. Rosenbaum MB, Elizari MV, Lizzari JQ et al: The differential electrocardiographic manifestations of hemiblock, bilateral bundle branch block and trifascicular blocks. In: Schlant RC, Hurst JW (Eds): *Advances in Electrocardiography*. New York: Grune and Stratton, 1972.

8. Schamroth L: *An Introduction to Electrocardiography* (7th ed). Blackwell Science Inc, 1990.

9. Scott RC: The electrocardiogram in ventricular septal defect. *Am Heart J* **62**: 842, 1961.

10. Sodi-Pallares D, Marsico F: The importance of electro-cardiographic patterns in congenital heart disease. *Am Heart J* **49**: 587, 1955.

11. Waldo AL, Pacifico AD, Bargeron LM Hr, James TN, Kirklin JW: Electrophysiological delineation of specialised AV conduction system in patients with corrected transposition of great vessels and ventricular septal defect. *Circulation* **52**: 43, 1975.

21

Heredofamilial Prolonged Q-T Syndromes

- *Heredofamilial prolonged Q-T (The Jervell-Lange-Nielsen and Romano-Ward) syndromes*
  - *The electrocardiographic characteristics, clinical significance and mechanism of tachyarrhythmias*
- *Acquired prolonged Q-T syndrome – clinical conditions, the electrocardiogram and its significance*

The prolonged Q-T syndrome is a functional abnormality, perhaps, associated with neurogenic influences, that may cause serious arrhythmias.

The hereditory long Q-T interval syndrome is an idiopathic prolongation of Q-T interval more than 0.44 sec in individuals with normal hearts. There are two identified syndromes which are seen in young individuals especially women. These are;

1. The Jervell-Lange-Nielsen Syndrome (Figs 21.1 and 21.2)

It is inherited by an autosomal recessive trait. In addition to long Q-T interval, these patients have congenital deafness and positive family history of long Q-T syndrome. It is characterised by syncopal attacks, paroxysmal tachyarrhythmias (polymorphic ventricular tachycardia or torsade de pointes or ventricular fibrillation) or sudden death. It is mostly familial and may be asymptomatic in certain members of the family.

2. The Romano-Ward Syndrome

It is inherited by an autosomal dominant trait. There is no associated deafness in these patients.

Clinical Significance

Some patients have prolonged Q-T intervals throughout their life without any manifest arrhythmias; while

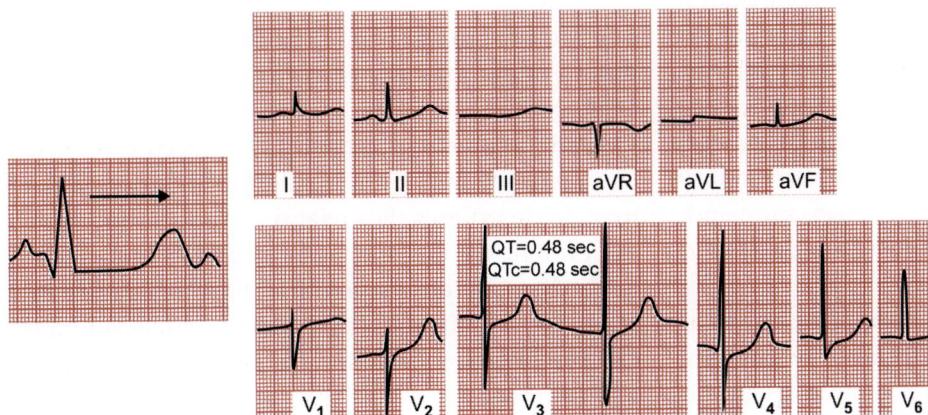

Fig. 21.1: Prolonged QTc syndrome of undetermined organ. It was recorded from a patient who complained of syncope. There was no history of drug intake and electrolytes were normal. There was neither family history nor history of deafness. The QT and QTc are 0.48 sec respectively because HR is 60/min

QT=0.48 sec
QTc=0.48 sec

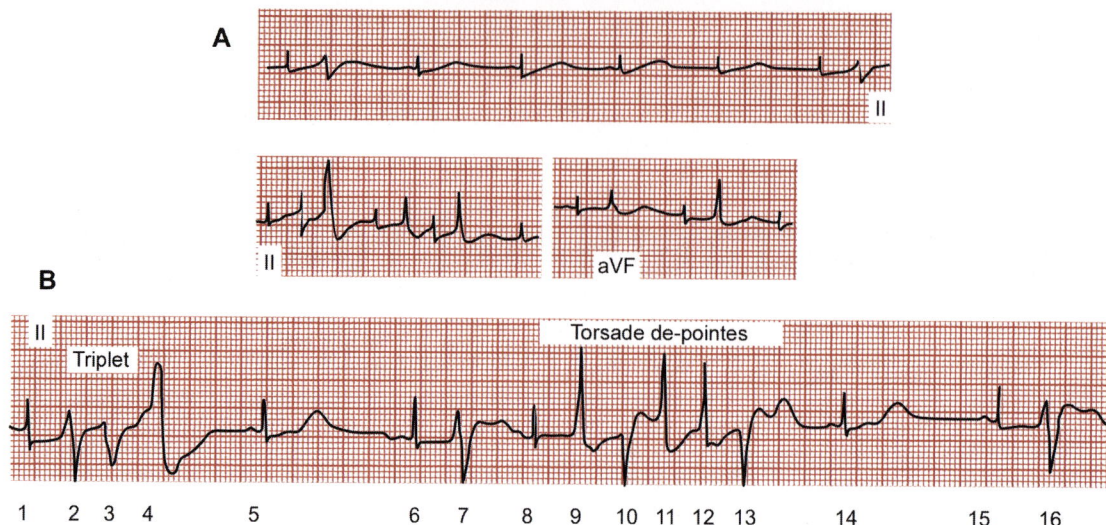

Fig. 21.2: A congenitally prolonged QTc syndrome. **A:** *Upper strip* (lead II). QTc is prolonged (QT = 0.68 sec, R-R = 1.44, QTc = 0.56 sec). There are two VPCs seen. *Lower strip* (leads II, aVF). VPCs are seen mostly in bigeminal fashion. **B:** The continuous strip (lead II) shows a polymorphic triplet (non-sustained polymorphic VT) in the beginning and a run of torsade de pointes in the middle (labelled) in addition to isolated VPCs

Note: The mother of the patient though asymptomatic had prolonged Q-T syndrome.

others are highly susceptible to symptomatic and potentially fatal ventricular arrhythmias.

The clinical studies have documented that these individuals with long Q-T interval, are prone to develop symptoms of syncopal attacks due to the development of tachyarrhythmias, i.e. ventricular tachycardia, torsade de pointes (Fig. 21.2) or ventricular fibrillation under the effect of vigorous excercise, intense emotional upset or any startle stimulus.

Mechanism of Tachyarrhythmias

QT dispersion (QTd): The QT interval on 12 lead surface electrocardiogram measures electrical depolarisation and repolarisation. Prolonged repolarisation (delayed recovery time) predisposes to ventricular excitability. Experimental studies have provided strong evidence of dispersion of ventricular recovery time for genesis of malignant ventricular arrhythmias. The excitability is proportional to the duration of repolarisation and, thus, dispersion of refractoriness is parallel to dispersion of repolarisation.

The increased QTd (QT maximum-QT minimum) means interlead variation of QT, indicates variability in ventricular recovery time, hence, predisposes to ventricular arrhythmias. The increased QT dispersion is known to occur in patients with prolonged QT syndrome (Fig. 21.3), explains the genesis of arrhythmias in these patients.

> *Every long QT interval is not associated with ventricular arrhythmias though it predisposes an individual to them. Neither the severity nor the cut off point of QT prolongation that predispose to ventricular arrhythmias have been defined. It is now postulated that; the more is the QT dispresion (QTd), the more are the chances of an arrhythmia.*

ACQUIRED PROLONGED Q-T SYNDROME

The acquired form of prolonged Q-T interval may be due to many reasons which are summarised in the Table 21.1.

Drug interactions recently have been recognised as a mechanism of prolongation of Q-T interval and torsade de pointes. For example, terfenadine which can prolong the Q-T interval is normally metabolised in the liver by an enzyme P_{450} to a metabolite that retains its antihistaminic property but does not cause Q-T prolongation. Therefore, terfenadine may become arrhythmogenic when the metabolising hepatic

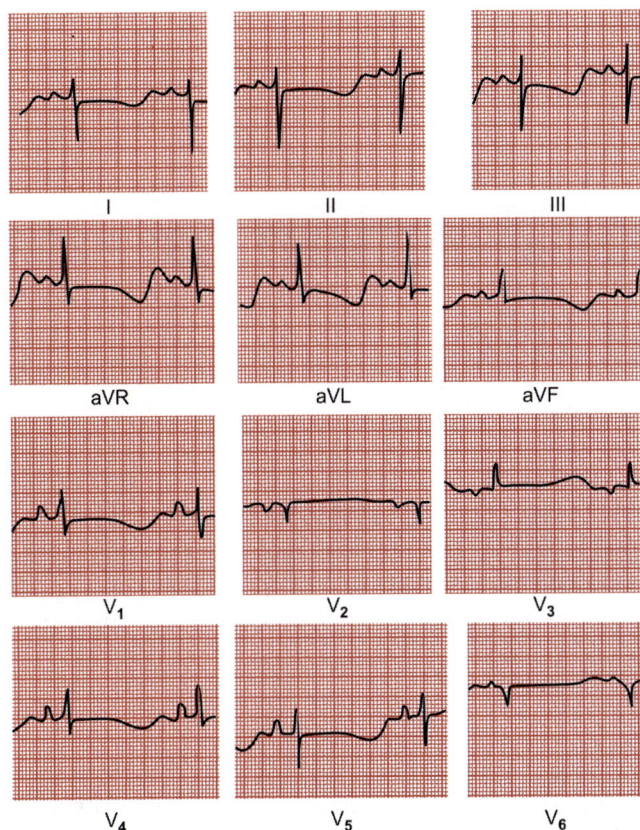

Fig. 21.3: The QT dispersion (QTd) in a patient with prolonged QTc syndrome. The ECG shows variable QT interval from 0.60 sec(lead III, aVF) to 0.80 sec (V₁-V₆), hence there is wide QT dispersion (interlead variation of QT). The T wave is biphasic in most of the leads

enzyme is blocked by an another substance such as ketoconazole, hence, both should not be combined.

CLINICAL SIGNIFICANCE

Acquired prolonged Q-T syndrome like congenital form, carry a risk of serious arrhythmias and sudden cardiac death, but the risk is eliminated when the initiating factor is found out and removed. In this syndrome also, torsades de pointes-a form of ventricular tachycardia is the commonest and it may trigger or degenerate into lethal ventricular fibrillation.

Table 21.1: Conditions responsible for acquired prolongation of Q-T (QTc) interval

- Drug idiosyncrasies (antiarrhythmic and psychotropic drugs) and drug interactions (e.g. terfenadine and ketoconazole)
- Hyponatraemia
- CNS injury
- Anorexia nervosa
- Electrolyte abnormalities, e.g. hypokalaemia, hypomagnesaemia, etc.
- Toxic substances
- Weight reduction by liquid protein diets
- Lithium carbonate

Suggested Reading

1. Bhandari AK, Scheinman M: The long Q-T syndrome. *Mod Concepts Cardiovascular Dis* **54**:45,1985.
2. Day CP, McComb JM, Compbell RWF: QT dispersion: An indication of arrhythmia risk in patients with long QT intervals. *Br Heart J* **63**:342-44,1990.
3. Fraser GR, Froggatt P, James TN: Congenital deafness associated with electrocardiographic abnormalities, fainting attacks and sudden death. *Quart J Med* **33**:362, 1964.
4. Garza LA, Vick RL, Nora JJ, et al: Heritable Q-T prolongation without deafness. *Circulation*, **41**:39,1970.
5. Isner JM, Sours HE, Pris AL et al: Sudden, unexpected death in avid dieters using liquid - protein - modified fast diet. Observations in 17 patients and the role of prolonged Q-T interval. *Circulation* **60**:1401, 1979.
6. Keating MT, Atkinson D, Dunn C, et al: Linkage of a cardiac arrhythmia, the long Q-T syndrome and the Harvey - ras -1 gene. *Science* **252**:704, 1991.
7. Moss AJ, Schwartz PJ, Crampton RS et al: The long Q-T syndrome: A prospective international study. *Circulation* **71**:17, 1985.
8. Schwartz PJ, Periti M, Malliani A: The long Q-T syndrome. *Am Heart J* **89**:378, 1975.
9. Schwartz PJ: The idiopathic long QT syndrome. *Ann Intern Med* **99**:561, 1982.
10. Smith WM, Gallaghar JJ: Les torsades de pointes. *Ann Intern Med* **93**: 578, 1980.
11. Wang O, Shen J, Splawski J, et al: SCN5A mutations associated with an inherited cardiac arrhythmia, long Q-T syndrome. *Cell* **80**:805, 1995.

22

Accelerated Conduction or Pre-excitation

- Accelerated conduction—definition and electrocardiographic patterns
- Wolff-Parkinson-White syndrome – definition, electrocardiographic characteristics, mechanisms, types, localisation of an accessory pathway and decision making
- Wolff-Parkinson-White syndrome variants – conduction through James fibre (Lown-Ganong-Levine syndrome) and conduction through unusual Mahaim fibres

Definition

It is an electrocardiographic term used to denote conduction through an anomalous pathway (accessory pathway) resulting in ventricular activation earlier than expected via the AV node-His-Purkinje pathway and is used to identify the following electrocardiographic patterns or syndromes;

1. Wolff-Parkinson-White (WPW) syndrome (conduction through Kent's bundle)
2. WPW variants:
   a) Lown-Ganong-Levine (LGL) syndrome (conduction through James bundle)
   b) Conduction through unusal Mahaim fibres producing fascicular tachycardia.
3. Isolated accelerated conduction beats.

WOLFF-PARKINSON-WHITE (WPW) SYNDROME

It is an electrocardiographic syndrome that results due to conduction through an anomalous atrioventricular pathway usually congenital in origin. The prevalence of WPW syndrome in the general population is approximately 3 per 1000. This pathway acts as a bypass tract between atria and ventricles. As the AV node, bundle of His and distal conducting system are bypassed, a sinus or supraventricular impulse reaches one of the ventricles earlier than the beat conducted through normal pathway, hence, excite the ventricle prematurely called *pre-excitation*.

The anomalous bypass tract in WPW syndrome is a bundle of Kent, while James bundle or fibres of Mahaim constitute an accessory pathway for WPW variants. All of them are situated ectopically any where along the AV ring. The Kent's bundle forms an accessory pathway between atria and the ventricles and bypasses the AV node in the classic WPW syndrome characterised by short P-R interval. The term 'syndrome' is attached to this disorder because frequently tachyarrhythmias due to accessory pathway occur.

The Electrocardiographic Pattern–Bundle of Kent

1. *A short P-R interval* less than 0.12 second is a characteristic feature, but it may be of any length shorter than that of normally conducted sinus beat in the same individual.
2. *QRS interval* is widened (> 0.12 sec).
3. *P-J interval* [interval between onset of P wave to junction (J) of QRS with ST segment is normal

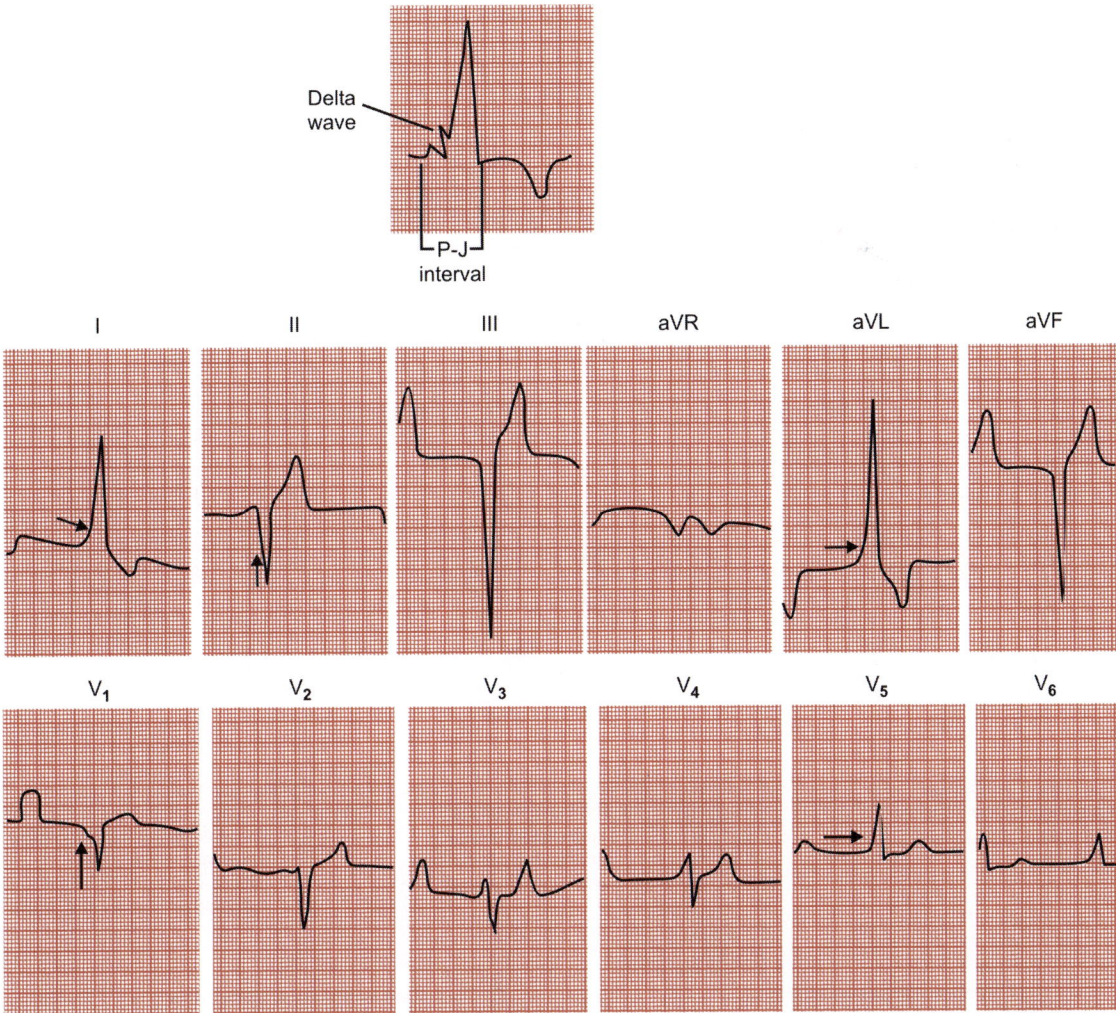

Fig. 22.1: Wolff-Parkinson-White (WPW) syndrome. **A:** Diagrammatic illustration of basic electrocardiographic deflections. A P-QRS-T complex drawn shows a short P-R interval, a delta wave on the upstroke of R wave, wide QRS and normal P-J interval. **B:** The ECG shows a short P-R interval (<0.10 sec), a positive delta wave on positive QRS ($\rightarrow$) in leads I, aVL, V_5-V_6. There is negative delta waves on negative QRS ($\uparrow$) in leads II,III, aVF and V_1-V_2. The QRS is wide (>0.12 sec). The ST-T vector is opposite to QRS, hence, the leads showing upright QRS have negative T waves and *vice versa*. The high voltage in leads I and III (R_I + S_{III} >21 mm) is due to WPW syndrome and not due to LVH

(< 0.26 sec)]. This implies that widening of QRS occurs at the expense of P-R interval.

4. *Delta wave or pre-excitation wave.* Notching or slurring of the QRS deflections by delta wave occurs on its ascending limb if the major deflection is upward or on its descending limb if the major deflection is downward (Fig. 22.1).

5. Secondary ST-T changes are frequently seen. They are generally directed opposite to the major delta wave and QRS complex. The electrocardiographic deflections in classic WPW syndrome are diagrammatically represented in Figure 22.1A.

6. The presence of associated supraventricular tachycardia is a common finding (50% cases).

7. The characteristic pattern of WPW syndrome can be altered by abnormalities of AV and intraventricular conduction delay.

Mechanisms of Pathogenesis

The ventricular activation takes place in two phases, i.e. pre-excitation and terminal ventricular activation.

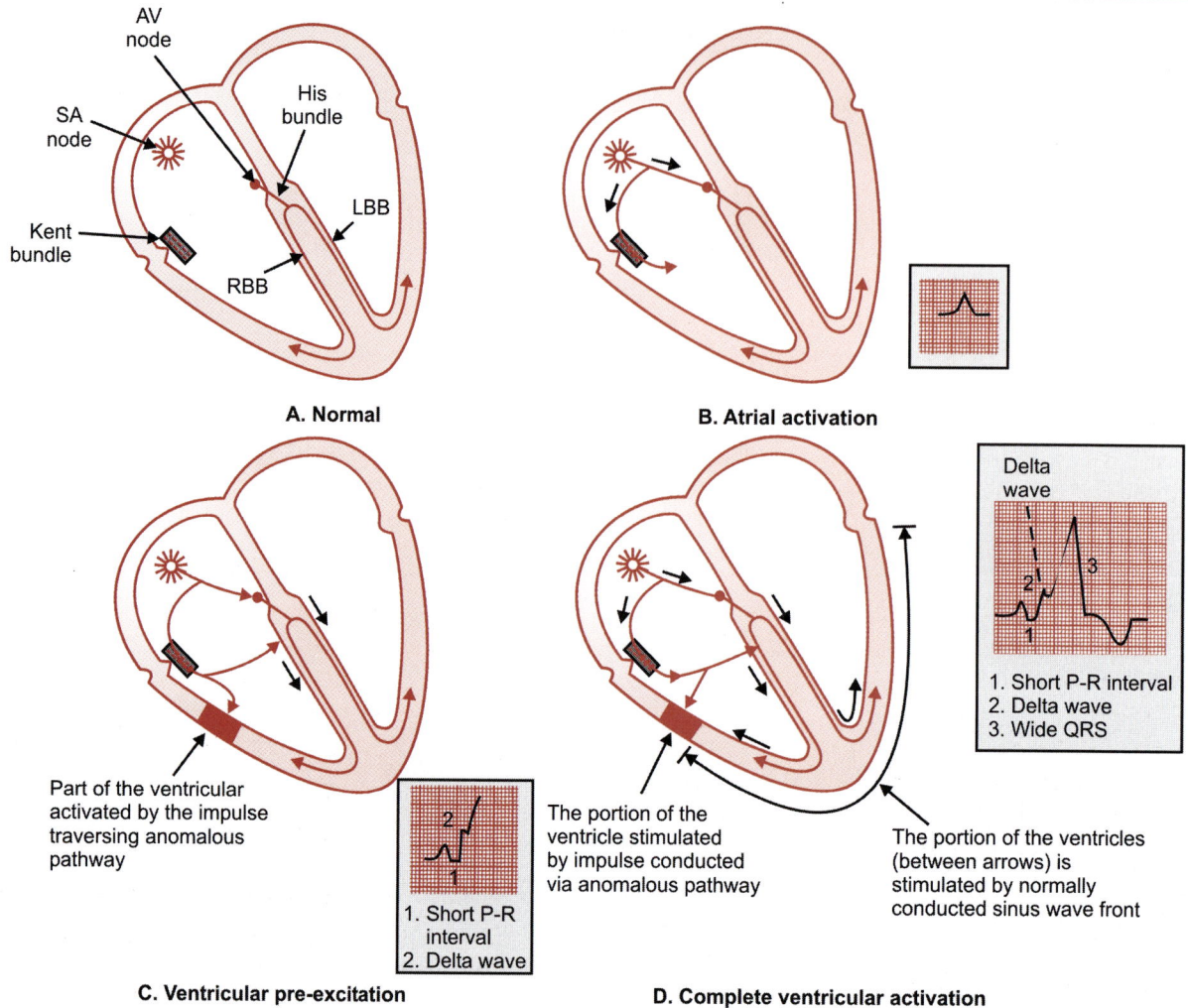

A. Normal

B. Atrial activation

C. Ventricular pre-excitation

Part of the ventricular
activated by the impulse
traversing anomalous
pathway

1. Short P-R
   interval
2. Delta wave

D. Complete ventricular activation

The portion of the
ventricle stimulated
by impulse conducted
via anomalous pathway

The portion of the ventricles
(between arrows) is
stimulated by normally
conducted sinus wave front

Delta
wave

1. Short P-R interval
2. Delta wave
3. Wide QRS

Fig. 22.2: A classic WPW syndrome pathogenesis (diagram). The conduction proceeds through anomalous pathway. **A:** Anatomy of basic anomalous pathway. **B:** *Atrial activation* producing a normal P wave. **C:** *Ventricular activation (pre-excitation).* A part of the ventricle (shaded) is activated prematurely by a part of activation front that has traversed the anomalous tract to reach the ventricle earlier than normal sinus activation front. The short P-R interval and delta wave indicate premature excitation of ventricle through the accessory pathway. **D:** *Completed activation of ventricles.* The unshaded part of the ventricles is activated by the normally conducted sinus impulses, thus ventricular activation process is completed leading to wide QRS

Therefore, the whole cardiac activation takes place in three phases as follows;

1. Atrial activation
2. Ventricular pre-excitation
3. Terminal ventricular activation after initial pre-excitation to complete the process of activation.

1. *Atrial activation:* Atrial activation is normal from SA node to atria resulting in normal P waves (Fig. 22.2B).

2. *Ventricular premature excitation or pre-excitation:* In classic WPW syndrome (bundle of Kent); the

sinus beat or activation front arbitrarily splits into two fronts; one passing through the anomalous tract and the other passing through the normal conduction pathway. The conduction occurs simultaneously through both the pathways. The part of activation front passing through the bypass tract reaches the ventricles earlier than the front travelling through normal pathway. This is because of the fact that anomalous pathway does not delay the impulse; while AV node delays the other activation front due to its inherent property - the net result is a short P-R interval.

Once the impulse conducted through the anomalous pathway reaches one of the ventricles earlier and excites it prematurely, the onward activation of the ventricle occurs through normal ordinary myocardial tissue which is poor and slow conducting medium than the highly specialised normal Purkinje system. Pre-excitation is, therefore, slow and bizarre which inscribes a bizarre delta wave on QRS complex (Fig. 22.2C), the amplitude of which varies depending on the size of the ventricular muscle mass activated by the impulse reaching through the bypass tract.

3. *Terminal ventricular activation:* The initial ventricular activation by pre-excitation wave is completed by activation front that has passed normally through the AV node, bundle of His and Purkinje system. In this way, the terminal part of ventricular activation occurs normally, hence, QRS deflection is wide due to fusion of normal and abnormal activation fronts (Fig. 22.2D).

To summarise, the QRS in classic WPW syndrome is, thus, a form of fusion complex – a complex resulting from a part activation of the ventricles by an impulse conducted through an anomalous pathway and a part activation of the ventricles by the impulse conducted through the normal pathway. In some instances, especially in the presence of AV conduction delay, the entire ventricular mass may be activated by the impulse travelling through the accessory pathway, and the entire QRS complex then becomes essentially a delta wave (Fig. 22.3B).

Diagnostic Clues to Classic WPW Syndrome

- A short P-R interval (< 0.12 sec)
- A wide QRS complex (> 0.12 sec)
- A delta wave (positive or negative) depending on the orientation of QRS
- A normal P- J interval.

Variations in ECG Pattern of WPW Type of Conduction

Two variations which commonly occur are;

1. *Short P-R Interval with Wide QRS and Shortened P-J Interval (Atrioventricular Conduction)*

It is postulated that the pre-excitation wave in this type stimulates the ventricles and process of ventricular activation is completed before the sinus conducted beat reaches the ventricles through the normal pathways. This explains the short P-R interval, wide QRS complex and shortened P-J interval. In this variation, the entire QRS complex becomes essentially a delta wave (Fig. 22.3B).

2. *Short P-R Interval, Normal QRS Complex and Short P-J Interval (Atrionodal or Atrio-His Conduction)*

It can be explained when conduction occurs through the fibres that bypass the AV node, enter and activate the bundle of His (atriohistian pathway) prematurely

SECTION EIGHT

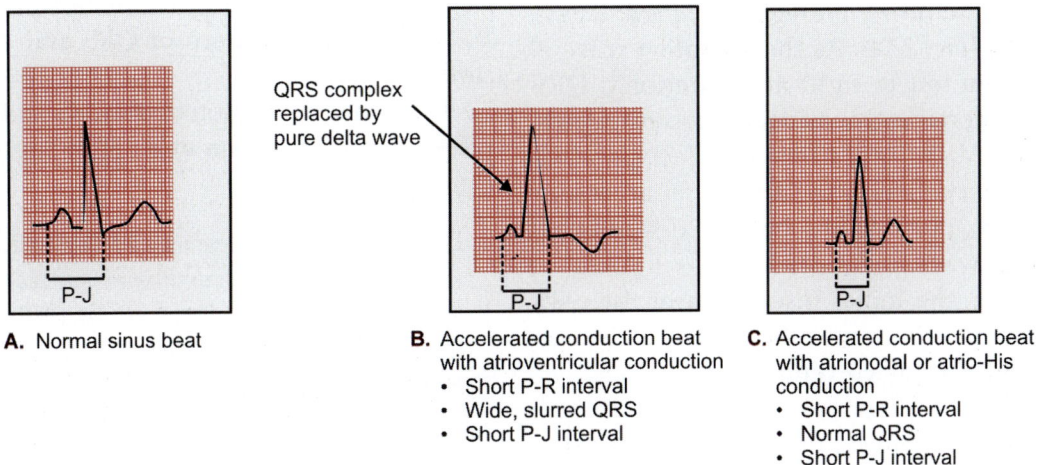

QRS complex replaced by pure delta wave

A. Normal sinus beat

B. Accelerated conduction beat with atrioventricular conduction
- Short P-R interval
- Wide, slurred QRS
- Short P-J interval

C. Accelerated conduction beat with atrionodal or atrio-His conduction
- Short P-R interval
- Normal QRS
- Short P-J interval

Fig. 22.3: Variations in electrocardiographic patterns of WPW syndrome

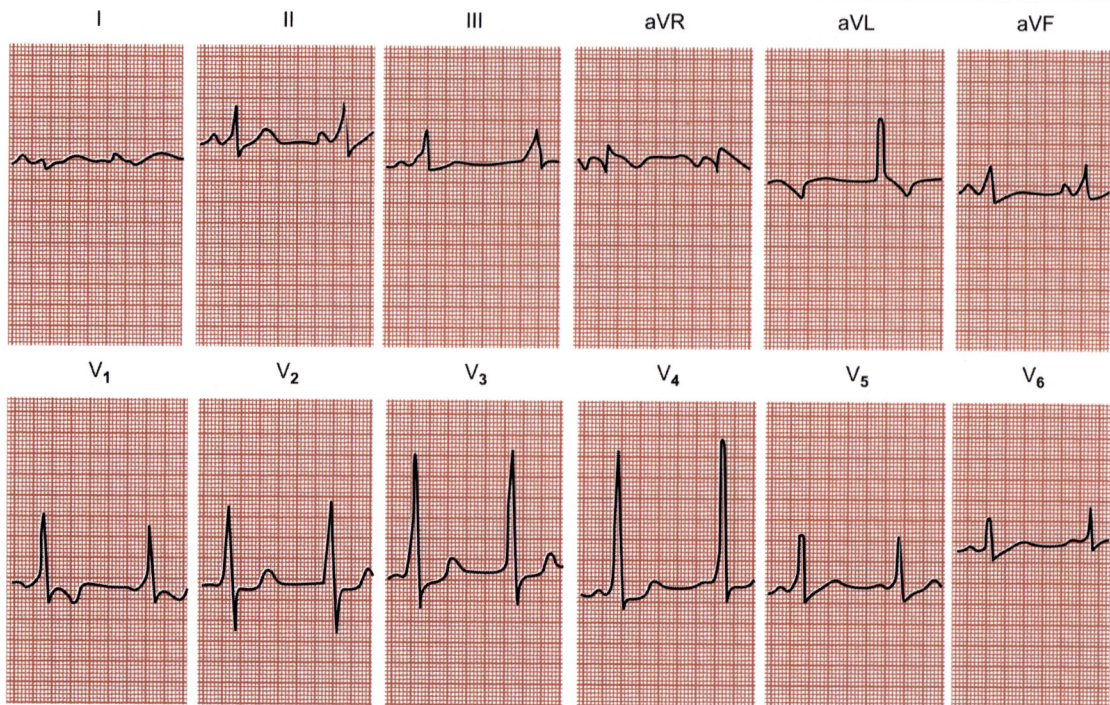

Fig. 22.4: WPW syndrome (Type A). The ECG shows: (i) left axis deviation (The lead II has equiphasic complex and aVL has maximum positive deflection) (ii) tall R waves in right precordial leads (V$_1$-V$_3$) indicating left to right ventricular activation (left sided accessory pathway), (iii) short P-R interval (0.10 sec), (iv) wide QRS (>0.12 sec) and (v) initial slurring of R waves in leads, II, III, aVF and V$_1$-V$_5$ due to presence of delta wave

and ventricular activation is completed in a normal fashion. The P-QRS-R complexes are normal except short P-R interval (Fig. 22.3C). This type of conduction occurs in Lown-Gonong–Levine syndrome-A WPW variant.

Rosenbaum Classification of WPW Syndrome

1. *Type A pre-excitation through left lateral accessory pathway (Fig. 22.4).* As the excitation wave is spreading from left to right and anteriorly, QRS complexes are dominantly positive in precordial leads V$_1$-V$_3$. Leads V$_4$-V$_6$ will always reflect positive deflection irrespective of the site of an accessory pathway, hence, there will be positive deflection of QRS and delta wave from V$_1$ to V$_6$.

In this type, the initial inscription of the QRS complex and the delta wave reflects early activation of the posterior part of left ventricle.

In type A WPW syndrome, the QRS complexes and delta waves are positive in leads V$_1$ and V$_2$

2. *Type B pre-excitation through right lateral accessory pathway (Fig. 22.5).* The pre-excitation wave and QRS forces in this type of WPW syndrome are oriented to the left and superiorly due to their respective axis deviation, therefore;

Superior deviation of both axes (QRS and delta wave axis) results in main negative deflection of QRS from V$_1$ to V$_3$ with negative delta wave. The leads V$_4$–V$_6$ will have pattern of QRS and delta waves similar to type A.

The initial inscription of the QRS and delta wave reflects early activation of anterior-superior part of right ventricle.

Due to superior axis deviation of QRS and delta wave in both types of WPW syndrome (type A and B), their orientation in standard leads (II, III, aVF, I and aVL) is more or less similar. The only differentiating feature between the two is; positive QRS and delta wave deflections in type A and negative in type B in leads V$_1$ or V$_1$-V$_3$. The pattern in leads V$_4$-V$_6$ remains constant in both the types.

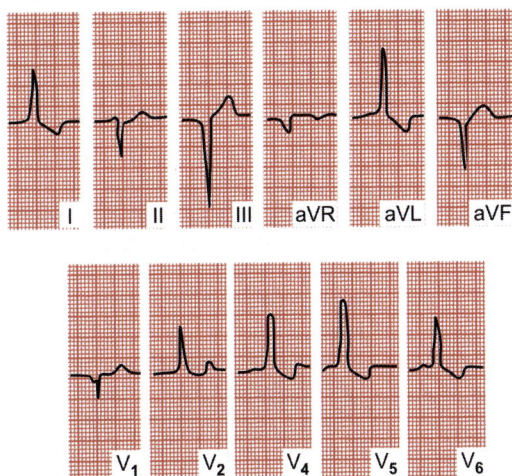

Fig. 22.5: WPW syndrome (type B). The ECG shows: (i) left axis deviation of > −30°, (ii) upstroke of R waves is slurred in leads I, aVL and V_2-V_6 due to presence of delta waves, (iii) there is positive deflection of both QRS and delta wave from V_2-V_6 with negative deflection in V_1 which indicates right sided accessory pathway and lead V_1 is situated lateral to it, (iv) a short P-R interval (0.10 sec) and (v) associated ST-T changes—ST depression and T wave inversion in leads with positive QRS deflection, i.e. leads I, aVL, V_2-V_6 and ST elevation with upright T wave in leads with negative QRS (leads II, III, aVF and V_1) due to orientation of ST-T vectors opposite to QRS in WPW syndrome

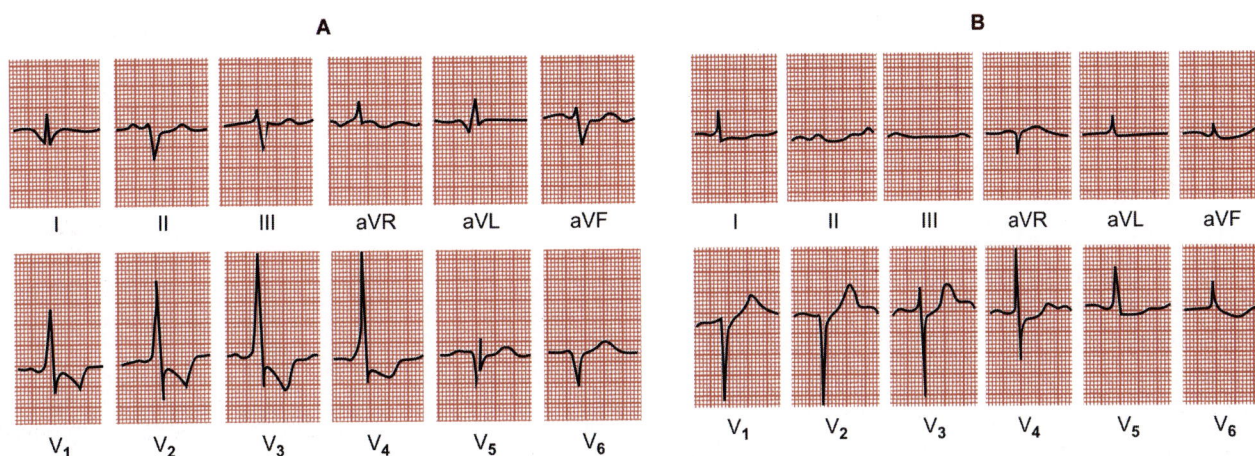

Fig. 22.6: WPW syndrome (Type C) simulating posterolateral infarction.

A: WPW conduction. The ECG shows a short P-R interval, wide QRS and delta waves on upstroke of R waves—WPW conduction. Type C is characterised by a negative delta wave (simulating q wave in lateral leads I, aVL, V_5-V_6, indicating pre-excitation of lateral wall of left ventricle. Right precordial leads (V_1-V_2) show tall wide R waves which pass through V_3-V_4. This pattern reflects spread of excitation forces from left to right side. The ST segment depression and T waves inversion in leads V_1-V_4 indicates a secondary change due to pre-excitation itself.

Note: The ECG can be confused with posterolateral infarction itself if negative delta waves in V_5-V_6 are misinterpreted as q waves of lateral infarction and tall R waves in right precordial leads may be misdiagnosed as posterior wall infarction. Remember, the tall R waves of posterior wall infarction are just limited to V_1 or maximum to lead V_2 but not beyond that. Secondly tall R wave of infarction will have upright tall T wave rather than inverted T wave seen in this ECG. Similarly, there are no evolutionary ST-T changes (ST elevation and T inversion) suggestive of lateral wall infarction.

B: The ECG recorded at different time from the same patient during resumption of sinus rhythm shows disappearance of delta waves (misinterpreted as q waves) which were seen in Figure 22.6A. There is normal R wave progression from V_1-V_4, i.e. tall R waves seen in A have also disappeared. The T wave inversion is seen in leads I, aVL, V_5-V_6, which is probably due to primary myocardial disease, which were earlier masked in previous ECG (A) by upright T waves in these leads.

All these features suggest WPW syndrome (type C) simulating pattern of posterolateral infarction, can lead to wrong diagnosis if serial ECGs are not recorded

3. Type C WPW syndrome (Fig. 22.6): This was not included in Rosenbaum classification but has been described. It is characterised by a negative delta wave in left lateral leads.

Various Accessory Pathways

Studies using surface potential mapping, epicardial mapping during surgery and various electrophysiological studies have identified a number of accessory pathways. Presence of more than one QRS pattern in an individual patient suggests the possibility of multiple bypass tracts. A short P-R interval with a normal QRS complex accompanied by paroxysmal supraventricular tachycardia has been suggested as a variant of WPW syndrome (Lown - Ganong - Levine syndrome).

It has become clear that bypass tract (bundle of Kent) in WPW syndrome may be situated any where along the AV ring. Rosenbaum and his associates (1945) first attempted to localise bypass tracts, separating them into type A- a left bypass tract and type B -a right bypass tract. The classification proposed by Rosenbaum is nowadays no longer acceptable because recent advances in electrophysiology and epicardial mapping have suggested many other accessory pathways which can be localised on surface 12 lead ECG. More than 90% bypass tracts, however, occur at 4 main sites;
1. Right lateral pathway (13%)
2. Left lateral pathway (45%)
3. Posteroseptal pathway (right or left). These two groups constitute 30-35% cases
4. Anteroseptal pathway (right or left). These are least common.

The electrocardiographic patterns in relation to different main sites of an accessory pathway (Kent bundle) are tabulated (Table 22.1).

Decision Making Leads and Parameters in Localisation of an Accessory Tract (Fig. 22.7)

Polarity of QRS in leads V_1 to V_3 and axis deviation of QRS and delta wave are helpful in diagnosing the direction of conduction through the accessory pathway.
1. Negative deflection of QRS and delta waves in leads V_1-V_3 with left axis deviation of QRS on frontal plane indicates right lateral accessory pathway. If there is normal QRS axis, then it indicates right anteroseptal pathway (Table 22.2).
2. Positive QRS in leads V_1-V_3 with left axis deviation of QRS on frontal plane indicates left posteroseptal accessory pathway. When QRS axis is deviated to left and inferiorly, it indicates left lateral pathway (Table 22.2).

Table 22.1: The location of various accessory pathways and their electrocardiographic patterns

Accessory pathways	ECG patterns
1. Left lateral	The QRS and the delta wave axes are deviated rightwards and inferiorly, hence, leads I and aVL will record negative QRS and delta waves, while leads II, III and aVF will record positive QRS deflections with positive delta waves. Leads V_1-V_3 will register upward QRS deflections with positive delta waves. As pattern of leads V_4-V_6 does not change during the conduction through the accessory pathway, therefore, there will be positive deflections of QRS and delta wave from V_1 to V_6
2. Right lateral	This is equivalent to type B WPW syndrome as already discussed (Fig. 22.5)
3. Right anteroseptal	There is normal to inferior axis. The delta waves and QRS complexes are upright in leads I, II, aVL, aVF, isoelectric in lead III and negative in aVR. The QRS and delta waves are negative in leads V_1 and V_2
4. Right posteroseptal	The main pre-excitation front is travelling from right to left, it produces left axis deviation of QRS and delta wave. There will be negative QRS deflections with negative delta waves in leads II, III and aVF, with positive deflections in leads I and aVL. As the lead V_1 is situated just right to the accessory pathway, hence, it will record either negative or equiphasic QRS and delta waves (an important diagnostic feature). The rest of the precordial leads from V_2 to V_6 will show positive QRS and delta waves (Fig. 22.8)
5. Left posteroseptal	The left posteroseptal pathway conduction is equivalent to type A WPW syndrome as already discussed (Fig. 22.4)

Comment: Dominantly negative QRS in V_1 and dominantly positive QRS in V_2 indicates right posteroseptal pathway; while main positive deflection in both V_1 and V_2 indicates left posteroseptal accessory

Table 22.2: Main QRS deflections in leads V_1 to V_3 and polarity of QRS and delta waves axes in different accessory pathway

Site of accessory pathway	Main QRS deflection			QRS and delta waves axes	
	V_1	V_2	V_3		
Anteroseptal	(−)	(−)	(−)	Normal	
Right lateral	(−)	(−)	(−)	Left	
Right posteroseptal	(−)	(+)	(+)	Left	The differentiating feature between the two is QRS deflection in V_1 (Read comments)
Left posteroseptal	(+)	(+)	(+)	Left	
Left lateral	(+)	(+)	(+)	Left, inferior	

(−) Negative   (+) Positive

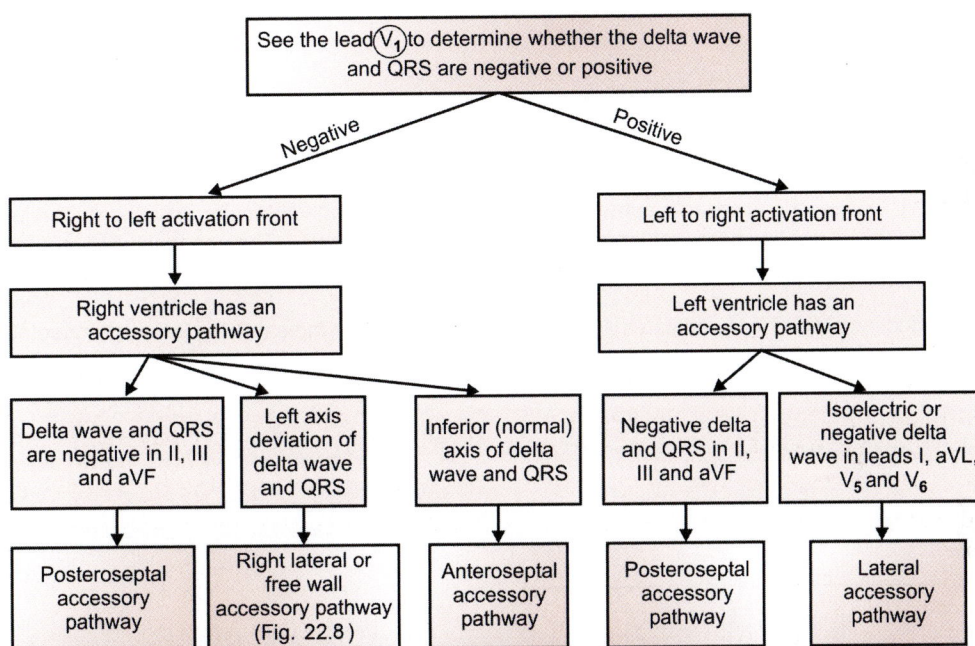

Fig. 22.7: Flow chart for localisation of accessory pathway

pathway. Therefore, V_1 and V_2 are decision making leads in right and left posteroseptal pathways. For quick decision making process in localisation of an accessory pathway, read the flow chart (Fig. 22.7).

Intermittent WPW syndrome (Fig. 22.9)

The WPW syndrome may be permanent or intermittent. The intermittent WPW syndrome may occur periodically in a haphazard fashion or it may occur regularly. For example, a WPW syndrome with 2:1 conduction will be regular where every alternate beat reflects WPW pattern.

Complications

1. Reciprocating tachycardia
2. Atrial fibrillation

1. *Reciprocating Rhythm and Tachycardia (Read Chapter 36)*

The wide QRS tachycardia in patients with pre-excitation syndrome can be due to multiple mechanisms;

(i) Sinus or atrial tachycardia, AV node re-entry, atrial flutter or fibrillation with antegrade conduction over the accessory pathway

SECTION EIGHT

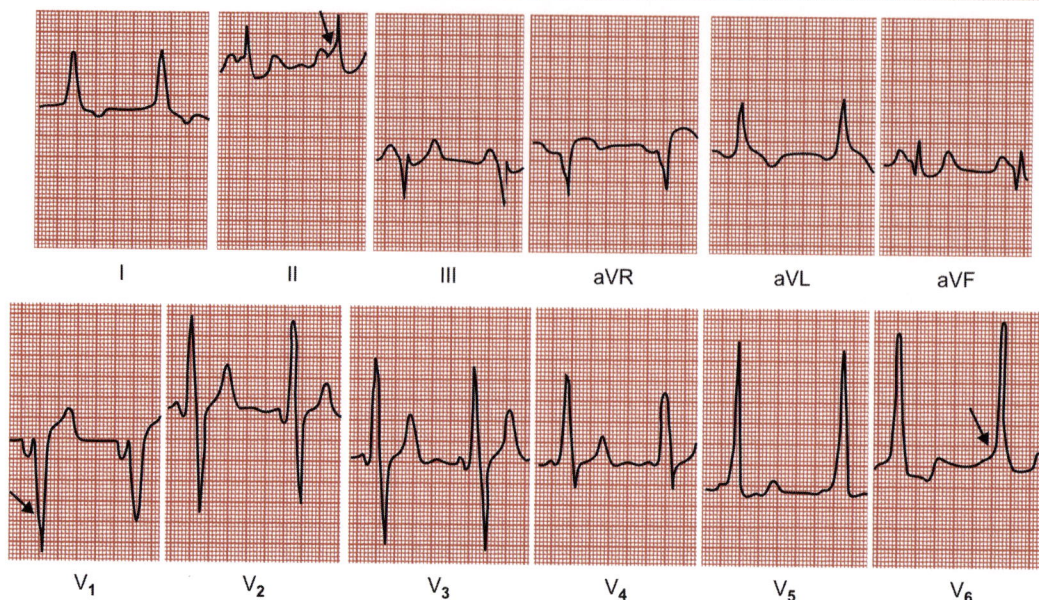

I II III aVR aVL aVF

V$_1$ V$_2$ V$_3$ V$_4$ V$_5$ V$_6$

Fig. 22.8: WPW conduction through the right posteroseptal accessory pathway. The ECG shows, (i) Left axis deviation of QRS, (ii) A short P-R interval, wide QRS and delta waves (some delta waves are indicated by arrows) seen in most of the leads indicate WPW conduction. The negative QRS and negative delta waves in leads III and aVF (inferior leads) and positive QRS and delta waves in leads I and aVL localise the accessory pathway to right side (right to left ventricular activation). The left axis deviation of QRS and delta wave suggest right posteroseptal/right free wall accessory pathway. The negative QRS in V$_1$ (decision making lead) and positive QRS from V$_2$-V$_6$ indicate right posteroseptal pathway activation and lead V$_1$ is situated just right to the accessory pathway.

Note: The negative deflection of QRS in V$_1$ indicates right, and positive deflection indicates the left posteroseptal pathway (Table 22.2)

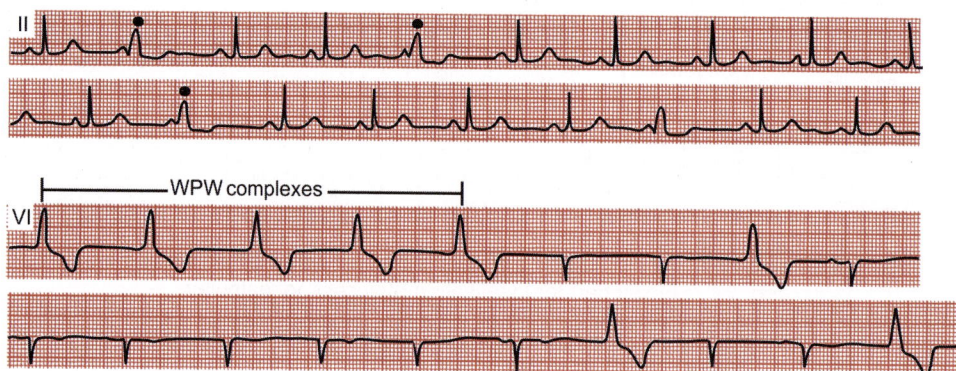

Fig. 22.9: Intermittent WPW syndrome. The continuous ECG leads (II and V$_1$) show a normal sinus rhythm (normal P wave, P-R interval followed by narrow QRS), and interspersed wide QRS complexes with delta wave, a short P-R interval (<0.10 sec) and inverted T waves suggest intermittent WPW syndrome. Some of WPW complexes are indicated by black dot at the top. The lead V$_1$ in the beginning shows 5 consecutive complexes with WPW conduction

(ii) Orthodromic reciprocating tachycardia with functional or pre-existing bundle branch block

(iii) Antidromic reciprocating tachycardia

(iv) Reciprocating tachycardia with antegrade conduction through one accessory pathway and retrograde conduction through another accessory pathway (multiple accessory pathways present).

2. Atrial Fibrillation in WPW Syndrome (Fig. 22.10)

The retrograde return of the impulse through the accessory pathway, on an occasion, may be so rapid

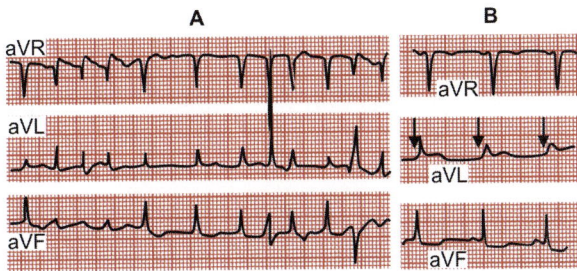

Fig. 22.10: WPW syndrome with atrial fibrillation. The ECG leads (aVR, aVL and aVF) show: **A:** There is variable P-R intervals indicating atrial fibrillation. No fibrillation waves are seen. The ventricular rate at times, is fast (>200/min) and no delta wave is seen indicating direct transmission of atrial impulses to ventricles via bypass tract. **B:** The ECG taken after resumption of normal rhythm shows QRS complexes with WPW conduction (short P-R, delta waves indicated by arrows) suggesting that WPW syndrome was the underlying cause of atrial fibrillation in this case

that the atria are stimulated for the second time before they have completely recovered from their antegrade activation by the sinus impulse. In other words, if the atria are stimulated repeatedly during the end period of recovery, atrial fibrillation results. Once the atrial fibrillation has been precipitated, then, an antegrade conduction to the ventricle occurs rapidly through the accessory pathway leading to a rapid ventricular rate of more than 200 bpm (most common). Antegrade conduction through the normal AV nodal pathway, in such a situation will be rare.

Differential Diagnosis of WPW Syndrome on ECG

The WPW syndrome may mimic electrocardiographically with other diseases, some of which are considered below with their main differentiating features:

1. *Right ventricular hypertrophy:* The tall R wave in right precordial leads (V_1 and V_2) occurs both in WPW syndrome and right ventricular hypertrophy. The distinguishing features of right ventricular hypertrophy are;
   i) There may be clinical evidence of right ventricular hypertrophy (RVH)
   ii) Invariably, there is a right axis deviation in RVH which is less common in WPW syndrome
   iii) There may be concomitant right atrial hypertrophy (P pulmonale) in RVH
   iv) Normal P-R interval
   v) Absence of delta waves.

2. *Posterior wall myocardial infarction:* True posterior wall myocardial infarction leads to tall R waves in right precordial leads which may simulate some forms of WPW syndrome. The distinguishing features of posterior wall infarction are;
   i) Associated tall upright symmetric T waves in leads showing tall R waves (V_1 and V_2)
   ii) Evidence of associated lateral wall or inferior wall infarction (ST segment depression/elevation and T wave inversion)
   iii) Normal P-R interval
   iv) Absence of delta wave
   v) A clinical evidence of myocardial infarction.

3. *Anterolateral and inferior wall infarction:* The negative delta wave of WPW syndrome may simulate q wave of infarction. The negative delta waves, if appear in leads I and aVL, simulate anterolateral infarction and, if present in leads II, III and aVF, simulate inferior wall infarction (Fig. 22.11). In such a situation, the typical ST-T changes of infarction (ST elevation with T inversion) with clinical history of myocardial infarction and raised myocardial enzymes help to distinguish it from WPW syndrome.

4. *Bundle branch block:* The initial positive delta waves in some leads may be so distinct and separated from QRS by a distinct notch, thereby producing QRS complexes resembling bundle branch block, particularly right bundle branch block. The shortened P-R interval, classical delta waves slurring in other leads, absence of a heart disease and normal terminal part of QRS differentiates WPW syndrome from bundle branch block.

5. *Ventricular tachycardia:* When supraventricular tachycardia or atrial fibrillation shows aberrant intraventricular conduction in WPW syndrome, it gives rise to a series of bizarre QRS complexes which resemble ventricular tachycardia. The characteristic features of atrial fibrillation or supraventricular tachycardia with aberration in WPW syndrome which differentiate it from ventricular tachycardia are;
   i) The rhythm is completely irregular if atrial fibrillation is the underlying rhythm
   ii) The presence of isolated normal QRS complexes

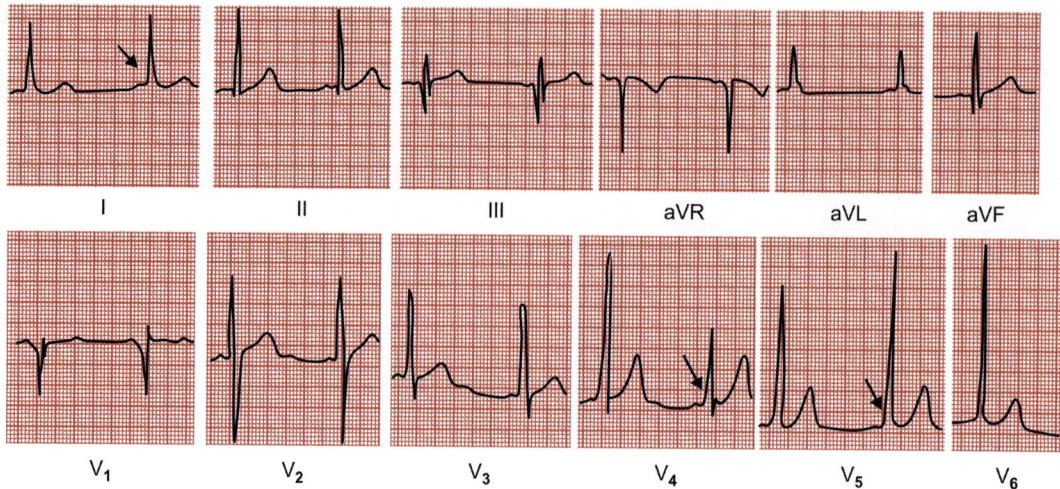

Fig. 22.11: WPW syndrome simulating inferior wall infarction. The ECG shows a short P-R interval, wide QRS and delta waves in leads I, V_4-V_6 (some of them are indicated by arrows) indicating WPW syndrome, the negative delta waves seen in II, III and aVF may be confused with q waves of inferior infarction. The T wave is upright in these leads which negate the existence of infarction. The negative delta wave in V_1 and leads II, III and aVF suggest right free wall accessory pathway. The detailed conduction studies are needed to confirm pre-excitation and localisation of the bypass tract

iii) The presence of occasional WPW fusion complexes

iv) In fact, there will be two types of wide QRS complexes. Some wide complexes will exhibit bundle branch block pattern due to aberrant conduction, while other complexes may exhibit WPW type of pattern. These complexes will be easily recognised if a beat or few beats show normal conduction

v) Rapid ventricular rate (> 200 bpm)

vi) The QRS morphology of bizarre complexes due to WPW conduction will be upright in leads V_1 and V_2 as well as in V_5-V_6.

WPW VARIANTS

1. WPW Syndrome with Normal P-R Interval (Mahaim Fibres Pre-excitation)

Two varieties of congenital Mahaim fibres (Fig. 22.12) include;

A. Nodoventricular or nodofascicular fibres: These arise from the AV node and get inserted either into the ventricle (nodoventricular) or into right bundle branch (nodofascicular). Nodoventricular connections can be involved in tachycardias (Fig. 22.13).

Mechanism of pre-excitation: A normal sinus beat passes through the AV node and bundle of His with physiological delay in the AV node, now passes

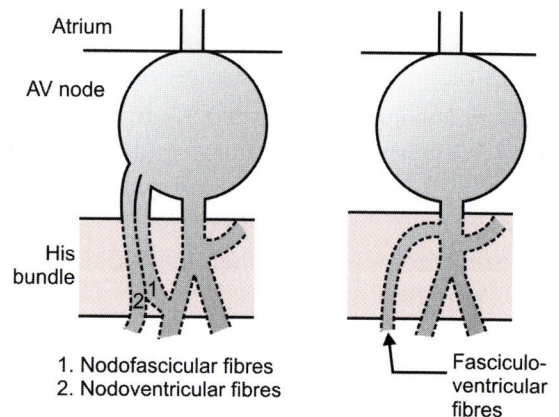

Fig. 22.12: Schematic representation of two types of congenital Mahaim fibres with pre-excitation.

A. *Nodofascicular or nodoventricular pathway.* The impulse in this type of fibre travels down the ventricle through the accessory pathway with retrograde conduction to atrial through bundle branches, bundle of His and AV node. The conduction sequence is: Bundle branch—His bundle—AV node—atria.

B. *Fasciculoventricular pathway.* The impulse travels down through the normal pathway to the ventricle with retrograde conduction to the fascicle. This pathway rarely produce tachycardia

rapidly through the nodoventricular fibres of Mahaim to the ventricles, exciting them prematurely (pre-excitation). The P-R interval in this type of pre-excitation will be normal because conduction upto the bundle of His occurs through the normal pathway.

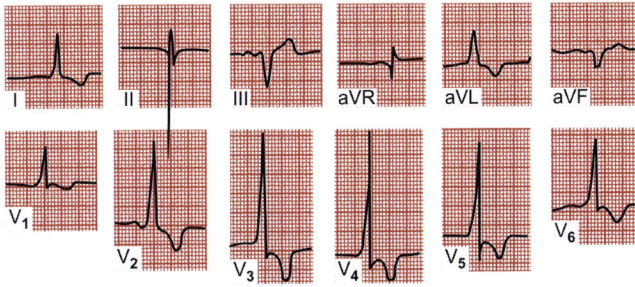

Fig. 22.13: Accelerated condition through nodofascicular (Mahaim) fibres. The ECG shows (i) A positive delta wave (pre-excitation wave) on the upstroke of R waves in leads I, aVL and V₁-V₆, (ii) A negative delta wave in leads II, III and aVF simulating q waves of infarction but there are no evolutionary changes of infarction, (iii) The P-R interval is normal indicating normal conduction from SA node to AV node and (iv) The WPW complexes are wide due to fusion of delta wave with QRS. *Conclusion:* The presence of delta wave indicates pre-excitation through a bypass tract. The superior orientation of delta wave (negative in II,III and aVF) indicates excitation front away from AV node. The normal P-R interval indicates that AV is not bypassed. All these suggest that there is abnormal connection between AV node and ventricles (nodoventricular fibre)

There will be a delta wave on QRS with normal P-J interval in this type of Mahaim fibres conduction because QRS complex is a fusion complex similar to WPW syndrome.

This Mahaim type of pre-excitation is appreciated in the presence of first and second degree AV block with prolonged P-R intervals. If any beat has normal P-R interval where other sinus conducted beats have prolonged P-R intervals, indicates Mahaim type of conduction.

Recent successful surgical interruption of accessory pathway in patients with apparent nodoventricular or nodofascicular pathways has led to a reappraisal of the anatomy with the suggestion that there are right atrioventricular accessory pathway with AV node like conduction properties.

B. *Fasciculoventricular fibres:* The fibres arise in His bundle or bundle branches and get inserted into the ventricular myocardium. Fasciculoventricular fibres generally are not involved in tachycardia. These types of Mahaim fibres produce a normal P-R interval and a fixed anomalous QRS complexes.

2. The Lown-Ganong-Levine (LGL) Syndrome (James bundle pre-excitation)

The LGL syndrome, a variant of WPW syndrome, is characterised by normal P waves, short P-R intervals and normal QRS complexes without delta waves. This syndrome is due to presence of James bundle as an accessory pathway which arises in the atria, bypasses the AV node and main bundle of His and joins the distal end of His bundle (Fig. 22.14).

Mode of conduction: The sinus beat passes through the atria normally and produces normal P wave. It now bypasses the AV node and enters the bundle of His distally, hence, produces a short P-R interval. Subsequent conduction to the ventricles is through normal pathway, hence, QRS complexes are normal. As the impulses passing through the James bundle do not reach the ventricle early, premature excitation of ventricles does not occur, therefore, there are no delta waves.

However, like WPW syndrome, it can induce reciprocating tachycardia or atrial fibrillation due to the presence of a facility for retrograde conduction (Fig. 22.15).

Summary

The electrocardiographic features of ventricular pre-excitation syndromes are summarised in Table 22.3.

SECTION EIGHT

Table 22.3: ECG findings in ventricular pre-excitation syndromes			
ECG finding	*WPW conduction*	*Intra-AV nodal atrionodal or atrio-His conduction (LGL syndrome)*	*Nodoventricular nodofascicular conduction (Mahaim fibre conduction)*
1. P-R interval	Short (<0.12sec)	Short	Normal
2. QRS duration	Wide (>0.12 sec)	Normal	Wide
3. Secondary ST-T changes	Yes	No	Yes
4. Delta wave	Yes	No	Yes

SECTION EIGHT

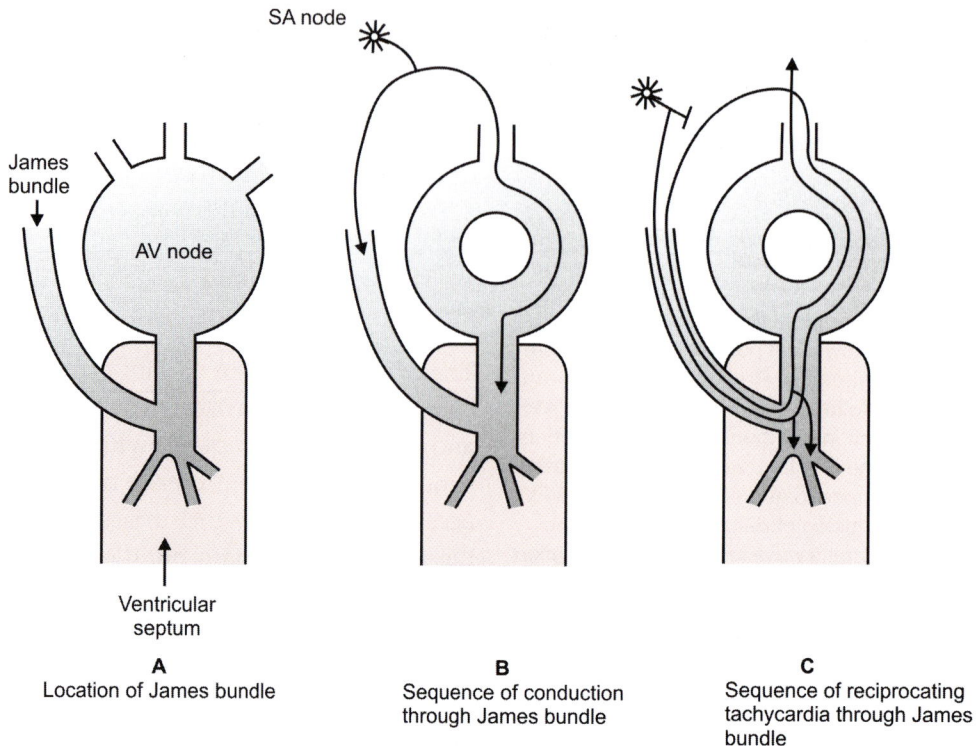

Fig. 22.14: Schematic representation of pre-excitation through a James bundle—an accessory (Atriohistian) pathway in Lown-Ganong-Levine syndrome. **A:** Location of James bundle. **B:** Sequence of conduction through James bundle. **C:** Conduction sequence through James bundle in Lown-Ganong-Levine syndrome (Atriohistian conduction)

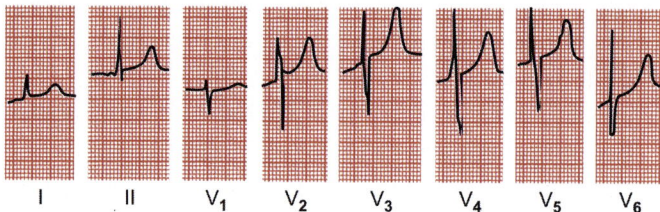

Fig. 22.15: Lown-Ganong-Levine syndrome. The ECG (leads I, II and V_1-V_6) shows a short P-R interval, normal QRS with no delta wave

Suggested Reading

1. Braunwald E: A Text book of Cardiovascular Medicine, 4th edn, Philadelphia: WB Saunders Publication 1992.
2. Wolff L, Parkinson J, White PD: Bundle branch block with short P-R interval in healthy young people prone to paroxysmal tachycardia. *Am Heart J* **5**: 685, 1930.
3. Rosenbaum FF, Hecht HH, Wilson FN et al: The potential variations of the thorax and the oesophagus in anomalous atrioventricular excitation (Wolff-Parkinson-Whole syndrome). *Am Heart J* **29**: 281, 1945.
4. Mangiafico RA, Petralito A, Grimoldi DR: Alternating WPW syndrome associated with an attack of angina. *J Electrocardiol* **23**:255, 1990.
5. Giorgi C, Ackaoni A, Nadean R et al: Wolff–Parkinson–White: VCG patterns that mimic other cardiac pathologies: A correlative study with the pre-excitation pathway localisation. *Am Heart J* **111**: 891, 1986.
6. Kent AFS: Observation on the auriculo-ventricular function of the mammalian heart. *Quart J Exp Physiol* **7**: 193, 1913.
7. Klein GJ, Guiraudon GM, Kerr CR et al: Non-ventricular accessory pathway: Evidence for a distinct accessory atrioventricular pathway with atrioventricular node like properties. *Angiology* **39**: 307, 1988.
8. Tchon P, Lehmann MH, Jazayeri M et al: Atrio fascicular connection or a nodoventricular Mahaim fibre? Electrophysiologic evolution of the pathway and associated reentrant circuit. *Circulation* **77**: 837, 1988.
9. Leitch J, Klein GL: New concepts on nodoventricular accessory pathways. *J Cardiovascul. Electrophysiol* **1**: 220, 1990.
10. Wellens HJJ, Brugada PC, Penn OC et al: Pre-excitation syndrome. In Zipes DP, Jalife J (Eds): Cardiac electrophysiology from cell to bed side. Philadelphia: WB Saunders Company 691, 1990.

11. Szabo TS, Klein GJ, Guirandon GM et al: Localisation of accessory pathway in the Wolff-Parkinson-White syndrome. PACE, **12**: 1691, 1989.

12. Yuan S, Iwa T, Bando T, Bando H: Comparative study of eight sets of ECG criteria for localisation of the accessory pathway in Wolff-Parkinson-White syndrome. *J Electrocardiol* **25**: 203, 1992.

13. Fisch C: Electrocardiography. In Braunwald - 'Heart Disease' - A Textbook of Cardiovascular Medicine, 5th edn. Vol I, Philadelphia: WB Saunders Company 1997, 4, 126.

14. Shir HT, Miles WM, Klein LS et al: Multiple accessory pathways in permanent forms of junctional reciprocating tachycardia. *Am J Cardiol* **73**: 396, 1994.

15. Xie B, Heald SC, Bashir V et al: Localisation of accessory pathways from the 12 lead electrocardiogram using a new algorith. *Am J Cardiol* **74**: 161, 1994.

16. Rodriguez LM, Smeets JL, deChillou C et al: The 12 lead ECG in midseptal, anteroseptal, posteroseptal and right free wall accessory pathways. *Am J Cardiol* **72**: 1274, 1993.

23

Hypertrophic Cardiomyopathy

- *Definition and aetiology*
- *Subtypes*
- *Pathogenesis of electrocardiographic manifestations*
- *The electrocardiogram in various subtypes of hypertrophic cardiomyopathy*

SECTION EIGHT

Although first described about a century ago but its unique features were not studied systematically until 1950s. Earlier, it was defined as an inappropriate hypertrophy of the myocardium that occurred in the absence of an obvious cause (e.g. aortic stenosis or systemic hypertension), predominantly involving the interventricular septum (asymmetric hypertrophy) of a nondilated left ventricle that showed hyperdynamic functions. A dynamic pressure gradient was demonstrated in the subaortic area that divided the left ventricle into high pressure apical region and low pressure subaortic area. At that time, many popular terms were used out of curiosity, the commonly employed were idiopathic hypertrophic subaortic stenosis (IHSS) and muscular subaortic stenosis. Subsequent studies have revealed that outflow gradient occurs just in a minority of patients. Nowadays, hypertrophic cardiomyopathy is preferred term because majority of patients do not have an outflow gradient or stenosis of left ventricular outflow tract. The hypertrophic cardiomyopathy produces diastolic rather than systolic dysfunction, characterised by abnormal stiffness of left ventricle with resultant impaired ventricular filling.

Definition

A heredofamilial disorder of autosomal dominant type, is characterised by asymmetric hypertrophy of the ventricular myocardium; predominantly of the left ventricle and rarely of the right ventricle. Hypertrophy of left ventricle may involve frequently the interventricular septum and/or the free wall of the left ventricle leading to reduction in the size of left ventricular cavity. The hypertrophy, uncommonly, may involve apical region and/or parabasal regions. The hypertrophy may be symptomatic or asymptomatic, and may or may not produce obstruction to the left ventricular outflow.

Aetiology

The cause of myocardial hypertrophy in HCM is still ambiguous. Various mechanisms proposed are:

1. *Abnormal calcium fluxes.* There is increased in number of calcium channels leading to abnormal calcium fluxes with resultant increase in intracellular calcium concentration.
2. *Abnormal sympathetic stimulation.* It may be due to both increased responsiveness of myocardium to catecholamines and excessive production of catecholamines.
3. *Abnormal thickening of intramural coronary arteries.* Thickening of coronary arteries leads to relative myocardial ischaemia resulting in fibrosis and compensatory ventricular hypertrophy.
4. *Subendocardial ischaemia.* It stimulates the hypertrophy of the cells of myocardium.

Subtypes

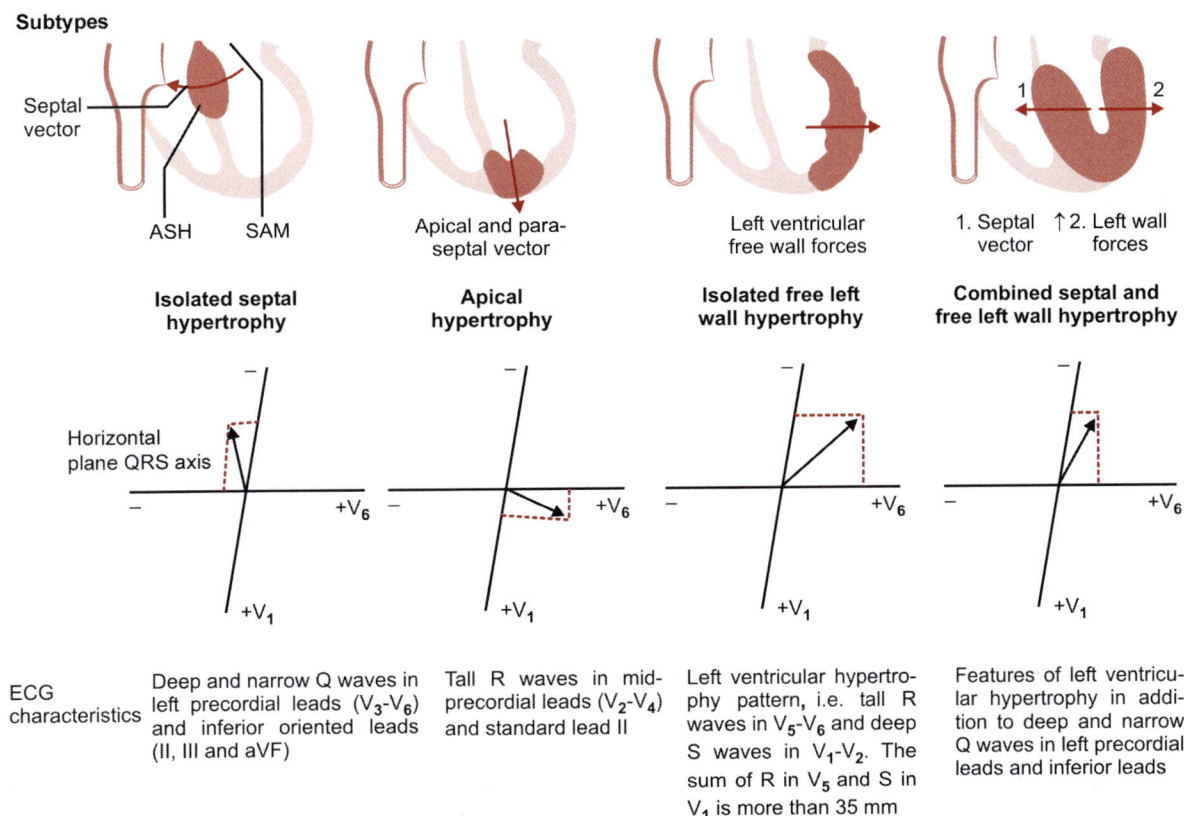

| ECG characteristics | Deep and narrow Q waves in left precordial leads (V_3-V_6) and inferior oriented leads (II, III and aVF) | Tall R waves in mid-precordial leads (V_2-V_4) and standard lead II | Left ventricular hypertrophy pattern, i.e. tall R waves in V_5-V_6 and deep S waves in V_1-V_2. The sum of R in V_5 and S in V_1 is more than 35 mm | Features of left ventricular hypertrophy in addition to deep and narrow Q waves in left precordial leads and inferior leads |

Fig. 23.1: Diagrammatic illustration of sites of hypertrophy, QRS axis on horizontal plane and electrocardiographic characteristics of subtypes of hypertrophic cardiomyopathy

SECTION EIGHT

5. **Structural abnormalities.** The structural abnormalities of the septum may lead to myocardial cells hypertrophy.

Macroscopic Subtypes

1. **Left ventricular hypertrophy** (Fig. 23.1)
   A. *Asymmetric interventricular septal hypertrophy*
   B. *Hypertrophy of free walls of left ventricle*
   C. *Hypertrophy of apical and parabasal areas of left ventricle*
   D. *Combined interventricular septum and free left wall hypertrophy*
2. **Right ventricular hypertrophy** . It is rare.

The pathogenesis of electrocardiographic features
   The electrocardiographic manifestations are due to:
   (i) A mass effect (increased left or right ventricular mass)

(ii) Relative myocardial ischaemia and
(iii) Pressure effect on the conduction tissue.

The electrocardiographic manifestations. They include:

1. Ventricular hypertrophy (left common, right rare)
2. Intraventricular conduction defects, i.e. left anterior fascicular block (abnormal left axis deviation) and bundle branch blocks. These are similar to dilated cardiomyopathy.
3. Arrhythmias. Ventricular arrhythmias are more common that supraventricular.
4. Atrial hypertrophy (left and/or right)
5. A short P-R interval
6. An electrocardiographic pattern resembling WPW syndrome.
7. Prolongation of QT (QTc) interval and increased QT dispersion (QTd).

The Electrocardiogram

1. *Left Ventricular Hypertrophy*

a) *Asymmetric interventricular septal hypertrophy (Fig. 23.2)*

Due to hypertrophy of interventricular septum (mass effect), there is an increase in the magnitude of left to right septal vector resulting in prominent, deep but narrow Q waves in midprecordial (V_2–V_4) and/or left precordial leads (V_5-V_6) and/or inferior oriented leads (II, III and aVF). These changes may mimic anterior or inferior wall infarction.

b) *Free left walls hypertrophy (Fig. 23.3)*

The hypertrophy of free walls of left ventricle results in augmentation of free wall forces leading to left ventricular hypertrophy due to systolic overload. Left ventricular hypertrophy is reflected by tall R waves in V_5-V_6 with corresponding deep S waves in leads V_1-V_2. The voltage criteria of left ventricular hypertrophy are present. Due to systolic overload, the inversion of T wave with ST segment depression occurs due to relative ischaemia.

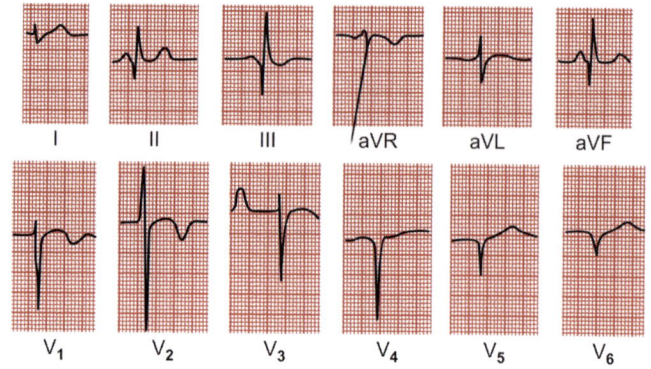

Fig. 23.2: Hypertrophic cardiomyopathy (asymmetric septal hypertrophy). The electrocardiogram shows narrow deep q waves in leads II, III, aVF and V_4-V_6. The q wave axis is superior -110° approx. The initial prominent r wave in V_1 indicates that initial QRS vector is directed superiorly, to the right and anteriorly. The S wave in V_1 is of not increased amplitude and the R wave in precordial leads is of low amplitude, i.e. there is no associated LVH.

The manifestation of abnormal q wave in inferior and lateral leads in the absence of any evidence of LVH indicates increased magnitude of L → R septal vector due to dominant septal hypertrophy.

Note: This pattern may be misinterpreted as inferolateral infarction but absence of evolutionary change negate that fact.

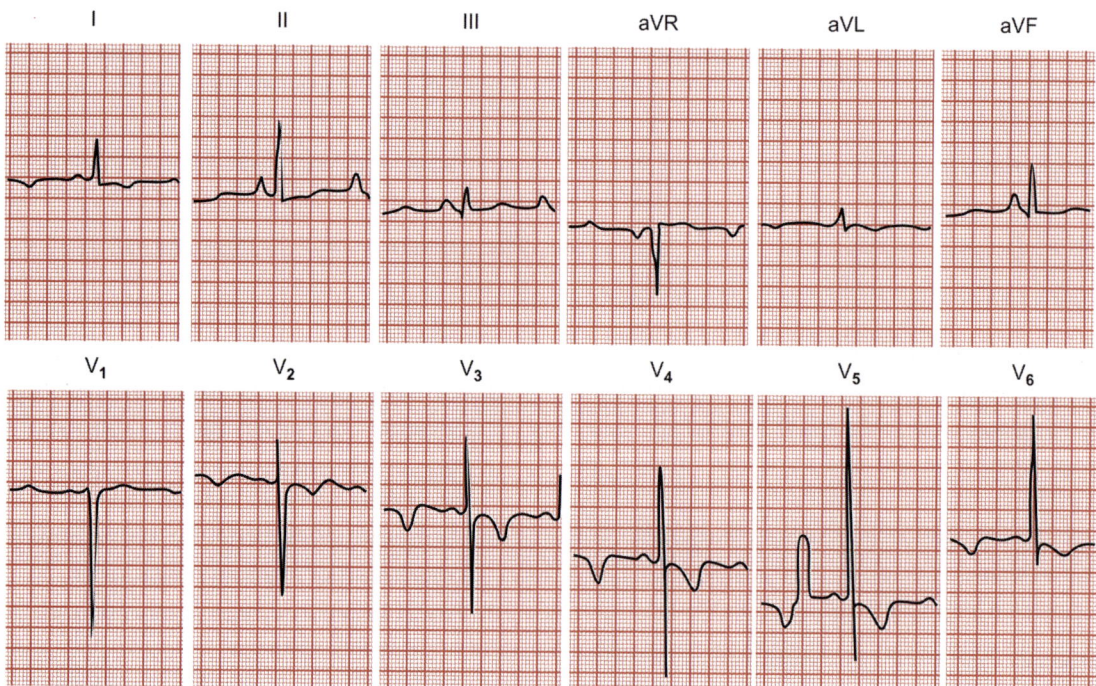

Fig. 23.3: Hypertrophic cardiomyopathy (left ventricular free walls). The ECG shows (i) *Left ventricular hypertrophy*—tall R waves in V_5-V_6 (R in V_6 > 27 mm) with deep S wave in leads V_1-V_2 and RV_5 + SV_1 is 55 mm. There are associated ST segment depression and T wave inversion in leads I, aVL, V_4-V_6 (note shelf like angulation of ST segment in V_5-V_6 seen in LVH). (ii) *Right atrial hypertrophy*—tall peaked P waves in leads II, III and aVF and (iii) *Probable right ventricular hypertrophy*—normal QRS axis and prominent R wave in V_2-V_4 with ST depression and T wave inversion.

Note: The combination of LVH with right atrial hypertrophy is characteristically seen in hypertrophic cardiomyopathy

SECTION EIGHT

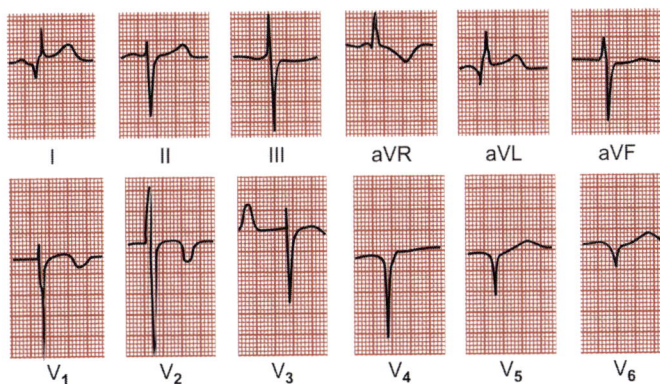

Fig. 23.4: Hypertrophic cardiomyopathy (apical) simulating anterior wall MI. The ECG recorded from 16 yrs male shows narrow, deep Q waves in leads I, aVL and V_4-V_6 with ST elevation with concavity upwards in leads I and aVL but T waves are upright. The T waves are inverted in V_1-V_2, indicate juvenile pattern.

These changes can stimulate anterior myocardial infarction (MI) but Q waves are neither wide nor deep in lateral precordial leads. There are no evolutionary changes of MI

Fig. 23.5: Hypertrophic cardiomyopathy (Combined septal and free walls of left ventricle). The ECG shows a q wave in left oriented leads (I, aVL, and V_5) which is more than normal (accentuated).
(ii) *Left ventricular hypertrophy*—tall R waves in V_5 (28 mm) and deep S in lead V_1 and RV_5 + SV_1 = 40 mm indicate LVH.
(iii) There is ST segment depression in leads I, aVL, V_5-V_6 and T is inverted in lead I and aVL (Shelf like angulation of ST segment in aVL) with biphasic T in V_5-V_6.

All these features can be seen in left ventricular volume overload from which it has to be differentiated

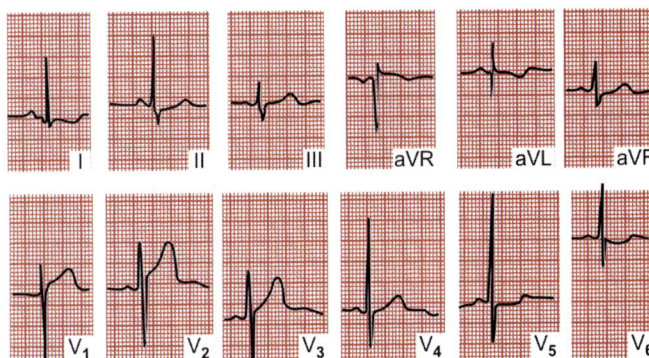

c. *Hypertrophy of apical and parabasal areas (Fig. 23.4)*
Due to hypertrophy of apical and parabasal areas, there is increased magnitude of apical and parabasal forces resulting in orientation of resultant QRS vector to midprecordial region on horizontal plane, therefore, there are tall R waves in mid-precordial leads (V_2-V_4) and standard lead II. The R wave is usually taller in lead V_4 than in lead V_5; and taller in lead V_5 than lead V_6.

The associated ST-T changes, i.e. ST segment depression and T wave inversion are seen in mid-precordial leads forming a shelf like appearance of ST segment.

d. *Combined hypertrophy of the interventricular septum and free walls of left ventricle (Fig. 23.5)*
(i) The asymmetric septal hypertrophy is reflected by q waves in left precordial and inferior oriented leads as already discussed.
(ii) The left ventricular free wall hypertrophy is reflected on ECG by tall R waves in left precordial leads and concomitant deep S waves in right precordial leads.

The associated ST-T changes, i.e. ST segment depression with convexity upwards and T wave inversion forming a shelf like appearance are characteristically seen.

B. Right Ventricular Hypertrophy

The right ventricular involvement in hypertrophic cardiomyopathy is uncommon, when it occurs, it may involve septum as well as free walls of right ventricle which may be reflected electrocardiographically by:
i) Right axis deviation: The mean frontal plane QRS axis lies in right inferior quadrant and may even touch the region of ± 180°.
ii) Right ventricular hypertrophy is reflected by tall R waves in right precordial leads (V_1-V_2) with persistence of S waves in left precordial leads (V_5-V_6). The T wave is inverted in right precordial leads.
iii) Right atrial hypertrophy which concomitantly occurs, is reflected by tall peaked P waves in leads II, III and aVF.

SECTION EIGHT

iv) Complete or incomplete right bundle branch block (RBBB) occurs due to pressure effect on conduction tissue.

2. Conduction Defects

Hypertrophic cardiomyopathy may be associated with left anterior fascicular block and left bundle branch block (LBBB).

i) *Left anterior fascicular block:* It occurs in about one-third of patients and is reflected by leftwards mean frontal plane QRS axis deviation usually to the region of −30° or more. The left axis deviation is even more significant sign of hypertrophic cardiomyopathy in children.

ii) *Left bundle branch block (LBBB):* Both complete and incomplete left bundle branch block can occur infrequently, more commonly in symptomatic patients without outflow tract obstruction. Complete bundle branch involvement is more common after surgery. The electrocardiographic manifestation of incomplete left bundle branch block is disappearance of q wave in leads V_5-V_6; this may be the reason why the deep Q waves do not manifest in all cases of hypertrophic cardiomyopathy.

3. Atrial Hypertrophy

Both right and/or left atrial enlargement may occur consequent to ventricular hypertrophy and manifest electrocardiographically by respective P wave abnormalities. Biatrial hypertrophy/enlargement will produce tall as well as wide and notched P waves in lead II. The right atrial hypertrophy in the presence of left ventricular hypertrophy and strain is highly suggestive of hypertropic cardiomyopathy (Fig. 23.3).

4. Short P-R Interval (Fig. 23.6)

A short P-R interval of < 0.12 sec can occur in some cases, the mechanism of which is not known.

5. WPW Syndrome

It is uncommonly associated with hypertrophic cardiomyopathy. It has also been reported that patients whose electrocardiogram show delta waves or delta like waves tend to have more severe outflow

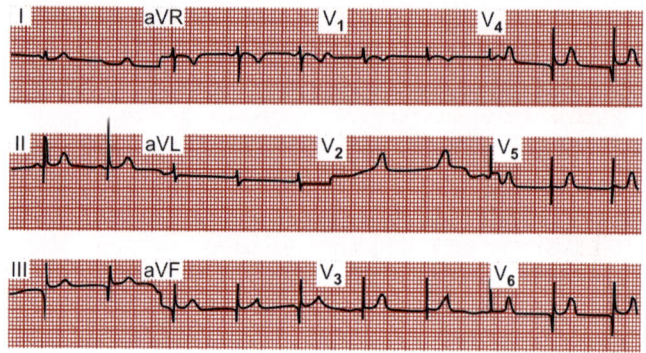

Fig. 23.6: Hypertrophic cardiomyopathy with short P-R interval. The ECG shows;
i. Sinus bradycardia (heart rate is 60 bpm)
ii. P-R interval is short (<0.12 sec). There is no evidence of WPW syndrome to explain it.
iii. Deep, narrow Q waves are seen in leads II, III, aVF and V_3-V_6 with a tall R wave in lead V_1 are suggestive of postero-inferolateral infarction but Q waves are deep but narrow in inferior and lateral leads and T wave is characteristically upright, these finding negate the possibility of old postero-inferolateral infarction. All these changes along with unexplained short P-R interval and slow heart rate can occur in hypertrophic obstructive cardiomyopathy (septal hypertrophy)

tract obstruction. Some of the case reports attribute delta waves or delta like waves to incomplete left bundle branch block due to pressure effect rather than actual WPW syndrome.

6. Prolonged QT and Increased QT Dispersion

Prolongation of QT and increased QT dispersion (QTd) at times, may be associated with hypertrophic cardiomyopathy. The increased QT dispersion is attributed underlying mechanism for malignant ventricular arrhythmias and sudden death in patients of hypertrophic cardiomyopathy.

7. Arrhythmias

Ventricular arrhythmias are more common both in symptomatic and asymptomatic patients than supraventricular arrhythmias. The ventricular arrhythmias include ventricular ectopics, ventricular tachycardia and ventricular fibrillation. The supraventricular arrhythmias commonly include supraventricular tachycardia. Atrial fibrillation (Fig. 23.7) is uncommon and occurs only in 10% cases.

| I | II | III | aVR | aVL | aVF |

| V₁ | V₂ | V₃ | V₄ | V₅ | V₆ |

II

V₁

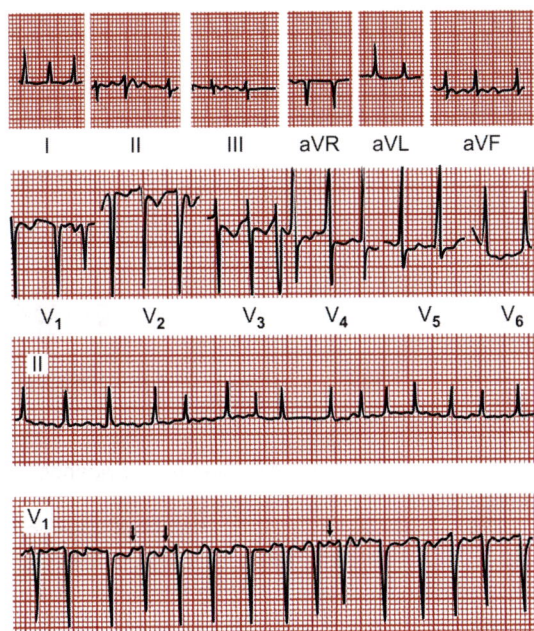

Fig. 23.7: Hypertrophic cardiomyopathy (left ventricular free walls) with atrial fibrillation. The electrocardiogram shows;

i. Normal QRS axis

ii. Left ventricular hypertrophy. There is tall R wave in V_5 (>27 mm) and V_6 with deep S wave in V_1 ($RV_5 + SV_1 = 50$ mm)

iii. Atrial fibrillation. The indulation of baseline with irregular R-R intervals (continuous leads II and V_1) suggests atrial fibrillation. Occasionally fibrillatory waves simulating P waves (↓) are also seen.

This episode of atrial fibrillation was recorded during tachycardia in a patient of hypertrophic cardiomyopathy. There was no evidence of any short P-R interval during normal sinus rhythm in this patient, hence does not indicate WPW conduction

Clinical Significance

1. The q wave in anterior chest leads (V_2–V_6) or in inferior leads or in both, may simulate anterior, inferior or inferolateral infarction. These q waves -so called non-infarction q waves are deep and narrow but not wide. They are not associated with evolutionary changes of infarction. They are usually associated with tall R waves in left precordial leads.

2. The changes of hypertrophic cardiomyopathy may simulate diastolic overload of left ventricle due to any cause, from which it has to be differentiated by clinical, echocardiographic and vectorcardiographic findings.

Suggested Reading

1. Buja G, Miorelli M, Turrini P et al. Comparison of QT dispersion in hypertrophic cardiomyopathy between patients with or without ventricular arrhythmias and sudden death. *Am J Cardiol* **72**: 973, 1993.

2. Cohen J, Effect H, Goodwin JF et al: Hypertrophic obstructive cardiomyopathy. *Brit Heart J* **26**: 16, 1964.

3. Frank S, Braunward E: Idiopathic hypertrophic subaortic stenosis. *Circulation* **37**: 759, 1968.

4. Goodwin JF: Prospects and predictions for cardiomyopathies. *Circulation* **50**: 210, 1974.

5. Henry WL, Clerk CE, Epstein SE: Asymmetric septal hypertrophy-echocardiographic identification of pathognomonic anatomical abnormality of IHSS. *Circulation* **47**: 225, 1973.

6. Kowey PR et al: Sustained arrhythmias in hypertrophic obstructive cardiomyopathy. *N Eng J Med* **310**:1566, 1984.

7. McKenna NJ: Arrhythmias and prognosis in hypertrophic cardiomyopathy. *Eur Heart J* **4**: 225, 1983.

8. Perosio AM, Suarez LD, Bunster AM et al: Pre-excitation syndrome and hypertrophic cardiomyopathy. *J Electrocardiol* **16**: 29, 1983.

9. Teare RD: Asymmetrical hypertrophy of the heart in young adults. *Brit Heart J* **20**: 1, 1958.

10. Westlake RE, Cohen W, Willis WH: WPW syndrome and familial cardiomegaly. *Am Heart J* **64**: 314, 1962.

11. Yamaguchi H, Ishimura T, Nishiyams S et al: Hypertrophic nonobstructive cardiomyopathy with giant negative T waves (apical hypertrophy), Ventriculographic and echocrdiographic features in 30 patients. *Am J Cardiol* **44**: 401, 1979.

SECTION EIGHT

Acquired Heart Disease

SECTION NINE

24

Rheumatic Heart Disease

■ *Acute rheumatic carditis—electrocardiographic presentations.*
■ *The electrocardiogram in mitral, aortic, pulmonary and tricuspid valvular diseases*
■ *The electrocardiogram in combined valvular lesions.*
■ *Floppy mitral valve (mitral valve prolapse) syndrome—The electrocardiographic characteristics*

Clinical presentations are;
1. Acute rheumatic carditis
2. Chronic rheumatic valvular heart disease (RHD)

ACUTE RHEUMATIC CARDITIS (FIG. 24.1)

Carditis during acute rheumatic fever is called *acute rheumatic carditis,* may manifest clinically as an endocarditis, myocarditis or pericarditis or pancarditis (involvement of all the three layers of the heart), the last being more common in children.

The Electrocardiogram

Acute rheumatic carditis may manifest electrocardiographically in several ways;

i) *Sinus tachycardia.* It is a common manifestation and is disproportionate to the degree of fever

ii) *Prolongation of P-R interval.* It is included in John's minor criteria for diagnosis of rheumatic fever. First degree AV block (P-R > 0.20 sec) is a common finding. However, at rapid heart rate, P-R interval may remain within normal range (< 0.20 sec). Second degree AV block may infrequently be seen

iii) *AV dissociation* is not infrequent

iv) *Feature suggestive of acute pericarditis.* Raised ST segment with concavity upwards in majority of the leads suggest acute pericarditis.

v) *Features of myocarditis:* They may be present in majority of the leads in the form of;
   a) Depression / elevation of ST segment
   b) Nonspecific T wave changes, i.e. upright or inverted T waves
   c) Prolongation of QT (QTc) interval
   d) Widening of QRS complexes due to intra-ventricular conduction delay.
   e) An arrhythmia in the form of an ectopic beat or beats. Nonparoxysmal AV nodal (idionodal tachycardia) may occur.

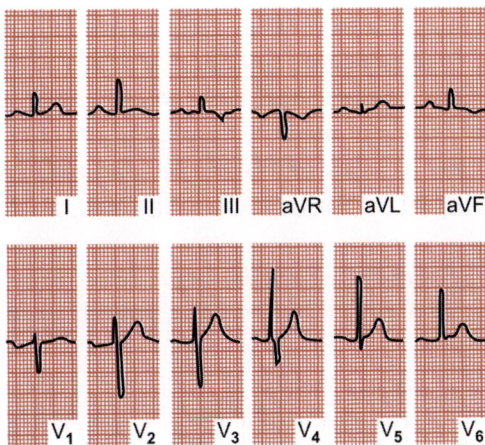

Fig. 24.1: Acute rheumatic myocarditis. The electrocardiogram shows decreased voltage in standard leads. It is not low voltage as leads II and aVR has voltage > 5 mm. The P-R interval is prolonged 0.24 sec. The ST segment is minimally elevated in leads III and aVF with asymmetric T wave inversion. The ST segment is minimally elevated with concavity upwards and upright T waves in leads I, II, aVL and V_2-V_6. The QTc is normal. The QRS complexes are also normal

Sinus tachycardia, nonparoxysmal AV nodal tachycardia, conduction blocks (first and second degree AV block), prolongation of QTc interval and nonspecific ST-T changes suggest myocarditis of any origin, hence, are not specific to rheumatic carditis.

2. CHRONIC RHEUMATIC VALVULAR HEART DISEASE

Mitral Stenosis (MS)

It is mostly rheumatic, rarely congenital (Lutembacher's syndrome) in origin. Pure or predominant mitral stenosis occurs in 40% cases of rheumatic heart disease. It is more common in middle-aged females and even in children. Sex ratio is 2: 1.

Haemodynamic Alterations

The mitral valve orifice is 4-6 cm^2 (average 5 cm^2) in diastole in health. Significant obstruction to the inflow of blood through mitral valve occurs when its orifice is reduced to half of its normal size. When mitral valve orifice is reduced to 1 cm^2, the left atrial pressure rises significantly and may reach upto 25 mm Hg in an effort to maintain normal cardiac output. Therefore, left atrial hypertrophy is the haemodynamic hallmark of mitral stenosis. It must be stressed here that large or huge enlargement of left atrium (*giant left atrium*) is a hallmark of mitral regurgitation rather than mitral stenosis due to volume overload. The elevated left atrial pressure consequent to mitral stenosis results in pulmonary venous and arterial hypertension, which in sequence, leads to right ventricular hypertrophy or dilatation. Right ventricular dilatation (enlargement) with some degree of hypertrophy is more common than pure right ventricular hypertrophy.

The Electrocardiogram (Fig. 24.2)

The electrocardiographic findings in mitral stenosis occur due to above mentioned haemodynamic alterations. These are as follows:

1. *Left atrial enlargement.* The width of P wave is slightly increased (> 2.5 mm) and P waves are notched in standard leads I, II, III and aVF. In lead V$_1$, the P wave is biphasic, the negative component representing left atrium will be more prominent > 0.04 sec. The P wave abnormality of mitral stenosis depends on the mitral valve orifice area, the gradient across the valve, left atrial pressure and size. The so called *P mitrale*–characteristically seen in left atrial enlargement due to mitral stenosis with sinus rhythm; is notched (duration of notch is 0.04 sec) and widened P wave (> 0.12 sec) in standard leads and biphasic P waves in V$_1$ whose terminal negative deflection is > 0.04 sec. This is due to left axis deviation of P wave (+ 45º to –30º). The P vector is oriented to the left and posteriorly–an early sign of left atrial enlargement. The ECG signs of left atrial enlargement correlate well with left atrial volume than left atrial pressure and often regress following successful valvotomy. If pulmonary hypertension develops and biatrial enlargement occurs then a bifid P appears. This is M-shaped wave in which initial positive deflection is due to right atrial hypertrophy and terminal positive deflection is due to left atrial hypertrophy. This bifid P wave indicates increased both anterior and posterior P wave forces.

2. *Right axis deviation of QRS.* There is a right axis deviation of QRS in the region of + 80° to + 120° but may be more in severe cases. This is due to right ventricular hypertrophy, and at times, may be the only evidence of right ventricular hypertrophy. Right axis deviation roughly correlates with the degree of mitral stenosis.

3. *Clockwise rotation.* There may be clockwise rotation of heart on horizontal plane with slight shifting of transition zone to the left, i.e. towards V$_5$-V$_6$.

4. *Changes in QRS morphology.* These depends on severity of mitral stenosis and dominance of right ventricle

   A. *Mild mitral stenosis.*

   i) Right precordial leads (V$_1$-V$_2$). The QRS complexes reflect moderate degree of right ventricular hypertrophy in the form of low amplitude of the complexes with neither positive or negative predominance

   ii) Left precordial leads (V$_5$-V$_6$) tend to be normal (qR or QRS configuration)

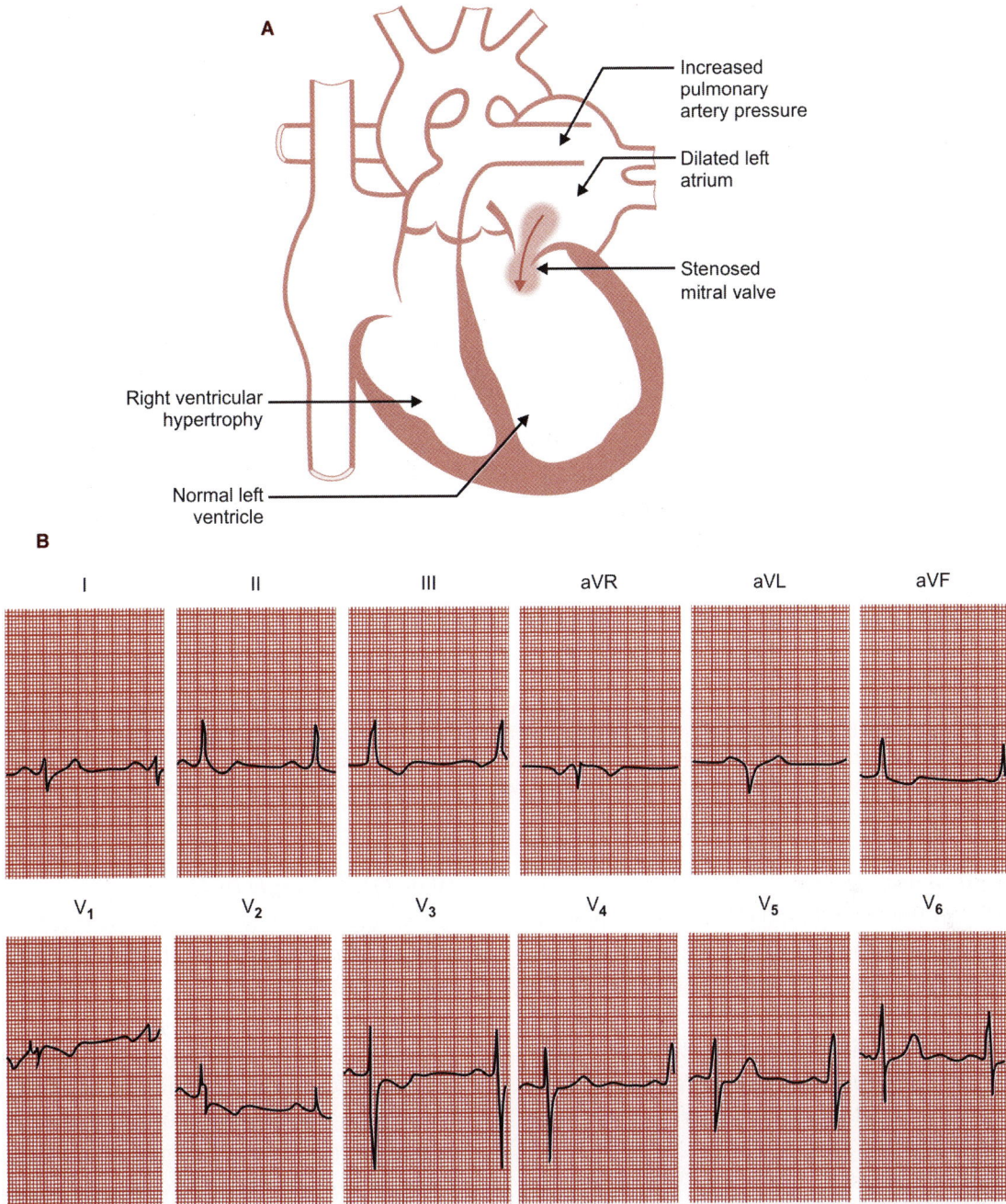

Fig. 24.2: Rheumatic heart disease with mitral stenosis resulting in left atrial enlargement and right ventricular hypertrophy.

A: The left atrial and right ventricular hypertrophy are its immediate consequences (diag). The dotted lines indicate the chamber enlarged. RA = right atrium, RV = right ventricle, LA = left atrium, LV = left ventricle, MS = mitral valve stenosis.

B: The ECG shows the following characteristics:
  i. Right axis deviation of QRS on frontal plane (+100°).
  ii. *Left atrial hypertrophy* is evident by P mitrale (wide notched P wave—M shaped) in leads I, II, and aVL, and P is inverted in III and aVF due to left axis deviation of P wave. The P wave is biphasic in lead V_1 where negative terminal deflection is prominent and wide
  iii. *Right ventricular hypertrophy*—A small complex in lead V_1 and a large R wave is especially seen in V_2 (R>S) with T wave inversion. There is marked clockwise rotation—transition zone is seen in V_5. Persistence of S wave in V_5-V_6 with above mentioned features indicate right ventricular hypertrophy. The ST segment in depressed in leads II, III and aVF due to RVH

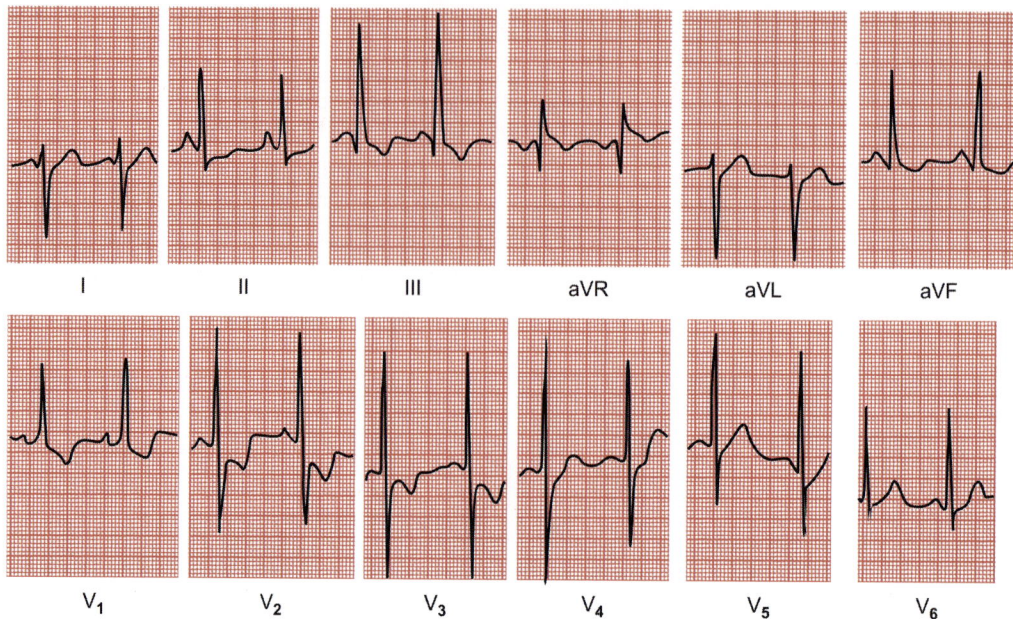

Fig. 24.3: Rheumatic heart diseases with severe mitral stenosis. The ECG shows;
  i. Right axis deviation of QRS on frontal plane. Heart rate is 110/min regular
  ii. Vertical heart position with marked clockwise rotation (a large qR pattern in aVR) with shifting of transition zone leftwards between V_4-V_5
  iii. *Biatrial hypertrophy.* Tall and wide P waves (>2.5 mm) in leads II, III and aVF. The lead V_1 shows biphasic P wave with prominent and wide both positive and negative components. There is right axis deviation of P wave
  iv. *Right ventricular hypertrophy.* There are tall R wave with small or rudimentary S wave in leads V_1-V_3 and significant depression of ST segment with deep symmetric T wave inversion indicating right ventricular hypertrophy with strain (relative ischaemia). There is RS pattern in V_5-V_6.

B. *Moderate mitral stenosis*
  i) Right precordial leads (V_1-V_2). There is an increase in the height of R wave which may become equal to S wave. The width of RS complex is increased but does not exceed 0.12 second, is common due to right ventricular hypertrophy cum dilatation. There is clockwise rotation of the heart with shifting of transition zone towards left (V_5-V_6).
  ii) Left precordial leads (V_5-V_6). There is diminution of R wave and prominence of S wave due to clockwise rotation.

C. *Severe mitral stenosis* (Fig. 24.3)
  i) Right precordial leads (V_1-V_2). Tall R waves or qR pattern are seen in these leads. The R: S ratio in lead V_1 is more than 1. The T waves are inverted in V_1-V_3 and leads II, III and aVF.
  ii) Left precordial leads (V_5-V_6). These leads reflect rS or RS pattern. The deep S wave persists in V_5-V_6.

5. *Wide QRS-T angle (> 45°).*
  As QRS axis is deviated to the right but T wave axis on frontal plane is shifted to the left resulting in wide QRS-T angle.

6. *Atrial fibrillation* (Fig. 24.4)
  It is a common complication of mitral stenosis. The manifestation of atrial fibrillation together with right axis deviation of QRS on frontal plane in a relatively young patients under the age of 40 years is highly suggestive of underlying mitral stenosis. Atrial fibrillation develops due to chronic left atrial enlargement.

7. *The associated ST–T changes*
  Due to right ventricular hypertrophy, the mean QRS axis on the frontal plane is directed anteriorly and to the right, the mean T wave axis is directed opposite to it, i.e. (i) posteriorly resulting in inverted T waves in the right precordial leads (V_1-V_3) that register tall R waves and (ii) superiorly and to the left resulting in T wave inversion in inferior leads (II, III and aVF).

SECTION NINE

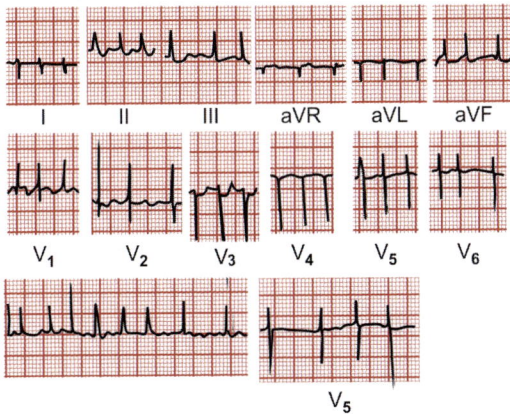

Fig. 24.4: Rheumatic mitral stenosis with atrial fibrillation. The ECG shows;

i. *Right ventricular hypertrophy.* It is manifested by RS pattern in V_1-V_2 with persistence of large S wave (rS pattern) in V_5-V_6 due to clockwise rotation. There is right axis deviation and vertical heart position

ii. *Atrial fibrillation* is evidenced by fibrillatory (f) waves producing undulation of baseline and variable R-R intervals (lower strip—leads V_1 and V_5). The ventricular rate is fast

The ST segment is minimally depressed in V_1-V_3 with convexity upwards indicating right ventricular systolic overload. In long standing cases, the ST segment may be depressed with T wave inversion in the right precordial leads indicating right ventricular strain–an expression of relative ischaemia of right ventricle due to its hypertrophy.

Mitral Regurgitation

The isolated mitral regurgitation is commonly of nonrheumatic than rheumatic origin. In rheumatic heart disease, combined mitral stenosis and regurgitation is more common than isolated mitral stenosis or regurgitation.

Haemodynamic Alterations

The resistance to left ventricular emptying is reduced due to double outlet in mitral regurgitation. Both aortic and mitral orifices share the left ventricular output. As a consequence of incompetence of mitral valve, the left ventricle releases its tension by pushing the blood into left atrium in addition to its ejection into aorta. Thus, the initial compensation of mitral regurgitation consists of complete systolic emptying of left ventricle.

However, a progressive increase in left ventricular end-diastolic volume occurs as the severity of mitral regurgitation increases and left ventricular function deteriorates. With the onset of decompensation, left ventricle dilates and ultimately fails. The left atrium becomes enlarged and may *become giant* due to volume overload. Atrial fibrillation may occur but is less common than isolated mitral stenosis.

Causes

The conditions associated with mitral regurgitation are;

1. It may be an associated congenital anomaly in certain congenital heart diseases; such as endo-cardial cushion defect, corrected transposition, endocardial fibroelastosis, 'parachute' mitral valve deformity, septum primum defect, etc.
2. Acute rheumatic carditis.
3. Chronic rheumatic heart disease
4. Mitral valve prolapse (Floppy mitral valve)
5. Infective endocarditis.
6. Cardiomyopathies, i.e. dilated or hypertrophic. In hypertrophic cardiomyopathy, the anterior leaflet of mitral valve gets displaced anteriorly during systole.
7. Massive idiopathic calcification of mitral annulus.
8. Acute myocardial infarction with rupture of papillary muscle producing an acute mitral regurgitation.
9. Cardiac surgery.
10. Ventricular aneurysm involving the base of a papillary muscle.
11. Systemic lupus erythematosus (Libman-Sach's endocarditis), rheumatoid arthritis, ankylosing spondylitis, etc.
12. A healed myocardial infarction with papillary muscle dysfunction. The transient mitral regurgitation may occur during ischaemia of a papillary muscle.
13. Left ventricular dilatation including valve ring dilatation due to any cause.
14. Rarely due to lung carcinoid.

The Electrocardiogram (Figs 24.5A and B)

Mitral regurgitation, irrespective of its cause, presents with following electrocardiographic characteristics;

SECTION NINE

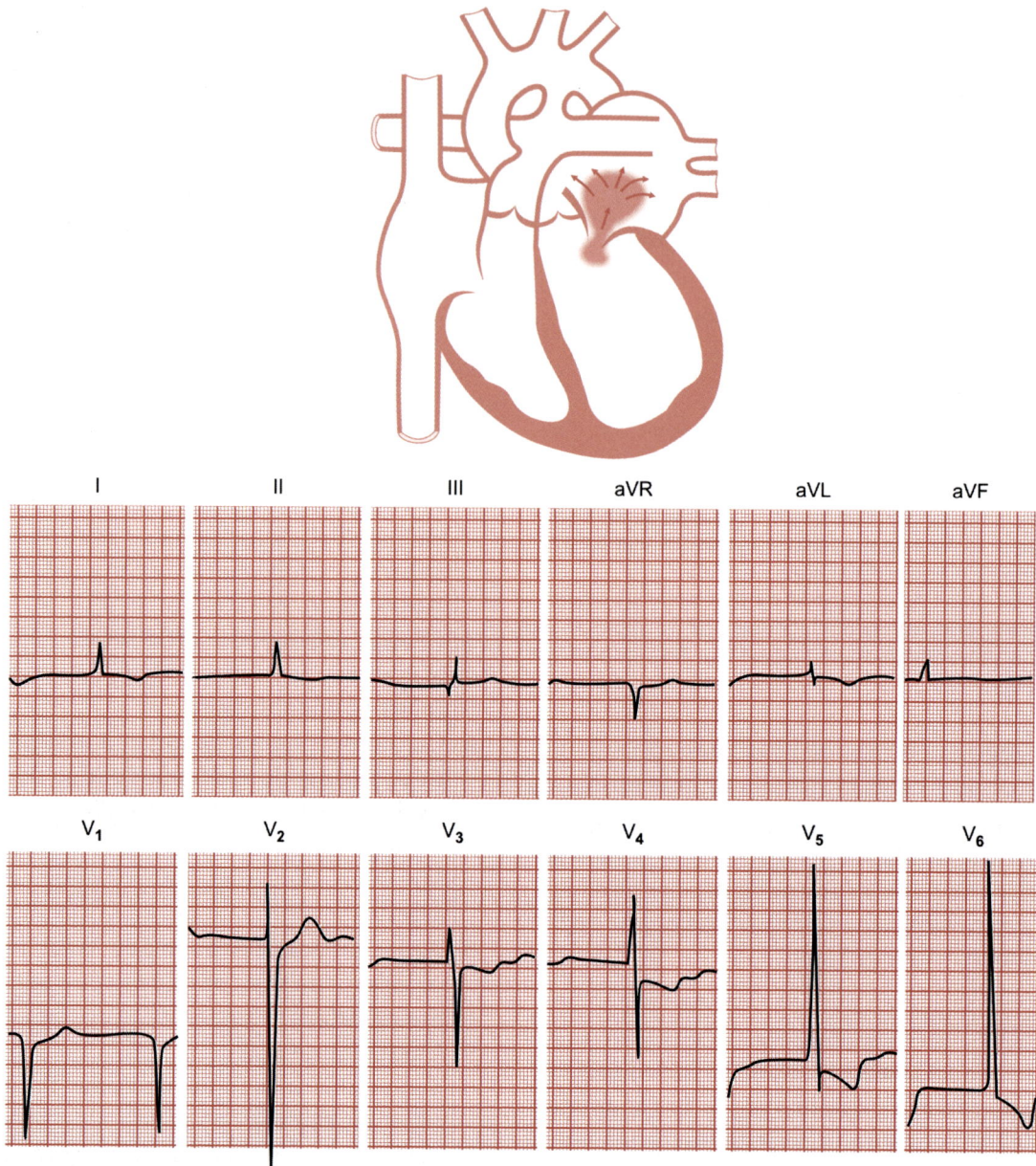

Fig. 24.5: Rheumatic mitral regurgitation.

A. Diagrammatic illustration of left atrial and left ventricular enlargement. The dotted lines indicates chambers enlarged. LA = left atrium, MR = mitral regurgitation. LV = left ventricle

B. The ECG recorded from mitral regurgitation with digitalis toxicity shows;

   i. Left ventricular hypertrophy in evident by voltage criteria: i.e. $RV_5 > 27$ mm, $RV_6 > 26$ mm, and $SV_1 + RV_5 > 35$ mm
   The T wave inversion in leads I, aVL and V_3-V_6 with ST segment depression in V_3-V_6 is due to LVH. The QRS axis is $+45°$ and ST and T axes are $\pm 180°$, i.e. ST segment and T is upright in aVR which are quite opposite to LVH, raise the possibility that something else in addition to LVH is present that is modifying repolarisation.

   ii. Junctional rhythm—P waves are absent. The patient had symptoms of digitalis toxicity—nausea, vomiting. The ST-T changes could also be due to added effect of digitalis

1. *A normal frontal plane QRS axis.* A normal axis on frontal plane is common in rheumatic mitral regurgitation. Left axis deviation in rheumatic mitral regurgitation is uncommon, however, occurs commonly when mitral regurgitation is due to nonrheumatic origin, i.e. dilated cardiomyopathy or myocardial fibrosis in long standing heart failure.

2. *Left atrial enlargement.* The giant left atrium is common, which facilitates the development of atrial fibrillation. Otherwise, P wave may show widening (> 2.5 mm) in all the leads. P mitrale or bifid P wave occurs if there is left atrial or biatrial hypertrophy.

3. *Left ventricular diastolic overload.* This is reflected by tall R waves with an initial prominent, deep but narrow q waves in leads V_5-V_6. The sum total of R wave in V_5 and S wave in V_1 exceeds 35 mm ($RV_5 + SV_1 > 35$ mm). Sometimes, due to diastolic overload, S wave in V_1 may be of small magnitude. The associated T waves in V_5-V_6 are upright, sharp pointed and tall. The ST segment may be elevated minimally with concavity upwards in the same leads. Left ventricular hypertrophy / enlargement on ECG is mostly not seen in acute mitral regurgitation.

4. *Right ventricular hypertrophy:* Approximately 15% patients may exhibit electrocardiographic evidence of right ventricular hypertrophy, a change that reflects the presence of pulmonary hypertension of sufficient severity to counterbalance the hypertrophied left ventricle of mitral regurgitation.

5. *Atrial fibrillation* (Fig. 24.6). It is less common but may be present.

Combined Mitral Stenosis and Regurgitation (MS and MR)

The combined mitral stenosis and regurgitation is mostly due to rheumatic heart disease.

The Electrocardiogram (Figs 24.7 and 24.8)

The electrocardiographic manifestations are variable and depend on the dominance of valvular lesion. Therefore, the ECG findings fall into two combinations;

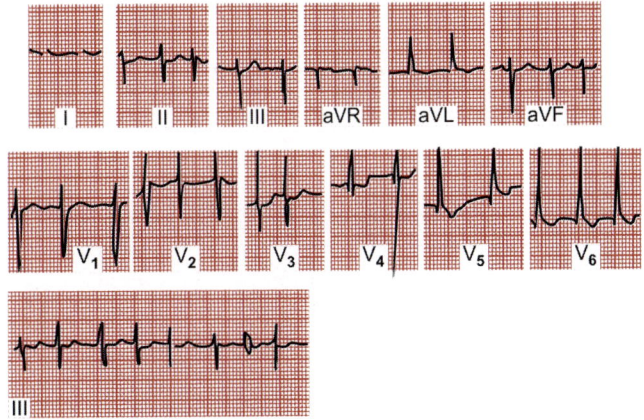

Fig. 24.6: Rheumatic mitral regurgitation with atrial fibrillation. The electrocardiogram recorded from a 20 yr female shows;

  i. *Left ventricular volume overload.* There is q wave in leads V_4-V_6, I and aVL. The R wave is tall > 27 mm in V_6 and $RV_5 + SV_1 = 40$ mm. There is left axis deviation and counterclockwise rotation with transition zone in V_2. The ST segment is depressed in leads I, aVL, V_4-V_6 with T wave inversion.

  ii. *Atrial fibrillation.* The P waves have been replaced by fibrillatory (f) waves which produce a fine wavy undulating baseline. The R-R interval is irregular with change in amplitude of R waves in same lead. The ventricular rate is rapid (100 bpm approx). The atrial fibrillation is best demonstrated in the lower most rhythm strip (lead II) which shows no P wave and irregular R-R intervals

1. *Dominant mitral regurgitation.* If mitral regurgitation is dominant, then there will be left atrial enlargement (P wave is wide > 2.5 mm and notched-P mitral), left ventricular volume (diastolic) overload (tall R waves in V_5-V_6; sum of R wave in V_5 and S wave in V_1 is more than 35 mm) and right axis deviation. The right axis deviation may be the only electrocardiographic finding of mitral stenosis. Atrial fibrillation may be an associated finding or there may be sinus rhythm.

2. *Dominant mitral stenosis.* If mitral stenosis is dominant, then P wave morphology is similar to isolated mitral stenosis i.e. P wave of left atrial enlargement (wide or broad bifid P waves called P mitrale). In addition to this, there will be features of right ventricular hypertrophy and left ventricular diastolic overload. Atrial fibrillation may be associated.

3. *Both mitral lesions dominant.* When both mitral stenosis and mitral regurgitation are dominant

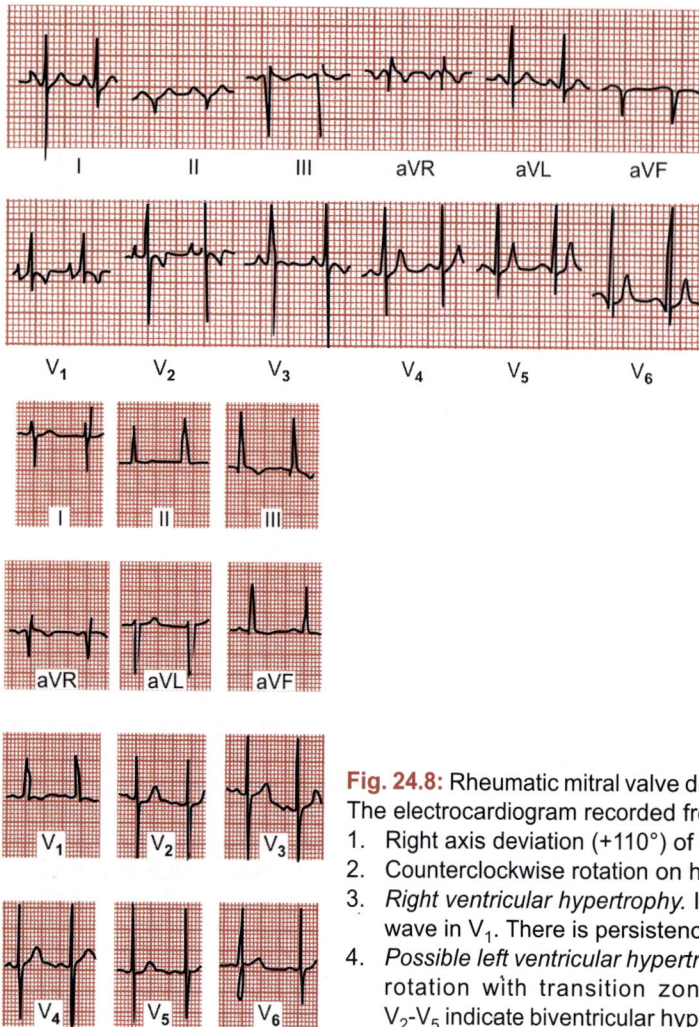

Fig. 24.7: Rheumatic mitral stenosis and mitral regurgitation (double mitral valve lesion) in an adult. The electrocardiogram recorded from a 30 year male with double mitral valve disease with pulmonary hypertension shows;
1. Left axis deviation of QRS on frontal plane (-20°)
2. Counterclockwise rotation of QRS on horizontal plane, i.e. transition zone lies in lead V_2.
3. *Biatrial hypertrophy.* The P waves are tall and wide in leads I, II, aVL and aVF. There is biphasic P wave in V_1 which shows peaking of initial upright component (right atrial hypertrophy) and widened and prominent terminal negative component (left atrial hypertrophy)
4. *Right ventricular hypertrophy.* It is evident by tall R waves in lead V_1 with prominent S wave (R:S > 1). There is persistence of deep S wave in V_5-V_6. There is inversion of T waves in leads V_1-V_2 indicating posterior deviation of T wave axis (wide QRS-T angle) due to hypertrophied and strained right ventricle.
5. *Left ventricular volume overload* is suggested by prominent q waves and tall R wave (>27 mm) in leads V_5-V_6 with upright tall T waves.
6. *Biventricular hypertrophy* is suggested by tall equiphasic QRS in mid-precordial leads V_2-V_4

Fig. 24.8: Rheumatic mitral valve disease (dominant mitral stenosis with mitral regurgitation). The electrocardiogram recorded from a 17 yrs girl shows;
1. Right axis deviation (+110°) of QRS of frontal plane
2. Counterclockwise rotation on horizontal plane—transition zone lies between V_2-V_3
3. *Right ventricular hypertrophy.* It is evident from tall monophasic R wave with inverted T wave in V_1. There is persistence of large S wave in V_5-V_6
4. *Possible left ventricular hypertrophy.* The good voltage of R wave with counterclockwise rotation with transition zone between V_2-V_3 and large R and S waves from V_2-V_5 indicate biventricular hypertrophy rather than isolated right ventricular hypertrophy

then there will be hypertrophy/enlargement of all the four chambers with some variations. The ECG will show;
1. *Biatrial hypertrophy:* The P waves are tall (> 2.5 mm) and wide (> 2.5 mm) seen in most of the leads.
2. *Biventricular hypertrophy:* Right ventricular hypertrophy is reflected by tall R wave (R: S ≥ 1) in leads V_1-V_3 with T wave inversion. The left ventricular volume overload is reflected by tall R wave > 26 mm in lead V_5-V_6 with prominent q waves and upright T waves. Due to balance of right ventricular and left ventricular forces, the transition zone remains in leads V_3-V_4 but reflects large equiphasic complexes.

The important diagnostic clues are given in the box.

B. Aortic Stenosis (Read Congenital Aortic Stenosis in Chapter 20)

Rheumatic aortic stenosis as an isolated lesion is rare. Aortic stenosis is usually associated with mitral valve lesion in rheumatic heart disease. Isolated aortic stenosis is mostly congenital (bicuspid aortic valve)

Haemodynamic Alterations

The haemodynamic alterations are limited to left side of the heart, i.e. left ventricle and left atrium. Due to obstruction to the outflow from the left ventricle, concentric hypertrophy of left ventricle results as a

ECG clues to double mitral valve lesions

Double mitral lesions should be suspected;

(i) If there are features of left atrial enlargement (wide, notched P wave) *in combination with* left ventricular overload (tall R waves in V_5-V_6 with prominent deep and narrow q waves) with right axis deviation or a tall or relatively tall R waves in V_1.

or

(ii) If there are features of left atrial enlargement *in combination with* right ventricular hypertrophy with left axis deviation (> 0 to −30°) and tall R waves in V_5–V_6.

or

(iii) If there are features of biatrial enlargement *in combination with* biventricular hypertrophy - Tall R wave in V_1-V_2 with tall R wave in V_5-V_6 (qR or qRS pattern) with a transition zone in V_3-V_4 depicting both tall and equal R and S).

(iv) Rhythm in double mitral lesion may be sinus or atrial fibrillation.

marker of systolic overload. As a consequence, there is first enlargement/hypertrophy of left ventricle followed by an enlargement of left atrium.

Causes

Aortic stenosis may be subvalvular, valvular and supravalvular.

1. *Valvular.* It may be due to a congenital anomaly (bicuspid aortic valve), rheumatic heart disease or idiopathic calcification of aortic valve.

2. *Subvalvular.* It may be due to hypertrophic cardiomyopathy or a membranous diaphragm or a fibrous ring encircling the left ventricular outflow tract just beneath the base of aortic valve.

3. *Supravalvular.* It may be due to localised or diffuse narrowing of aorta just above the level of coronary arteries. It may be a part of William's syndrome. Other features of this syndrome include infantilism, hypercalcaemia, '*elfin facies*', mental retardation, craniostenosis, squint, narrowing of systemic and pulmonary arteries, inguinal hernia, abnormality of dental development, auditory hyperacuesis and cryptorchidism in males. Supravalvular stenosis may be familial and transmitted as an autosomal dominant trait.

The Electrocardiogram (Fig. 24.9)

The electrocardiogram may be normal but when abnormal, the manifestations are due to left ventricular systolic overload. These include:

1. *A normal frontal plane QRS axis is common.* Left axis deviation is uncommon, occurs only when aortic stenosis is either associated with myocardial fibrosis following hypertrophy of left ventricle or in long standing disease associated with heart failure or when calcific aortic stenosis encroaches on the left anterior division of left bundle branch producing left anterior hemiblock.

2. *Left atrial enlargement.* This is reflected by wide and notched P waves but this is not a marked feature.

3. *Left ventricular systolic (pressure) overload.* There will be features of left ventricular hypertrophy, i.e.

   i) Right precordial leads (V_1-V_2) will register deep S wave with upright T waves. The ST segment in these leads is normal.

   ii) Left precordial leads (V_5-V_6) will show tall R waves. The R wave in V_6 may be more than 27 mm. eIt may be taller than V_5. The q wave in these leads is attenuated. The ST segment depression may be observed in these leads. Pattern of incomplete left bundle branch block with left axis deviation may be present, and in that situation, there will be loss of q waves in the left precordial leads. Ventricular activation time is increased in these leads.

4. *Atrial fibrillation.* It is rare in isolated aortic stenosis, if present, indicates concomitant mitral stenosis.

5. *Associated changes of myocardial ischaemia* may occasionally complicate aortic stenosis. These are

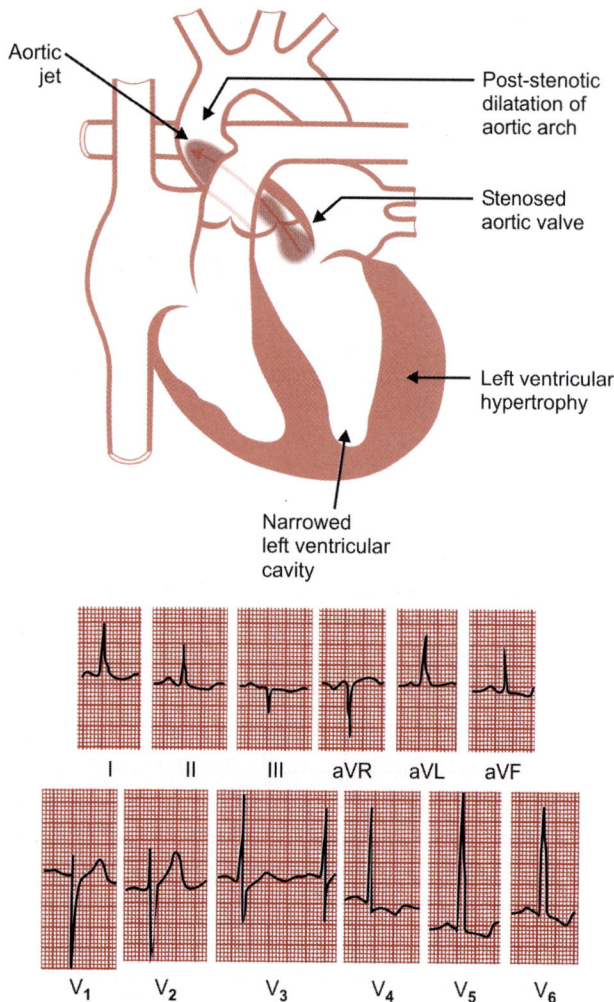

Fig. 24.9: Aortic stenosis. The electrocardiogram shows left axis deviation, counterclockwise rotation (transition zone lies between V_2 and V_3) and left ventricular hypertrophy (R in V_5 > 27 mm, $RV_5 + SV_1$ > 35 mm) with strain (ST segment depression and T wave inversion in leads V_4-V_6). All these suggest pressure overload on left ventricular due to aortic stenosis

in the form of ST depression and T wave inversion in left precordial leads in young persons.

Aortic Regurgitation (AR)

Isolated aortic regurgitation is usually of non-rheumatic origin. When it occurs in rheumatic heart disease, then it is mostly associated with either mitral valve lesion or aortic stenosis.

Haemodynamic Alterations

Regurgitation of a large volume of blood through the incompetent aortic valve into left ventricle results in diastolic overloading of left ventricle. This causes hypertrophy of interventricular septum as well as free walls of left ventricle. There is an associated enlargement of left atrium consequent to rise in left ventricular end-diastolic pressure. There may be improper filling of coronary arteries in severe aortic regurgitation resulting in myocardial ischaemia.

Causes

The nonrheumatic causes of aortic regurgitation are;
1. Congenital. It may be due to bicuspid aortic valve, due to leakage of membranous subaortic stenosis, prolapse of aortic cusp in ventricular septal defect or congenital fenestrations of aortic valve.
2. Infective endocarditis.
3. Traumatic nonpenetrating cardiac injuries.
4. Syphilitic aortitis or aneurysm of the ascending aorta.
5. Ankylosing spondylitis.
6. Cystic medial necrosis of ascending aorta.
7. Marfan's syndrome, idiopathic dilatation of aorta.
8. Aortic dissection.
9. Severe hypertension.

The Electrocardiogram (Figs 24.10 and 24.11)

The electrocardiographic manifestations are as a result of left venricular diastolic overload (volume overload) and associated enlargement of left atrium. Changes of myocardial ischaemia occur in severe aortic regurgitation. The changes in chronic aortic regurgitation are;
1. *Left ventricular diastolic overload.* This is reflected on ECG in the form of;
   a) Tall R wave in left oriented leads (1, aVL, V_5-V_6) with deep S wave in right precordial leads (V_1-V_2). The voltage criteria of left ventricular hypertrophy (R in V_6 > 27 mm and R V_5 + S V_1 > 35 mm) may be present.
   b) A prominent well-developed q waves in leads 1, aVL, V_5 and V_6 due to septal hypertrophy
   c) Tall symmetric upright T waves.
   d) Increased ventricular activation time in left precordial leads.
2. *Frontal plane QRS axis.* In about two-third patients, the frontal plane QRS axis is normal. In rest one-third patients, there is left axis deviation.

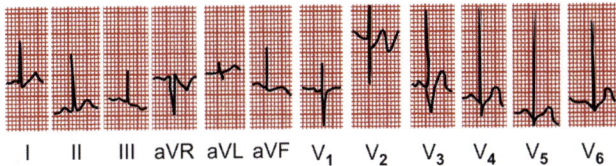

Fig. 24.10: Aortic regurgitation. The ECG shows;
1. Normal axis of +60° (aVL has an equiphasic complex)
2. *Counterclockwise* rotation leading to shifting of transition zone to V_2
3. Left ventricular hypertrophy (volume overload) is reflected by R wave in V_5 or V_6 > 26 mm; RV_5 + SV_1 = 40 mm. There is prominent q wave in V_5-V_6 and T is upright in left precordial leads indicating volume overload on left ventricle

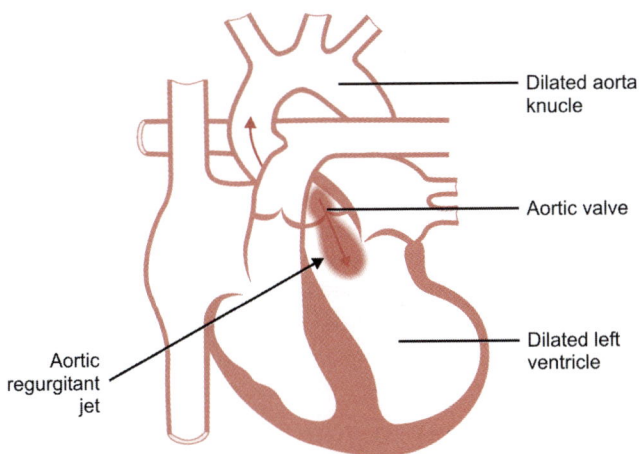

Dilated aorta knucle

Aortic valve

Aortic regurgitant jet

Dilated left ventricle

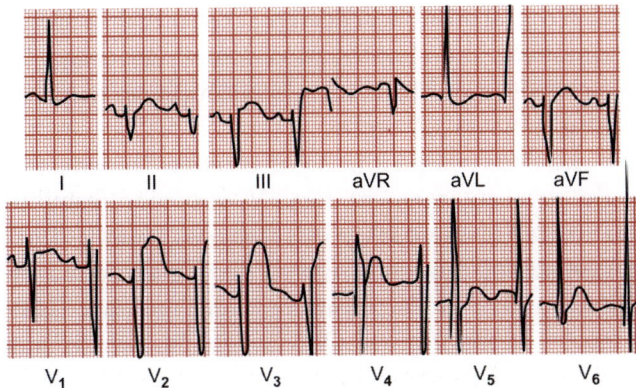

Fig. 24.11: Aortic regurgitation with aortic stenosis. The ECG shows;
  i. Left axis deviation of QRS
 ii. *Left ventricular volume overload.* There is a large narrow q wave in leads V_4-V_6 and lead aVL. There is evidence of LVH by voltage criteria, i.e. RV_5 + SV_1 = 48 mm. The ST segment is upsloping with upright T wave but is depressed in aVL and lead I
iii. Sinus tachycardia. The heart rate (R-R interval) is regular at a rate of 100/min.

Left axis deviation occurs in those patients who have severe aortic regurgitation with congestive heart failure. The left axis deviation is mostly due to left anterior hemiblock produced by fibrosis due to long standing aortic disease.

3. *Left atrial enlargement.* It is reflected by wide notched P waves.
4. *Inversion of U waves.* This is a sensitive sign of left ventricular enlargement, occurs both in aortic stenosis and aortic regurgitation.
5. *P-R interval prolongation.* When AR is caused by inflammatory process, the P–R interval may be prolonged.
6. *Changes of myocardial ischaemia.* Due to reduced coronary filling in aortic regurgitation, there may be changes of myocardial ischaemia/infarction in the form of ST depression or elevation with or without T wave inversion. They occur in young persons with long standing severe disease.
7. *Atrial fibrillation may be present.*

In acute aortic regurgitation, the ECG may or may not show left ventricular hypertrophy despite the presence of left heart failure and severe regurgitation. However, nonspecific ST segment and T wave changes are common.

Tricuspid Stenosis

It is uncommon in rheumatic heart disease but when present is usually of rheumatic origin and is always associated with rheumatic mitral valve disease (stenosis or regurgitation) or aortic valve disease.

Haemodynamic Alterations

Since mitral valve disease especially mitral stenosis generally precedes the development of tricuspid stenosis of rheumatic origin, therefore, patient will have biatrial enlargement/hypertrophy with moderate degree of right ventricular hypertrophy because tricuspid stenosis relieves right ventricular hypertrophy, which is primarily due to mitral valve disease.

The Electrocardiogram (Fig. 24.12)

The electrocardiographic findings are due to haemodynamic disturbances and include;

SECTION NINE

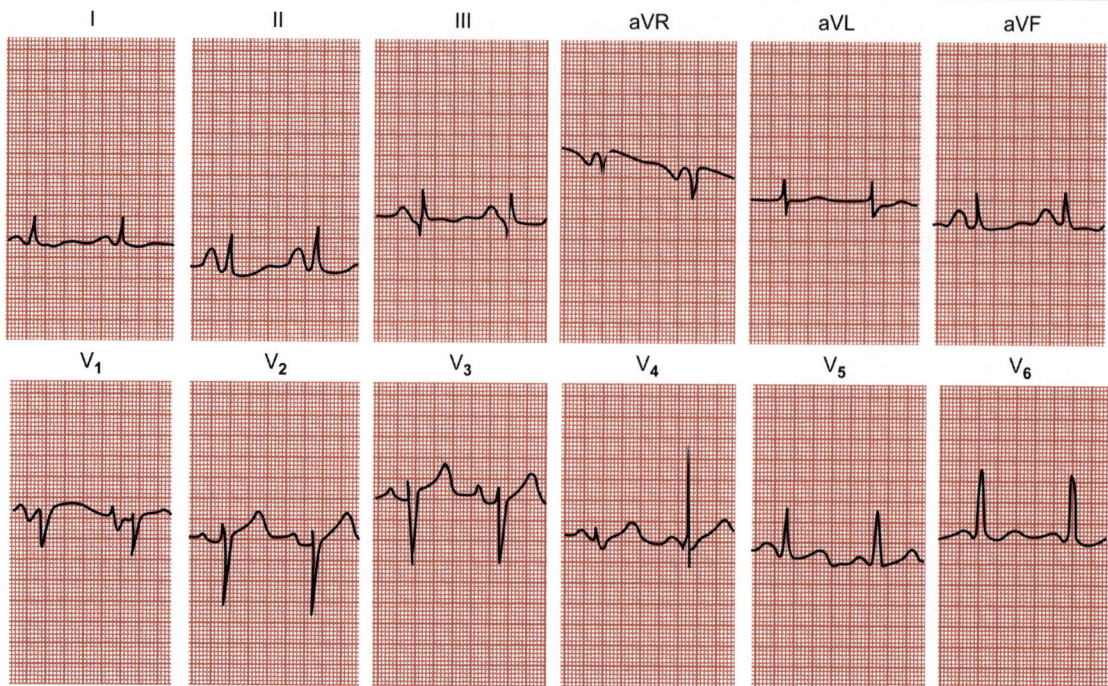

Fig. 24.12: Rheumatic mitral and tricuspid stenosis. The ECG taken from 46-yr-old woman shows biatrial enlargement, i.e. The P waves are tall (>2.5 mm) and wide (>2.5 mm) in leads II, III and aVF. *Right atrial hypertrophy* is reflected by tall peaked P wave (3.5 mm) in leads II and aVF. *Left atrial hypertrophy* is evidenced by notched P waves in leads II, III and aVF. The negative component of biphasic P wave in lead V_1 is also broad and prominent. There are nonspecific ST-T changes in leads II, III and aVF. The mean QRS axis is + 45°

1. Features of biatrial enlargement.
2. Features of moderate right ventricular hypertrophy.

1. *Biatrial Enlargement:*

Left atrial enlargement is reflected as P wave abnormality. P waves are widened (>2.5 mm) on frontal plane axis and there is an accentuation and delay in the terminal negative component of biphasic P wave in lead V_1. Both these signs indicate left atrial hypertrophy due to associated mitral valve disease in tricuspid stenosis of rheumatic origin.

Right atrial hypertrophy is reflected in marked increase in amplitude of P waves (> 2.5 mm) on frontal plane axis and there is an accentuation of initial component of bifid P wave on frontal plane and accentuation and peaking of initial positive component of biphasic P wave in lead V_1. P wave abnormalities are best seen in leads II, III and aVF and are due to rightwards shift of P wave axis.

In nutshell P waves in tricuspid stenosis are tall as well as wide and become notched or 'M-shaped' in which initial positive deflection is taller than terminal component, the manifestation sometimes called 'P-tricuspidale', indicates biatrial hypertrophy in tricuspid stenosis, hence, the name.

The QRS complex in V_1 also reflect the effect of right atrial enlargement. Lead V_1 may manifest with an initial q wave of a qR complex, may mimic anteroseptal infarction which can be excluded on clinical and other electrocardiographic findings. There may be attenuation of QRS in lead V_1 which gets suddenly increased in lead V_2.

2. *Moderate Right Ventricular Hypertrophy*

The electrocardiographic findings are either minimal or absent and are masked by biatrial enlargement. These may be in the form of right axis deviation and small amplitude of R waves in right precordial leads. Leads V_1 and V_2 may reflect rs, rsr' or qrs or QR complex. Incomplete right bundle branch block is not uncommon. Standard lead I and lead V_1 reflect qrs complex.

The diagnostic clues to tricuspid stenosis on ECG are listed in the box.

ECG clues to Tricuspid Stenosis

* *P wave:* Both amplitude and duration of P wave are increased. P waves are notched or 'M-shaped' called *P-tricuspidale*, seen in leads II, III and aVF due to right axis of P wave.
* *The QRS complexes:* They are short in amplitude. The QRS axis is deviated rightwards, which may be the only evidence of right ventricular hypertrophy. The lead V_1 has rs or rsr' or qrs or QR complex.

Tricuspid Regurgitation

Isolated tricuspid regurgitation due to rheumatic heart disease is rare. It is functional and always secondary to marked dilatation of right ventricle and tricuspid valve annulus. Organic tricuspid regurgitation, if at all occurs in rheumatic heart disease is associated with tricuspid stenosis.

Causes

Functional tricuspid regurgitation occurs as a consequence to;
1. It may complicate right ventricular failure of any cause, i.e. right ventricular infarction, rheumatic or congenital heart diseases with severe pulmonary hypertension, ischaemic heart disease, cardiomyopathies and cor pulmonale.
2. Less commonly, it results from congenitally deformed tricuspid valve, atrioventricular canal defects and Ebstein's anomaly.
3. Infarction of papillary muscles of right ventricle.
4. Tricuspid valve prolapse.
5. Carcinoid syndrome
6. Endomyocardial fibrosis
7. Infective endocarditis
8. Trauma

The Electrocardiogram

The sole ECG finding suggesting tricuspid regurgitation is a small q wave followed by a tall or relatively tall R wave, i.e. a qR complex in lead V_1.

Pulmonary Stenosis

Read Chapter on Congenital Heart Disease.

Pulmonary Regurgitation

ECG findings are similar to tricuspid regurgitation.

FLOPPY MITRAL VALVE (MITRAL VALVE PROLAPSE) SYNDROME

It is a condition in which mitral valve leaflets billow or bulge or prolapse into left atrium during ventricular systole producing mitral regurgitation. Posterior leaflet prolapse is commoner than anterior. The syndrome is called by many names as *mid-systolic click-murmur, billowing mitral leaflet, Flail mitral valve or Barlow's syndrome, etc.* The syndrome was first described by Barlow and Pocock, since then it has evoked much interest and has received important considerations as a clinical entity during the last two decades. The primary mitral valve prolapse appears to be a degenerative condition involving the valve and its supporting tissue resulting in the lengthening and attenuation of chorda tendinea.

Causes

1. *Primary*—A degenerative condition.
2. *Secondary*—It occurs in following conditions;
   i) Papillary muscle dysfunction in coronary artery disease.
   ii) Hypertrophic cardiomyopathy
   iii) Marfan's syndrome or cystic medial necrosis.
   iv) The Wolff-Parkinson-White (WPW) syndrome.
   v) The hereditary prolonged Q-T syndrome.
   vi) Following mitral valvotomies
   vii) Acute rheumatic fever.
   viii) Ostium primum atrial septal defect.
   ix) Chronic rheumatic heart disease.

Haemodynamic Alterations

Mitral valve prolapse is usually a benign condition, occurs in 2nd and 3rd decade of life, commonly in females. It is mostly asymptomatic and detected on routine examination. Symptomatic patients have significant mitral regurgitation and ventricular dilatation. The prolapse of mitral valve puts traction on the papillary muscles and left ventricular

SECTION NINE

myocardium leading to their dysfunction, ischaemia, and rupture of chorda tendinea, etc. Frank valvular regurgitation results in ventricular dilatation. The ECG changes and ventricular arrhythmias result from regional myocardial dysfunction as a result of increased stress on the papillary muscles.

The Electrocardiogram (Figs 24.13 and 24.14)

The electrocardiographic manifestations occur in 37% cases as reported by Barlow and Pocock. These manifestations vary spontaneously, may get exacerbated after an effort. These include;

1. T Wave Abnormality

i) *T wave inversion in inferior leads (II, III and aVF).* The mean frontal plane QRS axis is usually in the region of +80° to +100°, while T wave axis is around – 40°, thus, there is widening of QRS-T angle. As QRS axis is oriented towards inferior leads, tall R waves appear in leads II, III and aVF. The T wave axis is away from these leads, hence, T wave inversion is observed in these leads (Fig. 24.13). The distribution of T wave and QRS axes form a 'half past two' pattern of a clock as shown in the diagram (Fig. 24.14). The peculiar presentation of QRS and T wave axes is characteristically seen in this syndrome.

ii) *T wave inversion in mid-precordial leads (V_3-V_4).* The T wave inversion may occur in all precordial leads, but more common in mid-precordial leads (V_3-V_4). These changes may normalise spontaneously after an effort. Grant in 1957 termed this phenomenon as 'isolated T wave negativity syndrome' and observed it in healthy young adults. He did not recognise it as being associated with mitral valve prolapse.

2. The ST Segment Abnormalities

The ST segment abnormalities may resemble myocardial ischaemia. The abnormal manifestations include horizontal depression of ST segment with sharp angled ST-T junction. In some cases, there may be plane depression of ST segment which may be increased on effort. These changes are best seen in inferior oriented leads (II, III & aVF) and/or

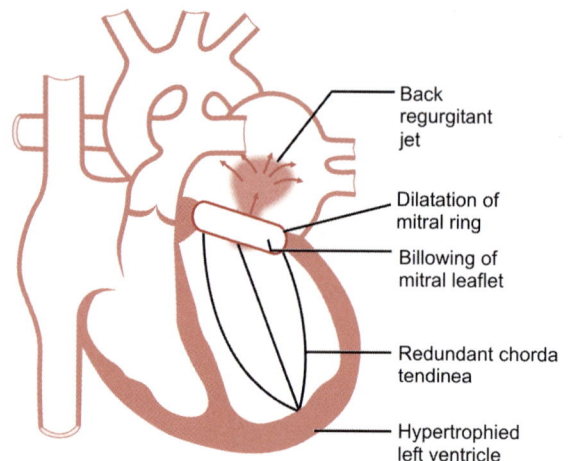

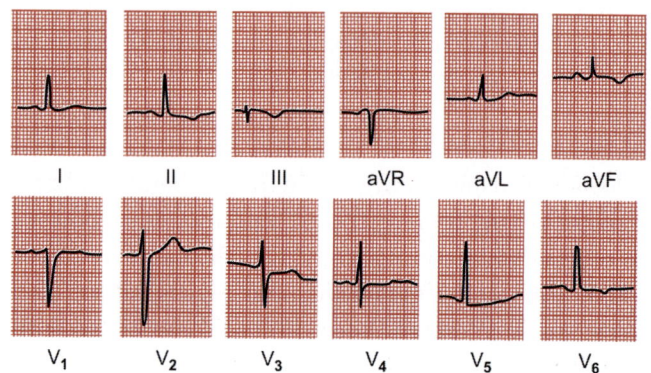

Fig. 24.13: Floppy mitral valve syndrome. The ECG was recorded from a 25 yrs female with mitral regurgitation proved to be having prolapse of mitral leaflet. Note the following features;

i. There is ST depression in leads II, III and aVF (inferior leads) and lateral leads V_5-V_6 due to traction on the myocardium by prolapsed posterior mitral leaflet.

ii. The QRS axis is normal and T wave axis is around –40°

iii. There is T wave inversion in leads V_4-V_6

There is no evidence of left ventricular hypertrophy or strain or coronary artery diseases to explain these findings

anterolateral leads. Sometimes evolutionary pattern starting from a normal ST segment to a depressed ST segment then inversion of T wave, and its subsequent disappearance may be seen.

3. Prolongation of QT Interval and Increased QT Dispersion (QTd)

Although prolongation of QT interval has been reported but is rare. There is also an increased association between mitral valve prolapse and prolongation of QT interval and QT dispersion, which

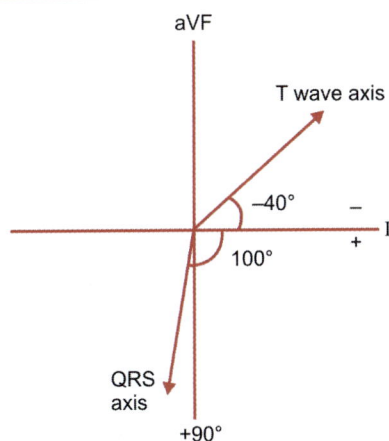

Fig. 24.14: Diagrammatic illustration of QRS and T wave axis on frontal plane in Floppy mitral valve syndrome

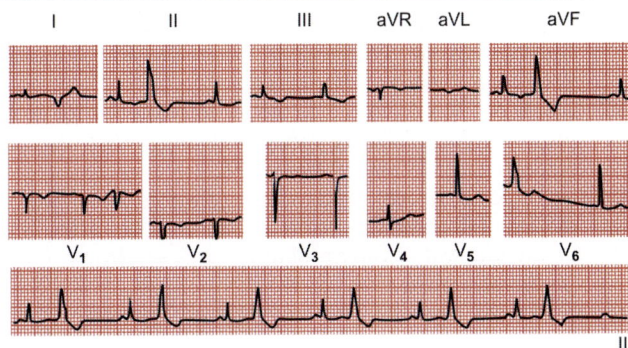

Fig. 24.15: Mitral valve prolpase with an arrhythmia. The ECG recorded from a 18 yr F with mitral valve prolapse proved by echocardiography shows;

  i. The ST segment depression and T wave inversion in inferior leads (II, III and aVF) suggestive of ischaemia of inferior wall. The ST segment and T wave changes seen in V_1-V_2 (suggest persistent juvenile pattern)
  ii. VPCs. There are frequent VPCs, one seen in each lead I, II, aVF, V_1 and V_6
  iii. Ventricular bigeminy rhythm. The lower strip recorded from the same patient at different interval showed a normal sinus beat alternating with a VPC constituting ventricular bigeminy rhythm

play a significant role in the genesis of arrhythmias and sudden death.

Paroxysmal supraventricular tachycardia is most common sustained tachyarrhythmia in patients with mitral valve prolapse and may be related to an increased incidence of atrioventricular bypass tract in this condition. Conversely, there is evidence that incidence of mitral valve prolapse among patients of WPW syndrome is increased. The patients of MVP who develop PSVT should be subjected to electrophysiological studies for demonstration of pre-excitation. This is important because digitalis and propranolol which may be useful in re-entrant tachycardia may be hazardous in the presence of antegrade conduction over an atrioventricular bypass tract.

4. Arrhythmias (Fig. 24.15)

Ventricular ectopics (spontaneous or excercise induced), unifocal or multifocal or ectopics with short coupling interval resulting in R on T phenomenon may be observed. These ectopics may vary with posture and may in fact disappear with upright posture. Ventricular tachycardia is uncommon.

The ventricular arrhythmias are as a result of abnormal traction on the papillary muscles leading to focal ischaemia of myocardium. Conduction blocks (sinoatrial, bundle branch block, left anterior hemiblock, etc) have been observed but their relationship to this syndrome is still ambiguous.

Suggested Reading

  1. Barlow JB, Pocock WA: The problem of non-ejection clicks and associated mitral systolic murmurs, emphasis on the billowing mitral leaflets syndrome. *Am Heart J* **97**: 277, 1975.
  2. Barlow JB, Pocock WA: Mitral valve prolapse, the athlete's heart, physical activity and sudden death. *Int J Sports Cardiol*, **1**: 9, 1984.
  3. Barlow JB: Prospective on mitral valve prolapse. Philadelphia; FA Davis Co., 1987.
  4. Barlow JW, Pocock WA, Obel EWP: Mitral valve prolapse, primary, secondary, both or neither. *Am Heart J* **102**: 140, 1981.
  5. Braunwald E: Valvular heart disease. In *Harrison's Principles of Internal Medicine*, 14th edn. McGraw Hill Inc. 1997.
  6. Burch GE, De Pasquale NP, Philip JH: The syndrome of papillary muscle dysfunction. *Am Heart J* **75**: 399, 1968.
  7. Cooksey JD, Dunn M, Massie E: Clinical vectorcardiography and electrocardiography. 2nd ed Chicago, Year Book Medical Publishers, 1977.
  8. Cueto J, Toshima J, Asmyo G, et al: Vectorcardiographic studies in acquired valvular disease with reference to the diagnosis of RVH. *Circulation* **35**:588,1967.
  9. Demaria AN, Amsterdam EA, Vismara LA: Arrhythmias in the mitral valve prolapse syndrome, *Ann Intern Med* **84**: 656, 1976.
  10. Ehler KH, Engle MA, Levine AR et al: Left ventricular abnormality with late mitral insufficiency and abnormal electrocardiograms. *Am J Cardiol* **26**: 333, 1970.

SECTION NINE

11. Gallagher JJ, Gilbert M, Svenson RH: Wolff-Parkinson-White syndrome. The problem evaluation and surgical correlation. *Circulation* **57**:767,1975.

12. Gooch AS, Viscencio F, Maranhao, V: Arrhythmias and left ventricular asynergy in prolapsing mitral leaflet syndrome. *Am J Cardiol* **29**: 611, 1972.

13. Grant RP: Clinical electrocardiography, New York: McGraw Hill 1957.

14. Jersaty RM: Mitral valve prolapse—click syndrome. *Prog Cardiovascular Dis* **15**: 623, 1973.

15. Liedtke AJ, Gault JH, Leaman DM et al: Geometry of left ventricular contraction in the systolic click syndrome, characterisation of a sequential myocardial abnormality. *Circulation* **47**: 27, 1973.

16. Lobstein HP, Horwitz LD, Curry JE et al: Electrocardiograhic abnormalities and coronary angiograms in mitral click-murmur syndrome. *N Eng J Med* **289**: 127, 1973.

17. Morris JJ, Estes EH, Wholen RE, et al: P wave analysis in valvular heart disease. *Circulation* **29**:242;1964.

18. Pocock WA, Barlow JB: Aetiology and electrocardiographic features of the billowing mitral leaflet syndrome. *Am J Med* **51**: 731, 1971.

19. Pocock WA, Barlow JB: Post-excercise arrhythmias in the billowing posterior mitral leaflet syndrome. *Am Heart J* **80**: 740, 1970.

20. Roberts WC, Day PJ: Electrocardiographic observations in clinically isolated, pure and chronic severe aortic regurgitation. Analysis of 30 necropsy patients aged 19 to 65 yrs. *Am J Cardiol* **55**:43;1985.

21. Schamroth L: Electrocardiographic excursions. Oxford: Blackwell Scientific Publications, 1975.

22. Schamroth L, Schamroth CL, Sareli P et al: Electrocardiographic differentiation of causes of left ventricular overload. *Chest* **85**: 95, 1986.

23. Siegel RJ, Roberts WC: Electrocardiographic observations in severe aortic stenosis: Correlative necropsy study of clinical, haemodynamic, and ECG variables demonstrating relation of 12-lead QRS amplitude to peak systolic transaortic pressure gradient. *Am Heart J* **103**:210;1982.

24. Sodi-pallares D, Bisteni A, Hermann GR: Some views on the significance of qR and QR type of complexes in the right precordial leads in the absence of myocardial infarction. *Am Heart J* **43**: 716, 1986.

25. Stich KM, Borer JS, Hochreiter C, et al: Prognostic value and physiological correlates of heart rate variability in chronic severe mitral regurgitation. *Circulation* **88**: 127,1993.

25

Myocarditis and Cardiomyopathies

- ■ *Myocarditis—aetiology, pathogenic mechanisms and electrocardiographic features*
- ■ *Dilated cardiomyopathy—the ECG characteristics*
- ■ *Restrictive cardiomyopathy—causes and ECG features*

SECTION NINE

MYOCARDITIS

Inflammation of myocardium is called *myocarditis*. It may be acute or chronic. Chronic myocarditis occurs in Chagas' disease.

Causes

Any acute and chronic disease can involve the myocardium. Myocarditis is commonly due to infections and may be associated with pericarditis (myopericarditis). It may also be present in hypersensitivity states such as acute rheumatic fever or may be caused by radiations, chemicals, physical agents and drugs. Almost every infectious agent is capable of producing myocarditis. In an unknown number of cases, acute myocarditis progresses to chronic dilated cardiomyopathy. The causes are given in the Table 25.1.

Table 25.1. Aetiology of myocarditis

1. *Viral*
    Coxsackie B and A, influenza, adeno, echo, rubeola
2. *Bacterial*
    - A complication of bacterial endocarditis
    - Diphtheria
    - Focal suppurative myocarditis
    - Granulomatous myocarditis (tubercular, syphilis)
    - Typhoid fever
    - Brucellosis
    - Mycoplasma infection
    - Legionnaire's disease
3. *Rickettsial*
    - Scrub typhus
4. *Fungal*
    - Histoplasmosis
    - Blastomycosis
    - Actinomycosis
5. *Parasitic*
    - Trypanosomiasis (Chagas' disease)
    - Toxoplasmosis
6. *Hypersensitivity*
    - Acute rheumatic fever
7. *Miscellaneous*
    - Radiations
    - Chemicals
    - Physical agents
    - Drugs

Pathogenic Pathophysiology

Acute myocarditis results in a widespread but patchy distribution of multiple foci of inflammatory tissue resulting in myocardial ischaemia and/or myocardial injury and/or myocardial necrosis. The myocarditis affects atria, ventricles and conduction tissue. Due to patchy involvement, one region may be affected more than the other. It is not necessary that all the three pathological processes (ischaemia, injury, necrosis) may be present at the same time because they have different evolutionary pathological phases; for example, some foci may be in the ischaemic phase; whereas others have progressed to injury and necrosis phase. Acute myocarditis is commonly associated with ventricular dilatation without hypertrophy.

The Electrocardiogram

The electrocardiographic features are due to ischaemia, injury and necrosis of the myocardium. The electrocardiographic findings in acute myocarditis are nonspecific and bizarre. The abnormalities may involve electrocardiographic deflections (P-QRS-T) and may also manifest as a disturbance of impulse formation and conduction. The ECG changes include;

A. Abnormalities of QRS (Fig. 25.1)

 (i) *Low voltage of QRS complexes*: The height of QRS may be decreased due to loss of functional ventricular mass. At times, low voltage of QRS deflections may be observed if chronic cardiomyopathy develops (Fig. 25.1)

 (ii) *Increase in ventricular activation time (VAT)*. This is due to injury block, i.e. slowing of conduction through the injured or inflamed myocardium.

 (iii) *Irregular QRS deflections (notchings and slurrings)* These are due to impedance of activation front through the injured/inflamed ventricular wall (Fig. 25.2)

 (iv) *Pathological Q waves and/or loss of R wave magnitude*. If myocarditis is severe enough to produce

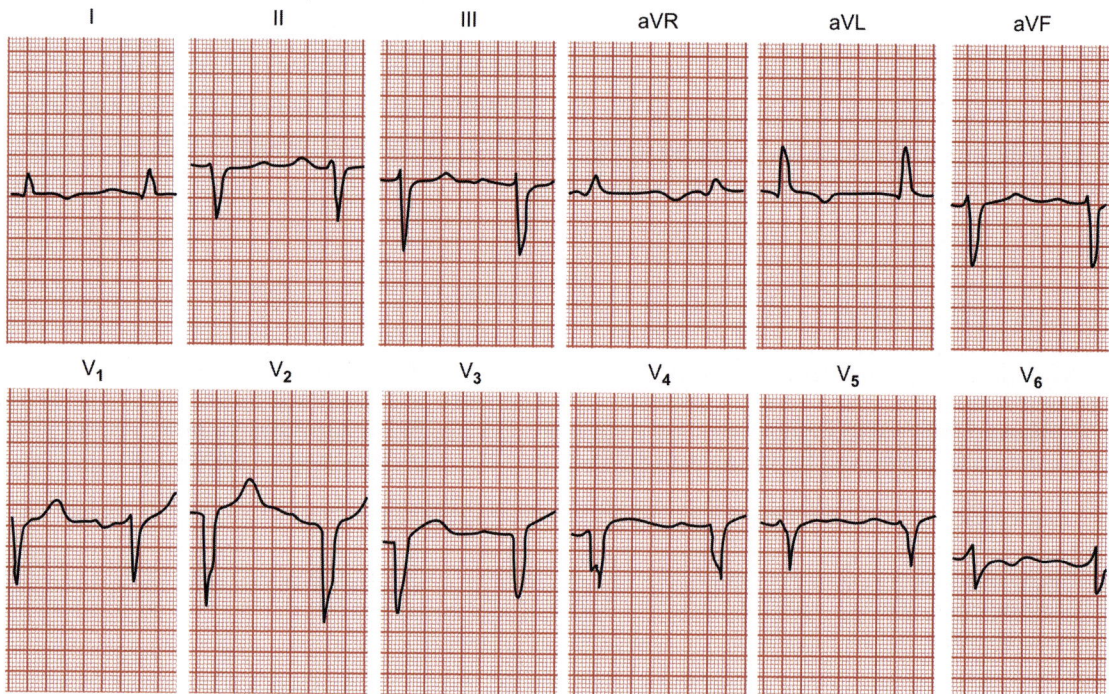

Fig. 25.1: Myocarditis. The ECG shows;
   i. First degree AV block (P-R interval is 0.24 sec)
   ii. Wide QRS (>0.10 sec but < 0.12 sec) complexes with notchings and slurrings
   iii. Left axis deviation > -70° is due to combined effect of left anterior hemiblock plus delayed indeterminate intraventricular conduction
   iv. Nonspecific ST-T changes. The ST segment is minimally elevated with T wave inversion in leads I, aVL, V$_6$

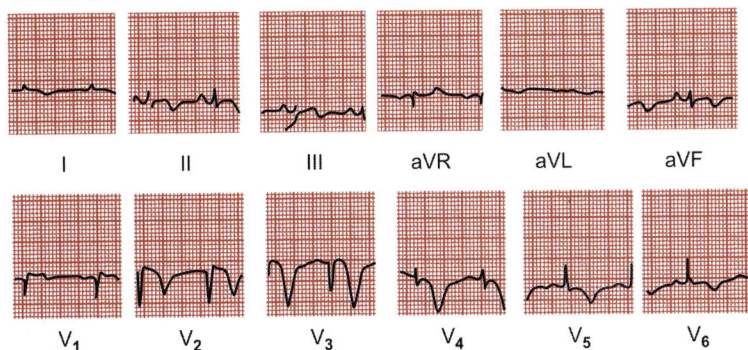

Fig. 25.2: Myocarditis. The electrocardiogram was recorded from a patient admitted with aluminium phosphide poisoning (toxic myocarditis). Note the following characteristics;
  i. Low voltage graph in the standard leads
  ii. T wave inversion in leads I, II, III, aVL, aVF and V_1-V_6
  iii. Height of R wave is reduced in precordial leads
  iv. QTc is prolonged (R-R = 0.64 sec QT = 40 sec, thus QTc is 0.50 sec).

Note: All these changes reversed with full recovery of the patient without any residual damage

Fig. 25.3: Acute myocarditis simulating acute pericarditis. Note the following features on electrocardiogram:
  i. Decreased height of R wave in standard leads but it is not low voltage graph as some complexes are >5 mm. There is elevation of ST segment with concavity upwards in leads II, III, aVF, and V_2-V_6. The T wave is upright in all these leads. Reciprocal ST depression is seen in aVR
  ii. The QT and QTc intervals are not prolonged
    All these feature can be seen in acute pericarditis, hence, at times may be impossible to differentiate between them

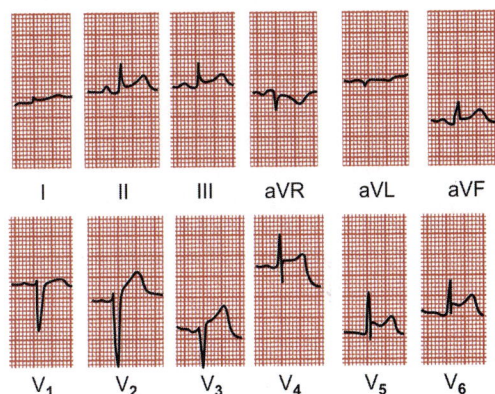

necrosis, then pathological Q waves will appear. The location of Q waves is unpredictable. There is decrease in the height of R wave due to loss of some functional myocardial tissue.

(v) *Left anterior hemiblock.* It may occur due to compression of anterior fascicle by inflamed or oedematous myocardial tissue. This presents as left axis deviation > – 30° (Fig. 25.3).

(vi) *Increased QRS duration.* The prolongation or widening of QRS may be marked and may range from 0.10 sec. to 0.12 sec. This is due to slow and delayed endocardial to epicardial activation through oedematous and inflamed myocardium.

(vii) *Intraventricular conduction defect.* Bizarre, irregular intraventricular conduction neither fitting into RBBB nor into LBBB may be seen. In Chagas' disease, right bundle branch block (RBBB) is more common.

B. The ST Segment Change (Figs 25.2 and 25.3)

Both the depression and elevation of the ST segment may occur depending on the subendocardial or subepicardial injury. When ST segment is elevated, it shows a rapid descent with inverted T wave (Fig. 25.2). The ST change may, sometimes, resemble acute pericarditis, i.e. ST is elevated with concavity upwards (Fig. 25.3).

C. The T Wave Change (Fig. 25.4)

Abnormalities of T waves are frequent. The abnormality usually manifests as low to inverted T waves in standard and left precordial leads. The T wave changes constitute sensitive but nonspecific diagnostic criteria.

D. Prolongation of QTc (Fig. 25.4)

A prolonged QTc is common due to slow depolarisation cum repolarisation. QTc interval of 0.60 to 0.70 seconds has been reported in the literature.

E. Arrhythmias/AV Blocks

Both atrial and ventricular extrasystoles may occur. Sinus tachycardia is a usual and expected manifestation of acute myocarditis. Idionodal tachycardia is

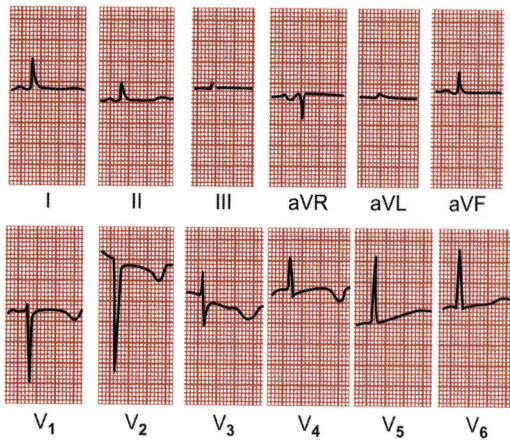

Fig. 25.4: Myocarditis. The electrocardiogram shows;
  i. Low voltage QRS complexes (< 5 mm) in standard leads.
 ii. Prolonged QT interval is seen where T wave is best visible (II, V_1-V_6). The QT interval is 0.52 seconds
iii. The ST-T change: There is minimal ST segment depression in precordial leads. The T wave is inverted from V_1-V_4 with flat to low T wave in V_5-V_6 and all standard leads

also common. Prolonged P-R interval (first degree AV block) is common but other AV blocks are uncommon. Atrial fibrillation is also uncommon.

The Evolution of Myocarditis

While the QRS and ST segment changes usually regress as the disease process subsides but T wave inversion in left precordial leads may persist for weeks and even months after acute myocarditis. Recovery is the rule in most instances of myocarditis, but persistent abnormal electrocardiograms are common following diphtheric myocarditis. If acute myocarditis passes on to chronic myocarditis, then changes similar to dilated cardiomyopathy will manifest.

CHAGAS' MYOCARDITIS

It may be acute or chronic. Acute myocarditis in Chagas' disease is related largely to immune lysis by antibody and cell mediated immunity directed against antigens released from *T. cruzi*–infected cells. At an average of 20 years after initial (usually unrecognised) infection, about 30% develop chronic Chagas' disease including myocarditis. Autoimmune mechanism has been proposed to be the underlying pathogenic process.

The Electrocardiogram

The electrocardiographic features are the rule, appear late in the course of the disease due to dilated cardiomyopathy and autonomic dysfunction. These include;

1. *Conduction defects.* Right bundle branch block, left anterior hemiblock are common; while AV blocks are less frequently observed. Sinus bradycardia and SA blocks may occur due to SA node dysfunction.

2. *Rhythm disturbance.* Both atrial and ventricular arrhythmias are common in the form of; atrial fibrillation with slow ventricular response, VPCs (monomorphic, polymorphic) and bouts of ventricular tachycardia during and following exercise. Idionodal or idioventricular escape rhythm may occur.

3. *The ST-T changes.* Elevated ST segment with coving and T wave inversion may be seen in most of the leads. The Q waves may also be observed.

4. *The P wave.* The wide and notched P waves due to left atrial enlargement may also be seen frequently.

REVIEW AT GLANCE

The Electrocardiographic Changes in Acute Myocarditis

The changes are due to slow depolarisation and repolarisation.

1. *Abnormalities of QRS*
   - Widened QRS complexes
   - Irregular QRS deflections (notchings and slurrings)
   - VAT is increased
   - Pathological Q waves / loss of R wave magnitude.

2. *The ST segment change*
   - Depression/elevation depending on subendocardial / subepicardial injury
   - If ST segment is elevated, it shows coving with rapid descent and inverted T waves.
   - Occasionally, pattern simulating myocardial infarction may be present.

3. *The T wave abnormalities*
   - Low to inverted T waves in standard and precordial leads.
4. *Conduction disturbances*
   - Pattern of left anterior hemiblock, i.e. left axis deviation (> – 30º)
   - *Intraventricular* conduction delay with wide, bizarre QRS complexes.
   - Prolonged P-R and QTc intervals.
5. *Arrhythmias /AV blocks*
   - Both atrial and ventricular ectopics common
   - Sinus tachycardia
   - Idionodal tachycardia
   - Atrial fibrillation is uncommon
   - First degree AV block common.

CARDIOMYOPATHIES

The cardiomyopathies constitute a group of diseases involving the heart muscle itself and are distinct entities because they are not the result of pericardial, hypertensive, congenital, valvular or ischaemic heart diseases. The term ischaemic cardiomyopathy refers to a condition in which multiple infarcts or diffuse fibrosis leads to dilatation of left ventricle and congestive heart failure. It may or may not be associated with angina pectoris.

Clinical or Functional Types

Depending on the functional impairment, three basic types are;

1. Dilated cardiomyopathy or congestive cardiomyopathy
2. Hypertrophic cardiomyopathy. It has been discussed as a separate Chapter 23.
3. Restrictive cardiomyopathy.

Dilated (Congestive) Cardiomyopathy

Dilated or congestive cardiomyopathy is a patchy disease involving the myocardium; manifests clinically with dilated heart, murmurs due to valvular incompetence and arrhythmias. It results from a wide variety of toxic and metabolic insults. Alcoholism may be an important cause. Postpartum cardiomyopathy is also a dilated cardiomyopathy. Ischaemic cardiomyopathy due to multiple infarcts and fibrosis also leads to dilated cardiomyopathy especially involving the left ventricle.

The Electrocardiogram (Figs 25.5 and 25.6)

The electrocardiogram is usually abnormal and nonspecific. The ECG changes include:

A. *Changes due to atrial enlargement:* Atrial enlargement on ECG is reflected in increased voltage or height of P waves in leads which normally record the good P waves, i.e. leads I, II, III, aVF and V_1.

B. *The QRS abnormalities*
   1. Generalised low voltage of QRS complexes in frontal plane leads with poor R wave progression in precordial leads is not uncommon. This is due to loss of functional muscle mass and fibrosis (Fig. 25.5).

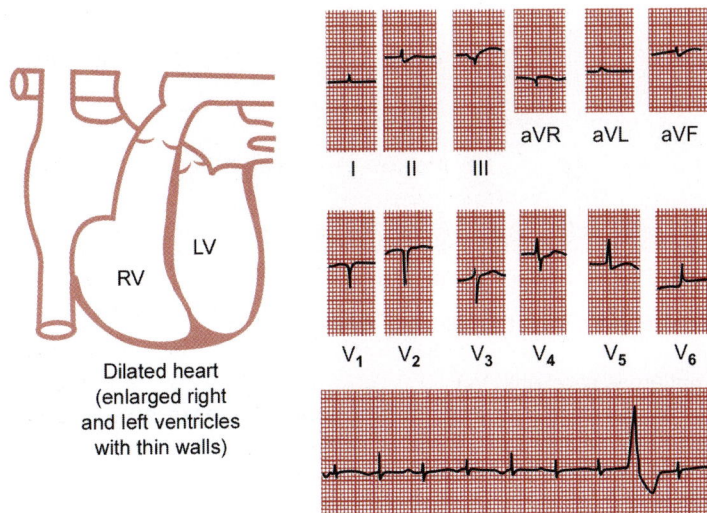

Dilated heart (enlarged right and left ventricles with thin walls)

Fig. 25.5: Dilated cardiomyopathy: The electrocardiogram was recorded from a 40 years female admitted with gross congestive heart failure proved to be dilated cardiomyopathy on echocardiogram. Note the following characteristics:
   i. Low voltage graph—All the standard leads show QRS deflections <5 mm and all the precordial leads record QRS deflections < 10 mm. There is coving of ST segment in leads II, III, aVF and V_2-V_6. The T wave is low to flat in all the leads.
   ii. Lower strip (rhythm strip II) shows multifocal atrial tachycardia and a ventricular ectopic

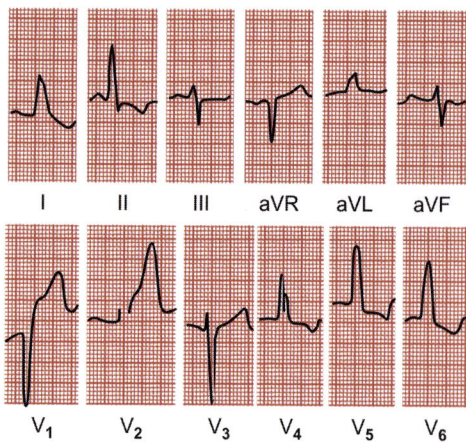

Fig. 25.6: Left bundle branch block in a patient with dilated cardiomyopathy. The electrocardiogram was recorded from a 45 yrs female admitted with congestive heart failure, proved to be cardiomyopathy on echocardiography, showed pattern of left bundle branch block evidenced by:
- i. Left axis deviation
- ii. Wide R wave with small S wave without q wave in leads V_4-V_6, I and aVL. There is slurring of R in leads aVL and V_4.
- iii. rS pattern in leads V_1-V_3
- iv. Associated ST-T changes, i.e. ST depression with convexity upwards V_4-V_6 and elevation of ST segment with concavity upwards in leads V_1-V_3

2. Left axis deviation (>-30°) due to left anterior hemiblock is a common manifestation.
3. Right axis deviation (> + 120°) due to involvement of left posterior fascicle is less common.
4. *Left bundle branch block (LBBB)*. This is also common. It may be incomplete with loss of q waves in left precordial leads due to septal fibrosis, or may be complete with its typical pattern and left axis deviation (Fig. 25.6). LBBB with right axis deviation is commonly seen in dilated cardiomyopathy.
5. *Right bundle branch block* (Fig. 25.7). This is uncommon. RBBB with left axis deviation (bifascicular block) has also been reported in dilated cardiomyopathy.
6. *Biventricular hypertrophy*. This is less common. There can be associated atrial (left or right) hypertrophy especially if patient is in

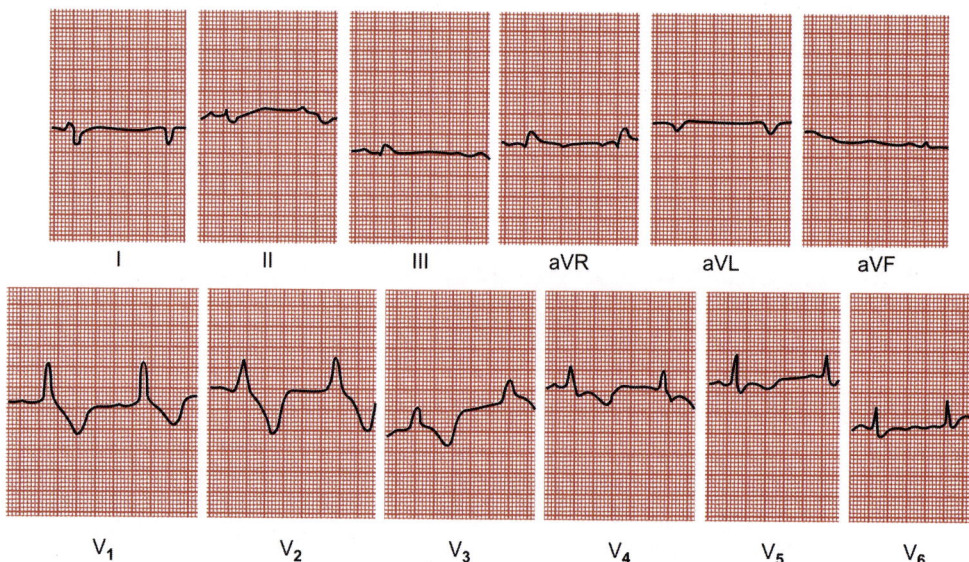

Fig. 25.7: Right bundle branch block pattern in dilated cardiomyopathy. Note the following characteristics;
- i. Low voltage graph
- ii. Right axis QRS deviation and clockwise rotation (RS pattern is seen upto V_6)
- iii. RBBB pattern: A wide slurred R wave from V_1-V_3 with RS pattern in V_4-V_6 with slurred S waves in these left side leads. There is associated minimal depression of convex upward ST segment with T wave inversion in all precordial leads

Note: This type of pattern in precordial leads can be seen in left sided accessory pathway but low voltage of the complexes without delta wave and normal P-R interval rules out the possibility

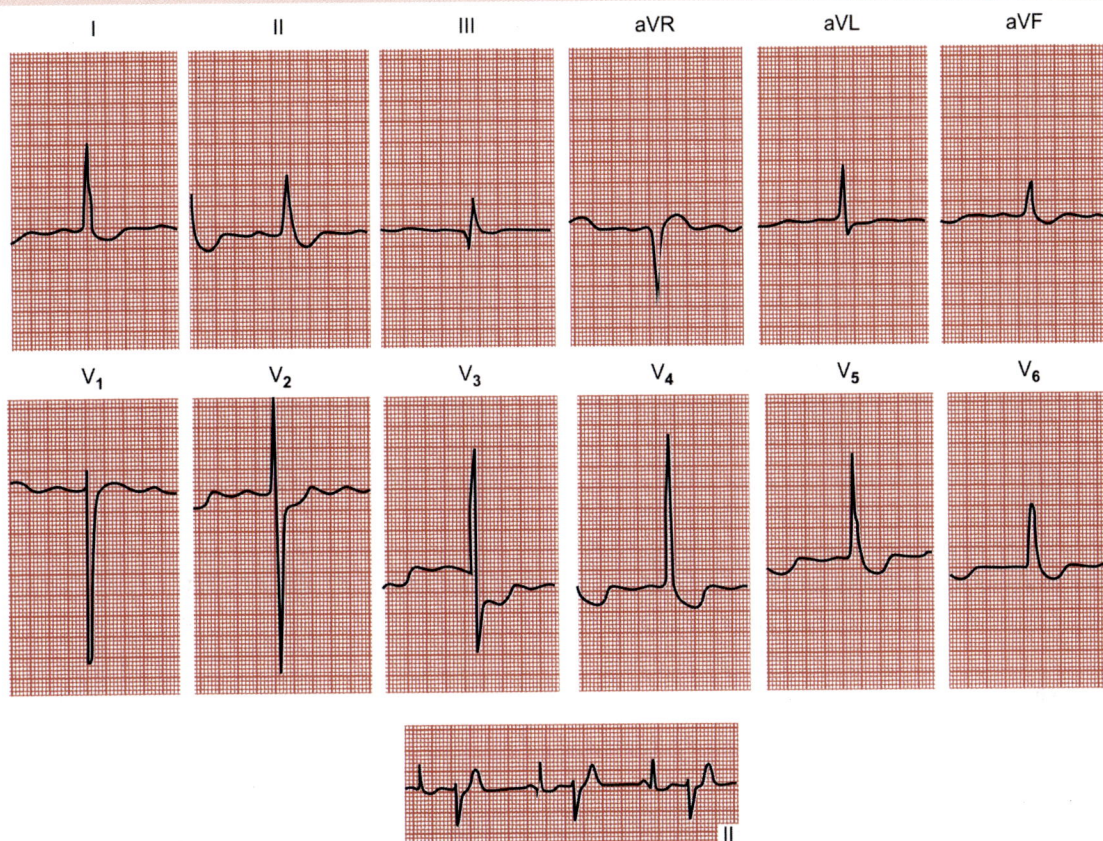

Fig. 25.8: Dilated cardiomyopathy. The 12 leads electrocardiogram (A) shows;

A: 1. *Left ventricular hypertrophy:* It is characterised by voltage criteria i.e. $SV_1 + RV_5 = 42$ mm with ST segment depression and T wave inversion in leads V_3-V_6

2. *Probable right ventricular hypertrophy:* The tall R waves in V_2-V_3 and ST segment depression and T wave inversion in these leads show anterior orientation of ST-T forces which is not expected with LVH alone

3. The P waves are normal. There is no evidence of atrial hypertrophy.

B: The lower strip (lead II) shows ventricular bigeminy rhythm

congestive failure (Fig. 25.8). The left atrial type of P waves (wide P waves) are more common.

7. *Left ventricular hypertrophy* (Fig. 25.8). The ECG changes of left ventricular hypertrophy (voltage criteria) are common in dilated cardiomyopathy. The associated ST changes (depression of ST segment with convexity upward) and inverted T waves are seen in left precordial leads, i.e. V_5-V_6.

8. *Pathological Q waves:* These are of no consequence because they reflect areas of inert necrotic myocardial tissue. These Q waves are seen infrequently in left oriented or inferiorly oriented (II, III, aVF) leads.

C. **ST segment and T wave abnormalities:** The ST segment depression and T wave inversion in left precordial and inferiorly oriented leads reflect primarily myocardial involvement, hence, form an important diagnostic criteria in patients with clinically diagnosed dilated cardiomyopathy.

D. **The wide QRS–T angle:** A wide QRS - T angle (>45°) is common.

E. **Conduction disturbances and arrhythmias:**

I. *Prolongation of P-R interval* (first degree AV block) is a common manifestation; while other grades of AV blocks are rare.

II. *Atrial and ventricular* ectopics are common (Figs 25.5 and 25.8). Atrial fibrillation is also a common rhythm disturbance seen in dilated cardiomyopathy. Frequent ventricular ectopics even of complex morphologies and ventricular tachycardias have been observed terminally. Supraventricular tachycardia occurs occasionally.

Restrictive Cardiomyopathy

Out of the three major categories of cardiomyopathies (dilated, hypertrophic and restrictive), the restrictive cardiomyopathy is least common. Primary form of restrictive cardiomyopathy is inherited and is rare. The secondary forms of restrictive cardiomyopathy occur due to variety of reasons and are common in certain geographic regions. The hallmark of the restrictive cardiomyopathy is abnormal diastolic function, rigid and non-compliant ventricular walls and impaired left ventricular filling. The systolic function of the heart is maintained even in spite of extensive infiltration of the myocardium. The restrictive cardiomyopathy bears some functional resemblance to constrictive pericarditis, from which it has to be differentiated because there is potential for successful treatment of constrictive pericarditis.

Causes

Although a variety of specific pathological conditions may result in restrictive cardiomyopathy yet the cause remains unknown in significant number of cases. Myocardial fibrosis, infiltration and myocardial scarring are the pathogenic mechanisms responsible for restrictive cardiomyopathy. The causes are divided into two groups and are given in Table 25.2.

Table 25.2: Classification of restrictive cardiomyopathies

1. *Myocardial causes*
   A. *Non-infiltrative*
   - Idiopathic
   - Scleroderma
   B. *Infiltrative*
   - Amyloidosis
   - Sarcoidosis
   - Gaucher's disease
   - Myxoedema
   C. *Storage diseases*
   - Haemochromatosis
   - Glycogen storage disease
   - Fabry's disease
2. *Endomyocardial causes*
   - Endomyocardial fibrosis
   - Hypereosinophilic syndromes
   - Carcinoid syndrome
   - Metastasis
   - Radiation injury

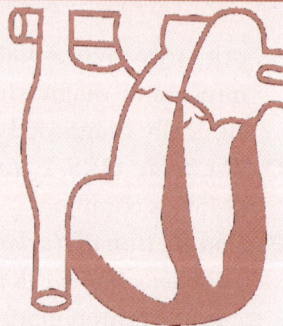

Restrictive cardiomyopathy

Haemodynamic Alterations

Three typical haemodynamic alterations occur in restrictive cardiomyopathy and form the basis of differentiation from constrictive pericarditis; but still at times (25% cases) it is difficult to differentiate. The alterations are;

1. The dip and plateau appearance in ventricular pressure, called the *square root sign* seen in constrictive pericarditis is absent.
2. Pressure in both ventricles is elevated but left ventricular pressure exceeds right ventricular pressure by 5 mm or more.
3. The pulmonary artery systolic pressure is > 50 mm Hg.

The Electrocardiogram

1. Amyloid Heart Disease (Fig. 25.9)

The electrocardiographic manifestations include:
1. Diminished voltage of QRS complexes.
2. Small or absent R wave in right precordial leads, may simulate anterior wall infarction. Presence of Q waves in inferior leads may simulate inferior wall infarction.
3. Arrhythmias. Atrial fibrillation is common. Complex ventricular arrhythmias are less common.
4. Conduction defects. Various types of AV conduction defects are seen. Sinus node dysfunction is also common.

2. Sarcoid Heart Disease

Sarcoidosis appears to have an affinity for involvement of AV junction and bundle of His. Diffuse myocardial involvement is less common. The electrocardiographic features include;
1. Varying degree of AV blocks and intraventricular conduction defects.
2. Pathological Q waves may appear when there is diffuse myocardial infiltration and may simulate myocardial infarction.

3. Haemochromatosis

Due to deposition of iron in the myocardium, there are changes in repolarisation in symptomatic patients

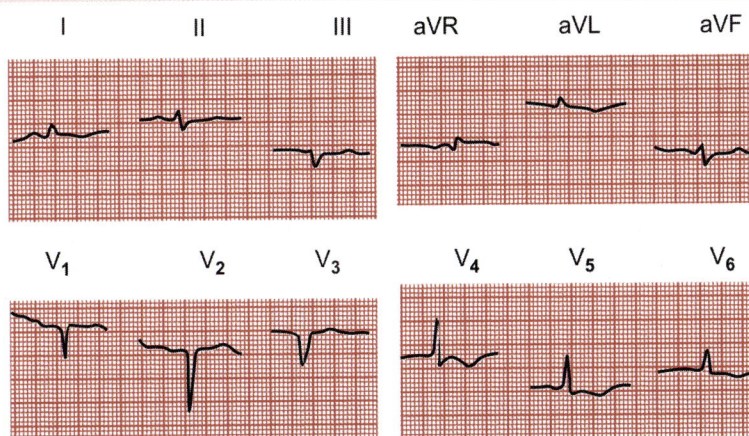

Fig. 25.9: *Cardiac amyloidosis.* The ECG was recorded from a 33 yrs old man with systemic amyloidosis and congestive heart failure, who died and subsequently autopsy proved amyloidosis. Note the following characteristics:
  i. Low voltage graph in standard and precordial leads
  ii. Left axis deviation
  iii. QS pattern in leads V_1-V_3 simulating the anteroseptal infarction. There is diminution of R wave in V_5-V_6. These changes in amyloidosis are common; and are due to infiltration of myocardium with the electrically inert substance. There is ST segment depression and T wave inversion in anterolateral leads (I, aVL, V_4-V_6)

in the form of ST-T wave abnormalities. Supraventricular arrhythmias are also common. These electrocardiographic features correlate with the degree of iron deposits in the heart.

4. Hypereosinophilic Syndromes
(Idiopathic and Loffler's Myocarditis)

Due to diffuse eosinophilic infiltration of the myocardium and especially the endocardium, there is inflammatory myocarditis and endocarditis. The electrocardiographic manifestations are usually nonspecific and include:
  1. Nonspecific ST-T abnormalities
  2. Arrhythmias especially atrial fibrillation
  3. Conduction defects particularly right bundle branch block may be present.

5. Carcinoid Syndrome

The carcinoid syndrome is caused by metastasising carcinoid tumour. The cardiac involvement may occur in addition to lungs, skin and GI tract, is commonly related to large circulating quantities of serotonin, bradykinin or other substances secreted by the tumour. There are no specific electrocardiographic changes in carcinoid heart disease; Therefore:
  1. Nonspecific ST-T abnormalities are common.
  2. Sinus tachycardia is frequently present.

3. Low QRS voltage may be seen in symptomatic patients
4. Right atrial enlargement without right ventricular hypertrophy may occasionally be seen.

Endomyocardial Fibrosis (EMF)

Endomyocardial fibrosis occurs most commonly in tropical and subtropical Africa, particularly Uganda and Nigeria, but is also found in tropical and subtropical regions in the rest of the world including India. The cardiac involvement may be right sided (right ventricular EMF) or left sided (left ventricular EMF) or biventricular EMF.

The Electrocardiogram

1. *Right ventricular EMF:* There may be diminished QRS voltage due to pericardial effusion, if present. There may be ST-T wave abnormalities and findings of right atrial enlargement producing a qR pattern in lead V_1. Atrial fibrillation may occur.
2. *Left ventricular EMF.* There may be diminished QRS voltage due to pericardial effusion, if present. Left ventricular hypertrophy may be present. There may be findings of left atrial hypertrophy (widened P waves). As with right sided involvement, atrial fibrillation may also occur.

SECTION NINE

3. *Biventricular EMF.* This is most common form of EMF. The electrocardiographic manifestations occur in the form of; low voltage graph due to presence of pericardial effusion, ventricular hypertrophy especially left, arrhythmias (atrial fibrillation is common), conduction defects (wide, bizarre QRS complexes) and loss of R wave progression in precordial leads.

Arrhythmogenic Right Ventricular Dysplasia

Patients with arrhythmogenic right ventricular dysplasia present with VT having a LBBB pattern (since tachycardia arises in right ventricle) often with right axis deviation and T waves inversions over the right precordial leads (V_1-V_2). The VT may be due to re-entry. Supraventricular arrhythmias can occur. In some patients, exercise can induce the VT.

Arrhythmogenic right ventricular dysplasia is actually a right ventricular type of cardiomyopathy possibility of familial origin. In the familial form, genetic abnormality has been located to chromosomes 1, 14 and 10. Most cases show abnormal inflow and outflow tract of right ventricle on echocardiography, CT and MRI.

Clinical Significance

It can be an important cause of ventricular arrhythmia in children and young adults with apparently normal hearts as well as older male patients.

The ECG (Fig. 25.10)

The ECG during sinus rhythm may exhibit complete or incomplete RBBB pattern with T wave inversion, in leads, V_1 to V_3. A terminal notch in the ORS (*called an epsilon wave*) may be present due to slow intraventricular conduction. The signal averaged ECG may be abnormal. During an episode of tachycardia, LBBB pattern is seen in leads V_1-V_3.

The treatment is conventional pharmacological therapy. Surgical manipulations and AICD have been successful in some patients. Radiofrequency ablation has been found unsuccessful.

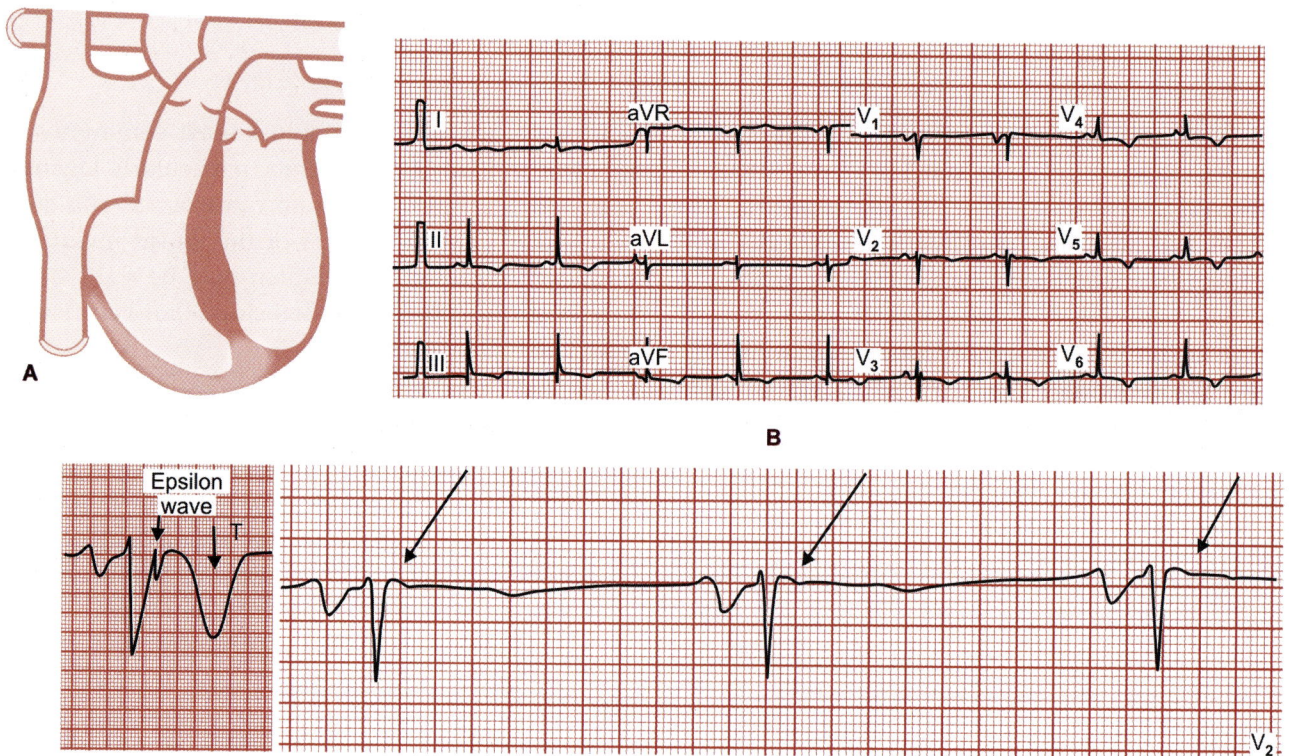

Fig. 25.10: Arrhythmogenic right ventricular dysplasia. **A:** Diagrammatic illustration. **B:** The ECG show depression with T wave inversion in leads I, II, III, V_1-V_5. The V_1 shows late right ventricular activation wave called epsilon wave (indicated by arrow)

REVIEW AT GLANCE

The ECG changes in cardiomyopathies

1. *Dilated cardiomyopathy:*
   a) P wave change – low voltage of P waves
   b) QRS abnormalities
      - Low voltage and poor progression of R wave in precordial leads.
      - Patterns of fascicular/bundle branch/bifascicular blocks are frequently seen.
      - Pathological Q waves are infrequent
   c) ST-T abnormalities, ST segment depression and T wave inversion is frequent.
   d) Wide QRS - T angle
   e) Conduction defects and arrhythmias.

2. *Restrictive cardiomyopathies*
   - Intraventricular conduction defects with bizarre QRS complexes.
   - Low voltage of QRS complexes (< 10 mm) in precordial leads.
   - Poor R wave progression across the precordial leads.

Suggested Reading

1. Arnold M, MeGuiro L, Lea JC: Loeffler's fibroplastic endocarditis. *Pathology* **20**: 79, 1988.
2. Bashour TT, Fadul H, Cheng TO: Electrocardiographic abnormalities in alcoholic cardiomyopathy. *Chest* **68**: 24, 1975.
3. Burstow DJ, Tajik AJ, Bailay KR et al: Two dimensional echocardiographic findings in systemic sarcoidosis. *Am J Cardiol* **63**: 478, 1989.
4. Corrado D, Basso C, Thieme G et al: Spectrum of clinicopathologic manifestations of arrhythymogenic right ventricular cardiomyopathy/dysplasia. A ventricular study. *J Am Coll Cardiology* **30**:1512-20,1997.
5. Casado J, Davila DF, Donis JH et al: Electrocardiographic abnormalities and left ventricular systolic function in Chagas' heart disease. *Int J Cardiol* **27**: 55, 1990.
6. Ceccjetti G, Binda A, Piperno A et al: Cardiac alterations in 36 consecutive patients with idiopathic haemochromatosis. Polygraphic and echocardiographic evaluation. *Eur Heart J* **12**: 224, 1991.
7. Chen CH, Nobuyoshi M, Kawai C: ECG pattern of left ventricular hypertrophy in nonobstructive hypertrophic cardiomyopathy; the significance of the mid-precordial changes. *Am Heart J* **97**: 687, 1979.
8. Dec GW, Fuster V: Medical progress: Idiopathic dilated cardiomyopathy. *N Engl J Med* **331**: 1564, 1994.
9. Dec GWJ, Waldman H, Southern J, et al: Viral myocarditis mimicking acute myocardial infarction. *J Am Coll Cardiol* **20**: 85, 1992.
10. Gertez MA, Kyle RA, Thibodeau SN: Familiar amyloidosis: A study of 52 North American born patients examined during a 30 yrs period. *Mayo Clin Proc* **67**: 428, 1992.
11. Goodwin JF: Congestive and hypertrophic cardiomyopathies: A decade of study. *Lancet* **i**: 731, 1970.
12. Haqor JM, Rashimtoola SH: Chagas' heart disease. *Curr Probl Cardiol* **20**: 825, 1995.
13. Karjalainen J: Functional and myocarditis-induced T wave abnormalities: Effect of orthostasis, betablockade and epinephrine. *Chest* **83**: 868, 1983.
14. Khosla SN, Chugh SN, Mehta HC, Chugh K: Serum transaminases in enteric myocarditis. *J Assoc Phy India* **29**: 11, 1981.
15. Martinez EE, Venturi M, Buffolo E et al: Operative results in Endomycardial fibrosis. *Am J Cardiol* **63**: 227, 1989.
16. Matsuura H, Palacios IF, Dec GW, et al: Intraventricular conduction abnormalities in patients with clinically suspected myocarditis are associated with myocardial necrosis. *Am Heart J* **127**: 1290, 1994.
17. Morgera T, DiLenarda A, Dreas L et al: Electrocardiography of myocarditis revisited: Clinical and prognostic significance of ECG changes. *Am Heart J* **124**: 455, 1992.
18. Nikolic G, Marriott HJL: LBBB with right axis deviation-a marker of congestive cardiomyopathy. *J Electrocardiol* **18**: 395, 1985.
19. Pellikka PA, Tajik AJ, Khandheria BK, et al: Carcinoid heart disease: Clinical and echocardiographic spectrum in 74 patients. *Circulation* **87**: 1188, 1993.
20. Peters NS, Poole-Wilson PA: Myocarditis-continuing clinical and pathologic confusion. *Am Heart J* **121**: 942, 1991.
21. Rosenbaum MB: Chagasic myocardiopathy. *Prog Cardiovas Dis* **7**: 199, 1964.
22. Rosenbaum MB: Myocardiopathy. *Prog Cardiovasc Dis*: **7**:142, 1964.
23. Schamroth L, Blumsohn D: The significance of left axis deviation in heart disease of Africans. *Br Heart J* **23**: 405, 1961.
24. Spyrou N, Foale R: Restrictive cardiomyopathies. *Curr Opin Cardiol* **9**: 344, 1994.
25. Wilensky RL, Yudelman P, Cohen AL et al: Serial ECG changes in idiopathic dilated cardiomyopathy confirmed at necropsy. *Am J Cardiol* **62**: 276, 1988.

SECTION NINE

26

Pericarditis

- *Acute pericarditis - definition, causes and evolution of electrocardiographic patterns during different stages*
- *Pericarditis with effusion - electrocardiographic patterns and their mechanisms*
- *Chronic constrictive pericarditis - electrocardiographic features*

PERICARDITIS

Inflammation of pericardium is called *pericarditis*. It may be acute, chronic or may be associated with effusion. Chronic pericarditis and pericardial effusion may be the end result of certain forms of acute pericarditis. Chronic pericarditis may occur with preceding acute phase and may lead to adhesions (adhesive or constrictive pericarditis) with or without effusion.

Aetiology

The causes of acute and chronic pericarditis with or without effusion are give in the Table 26.1.

The Electrocardiographic Abnormalities and their Pathogenesis

The acute pericarditis results in acute pericardial injury due to irritation by surrounding fluid or fibrin. There is, thus, a zone of injured tissue surrounding

---

Table 26.1: Causes of pericarditis

1. *Acute pericarditis*
   A. *Infective*
      - Viral, tubercular, pyogenic, fungal or parasitic
   B. *Non-infective*
      - Acute myocardial infarction
      - Uraemia
      - Neoplasia
      - Hypothyroidism
      - Trauma to pericardium (penetrating or non-penetrating injuries)
      - Post-radiation
      - Sarcoidosis
      - Acute idiopathic
   C. *Pericarditis due to hypersensitivity or autoimmunity*
      - Rheumatic fever
      - Collagen vascular disorders
      - Drug induced (procainamide, hydralazine, emetine, methysergide and others)
      - Postcardiac injury (postmyocardial infarction, i.e. Dressler's syndrome or following cardiac surgery)

2. *Chronic pericarditis (constrictive pericarditis)*
   - Viral or idiopathic
   - Tubercular, pyogenic or fungal
   - Myxoedema or hypothyroidism
   - Malignancy involving pericardium
   - Trauma
   - Chronic renal failure treated with haemodialysis.
   - Collagen vascular disorders
   - Following cardiac surgery
3. *Pericarditis with effusion*
   - Tuberculosis
   - Myxoedema
   - Cholesterol induced pericarditis
   - Neoplasms involving pericardium
   - Miscellaneous
     - Collagen vascular disorders
     - Pyogenic infections
     - Mycotic infections
     - Post-radiation
     - Uraemia
     - Slow leakage from ventricular aneurysm

the heart which is most marked in the apical region. There may also be associated epicardial ischaemia. *Mechanisms:* There are three basic mechanisms, i.e. acute pericardial injury, epicardial ischaemia and short circuiting effects that produce ECG abnormalities in pericarditis with or without effusion.

1. Acute Pericardial Injury and its Effect on ECG

In pericarditis, there is a zone of injured tissue surrounding the heart, the burnt of which affects the apical region. This manifests as ST segment deviation towards the injured surface.

2. Effects of Epicardial Ischaemia

This affects repolarisation of the heart, manifests by T wave deviation away from the ischaemic area.

3. Short-circuiting Effect

It is seen in pericardial effusion where fluid causes short-circuiting of electrical impulses generated by the myocardium. The low amplitude of P-QRS-T deflections and electrical alternans seen in pericardial effusion are due to this effect. This effect is seen commonly in large pericardial effusion with cardiac temponade. The voltage of the complexes return to normal or near normal after removal of fluid due to elimination of this effect.

The Electrocardiogram in Acute Pericarditis

The ECG patterns of acute pericarditis include:
1. The ST segment and T wave changes
2. The PR segment change

3. Sinus tachycardia.

Evolution of Electrocardiographic Changes during Acute Pericarditis (Table 26.2)

Serial electrocardiograms are extremely helpful in the diagnosis of acute pericarditis. The ECG changes can occur within few hours or days after acute pericardial pain and electrocardiographic diagnosis is made by detecting serial appearance of 4 stages of abnormalities of the ST segment and T wave (Table 26.2). These changes represent a current of injury pattern generated by inflamed pericardium leading to changes during repolarisation (ST-T changes). This epicardial or pericardial injury does not cause enough loss of myocardial potential, hence, abnormal Q waves are not seen in pericarditis.

Acute pericarditis affects only the repolarisation process leading to changes in ST segment and T wave

The evolution of ST segment and T wave change is described under four stages:

1. The ST Segment and T Wave Changes

Stage I (ST segment elevation with concavity upwards and upright tall T wave Fig. 26.1)

These changes occur early in pericarditis during pain and are diagnostic of it. These electrocardiographic changes include ST segment elevation with concavity upwards which is in contrast to ST elevation with convexity upwards seen in myocardial infarction; occur in all leads except aVR and V_1. The ST segment

SECTION NINE

Stages	Leads reflecting epicardial injury potentials (I,II,aVL,aVF, V_2-V_6)			Leads reflecting endocardial potentials (aVR, V_1)		
	J point and ST segment	T waves	P R segment	ST segment	T waves	P R segment
I	Elevated with concavity up-wards	Upright and may be tall	Isoelectric or depressed	Depressed	Inverted	Isoelectric or elevated
II	Isoelectric	Low to flat or may show inversion	Isoelectric or depressed	Isoelectric	Shallow to flat, to upright	Isoelectric or elevated
III	Isoelectric	Inverted	Isoelectric	Isoelectric	Upright	Isoelectric
IV	Isoelectric	Upright	Isoelectric	Isoelectric	Inverted	Isoelectric

Table 26.2: Evolution of ECG changes during different stages of pericarditis

A

aVR

II

aVF

V₁

V₂

V₃

V₄

V₅

V₆

III

I

(−)   (+)

ST-T

B

I   II   III   aVR   aVL   aVF

V₁   V₂   V₃   V₄   V₅   V₆

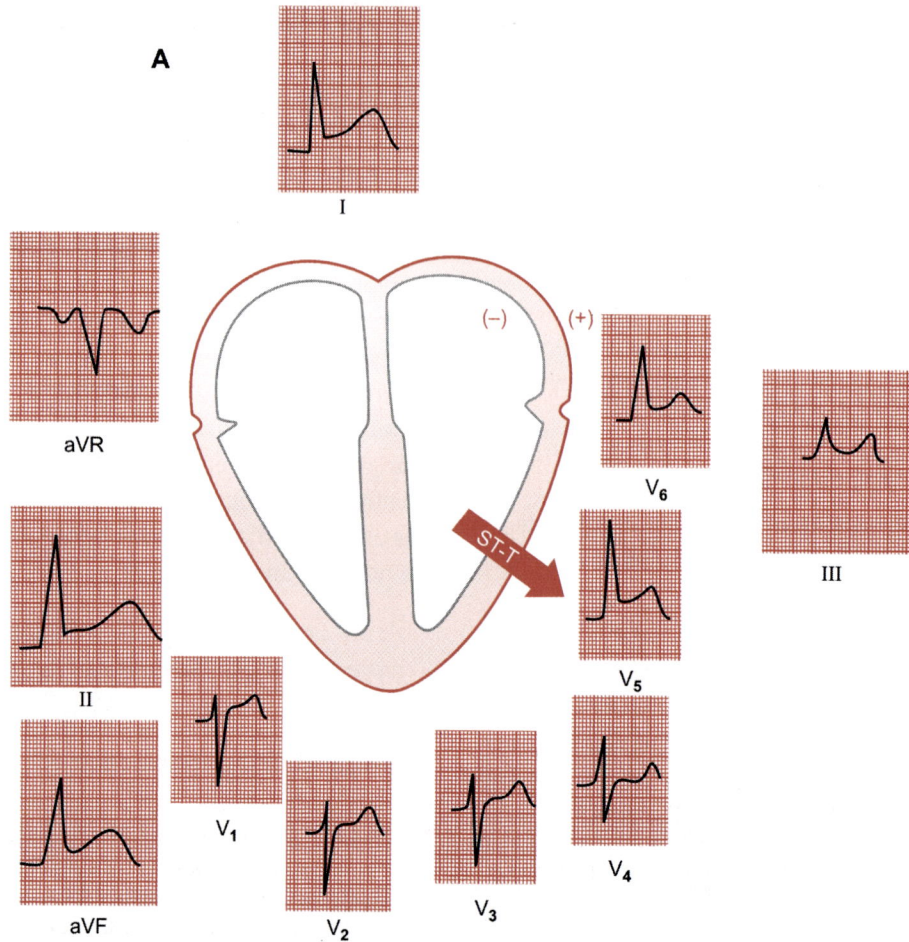

Fig. 26.1: Acute pericarditis

A: Genesis of ST segment elevation in all leads except aVR and V_1 due to epicardial current of injury (diagram)

B: The electrocardiogram recorded from a patient with pain and pericardial rub shows;

   i. Low voltage of QRS in standard leads. This is usually an effect recorded in pericardial effusion but may be seen in acute fibrinous pericarditis (an short circuiting effect).

   ii. The mean frontal plane QRS axis and ST vector is directed downwards towards positive pole of lead II and negative pole of aVR, hence ST segment is elevated in leads I, II, III, aVL and aVF and ST depression in aVR

   iii. There is good voltage of QRS in precordial leads. The ST segment is elevated with concavity upwards in leads V_2-V_6; while there is ST depression in lead V_1

   iv. The T waves are upright and tall in precordial leads. These T waves resemble T waves of early repolarisation

    All these changes in a symptomatic patient suggest pericarditis

axis in frontal plane is in the range of +30° to +60°. Since there is no myocardial ischaemia, the T waves remain upright and there are no q waves.

In horizontal plane, the leads V_2-V_6 are mostly oriented to injured surface, hence, record ST elevation. Since lead V_1 like aVR tends to be oriented towards cavity of the heart, records ST segment depression and T wave inversion.

As both the axes (ST and T) become aligned with and are dominantly directed downwards towards positive pole of lead II and/or negative pole of aVR or midway between them, hence, ST segment elevation with upright T wave occurs in leads oriented to injured surface, i.e. leads reflecting epicardial potentials (I, II, aVL, aVF, V_2-V_6) and ST depression occurs in leads reflecting endocardial potentials (aVR and V_1 Fig. 26.1.A).

Stage II. It occurs several days later and represents return of ST segment to the baseline accompanied by T wave flattening. This change in the ST segment usually occurs prior to apperance of T wave inversion. In contrast, T wave in myocardial infarction often becomes inverted before the ST segment returns to the baseline.

ST segment returns to the baseline with flattening of T wave

Stage III. It is characterised by frank inversion of T waves because T wave vector becomes opposite to ST vector. T wave inversion is generally seen in all the leads and is not associated with diminution or loss of R wave amplitude or appearance of Q wave. These features help to differentiate this stage of nonspecific T wave inversion from changes associated with evolution of myocardial infarction (Fig. 26.2).

Nonspecific T wave inversion without diminution or loss of R wave and without apperance of Q wave indicates acute pericarditis (Fig. 26.3).

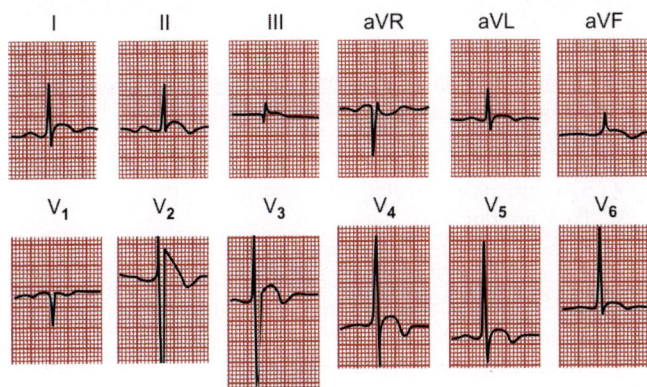

Fig. 26.2: Idiopathic acute pericarditis simulating acute myocardial ischaemia. The ECG was recorded from a 28 yrs male admitted with pericarditis. Note the following features:
Diffuse ST elevations (leads I, II, III, aVL, aVF and V_2-V_6) with ST depression in aVR and V_1 with deep T wave inversion with cove-plane configuration without reduction in the height of R wave and absence of Q wave indicate these changes to be due to pericarditis (myocardial injury current) rather than myocardial infarction

Stage IV. This occurs weeks to months later. During this stage, T waves become reversed, i.e. become upright. T wave inversion may occasionally persists indefinitely in patients with pericarditis due to tuberculosis, uraemia and neoplastic pericardial disease, indicates a chronic change.

The inverted T waves become upright during evolution of acute pericarditis but occassionally T waves inversion may persist indefinitely indicating chronic pericarditis

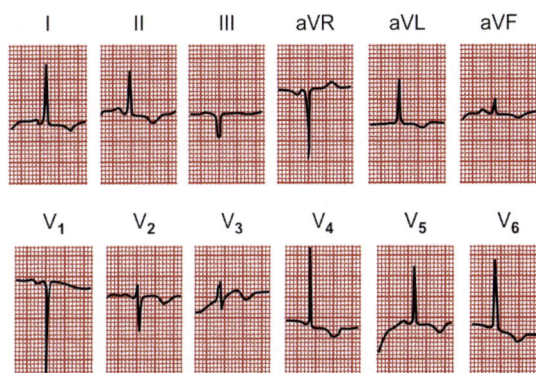

Fig. 26.3: Pericarditis simulating global myocardial ischaemia. The ECG was recorded from a 33 yrs old female admitted with acute myopericardial disease. Note the diffuse symmetric T wave inversion in all leads except aVR, which look like ischaemic. Remember that the coronary T are deeply inverted (> 5 mm) and are usually associated with Q wave or QS pattern

Electrocardiographic abnormalities appear in about 90% cases of acute pericarditis. All four stages are detected in 50% patients with acute pericarditis.

2. Changes in P-R Segment

Depression of PR segment is common with acute pericarditis simulating the pattern of acute atrial infarction. Depression of P-R segment occurs during the early stages of ST elevation or T wave inversion, is usually seen both in limb leads and precordial leads; and may reflect abnormal atrial repolarisation due to atrial inflammation.

3. Sinus Tachycardia

Sinus tachycardia is common and may be present in the absence of other contributory factors, such as fever or haemodynamic consequences. Other atrial arrhythmias are infrequent in uncomplicated acute pericarditis and suggest the presence of underlying heart disease. Atrioventricular block, bundle branch block and ventricular tachycardia are not features of acute pericarditis, their presence suggest the co-existence of extensive myocardial inflammation or fibrosis or acute ischaemia.

Differential Diagnosis

The ST segment elevation in pericarditis may be confused with early repolarisation changes seen in normal persons. However, the ST segment depression in aVR and V_1 seen in pericarditis is not seen in normal persons with early repolarisation syndrome. Secondly, the resolution of ECG changes occur in pericarditis; while they remain stable and permanent in normal persons (early repolarisation syndrome).

The ECG changes of acute pericarditis may mimic changes of myocardial infarction but distinguishing features given in the Table 26.3 help to differentiate between the two.

PERICARDITIS WITH EFFUSION

The characteristic features on ECG are:
1. Low voltage of P-QRS - T deflections (low voltage graph)

2. Low to inverted T waves
3. Electrical alternans.

The Genesis of Electrocardiographic Features (Fig. 26.4)

With the evolution of acute pericarditis to chronic pericarditis with effusion, the magnitude of all the ECG deflections become diminished. This is due to short-circuiting of electrical impulses by the surrounding fluid or thick layer of fibrin as already discussed. The ECG shows low voltage of all the components of the electrical excitation (P-QRS-T). The sum of QRS complexes in all the three standard leads (I,II,III) does not exceed 15 mm (Fig. 26.5).

Low to inverted T waves in most of the leads in chronic pericarditis with or without effusion is due to epicardial current of injury of acute pericarditis and / or epicardial ischaemia or associated myocarditis near the epicardial surface (Fig. 26.5). Due to epicardial injury / ischaemia, the T wave axis deviates away from the ischaemic region as it occurs with myocardial ischaemia any where in the heart (Law of myocardial / epicardial injury / ischaemia). The T waves will be inverted in all the leads except aVR where it will be upright. Since T wave vector is directed away from the apex of the heart, hence, T wave inversion is most marked in leads V_5-V_6. Lead V_1 show upright T wave like aVR. The end of chronic stage is characterised by a gradual return of the low to inverted T waves to normal.

Electrical alternans (Fig. 26.6) in which the height of the complexes (QRS-T) alternates, is seen in massive pericardial effusion with cardiac temponade. This is seen in mid-precordial leads (V_3-V_4). The genesis of electrical alternans is not well understood. Electrical alternans should not be confused with pulsus

Table 26.3: Distinguishing ECG features between myocardial infarction and pericarditis	
Acute myocardial infarction	*Acute pericarditis*
• ST segment is elevated with convexity upwards.	• ST segment is elevated with concavity upwards.
• Pathological Q waves are seen in area of infarction.	• They are not seen.
• T waves are inverted in area infarcted. underlying myocardium is involved.	• T waves are usually tall and upright unless.
• ECG changes are confined to the area of infarction (in leads overlying the area of infarction)	• ECG changes are widespread, seen in all the leads except aVR and V_1.
• Reciprocal changes are frequently seen.	• No reciprocal change is seen.

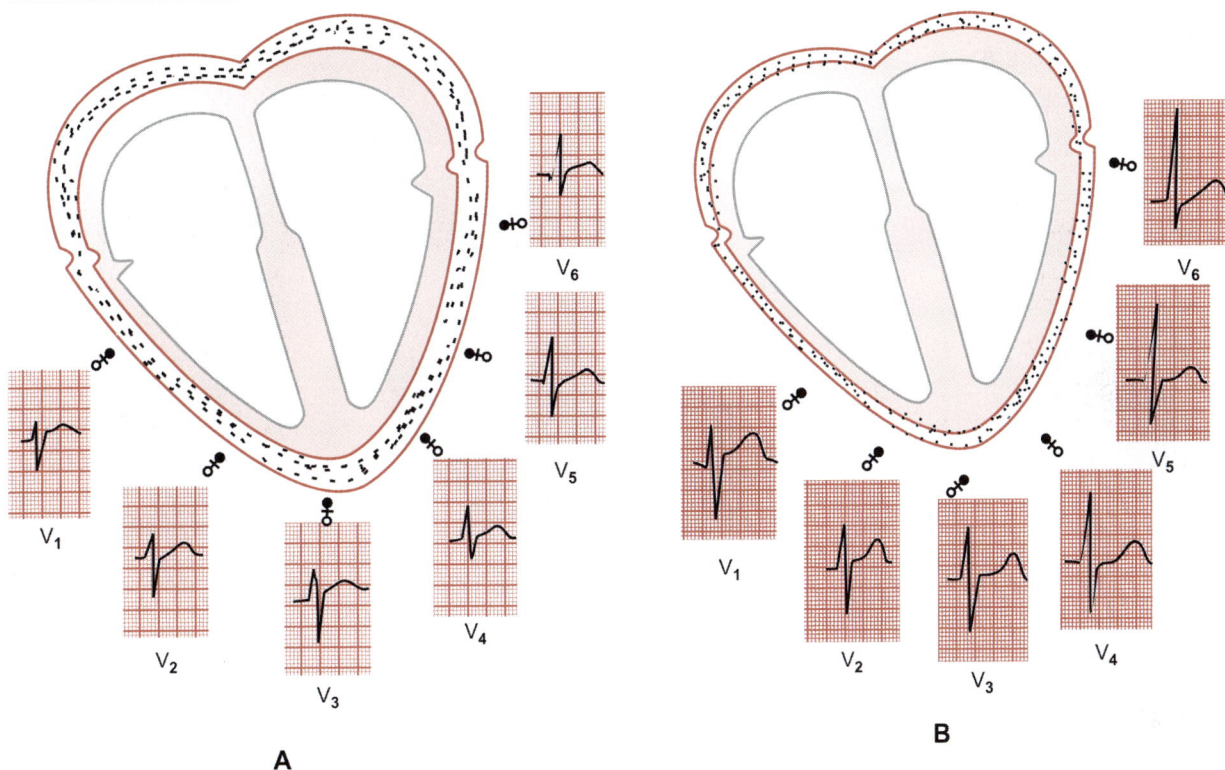

Fig. 26.4: Pericardiac effusion with cardiac temponade
A: *Before paracentesis.* Diagram illustrating the short-circuiting effects of fluid in the genesis of low voltage of P-QRS-T deflections in precordial leads.
B: *After paracentesis.* Now the short-circuiting effect of fluid is minimal or totally eliminated explains the return of voltage of P-QRS-T complexes

alternans in which ventricular contractions of alternate force produce alternation of pulse of good and low volume due to changes in blood pressure.

Electrical alternans is a specific indicator of pericardial effusion and reflects pendular swinging of the heart within pericardial cavity and is related to beat to beat alteration of right and left ventricular filling.

Electrical alternans may also occur in constrictive pericarditis, in tension pneumothorax, after myocardial infarction with severe cardiac muscle dysfunction and supraventricular tachycardia (Fig. 26.7).

Electrical alternans of QRS complex may occur in a 2:1 or 3:1 pattern. Alternans is usually limited to the QRS complex, but alternans of P wave, QRS complex and T wave-total electrical alternans may rarely occur in extreme cardiac temponade. There may

alteration of polarity of QRS complex (a positive QRS complex alternates with negative QRS (Fig. 26.6).

Due to disappearance of abnormal heart motions within the pericardial sac, the electrical alternans disappears when the pericardial fluid is removed. The voltage of P-QRS-T also improves.

CHRONIC CONSTRICTIVE PERICARDITIS

The electrocardiographic changes of chronic constrictive pericarditis are similar to chronic pericardial effusion (low amplitude of QRS complexes with low to inverted T waves). Electrical alternans may occur but is rare. In addition to above changes, there may be enlargement of left atrium in chronic constrictive pericarditis due to constriction around the atrioventricular groove which results in wide, notched P waves (P mitrale) in frontal plane leads, and a delayed and widened terminal negative component of

SECTION NINE

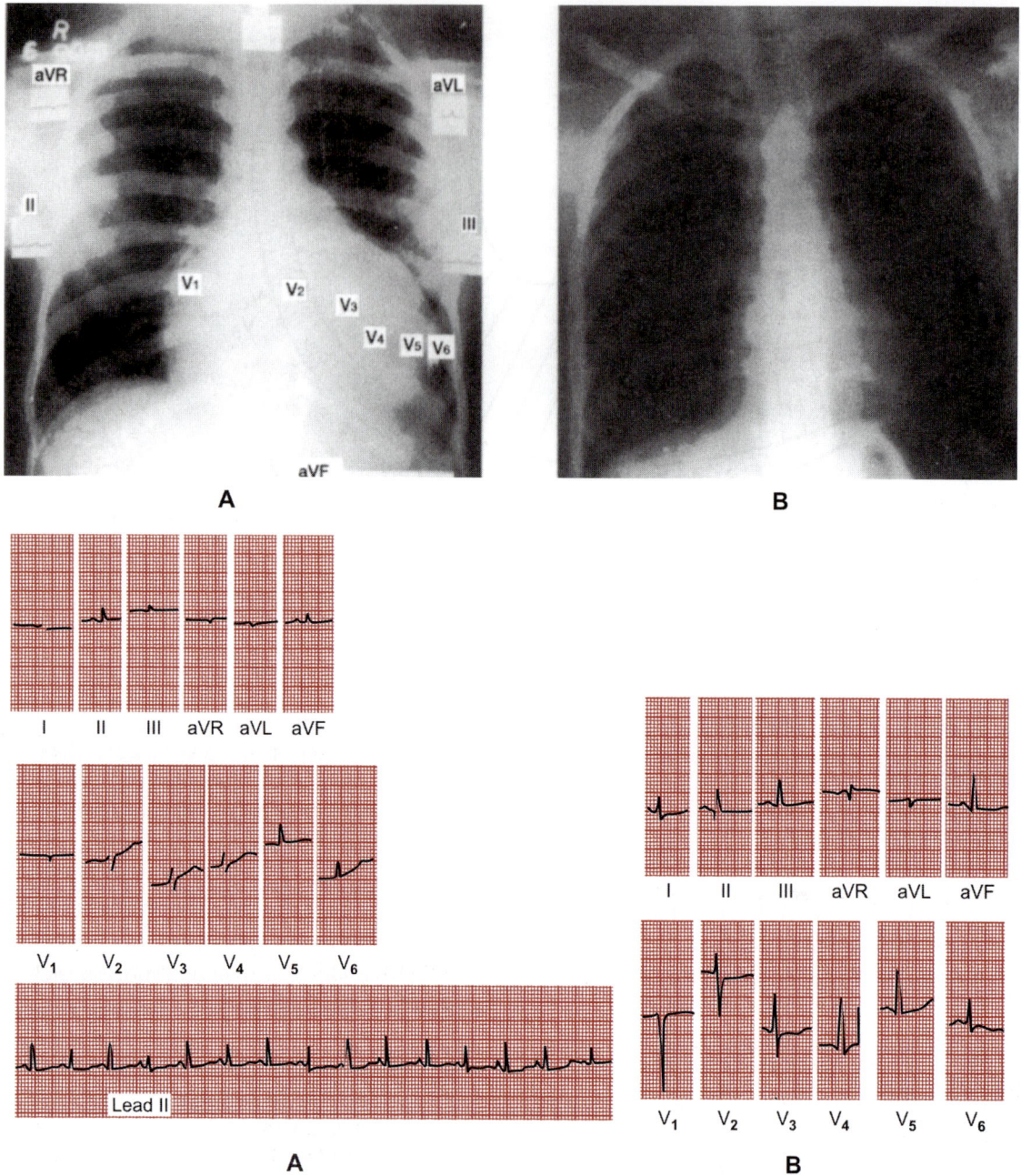

Fig. 26.5: Cardiac temponade due to massive pericardial effusion.

1. X-rays chest (PA view). **(A)** massive pericardial effusion with placement of leads. **(B)** After paracentesis(500 ml of fluid was removed)
2. The electrocardiograms.
    A: Before paracentesis. The ECG shows low voltage of P-QRS-T complexes in all leads. Lower rhythm strip (lead II) shows an electrical alternans—a characteristic electrocardiographic feature of cardiac temponade but can be seen in supraventricular tachycardias and myocardial infarction.
    B: After paracentesis. There is normal or near normal voltage of P-QRS-T complexes. The electrical alternans has disappeared. There is ST segment depression with low to flat T waves in all leads except aVR and V_1 indicates associated underlying myocarditis

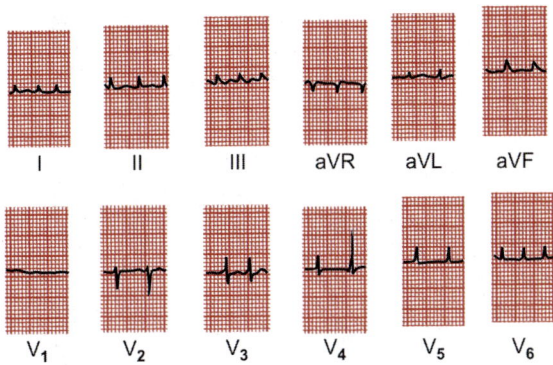

I II III aVR aVL aVF

V₁ V₂ V₃ V₄ V₅ V₆

Fig. 26.6: Pericarditis with effusion and atrial fibrillation. Atrial fibrillation with a ventricular rate of about 150 per minute. Small QRS complexes suggest the presence of a pericardial effusion

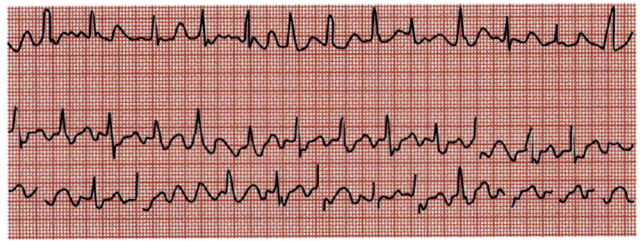

II

Fig. 26.7: Electrical alternans in supraventricular tachycardia. The ECG lead II shows proxysmal supraventricular tachycardia at a rate of 166/min and is slightly irregular. There is alternation of small QRS with large QRS intermittently indicating electrical alternans

biphasic P wave in lead V_1. Atrial fibrillation occurs in 30% cases. This is due to atrial dilatation and stress.

Atrioventricular blocks, intraventricular conduction defects, and pseudoinfarction pattern with deep and wide Q waves have been reported and seemed to be related to extension of calcification into the myocardium and around the coronary arteries compromising coronary blood flow. A pattern of right ventricular hypertrophy with right axis deviation may be present in 5% cases and, is due to dense pericardial sac overlying the right ventricle in association with its compensatory dilatation due to constriction around the mitral atrioventricular ring and hypokinesis of the outflow tract.

Suggested Reading

1. Bashour FA, Cochran PW: The association of electrical alternans with pericardial effusion. *Dis Chest* **44**: 146, 1963.
2. Dalton JC, Pearson RJ, White PD: Constrictive pericarditis; A review and long-term follow-up of 78 cases. *Ann Int Med* **45**: 445, 1956.
3. Fukuda K, Nakmura Y, Ogawa S et al: Constrictive pericarditis with electrocardiographic evidence of right ventricular hypertrophy. *Chest* **96**: 691, 1989.
4. Ginzton LE, Laks MM: The differential diagnosis of acute pericarditis. *Circulation* **65**: 1004, 1982.
5. Kouvaras G, Soufras G, Chronopoulos G, et al: The ST segment as a different diagnostic feature between acute pericarditis and acute anterior myocardial infarction. *Angiology* **41**: 207, 1990.
6. Levine HD: Myocardial fibrosis in constrictive pericarditis: Electrocardiographic and pathologic observations. *Circulation* **48**: 1268, 1973.
7. Lorell BH: Pericardial disease 'in Braunward Heart disease—A Text book of Cardiovascular Medicine, 5th edn. Vol. 2, WB Saunders Company 1478, 1997.
8. Nizet PM, Marriott HJL: The electrocardiogram and pericardial effusion. *JAMA* **198**: 169, 1966.
9. Spodick DH: Diagnostic electrocardiographic sequences in acute pericarditis. Significance of PR segment and P-R vector changes. *Circulation* **48**: 575, 1973.
10. Spodick DH: Differential characteristics of electrocardiogram in early repolarisation and acute pericarditis. *N Engl J Med* **295**: 523, 1976.
11. Spodick DH: Frequency of arrhythmias in acute pericarditis determined by Holter monitoring. *Am J Cardiol* **53**: 842, 1994.
12. Surawicz B, Lasseter KC: Electrocardiogram in pericarditis. *Am J Cardiol* **26**: 471, 1970.
13. Teh BS, Walsh J, Bell AJ, et al: Electrical current paths in acute pericarditis. *J Electrocardiol* **26**: 291, 1993.
14. Toriya Martinez RN, Gonzaledz Hermosillo JA: Acute nonspecific pericarditis. *Arch Inst Cardiol Mex* **57**: 307, 1987.
15. Usher BW, Popp RL: Electrical alternans: Mechanism in pericardial effusion. *Am Heart J* **83**: 459, 1972.

27

Acute Pulmonary Thromboembolism (Acute Cor Pulmonale)

- ECG manifestations of acute cor pulmonale (thromboembolism)
- ECG patterns in acute pulmonary thromboembolism (acute cor pulmonale) versus acute inferior wall infarction

Definition

It is defined clinically as right ventricular hypertrophy or dilatation secondary to acute pulmonary hypertension, often due to massive pulmonary embolism.

Pathogenesis

Massive acute pulmonary embolism results in reduction of cross-sectional area of pulmonary vasculature and subsequent vasoconstriction of pulmonary arterioles leading to pulmonary arterial hypertension which, in turn, leads to right ventricular and right atrial hypertrophy/dilatation as a haemodynamic consequence. The pulmonary arterial hypertension also results in diminished cardiac output and reduced coronary blood flow leading to myoepicardial ischaemia.

The Electrocardiographic Manifestations

The following electrocardiographic disturbances in cases of acute cor pulmonale (thromboembolism) result from haemodynamic consequences as well as from myocardial ischaemia/injury and hypoxia.

1. *Low amplitude of deflections.* It may be seen mostly in all the leads, but the genesis is not understood.

2. *Right atrial and right ventricular dilatation or hypertrophy*
3. *Right ventricular ischaemia/injury*
4. *Complete or incomplete right bundle branch block*
5. *Atrial arrhythmias.* All types of atrial arrhythmias (atrial ectopics, atrial tachycardia, atrial fibrillation, chaotic atrial or multifocal atrial tachycardia) can occur. These are due to acute atrial dilatation coupled with atrial myocardial ischaemia.

The Electrocardiogram (Figs 27.1 to 27.4)

A. Frontal Plane Leads (I, II, III , aVR, aVL and aVF)

(i) S_I, Q_{III}, T_{III} *pattern* (Fig. 27.1). This pattern was first described by McGinn and White in 1935. This triad consists of prominent S waves in lead 1, Q waves and inverted T waves in lead III. The S wave in lead 1 and aVL > 1.5 mm, Q wave and T wave inversion in lead III appear within 24 hours of acute thromboembolism and undergo resolution. The Q waves in lead III are not pathological (duration < 0.04 sec and depth is < 25% of R wave). These insignificant q waves may also appear in leads II and aVF simulating

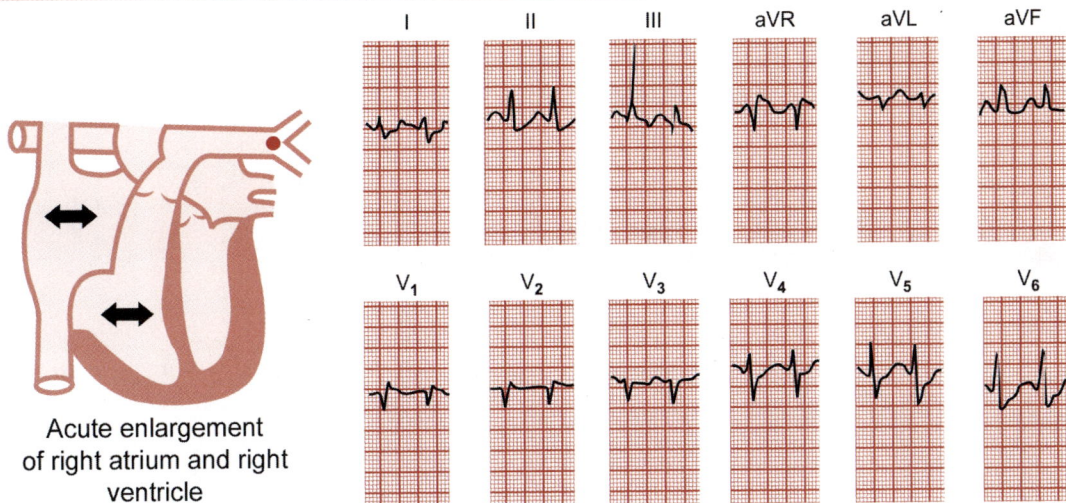

Fig. 27.1: S$_I$, Q$_{III}$, T$_{III}$ syndrome in acute pulmonary embolism. The ECG shows;
  i. Prominent S wave in lead I having rS pattern with ST depression
  ii. Prominent q wave with T inversion in lead III
  iii. There is ST depression in lead II
  iv. A prominent R wave in aVR indicates rightward shift of QRS
  v. A QR pattren in V$_1$-V$_2$ indicates right atrial cum right ventricular enlargement
  vi. Right ventricular hypertrophy. The right axis deviation, qR pattern in V$_1$-V$_2$ and persistence of deep wide S wave in V$_5$-V$_6$ indicates right ventricular hypertrophy

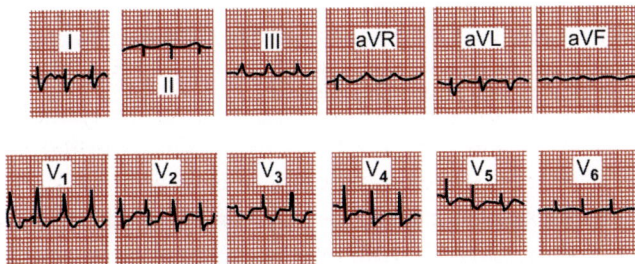

Fig. 27.2: Transient right bundle branch block with S$_I$, Q$_{III}$, T$_{III}$ syndrome in a patient with acute pulmonary embolism proved on lung scan. The electrocardiogram shows;
  i. Prominent S wave in lead I having rS pattern
  ii. Prominent q wave in lead III having qR pattern
  iii. T wave is inverted in leads III and aVF due to left axis deviation of T wave axis (−30°). T wave is biphasic in lead II
  iv. ST depression is seen in lead II
  v. A prominent R wave is seen in aVR due to rightward QRS axin on frontal plane
  vi. Right bundle branch block is revealed by rSR' pattern in leads V$_1$-V$_2$ with ST depression and persistence of wide S wave in leads V$_5$-V$_6$
  vii. T is inverted in right precordial leads V$_1$-V$_3$
   All these features transiently occur in acute pulmonary embolism

inferior wall infarction. Similarly, T wave inversion may also be present in leads II and aVF which further confuse it to be due to inferior wall ischaemia/infarction. The absence of ST segment changes of infarction (ST segment coving/elevation) makes them unlikely due to infarction.

(ii) The ST segment depression in leads I and II may occur. A 'stair-case' ascent of ST segment (flattening of the initial part of ST segment and T wave, followed by a more or less sharp rise and then flattening of terminal portion of the T wave) may be seen. Elevated ST segment is seen in leads III and aVF.

(iii) Right QRS axis deviation of + 120° or more.

(iv) A prominent R wave in lead aVR. It is due to right axis deviation and right ventricular hypertrophy.

(v) *Transient right bundle branch block.* Incomplete or complete right bundle branch block can occur (Fig. 27.2.) due to compression effect of hypertrophied right ventricle on the right bundle. It will be reflected in standard leads recording the

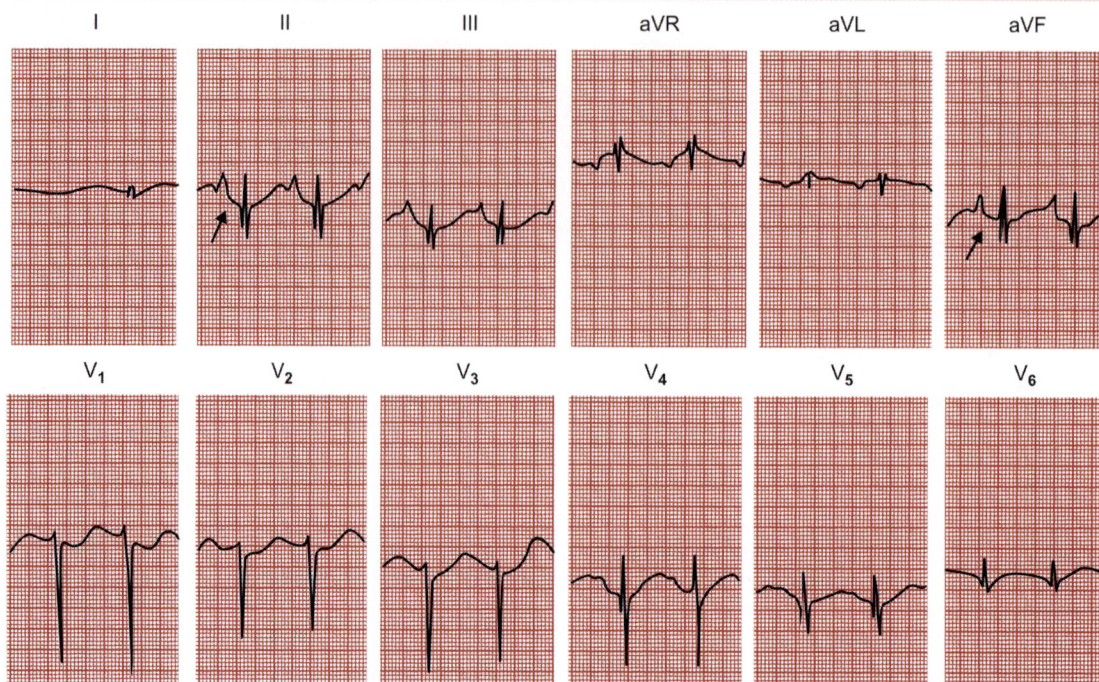

Fig. 27.3: Acute cor pulmonale due to thromboemobolism proved on lung scan. The ECG shows;
  i. The mean frontal QRS axis is +90°
 ii. *Right atrial hypertrophy.* The tall peaked P waves II, III, aVF indicate right atrial enlargement. The sagging P-R segment and rising S-T segment in the same leads reflect Ta waves of atrial repolarisation (indicated by arrow ↗)
iii. *Right ventricular hypertrophy.* The clockwise rotation with rS complex in V₁-V₄ with deep S wave in V₅-V₆ is suggestive of RVH indirectly. The terminal QRS forces are negative in lead I, II, III, thus QRS terminal vector is directed superiorly and to the right which favours RVH due to any cause. Therefore, clear evidence of RAH with suggestive criteria for RVH makes the diagnosis of acute cor pulmonale in presence of thromboembolism proved on lung scan

right ventricular epicardial complex and right precordial leads (V₁-V₂).

(vi) Tall, peaked P waves (P-pulmonale) are seen in standard leads due to right atrial dilatation. These are best visible in leads II, III and aVF. In lead V₁, P wave is upright or biphasic. If P is biphasic in V₁, then the initial upright component is prominent (Figs 27.3 and 27.4.) Low upright P waves are seen in leads I and aVL.

B. Horizontal Plane Leads (V₁ to V₆)

(i) *Clockwise rotation of heart.* There is clockwise rotation of electrical forces on horizontal plane leading to shift of transition zone from V₃ leftwards to V₅ or V₆. Consequent to this, rS or Rs complexes will be seen in all precordial leads. This is a common change seen on ECG.

(ii) *Increase in height of R wave in right precordial leads (V₁-V₃).* Due to right ventricular hypertrophy,

there is increase in height of R wave from V₁ to V₃ resulting in R:S > 1 in leads V₁ and V₂, and may extend upto V₃-V₅ if there is marked clockwise rotation.

(iii) *A qR complex in lead V₁.* A small q wave followed by a large R wave reflects right atrial and right ventricular hypertrophy/enlargement.

(iv) Acute pulmonary embolism may manifest as a diminution in the amplitude of the S wave, with slurring of the ascending limb or flattening of the nadir in the right precordial leads (V₁-V₃). This manifestation indicates development of right ventricular dominance or more probably the early manifestation of RBBB. This change may be associated with tall R wave (R≥S)in leads V₁-V₂.

(v) *Prominent S wave is seen in V₅-V₆.* It is due to orientation of QRS vector superiorly and to the right.

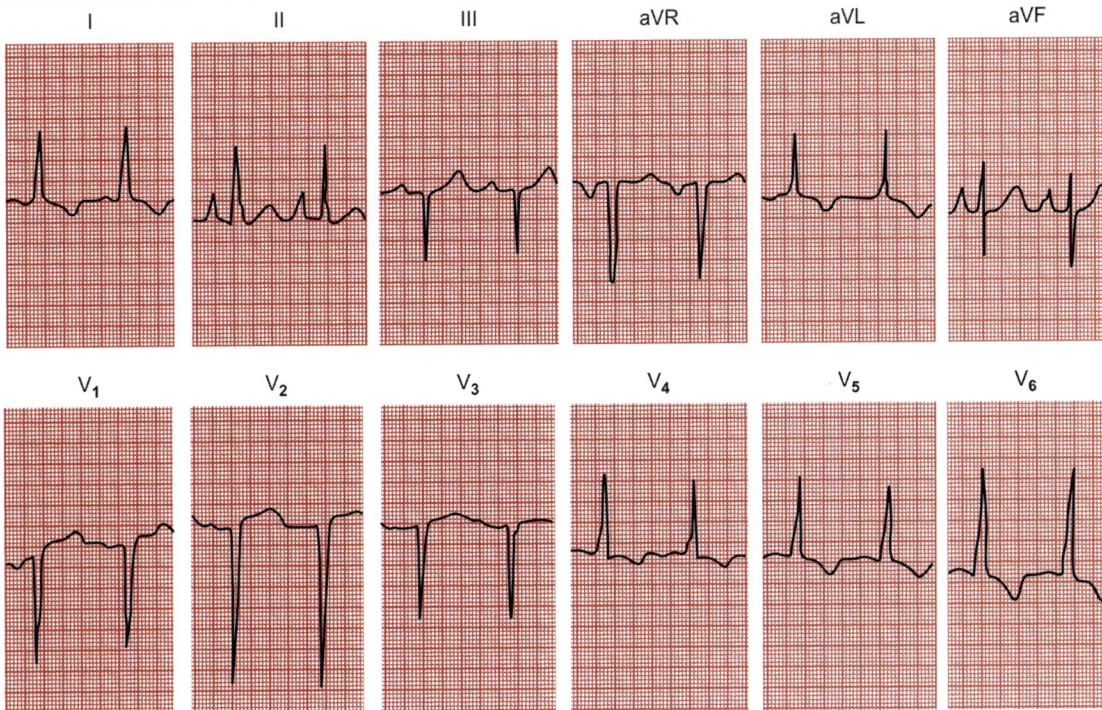

Fig. 27.4: Right atrial hypertrophy due to acute pulmonary embolism in a patient with systemic hypertension and congestive heart failure. The electrocardiogram shows;

i. Right atrial hypertrophy. It is evidenced by tall peaked P waves > 2.5 mm in leads II, III and aVF with P wave axis of + 75°

ii. Left ventricular hypertrophy due to systemic hypertension is evident by voltage criteria ($RV_6 + SV_1 = 38$ mm) with left axis deviation. T wave inversion in leads I, aVL, V_4-V_6 are due to left ventricular hypertrophy

Note: Right atrial hypertrophy in the absence of left atrial hypertrophy in systemic hypertension suggests acute pulmonary embolism.

(vi) The *ST segment change.* The ST segment is elevated with coving in right precordial leads (V_1-V_3), while ST segment is depressed in left precordial leads V_5-V_6 in the form of horizontality or plain depression of ST-T junction.

(vii) The T wave may be inverted in right pericardial leads (V_1-V_4) indicating acute right ventricular strain. The T wave is upright in left precordial leads (V_4-V_6). This T wave change is persistent and may take 3-4 weeks to become upright again.

(viii) *The U wave change.* If U wave is present, then it may also be inverted.

(ix) Transient right bundle branch block pattern. This is reflected in the form of rSR' or wide RsR' complexes in leads V_1-V_2 (Fig. 27.2) and wide S waves in V_5-V_6.

(x) *Atrial arrhythmias.* All types of atrial arrhythmias can occur but multifocal atrial tachycardia is the commonest arrhythmia seen. Other atrial arrhythmias noticed include; atrial ectopics, paroxysmal atrial or junctional tachycardia, atrial fibrillation or flutter.

The ECG changes in acute cor pulmonale (thromboembolism) are transient and nonspecific. As a general rule, the ST segment and T waves changes last only for few days or even for briefer duration; while rotational QRS changes can persist for 1-3 weeks after the acute episode.

Diagnosis and Differential Diagnosis

The electrocardiogram is useful not only to exclude acute myocardial infarction but to identify some patients with large pulmonary embolism leading to haemodynamic consequences, for example, acute right atrial and ventricular strain. The most

SECTION NINE

Table 27.1: Differentiating features between acute thromboembolism and inferior wall infarction

Acute thromboembolism	Acute inferior wall infarction
• Sinus tachycardia is invariably present	• Sinus bradycardia is more frequent than sinus tachycardia.
• The q waves are deeper in lead III and shallow or small in leads II and aVF.	• The Q waves in leads II, III and aVF are wide (>0.04 sec) and deep (>25% of R wave).
• Tall R waves with inverted T waves in V_1-V_2 is commonly observed pattern.	• This pattern is not seen. Even T wave inversion of anteroseptal infarction in V_1-V_4 if associated with inferior wall infarction may not be seen.
• The ST segment is either isoelectric or elevated in III and aVF but depressed in lead II.	• ST segment elevation with coving is characteristically seen in leads II, III and aVF.
• Changes are transient and shortlived.	• Changes are protracted and take some time to resolve.

characteristic feature of this disorder on ECG is the transient nature of the changes, hence, serial ECG recordings are most helpful. Despite the high incidence of abnormal tracing (70-75%), the diagnosis is still difficult because of transient and nonspecific nature of ECG changes. While a single ECG tracing is rarely helpful, a comparison with a tracing obtained before the onset of pulmonary embolism with serial tracings after the episode increase the sensitivity of ECG significantly. There is no single diagnostic ECG pattern for acute pulmonary embolism, therefore, combinations of various electrocardiographic patterns may be helpful in patients suspected of pulmonary embolism. Efforts have been made to correlate the ECG findings with pulmonary embolism but without much success. In a significant study, three or more of the ECG findings given in the box have been correlated with sensitivity of 76% on single ECG.

ECG Findings in Acute Pulmonary Thromboembolism

- Incomplete or complete RBBB
- S wave in leads I and aVL > 1.5 mm
- Leftwards shift of transition zone, i.e. to V_5
- QRS axis > +90° or more or indeterminate axis
- Low voltage of P- QRS-T in limb leads
- Q wave in leads III and aVF (Qs pattern) but not in lead II
- T wave inversion in precordial leads (V_1-V_4) and standard leads III and aVF

The ECG patterns in acute thromboembolism may simulate inferior wall infarction. The distinguishing features between the two are summarised in the Table 27.1.

REVIEW AT GLANCE

ECG changes in acute cor pulmonale

- Low amplitude of P-QRS-T deflections may be seen for unknown reasons.
- Right axis deviation due to right ventricular dominance. Due to this effect, R wave appears in aVR.
- Clockwise rotation and shift of transition zone leftwards to V_5-V_6 on horizontal plane. This effect results in rS or Rs pattern in all precordial leads. This is quite a frequent change.
- S_I, Q_{III}, T_{III} pattern is an important triad of acute thromboembolism.
- Tall, peaked P waves in leads II, III and aVF appear due to right atrial hypertrophy.
- Right ventricular dominance/hypertrophy results in an increase in R wave amplitude in right precordial leads. There is increase in R : S > 1 in leads V_1-V_2. As a result of right ventricular dominance, there is decrease in the amplitude of S wave in these leads. Sometimes, there may be qR pattern in V_1 due to right ventricular pressure exceeding the left ventricular pressure.
- ST segment elevation and T wave inversion may be seen in V_1-V_3 due to right ventricular strain, and occassionally, there may be ST segment depression in left precordial leads. The ST segment depression is common in leads II and I.
- The T wave inversion in standard leads III and aVF and precordial leads V_1-V_4.

- Right bundle branch block pattern (rsR' or RsR') may be seen transiently.
- Arrhythmias - Atrial arrhythmias are common.

Suggested Reading

1. Berman H, Schamroth L: Acute pulmonary embolism. *Heart and Lung* **8**: 1146, 1979.
2. Goldberger AL: Myocardial infarction 3rd edn. ST Louis: CV Mosby Co. 1984.
3. Goldhaber SZ, Morpurgo M: For the WHO/ISFC Task Force on Pulmonary Embolism: Diagnosis, treatment and prevention of pulmonary embolism. Report of the WHO/International Society and Federation of Cardiology Task Force. *JAMA* **268**:1727, 1992.
4. Lynch RE, Stein PD, Bruce TA: Leftword shift of frontal plane QRS axis as a frequent manifestation of acute pulmonary embolism. *Chest* **61**: 443, 1972.
5. McGinn S, White PD: Acute cor pulmonale resulting from pulmonary embolism; its clinical recognition. *JAMA* **104**: 1473, 1935.
6. Smith M, Ray CT: Electrocardiographic signs of early right ventricular enlargement in acute pulmonary embolism. *Chest* **58**: 205, 1970.
7. Sreeram N, Cheriex E, Smeets JLRM, et al: Value of the 12-lead ECG at hospital admission in the diagnosis of pulmonary embolism. *Am J Cardial* **73**: 298, 1994.
8. Tighe DA, Chung EK, Park CH: Electrical alternans associated with acute pulmonary embolism. *Am Heart J* **128**:188, 1994.
9. Weber DM, Philips JH: A re-evaluation of electrocardiographic changes accompanying acute pulmonary embolism. *Am J Med Sci* **251**: 381, 1967.

SECTION NINE

28

Chronic Obstructive Pulmonary Disease (COPD) and Chronic Cor Pulmonale

- *Electrocardiographic characteristics of emphysema and their possible pathogenic mechanisms*
- *Chronic cor pulmonale—The electrocardiographic characteristics*
- *Distinctive and comparative electrocardiographic features of acute and chronic cor pulmonale*

CHRONIC COR PULMONALE

It is defined as right ventricular hypertrophy or dilatation secondary to diseases of the lung parenchyma, pulmonary vasculature, thoracic cage and ventilatory control.

Chronic Obstructive Pulmonary Disease-Emphysema and Chronic Cor Pulmonale

Hypertrophic emphysema due to chronic obstruction of the bronchi, results in hyperinflation of the lungs, distorts the pulmonary vasculature and leads to development of pulmonary arterial hypertension and chronic cor pulmonale. The hyperexpanded lungs influence the cardiac electrical events in the following ways:

1. *An insulating effect:* The hyperinflated voluminous lungs have an insulating effect on the transmission of electrical impulses across the chest, hence, low voltage of ECG complexes may be noticed in all the leads. Other causes of low voltage of P-QRS-T deflections are given in the box.

2. *Lower position of the heart:* Due to lowering of both domes of the diaphragm by the hyperinflated lungs, the heart tries to descend downwards and occupies a central position (tubular heart). This will change the position of the heart with respect to precordial leads. This also contributes to low voltage of ECG deflections in precordial leads because they are placed relatively higher with respect to the heart (Figs 28.1A and B). Sometimes in hypertrophic emphysema there is poor progression of R wave in

Causes of low voltage of P-QRS-T (low voltage graph)

- Obesity
- Myxoedema
- Massive bilateral or left sided pleural effusion
- Left pneumothorax
- Generalised anasarca (oedematous chest)
- Pericardial effusion
- Gross congestive heart failure due to dilated cardiomyopathy
- Acute pulmonary thromboembolism

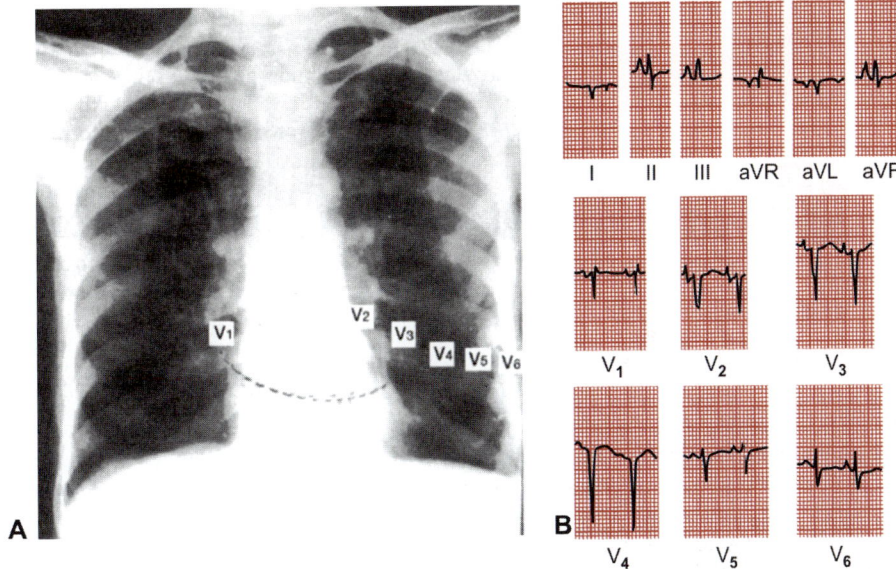

Figs 28.1A and B: Chronic obstructive pulmonary disease (COPD).

A: X-ray chest (PA view) demonstrates hyperinflated lungs and tubular heart resulting in low position of the heart with the result precordial leads (V_1-V_6) when placed at normal positions (drawn) reflect the basal portion of the heart.

B: The electrocardiogram recorded from the same patient whose X-ray is displayed shows;

   i. *Low voltage graph* due to diminished amplitude of QRS-T deflections. This is due to hyperinflation of lungs resulting in poor electrical transmission as a result of higher placement of electrodes with respect to heart.

   ii. Right axis deviation > +120° of both P and QRS axes on frontal plane

   iii. Right atrial hypertrophy. Tall peaked P waves are present in leads II, III and aVF. The positive initial deflection of biphasic P is also tall in leads V_1-V_3.

   iv. Incomplete right bundle branch block. There is rSr' pattern in V_1 and rS pattern in V_2-V_3 with slurred S and this pattern persists upto V_5 and R:S is equal to 1 in V_6 due to marked clockwise rotation. The rSr' pattern could also be due to large posterobasal segment activation in normal persons, but in this patient, the sudden change from rSr' pattern to rS (V_2-V_6) indicated transient phenomenon probably due to oxygen desaturation as it disappeared subsequently.

precordial leads resulting in rS or rS complex. This is due to lower placement of the heart with respect to placement of precordial electrodes. The ECG recorded one space lower down may show normal progression or diminished progression of R wave (Figs 28.2A and B).

3. *Rotational effect:* There is a marked clockwise rotation of the heart on horizontal plane especially when pulmonary arterial hypertension develops resulting in right ventricular hypertrophy and chronic cor pulmonale. The presence of rS complex in left precordial leads suggests a rotational effect. The transition zone is displaced leftwards to V_5-V_6 resulting in rS complex in these leads.

4. *Right ventricular and atrial hypertrophy:* When pulmonary arterial hypertension becomes evident in chronic obstructive pulmonary disease, the right ventricle becomes hypertrophied and ultimately may show dilatation, a condition called '*chronic cor pulmonale*'. Right axis of P waves and *P-pulmonale* indicate right atrial hypertrophy. The ratio of R wave to S wave more than 1 (R: S > 1) in leads V_1 and V_2, clockwise rotation and persistence of large S waves in V_5-V_6 indicate right ventricular hypertrophy, are characteristically seen in chronic cor pulmonale.

5. *Right bundle branch block:* Complete and incomplete right bundle branch block may accompany chronic obstructive lung disease especially if the disease is severe enough to produce right ventricular hypertrophy that puts pressure on right bundle.

6. *Right P wave axis:* The P wave axis in chronic obstructive pulmonary disease is always directed to the right (+60° to +90°) and form an important diagnostic criteria. The P pulmonale best seen in leads

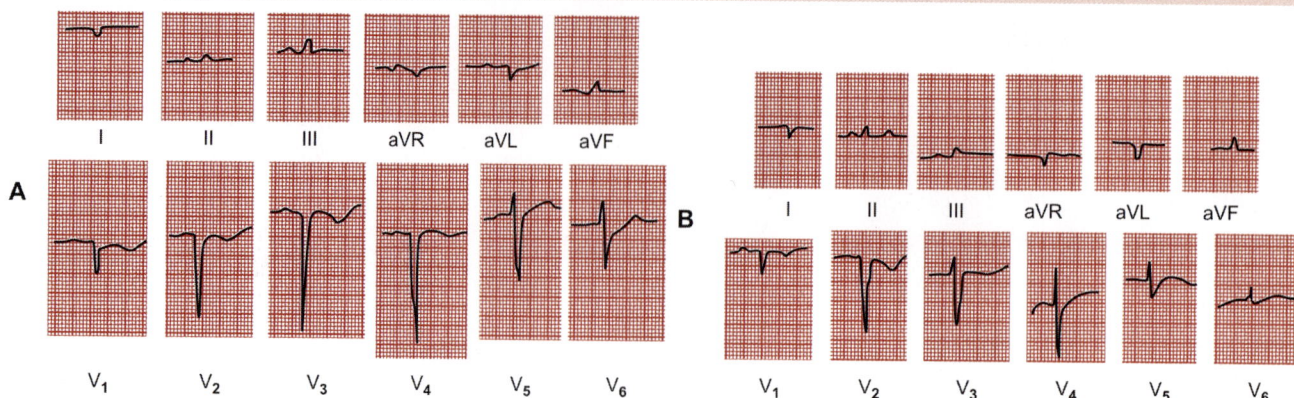

Fig. 28.2: Chronic obstructive pulmonary disease (hypertrophic emphysema).

A. The ECG taken shows low voltage graph in precordial leads. There is poor progression of R wave in precordial leads. There is rudimentary r from V_1-V_4 with ST depression and T wave inversion, may be misinterpreted as anteroseptal infarction but presence of rS pattern in V_5-V_6 with upright T excludes infarction

B. The ECG taken from the same patient one space lower down shows low voltage graph with normal or good progression of R wave from V_1-V_6. The ST segment depression and T wave change is now limited to V_1-V_3. The transition zone lies in V_5 or beyond it.

The ECGs demonstrate the rotational effect of hypertrophic emphysema which can produce QS pattern from V_1-V_4 simulating anteroseptal myocardial infarction which can be excluded by taking ECG one space lower down in case of doubt

II, III and aVF is the result of this right axis deviation of P wave.

7. **Variation in QRS axis.** There is variation in QRS axis. 90% cases show right axis deviation; while 10% cases have left axis deviation. Right axis deviation corresponds well to the severity of the disease. Usually, right axis deviation is between +80° to +90° but marked right axis deviation beyond +90° to +120° or more indicates severe disease and results in S_I, Q_{III}, R_{III} pattern. In severe cases, QRS axis may touch North-West region, i.e., right superior quadrant. This will result in deep S waves in leads II, III and aVF. The lead I may also reflect a small 's' wave resulting in S_I, S_{II}, S_{III} syndrome (Read Chapter on S_I, S_{II},S_{III} syndrome). Occasionally, left axis deviation may occur beyond – 30° upto – 60°, the mechanism of which is still elusive.

Sometimes, the QRS may be deviated somewhat posteriorly so that it tends to become more oblique to the leads on the horizontal plane leading to low QRS deflections in all precordial leads.

The frontal plane T wave axis follows QRS (+80° to +90°) resulting in tall 'T' waves in lead III than in lead 1. Otherwise, T waves are of low amplitude in all the precordial leads. The T wave inversion may

occur in right precordial leads due to right ventricular hypertrophy leading to cor pulmonale.

The Electrocardiogram

The abnormalities seen on ECG in P-QRS-T complexes due to above described mechanisms are;

A. *The P Wave Abnormality (Figs 28.3 and 28.4)*

    i)   Frontal plane P wave axis is directed to the right +80° to + 90°.

    ii) P pulmonale may appear, best seen in leads II, III and aVF and is due to rightward orientation of P wave axis. The P pulmonale indicates right atrial hypertrophy.

    iii) P wave in V_1 may be upright and tall or may be biphasic in which the initial upward deflection of P wave is accentuated and prominent (>1.5 mm) than terminal downward deflection.

B. *The QRS Abnormality (Figs 28.5 and 28.6)*

    i)   Frontal plane QRS axis is directed to right, i.e. +90°, hence, there is good voltage of QRS in leads III and aVF.

    ii) Marked right axis deviation results in deep S wave in lead 1 and tall R wave in lead III.

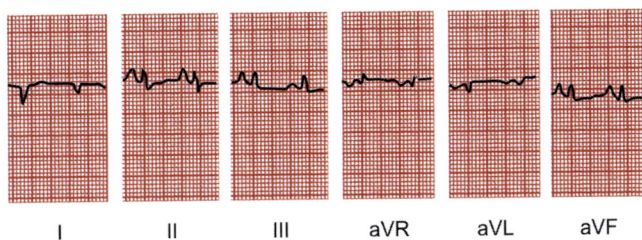

Fig. 28.3: The P wave abnormality in chronic obstructive pulmonary disease (COPD). The electrocardiogram (standard leads) shows;

i. Low voltage graph. All the complexes in standard leads are < 5 mm
ii. Right axis deviation of QRS
iii. P wave axis of +150° (P is inverted in aVL, tallest in lead III
iv. Right atrial hypertrophy. The P is tall (>2.5 mm in height) in leads II, III and aVF

All these features suggest emphysema (COPD).

iii) Low voltage of QRS may be seen in all the leads due to insulating affect of voluminous lungs, lowered position of the heart and, sometimes, to some extent by posterior displacement of QRS axis.

iv) S_I, S_{II}, S_{III} syndrome (Read Chapter 15). It means deep S wave in all the three standard leads. This is due to right superior orientation of QRS axis as well as due to posterior displacement of the apex of the heart so that QRS forces are away from these standard leads. The posterior apical displacement of heart produces deep S waves (RS pattern) in leads V_4-V_6. This is due to shifting of late forces of ventricular activation superiorly and to the left.

v) Shifting of transition zone leftwards resulting in RS or 'rs' pattern in left precordial leads. This is due to marked clockwise rotation on horizontal plane.

vi) There is good voltage of R wave in right precordial leads V_1 or V_2 and, even R and S ratio may be more than 1 (R:S > 1). This occurs due to right ventricular hypertrophy and cor pulmonale secondary to development of pulmonary arterial hypertension.

vii) Right bundle branch block (RBBB). This may appear transiently in cor pulmonale during acute exacerbation. It may be complete or incomplete (Fig. 28.7). Right bundle branch block is more

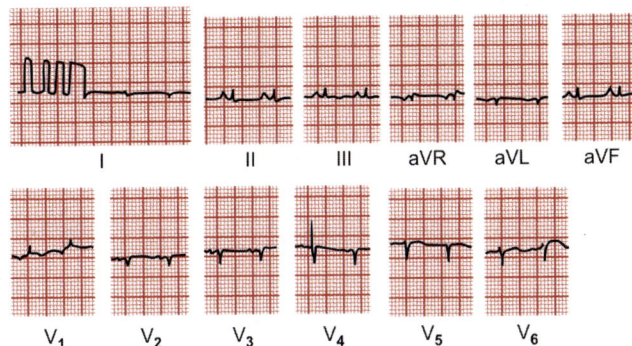

Fig. 28.4: Nonprogression of R wave and low voltage graph in chronic obstructive pulmonary disease (COPD). The electrocardiogram shows;

i. The frontal plane P wave axis is around + 80°
ii. Low voltage graph. All the QRS complexes in standard leads are< 5 mm and in precordial leads < 10 mm. This is due to impaired electrical transmission by voluminous lungs, low anatomical position of the heart and obliquity of QRS axis on horizontal plane
iii. Right atrial atrophy. This is evident by tall peaked P waves (> 2.5 mm) in leads II, III and aVF. This is due to rightward axis of P waves
iv. Right ventricular hypertrophy. The right axis deviation, clockwise rotation, the qR complex in V_1 but of low amplitude and persistence of rS pattern upto V_6 indicates right ventricular hypertrophy
v. Nonprogression of R wave in leads V_1-V_6. The rS pattern of < 5 mm is present in leads V_2-V_6; while there is qR complex in V_1 that indicates regression of R wave with further poor or nonprogression

common in acute thromboembolism than acute exacerbation of chronic cor pulmonale.

C. *The T Wave Abnormality*

i) Frontal plane T wave axis is to the right (+80° to +90°), hence, T wave is taller in lead III than lead 1 ($T_{III} > T_I$).
ii) T wave amplitude may be diminished in all the leads.
iii) The precordial leads show flat or low voltage of T waves but T wave inversion occurs in right precordial leads (V_1-V_3) when right ventricular hypertrophy and cor pulmonale develops.

D. *The ST Segment Changes (Fig. 28.7)*

The ST segment elevation may occasionally be seen in leads II, III and aVF during acute exacerbation of the disease due to increased oxygen desaturation and

SECTION NINE

SECTION NINE

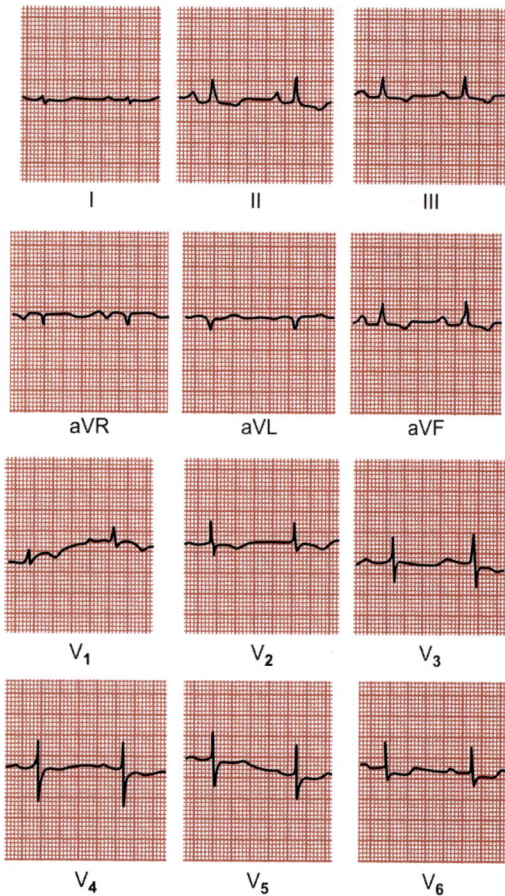

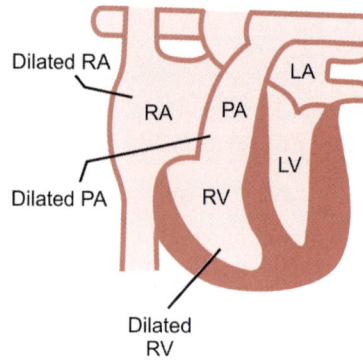

Fig. 28.5: Right atrial and right ventricular hypertrophy in COPD with chronic cor pulmonale. The electrocardiogram was recorded from a patient having congestive heart failure and type II respiratory failure. Note the following features:

i. *Right axis deviation.* There is marked right axis deviation leading to cavity pattern in leads aVR and aVL (P, QRS and T are negative)
ii. *Low amplitude of QRS* in standard leads (I, II, III, aVR, aVL and aVF) and precordial leads (V_1-V_6)
iii. *Right atrial hypertrophy.* Tall peaked P waves > 2.5 mm in height in leads II, III and aVF suggest right atrial hypertrophy. There is right axis deviation of P wave
iv. *Right ventricular hypertrophy.* The right axis deviation, clockwise rotation, the R wave >S wave in lead V_1 (R:S>1) with persistence of S wave in V_5-V_6 suggest right ventricular hypertrophy
v. *ST-T changes.* There is ST segment depression in leads I, II, III, aVF and V_1-V_6 indicate generalised myocardial hypoxia due to advanced lung disease and respiratory failure

is reversible. Sometimes, ST segment depression may be observed in most of the precordial and standard leads and is due to global hypoxia of acute pulmonary insufficiency. The common ST segment change is depression of ST segment and inversion of T wave in right precordial leads V_1-V_2, indicates right ventricular hypertrophy.

E. *Arrhythmias*

Atrial arrhythmias are commoner than ventricular. Atrial arrhythmias include atrial ectopics usually of multifocal origin. Multifocal atrial tachycardia is common atrial arrhythmia seen in COPD. The ventricular arrhythmias occur in the form of multiple, multifocal VPCs.

CHRONIC COR PULMONALE WITHOUT OBSTRUCTIVE DISEASE OF THE AIRWAYS

Chronic cor pulmonale can occur in diseases other than chronic obstructive pulmonary disease (COPD)

such as neuromuscular diseases, thoracic cage deformaties and diseases of the ventilatory control (Table 28.1). Alveolar hypoxia secondary to hypo-ventilation is the primary cause of pulmonary hypertension and development of chronic cor pulmonale. Alveolar hypoxia is a potent stimulus for pulmonary vasoconstriction. Sustained vasoconstriction resulting from chronic hypoxia leads to structural alterations in the pulmonary vasculature that contribute to pulmonary arterial hypertension.

The Electrocardiogram

The electrocardiographic findings in cor pulmonale without obstructive pulmonary disease and cor pulmonale due to pulmonary disease are similar except few. The ECG findings of an insulating effect and lowered position of the heart with respect to electrodes due to hyperinflated lungs, i.e. low voltage graph, and findings of acute ventricular stress, e.g. incomplete or complete bundle branch block are

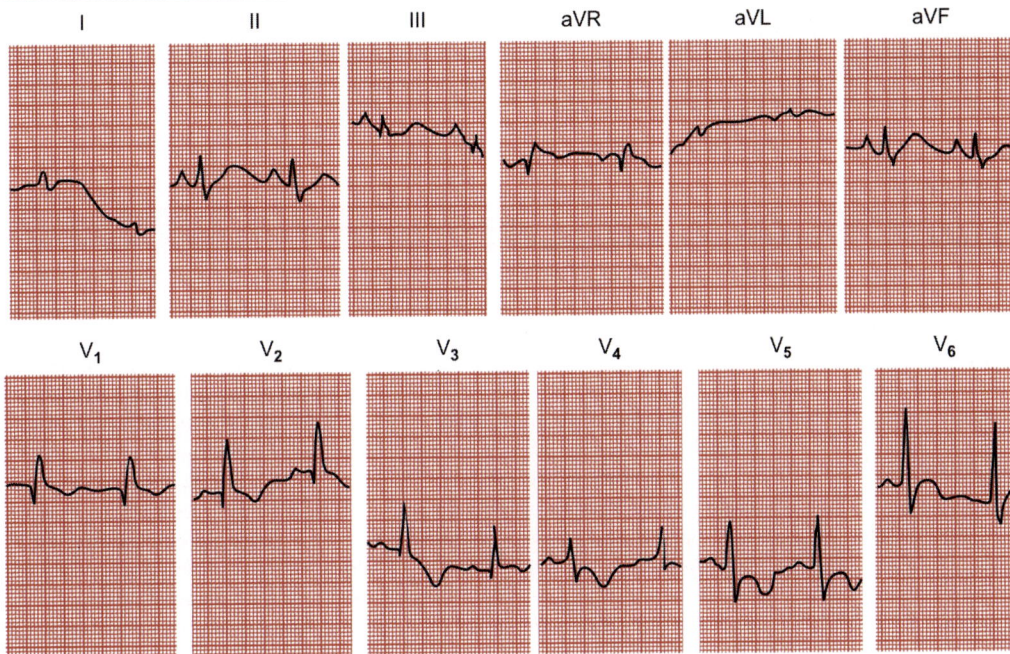

Fig. 28.6: Right atrial and right ventricular hypertrophy in chronic cor pulmonale. The ECG was recorded from a patient with chronic obstructive pulmonary disease with chronic cor pulmonale. Note the following features

   i. Low amplitude of QRS in some standard leads
  ii. Marked clockwise rotation
 iii. *Right atrial hypertrophy.* The P waves are tall and peaked in leads II, III and aVF indicating right axis deviation of P waves and right atrial hypertrophy
  iv. *Right ventricular hypertrophy.* The qR pattern in lead V_1-V_3 and persistence of wide deep S wave in leads V_5-V_6 suggest right ventricular hypertrophy. The ST segment depression and T wave inversion in leads V_1-V_6 indicates combined effect of right ventricular hypertrophy and hypoxaemic effect of basic lung disease.

Note: The pattern can be confused with anterior wall myocardial infarction but actually it is not because in anteroseptal infarction involving the lead V_1-V_3, there will be QS pattern rather than qR. Secondly ST segment is depressed with inverted T waves. Thirdly associated right atrial hypertrophy indicates the qR pattern due to right ventricular hypertrophy—a rotation effect when right ventricular pressure equals or exceeds left ventricular pressure. All these features suggest it to be combined right atrial and right ventricular hypertrophy

SECTION NINE

Table 28.1: Causes of cor pulmonale other than COPD	

I. Diseases affecting the pulmonary vasculature
   A. Primary diseases of the vessel wall
      • Primary pulmonary hypertension
      • Granulomatous pulmonary arteritis
      • Toxin-induced pulmonary hypertension
      • Peripheral pulmonary artery stenosis
   B. Thrombotic disorders
      • Sickle cell anaemia
      • Pulmonary microthrombi
   C. Embolic disorders
      • Repeated thromboembolism or tumour embolism or other embolisms (amniotic fluid, fat, air)
      • Parasitic diseases such as schistosomiasis
	II. Compression of pulmonary arteries
	      • Mediastinal tumours
	      • Aneurysms
	      • Granulomata
	
	III. Neuromuscular disorders and chest wall abnormalities
	      • Neuromuscular weakness
	      • Kyphoscoliosis
	      • Thoracoplasty
	      • Pleural fibrosis
	      • Sleep apnoea syndrome
	      • Idiopathic hypoventilation

Table 28.2: Comparison of ECG characteristics in acute (thromboembolism) and chronic cor pulmonale due to COPD

ECG change	Acute thromboembolism (acute cor pulmonale)	Chronic cor pulmonale due to COPD
1. *Frontal plane leads* (I,II,III,aVR, aVL and aVF)		
• Amplitude of P	Tendency to a generalised low amplitude of all ECG deflections	Low amplitude of only QRS-T deflections. P wave amplitude is increased in leads II, III and aVF.
• P wave axis in lead II	Right axis with tall, peaked P wave (>2.5 mm in height).	Right axis with P pulmonale in leads II, III and aVF. A pronounced T_a wave may develop in these leads.
• QRS axis	– Right axis. A prominent R wave in aVR. – S_I, Q_{III}, T_{III} pattern is common. – Right bundle branch block pattern (rSR' or RsR') occurs acutely and commonly.	– Right axis with prominent R(qR) in aVR. – S_I, S_{II}, S_{III} pattern is common. – Right bundle branch block (complete or incomplete) is uncommon and occurs during acute exacerbation.
• ST segment	ST segment depression in leads I and II. A 'staircase' ascent of ST segment.	During acute exacerbation of the disease, there may be ST elevation in standard leads II, III and aVF due to acute ischaemia/injury and is reversible.
• T wave	T wave inversion in II, III and aVF, is associated with S_I, Q_{III} abnormality, hence, these changes may simulate inferior wall infarction.	The T wave is diminished in amplitude in all the leads. It is upright in standard leads. Due to right axis deviation of T wave, it is larger in lead III than lead I ($T_{III}>T_I$).
2. *Horizontal plane leads* (V_1 to V_6)		
• Clockwise rotation	It is frequent. It leads to shifting of the transition zone leftwards to V_5-V_6 resulting in rS or Rs pattern in all precordial leads. R wave height is less frequently diminished.	There is marked clockwise rotation with shifting of transition zone leftwards to V_5-V_6 and even V_7-V_8. There is diminished height of R wave, hence, complexes are usualy rS or Rs type. Sometimes, an initial r wave in right precordial leads (V_1-V_3) is absent resulting in QS pattern.
• Low amplitude of QRS	Uncommon	Low amplitude of QRS is common. In severe cases, R wave in V_6 may be less than 5 mm, the reasons have been discussed in the text.
• Right ventricular hypertrophy pattern	Common. The R wave in right precordial leads is increased resulting in R:S>1 in leads V_1-V_2	Less common. There is diminution of R wave amplitude in all precordial leads especially, in left precordial leads. But R: S > 1 is also seen in leads V_1-V_2 which may extend upto left precordial leads
• T wave (V_1-V_2)	Inverted in right precordial leads	T is upright in COPD but of decreased amplitude, gets inverted in V_1-V_2 in chronic cor pulmonale.
• Arrhythmias	Atrial arrhythmias are common	Both atrial and ventricular tachyarrhythmias occur.

SECTION NINE

I	II	III	aVR	aVL	aVF

V_1	V_2	V_3	V_4	V_5	V_6

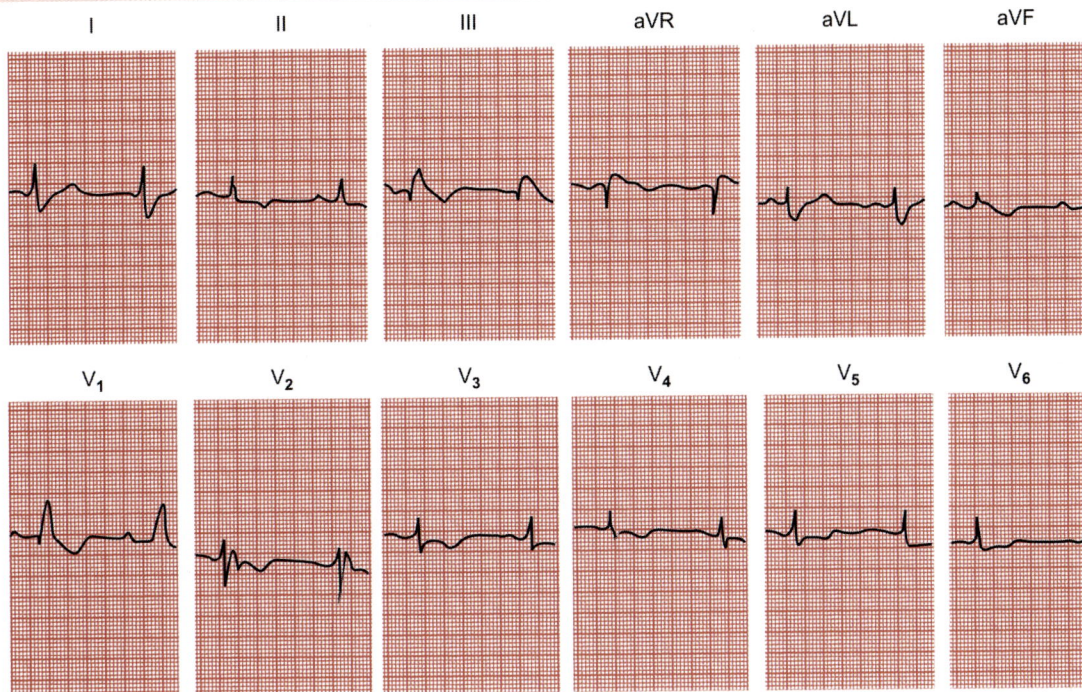

Fig. 28.7: Right bundle branch block in a patient with COPD with chronic cor pulmonale. Note the following characteristics on electrocardiogram;

  i.   Mean frontal plane QRS axis + 70°
  ii. *Right bundle branch block.* It is evident by wide rSR' pattern in V_1 and rSr' in V_2 with ST-T changes and presence of wide S wave in leads I, aVL, V_4-V_6
  iii. *Chronic obstructive pulmonary disease* is evidenced by poor voltage of QRS deflections and nonprogression of R wave in precordial leads. The T wave inversion in leads II, III, aVF and V_3-V_6 is due to global hypoxia due to chronic pulmonary disease
  iv. This pattern in V_1-V_2 may be seen in RVH, but absence of P pulmonale and rSr' pattern in V_2 negate the possibility of RVH either alone or combined with RBBB

Note: RBBB in chronic pulmonary disease is rare and is transient. It could well be due to an isolated congenital abnormality in a patient with COPD. If is persists permanently then it is congenital rather than acquired

usually not seen in cor pulmonale without COPD. The ECG findings in cor pulmonale due to causes other than COPD include;

1. Right axis deviation (mean QRS axis is around + 110°)
2. R : S in lead V_1 > 1
3. R : S in lead V_6 < 1
4. Clockwise rotation of the electrical axis resulting in shifting of transition zone leftwards
5. P pulmonale
6. $S_I Q_{III}$ or S_I, S_{II}, S_{III} pattern
7. Normal voltage of QRS

The ECG changes both in acute and chronic cor pulmonale are compared in Table 28.2.

Suggested Reading

1. Delise P, Piccolo E, O'Este D et al: Electrogenesis of S_I, S_{II}, S_{III} electrocardiographic pattern. *J Electrocardiol* **23**: 23, 1990.
2. Goodwin JF, Abdin ZN: The cardiogram of congenital and acquired right ventricular hypertrophy. *Br Heart J* **21**: 523, 1954.
3. Grant RP: Left axis deviation. A electrocardiographic–pathological correlation study. *Circulation* **14**: 233, 1956.
4. Ikeda K, Kubota I, Takahshi K et al: P wave changes in obstructive and restrictive lung diseases. *J Electrocardiol* **18**: 233, 1985.
5. Kamper D, Chou TD, Fowler NO et al: The reliability of electrocardiographic criteria of chronic obstructive pulmonary disease. *Am Heart J* **80**: 445, 1970.
6. Kilcoyne MM, Davis AL, Ferrer I: A dynamic electrocardiographic concept useful in diagnosis of cor pulmonale. *Circulation* **42**: 903, 1970.

SECTION NINE

7. Schmock CL, Pomerantz B, Mitchell RS et al: The ECG in emphysema with and without chronic airway obstruction. *Chest* **60**: 328, 1971.

8. Selvester RH, Rubin HB: New criteria for ECG diagnosis of emphysema and cor pulmonale. *Am Heart J* **69**: 437, 1965.

9. Shah NS, Velury S, Mascarenhas D et al: Electrocardiographic features of restrictive pulmonary disease and comparison with those of obstructive pulmonary disease. *Am J Cardiol* **70**: 394, 1992.

10. Silver HM, Calatayud JB: Evaluation of QRS criteria in patients with chronic obstructive pulmonary disease. *Chest* **59**: 153, 1971.

11. Spodick DH: Electrocardiographic studies in pulmonary disease. Electrocardiographic abnormalities in diffuse lung disease. *Circulation*, **20**: 1067, 1959.

12. Wiedermann HP, Matthay RA: Cor pulmonale. In Braunwald E (Ed): Heart Disease, 5th edn. Philadelphia, WB Saunders Company 1604, 1997.

29

Systemic Hypertension

Blood pressure of 140/90 mm Hg is considered to be upper limit of the normal in an adult beyond 18 years.

An elevated arterial pressure is probably the most common and important health problem in the developing countries. It is commonly asymptomatic, readily detectable, usually treatable and often lead to lethal complications, if left untreated.

Haemodynamic Alterations

Systemic hypertension acts as systolic overload on the left ventricle and is initially overcome by sustained concentric hypertrophy of left ventricle, characterised by an increase in free wall thickness and ventricular muscle mass of the left ventricle. This is stage of cardiac compensation. Ultimately, sustained hypertension leads to left ventricular dysfunction resulting in its enlargement. Left ventricular dilatation leads to symptoms and signs of left heart failure. Angina pectoris may also occur due to combined effect of acceleration of coronary artery disease and increased oxygen myocardial demands due to increased ventricular mass of hypertrophied left ventricle. The majority of deaths due to hypertension result from myocardial infarction or congestive heart failure.

The Electrocardiogram (Fig. 29.1)

Systemic hypertension may manifest electrocardiographically in following manners.

A. Left Ventricular Hypertrophy (LVH)

The ECG characteristics of LVH have already been discussed in Chapter 9. The voltage criteria of QRS abnormality and frank T wave inversion occur in established hypertension of long duration, therefore, the following criteria may help in early diagnosis.

i) *Wide QRS-T angle and deviation of T wave axis from the left towards right.* This results in tall T wave in V_1 than V_6 before it gets inverted in left precordial leads in sustained hypertension. The frontal plane QRS-T angle begins to increase and usually falls between 45° to 60° but does not reach beyond 150°.

ii) *Presence of left atrial enlargement* in the absence of criteria for left ventricular hypertrophy.

iii) *Ventricular activation time (VAT)* in left precordial leads is increased (> 0.06 sec).

iv) *The small initial q wave in left oriented leads (V_5-V_6)* may disappear with development of left ventricular hypertrophy. Mostly, it is due to expression of left hemiblock and is mostly due to increased tension on the interventricular septum and the left bundle branch by the hypertrophied left ventricle. It could also be due to fibrosis of the left side of interventricular septum in long standing hypertension.

The term left ventricular *'strain'* is used to denote ST-T changes of left ventricular hypertrophy or systolic overload. It is useful but non-committal term used in electrocardiography.

B. Left Atrial Enlargement

The electrocardiographic criteria of left atrial enlargement have been already described (Chapter 8).

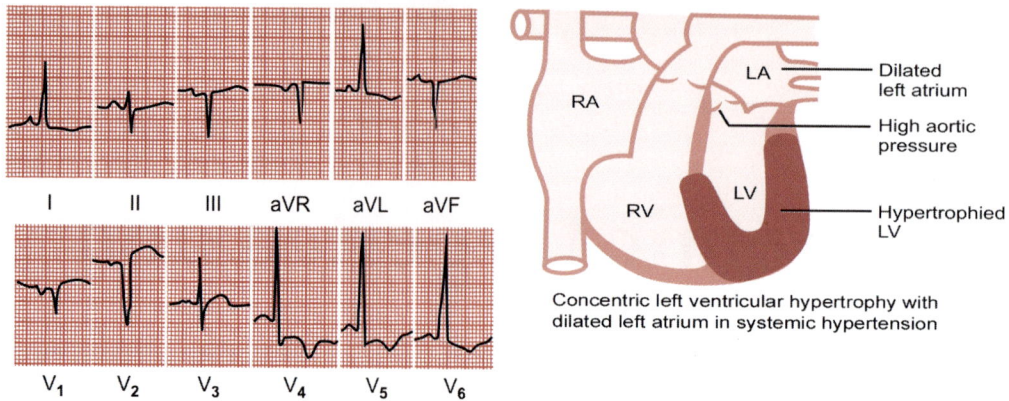

Fig. 29.1: Systemic hypertension. The electrocardiogram recorded from a patient whose BP at that time was 170/110 mm. Note the following characteristics:

   i. Left axis deviation -15° (R wave in lead I and aVL is of equal magnitude)
   ii. Horizontal heart (right ventricular epicardial complex rS in aVF and left ventricular epicardial complex qRS in aVL)
   iii. Counterclockwise rotation—transition zone lies between V_2-V_3
   iv. Voltage criteria of LVH: $RV_5 + SV_1 = 44$ mm and R wave in V_5 or V_6 is > 27 mm
   v. ST T changes. There is ST segment depression and T inversion in leads I, aVL V_4-V_6.
   vi. *Left atrial enlargement.* The P wave is tall and peaked in leads II, III and aVF. In lead V_1, the negative component of biphasic P is prominent.

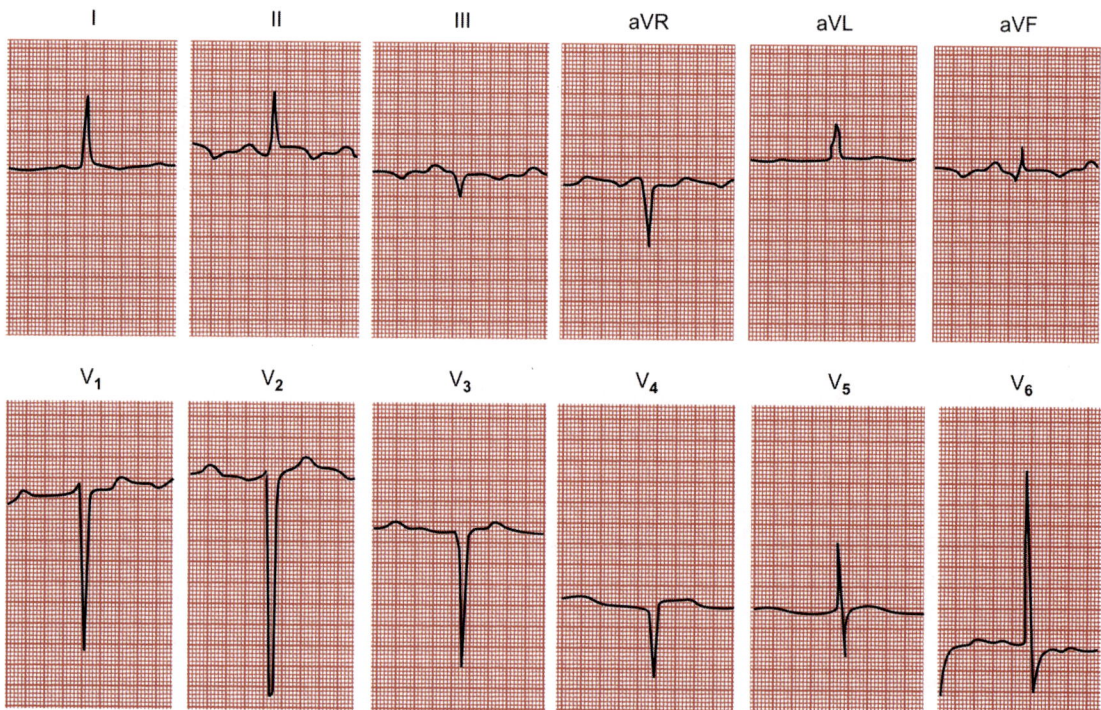

Fig. 29.2: Inferior wall infarction in a patient with systemic hypertension. The patient was admitted with retrosternal and epigastric pain which radiated to back between interscapular blades. Note the following characteristics on ECG;

   i. Left axis deviation
   ii. *Inferior wall infarction* was evident by q waves in leads II and aVF with QS pattern in lead III with ST segment elevation and T wave inversion. Reciprocal change in anterior leads is not present
   iii. *Left ventricular hypertrophy* was established by voltage criteria ($RV_6 + SV_1 = 54$ mm and R wave in $V_6 = 29$ mm). There is T wave inversion in V_5-V_6

There is poor progression of R wave from V_1-V_4 which is not due to anterior wall infarction but is due to LVH, because one would expect QS pattern in these leads to be associated with obliteration of voltage criteria of LVH and reduction in voltage in lead V_6 in anterior myocardial infarction

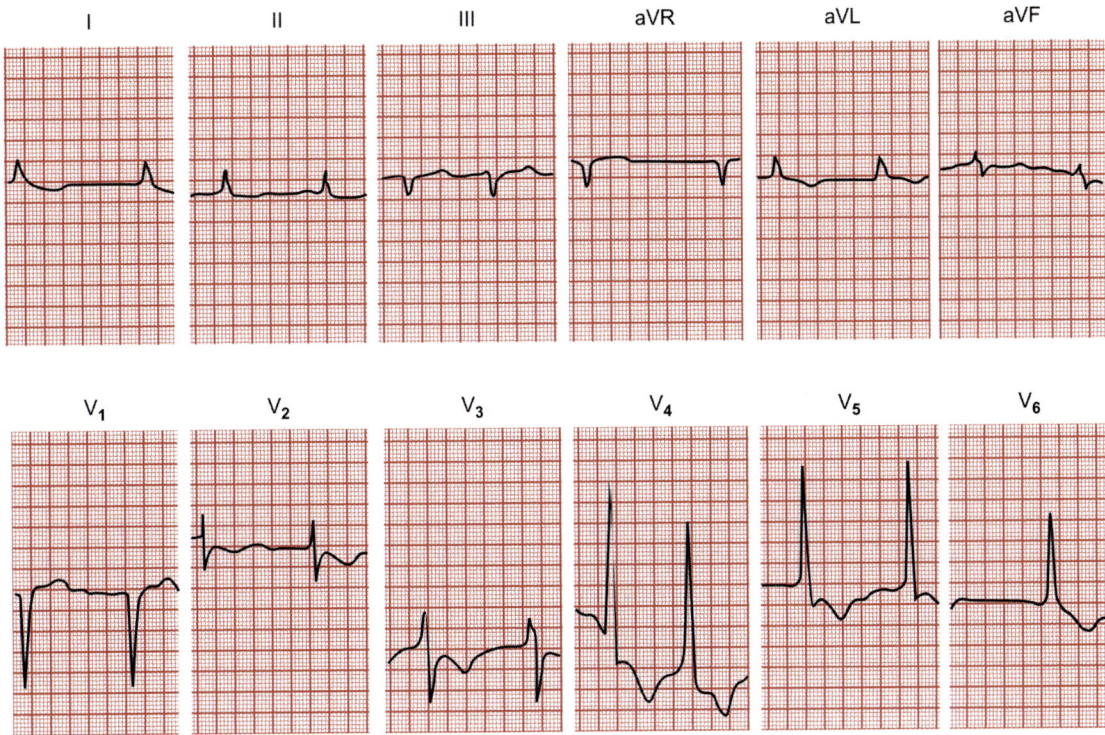

Fig. 29.3: Systemic hypertension with myocardial ischaemia and atrial fibrillation. The electrocardiogram shows;

1. *Left ventricular hypertrophy*. It is revealed by voltage criteria (SV_1 + RV_5 = 35 mm exactly in a 40 yr male patient) with associated ST-T changes in V_5-V_6. The QRS is wide in leads I, aVL, V_4-V_6 and VAT is increased.

2. *Myocardial ischaemia*. It is evident by deep symmetrical inversion of T wave in leads I, aVL, V_2-V_6. These could well be due to LVH with strain pattern, but the presence of inversion of T wave in V_2 indicates anterior orientation of T wave axis that is not expected in LVH. The presence of atrial fibrillation further strengthens it to be due to anterior wall ischaemia.

3. *Atrial fibrillation*. Though a long rhythm strip is not depicted but two complexes in each lead have been shown, which reveal no P wave but fibrillatory (f) waves causing wavy baseline (seen in II and aVF) and R-R interval is variable

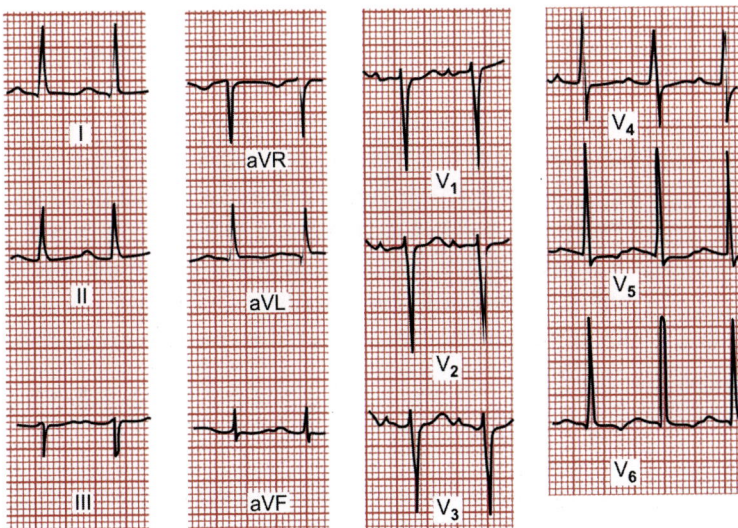

Fig. 29.4: Systemic hypertension with first degree AV block. The ECG shows;

i. Left axis deviation

ii. *Left ventricular hypertrophy*. The R wave in V_5 is > 27 mm and RV_5 + SV_1 is > 35 mm. There is associated ST segment depression and T inversion in leads V_5-V_6

iii. *First degree AV block.* The P-R interval is 0.24 sec.

SECTION NINE

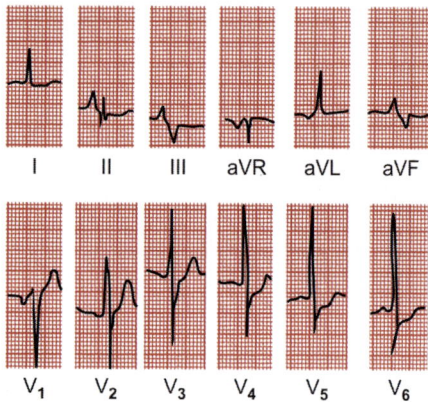

Fig. 29.5: Biatrial and biventricular hypertrophy in a patient with COPD and systemic hypertension (combined effect). Note the following features on ECG;

i. Left axis deviation of QRS on frontal plane
ii. *Right atrial hypertrophy* (Tall peaked P waves in leads II, III and aVF)
iii. *Left atrial hypertrophy* (the negative component of biphasic P in V_1 is deep and sharp)
iv. *Biventricular hypertrophy.* The tall R waves in V_5 and V_6 and deep S wave in V_1 and $RV_5 + SV_1 > 35$ mm indicate LVH. The good voltage of R wave in V_2 and V_3 and it becomes equal to S in V_3 and persistence of deep S wave in V_4-V_6 indicate right ventricular hypertrophy. Biventricular hypertrophy otherwise can also be diagnosed by too tall R and S waves in mid-precordial leads.

The left atrial enlargement on ECG is the sensitive, frequent and probably the earliest and the only change of left ventricular hypertrophy. The electrocardiographic manifestations of left atrial enlargement in the presence of left bundle branch block is most useful pointer to the potential presence of left ventricular hypertrophy due to systolic overload or so called systemic hypertension. It must be stressed that transient left atrial enlargement in acute pulmonary oedema is usually due to left ventricular failure.

C. Left Axis Deviation

Left axis deviation is invariably associated with left ventricular hypertrophy due to hypertension; when present along with other criteria of LVH, it usually indicates left ventricular hypertrophy of long standing duration. The left axis deviation in left ventricular hypertrophy indicates myocardial disease over and above the simple left ventricular hypertrophy.

D. Myocardial Ischaemia/Infarction Pattern

Long standing hypertension may lead to changes of myocardial ischaemia or infarction, may be misconceived due to left ventricular strain. Myocardial ischaemia produces changes in all the leads irrespective of any localisation; while strain pattern is limited to left precordial leads. Hypertension, otherwise predisposes to myocardial infarction (Fig. 29.2).

The following electrocardiographic signs are pointers to the associated presence of myocardial ischaemia most probably due to coronary artery disease (Fig. 29.3).

a) Deep symmetrical inversion of T waves in left precordial leads (V_4-V_6), leads I and aVL.
b) Presence of left bundle branch block or AV blocks.
c) Atrial fibrillation.

E. Arrhythmia/AV Blocks

Long standing hypertension may manifest as an arrhythmia mostly ventricular (ventricular ectopics) or rarely atrial (atrial fibrillation). First degree AV block (Fig. 29.4) is commoner than other grades of AV block.

Hypertension Associated with Other Conditions

On one hand, hypertension predisposes to myocardial ischaemia or infarction and on the other hand, it may be associated with other conditions. Hypertension of long duration usually expresses electrocardiographically by left ventricular hypertrophy and left atrial enlargement. If there are features of right atrial or right ventricular hypertrophy in addition to left ventricular and left atrial hypertrophy, then there must be some other cause to explain the right sided events such as valvular lesions, acute pulmonary embolism or chronic obstructive or interstitial pulmonary disease (Fig. 29.5)

Effect of Treatment

The increased QRS voltage manifestation as well as ST-T changes of left ventricular systolic overload may readily respond to antihypertensive therapy. Thus, while ECG signs of LVH tend to regress following control of hypertension, the signs of left atrial enlargement tend to persist, hence, are useful characteristics for diagnosing left ventricular hypertrophy in early stages of hypertension as well as treated or controlled patients of hypertension.

Suggested Reading

1. Dahlof B, Pannert K, Hansson L: Reversal of left ventricular hypertensive patinets: A meta-analysis of 109 treatment studies. *Am J Hypertens* **5**:95,1992.
2. Das G, Collins J, Weissler AM: Natural history of electrical interventricular septal force in the course of left ventricular hypertrophy in man. *J Electrocardiol* **14**:109,1981.
3. Ghali JK, Liao Y, Simmons B, et al: The prognostic role of LV hypertrophy in patients with or without coronary artery disease. *Am Inter Med* **117**:831,1992.
4. Piccolo E, Revicle A, Delise P, et al : The role of left ventricular hypertrophy. An electrophysiologic study in man. *Circulation*, **16**: 1044, 1979.
5. Romilt DW, Scott RC: Left atrial involvement in acute pulmonary oedema. *Am Heart J* **83**: 328, 1972.
6. Schmicder RE, Messeli FM: Determinants of ventricular ectopy in hypertensive cardiac hypertrophy. *Am Heart J* **123**: 89, 1992.
7. Schneider JF, Thomas HE Jr, McNamara PM, et al : Clinical electrocardiographic study of newly acquired left bundle branch block. The Framingham Study. *Am J Cardiol* **85**: 1332, 1985.
8. Tarazi RC, Miller A, Frohlich E, et al : Electrocardiographic changes reflecting left atrial abnormalities in hypertension. *Circulation* **34**: 818-22, 1966.

The Disorders of Cardiac Rhythm

SECTION TEN

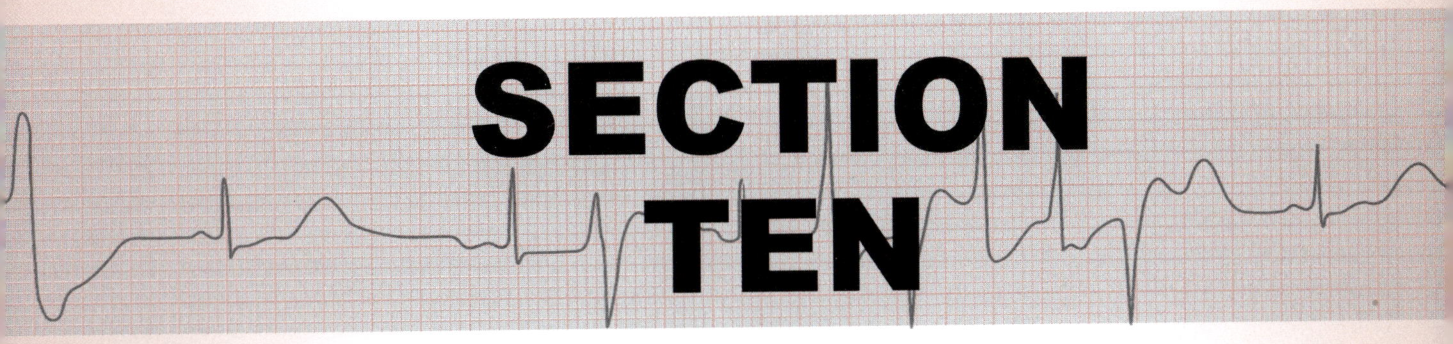

30

Basic Physiopathologic Considerations

- ■ *Anatomy and physiology of conduction system*
- ■ *Classification of arrhythmias*
- ■ *Fundamentals for description of abnormal cardiac rhythm*
- ■ *Arrhythmogenesis (mechanisms of production of tachyarrhythmias)*

ANATOMY AND PHYSIOLOGY OF CONDUCTION SYSTEM

It has been discussed in details.

Natural Pacemakers of Heart and their Rates

The pacemaker cells are present throughout the conduction system but their discharge rate varies. More distally a pacemaker is situated from the SA node, the slower is its inherent discharge rate. The potential pacemakers and their approximate discharge rates are given in the box.

Normally, there is only one pacemaker that controls the heart rate; otherwise chaos will supervene. This concept of protection is one of the most important principle governing electrophysiology of the heart. Normally, fastest pacemaker (SA node) controls the heart and other pacemakers—called

subsidiary pacemakers remain dormant. It is also an intrinsic property of the heart which permits a subsidiary pacemaker (slower pacemaker) to take over the function of control of the heart when fastest pacemaker fails or defaults. Thus, if sinus pacemaker fails, nodal pacemaker will discharge the function of producing nodal rhythm, hence, in ECG, the presence of nodal rhythm indirectly reveals the failure of the sinus pacemaker. In case of complete heart block, the sinus beats are not conducted to the ventricles, in such a situation, pacemaker function of ventricular activation will be taken up by AV node below the site of block or Purkinje system, manifesting as an *idionodal* or *idioventricular escape rhythm* respectively. If sinus rate slows down as in sinus bradycardia or SA blocks, then AV node or one of the ventricles may also produce the escape beat or beats occasionally or intermittently.

Discharge rates of potential pacemakers of the heart

Pacemaker	Discharge rate per minute
1. SA node	75-80 approximate
2. AV node	50-60 approximate
3. Bundle of His	40-50 approximate
4. Purkinje cells of ventricular mass	15-40 approximate

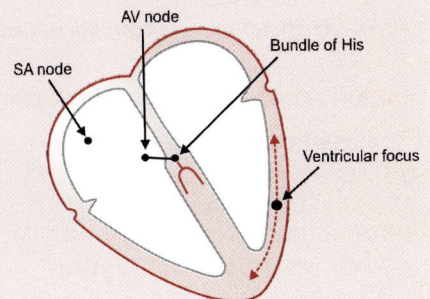

Table 30.1: Classification of arrhythmias

1. **Primary disorders of rhythm**
A. *Disturbances of impulse formation*
   a. *Sinus rhythms*
      - Sinus premature beats
      - Sinus tachycardia
      - Sinus bradycardia
      - Sinus arrhythmia (respiratory and nonrespiratory)
      - Sinus arrest (pause or standstill) or vagotonic block
   b. *Atrial rhythms*
      - Atrial premature beats
      - Paroxysmal atrial tachycardia
      - Multifocal chaotic atrial tachycardia
      - Wandering atrial pacemaker
      - Atrial flutter
      - Atrial fibrillation
   c. *AV nodal (junctional) rhythms*
      - AV nodal ectopics or premature complexes
      - AV nodal tachycardia (paroxysmal and nonparoxysmal)
      - Extrasystolic AV nodal (idionodal) tachycardia
   d. *Ventricular rhythms*
      - Ventricular premature complexes or ectopics
      - Idioventricular rhythm
      - Accelerated idioventricular rhythm
      - Ventricular tachycardia
      - Torsade de pointes
      - Ventricular flutter
      - Ventricular fibrillation
      - Chaotic rhythm
      - Ventricular parasystole
      - Ventricular asystole
B. *Conduction defects*
   a. *SA blocks*
      - First degree
      - Second degree
      - Third degree
   b. *Intra-atrial blocks*
   c. *AV blocks*
      - First degree
      - Second degree (Mobitz type I and II)
      - Complete AV block
      - Dual AV conduction
      - Supernormal AV conduction
   d. *Intraventricular blocks*
      - Right bundle branch block (complete or incomplete)
      - Left bundle branch block (complete or incomplete)
      - Bilateral bundle branch block
      - Intermittent bundle branch block (right or left)
      - Peri-infarction block
   e. *Exit block*
C. *Miscellaneous disturbances (disturbance of both impulse formation and conduction)*
   a. AV dissociation (complete or incomplete)
   b. Pre-excitation syndromes
   c. Reciprocal beats, rhythm and tachycardia
   d. Parasystole (atrial, AV nodal and ventricular)
   e. Electrical alternans
   f. Slow atrial rhythm
   g. Left atrial rhythm
   h. Coronary sinus rhythm
   i. Concealed conduction
   j. Phasic aberrant intraventricular conduction
D. *Artificial pacemaker induced arrhythmias*

Classification of Cardiac Arrhythmias

The classification of arrhythmias is given in the Table 30.1.

Fundamentals for Description of an Abnormal Cardiac Rhythm

For description of a cardiac rhythm, three things are essential;

1. *Anatomical site:* The rhythm may arise either from SA node, atria, AV node, bundle of His, bundle branches or ventricles. They are recognised by their characteristics.
2. *Discharge sequence:* Every rhythm has a discharge sequence; such as, normal sinus rhythm or an escape rhythm or idionodal or idioventricular rhythm. Bradycardia, tachycardia, extrasystoles,

flutter, fibrillation also indicate the discharge sequence of a rhythm.

3. *Conduction sequence :* Conduction sequence must be described while interpreting a rhythm strip, i.e. 2:1 AV block, 3:2 SA or AV block, complete heart block, atrial flutter with 3:1 block, etc.

Any description of a cardiac rhythm without reference to all the three above fundamental facts is considered to be incomplete. For example the term 2:1 AV block is incomplete unless or until you describe the basic rhythm. The 2:1 AV block with sinus rhythm is complete description and indicates a pathological disease of AV node resulting in increased refractoriness of AV node. On the other hand, atrial flutter with 2:1 block indicates that block is a physiological barrier to put hurdle to a rapid atrial rate so as to relieve ventricles from excessive discharge or burden. Therefore, just writing 2:1 AV block is unqualified statement and is misleading. Similarly, tachycardia, flutter, fibrillation are unqualified statements unless you point out the origin of basic rhythm. For example, atrial flutter is a qualified term to be used in electrocardiography, but it becomes more informative if conduction sequence is also mentioned, i.e. 1:1, 2:1, 4:1 conduction. This conduction sequence will indicate whether ventricular response is slow or rapid. This point has haemodynamic and clinical significance. Therefore, for all practical purposes, a rhythm strip should be interpreted with full description of origin, discharge and conduction sequence of the rhythm.

Description of Dual Rhythm

Dual rhythm means presence of two pacemakers for the control of the heart. A dual rhyhm is always present in AV dissociation and complete heart block; one pacemaker for atrial activation and other for the ventricular activation. When such dual rhythm is present, description of both the dissociated rhythms must be stated. For example, sinus rhythm with complete heart block and an idioventricular escape rhythm is a full description of dual rhythm in complete heart block.

THE BASIC APPROACH FOR ANALYSIS OF CARDIAC RHYTHM

The basic approach to analyse the cardiac rhythm based on the fundamentals of electrocardiography are given in the box.

Graphic Representation (Ladder Diagram) for Intracardiac Conduction

Ladder diagram is frequently used for graphic representation of anatomic levels of SA node, atria, AV node and ventricles as ordinates and the abscissa represents time (Fig. 30.1).

Points for Analysis of Cardiac Rhythm (See Appendix)

1. *Define the atrial deflection (P wave) and analyse it to know whether it is?*
   a) A normal P wave
   b) An ectopic P wave (an abnormal shape of P wave)
   c) A flutter 'F' wave
   d) A fibrillation 'f' wave.
2. *Calculate atrial rate, i.e. P-P interval.*
3. Determine whether atrial rhythm is regular (regular P-P intervals) or irregular (irregular P-P intervals)
4. The relationship of atrial deflection (P wave) to QRS complex of ventricular deflection
5. Shape of QRS complex—narrow or wide.

ARRHYTHMOGENESIS (FIGS 30.2 TO 30.4)

The genesis of abnormal cardiac rhythm is divided into two main categories.

1. *Abnormalities of automaticity*: The abnormal automaticity, theoretically, arises from a single disordered cell or an ectopic focus of few cells.
2. *Abnormalities of conduction*: The abnormalities in conduction arise due to abnormal interactions between the cells.

The three mechanisms of arrhythmias include;

A. *Accelerated automaticity*
B. *Triggered activity* - Triggered activity is pacemaker activity that results consequent to a preceding impulse or series of impulses without which electrical quiescence occurs.
   i) Triggered activity due to early afterdepolarisations (EADs) called reflection.
   ii) Triggered activity due to delayed afterdepolarisations (DADs)
C. *Re-entry (circus movement)*

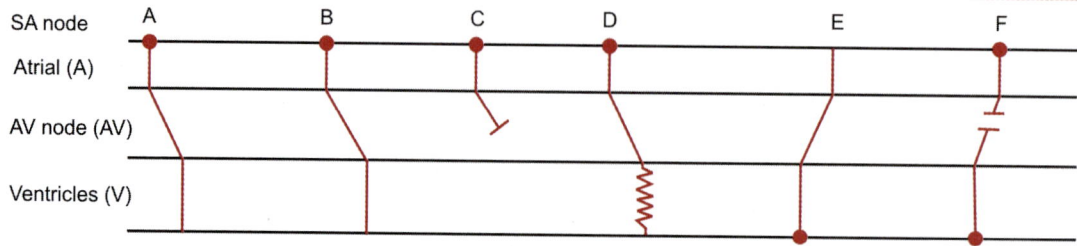

Fig. 30.1: Graphic representation for intracardiac conduction using ladder diagram during analysis of arrhythmias. The ordinate reflects the anatomical levels while the abscissa reflects time.

　　The black dot reflects impulse origin.

A: *Normal conduction.* It demonstrates normal conduction of a sinus impulse. The black dot indicates the origin of impulse from SA node which is conducted quickly through atria (A) as shown by relatively steep slope. The impulse is delayed in AV node as shown by relatively gradual slope and finally conducted to the ventricles quickly as reflected once again by the relatively steep slope.

B: *Delayed AV conduction.* It represents first degree AV block. A shallower slope at the level of AV node indicates delay in intranodal conduction

C: AV block. There is interruption of conduction within AV node (a barrier is put to denote it).

　　A, B and C (combined) shows Wenckebach 3:2 AV block in which A shows normal sinus conducted beat, B shows a beat with prolonged P-R interval and C shows blocked sinus beat.

D: Aberrant intraventricular conduction. It represent phasic aberrant ventricular conduction (it is denoted by wavy line)

E: Ectopic ventricular impulse. The black dot at ventricular level indicates the site of origin of impulse, which gets conducted retrogradely to the atria (VA conduction)

F: AV dissociation with interference within AV node. The two black dots represent the site of origin of two impulses which collide and interfere with each other's progress within AV node (indicated by two barriers)

1. Abnormal Automaticity

The ionic basis of automaticity is explained by a net gain in intracellular positive charges during diastole. The normal mechanism of cardiac rhythmicity is slow depolarisation of the membrane during diastole until the threshold potential is reached and the pacemaker fires. This mechanism can be accelerated by increasing the rate of diastolic depolarisation or changing the threshold potential. Such changes are thought to produce sinus tachycardia, escape rhythms and accelerated AV nodal rhythms; and are possibly due to depolarisation induced abnormal automaticity (Fig. 30.2).

2. Triggered Activity (Fig. 30.2B)

A. *Triggered activity due to early afterdepolarisations (EADs-called reflection)*

　　The term *early afterdepolarisation (EAD)* means depolarisation that occurs before full repolarisation of the fibre. The early afterdepolarisations arise from a reduced level of membrane potential during phase 2 (type 1) and 3 (type 2) of the cardiac action potential. Therefore, if adjacent cells repolarise at different rates; the cells that repolarise more quickly may be restimulated by those cells that have not been yet depolarised. EADs may be responsible for lengthened depolarisation and predisposition to ventricular tachyarrhythmias in several clinical situations; such as congenital and acquired forms of long Q-T syndrome.

　　Patients with idiopathic Q-T syndrome may have myocardial defect in repolarisation or a sympathetic imbalance. Sympathetic stimulation could periodically increase the EADs amplitude to provoke ventricular tachyarrhythmias.

B. *Triggered activity due to delayed afterdepolarisations (DADs)*

　　Myocardial damage can result in oscillations at the end of the action potential. These oscillations may reach threshold potential and produce an arrhythmia. The abnormal oscillations can be exaggerated by pacing and by catecholamines; and these stimuli can be used to trigger this abnormal form of automaticity.

　　Triggered activity due to delayed afterdepolarisations (DADs) arises after completion of repolarisation (phase 4), generally at a more negative

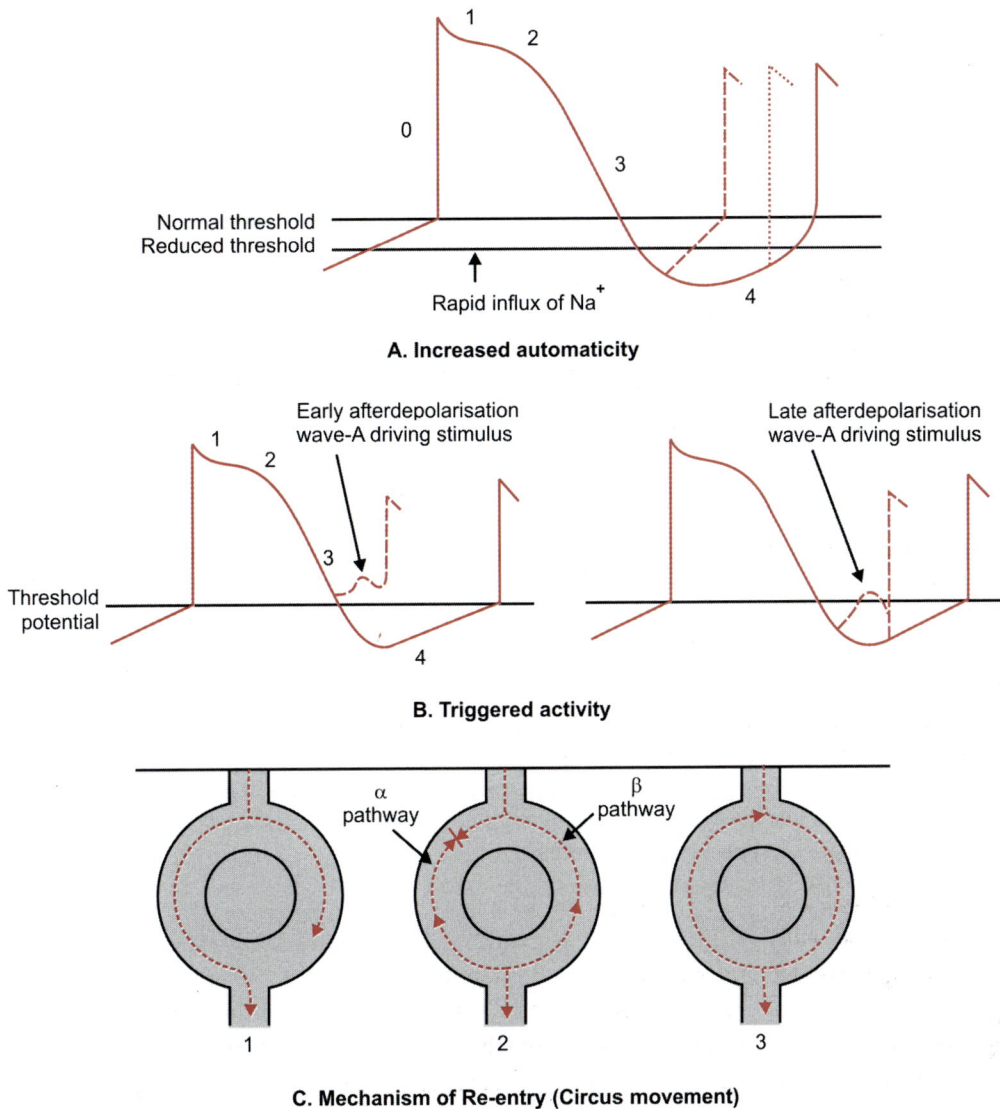

A. Increased automaticity

Normal threshold
Reduced threshold

Rapid influx of Na$^+$

Early afterdepolarisation
wave-A driving stimulus

Late afterdepolarisation
wave-A driving stimulus

Threshold
potential

B. Triggered activity

α pathway

β pathway

C. Mechanism of Re-entry (Circus movement)

Fig. 30.2: Mechanism of arrhythmogenesis

A. Increased automaticity. The diagram illustrates action potentials (i.e. the potential difference between intracellular and extracellular fluid) of myocardium after stimulation. The increased automaticity is due to a reduced threshold potential or an increased slope of phase 4 depolarisation.

B. Triggered activity: The diagram illustrates action potentials and triggered activity due to early afterdepolarisations (EADs) and late afterdepolarisations (DADs) reaching threshold potential

C. Re-entry (circus movement). The diagram (1) shows the impulses passing down both limbs of the potential tachycardia circuit. The diagram (2) shows that impulse is blocked in α pathway but proceeds slowly down the β pathway and returns along the α pathway. The diagram (3) shows the impulse travels so slowly along the β pathway that when it returns along the α pathway to its starting point, it is able to travel down the β pathway producing a circus movement tachycardia

membrane potential (Fig. 30.2) than from which early afterdepolarisations (EADs) arise. All afterdepolarisations may not reach threshold potential; but if they do, they can trigger another afterdepolarisation and, this then self-perpetuate to produce an arrhythmia. Some of the arrhythmias produced by digitalis toxicity are due to this type of triggered activity.

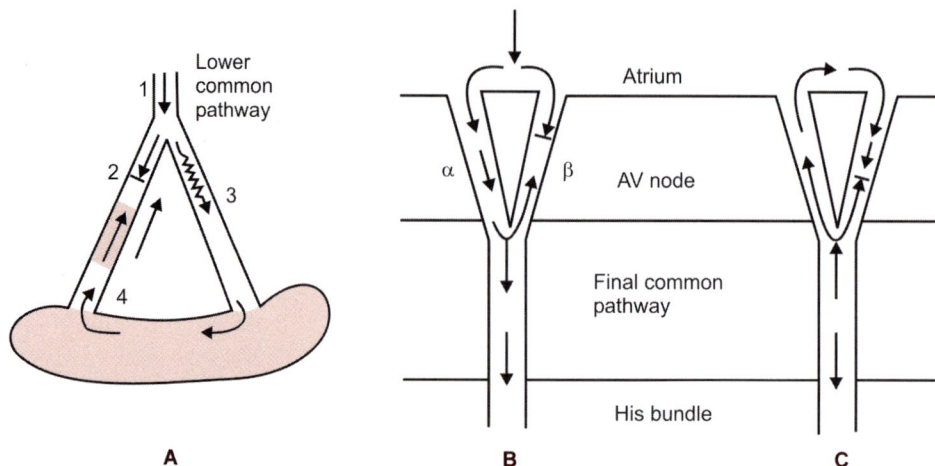

Fig. 30.3: Anatomical re-entry.

A: *Re-entry through Purkinje fibres leading to ventricular ectopics and tachycardia.* The Purkinje fibres splits into two pathways. An impulse travelling through lower common pathway (at I), gets blocked in antegrade conduction at site 2 (arrow followed by bar), but travels down slowly at 3 (serpentine arrow) to excite the ventricle. The impulse now re-enters the Purkinje system of myocardium, excites it and then re-enters at site 4 as a result of which ventricular extrasystole results. Continued re-entry in this manner produces ventricular tachycardia.

B: *Mechanism of atrial echo.* Schematic representation of anatomical intranodal pathway for an atrial echo. A premature atrial impulse (APC) exhibits unidirectional block, fails to get conducted through beta pathway, but gets conducted antegradely through alpha-pathway. While traversing through final common pathway, finding the beta pathway responsive, it gets conducted through this circuit producing an atrial echo resulting in nodal re-entrant tachycardias.

C: *Mechanism of ventricular echo.* A premature impulse from the His bundle traverses the final common pathway, encounters refractory beta-pathway (unidirectional block), reaches retrogradely to atrium through alpha-pathway and now returns through the recovered beta pathway to produce ventricular echo

3. Re-entry [Re-entrant Excitation, Circus Movement, Reciprocal Beats or Echoes, or Reciprocating Tachycardia (Figs 30.3 and 30.4)]

The SA node generates electrical activity during each cardiac cycle; which spreads throughout the heart and continues till the entire heart is activated. Each cell gets activated, turn by turn, and lastly the cardiac impulse dies out when all the fibres have been discharged; and then heart becomes completely refractory. During this refractory period, the electrical impulse has no place to go, hence, gets extinguished and activation restarted by the next sinus impulse. If, however, a group of contiguous fibres not activated during initial phase of depolarisation, recovers excitability in time, gets discharged by the same impulse before the impulse dies out is called *re-entry*. Re-entry also implies that an impulse can re-excite areas that were just discharged and have now recovered from the initial depolarisation. This may be explained as follows;

"A wave of depolarisation may be forced to travel in one direction around a ring of cardiac tissue. If the time to conduct around the ring is longer than the recovery period of any tissue within the ring, a circus movement results producing coupled ectopics and its self-perpetuation results in a tachycardia (Fig. 30.2C)."

The re-entry may be facilitated by anatomical pathways (Fig. 30.3) or can occur in contiguous fibres that exhibit functionally different electrophysiological properties or may occur randomly such as in atrial fibrillation.

The tachyarrhythmias due to re-rentry mechanism are given in the box; and they are diagrammatically illustrated in Figures 30.3 to 30.5.

OTHER ELECTROPHYSIOLOGICAL ABNORMALITIES LEADING TO CARDIAC ARRHYTHMIAS

1. Supernormal Conduction

The term is applied to situations when conduction is better than normal but is not effective as normal. This

A
B

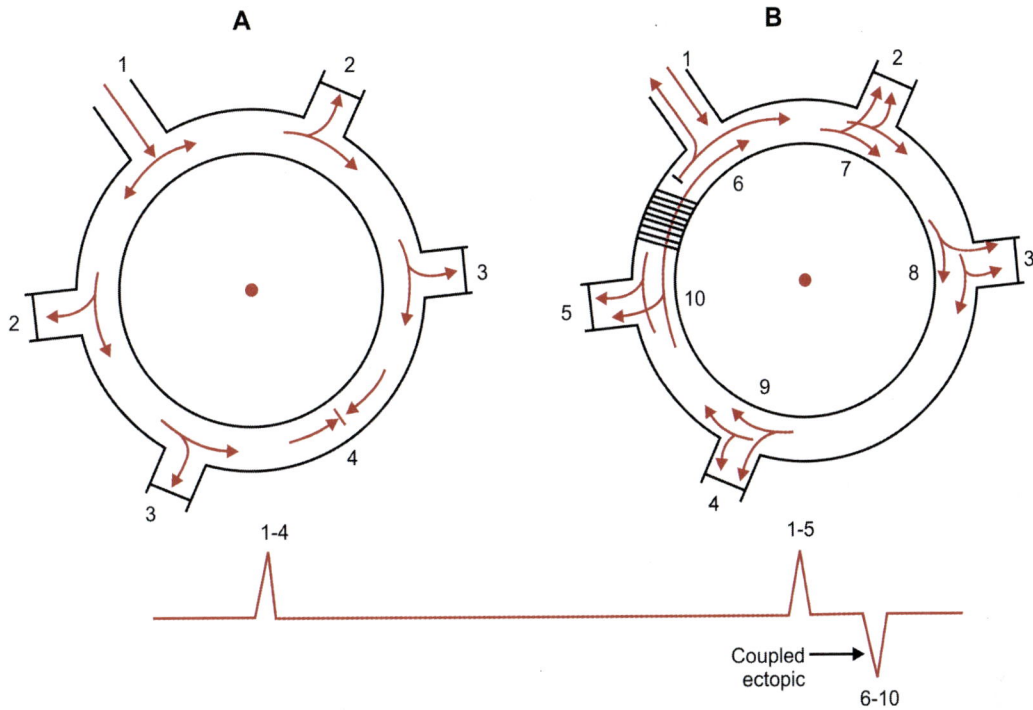

Fig. 30.4: Diagrammatic illustration of re-entry (circus movement) mechanism explaining the coupled ectopics.

A: A ring of conducting fibres and branches of the Purkinje system are shown. The excitation impulse is assumed to enter the conduction system at point 1, where it splits, one impulse passes in clockwise direction and other in anticlockwise direction. In their course around the ring, the impulse splits at points 2 and 3, from where excitation spreads via adjoining branches into other portions of Purkinje network. At the same time, the original impulses from both sides reach and finally meet and obliterate each other at point 4. In this way, the spread of excitation impulse through Purkinje fibre and syncytial network depolarise the ventricular myocardium producing ventricular deflection as shown below the diagram.

B: The circular pathway of the conduction system is same as in A except that one segment of myocardium is refractory (stippled). In this situation, the excitation impulses enters the circular ring of conducting fibres at point I, can be transmitted in only one direction (shown by arrows). Since spread in anticlockwise direction is prevented by refractory segment, the impulse enters in clockwise direction and produces a ventricular deflection (B1-5) after spreading through circular ring pathway and adjoining fibres of conduction at points, 2,3,4 and 5. By the time, the impulse arrives at the previously refactory segment of conduction pathway (stippled), the region becomes responsive and is able to conduct the impulse. Consequently the excitation impulse re-enters the circular ring of conducting fibres and traverses it for the second time to produce the coupled extrasystole (B6-10) as shown in the diagram below.

Tachyarrhythmias due to re-entry (Fig. 30.3)

SA node	*Atrial*	*Nodal*	*Ventricular*
• SA node tachycardia	• Atrial flutter • Atrial fibrillation	• AV nodal re-entrant tachycardia • Atrioventricular tachycardia (AVRT) • Pre-excitation syndrome with tachycardia	• Ventricular tachycardia • Ventricular fibrillation

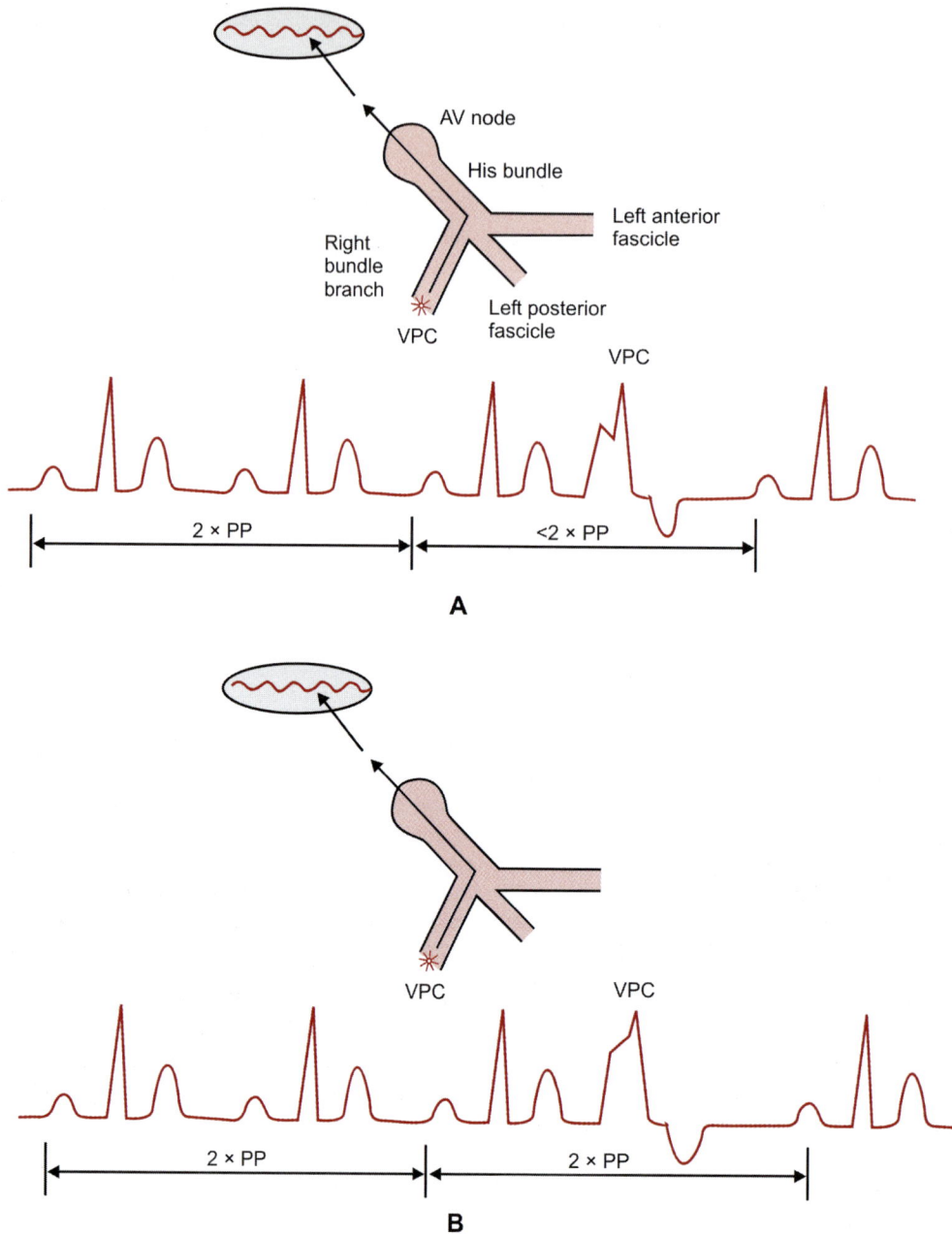

Fig. 30.5: Phenomenon of concealed conduction.

A: A ventricular premature impulse denoted (*) is conducted in the retrograde fashion to the atria through the AV node and penetrates the SA node and resets its timings, hence, the compensatory pause following the VPC is incomplete, i.e. less than two sinus cycles (< 2 x PP)

B: The ventricular premature impulse after reaching the atria retrogradely depolarises the atria but does not penetrate the SA node and does not reset its timing, therefore, next sinus beat occurs on time. The compensatory pause is complete, i.e. exactly twice the sinus cycle (2 x PP)

phenomenon always occurs when conduction is depressed, but has been observed in normal cardiac tissues as well. It takes place generally during the relative refractory period of the preceding complex, hence, called superconduction. The electrophysiological basis underlying supernormal conduction is supernormal excitation or some other mechanisms. Supernormal conduction is said to be present when AV nodal conduction is more rapid than expected or AV conduction results when AV block is expected.

2. Single Focus of Subthreshold Activity (Wedensky Facilitation)

In this phenomenon, presumably a localised metabolic or circulatory or electrolyte disturbance causes a subthreshold increase in focal excitability. If, on this subthreshold background, there is superimposed a further, *albeit* temporary, rise in focal excitability induced by the trigger impulse, the level of excitability in the ectopic centre becomes transiently superthreshold. This produces discharge of the ectopic impulse. The trigger impulse may be sinus or other ectopic impulse, initiates discharge of an ectopic focus of subthreshold activity. The mechanism by which this trigger impulse increases excitability of the ectopic focus is not known. One possible explaination is that initial beat alters the chemical environment of the ectopic centre by causing circulatory changes. The other view is that it may be due to Wedensky fecilitation, in which a segment of depressed Purkinje or muscle fibres blocks, completely or incompletely, the spread of the trigger impulse into this blocked area, with the result, blocked impulses cause a momentary increase in the excitability of the Purkinje or myocardial fibres distal to the site of block to suprathreshold level and discharge the ectopic focus.

3. Concealed Conduction (Fig. 30.5)

It describes a phenomenon during which an impulse penetrates the conduction tissue (AV node or other areas) without emerging from it. As the name suggests, the transmission of the impulse is concealed, hence, it is not visible on surface electrocardiogram, but its effect on the conduction and/or formation of subsequent complexes is seen. This phenomenon is best demonstrated during a ventricular premature complex (VPC). Partial or complete retrograde penetration of the SA node by a ventricular premature complex, resets its timing, resulting in production of a compensatory pause (i.e. following sinus conducted beat is delayed resulting in a pause) or the following sinus beat is conducted with a long P-R interval if the VPC is interpolated (Fig. 30.5). The slower ventricular response when atrial rate increases from atrial flutter to atrial fibrillation is again due to concealed conduction because a large number of atrial impulses bombard the AV node but cannot emerge from it. Concealed conduction occurs in WPW syndrome and can be manifested by unidirectional antegrade/retrograde block of the accessory pathway. Concealed conduction of nodal extrasystoles can produce electrocardiographic manifestation of an apparent or pseudo AV block.

4. Parasystole

Read the Chapter 38 on parasystole.

5. QT Dispersion (QTd)

The abnormal lead to lead variation of QT (QTd), predisposes to arrhythmias such as torsade de pointes or ventricular tachycardia. The proposed mechanism of arrhythmias demonstrated in experimental study revealed that large dispersion of repolarisation (QTd) facilitates the development of a conduction delay necessary to induce arrhythmia by an early premature stimulus applied at the site with a short monophasic action potentials (MAP). Read QT dispersion.

REVIEW AT A GLANCE

- These are 4 important sites of pacemakers, i.e. SA node, AV node, bundle of His and ventricle.
- SA node is the fastest pacemaker and ventricular pacemaker is the slowest. More distally a pacemaker is situated, the slower is its rate of discharge.
- SA node is an original pacemaker. The other pacemakers are subsidiary pacemakers.
- Normally heart is controlled by one pacemaker - SA node discharges at a highest rate

and thus other pacemakers normally remain suppressed or dormant. In case, the original pacemaker fails or becomes slow, then a subsidiary pacemaker may discharge intermittently or may take the complete control of the heart.

- Arrhythmias are classified into primary and secondary disorders. Primary disorders include arrhythmias due to impulse formation and impulse conduction.
- Fundamental description of a rhythm includes its anatomical site, sequence of discharge and conduction rate or ratio.
- The mechanisms of producing tachyarrhythmias include automaticity, triggered activity and re-entry.

Suggested Reading

1. Chan AQ, Pick A: Re-entrant arrhythmias and concealed conduction. *Am Heart J* **97**:644,1979.
2. Cranefield PF: Action potentials, afterpotentials and arrhythmias. *Circ Res* **41**:415, 1977.
3. Domato AN, Lau SH: Concealed and supernormal AV conduction. *Circulation* **43**:967, 1971.
4. El-Sherif N, Craelius W: Early afterdepolarisations and arrhythmogenesis. *J Cardiovasc Electrophsiol* **1**:145, 1990.
5. Fisch C, Greenspan K: Wendesky's observations (Edit). *Circulation* **35**:819,1967.
6. Fischer JD: Role of electrophysiological testing in the diagnosis and treatment of patients with known and suspected bradycardias and tachycardias. *Prog Cardiovasc Dis* **24**:25, 1981.
7. Hoffman BF: The genesis of cardiac arrhythmias. *Prog Cardiovasc Dis* **8**:319,1966.
8. January CT, Shorofsky S: Early afterdepolarisations: Newer insights into cellular mechanisms. *J Cardiovasc Electrophysiol* **1**:161, 1990.
9. Kuo CS, Munakata K, Reddy CP, Surawicz B: Characteristic and possible mechanism of ventricular arrhythmia on dispersion of action potential durations. *Circulation* **67**:1356, 1983.
10. Langendorf R: Concealed AV conduction. The effect of blocked impulses on the formation and conduction of subsequent impulses. *Am Heart J* **35**:542, 1948.
11. Langerdorf R, Pick A: Concealed conduction in AV junction. In: Dreifus, Likoff (Eds): *Mechanisms and Therapy of Cardiac Arrhythmias*. New York: Grune and Stratton.
12. Schamroth L: *An Introduction to Electrocardiography*, 7th ed. Blackwell Science publication, 1993.
13. Sicouri S, Aztzelevitch C: Drug induced afterdepolarisations and triggered activity in a discrete subpopulation of ventricular muscle cell (M cells) in the canine heart: Quinidine and digitalis. *J Cardiovasc Electrophysiol* **4**:48, 1993.
14. Wit AL, Rosen MR, Hoffman BF: Electrophysiology and pharmacology of cardiac arrhythmias II. The relationship of normal and abnormal electrical activity of cardiac fibres to the genesis of arrhythmias. *Am Heart J* **85**:515,1974.
15. Zipes DP, Miles WM, Klein LS: Assessment of the patient with a cardiac arrhythmia. In: Zipes DP, Jalife J (Eds): *Cardiac Electrophysiology: From Cell to Bedside*, 2nd ed. Philadelphia: WB Saunders Company 1009, 1994.
16. Zipes DP: Genesis of cardiac arrhythmias: Electrophysiological considerations. In: Braunwald Heart Diseases—*A Textbook of Cardiovascular Medicine*, 5th ed, 546, WB Saunders Company 1997.
17. Zipes DP: Monophasic action potentials in diagnosis of triggered arrhythmias. *Prog Cardiovasc Dis* **33**:385, 1991.

31

Sinus Rhythm and Its Manifestations

- Definition and characteristics of sinus rhythm
- Sinus arrhythmia—respiratory and nonrespiratory with ECG characteristics
- Sinus bradycardia—causes and electrocardiographic characteristics
- Sinus tachycardia—causes, mechanisms and its ECG characteristics
- Sinus node re-entrant tachycardia and its characteristics

SINUS RHYTHM

Definition

Rhythm is said to be normal sinus when impulses originating from the SA node at a rate of 60-100 bpm are conducted through atrial internodal pathways; and further there is a slight physiological delay at AV node, and ultimately are transmitted to the ventricles. The P waves are produced at a rate which varies from 60-100 bpm in an adult and reflect atrial depolarisation. The infants and children generally have faster heart rates than the adults. Impulses reaching the AV node proceed uninterruptedly through bundle of His, bundle branches and the Purkinje system to the ventricles. A narrow QRS complex results due to ventricular depolarisation and follows P wave at fixed P-R interval. Normally, there is an associated slight to moderate respiratory sinus arrhythmia. The sinus nodal discharge rate responds readily to autonomic stimulation and reflects the net effect of two opposing autonomic influences, i.e. vagus and sympathetic. The vagal stimulation decreases; while sympathetic stimulation increases the spontaneous sinus node discharge rate.

The Electrocardiogram

1. The P wave is usually upright in all standards leads (I, II, III, aVL, aVF) except aVR. The P wave vector lies between $+45°$ to $+65°$. It is best seen in leads II, and aVF. It is also upright in all precordial leads except V_1 where it may be biphasic. It is due to orientation of P wave vector anteriorly and to the left on horizontal plane.
2. P-R and R-R intervals remain constant.
3. Atrial and ventricular rates are identical and range between 60-100 bpm. The rate of sinus rhythm varies significantly depending an age, sex and physical activity.
4. There is no ectopic activity.

Sometimes, during sinus rhythm, the morphology of the P waves or QRS complexes will appear abnormal. The P-R and QRS intervals may also exceed the normal limits. In such cases, the label "*sinus rhythm*" still applies, but one would hesitate to call a rhythm as "normal" when abnormalities of waveform or interval exist. In electrocardiography, the sinus rhythm with abnormalities must be qualified as sinus beats/rhythm with AV block or sinus beats/rhythm

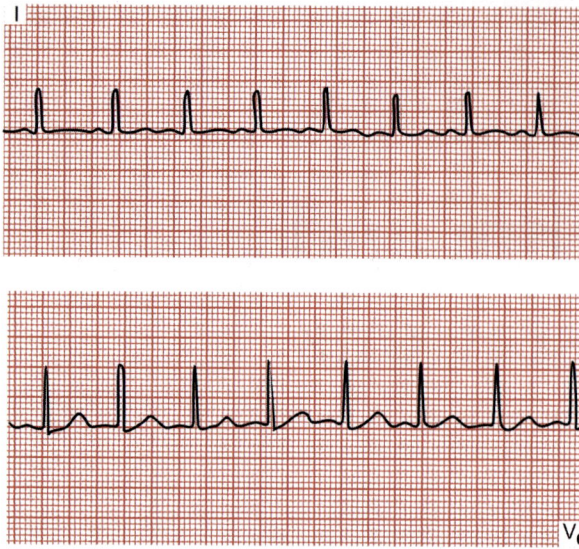

Fig. 31.1: Normal sinus rhythm. The electrocardiogram (leads I and V$_6$) shows;

i. Normal P waves and P-R intervals
ii. Normal QRS complexes and T waves
iii. Heart rate 90/min regular

with aberrant intraventricular conduction, etc. It has been discussed in previous chapter.

SINUS ARRHYTHMIA

Sinus arrhythmias is characterised by alternating periods of slow and rapid heart rates. It is due to fluctuating discharge of SA node due to phasic variations in the sinus cycle lengths (R-R intervals) during which maximum sinus cycle length minus minimum cycle length exceeds 0.12 sec or the maximum sinus cycle length minus minimum cycle length divided by the minimum sinus cycle length exceeds 10%. It is the most frequent arrhythmia and is considered to be a normal event.

Diagnostic Clues to Sinus Arrhythmia

1. Maximum R-R interval – minimum R-R interval in the same lead exceeds 0.12 sec.
2. Maximum R-R – minimum R-R ÷ minimum R-R interval exceeds 10% in the same lead.

TYPES

1. Respiratory Sinus Arrhythmia

The heart rate changes with respiration. The rate is faster during inspiration and slower towards the end of expiration. This is due to reflex stimulation of vagal receptors in the lungs. It is a benign condition.

The Electrocardiogram (Fig. 31.2)

In respiratory arrhythmia, the R-R interval shortens during inspiration and lengthens during expiration.

2. Nonrespiratory Sinus Arrhythmias

The change in heart rate is not related to respiration. This is observed during certain conditions where vagal tone fluctuates such as in persons with a cardiac disease or myocardial infarction especially in association with sinus bradycardia. Digoxin therapy or enhanced vagal tone can also give rise to this arrhythmia.

The Electrocardiogram (Fig. 31.3)

In nonrespiratory arrhythmia, there are alternate periods of lengthening and shortening of R-R intervals.

3. Ventriculophasic Sinus Arrhythmia

This arrhythmia occurs under the influence of autonomic nervous system in response to changes in ventricular stroke volume; is seen when ventricular rate is slow and change in stroke volume is marked. The most common example is complete heart block where P-P interval containing QRS is shorter than P-P interval without a QRS complex. Other example is a VPC with a compensatory pause.

SINUS BRADYCARDIA

It is defined as sinus rhythm with a rate less than 60 bpm in an adult.

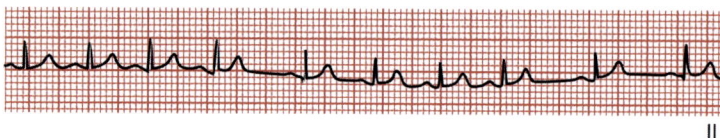

Fig. 31.2: Respiratory sinus arrhythmia. The variable R-R intervals are due to effect of respiration

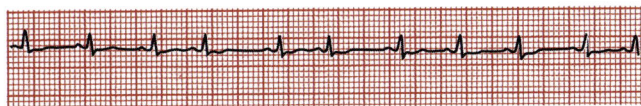

Fig. 31.3: Nonrespiratory sinus arrhythmia. The electrocardiogram was recorded from a patient with dilated cardiomyopathy. The lead II reveals variable R-R intervals, each QRS complex is narrow and preceded by a P wave. This is not atrial fibrillation known to occur in dilated cardiomyopathy as P wave preceding QRS complex are nicely seen with a fixed P-R interval. This is even not a multifocal atrial tachycardia because there is no change in P wave morphology

Causes

1. Physiological : Vagotonic persons, athletes and during sleep. It can be induced by carotid sinus compression.
2. Hypothyroidism.
3. Obstructive jaundice.
4. Hypothermia
5. Sick sinus syndrome
6. Electrolyte disturbance, i.e. hyperkalaemia, hypermagnesaemia, etc.
7. Inferior wall infarction
8. Drugs (digoxin, beta blockers, calcium channel blockers, etc.)
9. Second degree AV block.
10. Raised intracranial pressure.
11. Uraemia
12. Poisoning (organophosphorus, aluminium phosphide, scorpion sting bite, etc.)
13. Hyperactive carotid sinus.

The Electrocardiogram (Fig. 31.4)

1. Sinus rate is < 60 bpm.
2. The P wave has normal contour and precedes each normal QRS complex.

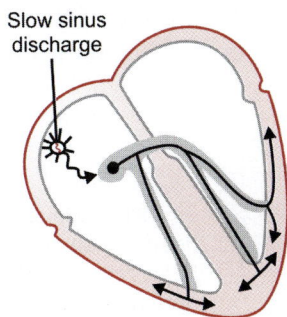

3. The R-R interval is constant unless concomitant AV block or sinus arrhythmia is present.
4. Sinus arrhythmia often coexists with sinus bradycardia.

By definition, any rhythm with a heart rate < 60 bpm is classified as a sinus bradycardia. Bradycardia with normal heart is tolerated well without any ill effect; however, in the presence of diseased heart, it may produce haemodynamic consequences and requires treatment.

> Note: In complete heart block, there is bradycardia with idioventricular rhythm but is not classified as sinus bradycardia because sinus beats are blocked at AV node.

Sinus bradycardia can persist with normal sinus rhythm, but at times; if rate falls below the inherent rate of discharge of AV node, AV nodal escape beat or beats or even AV nodal escape rhythm may arise. At slow heart rates, sinus beat/beats may also get aberrantly conducted producing wide QRS.

SINUS TACHYCARDIA

It is defined as sinus rhythm with a heart rate equal to or greater than 100 bpm in an adult. During sinus tachycardia, the sinus node can exhibit a discharge rate between 100-180 bpm during extreme exertion. The maximum rate achieved during strenuous physical excercise decreases with age from 200 bpm to 140 bpm, hence, upper limit is not fixed but varies. It has gradual onset and termination.

Mechanism

Accelerated phase 4 diastolic depolarisation of sinus nodal pacemaker cells is responsible for sinus tachycardia. Rate change can result if there is shift in

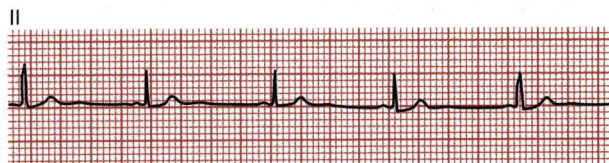

Fig. 31.4: Sinus bradycardia. The lead II shows regular normal sinus rhythm at a rate of 43/min. The QRS complexes are narrow preceded by normal P waves

Slow sinus discharge

pacemaker cells within the sinus node itself. Carotid sinus massage and Valsalva or other vagal manoeuvres gradually slow the sinus tachycardia which then accelerates to its previous level after cessation of enhanced vagal tone. More rapid sinus rates can fail to slow in response to a vagal manoeuvre.

Causes

1. Anxiety states, excessive use of tea, coffee, smoking, etc.
2. Hyperthyroidism
3. Acute pulmonary embolism.
4. Congenital heart disease
5. Drug induced (adrenaline, thyroid medications, nicotine or alcohol, atropine, caffeine, amylnitrate, nifedipine, etc)
6. Physiological in neonates and during REM sleep (heart rate varies between 100-160 bpm)

The Electrocardiogram

1. Heart rate is generally > 100 bpm. The P-P interval is constant but can vary slightly from cycle to cycle.
2. The P wave has normal configuration but can develop a large amplitude.
3. Each P wave precedes QRS complex with a stable P-R interval unless concomitant AV block ensues.
4. The R-R interval is also regular
5. The QRS complex is narrow and normal indicating normal intraventricular conduction.

SINUS NODAL RE-ENTRANT TACHYCARDIA (FIG. 31.6)

It is a supraventricular tachycardia with slower rate ranging between 80-200 bpm (average rate being 130-140 bpm) and accounts for 5-10% cases all supraventricular tachycardias. It occurs in all age groups without sex predilection. Patients with tachycardia are usually old and have a higher incidence of heart disease than patients with supraventricular tachycardia due to other mechanisms. Due to slow heart rate, many patients do not seek medical help as it does not cause serious symptoms. Sinus node re-entry may be responsible for apparent anxiety related sinus tachycardia. Drugs such as beta blockers, calcium channel blockers and digitalis may be effective in terminating and preventing recurrences of sinus node tachycardia. Surgery or radiofrequency catheter ablation to destroy all or a part of SA node is rarely needed.

Mechanisms

Electrophysiologically, sinus node behaves similar to AV node, i.e. there can be potential for dissociation of conductivity during which an impulse can be conducted through some nodal fibres but not in others, resulting in re-entry. The re-entrant circuit is located within sinus node itself or involves sinus node and the atrium.

The Electrocardiogram (Fig. 31.7)

1. Sinus rate varies between 80-200 bpm (average 130-140 bpm).
2. The P wave morphology during tachycardia is identical and similar to sinus P wave.
3. The P-R interval is related to the tachycardia rate but generally P-R interval is short and R-P interval is long.
4. AV block can occur without affecting the tachycardia. Vagal manoeuvres can slow and then abruptly terminate the tachycardia.
5. Electrophysiologically, the tachycardia can be initiated and terminated by a premature atrial and uncommonly ventricular excitation.
6. This tachycardia does not depend on the critical degree of intra-atrial or AV nodal conduction delay. This point differentiates it from AV nodal re-entrant tachycardia.

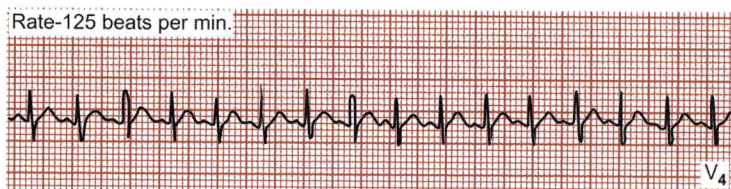

Rate-125 beats per min.

Fig. 31.5: Sinus tachycardia. The electrocardiogram (lead V_4) shows a normal regular sinus rhythm with heart rate of 125/min. The P-QRS-T complexes are normal

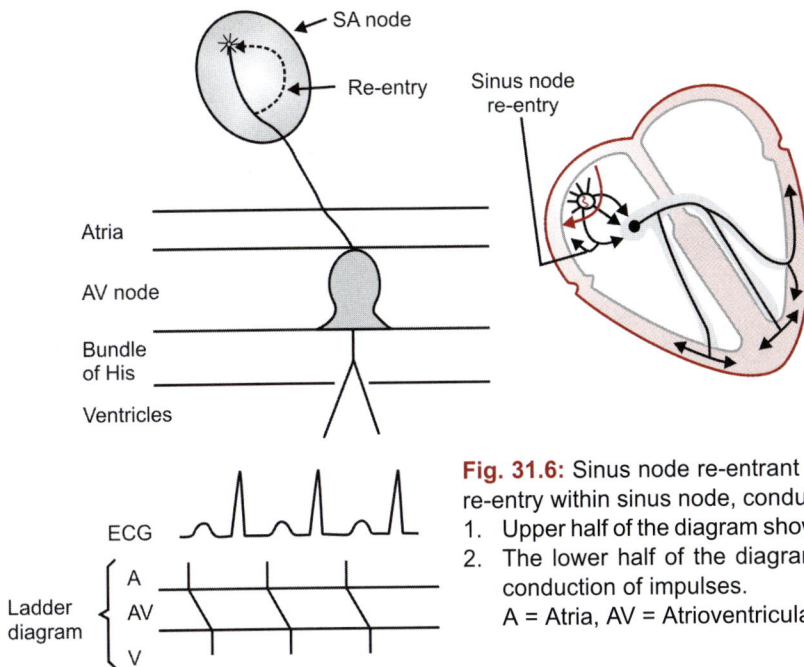

Fig. 31.6: Sinus node re-entrant tachycardia (diagram). The tachycardia is due to re-entry within sinus node, conducts normally to rest of the heart.
1. Upper half of the diagram shows a scheme of the presumed anatomical pathway
2. The lower half of the diagram shows ECG with ladder diagram showing the conduction of impulses.
A = Atria, AV = Atrioventricular node, V = Ventricle

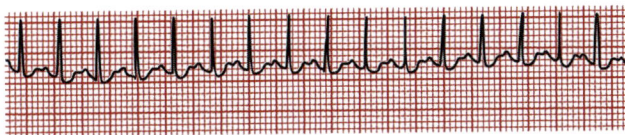

Fig. 31.7: Probable sinus node re-entrant tachycardia. The electrocardiogram (lead II), recorded from a 50 yrs female patient during acute anxiety state reveals;
   i. Regular heart rate of 125 bpm
   ii. The P wave precedes each QRS complex and occur near the descending limb of T wave. The morphology of P waves is exactly similar
   iii. The height of R wave is exactly similar. The QRS complexes are narrow
   iv. There is tachycardia induced ST depression
   v. P-R interval is 0.16 sec and R-P interval is longer

Note: It is difficult to differentiate between autonomic influenced tachycardia and re-entrant sinus tachycardia. Electrophysiological studies are needed to confirm it.

7. Prolongation of AV nodal conduction time or development of AV nodal block can occur prior to termination of the tachycardia, but does not affect the sinus node re-entry.

Suggested Reading

1. Fischer JD: Role of electrophysiological testing in the diagnosis and treatment of patients with known and suspected bradycardias and tachycardias. *Prog Cardiovasc Dis* **24**:25, 1981.
2. Narula OS: Sinus node re-entry: A mechanism for supraventricular tachycardia. *Circulation* **50**:114, 1974.
3. Naccarelli GV, Shih H, Jalal S: Sinus node re-entry and atrial tachycardias. In Zipes DP, Jalife J (Eds): *Cardiac Electrophysiology, From Cell to Bedside* (2nd ed). Philadelphia: WB Saunder Company 607, 1994.
4. Sperry RE, Ellenbogen KA, Wood MA, et al: Radio-frequency catheter ablation of sinus node re-entrant tachycardia. *PACE* **16**: 2202, 1993.
5. Zipes DP: Specific arrhythmias: Diagnosis and management. In Braunwald—Heart Disease - A Textbook of Cardiovascular Medicine (5th ed). Philadelphia: WB Saunders Company **1**: 649, 1997.

32

Abnormal Atrial Rhythm (Atrial Arrhythmias or Dysarrhythmias)

- ■ *Atrial ectopics or extrasystoles or premature beats-causes and electrocardiographic characteristics*
- ■ *Wandering atrial pacemaker rhythm - definition, causes, electrocardiographic characteristics*
- ■ *Atrial tachycardias - mechanisms and electrocardiographic characteristics of automatic, re-entrant and non-paroxysmal (digitalis induced) atrial tachycardia with block*
- ■ *Multifocal atrial tachycardia - causes and electrocardiographic characteristics along with its clinical significance*
- ■ *Atrial flutter - causes, electrocardiographic characteristics and differential diagnosis*
- ■ *Atrial fibrillation - mechanism, causes, electrocardiographic characteristics and Ashman's phenomenon*

ATRIAL ARRHYTHMIAS

ATRIAL ECTOPICS (EXTRASYSTOLES OR PREMATURE BEATS)

Definition

An atrial premature complex (APC) or a beat or an extrasystole or an ectopic is a premature discharge from an ectopic focus located somewhere in the atria outside the sinoatrial (SA) node.

Causes

1. Sometimes, a normal finding.
2. Stress, anxiety, coffee, tea and alcohol intake.
3. Heart diseases such as heart failure, myocardial ischaemia, valvular heart diseases, coronary artery disease, etc.
4. Chronic lung diseases such as COPD, cor pulmonale, etc.
5. Hyperthyroidism or thyrotoxic heart disease.
6. Systemic infections.
7. Electrolyte distubances such as hypokalaemia, hypomagnesaemia, etc.
8. Drug induced (digitalis intoxication).

The Electrocardiogram (Figs 32.1 and 32.2)

1. *Heart rate and rhythm:* Heart rate (R-R interval) is intermittently irregular. The premature beats disturb the regularity of underlying rhythm.
2. *Abnormal P (P') wave morphology:* The P wave of an atrial ectopic may be of low amplitude or pointed or notched orbiphasic or inverted due to conduction of the atrial ectopic impulse through unusual pathway. Being premature, it is recorded earlier than the next anticipated sinus P wave. The

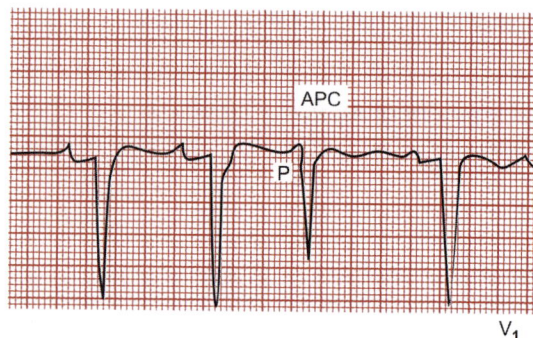

Fig. 32.1A: Atrial ectopic beat with no P-R interval. The P wave of ectopic falls on the beginning of small initial R wave and deforms it

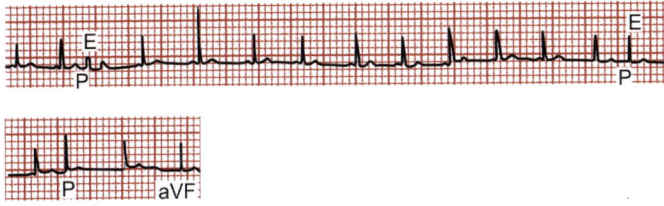

Fig. 32.1B: Multifocal atrial ectopics. The electrocardiogram (aVF) shows atrial ectopics of different origin. The first ectopic (E) has low amplitude of P wave with short P-R interval followed by narrow QRS complex indicating low atrial origin. The second atrial ectopic has merged P wave within QRS indicating atria and ventricular activation occurring simultaneously due to atrial focus being equidistant both from atria and ventricle. The third ectopic in lower strip has P wave just at onset of QRS without any P-R interval

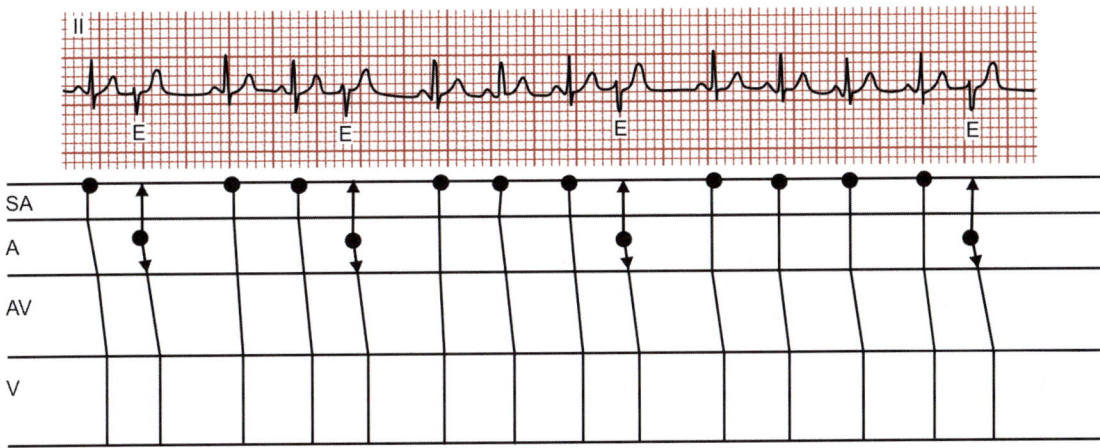

Fig. 32.1C: Atrial premature complexes (APCs). The electrocardiogram (lead II) shows rhythm intercepted irregularly by atrial premature complexes. The atrial premature complex (labelled as E) shows a small upright P wave with short P-R interval followed by a normal QRS complex indicating low or mid-atrial APC with normal intraventricular conduction. There is fixed coupling interval of 0.88 sec and there is a long compensatory pause. Below is shown a ladder diagram showing the site of origin of APC. SA—sinoatrial level, A—atrial level, AV—AV nodal level, V—ventricular level. The black dots on ladder diagram shows site of origin of impulse. The pre-ectopic and postectopic intervals are constant

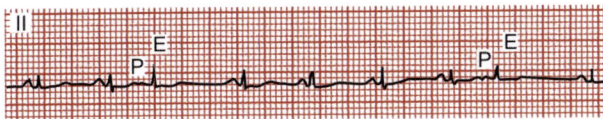

Fig. 32.1D: Atrial premature complexes with retrograde conduction. The ECG was recorded from 20 years old healthy person. The electrocardiogram shows constant R-R interval with heart rate of 60/min. This indicates vagotonic young man. Two atrial ectopics are seen. Each ectopic appears to originate either from low atrium or high AV node as there is inverted P wave with short P-R interval preceding each normal QRS. The normal QRS of ectopics indicates normal intraventricular conduction from AV node to ventricles. The pre-ectopic and post-ectopic intervals are fixed. There is a long compensatory pause

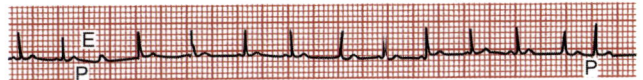

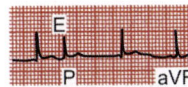

Fig. 32.1E: Atrial premature beats with normal and short P-R intervals. The leads aVF of ECG shows two types of atrial ectopics. The third beat of upper strip is an atrial premature beat with an abnormal upright P' wave with normal P-R interval and has a compensatory pause. The QRS of the ectopic is wide due to aberrant intraventricular conduction. At the end of upper strip and second beat of lower strip shows two atrial ectopics each having abnormal P' wave just preceding narrow QRS (very short P-R interval). Both are followed by a compensatory pause. The narrow QRS complex similar to sinus beat indicates its normal intraventricular conduction

morphology of P wave is similar in unifocal ectopics but varies in multifocal atrial ectopics (32.1B).

3. *Fixed coupling interval* (32.1C): The interval between an ectopic beat and the preceding sinus conducted beat is called coupling interval which is fixed for unifocal atrial ectopics. It may be variable in multifocal atrial ectopics.

SECTIONTEN

4. *A compensatory pause* (Fig. 32.1A): An atrial premature beat is followed by a long interval called *'postectopic interval' or 'compensatory pause'*. The pre-ectopic interval is shorter than postectopic interval or compensatory pause. The compensatory pause is said to be *incomplete* when the sum total of pre-ectopic and postectopic intervals is less than twice of the interval between two sinus beats and, if the compensatory pause is exactly twice of sinus cycle, then it is called complete. The mechanism of production of compensatory pause whether complete or incomplete is discussed with ventricular ectopics or VPCs (Read VPCs).

5. *Conduction*: The premature impulse (P' wave) is followed by a QRS if conducted to the ventricles (32.1D), and is not followed by QRS if it gets blocked within AV node (blocked P wave) producing a sinus pause on ECG. The atrial premature beat which gets conducted will produce an abnormal P (inverted or low upright P) wave.

6. *Shape of QRS*: The shape of QRS following an ectopic P wave depends on the mode of conduction to the ventricles;

   (a) The QRS is narrow and normal if conduction to the ventricles is undisturbed.

   (b) The QRS complex is wide and abnormal shaped if conduction through the ventricles is delayed or aberrant–called *an atrial ectopic with an aberrant intraventricular conduction*. The QRS complex, thus, produced by an atrial ectopic resembles the QRS complex of ventricular ectopic, from which, it has to be differentiated. In this type of aberration (Ashman's phenomenon), the premature impulse reaches the bundle branches when only one branch has recovered from previous excitation; while other is still refractory, hence, gets conducted through the bundle branch which has recovered resulting in a bundle branch block pattern usually a right bundle branch block pattern (rSR'). Thus, a bundle branch block pattern (rSR') of QRS following an ectopic P wave suggests an atrial ectopic with aberrant conduction rather than a ventricular ectopic.

7. *P-R interval*: It may be short, normal, prolonged or absent. The length of P-R interval depends on the ability of the AV node to conduct an atrial ectopic to ventricles:

   a) *Long P-R interval:* The long P-R interval will result when an atrial premature beat finds AV node partially refractory to conduction, hence, it has to encounter it and in the process gets delayed.

   b) *Relatively short P-R interval* (Fig. 32.1C): An atrial ectopic will have relatively short P-R interval than the normal sinus beat if ectopic focus lies near to AV node, i.e. it lies low or distally in the atria. This is due to the fact that the atrial ectopic reaches the AV node quicker than the sinus beat due to short distance.

   c) *Normal P-R interval:* The P-R interval of an ectopic and the sinus beat may be more or less equal if an ectopic focus in atria, and the SA node, are equidistant from AV node. The time taken by an ectopic to reach AV node is equal to the time taken by sinus beat (Fig. 32.1E).

   d) *No P-R interval* (Fig. 32.2): The blocked atrial premature or ectopic beat will not have any P-R interval as it is not followed by QRS. The abnormal P wave (P') may not be visible if it is

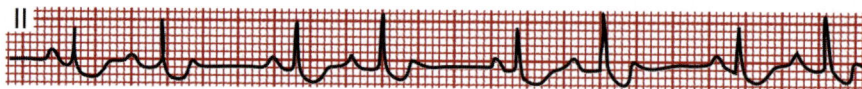

Fig. 32.2: Wenckebach's conduction with nonconducted P waves. The electrocardiogram (lead II) shows
  i. *Wenckebach's conduction:* The first P is conducted with normal P-R interval, second P has a longer P-R interval and third P is blocked; this sequence is being repeated indicating Wenckebach's type of conduction. This is not 3:2 Wenckebach's AV block because the third P is not a sinus P as it has a different shape and occurs prematurely.
  ii. *Nonconducted P' waves:* The third Ps is an abnormal P wave originating from ectopic atrial focus, being premature, gets blocked.
        This ECG highlights blocked atrial ectopics in Wenckebach's fashion.

superimposed on the preceding T wave of the sinus beat, with the result, the T wave becomes slightly deformed. If P wave is not visible at all, it will produce a pause on ECG which will resemble or look like a sinus pause of SA arrest. To differentiate between the two (pause produced by a blocked atrial ectopic and that produced by sinus arrest), the preceding T wave must be compared with other T waves for any slightest abnormality.

8. *Deformity of T wave:* The atrial ectopic beat may, sometimes, occurs so early that it distorts the T wave of previous QRS complex. An abnormal or notched T wave followed by an early QRS complex should arouse the suspicion of an atrial premature beat.

Clinical Significance

1. They must be recognised and interpreted correctly, otherwise, unnecessary confusion will prevail in the event of tachycardia resulting from them.
2. Frequent multifocal atrial ectopics (extrasystoles) predispose to atrial fibrillation.
3. Three or more consecutive atrial extrasystoles in a row constitute a paroxysmal atrial tachycardia.

ATRIAL BIGEMINY

When a normal sinus conducted beat is followed by an atrial premature beat, it is called *atrial bigeminy*. If atrial bigeminy occurs regularly and takes the form of a rhythm, it is called *atrial bigeminy* rhythm (Fig. 32.3). The most common cause of atrial bigeminy rhythm is digitalis.

ATRIAL INTERPOLATED BEAT

An atrial ectopic sandwitched between two sinus beats is called an *atrial interpolated beat*. There is no compensatory pause following an atrial interpolated beat.

ATRIAL ESCAPE BEAT

Sometimes, an atrial premature complex (APC) may penetrate the SA node and reset its timing and in the mean time, occasionally, an another atrial ectopic instead of a normal sinus beat may follow an APC called an *atrial escape beat* (Read Chapter on Escape Rhythm). The atrial escape beat is inscribed late while APC being premature occurs early—a distinguishing feature between the two. An atrial escape beat is not followed by a compensatory pause.

SECTION TEN

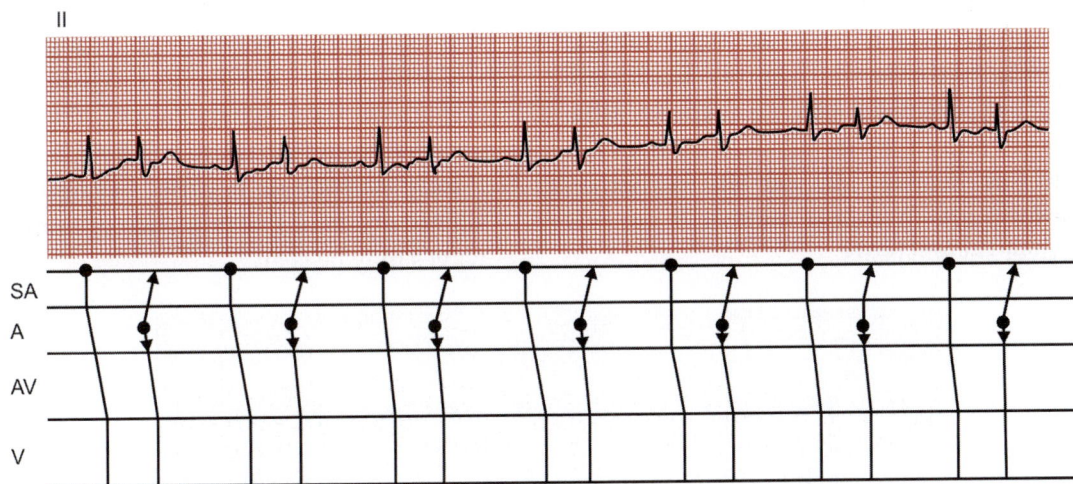

Fig. 32.3: Atrial bigeminy rhythm with aberrant conduction of atrial ectopics. The ECG (lead II) shows a normal sinus conducted beat with P-R interval of 0.16 sec followed by an atrial premature beat (abnormal P wave) with P-R interval of 0.08 sec regularly, constituting atrial begeminy rhythm. Sinus beats are followed by normal narrow QRS. The atrial ectopics are followed by slightly wider QRS with slurred S waves indicating aberrant intraventricular conduction.

The ladder diagram shown below depicts the site of origin of impulses. SA—sinoatrial level, A—atrial level, AV—AV nodal level, V—ventricular level. The black dots on ladder diagram show the origin of beats

Summary of Atrial Premature Beats

1. Timing
2. Conduction
   - Atrial conduction
   - AV conduction

   - Premature with a compensatory pause.

   - Abnormal —bizarre P; if retrograde then an inverted P (P') wave
   - Blocked (no P-R interval) or conducted antegradely

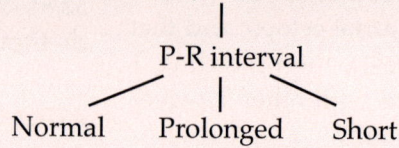

   P-R interval

   Normal   Prolonged   Short

   - Intraventricular conduction
   - Normal or aberrant (wide QRS)

ATRIAL PARASYSTOLE

Read the chapter on Parasystole.

Summary: The events associated with atrial premature beats are summarised in the box.

WANDERING ATRIAL PACEMAKER RHYTHM

This variant of sinus arrhythmia involves temporarily transfer of the dominant pacemaker (SA node) site to latent pacemaker site having the next highest degree of automaticity (atria or AV node). In this arrhythmia, only one pacemaker at a time controls the rhythm in sharp contrast to AV dissociation.

Wandering pacemaker in the atria produces a supraventricular rhythm in which impulses originate from two or more pacemaker sites, i.e. SA node, atria, AV node. The heart rate varies between 60-100 bpm due to shift of pacemaker from one site to another. The change from one rhythm to another is gradual and occurs over several beats.

Causes

1. Sick sinus syndrome
2. Chronic obstructive pulmonary disease
3. Valvular heart disease
4. Normal phenomenon that occurs in very young and particularly athletes (increased vagal tone).

The Electrocardiogram (Figs 32.4 and 32.5)

As pacemaker activity wanders between different sites of origin within atria, therefore, ECG characteristics include;

1. There is a cyclic increase in R-R and P-R intervals, that occurs gradually due to shift of pacemaker site and there is change in P wave morphology. Generally, these changes get reversed when pacemaker shifts back to sinus node.
2. *P wave morphology*: It varies because of different sites of origin of P waves. Two or more types of P waves may be seen.

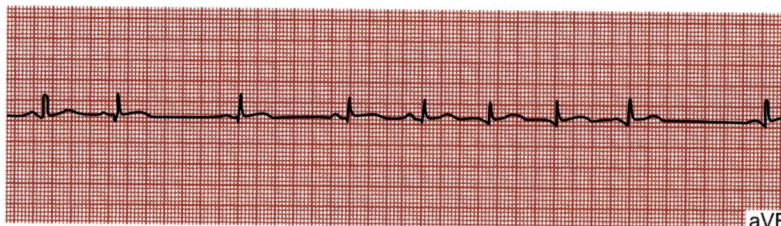

Fig. 32.4: Wandering atrial pacemaker. The electrocardiogram (lead aVF rhythm strip) shows a rapid heart rate with variable shapes of P waves, variable P-R and R-R intervals. The shape of QRS is normal indicating normal intraventricular conduction
Note: The P wave changes its shape as pacemaker wanders from one site to another between SA node and AV junction

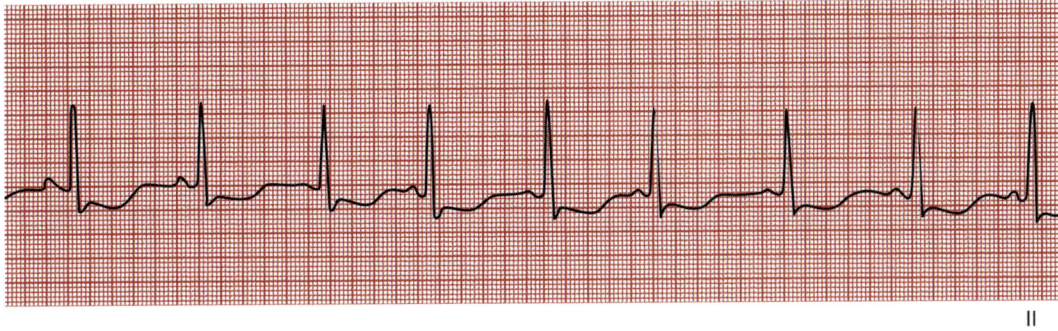

Fig. 32.5: Wandering atrial pacemaker with primary myocardial disease. The lead II shows ventricular rate of 90/min. There is variation in shapes of P waves (first three P have variable shapes indicating three different origin), P-R intervals and R-R intervals. The ST segment depression indicates the basic myocardial disease

3. P-P and R-R intervals also vary cyclically because each impulse travels through the atria via a different pathway.
4. Each P wave is followed by QRS complex, hence, there is one P wave for each QRS complex.
5. The relation of P wave with QRS varies, i.e. it may precede, follow or get superimposed on QRS.
6. The overall atrial and ventricular rates remain between 60-100 bpm. If heart rate is more than 100 bpm, then it automatically becomes a multifocal (chaotic) atrial tachycardia rather than wandering pacemaker.
7. The QRS complexes are narrow as ventricular depolarisation is usually undisturbed.

The wandering atrial pacemaker means the shift of pacemaker activity temporarily from SA node to other sites (atria or AV node) and then back to SA node, hence, there is a cyclic change of P wave morphology, P-R and R-R intervals over few beats followed by sinus beats, therefore, heart rate does not increase beyond 100 bpm.

ATRIAL TACHYCARDIAS

It is a supraventricular arrhythmia arising from the atria outside the SA node, discharges at a rate of 120-250 bpm and the P wave configuration is different from that of sinus P wave. The P waves are usually in the second half of tachycardia cycle (long R-P/short P-R tachycardia). Atrial tachycardia (nonparoxysmal) is mostly due to digitalis.

There are three underlying mechanisms reponsible for atrial tachycardia, i.e. automatic, triggered and re-entry (Fig. 32.6.). Entrainment, resetting curve pattern in response to overdrive pacing, recording monophasic action potential and response to adenosine may be useful to distinguish one from the other. However, there are no clearcut distinctions between atrial tachycardias due to different mechanisms.

Analysis of P wave configuration during tachycardia indicates that a positive or biphasic P wave in aVL predicts right atrial focus while a positive P wave in V_1 predicts left atrial focus.

Causes

They are given in the box.

Causes of Atrial Tachycardias

- Digitalis induced
- Coronary artery disease including myocardial infarction
- Cor pulmonale
- Acute metabolic disturbances
- Rheumatic heart disease
- Electrolyte imbalance
- Acute alcohol intoxication
- Idiopathic

1. Digitalis Induced Nonparoxysmal Atrial Tachycardia (Fig. 32.7)

It is an automatic atrial tachycardia. When tachycardia is due to digitalis toxicity, the atrial rate can increase gradually as the digitalis is continued; this increase may be associated with gradual prolongation of P-R interval. If atrial rate is not high and AV conduction

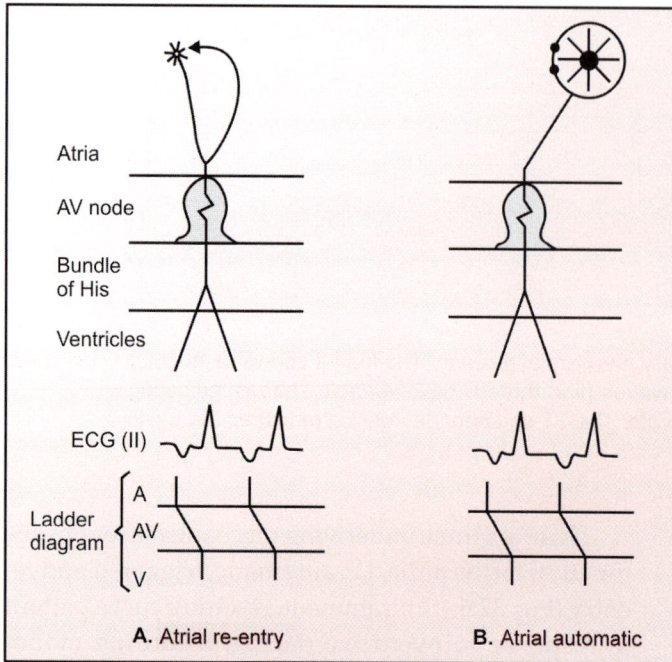

Fig. 32.6: Diagrammatic illustration of mechanisms of various atrial tachycardia.
A. Re-entry
B. Enhanced automaticity. At the top of each example, a schematic representation of anatomical pathway is drawn. In the lower half, ECG and explanatory ladder diagram are depicted

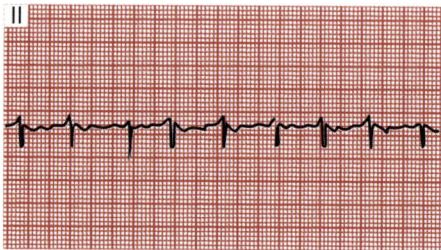

Fig. 32.7: Nonproxysmal atrial tachycardia with second degree AV block

Characteristic isoelectric intervals between P waves are usually present in all the leads in this arrhythmia which are not seen in atrial flutter - forms an important distinguishing feature. All these electrocardiographic features disappear after stopping digitalis and diuretics; with substitution of potassium, in case, hypokalaemia is present.

2. Automatic Ectopic Atrial Tachycardia (Paroxysmal Atrial Tachycardia)

It is characterised by a supraventricular tachycardia due to rapid discharge of an ectopic atrial focus, that accelerates its rate after initiation. Heart rate is less than 200 bpm. The P wave configuration is abnormal. The P-R interval is influenced by tachycardia rate. AV block can exist without affecting the tachycardia which continues uninterrupted. Vagal maneuvers generally do not terminate the tachycardia even though they can produce AV block. Initiation of tachycardia with premature atrial complex is not possible; but is independent of intra-atrial and intranodal conduction delay when it occurs. The first P wave of the tachycardia is same as subsequent P waves of tachycardia due to same focus of origin–in contrast to most forms of re-entrant supraventricular

is not suppressed by digitalis, then conduction ratio may be 1:1 (each P wave is conducted to the ventricles), hence, both atrial and ventricular rates are high.

If the atrial rate increases further and AV conduction gets suppressed by digitalis, the Wenckebach's (Mobitz type 1) second degree AV block can occur. This is commonly called *'atrial tachycardia with block'*– a characteristic feature of digitalis toxicity. In nearly half of cases of atrial tacycardia with block, atrial rate is irregular.

Frequently, other manifestations of digitalis toxicity such as ventricular premature complexes (VPCs) in isolation, or in bigeminy pattern may also be present. This tachycardia with block may resemble atrial flutter from which it has to be differentiated.

tachycardia in which initial and susequent P waves differ. The pacing does not terminate tachycardia. It is difficult to differentiate it from atrial re-entrant tachycardia (a rare form of tachycardia).

The Electrocardiogram (Fig. 32.8)

1. *Atrial rate*: It varies between 120-250 bpm.
2. *Heart rhythm*: It is regular, i.e. P-P and R-R intervals are constant and regular.
3. *AV conduction*: On reaching the AV node, the atrial impulse may be conducted as follows:

(i) *With normal P-R interval:* It indicates normal AV conduction.

(ii) *With short P-R interval:* The P-R interval may be short if conduction ratio is 1:1. The speed of conduction through AV node increases as the atrial rate increases, thereby, shortens P-R interval.

(iii) *With prolonged P-R interval (first degree AV block):* Because of rapid ectopic discharge and conduction ratio being 1:1, there may be insufficient time for the AV node to recover completely. The atrial impulse, is thus, conducted with prolonged P-R

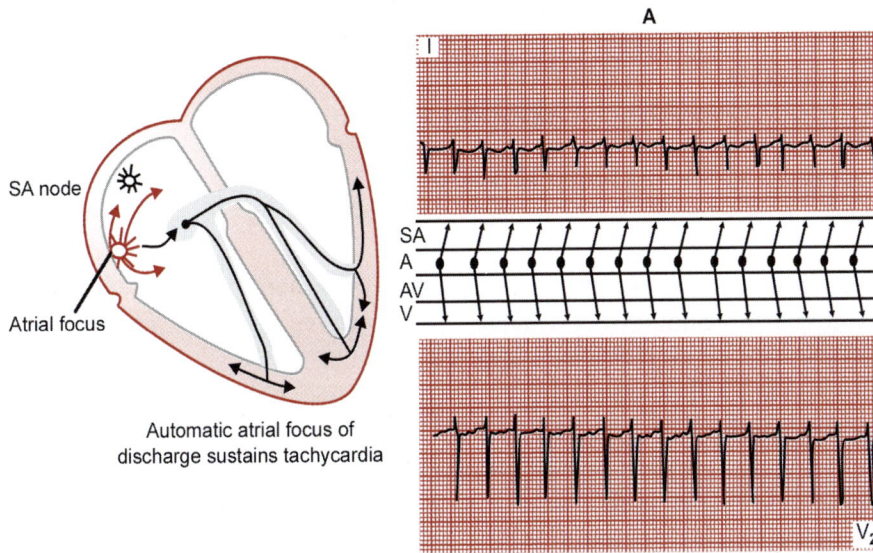

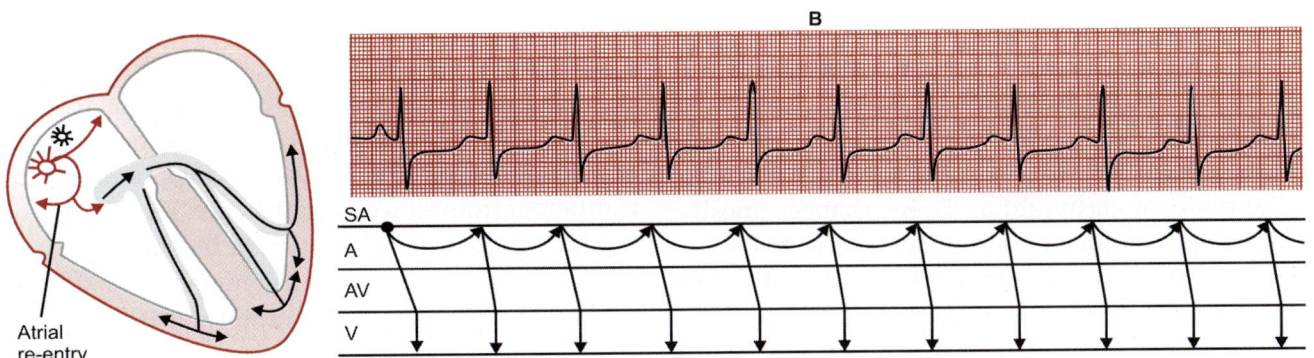

Figs 32.8A and B: A: Automatic proxysmal atrial tachycardia. The electrocardiogram (rhythm strip leads I and V₂) shows regular heart rate of 185/min approx. The R-R interval is regular. As rate is very fast, P waves are not clearly seen and distort the T wave of preceding beat. There is 1:1 conduction (one P wave is followed by a QRS complex). QRS is normal indicating normal intraventricular conduction. Due to fast rate, the origin of P wave and their conduction cannot be identified. The identical morphology of narrow regular QRS complexes indicate it to be automatic or ectopic atrial tachycardia. **B:** Atrial re-entrant tachycardia. First beat is preceded by P wave which is different from P' waves of tachycardia sequence

interval (first degree AV block) due to conduction delay in AV node.

(iv) *With second degree AV block.* If the ectopic tachycardia is too rapid to produce its cycle length shorter than the refractory period, then every second atrial impulse falls within the refractory period of AV node, hence, gets blocked resulting in 2:1 AV block. The tachycardia may be associated with various types of second degree AV block such as 3:2 Wenckebach's conduction or fluctuating ratio of conduction within second degree AV block (e.g. 3:2 and 2:1, 2:1 and 3:2, etc). The presence of second degree AV block in this tachycardia is conventionally called *paroxysmal arial tachycardia (PAT) with block.*

4. *Morphology of P waves:* The ectopic P wave (P' wave) morphology is quite different than the P wave of sinus beat due to different origin of P' wave (atrial origin). At faster rates P' waves (ectopic P' waves) may be difficult to see and may distort the preceding T wave. Leads II, III and aVF are best leads to study the morphology of P waves.

5. *Morphology of QRS:* The QRS complexes are supraventricular in nature, i.e. they are narrow because the conduction through the ventricles is undisturbed. Therefore, this tachycardia is *narrow QRS complex tachycardia.* The QRS complex becomes wider if conduction is aberrant through ventricles via one bundle branch only, resulting in a bundle branch block pattern (RBBB pattern more common than LBBB pattern).

6. *ST-T changes:* The ST segment depression and T wave inversion may appear in those leads where the QRS complexes are dominantly upright, indicate relative myocardial ischaema during the episode of tachycardia. These changes mostly disappear following termination of tachycardia, sometimes, may persist for hours or days after tachycardia has subsided—called post-tachycardia syndrome. These changes may occur in any type of tachycardia irrespective of its cause, hence, called—tachycardia induced ST-T changes.

7. *Carotid sinus massage* slows the atrial rate in automatic atrial tachycardia, by producing AV block but does not terminate it completely. In contrast to this, AV nodal tachycardia may be completely abolished by this maneuver, i.e. a point that differentiates between the two.

8. *Atrial tachycardia may occur in paroxysms (bursts);* when it terminates, there may be a long pause before normal sinus rhythm is restored.

REVIEW AT GLANCE

Paroxysmal Atrial Tachycardia

• Atrial conduction	Abnormal P' waves precede the QRS complexes.
• AV conduction	First degree or second degree AV block. Normal 1:1 conduction can occur but uncommon.
• Intraventricular	Normal (narrow QRS complex) or aberrant (wide QRS complex) conduction tachycardia.
• ST segment	Frequently depressed.
• T wave	Frequently inverted.

ATRIAL RE-ENTRANT TACHYCARDIA (FIG. 32.8B)

It is characterised by abnormal P (P') wave contour that is different from sinus P wave. The P-R interval depends on the tachycardia rate. AV block can develop without interrupting the tachycardia. Re-entry can exist in atria around surgical scar or atriotomy incision or through an anatomical defect.

Electrophysiologically, initiation of tachycardia occurs with a premature beat during the atrial relative refractory period resulting a critical degree of intra-atrial conduction delay. The atrial activation sequence is different from sinus rhythm, hence, first P wave of the tachycardia is different from the subsequent P waves of tachycardia. Vagal maneuvers do not terminate it. Electrocardiographically it resembles atrial automatic tachycardia except first P wave in tachycardia sequence is different from subsequent P' waves.

It is not a well recognised cause of atrial tachycardia because of infrequent occurrence (5-10%). The tachycardia can be initiated and stopped by an atrial extrasystole or extra-stimulus. Spontaneous stimulation can be sudden either with progressive slowing or with alternate long-short cycle lengths.

Electrocardiographically, it is difficult to differentiate atrial re-entrant tachycardia from atrioventricular nodal re-entrant tachycardia (AVNRT). Detailed electrophysiological studies are needed to localise the site of re-entry.

MULTIFOCAL ATRIAL TACHYCARDIA (MAT)

Multifocal atrial tachycardia (MAT), as the name suggests, is an ectopic supraventricular tachycardia that originates from three or more atrial foci. It has a rate of 100-150 bpm. Multifocal atrial ectopics can also occur without inducing tachycardia.

Causes

It most commonly occurs due to hypoxaemia irrespective of its cause or may be due to drugs.
1. Pulmonary diseases producing hypoxaemia;
    i) Chronic obsructive pulmonary disease and cor pulmonale
    ii) Acute respiratory distress or failure
    iii) Acute interstitial lung disease
    iv) Pulmonary embolism
    v) Pneumonias.

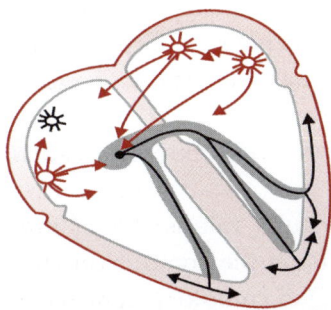

2. Congestive heart failure
3. Drugs. Theophylline is a common cause; but digitalis is an uncommon cause.

The Electrocardiogram (Fig. 32.9)

1. *Varying P wave contours*: There may be at least three or more P wave configurations due to three or more foci of origin.
2. *Intraventricular conduction*: There is always 1:1 conduction (one P wave is followed by an QRS complex).
3. *Irregular rhythm*: Heart rate is irregular. This arrhythmia is characterised by varying P-P and R-R intervals.
4. *Variable P-R interval*: There may be slight change in P-R interval from beat to beat.
5. *Heart rate* : It is more than 100 bpm. This arrhythmia is just like wandering atrial pacemaker but heart rate of more than 100 bpm differentiates it from wandering atrial pacemaker.
6. *The morphology of QRS*: The morphology of QRS complex is supraventricular (narrow QRS) due to normal pathway of intraventricular conduction. The QRS may become wide if there is an aberrant intraventricular conduction.

Multiple atrial foci of excitation sustain tachycardia

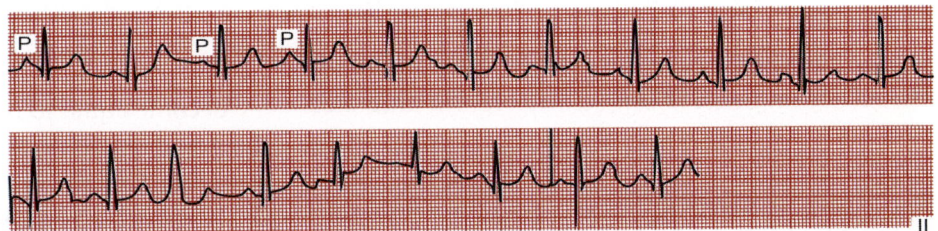

Fig. 32.9: Multifocal atrial tachycardia (MAT). The electrocardiogram (lead II) recorded from a patient with COPD and cor pulmonale shows:
   i. Variable morphology of P waves indicating their different foci of their origin
   ii. P-R interval is slightly variable from beat to beat
   iii. Irregular rhythm—There are varying P-P and R-R intervals but there is 1:1 conduction (one P wave for each QRS)
   iv. Rate is greater than 100/min, hence, it is multifocal atrial tachycardia rather than wandering atrial pacemaker where heart rate usually does not exceed 100/min
   v. QRS complexes are narrow and identical indicating normal intraventricular conduction
   vi. There is one ventricular ectopic (E) in the bottom strip
   vii. Lower voltage of QRS complexes is due to COPD.

In MAT, there should be at least three different configurations of P waves and atrial rate must be more than 100 bpm.

Clinical Significance

1. It is pertinent to recognise this arrhythmia as it is easily confused with atrial fibrillation due to variable morphologies of the P waves which may be confused with fibrillatory (f) waves. Atrial fibrillation needs digitalis to slow the ventricular rate, hence, if not differentiated from MAT, then unnecessary high doses of digitalis may be given, to which MAT does not respond and results in digitalis toxicity.
2. It may eventually develop into atrial fibrillation.

ATRIAL FLUTTER

Definition: It is an electrocardiographic expression of rapid and regular atrial excitation either due to intra-atrial re-entry (circus movement) of impulses or due to rapid discharge of an atrial focus (focal automatic discharge). *'Circus movement'* is the most common underlying mechanism of atrial flutter or fibrillation. It is defined as a supraventricular arrhythmia characterised by the appearance of 'saw-toothed shaped' regular flutter (F) waves at a rate of 250-350 bpm. Slow flutter rates can occur in patients with large or hypertrophied atria, and also in those receiving antiarrhythmic therapy (quinidine or procainamide). The most commonly observed atrial rate in untreated patients is 300 bpm and ventricular rate is half of the atrial rate, i.e. 150 bpm. A significantly slower rate in the absence of drugs indicates abnormal AV conduction. In children, in patients with pre-excitation syndrome and, occasionally in patients with hyperthyroidism, atrial flutter can conduct to the ventricles in a 1:1 fashion producing a rapid ventricular rate equal to atrial rate i.e. 300 bpm. The rate in atypical atrial flutter, also called flutter fibrillation (type II), is still higher, i.e. 350-450 bpm than type I (typical flutter).

Mechanism

Re-entry is probably the underlying mechanism for most atrial flutter.

Causes

1. Thyrotoxic heart disease
2. Valvular heart disease
3. Ischaemic heart disease
4. Pericardial disease
5. Acute pulmonary thromboembolism
6. Severe pulmonary disease
7. Congenital heart disease
8. Sick sinus syndrome
9. Pre-excitation syndrome
10. Idiopathic

The Electrocardiogram (Figs 32.10 to 32.13)

1. *Flutter waves*: Instead of P waves, identically re-curring regular flutter (F) waves representing abnormal atrial depolarisation and repolarisation are seen. These waves assume a 'saw toothed' or 'picket fence' appearance, are most easily seen and appreciated in inferior leads (II, III, aVF) and V_1. The 'F' waves are contiguous due to continued atrial activity and there is no visible isoelectric baseline between them. Some of the flutter waves are obscured by QRS complexes. Sometimes, flutter waves may be coarse and look like actual P waves (Fig. 32.11). The flutter waves may deform the ST segment in such a way that it may look like an elevated or depressed ST segment or may deform the R wave producing rSr' or rR' pattern, and sometimes, they may become so large to become equal to R(r) wave (Fig. 32.12).
2. *Atrial rate*: It varies between 250-350 bpm (average being 300 bpm).
3. *Ventricular rate*: Ventricular rate is slower than atrial rate and depends on the conduction ratio (ratio of 'F' waves to QRS complex). Ventricular rate is regular due to fixed conduction ratio; however, becomes irregular, in situations, where either the conduction ratio fluctuates or there is an associated atrial fibrillation (flutter fibrillation).
4. *Second degree AV block*: As already discussed, heart rate depends on the efficacy of AV conduction. The 1:1 conduction leads to very high ventricular rate, therefore, to reduce the ventricular rate, there is always a second degree AV block in ratio of 2:1, 4:1,

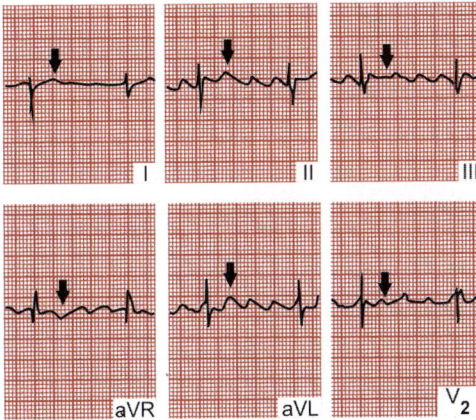

Fig. 32.10: Atrial flutter with 4:1 AV conduction. The electrocardiogram shows:
  i. Atrial rate is regular at 250/min
  ii. There is saw-tooth appearance of flutter waves (F waves) in leads II, III and aVF. Some of 'F' waves are indicated by arrows.
  iii. There is 4:1 conduction (one out of 4 consecutive flutter waves evokes a ventricular response)

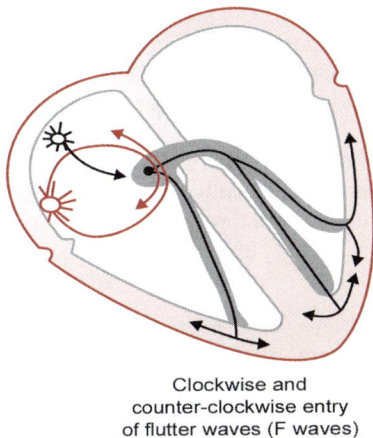

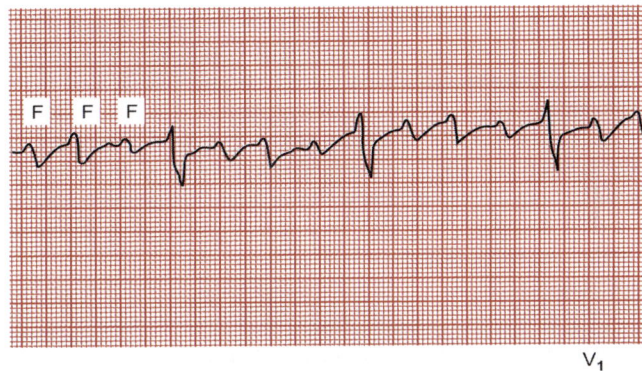

Clockwise and
counter-clockwise entry
of flutter waves (F waves)

Fig. 32.11: Atrial flutter. The flutter waves resemble or look like normal P waves. The atrial rate is 300/bpm. The ventricular rate is 75 bpm. The flutter waves labelled as 'F' are seen preceding each QRS complexes. These flutter (F) waves resemble normal to biphasic P waves seen in lead V₁. The 4th flutter wave is superimposed on QRS and distorts it. This is not 4:1 second degree AV block because atrial rate is high, atrial waves are dissimilar and every fourth presumed P is superimposed on QRS without any P-R interval. Hence, it is flutter with 4:1 conduction

6:1, 8:1 (even ratios). Usually ventricular rate is half of the atrial rate due to common 2:1 conduction. Even ratios are commoner than odd ratios (3:1, 5:1, etc.) Atrial flutter can be complicated by complete heart block.

Note: Ventricular rate is regular when conduction ratio is fixed. Sometimes, it is completely irregular due to fluctuation of conduction ratio from 4:1 to 6:1 or to 2:1 (Fig. 32.13). Regular 3:2 ratio will result in ventricular bigeminy rhythm. Similarly alternating 4:1 and 2:1 conduction will also result in bigeminy rhythm. Read chapter 39.

5. *Morphology of QRS complexes:* The QRS complexes are usually narrow as long as conduction to the ventricles is normal. Intraventricular conduction of flutter waves, at times, may be associated with aberrant ventricular conduction producing wide QRS complexes.

Types

The atrial flutter is divided into two types depending on the heart rate and electrocardiographic appearance.
1. *Type I* (pure atrial flutter). It is a classically described atrial flutter with a rate varying from 250-350 bpm (average 300 bpm). This produces a 'saw-toothed appearance' of the baseline on ECG.

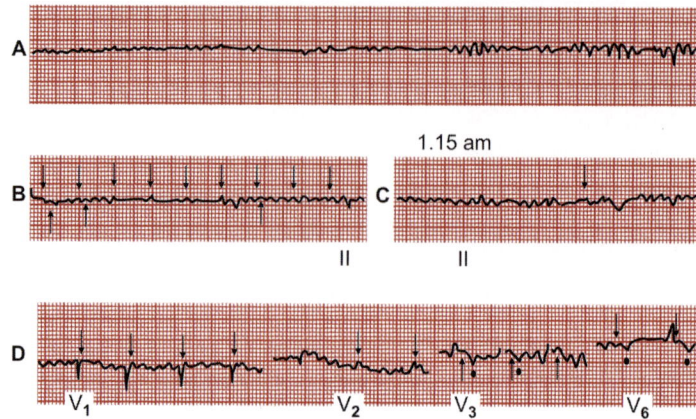

Fig. 32.12: The varied electrocardiographic pattern produced by atrial flutter;
A. Atrial flutter (lead II). There is typical saw-toothed pattern in the beginning of the strip. The atrial rate is about 300/min. The QRS complexes are so small that they resemble P wave or flutter waves but are so regular (see the scale above) that there is no confusion about their identity. This can be confused with an artifact which cannot be so regular.
B. The atrial flutter (F) waves deforming the ST segment (indicated by arrows below). The upper arrows show regular small QRS complexes.
C. The flutter waves are equal to QRS complexes, but careful inspection shows few clear small QRS complexes having same morphology as seen in A and B strips (one is indicated by an arrow). It can be confused with cardiac asystole.
D. Precordial leads from the same patient shows flutter waves producing rSr' pattern where r' wave is due to flutter wave. In V_3, it deforms the ST segment (indicated by arrows ↑) simulating ST elevation. In leads V_3 and V_6 flutter wave simulate T wave inversion (indicated by black dots below).

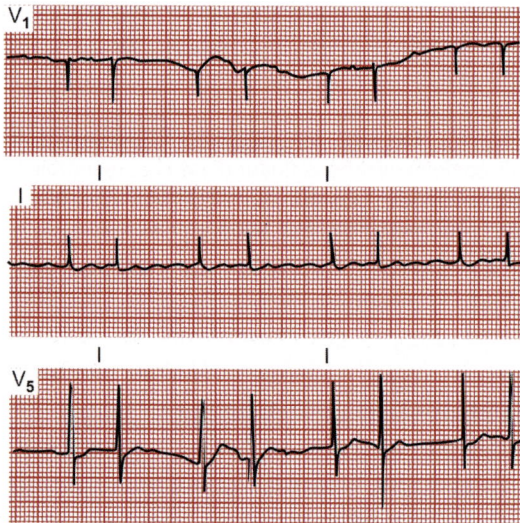

Fig. 32.13: Atrial flutter with alternating 4:1 and 2:1 conduction. The basic rhythm is atrial flutter. Note the regular irregularity of ventricular cycles—short and long R-R cycles. The long R-R cycle is < 2 × short R-R cycle. The short R-R cycle is longer than 2 flutter cycles. This ECG finding is suggestive of Wenckebach's AV conduction. There is slow atrial flutter cycle due to quinidine effect

2. *Type II* (impure flutter or flutter fibrillation). It occurs at a faster rate (350-400 bpm) which is more than pure atrial flutter but less than pure atrial fibrillation. The classic saw-toothed appearance is not seen. The flutter waves appear as upright deflections in leads II, III, aVF and V_1. Ventricular rate is irregular, but there is no undulation of baseline as seen in atrial fibrillation, hence, called as flutter-fibrillation (Fig. 32.14). This behaves as atrial fibrillation rather than atrial flutter in its response to treatment.

Differential Diagnosis

1. *Atrial tachycardia:* In this arrhythmia, the ectopic P waves simulating 'F' waves are separated by an isoelectric baseline, while no such baseline is visible in atrial flutter.

2. *Second degree AV block with variable conduction ratio (Mobitz type II):* Second degree AV block with variable conduction ratio (3:1, 4:1 or 5:1) will produce irregular heart rate (variable R-R intervals) but regular heart rate occurs if conduction ratio is fixed. The P waves may be confused with 'F' wave in second degree AV block in the absence of undulation of baseline. In such a situation, peaked tip of the P waves and normal baseline

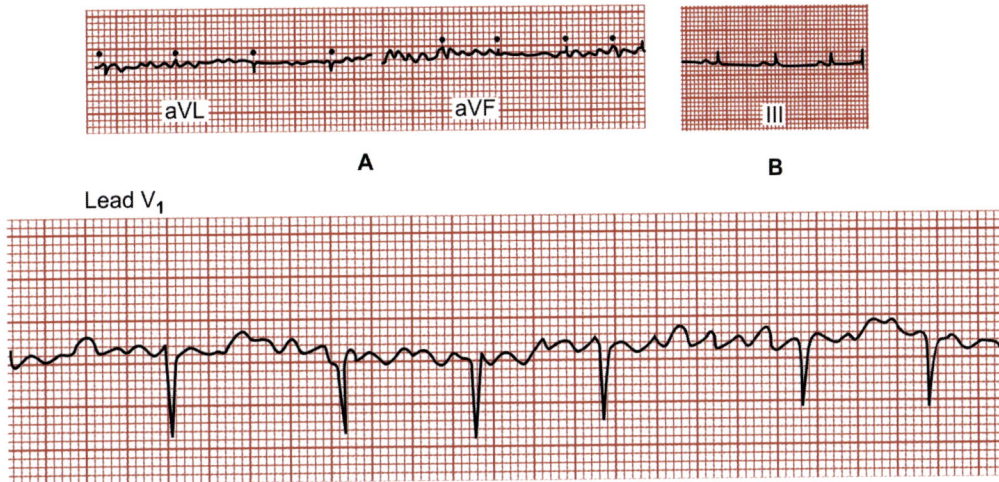

Fig. 32.14: Impure flutter or flutter fibrillation.
A. The electrocardiographic leads (aVL, aVF, V_1) show the following characteristics;
   i. Atrial rate is fast 375 bpm, i.e. faster than pure atrial flutter best seen in V_1
   ii. The flutter (f) waves are seen as upright irregularly placed waves having no fixed pattern or shape or conduction. There is slight undulation of baseline between ventricular complexes
   iii. R-R interval is variable indicating irregular ventricular response
B. The lead III is depicted after disappearance of atrial flutter. Note the normal P wave precedes a small qrs which confirms that small complexes (denoted by dots above) are actual qrs complexes and not an artifact

between P waves and fixed P-P intervals suggest AV block rather than atrial flutter.

Clinical Significance

1. Digitalis often converts atrial flutter to atrial fibrillation by shortening the atrial refractory period. This may be followed by conversion to normal sinus rhythm when the digitalis is stopped.
2. Succeeding attacks of atrial flutter tend to last longer and frequently lead to development of atrial fibrillation.
3. Atrial flutter responds rapidly and completely to electrical cardioversion.

REVIEW AT A GLANCE

Diagnostic Clues to Atrial Flutter on ECG

- Saw-toothed regular, identically recurring flutter waves-called 'F' waves at a rate of about 300/min.
- Regular rapid ventricular rate in pure atrial flutter (type 1) and irregular in flutter fibrillation

(type II). There is always a second degree AV block to reduce ventricular rate.
- F waves are contiguous with no isoelectric baseline visible between them.
- Carotid massage makes the flutters waves visible clearly by slowing the heart rate by increasing AV block.

ATRIAL FIBRILLATION (AF)

Definition: Atrial fibrillation is a supraventricular arrhythmia characterised by replacement of P waves by fibrillatory (f) waves, uncoordinated atrial contractions and a classically irregularly irregular ventricular rate. It can be intermittent or may become a chronic persistent condition. It is always organic in origin except lone (idiopathic) atrial fibrillation. The lone atrial fibrillation occurs in young individuals without an evidence of a heart disease. A familial preponderance has also been reported.

Mechanisms

Numerous excitatory impulses from multiple ectopic atrial foci or by atrial re-entry course irregularly through the atria and bombard the AV node at frequent and irregular intervals; the rate of such impulses reaching the AV node varies between 400-600 bpm. The AV node can only conduct some of them because following conduction of one impulse, it becomes refractory for a short period and blocks the impulses reaching to it during this period. As refractory period of AV node varies with factors such as vagal stimulation, respiration, emotion, excercise, partial penetration of impulses into AV node, etc. the conduction of atrial impulses to the ventricles is irregular, hence, there is usually an irregularly irregular ventricular rate—a hallmark of this condition. All cases of atrial fibrillation are thus accompanied by some form of AV block. Intra-ventricular conduction also sometimes becomes aberrant due to irregular conduction of these impulses–called *'Ashman's phenomenon'* leading to wide QRS complexes that can easily be mistaken for ventricular premature complexes (VPCs).

The phenomenon of lone atrial fibrillation is reported to be due to presence of a congenital quiescent anomalous or additional AV nodal bypass tract, that permits rapid reciprocal return of sinus impulses to the atria—a mechanism similar to WPW syndrome. The rapid return of impulses to atria produce premature atrial excitation and may precipitate AF.

Causes

1. Heart failure
2. Ischaemic heart disease
3. Thyrotoxic heart disease
4. Valvular heart disease especially mitral valve disease, e.g. mitral stenosis and mitral regurgitation
5. Congenital heart disease (atrial septal defect, WPW syndrome, Ebstein's anomaly)
6. Sick sinus syndrome—a structural nodal disease.
7. Acute and chronic cor pulmonale
8. Chronic constrictive pericarditis
9. Left atrial myxoma
10. Hypertensive heart disease
11. Heart surgery
12. Cardiomyopathies, alcohol induced ('Holiday heart syndrome')
13. Idiopathic (lone)

The Electrocardiogram (Figs 32.15 and 32.17)

1. *Fibrillatory (f) waves replace the normal P waves:* Instead of P waves, fibrillatory (f) waves are present. The 'f' waves are small, poorly defined and distort the baseline (undulations of baseline). Sometimes, they may be of low amplitude and the baseline may appear almost straight, or at times, they may be coarse like flutter waves (coarse atrial fibrillation or flutter fibrillation).

2. *Varying R-R interval:* Heart rate is irregularly irregular and R-R interval is variable from beat to beat. The rate of the heart may be fast or slow depending on conduction through AV node. Slowing of heart rate is a usual response after digitalis therapy. Digitalis slows the heart rate by increasing the refractory period of AV node (Fig. 32.16).

3. *Morphology of QRS:* The QRS complexes are narrow due to normal intraventricular conduction of the fibrillatory impulses. The QRS complexes may become wide and bizarre looking like ventricular ectopics due to aberrant conduction called Ashman's phenomenon (long and short cycle lengths). This is discussed in detail below.

4. *Atrial rate:* It is very high varying between 400-600 bpm and ventricular rate is usually one fourth of it, i.e. 100-160 bpm. In patients of WPW syndrome or thyrotoxic crisis with atrial fibrillation, the ventricular rate is high and, at times, can exceed 300 bpm. This is due to nonexistence of physiological AV block in these conditions. The physiological AV block is usual and must in AF to slow the ventricular rate.

The undulations of the baseline due to fibrillatory waves and beat to beat change in R-R interval with rapid ventricular rate are hallmarks of atrial fibrillation on ECG in untreated patients.

Slow Atrial Fibrillation (Fig. 32.17)

Slow atrial fibrillation means slow ventricular response, which in untreated patients, indicates either a high vagal tone (hypervagotonaemia) or an underlying conduction disturbance in the AV node or bundle of His.

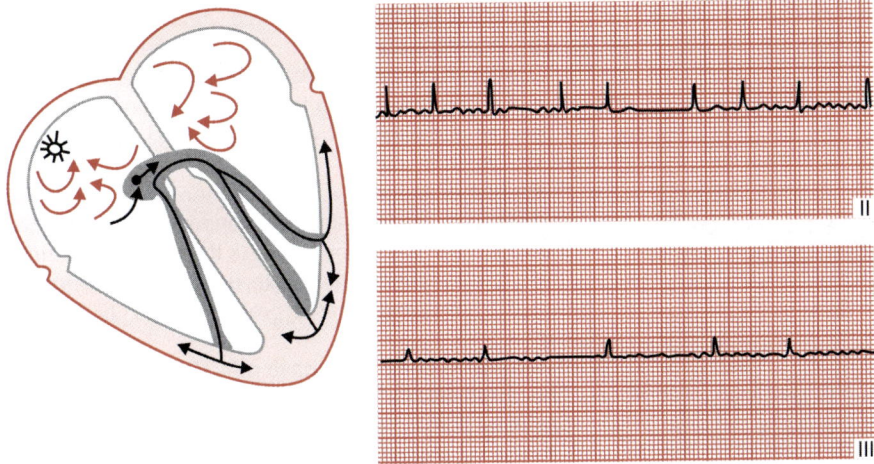

Fig. 32.15: Atrial fibrillation(AF). The electrocardiogram (leads II and III) shows;
  i. Instead of regular P waves, there are small fine, rapid, irregular fibrillatory (f) waves between R-R waves
  ii. Atrial rate is > 400 bpm
  iii. Ventricular rate is fast 108/min
  iv. R-R interval is irregular due to varied ventricular response

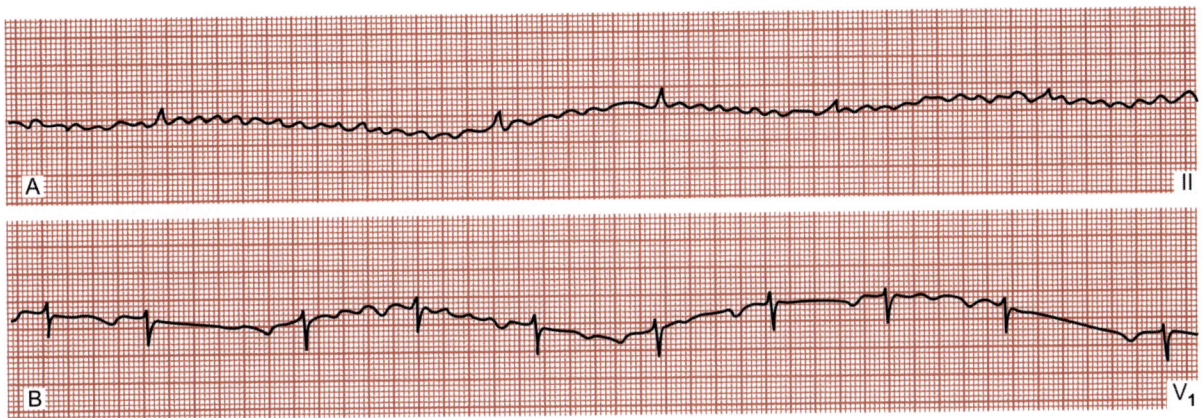

Fig. 32.16: Atrial fibrillation with slow ventricular response induced by digitalis. The electrocardiogram recorded before (A) and after digitalis (B) reveals;
A. Lead II rhythm strip shows atrial fibrillation (f waves are clearly seen with irregular R-R intervals) with heart rate (80/min)
B. Lead V$_1$ shows irregularly irregular heart rate of 62/min (digitalis effect). The digitalis increases the block to fibrillatory waves at AV node but does not revert it. Therefore, the slower ventricular response in atrial fibrillation could be due to digitalis or high vagal tone (slow atrial fibrillation). At slow ventricular rate, the fibrillatory waves are nicely seen

Fig. 32.17: Slow atrial fibrillation. The electrocardiogram (leads I, II) was recorded from a 40 yr male who did not receive any medication and did not have any cause to explain atrial fibrillation. *Note the following characteristics*
  (i) Lead II. The P waves are not visible. There are fibrillatory (f) waves seen between irregular R-R intervals. The QRS complex is narrow. The heart rate is slow.
  (ii) The lower strip (lead I) from same patient shows no fibrillatory waves in between irregular R-R interval (fine atrial fibrillation). The QRS complex is narrow. The heart rate is slow < 60 bpm.
The slow atrial fibrillation in this case could be due to high vagal tone inducing block at AV node.
The lower strip can be confused with AV nodal rhythm in the absence of P wave or f wave but irregular R-R interval excludes this possibility

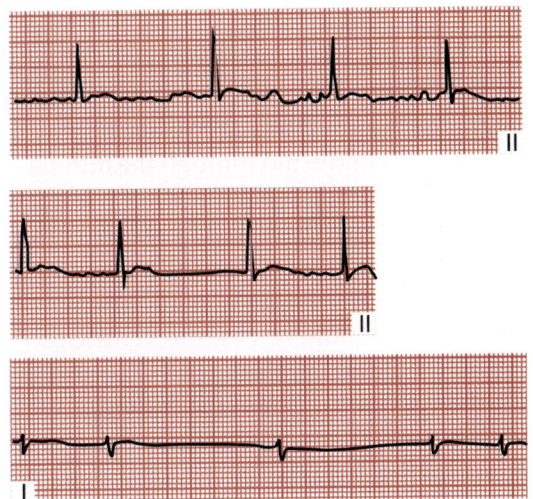

SECTION TEN

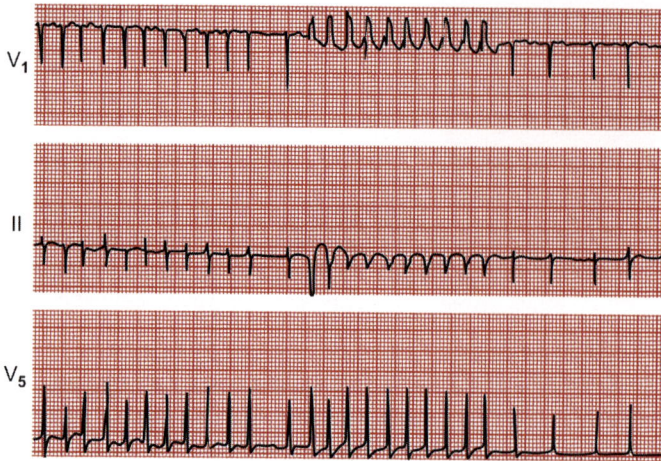

Fig. 32.19: Atrial fibrillation with a ventricular premature complex (VPC). The electrocardiogram (V$_1$) shows qR pattern with T wave inversion, could be due to right ventricular hypertrophy but is difficult to comment unless full 12 lead ECG is provided. Atrial fibrillation is evident from irregular wavy baseline between irregular R-R intervals (irregular ventricular response). The third beat from the beginning of the strip is a VPC due to the following reasons:
1. The initial vector is opposite to the normal conducted beat. Actually the whole QRS complex is opposite to normal beat.
2. There is a compensatory pause following this wide QRS complex
3. It is not related to change in cycle lengths.

Fig. 32.18: Atrial fibrillation with rapid ventricular response and phasic aberrant conduction. The short runs of phasic aberrant conduction resemble VT (paroxysmal VT). The diagnosis of VT is excluded on the basis of:
  i. Absence of post-ectopic pause following last wide QRS of tachycardia phase
  ii. Presence of Ashman's phenomenon (long and short cycle lengths leads to aberrant conduction). The longer the ventricular cycle, the longer is the refractory period; and shorter the ventricular cycle, is shorter the refractory period. The long RR interval precedes wide QRS tachycardia
  iii. Bizarre QRS complexes have rsR′ (RBBB) pattern
  iv. The atrial fibrillation (absent P waves, undulating baseline due to fibrillating waves and irregular R-R intervals) is present that predispose to aberrant conduction by producing variable R-R intervals (variable cycle lengths)

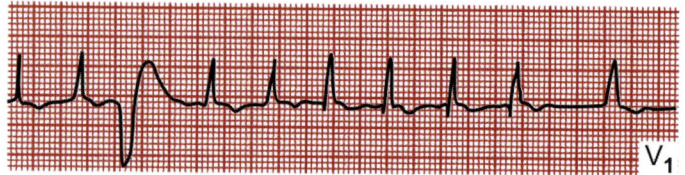

Aberration in Atrial Fibrillation—Ashman's Phenomenon (Figs 32.18 and 32.19)

Aberration refers to an abnormal intraventricular conduction of supraventricular impulses. The QRS complexes appear wide, bizarre and may resemble ventricular premature complexes (VPCs).

Normally, a supraventricular impulse after reaching the AV node, is delayed in it for a brief period, and then, is conducted through the bundle of His and its branches simultaneously to activate the ventricles producing a narrow and normal QRS. However, if one of the bundle branch is still refractory (not fully recovered from previous excitation) when the impulse reaches the bundle of His, the ventricles will not be depolarised normally; in such a situation, the impulse will be conducted down the fully recovered bundle branch to depolarise one of the ventricles in a normal fashion. The impulse then will spread abnormally through the adjacent muscle cells to depolarise the other ventricle, called sequential depolarisation. Because the total ventricular depolarisation takes longer time than normal, the resulting QRS will appear wider than normal or aberrant resembling a bundle branch block pattern. This aberration is called *Ashman's phenomenon*. The aberrant QRS resembles a VPC but it actually originates from a supraventricular site. The aberration - Ashman's phenomenon in atrial fibrillation is related to long and short cycle lengths due to varying R-R intervals. The change of long cycle length to short cycle length (R-R interval) predispose to aberrant intraventricular conduction due to differential refractoriness of bundle branches (Read also Chapter 39). The aberrant QRS complexes are frequently observed during atrial fibrillation because any premature supraventricular impulse or sudden rate acceleration can cause the aberration. The danger of aberration lies not in the phenomenon itself; but in misinterpretation which may lead to incorrect treatment.

The aberration of QRS in Ashman's phenomenon often assumes an rSR' pattern (RBBB pattern) in lead V$_1$. This is because of unequal refractoriness as well as recovery of bundle branches. Following excitation, the right bundle takes longer time to recover than the left bundle, hence, aberration leads to pattern of RBBB commonly because supraventricular impulses finding the right bundle branch refractory, pass through the recovered left bundle.

Caution: Aberrantly conducted supraventricular impulses are often mistaken for VPCs during atrial fibrillation. Do not jump to the use of xylocaine to treat such wide QRS complexes in atrial fibrillation. The abnormal complexes may simply represent aberrant conduction and do not require special treatment except treatment of the cause.

REVIEW AT GLANCE

Atrial Fibrillation at a Glance

- In atrial fibrillation, there is beat to beat change due to irregularly irregular ventricular response hence, R-R interval changes with each successive beat with no visible P waves.
- Replacement of P waves by fibrillatory 'f' waves that distort the baseline in the form of undulations is a characteristic feature on ECG.
- Sometimes, atrial fibrillation may be so fine that undulation of baseline is barely visible as wavy baseline, in such a situation, only variable R-R interval becomes only an important diagnostic clue.

Suggested Reading

1. Botteron GW, Smith JM: Spatial and temporal inhomogeneity of adenosine's effect on atrial refractoriness in humans using atrial fibrillation to probe atrial refractoriness. *J Cardiovas Electrophysiol* **5**: 477, 1994.
2. Cosio FG, Lopex-Gell M, Arribas F et al: Mechanism of entrainment of human common flutter studied with multiple endocardial recordings. *Circulation* **89**: 2117, 1994.
3. Coumel O: Paroxysmal atrial fibrillation. A disorder of autonomic tone. *Eur Heart J* **15**: 9, 1994.
4. Domanski MJ: The epidemiology of atrial fibrillation. *Coronary Artery Dis* **6**: 95, 1995.
5. Evans W, Swann P: Lone auricular fibrillation. *Brit Heart J* **16**: 189, 1954.
6. Falk RH, Podrid PJ (Eds): Atrial fibrillation : Mechanisms and management. New York Raven Press 1992.
7. Fuberg CD, Psaty BM, Manolio TA, et al: Prevalence of atrial fibrillation in elderly subjects (The Cardiovascular Health Study). *Am J Cardiol* **74**: 236, 1994.
8. Olshansky B, Wilber DJ, Hariman RJ: Atrial flutter. Update on the mechanism and treatment. *PACE* **15**: 2308, 1992.
9. Ruffy R: Atrial fibrillation. In Zipes DP, Jalife J (Eds). Cardiac Electrophysiology: From cell to Bed side, 2nd edn Philadelphia: WB Saunders Company 682, 1994.
10. Schamroth L, Krikler DM: The problem of lone atrial fibrillation. *South Afr Med J* **46**: 502, 1967.
11. Shine KI, Kastor JA, Yarchak PM: Multifocal atrial tachycardia. Clinical and electrocardiographic features. *N Engl J Med* **279**: 344, 1968.
12. Waldo AL: Atrial flutter-Mechanisms, clinical features and management. In Zipes DP, Jalife J (Eds), Cardiac Electrophysiology. From cell to Bedside, 2nd edn, Philadelphia, WB Saunders Company 666, 1994.
13. Waxman MB, Yao L, Cameron DA, et al: Effect of posture, Valsalva maneuver and respiration on atrial flutter rate. An effect mediated through cardiac volume. *J Am Coll Cardiol* **17**:1545, 1991.
14. Wells JL Jr et al: Characterisation of atrial flutter. Studies in man after open heart surgery using fixed atrial electrodes. *Circulation*, **60**: 665, 1979.
15. Woeber KA: Thyrotoxicosis and the heart. *N Engl J Med* **327**: 94, 1992.
16. Zipes DP, Garson A Jr: Twenty six Bethesda Conference: Recommendations for determining eligibility for competition in athletes with cardiovascular abnormalities. Task force 6: Arrhythmias. *J Am Coll Cardiol* **24**: 892, 1994.

33

Atrioventricular (AV) Nodal Disturbances

- ■ *AV nodal (junctional) escape beats—mechanisms and electrocardiographic characteristics.*
- ■ *Premature AV nodal (junctional) complexes—mechanisms and electrocardiographic characteristics.*
- ■ *AV nodal (junctional) rhythm, its acceleration and idionodal tachycardia—mechanism, causes and electrocardiographic characteristics.*

The dominant pacemaker that maintains the cardiac rhythm by suppressing other pacemaker sites by its inherent increased automaticity (rapid rate of discharge) is called *primary pacemaker;* that lies in the SA node.

There are other sites where automatic fibres or pacemaker cells are present; but they are prevented from taking part in normal depolarisation by primary pacemaker (SA node), hence, are called *latent or secondary pacemakers.* Normally they are suppressed by rapid inherent discharge of SA node (primary pacemaker). Such latent pacemakers are found in some parts of atrium, in the AV node, His bundle, in the bundle branches and in the peripheral conduction tissue (Purkinje fibres). Under usual conditions, automatic fibres are not found in the atrial or ventricular myocardium.

Electrocardiographic Characteristics of Nodal Rhythm/Beats

The electrocardiographic characteristics of an impulse/rhythm originating from the AV node depend on the conduction sequences;

1. *The nodal impulse or impulses may be conducted antegradely to the ventricles through the normal conduction pathways and retrogradely to the atria.*

When an AV nodal impulse or impulses are conducted to the atria and the ventricles concomitantly (Fig. 33.1), the conduction through the ventricles, if uninterrupted, proceeds through the normal AV conduction pathways producing normal or near normal narrow QRS complex with upright T waves. The atria being placed above the AV node, are depolarised in retrograde fashion, i.e. from below upwards, resulting in inverted P (P') waves in leads II, III and aVF and upright P waves in aVR and aVL and equiphasic P waves in standard lead I. This is due to the fact that P wave axis is directed superiorly to the region of −80° to −90° on the frontal plane which means it is towards the negative pole of leads II, III and aVF. The inverted P (P') in these leads is sharp, pointed and narrow while P waves are dominantly upright in lead V_1. The P is upright in all other precordial leads $(V_2$-$V_6)$.

The relationship of P wave to the QRS complex depends on the relative speed of antegrade and retrograde conduction. Therefore, the P wave may precede, get burried within QRS or may follow the QRS complex (Figs 33.2A and B):

(i) If retrograde activation of atria occurs earlier than the antegrade activation of the ventricles, then the retrograde P (inverted P') wave will

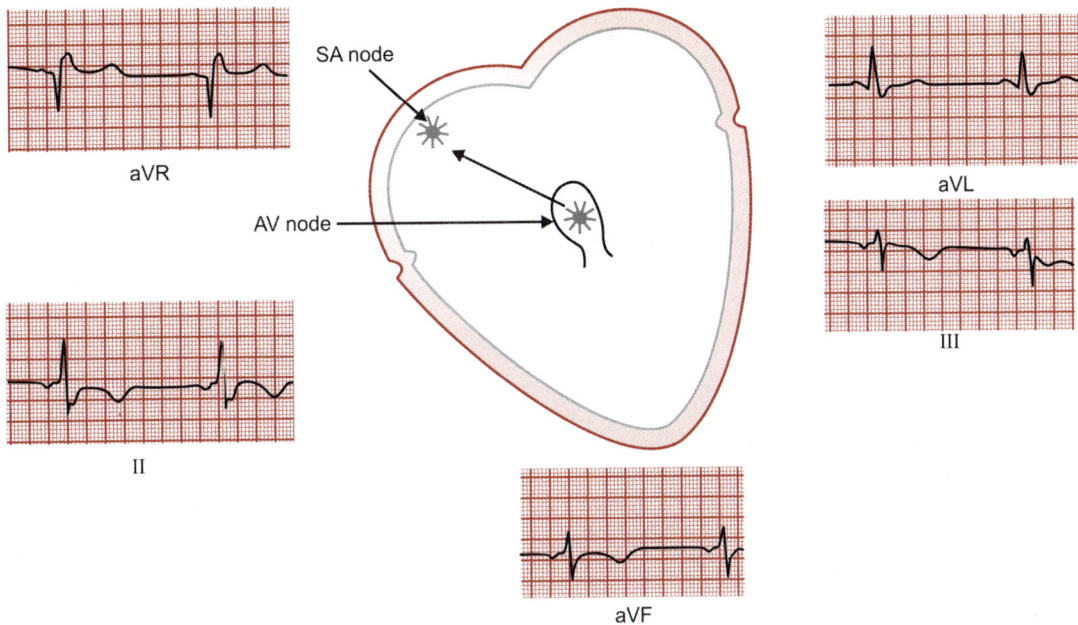

Fig. 33.1: AV nodal premature or escape beat/beats. The diagram shows retrograde activation of atria and normal antegrade conduction to the ventricles

precede the QRS complex. The P-R interval in this situation will be short.

(ii) If retrograde conduction to the atria and antegrade conduction to the ventricles coincides and occurs synchronously, then P′ waves will be burried within QRS and will not be visible.

(iii) If retrograde activation of the atria occurs later than antegrade activation of the ventricles, the retrograde P′ wave will follow the QRS. Such retrograde or inverted P′ wave are seen immediately after QRS distorting the ST segment, but can easily be recognised by their sharp pointed tip.

2. *AV nodal beats or rhythm with antegrade conduction to the ventricles only:*

The AV nodal impulses may be conducted to the ventricles only, resulting in normal QRS-T complex. The retrograde conduction to the atria does not occur because of one of the followings;

(i) There is true retrograde AV block

(ii) There is interference with the retrograde conduction of the AV nodal impulses to atria by concomitant sinus impulses called interference dissociation, is commonly seen in idionodal

tachycardia. This phenomenon has been discussed in Chap 8—AV dissociation.

Dissociation of sinus P waves from AV nodal complexes constitute AV dissociation–is an important ECG manifestation of accelerated AV nodal rhythm or idionodal tachycardia.

3. *Occasionally, antegrade conduction to the ventricles may be blocked or impeded by interference.*

The Types of AV Nodal Disturbance

1. AV nodal (junctional) escape beat/beats.
2. Premature AV nodal (junctional) complexes called junctional or nodal ectopics.
3. AV junctional rhythm
4. Nonparoxysmal AV nodal (junctional) tachycardia (idionodal tachycardia)
5. Tachycardias involving the AV node
   A. Extrasystolic or automatic ectopic focal discharge (enhanced focal automaticity)
   B. Re-entrant tachycardias or reciprocating tachycardias (they are discussed in details in Chapter 36)

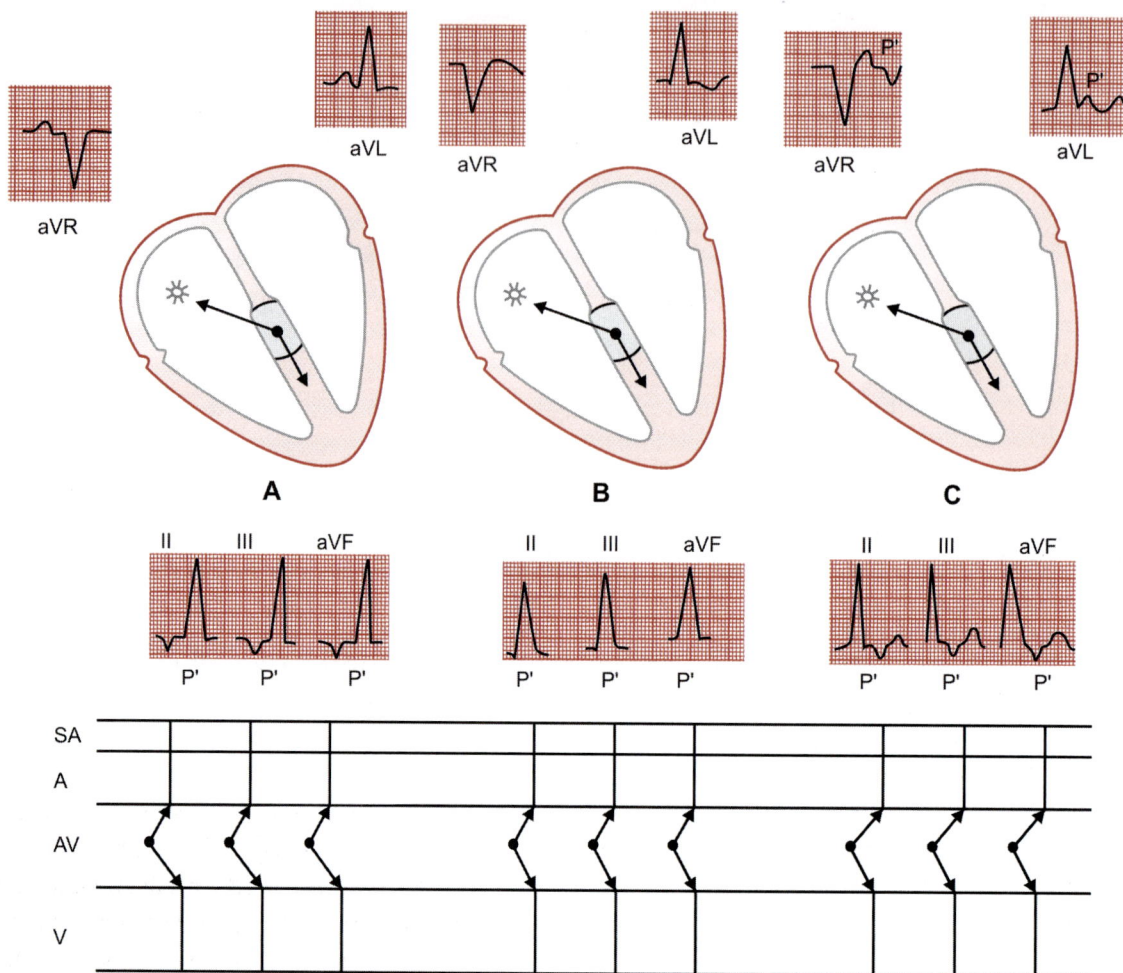

Fig. 33.2A: Diagrammatic illustrations showing various conduction mechanisms and relation of P' wave to QRS in AV nodal beats/rhythm (Leads II, III, aVR, aVL and aVF shown)

A: It illustrates AV nodal beats with earlier retrograde conduction to the atria than antegrade conduction to the ventricles resulting in inverted P waves (II, III, aVF) preceding normal QRS.

B: It illustrates simultaneous and synchronous retrograde atrial and antegrade ventricular activation resulting in P' waves burried within QRS

C: It illustrates the antegrade ventricular activation (conduction) earlier than retrograde atrial activation resulting in inverted P waves following the QRS in leads II, III and aVF.

Note: If P wave is inverted in leads II, III and aVF then P will be upright in leads aVR and aVL. This is due to superior orientation of P wave vector

Causes

1. Acute myocardial infarction especially inferior wall infarction.
2. Heart failure
3. Valvular (mitral and tricuspid valve) diseases
4. Cardiomyopathies
5. Sick sinus syndrome—a structural nodal disease
6. Myocarditis
7. Drug effect (digitalis and theophylline)
8. Electrolyte disturbance.

AV NODAL (JUNCTIONAL) ESCAPE BEATS (READ CHAPTER 40—ESCAPE RHYTHM)

Normally sinus node keeps a full control over AV node in the matter of discharge of impulses. It does not allow the AV node to escape from its control because

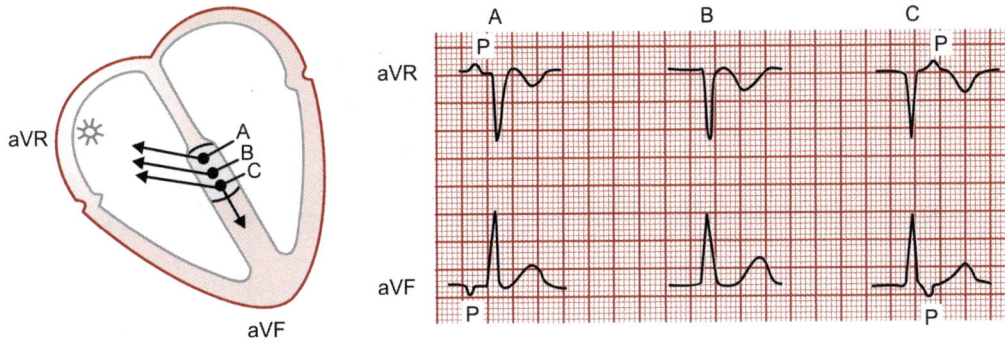

Fig. 33.2B: Electrocardiographic patterns of AV nodal ectopics originating from different sites in AV node:
A: Upper nodal region. The ectopic impulse originating from upper nodal region will have inverted P (P') in aVF and upright P in aVR preceding the QRS. This indicates retrograde atrial activation precedes antegrade ventricular activation
B: Mid-nodal region. The P wave will be invisible both in aVR and aVF indicating near synchronisation of activation of both atria and ventricles.
C: Lower nodal region. The inverted P of an ectopic impulse in aVF and upright P in aVR follows the QRS complex indicating antegrade ventricular activation precede retrograde atrial activation

SA node is *'the King of its own empire'*. The AV node can only escape and fire when the sinus discharge rate falls below the AV nodal inherent rate of discharge. Therefore, an AV nodal escape is only possible if there is decreased impulse formation from SA node due to any cause and/or the sinus impulse fails to reach the AV node due to interruption any where along its pathway of propagation from atria to AV node. Hence, a latent pacemaker becomes 'manifest' or 'dominant' pacemaker either by default or by usurpation.

Definition. AV nodal or junctional escape beats are defined as the beats produced by the AV node either by default or by usurpation. The interval between last conducted sinus beat and the AV nodal escape beat is the measure of the initial discharge rate of the AV nodal (junctional) focus, and generally lies between 40-60 bpm (inherent discharge rate of AV node).

The Electrocardiogram (Fig. 33.3)

1. *P wave configuration.* The configuration of P wave varies (Figs 33.2A and B) depending on the mechanism of conduction.
   a) A negative or inverted P wave (P' wave) may precede the narrow QRS complex indicating retrograde atrial activation earlier than antegrade ventricular activation. The P-R interval is short (< 0.12 sec) but can be normal. The inverted P' waves are seen in leads II, III and aVF. The P wave is upright in aVR and precordial leads.
   b) The P wave may not be visible due to its superimposition on QRS. This happens when AV nodal escape beat activates the atria and ventricles simultaneously due to focus of discharge in AV node being equidistant from atria and ventricles.
   c) A negative or inverted P (P') wave may follow a narrow QRS complex. This indicates antegrade ventricular activation is earlier than retrograde atrial activation.
   d) Absent P wave indicates retrograde AV block.
2. *Morphology of QRS complex.* An AV nodal escape beat being supraventricular in origin, has normal narrow QRS complex due to normal intraventricular conduction. Aberrant intraventricular conduction results in a wide QRS configuration.
3. *Fixed coupling interval.* AV nodal escape occurs only when sinus beat either does not reach or reaches later than expected, hence, AV nodal escape beat/beats are inscribed late. The distance between the sinus beat and an escape beat is slightly longer than normal, but subsequent escape beats constituting a rhythm will have fixed coupling interval.

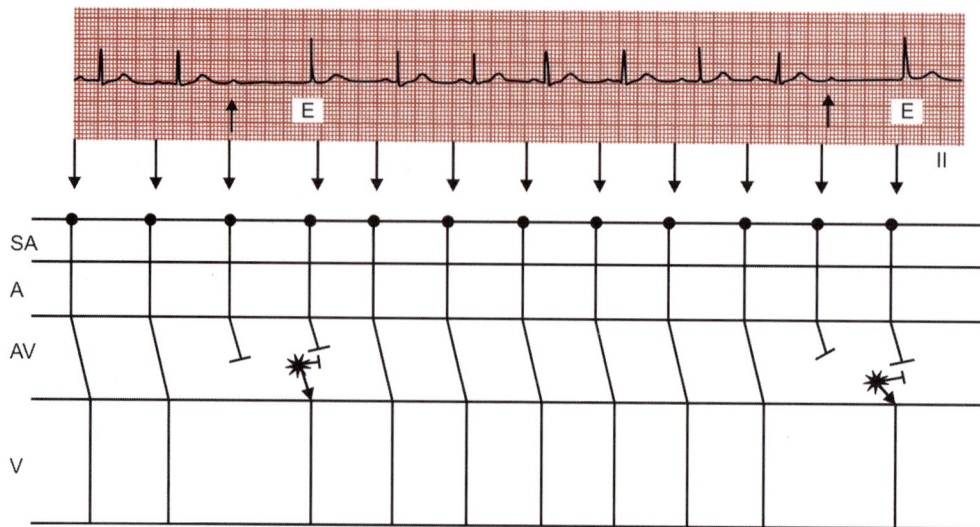

Fig. 33.3: Wenckebach conduction with AV nodal escape beats. The ECG lead II shows first and second sinus beats with P-R interval of 0.18 sec and 0.20 sec respectively followed by a blocked P wave indicating Wenckebach conduction. The blocked P (arrow ↑) is followed by an AV nodal escape beat (normal QRS with no visible P wave labelled as E). The Wenckebach period is terminated and started a fresh. The next 6 sinus beats show progressively lengthening of P-R interval followed by nonconducted P (arrow) wave. This is followed by another AV nodal escape beat (E).

Below is drawn a ladder diagram to show the pathway of conduction of impulses

SA = SA node, A = Atria, AV = Atrioventricular node, V = Ventricle

4. *Compensatory pause.* An AV nodal escape beat is not followed by a compensatory pause. On the other hand, AV nodal premature beat (ectopic) is followed by a compensatory pause–a feature that differentiates the two AV nodal beats.

5. They are occasional and disappear as sinus rate accelerates and reaches above the AV nodal discharge rate.

6. There must be some cause to explain the nodal escape beats/rhythm, hence, there may be an evidence of sinus arrhythmia or sinus bradycardia or intermittent sinus pauses on ECG. Remember, AV nodal escape beats occur by default and do not constitute primary AV nodal rhythm. They are always secondary to sinus nodal dysfunction/ disease.

A nodal escape beat is inscribed late as compared to AV nodal ectopic beat though both are premature complexes—Read chapter 40. AV nodal escape beat or beats are not followed by compensatory pause—a feature that distinguishes them from AV nodal ectopics.

PREMATURE AV NODAL (JUNCTIONAL) COMPLEXES/AV NODAL EXTRA-SYSTOLES OR ECTOPICS

An impulse arising from the AV node (the exact site, i.e. AN, N, NH region; low atrium or bundle of His - is not known) prematurely is called an *AV nodal (junctional) extrasystole or an AV nodal ectopic.* This beat attempts to get conducted antegradely to the ventricles and retrogradely to the atria. If uninterrupted in its course, the impulse discharges the atria to produce a premature retrograde P wave (inverted P' wave) and discharges the ventricles to produce a premature QRS complex of supraventricular configuration (narrow QRS). Alterations in the conduction time can influence P-R and R-P relationships without change in the site of origin of the impulses. An AV nodal extrasystole exhibiting aberrant conduction looks like a ventricular extrasystole from which it has to be differentiated (Read Chapter 39 on aberrant conduction).

The Electrocardiogram (Fig. 33.4)

1. They being premature occur earlier than anticipated sinus beats, hence, postectopic interval is longer than pre-ectopic interval.

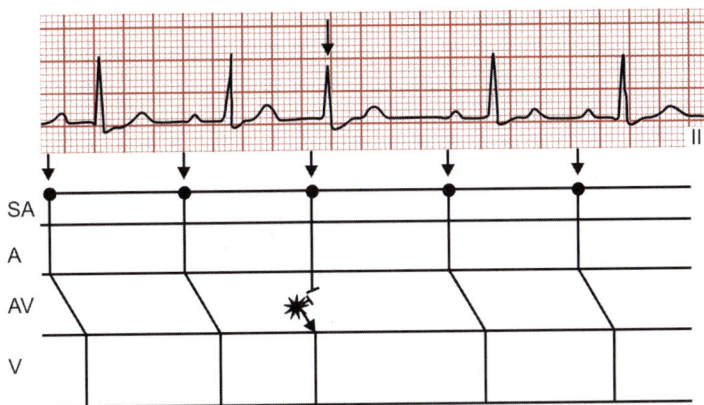

Fig. 33.4: An AV nodal ectopic beat. The lead II shows first two sinus complex conducted with first degree AV block (P-R interval is 0.24 sec). The third complex is a AV nodal ectopic (arrow) does not have visible P wave and QRS is slightly wider than the sinus beat, occurs prematurely and is followed by a compensatory pause. Following this beat, again sinus impulses are conducted with first degree AV block. Below is drawn a ladder diagram to show the site of origin and conduction of impulses at various levels. SA - Sinoatrial node; A - Atrial; AV - Atrioventricular node; V - Ventricle

2. The retrograde (inverted) P′ waves may occur before, during (superimposed on QRS) or after QRS complexes. They are best seen in leads II, III and aVF. The P wave of ectopics is upright in aVR and precordial leads.

3. The P-R interval varies depending on the conduction time of the extrasystole. It may be short (high nodal), or absent (mid nodal).

4. There is a compensatory pause following the extrasystole, which may be complete or incomplete depending on the interference of the sinus discharge. The mechanism of production of a compensatory pause has been discussed with concealed conduction (Fig. 33.5).

5. Sometimes, a nodal beat gets sandwitched between two sinus beat called a nodal interpolated beat. The pre-ectopic and post-ectopic intervals are more or less equal (Fig. 33.5).

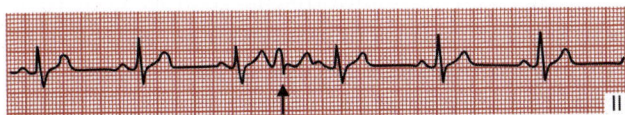

Fig. 33.5: AV nodal interpolated beat indicated by an arrow. The nodal complex (QRS with no visible P wave) is interposed between two sinus complexes

AV NODAL (JUNCTIONAL) RHYTHM

AV nodal rhythm is usually an escape rhythm, occurs when AV nodal extrasystoles or ectopics continue for sometime in the form of a rhythm. The rate of this rhythm is the actual inherent rate of AV nodal discharge, i.e. 40-60 bpm. This rhythm can occur only and if the sinus node fails to discharge its impulses and/or there is failure of conduction of these sinus impulses to AV node, thus, the nodal rhythm arises by default rather than primary in nature. Rarely, AV nodal extrasystolic focus may discharge at a slower rate to produce a nodal rhythm for some period. Usually, such an ectopic focus discharges at a faster rate to produce an AV nodal tachycardia rather than an AV nodal rhythm.

AV nodal rhythm is usually secondary to failure of sinus discharge for sometime, hence, is a secondary phenomenon rather than a primary rhythm disorder

Causes

1. As a normal phenomenon due to high vagal tone.
2. It can appear as an escape rhythm during profound sinus bradycardia.
3. It can appear during heart blocks.
4. Sick sinus syndrome.

The Electrocardiogram (Figs 33.6 and 33.7A to C)

1. Heart rate is regular at a rate of 40-60 bpm. The R-R intervals are also regular.
2. The retrograde (inverted) P′ waves may either precede or merge with or follow QRS. These inverted P′ waves are seen in leads II, III and aVF, but the P wave is upright in lead aVR and precordial leads.
3. The QRS complexes are narrow due to normal intraventricular conduction. These complexes may be followed by retrograde atrial discharge produc-

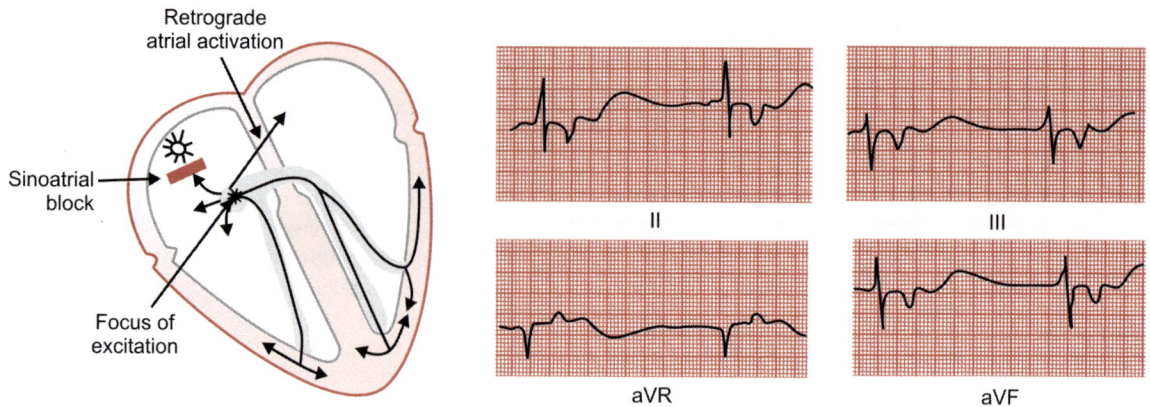

Fig. 33.6: AV nodal rhythm. Note inverted P follows QRS in leads II, III, aVF and P is upright in aVR. The nodal discharge rate is 50/min

ing inverted P′ wave or can occur independent of atrial discharge resulting in AV dissociation.

Clinical tip. *The escape rhythm in fact serves as a safety valve to prevent the occurrence of cardiac asystole. It does not require any treatment.*

ACCELERATION OF AV NODAL RHYTHM (ACCELERATED AV NODAL RHYTHM OR IDIONODAL TACHYCARDIA)

1. **Accelerated AV nodal escape rhythm:** The AV node can accelerate its rate beyond its inherent rate of 40-60 bpm and may take the full control of the rhythm of the heart. If the rate lies between 60-100 bpm (usual rate is 70-80 bpm), it is called an *accelerated AV nodal rhythm*. The electrocardiographic characteristics are same as described already under AV nodal escape rhythm.

2. **Nonparoxysmal idionodal tachycardia.** This is nothing but further augmentation of accelerated rhythm of AV node beyond 100 bpm. This is actually misnomer as a tachycardia because the usual rate in this tachycardia is 70-80 bpm but can go up further. This tachycardia can happen when AV node has taken full control of cardiac rhythm as a dominant pacemaker. The tachycardia is non-paroxysmal because it is gradual in its onset as well as in its termination. Occasionally, nonparoxysmal AV nodal tachycardia can manifest abruptly due to slowing of the dominant pacemaker.

Note: The accelerated AV nodal rhythm and idionodal tachycardia express electrocardiographically in a similar fashion, have same mode of initiation and termination. The only difference lies in the heart rate which in absolute term is not-hence, some consider them as one rather than separate entities.

Causes
1. Digitalis toxicity
2. Myocardial infarction.
3. Acute rheumatic fever.
4. Heart failure
5. Valvular heart disease
6. Myocarditis.

Mechanism
An accelerated automatic discharge of AV node (in or near to His bundle) is the underlying mechanism for this arrhythmia. It is hereby stressed that it may simulate paroxysmal AV nodal extrasystolic tachycardia which is due to an ectopic or an extrasystolic focus in the atrium or AV node.

The Electrocardiogram in Accelerated Nodal Rhythm/Idionodal Tachycardia (Figs 33.8 and 33.9)

1. *Heart rate.* It is more than AV nodal rhythm (> 60 bpm). In accelerated AV nodal rhythm it is between 70-80 bpm; while in idionodal tachycardia, it is usually in the range of 70-100 bpm but has a tendency to go up and may cross 100 bpm. Though,

P wave is embedded in QRS which is wider than normal

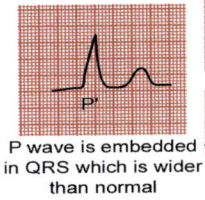

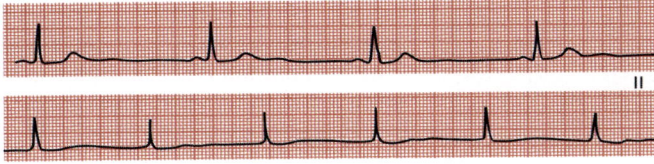

Fig. 33.7A: AV nodal escape rhythm. Sinus bradycardia with AV nodal escape rhythm. The leads II upper strip shows profound sinus bradycardia at 38/min regular. The lower strip continuous of lead II shows nodal rhythm (QRS complexes with embedded P waves) at a rate of 60/min. Falling sinus rate led to emergence of AV nodal rhythm

Fig. 33.7B: AV nodal escape rhythm. AV nodal escape rhythm following AV nodal delay. The first sinus beat is normal with normal P-R interval (0.16 sec). The second beat has prolonged P-R interval (0.24 sec), is followed by AV nodal rhythm (last 5 QRS complexes with no visible P waves)

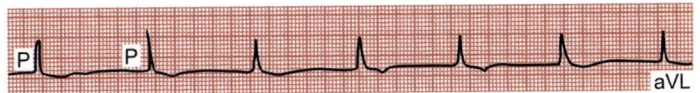

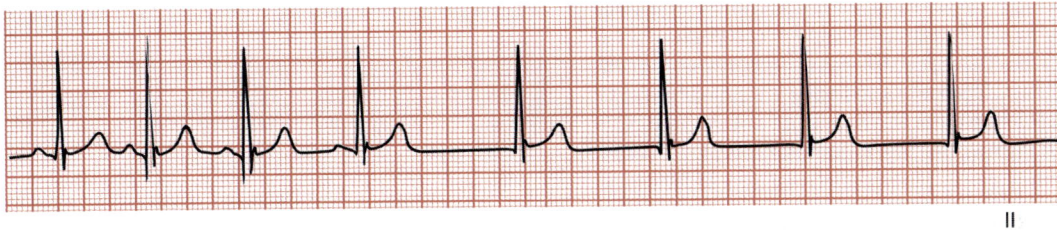

Fig. 33.7C: AV nodal escape rhythm following sinus arrhythmia. First 4 beats show marked sinus arrhythmia with emergence of nodal rhythm (↓)

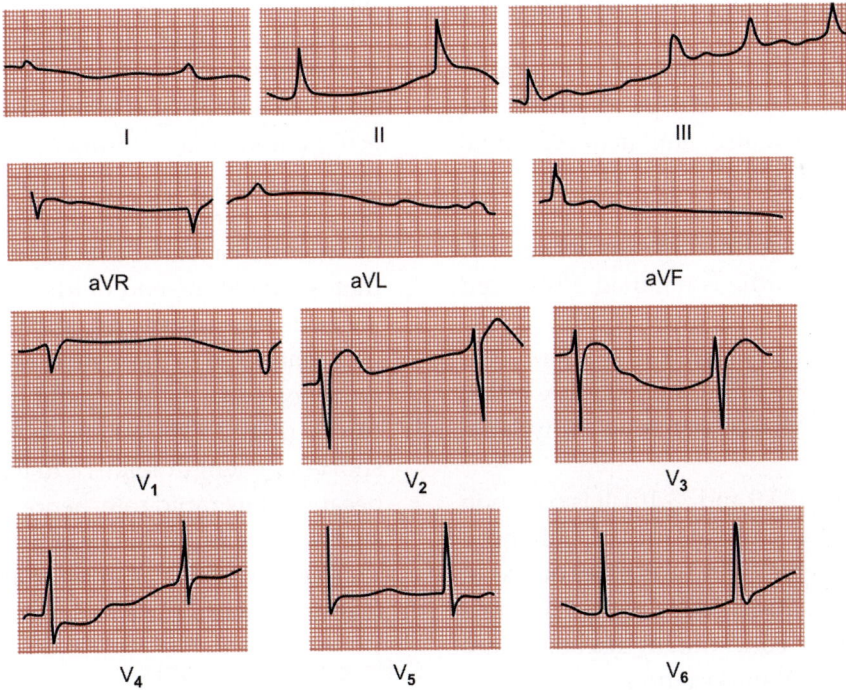

Fig. 33.7C: AV nodal arrhythmia in AV nodal escape rhythm—An autonomic phenomenon. The 12 lead ECG shows all characteristics of nodal rhythm (QRS with no visible P wave) at a rate of 60/min regular. **Note** the irregular R-R intervals in lead III, indicates nodal arrhythmia due to autonomic influence akin to sinus arrhythmia

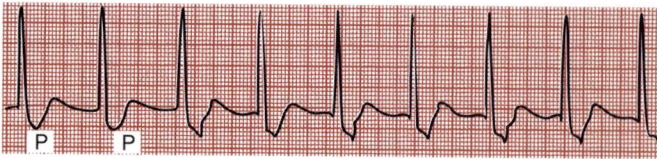

Fig. 33.8: Accelerated AV nodal rhythm at a rate of 96/min approx. The narrow QRS complexes are followed by inverted P waves (labelled P'). The rhythm is regular. The condition which led to this rhythm could not be ascertained as initial events are not recorded in this ECG

Fig. 33.9: Idionodal tachycardia with AV dissociation.

A: Idionodal tachycardia with AV dissociation. The lead II shows upright P preceding narrow QRS for first 7 beats, at more or less fixed interval suggesting normal AV association. The 8th and 9th QRS complexes (↑)have invisible P waves (P is embedded within QRS) and the last beat has upright P that follows QRS indicating AV dissociation

B: Idionodal tachycardia with AV dissociation and first degree AV block. The first, 4th and 7th complexes have small P wave with negligible P-R intervals, are unrelated to QRS. Rest QRS complexes have invisible P waves. The 9th QRS has clear P wave, is a capture beat (C). The last complex has QRS complex probably sinus with P-R interval of 0.24, indicating first degree AV block

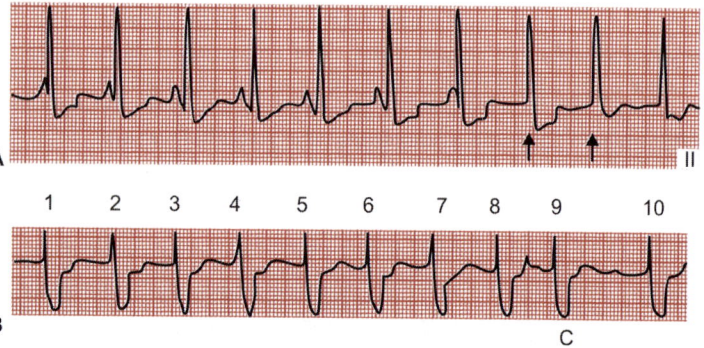

the term tachycardia is applied when heart rate goes beyond 100 bpm, but this is an exception where the term 'tachycardia' can be used at a heart rate of less than 100 bpm.

2. *The QRS complexes :* They are narrow and similar to that seen in AV nodal escape rhythm. The conduction sequence is also similar to AV nodal rhythm. The wide QRS complexes indicate aberrant conduction.

3. *Autonomic influence.* Autonomic influence over nodal rhythm/tachycardia is retained. Enhanced vagal tone can slow while vagolytic agents increase the discharge rate. Under autonomic influence, the R-R intervals may, sometimes, vary slightly called *'nodal arrhythmia'* which is akin to sinus arrhythmia (Fig. 33.7C).

4. *AV dissociation* (Figs 33.9 and 33.10). It is common due to the fact that the rate of an enhanced idionodal rhythm or tachycardia is more or less in the same range, i.e. 70-80 bpm as that of sinus discharge rate, hence, concomitant discharges are frequent producing AV dissociation.

5. *No protection to pacemaker activity.* AV nodal pacemaker is unprotected, hence, acceleration of sinus rate over and above the idionodal rate will terminate it. Similarly, there is dislocation of ectopic rhythm by a capture beat. This is due to the fact that ventricular capture beat penetrates the AV node and resets its ectopic cycle.

6. *Ventricular capture beats.* Idionodal rate being slow (70-80 bpm) as compared to extrasystolic/ectopic nodal tachycardia (> 100 bpm), results in long cycle length or diastolic period relative to refractory period of AV node. This facilitates the ventricular capture beats because an ectopic beat that occurs at the end of idionodal cycle will find AV node responsive and, under this circumstance, gets conducted to the ventricles. This phenomenon does not occur in AV nodal extrasystolic tachycardia (Fig. 33.11) which, in contrast, produces short cycle length relative to its refractory period because of its rapid rate, hence, under this circumstance, there is no chance of a ventricular capture. This constitutes an important distinguishing feature between the two.

Differential Diagnosis

The distinguishing features of idionodal and paroxysmal AV nodal extrasystolic tachycardia are given in the Table 33.1.

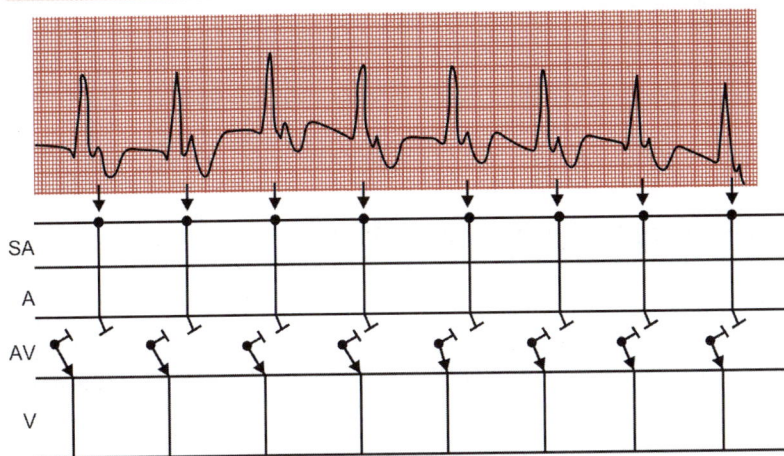

Fig. 33.10: Idionodal tachycardia. The lead II shows slightly wider QRS complexes than normal followed by upright P wave. The rate is more than 100/min

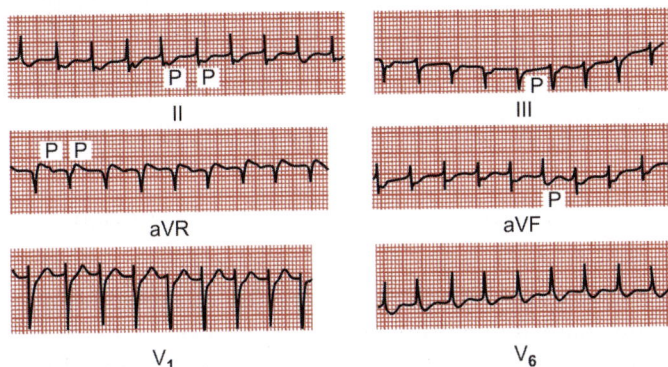

Fig. 33.11: Paroxysmal AV nodal extrasystolic tachycardia. The tachycardia rate is 188/min regular in which the narrow QRS complexes are followed by inverted P' waves at short fixed R-P interval in leads II, III and aVF. The P wave is upright in leads aVR, V_1 and V_6. The identical and fixed shape of P waves, rapid heart rate and narrow QRS complexes indicate nodal extrasystolic tachycardia but idionodal tachycardia can not be ruled out unless or until initial events of tachycardia are recorded, otherwise, both needs differentiation by detailed electrophysiological studies

SECTION TEN

Table 33.1: Distinguishing features of two AV nodal tachycardias	
Idionodal tachycardia	*Paroxysmal AV nodal extrasystolic tachycardia* (Fig. 33.10)
• It is due to an enhanced inherent automaticity, hence, is nonparoxysmal	• It is due to an extrasystolic focal nodal discharge (automatic focal AV discharge)
• Ventricular rate is between 70-80 bpm	• Ventricular rate is > 100 bpm
• Slow onset and persists after carotid massage with slowing of rate	• Abrupt onset and termination by certain manoeuvres, i.e. carotid massage
• Ventricular capture can occur	• It does not occur
• Commonly encountered clinically	• It is uncommon

Suggested Reading

1. Akhtar M, Jazayeri MR, Sra J, et al: Atrioventricular nodal re-entry. Clinical, electrophysiological and therapeutic considerations. *Circulation* **88**:282, 1993.
2. Burchell HB: Atrioventricular nodal (reciprocating) rhythm. *Am Heart J* **67**:391, 1964.
3. Janse MJ, Anderson RH, McGuire MA, et al: AV nodal re-entry:1. AV nodal re-entry revised. *J Cardiovasc Electrophysiol* **4**:561, 1993.
4. Josephson ME, Miller JM: Atrioventricular nodal re-entry: Evidence supporting an intranodal location. *PACE* **16**:599, 1993.
5. Nayebpour M, Billette J, Amellal F, et al: Effects of adenosine on rate-dependent atrioventricular nodal function: Potential role in tachycardia termination and physiological regulation. *Circulation* **88**: 2632, 1993.
6. Rosen KM: Junctional tachycardia: Mechanisms, diagnosis, differential diagnosis and management. *Circulation* **47**:654, 1973.

34

Paroxysmal Supraventricular Tachycardias

- *Current concepts, definition and mechanisms.*
- *Re-entrant or reciprocating tachycardias—atrioventricular nodal re-entrant (AVNRT) and atrioventricular re-entrant tachycardia (AVRT).*
- *AVNRT—dual concept of pathogenesis, typical and atypical re-entry and the electrocardiographic characteristics.*
- *AVRT—re-entry through an accessory pathway–antidromic and orthodromic circuit conduction and the electrocardiographic characteristics.*

Much confusion exists regarding the nomenclature of supraventricular tachycardias. It has now become apparent that a number of electrophysiological mechanisms operate for these tachycardias, hence, recently there has been an appraisal of the whole concept of supraventricular tachycardias;

1. The previously held view that the term is used for both atrial and nodal tachycardia where precise origin cannot be established is an oversimplification, which is no longer tenable nowadays.
2. Many supraventricular tachycardias which were previously thought to be an expression of an enhanced automaticity are now considered to be due to re-entry or reciprocating mechanism through reciprocal pathways.
3. Certain tachycardias where the mechanism involved is direct atrioventricular conduction with re-entry (AVRT) are as atrial in origin as ventricular, but are still retained in terminology of supraventricular tachycardias.

Therefore, it has become necessary while appraising the concept of supraventricular tachycardia; to determine not only the site of origin of the impulses but also whether tachycardia is an expression of an enhanced automaticity or a re-entry or a reciprocating mechanism (anatomical circuit)

Definition

Paroxysmal supraventricular tachycardia is defined as conduction of supraventricular impulses at a rate of more than 100 bpm with narrow QRS, regular R-R intervals and without an evidence of pre-excitation. It, if associated with wide QRS, is called paroxysmal supraventricular tachycardia with aberrant conduction.

Mechanisms

Paroxysmal supraventricular tachycardia describes two types of rhythm disturbances in which supraventricular impulses are conducted abnormally between atria and ventricles. Two mechanism involved are; (i) *an enhanced automaticity* and (ii) *an re-entry circuit (reciprocating mechanism)*. In both these forms, the heart rate is > 100 bpm. The re-entrant mechanism in supraventricular tachycardia may be intranodal (dual concept mechanism) or may be extranodal due to presence of an accessory pathway of conduction. In fact, the term paroxysmal supra-ventricular tachycardia is inappropriate where extranodal re-entry through an accessory pathway is present because tachycardia resulting from conduction through such pathways are no more supraventricular than they are ventricular in origin, since there is involvement of both atria and ventricles in the re-entry mechanism, but are still being retained under the head of supraventricular tachycardias. Depending on the mode of conduction, atrioventricular tachycardia (AVRT) may be orthodromic which simulate AVNRT or may be antidromic producing wide QRS. However, better term to be used in electrocardiography for such tachycardias is reciprocating tachycardias, but rising above the controversy in terminology, in this section, the descriptive titles will be used to make the subject clear and understandable.

ATRIOVENTRICULAR (AV) NODAL TACHYCARDIAS

They can occur due to an (i) enhanced automaticity or (ii) extrasystolic focal discharge or (iii) re-entry. The automatic enhanced nodal tachycardia (idionodal) or tachycardia due to extrasystolic focal discharge have been discussed in previous chapter. In this chapter re-entrant nodal tachycardias will be discussed.

The most common cause of paroxysmal AV nodal tachycardia is re-entry involving the low atrial or AV nodal fibres (typical conduction) or microentry circuit involving the concealed accessory pathway (atypical conduction) - called *atypical AV nodal tachycardia* in which normal antegrade conduction occurs through AV node to the ventricles and retrograde conduction occurs through AV nodal bypass tract (concealed accessory pathway).

1. AV Nodal Re-entrant Tachycardia (AVNRT)

This is most common cause of PSVT. A microentry circuit involving two pathways within AV node is the proposed mechanism for its pathogenesis. The onset of tachycardia is almost always associated with a supraventricular ectopic impulse showing prolongation of P-R interval due to marked AV nodal delay (prolonged A-H interval on bundle of His electro-cardiography is critical for genesis of this arrhythmia).

An atrial complex that conducts with a critical prolongation of AV nodal conduction time (long P-R and/or AH intervals) generally precipitates the re-entry. Premature ventricular stimulation also can induce AV nodal re-entry in one-third patients of this tachycardia. AVNRT occurs mostly in patients with no structural heart disease.

Pathogenesis—Dual Concept Mechanism Proposed for Re-entry

A dual concept mechanism consisting of fast and slow conducting pathways within the AV node is the proposed mechanism for its initiation. The prolonged P-R interval or prolonged A-H interval on bundle of His electrocardiography strengthens the concept of dual entry pathway within AV node. Therefore, the present concept is that the AV node is functionally split into two longitudinal pathways;
1. *Beta pathway (fast pathway)*. It exhibits rapid conduction and has a long refractory period.
2. *An alpha pathway (slow pathway)*. It conducts slowly and has a short refractory period.

These two pathways are connected above and below by a common pathway (Fig. 34.1) called proximal and distal pathways that are located within AV node and the whole circuit for circus movement lies in AV node.

Mode of Conduction Through These Pathways

It is discussed under three different situations;
A. *Normal sinus rhythm ;* A supraventricular impulse splits into two; one impulse travels down the beta pathway to produce a single narrow QRS with a normal P-R interval; the other impulse while passing down the alpha or slow pathway normally does not reach to the ventricles due to refractoriness of His bundle which has already been depolarised by the impulse that has reached to it earlier through beta pathway (Fig. 34.1). Normally there is no re-entry during sinus rhythm.
B. *Conduction of an atrial premature complex.* An atrial premature complex (APC) gets conducted in a typical and atypical manner
(i) Typical conduction (Figs 34.1 and 34.2A). In case of an atrial premature beat, the conduction pattern is just opposite to sinus rhythm as

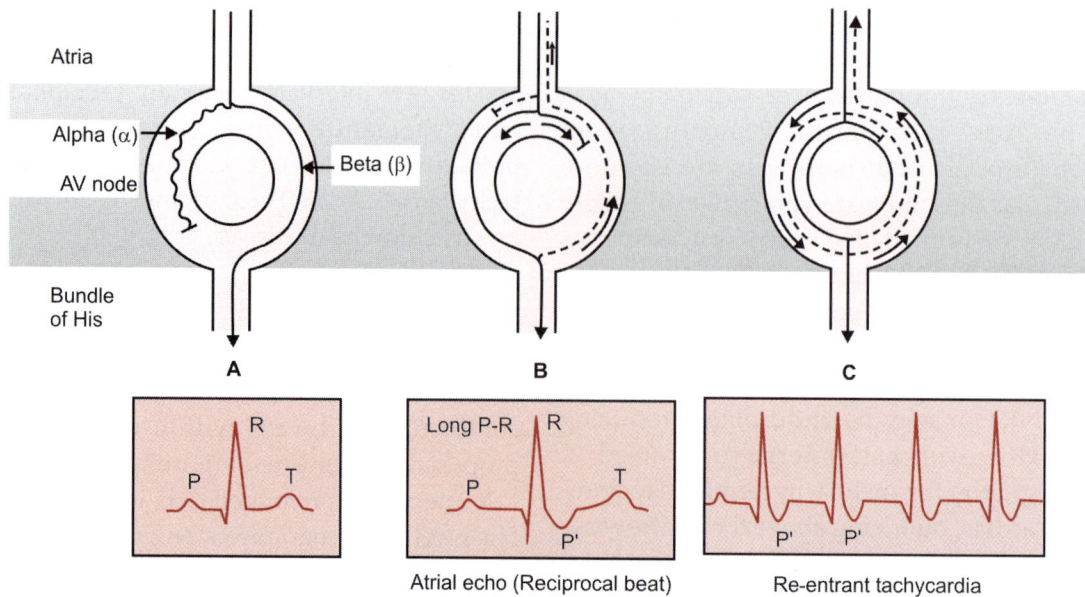

Fig. 34.1: Mechanisms of AV nodal re-entry and re-entrant tachycardia. The atria, AV node and His bundle are diagrammatically shown. The AV node is longitudinally split into two different functional pathways, alpha (α) and beta (β).

A: During sinus rhythm, the impulse passes down the beta (fast) pathway to produce normal P-R interval. Conduction through alpha pathway cannot pass down due to refractoriness of the bundle of His as shown

B: With a premature atrial beat, block occurs in fast beta pathways, hence, it passes down slowly through alpha pathway to the ventricles. It gets retrogradely conducted to atria again to produce an atrial echo (P', reciprocal beat). See the diagram below where inverted P' wave follows QRS. This has occurred after long P-R interval which is pre-requisite for retrograde conduction

C: When atrial premature beat is able to sustain circus movements through alpha and beta pathways, sustained AVNRT will result. The initiating event remains same, i.e. long P-R interval

discussed above. The atrial premature impulse or beat (APB) gets blocked in the beta pathway having a long refractory period, therefore passes down the alpha pathway slowly and slowly to the ventricles antegradely and while, in transition, finds the beta pathway responsive (refractory period is over) gets retrogradely conducted to the atria through the beta pathway producing an atrial echo (Fig. 34.1B). If this process of re-entry continues, tachycardia will result (Fig. 34.1C). In this type of re-entrant tachycardia, both the atria and ventricles are activated simultaneously by retrograde and antegrade conduction respectively, hence, P waves may not be visible on surface ECG as they get buried within QRS complex or follow QRS depending on the retrograde pathway used (Fig. 34.2). The P waves, if visible, are inverted in leads II, III and aVF, since atria are depolarised retrogradely. This is a typical (common) conduc-

tion pattern seen in 95% cases of AVNRT. The re-entrant loop of this tachycardia is given in the box.

> ### Re-entrant loop of typical AV nodal conduction pattern in AVNRT
> *An atrial premature complex (APC)* → *antegrade slow conduction (alpha pathway)* → *Final distal common pathway (distal AV node)* → *ventricle* → *retrograde re-entry through fast beta nodal pathway* → *retrograde atrial activation.*

(ii) Atypical AV nodal re-entry (Fig. 34.2B). In atypical nodal re-entry, the mechanism of conduction is opposite to typical re-entry and similar to entry as in the sinus rhythm, i.e. antegrade conduction proceeds over the fast pathways (beta pathway) and the retrograde conduction through slow (alpha) pathway. The tachycardia produced by this mechanism is rare (5-10% cases).

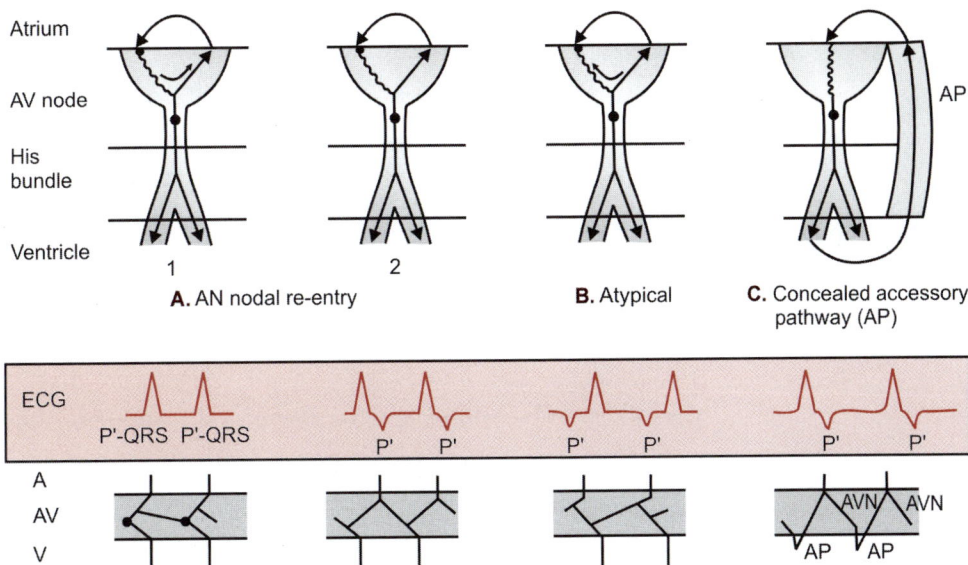

Fig. 34.2: Diagrammatic illustration of various paroxysmal supraventricular re-entrant tachycardias. The top portion of diagram represents the scheme of the presumed anatomical pathways. The lower half represents the ECG and the ladder diagram.

A: AV nodal re-entry: Left figure (1) shows retrograde atrial activation occurring simultaneously with antegrade ventricular activation through the slow nodal pathway and retrograde conduction through fast (beta) AV nodal pathway hence P' is merged with QRS. In the right figure (2), atrial activity occurs slightly later than ventricular activity due to retrograde conduction delay, hence, P' wave is inscribed after QRS

B: *Atypical conduction.* The AV nodal re-entry is just reverse to described above in A. AV nodal re-entry due to antegrade conduction over fast (beta) pathway and retrograde conduction over slow AV nodal pathway, hence P' precedes QRS

C: *Concealed accessory pathway (AP).* Reciprocating tachycardia is due to antegrade conduction over the AV node and retrograde conduction through accessory pathway. Inverted (retrograde) P' follows QRS

C. *AV nodal tachycardia with concealed accessory pathway of conduction* (Fig. 34.2C). It is possible to have tachycardia that uses either antegrade slow or fast pathway but gets conducted retrogradely over an concealed accessory pathway.

The ventricles are not needed to maintain AV nodal re-entry and spontaneous AV blocks can occur particularly at the onset of arrhythmia. Such blocks can take place in the AV node distal to re-entry circuit, between AV node and His bundle, within bundle of His or distal to it. Most commonly, when block occurs, it is below the bundle of His. Termination of this tachycardia, generally, results from block in the antegradely conducting slow pathways (a weak link) so that retrograde atrial response is not followed by a ventricular response.

The Electrocardiogram in AV Nodal Re-entrant Tachycardia (Fig. 34.3)

1. *Initiation and termination of tachycardia.* An atrial premature beat or complex (APB/APC) with a prolonged P-R interval initiates the re-entry process of AVNRT. The abrupt termination, usually with a retrograde P' wave, is sometimes followed by a period of asystole or bradycardia.

2. The P waves are inverted in leads II, III and aVF due to retrograde activation of the atria. They are upright in other leads.

3. The initiating P wave of an APC is followed by a QRS complex (atrioventricular conduction) but subsequent beats reveal either a QRS complex followed by an inverted P' wave (ventriculoatrial conduction) or a QRS complex with an imbedded P' wave leading to invisible P waves.

4. The QRS complexes are regular and narrow in AVNRT but may become widened due to aberrant intraventricular conduction. The aberrancy is more common in AVRT rather than in AVNRT due to rapid heart rate.

5. In AVNRT, the retrograde P (P') waves of the tachycardia are either burried within the QRS

SECTION TEN

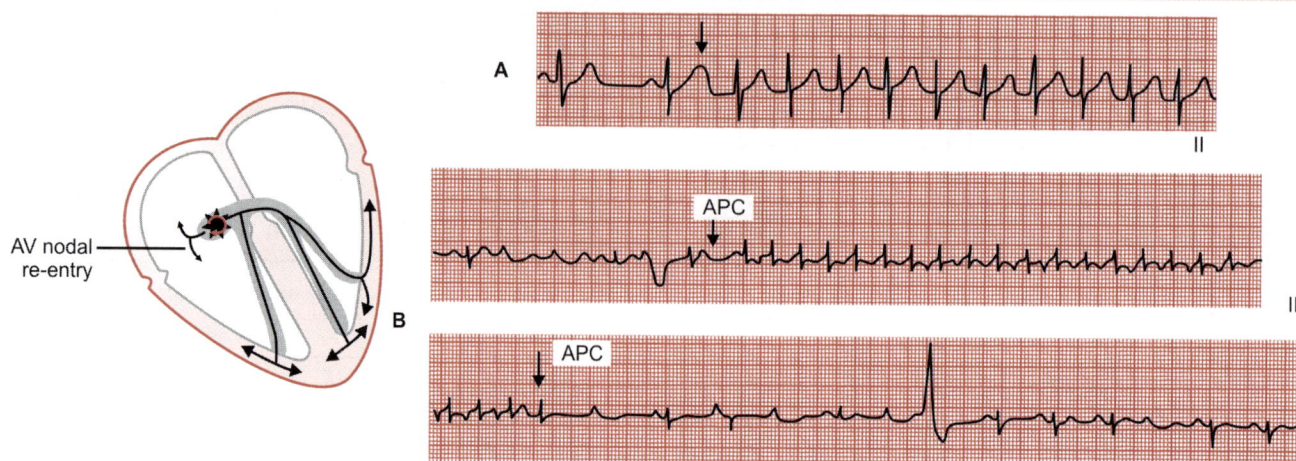

Fig. 34.3: Paroxysmal AV nodal re-entrant tachycardia (AVNRT)

A: Initiation via an atrial premature complex (APC) with prolonged P-R interval (AV nodal delay). The lead II shows first two sinus beats with normal P-R interval. The third complex is conducted with long P-R interval whose P distorts the preceding T wave (arrow and circle). This beat due to prolonged P-R interval initiates AV nodal re-entry leading to establishment of microentry circuit in AV node resulting in tachycardia. Note the QRS complexes have P wave embedded within them

B: Initiation and termination of paroxysmal AV nodal tachycardia. The upper strip (lead II) of ECG shows normal sinus rhythm in the beginning followed by a VPC and sinus beat, which is followed by an interpolated APC that initiates the tachycardia (↓) in which the narrow QRS complexes are followed by inverted P' waves at a rate of 186/min approx. The lower strip (continuous lead II) shows spontaneous termination of tachycardia by an APC having upright P wave (indicated by arrow) and is followed by a compensatory pause and then resumption of normal sinus rhythm. There is another VPC in the middle of strip

complex or barely visible distorting the terminal portion of QRS. This is due to more or less simultaneous activation of both the atria and the ventricles. Sometimes, the initiating event (an APC with long P-R interval) may not be seen on suface ECG, in such a situation, a narrow QRS tachycardia with invisible P′ waves or inverted P′ waves immediately following QRS, forms a diagnostic clue.

6. The conduction ratio (ventricle to atria) is 1:1. The ventricular rate is greater than 100 bpm. A rate of more than 200 bpm suggests AVRT rather than AVNRT.

7. There may be an associated ST-T changes (ST segment depression and T wave inversion) during tachycardia which reverts to normal after restoration of normal sinus rhythm.

2. Atrioventricular Re-entrant Tachycardia (AVRT)

This is less common form of PSVT. It uses a macro-entry circuit through an accessory pathway (bundle of Kent) that bypasses the AV node to form an accessory bridge between atria and the ventricles. AVRT is closely associated with WPW syndrome, a condition fully discussed in Chapter 22. Depending on the pathway in the circuit used by the supraventricular impulses, it is divided into;

*A. **Orthodromic AVRT** (Fig. 34.4A).* This is most common type of AVRT. In this type, the supraventricular impulses are conducted normally through the AV node, then quickly re-enter retrogradely into atria by travelling along the accessory pathway. The atria and ventricles are depolarised sequentially (Fig. 34.4A). As with AVNRT, the cycle in AVRT gets perpetuated itself as the impulses repeatedly travel the same pathway producing rapid ventricular rate with narrow QRS complexes (narrow QRS complex tachycardia).

*B. **Antidromic AVRT** (Fig. 34.4B).* The sequence of conduction of supraventricular impulses is reversed, i.e. they are conducted into the ventricles by an accessory pathway and then retrogradely into the atria through AV node. Rarely, these impulse instead of passing through AV node may get

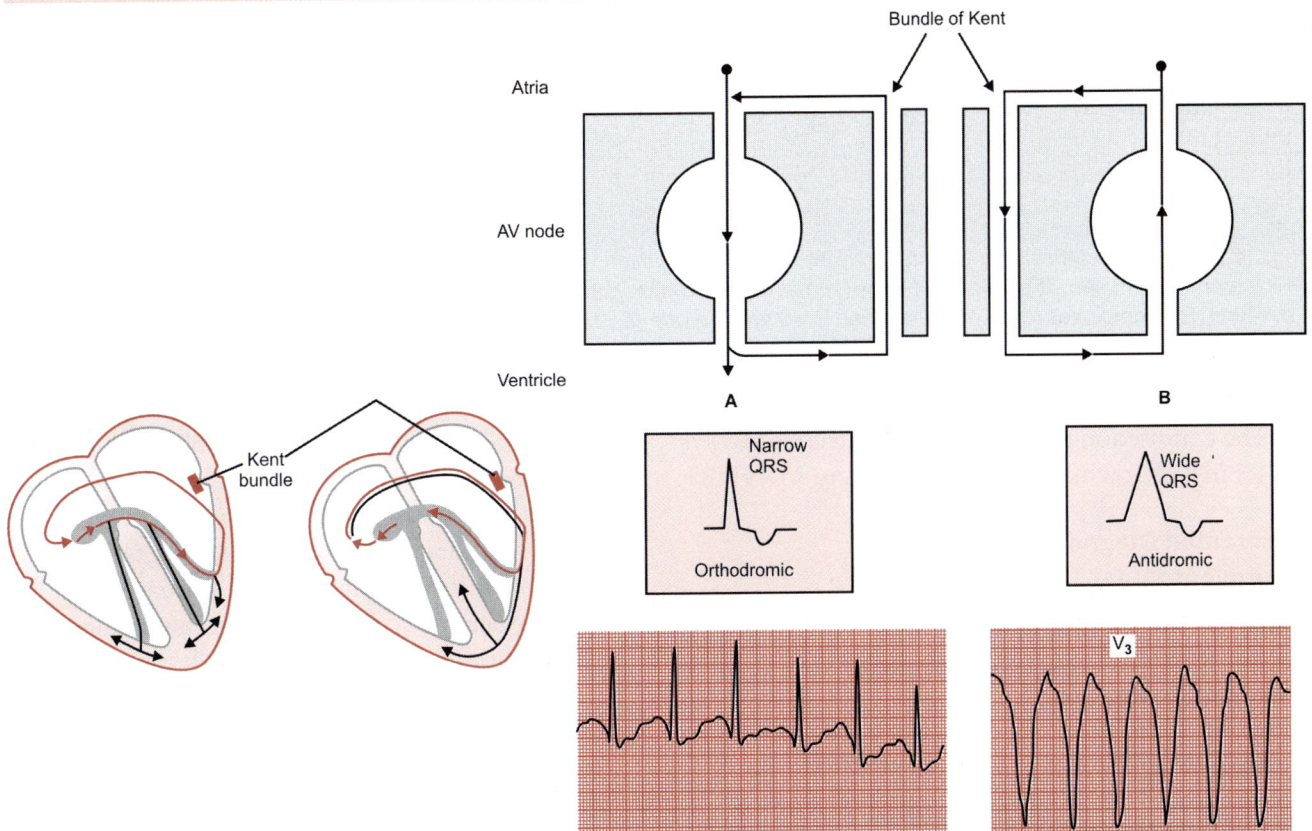

Fig. 34.4: An accessory pathway (Kent bundle) connecting the atria and ventricles in AVRT (diagrammatic representation)
A: Orthodromic AVRT: The impulse travels normally through AV node into ventricles and retrogradely to the atria through an accessory pathway resulting narrow QRS tachycardia
B: Antidromic AVRT. The impulse travels through the accessory pathway to the ventricles and then retrogradely into the atria via AV node resulting in wide QRS tachycardia
The lower half shows rhythm strips illustrating narrow and wide QRS complex tachycardia

conducted through another accessory pathway, if present. Antidromic AVRT is less common cause of PSVT and when present produces aberrantly conducted wide, bizarre QRS complexes simulating ventricular tachycardia.

- *Orthodromic AVRT produces narrow QRS complexes (narrow QRS tachycardia).*
- *Antidromic AVRT produces wide QRS complexes (wide QRS tachycardia) simulating ventricular tachycardia.*

The Electrocardiogram (Fig. 34.5)

1. An atrial premature complex (APC) initiates re-entry process similar to as in AVNRT. The initiating APC instead of having long P-R interval (a characteristic of AVNRT), has either a short or normal P-R interval indicating that AV nodal or intra-atrial delay is not necessary for initiation of AVRT.

2. Retrograde P' (inverted P) waves are commonly observed following the QRS–a sharp contrast to AVNRT in which the inverted P' waves are either burried in QRS or barely visible preceding or following QRS and distorting it.

3. The QRS complexes are narrow and regular in orthodromic AVRT similar to AVNRT. The QRS complexes are wide in antidromic AVRT simulating ventricular tachycardia.

4. The P wave are negative (inverted) in leads II, III and aVF similar to AVNRT.

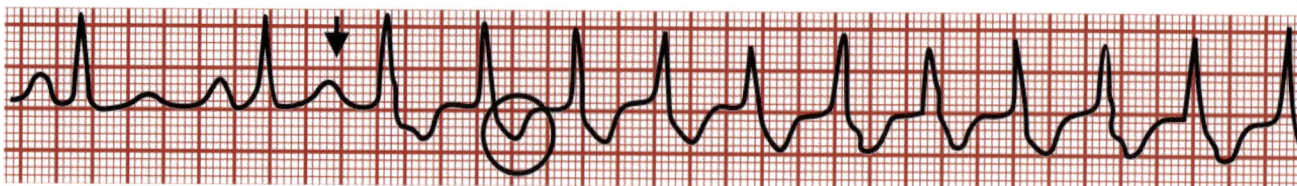

II

Fig. 34.5: The atrioventricular re-entrant tachycardia (AVRT). The lead II shows first two sinus complexes conducted with normal P-R interval of 0.16 sec. The third complex is normal QRS complex with normal P-R interval (arrow) that initiates the tachycardia, i.e. wide QRS complexes followed by inverted P waves at a rate of 214/min

5. The ventricular rate is higher in AVRT than AVNRT. The conduction ratio (ventricle to atria) is always 1:1 in AVRT; while AV blocks can occur in AVNRT.

Differential Diagnosis of Supraventricular Tachycardia

There are certain important clues on the ECG which permit differentiation among various supraventricular tachycardias.

1. Morphology of P Wave

- The P waves during tachycardia if identical to the sinus P waves and occurring with long R-P and short P-R intervals are most likely due to sinus node re-entry.
- If the abnormal P' wave of the first initiating premature atrial beat is the same as the ensuing P' waves of tachycardia, focal automaticity is the likely mechanism.
- Retrograde P (inverted P') waves in leads II, III and aVF generally represent re-entry involving the AV node (AVNRT) or atrioventricular pathway (AVRT).
- The tachycardia without visible P' waves is usually AV nodal re-entrant tachycardia. This is due to simultaneous or near simultaneous atrial and ventricular activation so that P' waves get burried within or get merged with QRS.
- The P' wave contour may at times suggest the mechanism.
  – For example inverted P' waves in leads 1, V_5 or V_6 suggest left sided accessory pathway (Kent bundle). This is because retrograde atrial activation through this pathway will be directed upwards and to the right, i.e. away from the positive pole of leads 1 and V_6.

- In tachycardia due to focal automaticity, the abnormal P' wave is usually well clear of QRS complex and initiating P´ waves and subsequent P waves have similar configuration. The P waves are also well clear of QRS in a reciprocating tachycardia due to WPW syndrome. In such a situation, see the relation between P-R and R-P intervals for diagnosis of the origin of PSVT (see the box). A critical prolongation of P-R interval is frequently associated with a reciprocating tachycardia due to AV nodal re-entry (AVNRT). No such prolongation is necessary for the initiation of focal tachycardia.

Supraventricular tachycardias: P-R and R-P relationship

1. *Short P-R / long R-P relationship.*
   - Atrial tachycardia
   - Atypical AV nodal re-entry
   - Sinus node re-entrant tachycardia
   - AVRT with slowly conducting pathway (permanent junctional reciprocating tachycardia)

2. *Long P-R/Short R-P interval*
   - AV nodal re-entry (AVNRT)
   - Atrioventricular re-entrant tachycardia

---

2. **AV block or AV dissociation.** One of the significant criteria to separate PSVT due to focal automaticity (focal discharge) from reciprocating AV nodal tachycardia is the presence of second degree AV block or AV dissociation. Reciprocating atrioventricular tachycardia (AVRT) due to functional accessory pathway presents rapid heart rate due to 1:1 conduction, because continuous reciprocating circuit producing tachycardia will get termi-

Table 34.1: Differentiation between two common types of paroxysmal supraventricular tachycardias

AV nodal re-entrant tachycardia (AVNRT)	Atrioventricular re-entrant tachycardia (AVRT-orthodromic conduction)
• Re-entry circuit is formed between fast and slow pathways within AV node (micro-re-entry circuit)	• Re-entrant circuit is constituted by the AV node and accessory pathway for reciprocation (macro re-entry circuit)
• P' waves are generally burried within QRS, hence, may not be visible	• Inverted visible P' waves generally follow narrow QRS. At times, they may be burried within QRS
• An atrial premature impulse that conducts with prolonged P-R interval initiates the tachycardia	• A sinus impulse or an atrial premature complex with normal or short P-R interval initiates the tachycardia by producing an atrial echo (reciprocal rhythm)
• QRS alternans (electrical alternans) and/or variation in cycle lengths can occur when rate is very fast	• No such alternation is seen
• Carotid sinus massage can slow the tachycardia slightly prior to its termination or, if termination does not occur, can produce only slight slowing of tachycardia	• There is either no effect or there may be slight slowing
• More common cause of PSVT	• Less common

nated automatically by any event that interrupts this circuit. Therefore, presence of AV block or AV dissociation in supraventricular tachycardia excludes the diagnosis of reciprocating tachycardia due to functional accessory pathway, since a single episode of AV block anywhere in the reciprocating circuit must terminate it.

C. QRS alternans. It is a feature of reciprocating tachycardia. It is probably rate-related phenomenon independent of tachycardia mechanism.

Narrow QRS Complex Tachycardia

The narrow QRS complex indicates normal intraventricular conduction. Therefore, tachycardia with narrow QRS complexes is always supraventricular in origin; may be due to focal automaticity or re-entry through SA node, atria, AV node or bundle of His. The types of atrial tachycardias (ectopic and re-entry) has been discussed in Chapter 32. The idionodal and extrasystolic junctional tachycardias producing narrow QRS complexes have been differentiated in Chapter 33. The other two common paroxysmal supraventricular tachycardias producing narrow QRS have been discussed in the beginning of this chapter. The common salient differentiating features between the two are summarised again in Table 34.1.

Suggested Reading

1. Bar FW, et al: Differential diagnosis of tachycardia with narrow QRS complex (< 0.12 sec). *Am J Cardiol* **54**: 555, 1984.
2. Chan AQ, Pick A: Re-entrant arrhythmias and concealed conduction. *Am Heart J* **97**: 644, 1979.
3. Cranefield PF: Action potentials, afterpotentials and arrhythmias. *Circ Res* **41**: 415, 1977.
4. Fisch C, Knoebel SB: Recognition and therapy of digitalis toxicity. *Prog Cardiovasc Dis* **13**: 71, 1970.
5. Godreyer BN, Bigger JT: Site of re-entry in paroxysmal supraventricular tachycardias. *Circulation* **43**: 679, 1971.
6. Josephson ME, Kastor JA: Supraventricular tachycardias; Mechanisms and management. *Ann Intern Med* **87**: 346, 1977.
7. Lown B, Wyatt NF, Levine HD: Paroxysmal atrial tachycardia with block. *Circulation* **21**: 129, 1960.
8. Obel OA, Camm AJ: Supraventricular tachycardias. ECG diagnosis and anatomy. *Eur Heart J* **18 (Suppl C)**: C2-11, 1997.
9. Pick A, Dominquez P: Nonparoxysmal AV nodal tachycardia. *Circulation* **16**: 102, 1957.
10. Rosen KM: Junctional tachycardia: Mechanism, diagnosis and differential diagnosis and management. *Circulation* **47**: 654, 1973.
11. Singer DH, Ten Erick RE: Pharmacology of cardiac arrhythmias. *Prog Cardiovase Dis* **11**: 488, 1969.
12. Wellen HJ: The value of the ECG in the diagnosis of supraventricular tachycardias. *Eur Heart J* **17 (Suppl C)**: 10-20, 1996.
13. Wit AI, Rosen MR: Electrophysiologic mechanism of cardiac arrhythmias. *Am Heart J* **106**: 798, 1983.

SECTION TEN

35

Ventricular Arrhythmias/ Dysarrhythmias

- *Ventricular premature complex (VPC)—ECG characteristics, types, morphology, origin, conduction, significance and pathogenesis*
- *Ventricular escape rhythm (idioventricular or accelerated idioventricular)—causes, ECG characteristics and significance*
- *Ventricular tachycardia (VT)—predisposing conditions, ECG characteristics and differential diagnosis of wide QRS complex tachycardia*
- *Ventricular flutter—causes, ECG characteristics*
- *Torsades de pointes—causes and ECG characteristics*
- *Ventricular fibrillation—causes and ECG characteristics*
- *Ventricular asystole—causes and ECG characteristics*
- *Dying heart—ECG characteristics of terminal events of the heart*
- *Other electrocardiographic techniques for arrhythmias—oesophageal electrocardiogram, cardiac mapping and signal—averaged ECG*

When pace of the heart is maintained by the ventricles, it is called *ventricular rhythm*. The ventricular rhythm is always abnormal, hence, called ventricular arrhythmia/dysarrhythmia and may manifest in many ways;

1. Ventricular extrasystoles or ectopics
2. Ventricular escape rhythm (idioventricular or accelerated idioventricular)
3. Ventricular tachycardia
4. Ventricular flutter
5. Ventricular parasystole.

VENTRICULAR ECTOPICS OR EXTRASYSTOLES

A premature discharge or an impulse arising from an ectopic ventricular focus is termed as a *'ventricular ectopic'*.

Causes

1. Sometimes, a normal finding.
2. Stress, exercise, etc.
3. Excessive intake of tea, coffee or alcohol.
4. Drugs - digoxin or other arrhythmogenic drugs.
5. Electrolytes disturbances (hypokalaemia or hypomagnesaemia).
6. Coronary artery disease (acute coronary insufficiency).
7. Acute myocardial infarction
8. Cardiomyopathies.
9. Pericardial diseases.
10. Hypoxaemia due to any cause.
11. Reperfusion (e.g. after thrombolytic therapy or angioplasty).
12. Following cardiac surgery or cardiac catheterisation.

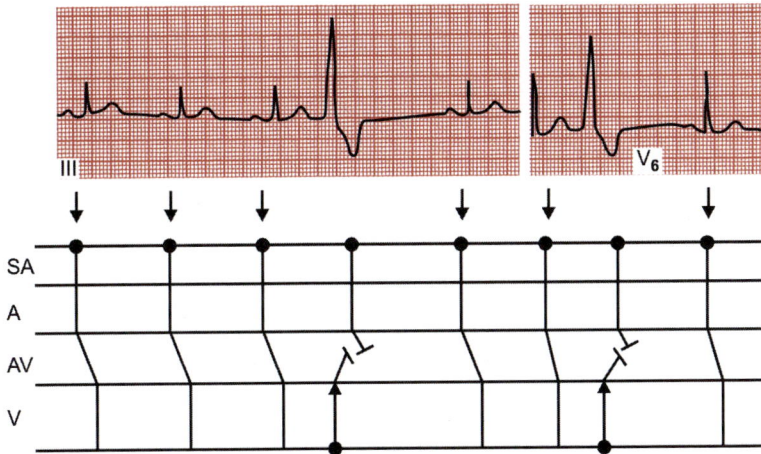

Fig. 35.1: A ventricular premature complex (VPC). The ECG (lead III and V₆) shows one premature ventricular complex in each lead. The ventricular premature complex is followed by a compensatory pause. Each ventricular premature complex (VPC) is followed by a sinus P wave which distorts the ST segment of VPC which becomes notched or peaked (indicated by ↑)

The ladder diagram below shows the site of origin of impulses (denoted by block dots).

SA—sinoatrial level, A—atrial level, AV—AV nodal level, V—ventricular level

13. Metabolic disorders.
14. Congenital cardiac disorders.
15. Poisoning-bites, aluminium phosphide intoxication, organophosphorus toxicity.
16. Idiopathic.

The Electrocardiogram

The ventricular ectopic is a premature beat that arises in the diastolic period of preceding sinus cycle, is recorded earlier than the anticipated sinus beat. The salient features are:

1. The R-R interval is irregular. The premature QRS complexes disturb the regularity of the underlying cardiac rhythm.
2. Morphologically, it is dissimilar to the sinus conducted beat. The QRS complex of an ectopic beat is wide and bizarre. The impulse originates from an ectopic focus in one of the ventricles, spreads abnormally through the ventricles and depolarise them sequentially; it takes longer than normal to do this, so the resulting QRS complex is wide and abnormal shaped. The duration of QRS is > 0.12 sec.
3. The ectopic beats may be unifocal or multifocal. The coupling interval (interval between an ectopic beat and preceding sinus beat) is constant if all the extrasystoles are unifocal. The shape and size of unifocal ectopics is also similar in the same lead. This is because the ectopic beats are, in the same way, related to, precipitated or forced by the preceding sinus beat.

4. The relationship of P wave with QRS complex varies under different situations depending on the timing of the ectopic and is discussed below;
   a) The ventricular ectopic may manifest just before the following sinus discharge. In this situation, the sinus P waves are either recorded after the bizarre QRS complex or may be superimposed on the ST segment of the ectopic (Fig. 35.1).
   b) The ventricular ectopic may manifest at the same time as the following sinus discharge. In such a situation, the P wave gets superimposed on QRS or gets hidden within it, thus, distorts the QRS complex of the ectopic (Fig. 35.2).
   c) The ventricular ectopic, although premature, may manifest late, i.e. after the sinus discharge but before the next sinus impulse reaches the ventricle. There is dissociation of sinus P wave from QRS of an ectopic, hence, P is recorded just before the bizarre QRS of an ectopic. The

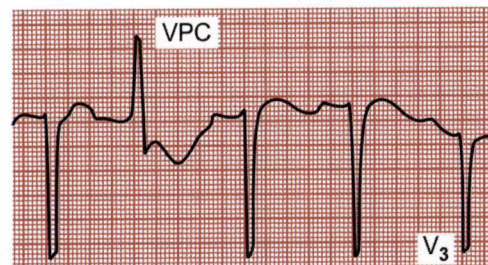

Fig. 35.2: The ventricular premature complex (VPC) with no visible P wave (P is completely burried within QRS due to near synchronisation of atria and ventricles

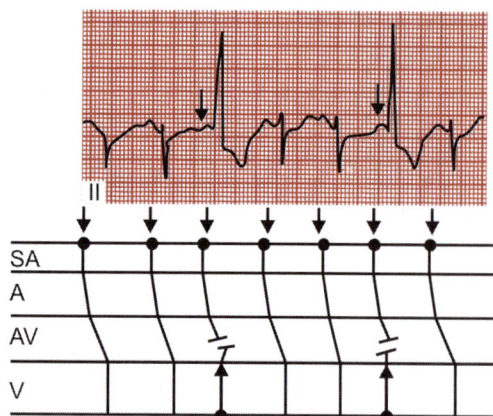

Fig. 35.3: End-diastolic VPC. The electrocardiogram (lead II) shows two ventricular extrasystoles which have discharged late in end-diastole, i.e. occur just after the following sinus discharge. The P wave with short P-R interval is thus recorded just before the wide, bizarre QRS complex of VPCs.

Note: It can be confused with sinus beat with aberrant conduction but normal P wave with short P-R interval favours end-diastolic VPC. Normal sinus beat with aberrant conduction will have normal P wave and normal P-R interval followed by QRS conforming to the pattern of one of bundle branch block. Below ladder diagram shows site of origin of impulses. SA—sinoatrial level, A—atrial level, AV—AV nodal level, V—ventricular level

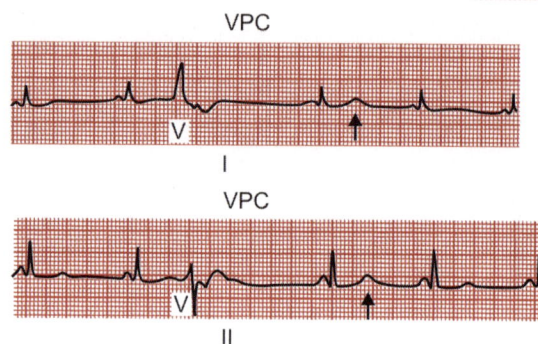

Fig. 35.4: The ventricular ectopics showing retrograde atrial activation (P′ wave). The leads I and II show a ventricular ectopic (wide QRS with a long compensatory pause) with retrograde P′ wave (inverted P′ follows QRS) indicating retrograde atrial activation. In addition, there is post-extrasystolic effect on the T wave of next sinus beat, i.e. the T wave of next sinus beat following the VPC is large and upright (↑) as compared to T wave of other normal sinus beats

P-R interval is short. This is called in end-diastolic ventricular ectopic (Fig. 35.3).

d) Occasionally, in the presence of sinus bradycardia or when ventricular ectopic is too premature to discharge long before the next scheduled sinus beat, consequently, the ectopic impulse reaches retrogradely to the AV node and atria earlier than they have been activated by the sinus beat. This ectopic impulse may reach the sinus node and delay its discharge (Fig. 35.4). The wide and abnormal QRS of ventricular ectopic is followed by a premature and inverted P wave due to retrograde conduction. This ventricular ectopic with retrograde conduction differs from nodal ectopic with retrograde conduction by wide and bizarre QRS complex.

In all the above described instances, the sinus and ectopic impulses meet and interfere with each other at the level of AV node, i.e. the sinus impulse is not allowed to pass to the ventricles and ventricular impulse is not allowed to pass to atria, hence, P wave may precede, gets superimposed or follow a wide QRS.

5. **The compensatory pause:** A long interval seen between the VPC and the next sinus beat is called '*compensatory pause*'. A compensatory pause is commonly observed following an VPC because VPC is unable to penetrate the AV node retrogradely and sinus discharge remains undisturbed, i.e. the next sinus beat occurs on schedule. The compensatory pause is assessed by measuring the interval between two sinus beats containing the VPC and is compared with the normal cycle length (baseline-R-R interval). The pause is said to be complete or full (Fig. 35.5) if the distance between two sinus beats that surround the VPC is exactly twice the normal cycle length (R-R interval). It is said to be incomplete if the interval between two sinus beats containing a VPC is less than the twice the normal cycle length (See Fig. 30.4 concealed conduction)

6. The pre-ectopic interval (interval between sinus beat and preceding ectopic beat) is shorter than post-ectopic interval (interval between an ectopic and next sinus beat) and is constant for all unifocal VPCs.

The pre-ectopic and post-ectopic intervals are constant and fixed for unifocal VPCs

7. **Secondary ST-T changes:** The ST segment and T wave slope is always in the opposite direction to the QRS complex of an ectopic. This is due to the

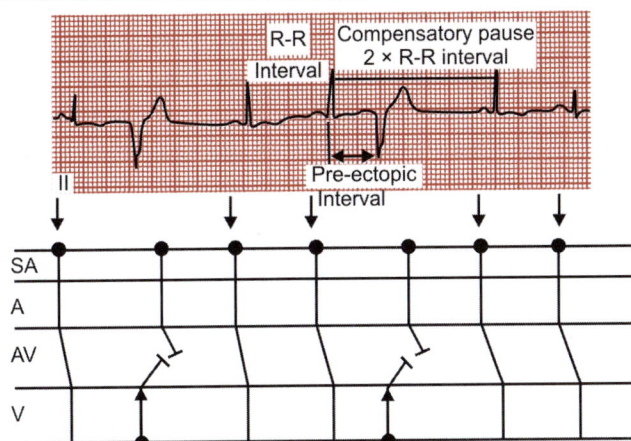

Fig. 35.5: Full compensatory pause following a VPC. The electrocardiogram (lead II) shows unifocal premature ventricular complexes There is a fixed coupling interval between a sinus conducted beat and ventricular premature complex (VPC). The compensatory pause between two sinus beats containing a VPC is full because it is equal to 2 × P-P or R-R intervals as labelled. The sinus (upright P) falls on T wave of ectopic complex due to which T wave appears peaked because ectopic ventricular discharge occurred earlier than the expected sinus discharge.

The ladder diagram is given to show the pathway of conduction of both sinus and ectopic beats (block dots indicate the site of discharge). SA = SA node, A = Atria, AV = AV node, V = Ventricles

fact that abnormal ventricular depolarisation is followed by an abnormal repolarisation. When the QRS complex of a VPC is dominantly upright, then there is associated ST segment depression with T wave inversion and, when it is dominantly negative, then ST segment is minimally elevated with concavity upwards and T is also upright. These changes are secondary to the abnormal depolarisation, and *per se* do not indicate myocardial ischaemia and are of no significance. These associated ST-T changes are similar to that seen in bundle branch blocks or fascicular blocks, etc.

Variants of Ventricular Premature Complexes (VPCs)

1. *An end-diastolic VPC:* It has already been discussed. It has a normal P wave that occurs in time, is just before the premature ectopic QRS complex with a short P-R interval. This late occurred VPC discharges after the atria have been depolarised by the sinus impulse but before the sinus impulse reaches the ventricle (Fig. 35.3).

2. *Ventricular fusion (Dressler's) beat:* When a sinus conducted impulse and a ventricular ectopic impulse reach the ventricles at the same time and both take part in depolarisation of the ventricles, a *fusion complex/beat* results. Therefore, the resulting QRS represents a blend or fusion of the normal and ectopic QRS morphologies. A fusion complex, in fact, is wider than normal QRS complex but narrower than a VPCs. The morphology of fusion complexes is highly variable depending on the part of depolarisation done by a normal sinus impulse and a part of depolarisation done by ventricular ectopic impulse. For diagnosis of ventricular fusion beat, the lead being analysed must show both normal and ectopic QRS complexes (Read Chapter 41 on fusion beats).

3. *An interpolated VPC* (Fig. 35.6): A VPC interposed or sandwitched between two normal sinus beats which does not significantly interrupt the underlying mechanism is called an *interpolated VPC*. The pre-ectopic and post-ectopic intervals are equal, hence, there is no compensatory pause. The characteristics of an interpolated beat are given in the box.

Characteristics of Interpolated VPCs

- They occur during slow sinus rhythm.
- The ectopic is sandwitched between two sinus beats and there is no compensatory pause.
- The R-R interval containing the interpolated VPC is slightly a longer than the R-R interval between two sinus beats (basic R-R interval).
- The sinus beat following an interpolated beat may show aberrant conduction due to partial refractoriness of AV node or may show prolonged P-R interval due to concealed conduction.

4. *Ventricular premature complexes (VPCs) with R on T phenomenon* (Fig. 35.7): The normal T wave represents the end part of ventricular repolarisation, the period during which the ventricles are still excitable, therefore, any ectopic beat falling on or coming near to T wave of the preceding beat is called 'A VPC with R on T phenomenon'. These VPCs predispose to the development of ventricular tachycardia or ventricular fibrillation, hence,

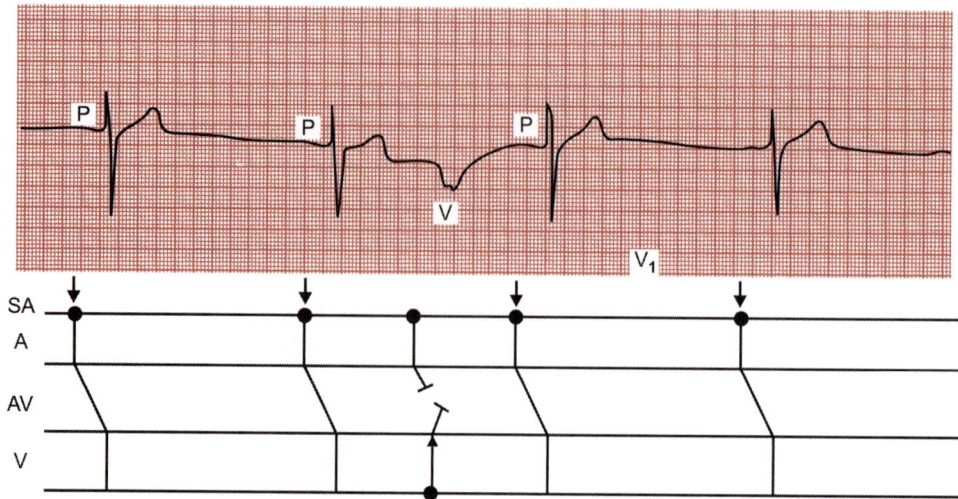

Fig. 35.6: An interpolated ventricular premature complex (VPC). The lead V_1 of the electrocardiogram shows sinus bradycardia at a rate of 46 bpm. There is an interpolated VPC in the middle of the strip. This is sandwiched between two normal sinus complexes and is not followed by a compensatory pause. Interpolated ventricular extrasystoles are mostly associated with sinus bradycardia

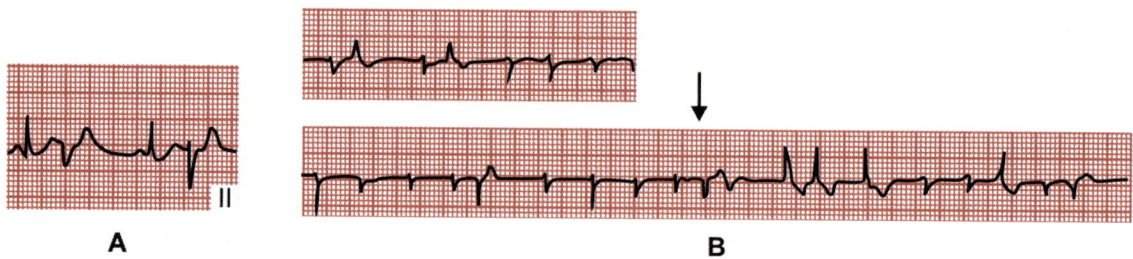

Fig. 35.7: A: Ventricular premature complexes (VPCs) with R on T phenomenon. The electrocardiogram (rhythm strip lead II shows two sinus conducted beats each followed by a ventricular premature complex (wide bizarre QRS complex) superimposed on the descending limb of T wave. These VPCs are consdered pre-malignant. **B:** R on T ventricular ectopic heralds the development of nonsustained ventricular tachycardia (↓). The electrocardiogram (continuous monitored lead II) shows two ventricular ectopics with R on T phenomenon (top strip). In the lower strip, there is an ectopic with different orientation after 4 normal beats, then there are again 4 normal beats followed by 5 VPCs in succession (nonsustained VT) in which first two have negative QRS and next 3 positive QRS deflection, which terminates spontaneously followed by frequent bidirectional VPCs seen towards the end of the strip

termed as 'premalignant' VPCs. These VPCs have shorter coupling intervals and almost invariably occur in the setting of acute catastrophic event in the heart such as acute myocardial infarction. It is further stressed that a coupling interval is indicative of refractoriness of myocardium to a VPC; if it is shortened, then, the heart becomes vulnerable to further excitation.

5. *Unifocal ventricular premature complexes (VPCs).* The VPCs that arise from the same ectopic focus, pass through the same pathway for conduction and produce QRS complexes of similar confi-guration in the same lead recorded at the same time are called *'unifocal ventricular premature complexes'* (Fig. 35.8).

6. *Multifocal (multiform) ventricular premature complexes (VPCs).* These VPCs take origin from different ectopic foci, but sometimes take origin from a single focus and are conducted to the ventricles through different pathways or routes. Therefore, the complexes are variable in configuration in the same lead recorded at the same time (Fig. 35.9).

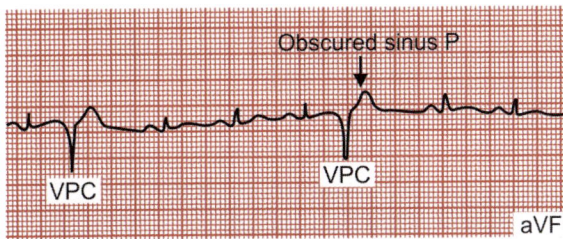

Fig. 35.8: Unifocal ventricular premature complexes (VPCs) or beats (VPBs). The electrocardiogram (lead aVF) shows two VPCs with same configuration and orientation indicating their origin from a single focus in one of the ventricles. It is difficult to ascertain the ventricle for their origin on a single lead

7. *Ventricular couplet or pair* (Fig. 35.10): A ventricular couplet or pair means two VPCs in a row, may be uniform or multiform. These VPCs may have similar orientation (unidirectional) or opposite orientation (bidirectional).

8. *Ventricular triplet* (Fig. 35.11): A ventricular triplet means three VPCs (uniform or multiform) in a row. By definition, three or more consecutive VPCs are termed as *'ventricular tachycardia'* (one normal followed by three successive VPCs).

9. *Ventricular bigeminy:* When a normal sinus beat alternates with a ventricular premature complex (VPC) in a repeating fashion whereby every second beat is a VPC, is called *'ventricular bigeminy'*. It is commonly seen in digitalis toxicity. The interval between a normal sinus beat and a VPC is called a coupling interval which remains fixed if VPCs are unifocal and are recorded in the same lead (Fig. 35.12). When an VPC alternates with a normal complex/beat for two or more times successively, it constitutes a ventricular bigeminy rhythm.

The rule of bigeminy: It states that a ventricular ectopic beat tends to follow a long R-R interval. This follows from the fact that a long R-R interval (long cycle length) precipitates an ensuing extrasystole. This phenomenon is best seen during irregular rhythms, i.e. sinus arrhythmias or atrial fibrillation. The compensatory pause of an ectopic or extrasystole,

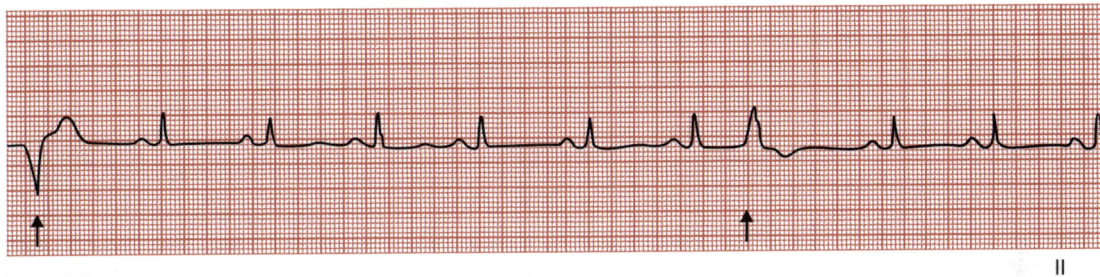

Fig. 35.9: Multiform ventricular premature complexes (VPCs). The electrocardiogram (lead II) shows two VPCs (indicated by ↑) having different orientations and configurations indicating either the different sites of origin or there is single site of origin with different mode of intraventricular conduction

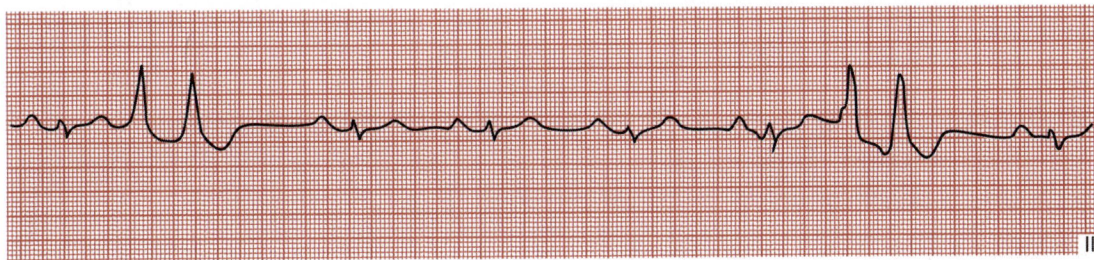

Fig. 35.10: A ventricular couplet. The electrocardiogram (lead II) was recorded from a patient of RHD who was on digitalis therapy. It shows:
   i. First degree AV block: The P-R interval of sinus conducted beat is 0.28 sec
   ii. Ventricular couplets (2 pairs): Two pairs of ventricular complexes (two successive ventricular premature complexes in a pair) are seen
     Both these findings on ECG suggest digitalis toxicity

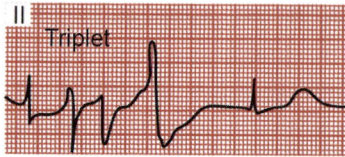

Fig. 35.11: A ventricular triplet or non-sustained ventricular tachycardia or ventricular quadrigeminy. The electrocardiogram (lead II a portion) shows ventricular triplet (3 VPCs in succession), each VPC has different configuration. The ECG was recorded from a patient with digitalis toxicity with hypokalaemia. In electrocardiography, 3 VPCs in succession is also called non-sustained ventricular tachycardia (VT). It can also be called ventricular quadrigeminy (one sinus beat followed by 3 successive VPCs). Out of all these terms, non-sustained VT is the conventional term to be used from diagnostic and therapeutic point of view

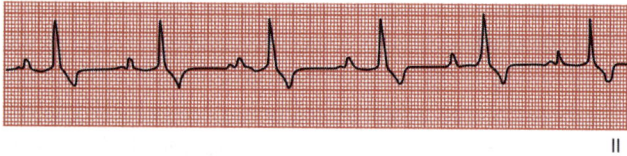

Fig. 35.12: Ventricular bigeminy recorded from a patient with dilated cardiomyopathy. The lead II of the electrocardiogram shows two types of QRS complexes. A short narrow QRS complex preceded by P wave indicates normal sinus complex. Each such complex is followed by a large and wide QRS complex without visible P wave and inverted T wave; that is ventricular premature complex (VPC). Alternation of normal QRS and VPC in a regular fashion suggests ventricular bigeminy rhythm

in turn, constitutes an another long R-R interval which tends to precipitate a further ectopic. This process becomes self-perpetuating resulting in the bigeminy rhythm (Fig. 35.13). All ventricular ectopics are not governed by this rule.

All ventricular premature complexes do not follow the rule of bigeminy.

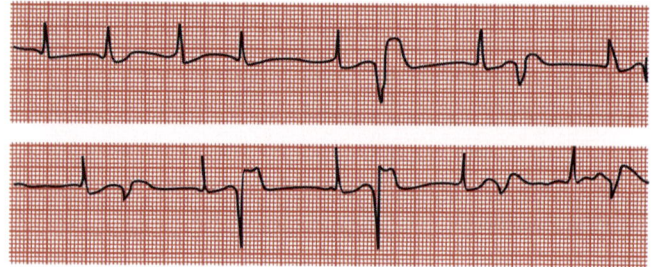

Fig. 35.13: Rule of ventricular bigeminy. The electrocardiogram (lead II) demonstrates 'rule of bigeminy'. Note the following characteristics;
1. *Sinus arrhythmia.* The first four beats in the upper strip show sinus arrhythmia characterised by varying R-R intervals
2. *Rule of bigeminy.* Between the 4th and 5th sinus beats there is a long R-R interval which precipitates the ventricular ectopic (↓)which perpetuates in the form of bigeminy rhythm seen at the end of upper and the whole of lower strip

10. *Ventricular trigeminy, quadrigeminy and pentageminy* (Figs 35.14 to 35.16): In trigeminy, every third complex is a uniform VPC and the same pattern is repeated in a rhythmic fashion (Fig. 35.14). In electrocardiography, one normal beat followed by two successive VPCs is also called ventricular trigeminy (Fig. 35.15) but better term is ventricular complete or pair.

In quadrigeminy, every fourth beat is a uniform VPC, occurring in rhythmic and cyclic fashion (Fig. 35.16). If one sinus beat is followed by three successive VPCs, then it may also be called *ventricular quadrigeminy,* or a ventricular triplet or non-sustained ventricular tachycardia, the last name is frequently used in electrocardiography due to its clinical significance.

In ventricular pentageminy (Fig. 35.17), every fifth complex is a uniform VPC and pattern is repeated cyclically.

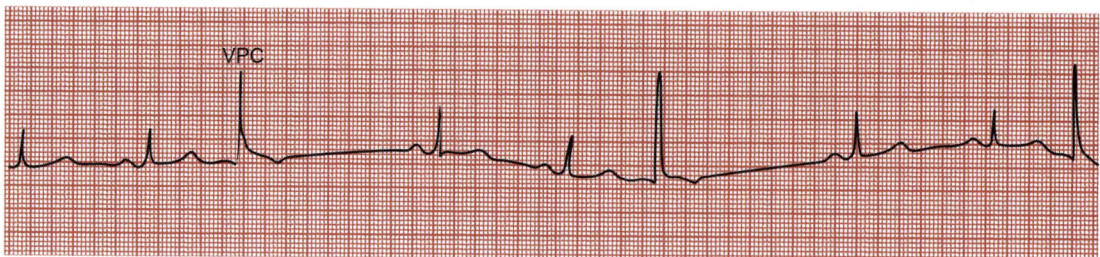

Fig. 35.14: Ventricular trigeminy: The leads II shows two sinus beats followed by a VPC in rhythmic fashion constituting a trigeminy rhythm

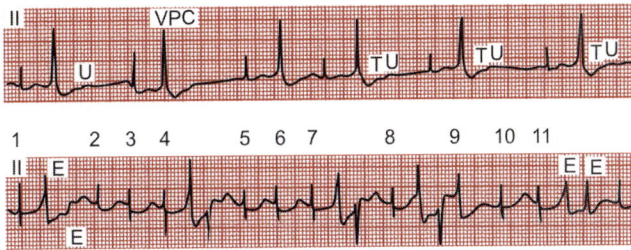

Fig. 35.15: Both ventricular bigeminy and trigeminy recorded from a patient with digitalis toxicity and hypokalaemia (serum K+ 2.3 mEq/L). The electrocardiogram (lead II) shows;
  i. Upper strip—There is regular bigeminy rhythm (one sinus beat alternates with a VPC regularly)
  ii. Lower strip—Ventricular trigeminy is revealed by first sinus conducted beat of the strip followed by two VPCs of different orientation—one with upward deflection and next with downward deflection called bidirectional VPCs. These bidirectional VPCs are seen following 4th, 7th and 8th sinus conducted beats. There is evidence of hypokalaemia by prolongation of Q-Tc interval and widening of T wave due to superimposition of U and P wave of next sinus beat (labelled as TUP waves) seen in 9th and 10th sinus beats. Again the 11th beat is followed by a coupled (two successive VPCs of same orientation) also called *trigeminy*.

All these features on ECG suggest digitalis induced arrhythmias potentiated by hypokalaemia

11. *Ventricular parasystole* (Read Chapter 38 on Parasystole)

Morphology of Ventricular Premature Complexes

Premature ventricular complexes (VPCs) may have an identical shape or may have different shapes in a given ECG lead.

1. ***Unimorphic or monomorphic VPCs***: Uniform or identical VPCs are called *unimorphic or monomorphic*. They may arise continuously from a single focus (unifocal) or may result from re-entry mechanism (Fig. 35.18).

2. ***Multimorphic or polymorphic ventricular premature complexes (VPCs)***: Premature ventricular complexes of varying configurations are called *multimorphic or polymorphic*. They may arise from multiple foci (multifocal), or more commonly, from a single focus but may get conducted through different pathways to depolarise the ventricles resulting in different QRS configurations (Fig. 35.19).

Therefore, in electrocardiography, the term monomorphic or polymorphic rather than unifocal or multifocal are appropriate terms to be used while describing VPCs in a given lead.

SECTION TEN

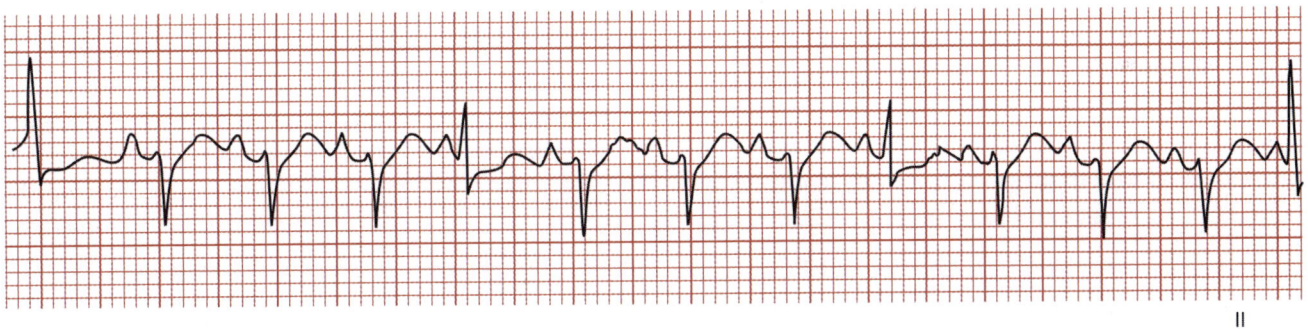

Fig. 35.16: Ventricular quadrigeminy rhythm. The electrocardiogram (rhythm strip lead II) shows three successive sinus beats followed by an end-diastolic interpolated VPC regularly constituting a regular rhythm called quadrigeminy rhythm

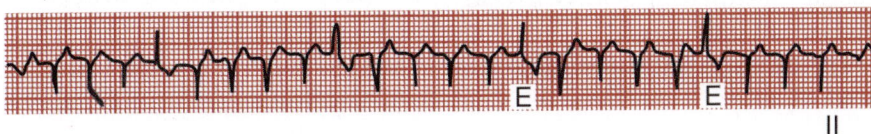

Fig. 35.17: Ventricular pentageminy. The electrocardiogram (lead II) shows a ventricular ectopic beat (E) occurring after every 4 sinus conducted beats regularly forming a pentageminy rhythm

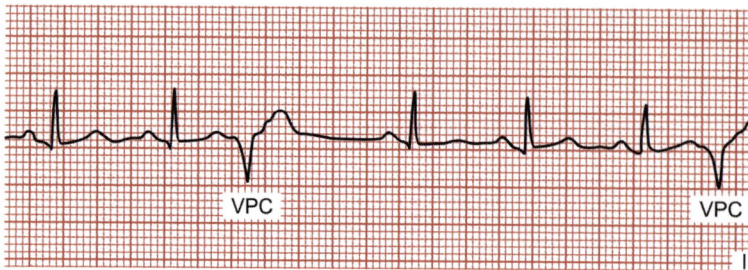

Fig. 35.18: Monomorphic ventricular premature complexes (VPCs). The electrocardiogram (rhythm strip—lead I) shows two VPCs having same configuration and direction indicating either arising from a single focus or from different foci with same mode of conduction or by re-entry mechanism. There is a fixed coupling interval between sinus beats and VPCs favouring re-entry as their mechanism of origin

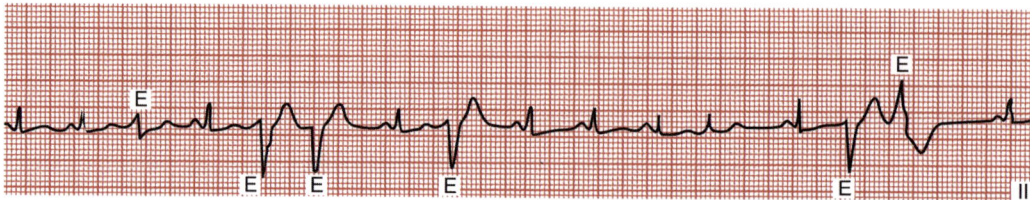

Fig. 35.19: Polymorphic ventricular premature complexes (VPCs). The electrocardiogram (rhythm strip lead II) shows ventricular premature complexes having different configuration and some have different direction in the same lead. The VPCs are labelled as 'E'. The second sinus beat in the beginning is followed by a nodal ectopic (E). The third sinus beats of the strip is followed by a couplet which is uni-directional, i.e. both VPCs have similar morphology and same direction. At the end also, a sinus conducted beat is followed by a couplet—the two successive VPCs having different morphology and opposite direction—bidirectional VPCs. AVPC is seen in the middle of strip.

Note: The different shapes of VPCs must be demonstrated in the single lead before labelling them as polymorphic

Origin of Ventricular Premature Complexes

For origin of a VPC, see the configuration of QRS complex in right oriented leads (V_1 or V_2) and left oriented leads (V_5 or V_6).

1. A right ventricular VPC: It arises from the right ventricle, has rS configuration similar to normal sinus conducted beat in lead V_1 or V_2 but the complex is wide (> 0.12 sec) and bizarre. It will have a QRS configuration in leads V_5-V_6 which is similar to the normal sinus beat in these leads, but the complex will be wider (>0.12 sec) and bizarre (Fig. 35.20).

2. Left ventricular VPCs: Orientation of VPCs arising from the left ventricle is just reverse to that described above in the right ventricular VPCs. The VPC will register qR or qRs complex resembling normal complex of V_5 or V_6 in lead V_1 or V_2 due to anterior orientation, and rS complex with deep S wave in lead V_5 or V_6 resembling normal pattern of V_1. The VPC will have wider (>0.12 sec) and bizarre conduction (Fig. 35.21).

Mechanism: The VPCs arising from left ventricle situated posterior to right ventricle are oriented

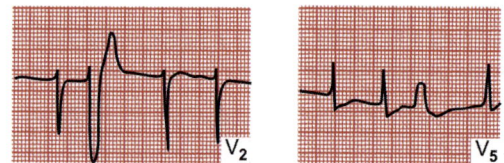

Fig. 35.20: Right ventricular premature complexes. The electrocardiographic leads show;
  i. Lead V_2: The configuration of a VPC resembles the normal sinus QRS except that it is wide (> 0.12 sec) and bizarre
  ii. Lead V_5: The VPC shows wide slurred R wave. The major deflection of VPC and sinus conducted beats is positive, i.e. same orientation

anteriorly towards leads V_1 and V_2, hence, qR complex (left ventricular epicardial complex) will be seen in these leads and consequent to it, there will be right ventricular epicardial complex (rS complex) of VPCs in leads V_5-V_6 representing the left ventricle. Reverse will happen in case VPCs arise from the right ventricle.

VPCs with posterior orientation (rS complex in V_1 and qR complex in V_5) originate from right ventricle; while VPCs with anterior orientation (qR in V_1 and rS in V_5) arise from the left ventricle.

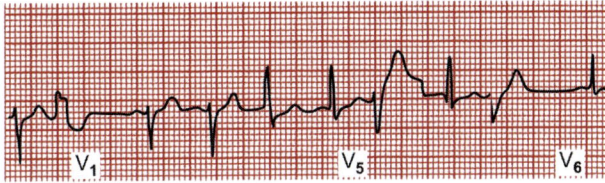

Fig. 35.21: Left ventricular premature complexes. The electrocardiographic leads show;
   i. Lead V_1. The configuration of a VPC in lead V_1 resembles normal pattern of V_5-V_6 (major positive deflection) but is wide and bizarre due to delayed activation of right ventricle.
   ii. Leads V_5 and V_6. The ectopic has right ventricular pattern (rS) resembling normal pattern in V_1 due to anterior orientation but the complex is wide (>0.12 sec) and bizarre

Conduction of Ventricular Premature Complexes (VPCs)

In all instances, where the P wave precedes, gets superimposed or follows QRS complex, the sinus and extrasystolic impulses meet and interfere with each other in the AV node. The sinus impulse is prevented from passing to the ventricles and the ventricular impulse is prevented from passing to the atria by AV node which acts as a formidable barrier. At times, the ventricular end-diastolic ectopic may reach the ventricles at the same time as the sinus impulse, thereby, resulting in a fusion complex or beat which shows the summation effect of both impulses.

Ventricular premature complexes (VPCs) with retrograde conduction: The VPCs may be conducted in retrograde fashion into the bundle of His and AV node, delaying or blocking the antegrade conduction of next sinus beat. They may get conducted to the atria in retrograde fashion producing an inverted P (P') waves in leads II, III and aVF. They may invade the sinus node, depolarise it, and reset its timing or they may just depolarise the atria without penetrating it or resetting its timing. If a SA node is penetrated and reset in timing, a full compensatory pause does not follow the VPC, but if SA node is not penetrated and its discharge is not interfered with, then a full compensatory pause follows the VPC (see the Fig. 30.5). A full compensatory pause is exactly twice the normal P-P or R-R intervals (2 × R-R or P-P interval).

Ventricular premature complexes with concealed conduction: Retrograde invasion of AV node by a VPC can result in delay in antegrade conduction of next sinus beat or total failure of conduction of the impulse. Since retrograde invasion of AV node is not recorded electrocardiographically but is recognised by its effect on subsequent electrocardiographic events, the phenomenon is called 'concealed conduction'. This is manifested by prolongation of P-R interval resembling first degree AV block or P wave is blocked, i.e. not followed by QRS complex resembling second degree AV block. These are actually *pseudo–AV block* due to concealed retrograde AV conduction.

Significance of Ventricular Ectopics

These are among the most common arrhythmias that occur in patients with or without heart disease. Although, isolated VPCs, may occasionally, occur in normal persons without heart disease, their presence should always be viewed with suspicion.

The VPCs are always significant if associated with heart ailment. Multifocal or polymorphic VPCs and VPCs occurring in couplets are always abnormal and indicate a serious myocardial disease. Unifocal or monomorphic VPCs are indicative of heart disease if;
a) They occur frequently (>10/min).
b) They follow bigeminal pattern or show R on T phenomenon.
c) They occur in setting of a heart disease.
d) They occur in patients above 40 years of age.
e) They are precipitated by excercise (exercise induced VPCs).

Frequent ventricular ectopics especially those arising in pairs or showing R on T phenomenon, often herald the onset of ventricular tachycardia or ventricular fibrillation. Therefore, a useful guide to decide about the benign or dangerous nature of the VPCs is to follow them, as subsequent evolution makes them more evident. Ventricular ectopics complicating myocardial infarction worsen its prognosis.

Note : Digitalis toxicity is the most common cause of VPCs especially of bigeminal pattern in a heart patient receiving digitalis, therefore, it must be stopped in such patients if they occur. It is clarified that digitalis will, rarely, if ever, cause VPCs of bigeminal pattern in a normal heart.

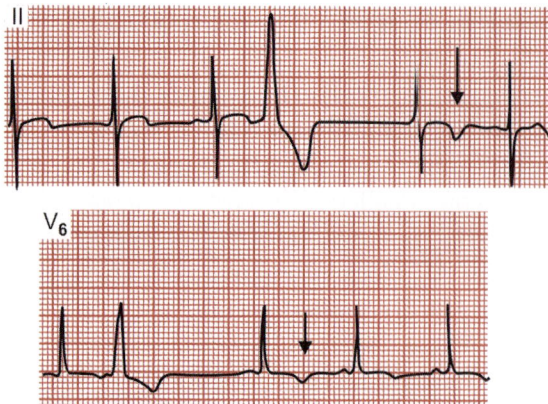

Fig. 35.22: Post-extrasystolic T wave change. The ECG (leads II and V$_6$) shows;

i. Lead II shows first three sinus complexes with biphasic T wave. The third sinus complex is followed by a VPC (wide QRS and inverted T) having a long compensatory pause. The next beat (beat following the VPC) shows a deep symmetric T wave inversion - post-extrasystolic T wave change (↓)

ii. The lead V$_6$ shows normal sinus rhythm with low inverted T waves indicating lateral wall ischaemia. A VPC (wide QRS and inverted T) falls on the ascending limb of inverted T of first sinus beat. The next sinus beat following the VPC shows wider and deeper T wave inversion as a post-extrasystole change (↓)

Premature Ventricular Complexes Originating from the Site of Myocardial Infarction

In the presence of myocardial infarction, VPCs may show some typical features of infarction pattern especially a qR or QR complex. When myocardial infarction cannot be diagnosed on the ECG such as in the presence of LBBB or WPW syndrome, then the presence of premature ventricular complexes of qR or QR (but not QS) configuration may confirm the diagnosis. The VPCs having qR configuration are presumed to be arising from the infarcted area in a setting of acute myocardial infarction.

Post-extrasystolic T wave change of following sinus beat (Fig. 35.22)

Occasionally, the T wave of next sinus conducted beat following a VPC becomes inverted or diminished in amplitude -once called *'The poor man's excercise test'*. It is not extrasystole as such which causes T wave inversion but is rather due to the pause which it produces. Although the ST-T changes following extrasystoles are commonly seen in patients with

coronary artery disease, but are nonspecific findings and, therefore, are of no clinical significance.

IDIOVENTRICULAR RHYTHMS

The intrinsic rhythm of the ventricles is called an *idioventricular rhythm.* Normally this rhythm is suppressed by the rhythm from the higher centres, hence, when present is always abnormal. It is usually an escape rhythm and may accelerate its rate due to an enhanced automaticity.

Electrocardiographic Manifestations

Depending on the heart rate; idioventricular rhythm manifests in following ways;

1. Idioventricular escape rhythm (rate 15-45 bpm)
2. Accelerated idioventricular rhythm (rate 45-100 bpm)

Idioventricular Escape Rhythm

It is a very slow escape rhythm originating in the ventricle at a rate of 15-45 bpm. It is actually an inherent ventricular rhythm (ventricle acts as a pacemaker). The appearance of this escape rhythm occurs when the higher pacemakers, i.e. SA node, atria or AV node become dysfunctional. This rhythm invariably occurs in patients with complete heart block (Read Chapter 41 on Escape Rhythm) or patients with structural nodal disease.

Causes

1. Acute myocardial infarction
2. Cardiomyopathy
3. Myocarditis
4. Drugs (e.g. digitalis)
5. Trauma
6. Dying heart
7. Following reperfusion.

The Electrocardiogram

1. The ventricular rate (i.e. R-R interval) is regular.
2. The ventricular rate is between 15-45 bpm.
3. The QRS complexes are wide, bizarre and all look alike.
4. The P waves may or may not be present. The presence of upright normal P waves indicate

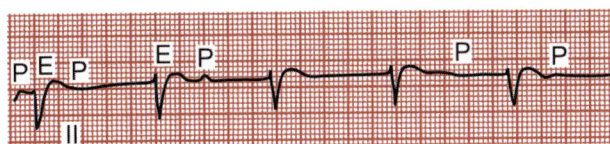

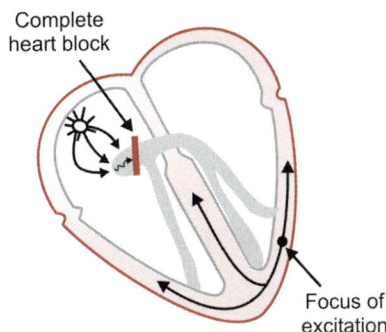

Fig. 35.23: Ventricular escape rhythm in complete heart block. The electrocardiogram shows P waves which have no relation to QRS (independent atrial rhythm). The escape beats have wide QRS (labelled as E) and occur at a rate of 42/min independently (idioventricular rhythm)

another independent supraventricular pacemaker (dual pacemaker rhythm) and supraventricular impulses are not able to reach or penetrate the ventricles. The two independent pacemakers rhythm (supraventricular and ventricular) are commonly seen in complete heart block. The P-P interval is regular like R-R interval but P waves are produced at higher rate than QRS, hence, the P waves are unrelated to QRS (Fig. 35.23). The absence of P waves suggest that higher pacemakers are not firing.

ACCELERATED IDIOVENTRICULAR RHYTHM

It is an ectopic ventricular rhythm with a rate of 45-100 bpm (usual rate is 70-80 bpm). It is faster than normal ventricular escape rhythm (15-45 bpm) but slower than ventricular tachycardia (> 100 bpm). Usualy the heart rate in this rhythm hovers within 10 bpm of sinus rate. This is the reason why cardiac rhythm is passed back and forth between two competing pacemakers (SA node and the ventricle). At times, it resembles slow ventricular tachycardia from which it has to be differentiated (Table 35.1) because an accelerated idioventricular rhythm is considered benign while slow ventricular tachycardia is not necessarily benign and may require urgent management.

Mechanism

Many characteristics of an accelerated idioventricular rhythm favour an enhanced automaticity of ventricular pacemaker as the responsible mechanism. Occasionally, the ectopic mechanism also can begin after a VPC or the ventricular focus can simply accelerate its rate sufficiently to overtake sinus rhythm.

Causes

1. Fever and acute carditis
2. Acute myocardial infarction
3. After reperfusion (following thrombolytic therapy or angioplasty)
4. Cardiomyopathy
5. Digitalis toxicity
6. May be observed during cardiac resuscitation.

The Electrocardiogram (Figs 35.24A and B, 35.25)

1. The QRS complexes are wide and all look alike. The ventricular rhythm is mostly regular but can be irregular, and occasionally shows sudden doubling due to presence of an exit block.
2. The ventricular rate is between 45-100 bpm. Because of slow heart rate, capture beats are common.
3. It emerges as a result of slight slowing of the sinus rate. The onset of arrhythmia is gradual via a fusion complex, and occurs when the rate of ventricular pacemaker exceeds the sinus rate because of sinus slowing or SA or AV blocks. The termination is also gradual via a fusion complex, and occurs when sinus rhythm accelerates or the ectopic ventricular rhythm decelerates. This is due to the fact that the ventricular rate in this rhythm is just around 10 bpm higher than sinus rate, hence, cardiac rhythm passes back and forth between the two competing pacemaker sites (SA node and the ventricle) through a fusion beat. A fusion beat occurs in transition during onset and offset of an accelerated idioventricular rhythm, i.e. from and to sinus rhythm–a characteristic electrocardiographic feature, indicates ventricular depolarisation partly by the sinus impulse and partly by the ventricular focal discharge.
4. It disappears as a result of an increase in sinus rate, hence, brief episodes of an accelerated idioventri-

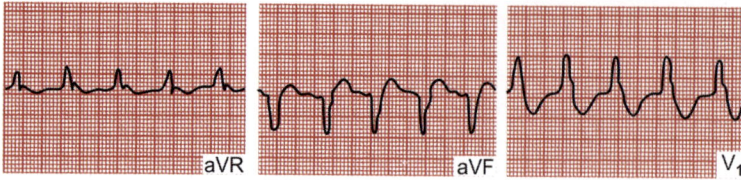

aVR　　　　aVF　　　　V₁

Fig. 35.24A: An accelerated idioventricular rhythm. The electrocardiogram (standard leads aVR, aVF and V₁) shows;
  i. Heart rate is regular at a rate of 100/min
  ii. There are wide QRS complexes unrelated to P waves

It has to be differentiated from slow ventricular tachycardia because it is a benign condition and does not require treatment

Fig. 35.24B: An accelerated ventricular rhythm (initiation and termination via a fusion complex). The electrocardiogram (lead II) shows;
  i. Beats no 1, 2, 14 and 15 are beats with sinus P wave and normal P-R interval
  ii. Beats no 3 and 13 show P wave with short P-R interval (↑) and wide QRS complex. These beats exhibit shape intermediate between beats with preceding P waves (sinus beats) and beats with wide QRS followed by inverted P waves (ectopic beats). These are fusion (F↑) complexes in which ventricular depolarisation is partly by sinus impulse and partly by ventricular ectopic
  iii. The beats 4 to 12 have wide QRS followed by inverted P waves occurring regularly at a rate of 75 bpm suggest an accelerated ventricular rhythm

Note: The fusion complex (3) heralds the onset of accelerated ventricular rhythm while a fusion complex (13) terminates it. The accelerated ventricular rhythm has onset and offset through a fusion complex indicates by arrows

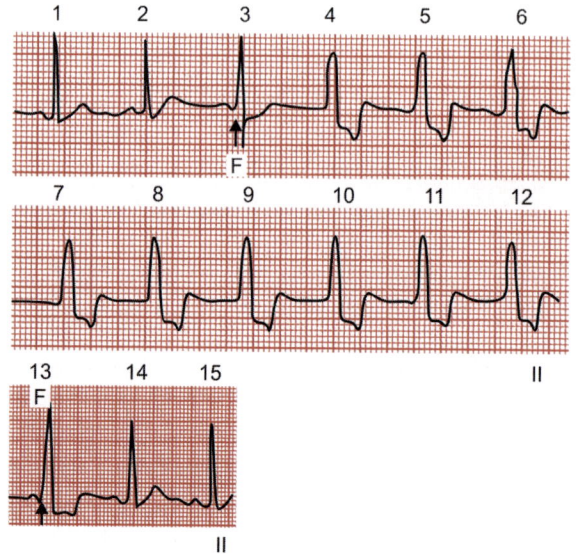

II

Fig. 35.25: An accelerated idioventricular rhythm with incomplete RBBB pattern in a patient with sick sinus syndrome. The ECG (leads II, V₁ and V₆) shows;
  i. *Sinus arrhythmia with SA arrest.* The last three beats in lead II are sinus conducted (↓) which show sinus arrhythmia and sinoatrial arrest indicating sick sinus syndrome
  ii. *An accelerated idioventricular rhythm.* The beginning of leads II, V₁ and V₆ shows wide QRS complexes without visible P waves indicating it to be either idionodal or idioventricular rhythm at a rate of 62 bpm. The presence of rSr' pattern in lead V₁ suggest the site of origin of the rhythm to be below AV node, hence, it is idioventricular rhythm.
  iii. *Incomplete bundle branch block pattern.* The narrow rSR' pattern in lead V₁ indicates the focus of origin in the one of the fascicles of left bundle as the QRS activation forces are directed anteriorly, and to the right

Therefore, the idioventricular rhythm which is an accelerated and has pattern of incomplete RBBB suggests ectopic fascicular nonparoxysmal tachycardia which gets self-terminated as revealed by normal sinus beats at the end of leads V₁ and V₆

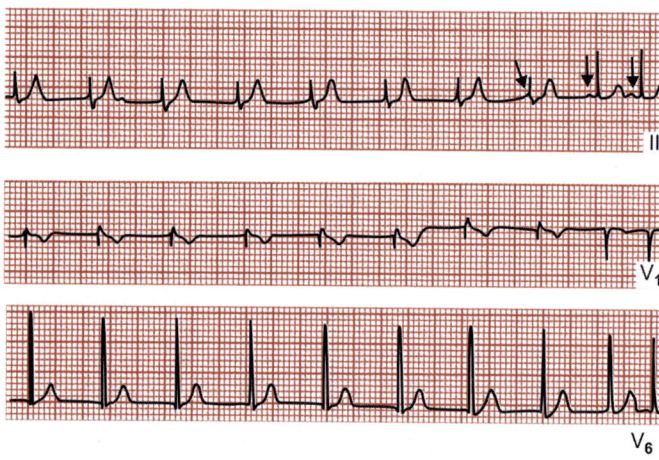

II

V₁

V₆

Table 35.1: Distinguishing electrocardiographic characteristics of an accelerated idioventricular rhythm from slow ventricular tachycardia	
An accelerated idioventricular rhythm (Fig. 35.25)	*Slow ventricular tachycardia (Fig. 35.26)*
• Ventricular fusion complex often heralds its onset. • Offset or termination is associated with a fusion beat or increase in sinus rate.	• The onset is via a premature ventricular complex (VPC) without prior fusion. • Offset is mostly spontaneous and is unrelated to an increase in heart rate.

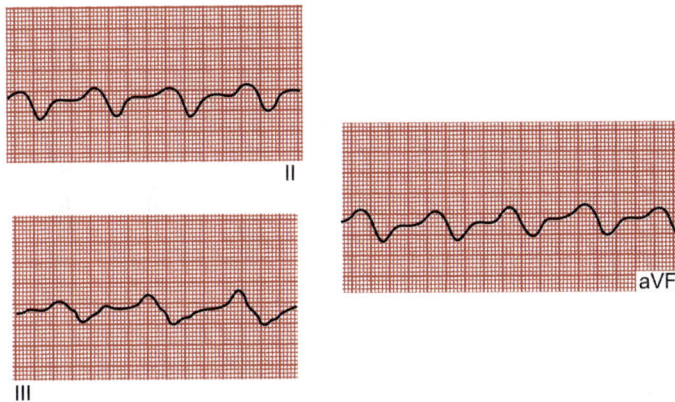

II

III

aVF

Fig. 35.26: Slow ventricular tachycardia. The electrocardiogram (leads II, III and aVF) shows;
  i. A wide QRS rhythm at a rate of about 83/min. The QRS complexes are small but more wide
  ii. The rhythm is regular (R-R interval is constant)
  iii. It got terminated spontaneously. It has to be differentiated from accelerated idioventricular escape rhythm—a benign condition

cular rhythm may alternate with periods of normal sinus rhythm. Accelerated idioventricular rhythm may persist for several minutes at a time, hence, an accelerated idioventricular rhythm is most often benign in nature.

5. Idioventricular rhythm may take origin from bundle of His (slight wide QRS) or bundle branch or a fascicle (Fig. 35.25) producing rSR' pattern or may take origin from ventricles (wide, bizarre QRS).

Clinical Significance

The rhythm is usually benign, does not require any treatment except for the underlying cause. If it produces haemodynamic disturbance, then attempts to be made to accelerate the sinus discharge rate above the rate of an idioventricular rhythm either by atropine or by temporary pacing (overdrive suppression). If digitalis is the cause, stop digitalis.

Caution. Treatment of an accelerated idioventricular rhythm with antiarrhythmic drugs such as xylocaine is not recommended, but if idioventricular rhythm degenerates into ventricular tachycardia, then conventional antiarrhythmic drugs or cardioversion should be attempted without delay.

VENTRICULAR TACHYCARDIA (VT)

Definition: It may be defined as a series of three or more consecutive ventricular ectopic beats which are recorded in a rapid succession. It is due to either rapid discharge of a ventricular ectopic focus or due to re-entry through a site distal to bundle of His, or in specialised conduction tissue / system, or in the ventricular muscle or in combination of both the sites. Nonre-entry mechanism can also occur in certain VTs. Unless invasive studies are undertaken, mechanism of tachycardia can only be conjectured.

Predisposing Conditions

1. Acute myocardial ischaemia or infarction
2. Cardiomyopathies (ischaemic or idiopathic)
3. Hypokalaemia and hypomagnesaemia
4. Drugs (digitalis and other proarrhythmic drugs)
5. Myocarditis

SECTION TEN

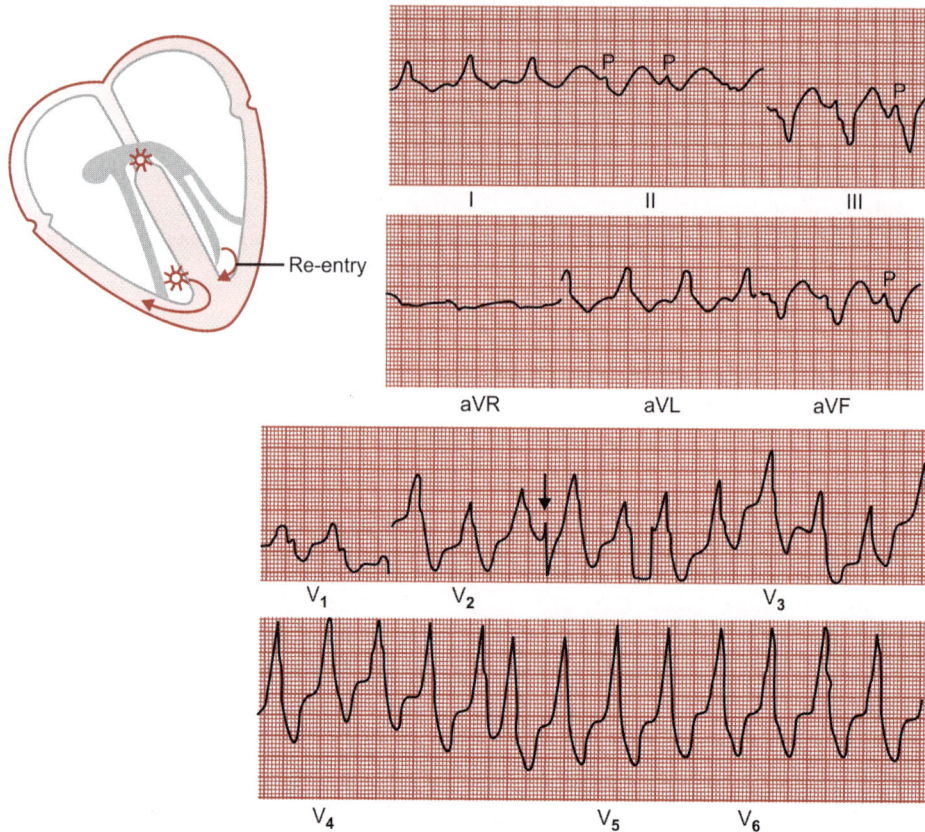

Fig. 35.27: Ventricular tachycardia (VT). The 12 leads electrocardiogram recorded shows;

i. Superior orientation of mean frontal QRS (wide rS pattern in II, III and aVF) which is directed anteriorly (wide R wave in V$_1$-Rabbit's ear appearance) and leftwards

ii. The QRS complexes are wide (>0.14 sec)

iii. Concordant pattern is seen in precordial leads (All QRS complexes show positive deflection in precordial leads)

iv. The heart rate is 136/min, regular (R-R interval is regular)

v. A capture beat is seen in lead V$_2$ indicated by an arrow (↓), which is a diagnostic sign of VT

vi. The QRS complex have only biphasic pattern (rS or Rs) in all leads which differentiates if from SVT with aberrant conduction where triphasic pattern of one of bundle branch block (rSR;' or qRS) is seen

vii. There is AV dissociation. Some of the upright P wave follows QRS and some precedes the QRS. The presence of capture beat in lead V$_2$ confirms AV dissociation.

6. Reperfusion
7. Ventricular aneurysm
8. Mechanically induced by a pacing catheter or flow directed pulmonary artery catheter, etc
9. Miscellaneous, i.e. sarcoidosis, idiopathic arrhythmogenic right ventricular dysplasia
10. Pacemaker mediated ventricular tachycardia (DDD pacemaker).

The Electrocardiogram (Figs 35.27 to 35.31)

1. **The QRS complexes**:
   - They are wide and bizarre due to slow and prolonged ventricular depolarisation.

- The QRS duration is > 0.14 sec.
- The QRS complexes usually look alike (monomorphic); on occasion, the QRS complexes have variable shapes (polymorphic), can vary in a more or less repetitive manner (torsades de pointes), can vary in alternate complexes (bidirectional) or can vary in a stable but changing contours (i.e. RBBB pattern changing to LBBB pattern) or may have a fixed bundle branch block pattern (RBBB or LBBB).

2. **The ventricular rate**: It is >100 bpm and regular but can slightly vary. Ventricular rate > 200 bpm

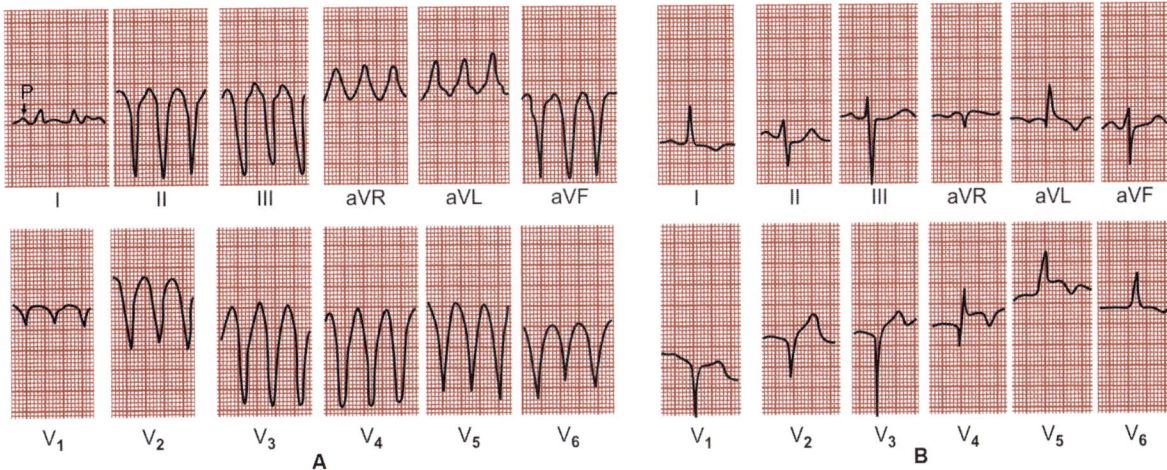

Fig. 35.28: Ventricular tachycardia. The electrocardiogram **A:** was recorded from a patient who landed in emergency department with chest pain and cardiovascular compromise. The electrocardiogram after cardiovascular resuscitation was also recorded as shown in **B.**

A: The ECG at admission showed ventricular tachycardia with following characteristics;
  i. Superior frontal plane axis around −140° (North-West zone)
  ii. Monomorphic QRS complexes with duration >0.14 sec but vary in amplitude
  iii. Precordial concordant pattern. All complexes have negative deflection in precordial leads.
  iv. Lead I shows P wave having no relationship to QRS, i.e. AV dissociation. AV dissociation is a characteristic feature but seen in 75% cases of VT
  v. Heart rate is 214/min regular

B: After successful resuscitation and termination of VT, the ECG revealed acute anterior myocardial infarction with left anterior hemiblock, the characteristic features being;
  i. QS pattern in leads V_1-V_3 with q wave in V_4-V_5 and aVL. The ST segment in elevated with convexity upwards in leads aVL, V_2-V_6 and T is inverted in leads I, aVL, V_4-V_6. The T wave in leads V_2-V_3 is upright and dragged up with ST segment.
  ii. Reciprocal ST segment depression in leads II, III and aVF.
  iii. Left axis deviation with rS pattern in leads II, III and aVF. The S wave is deepest in lead III indicating axis around −60°

Note: The tachycardia in an acute setting of myocardial infarction should always be considered ventricular tachycardia unless proved otherwise

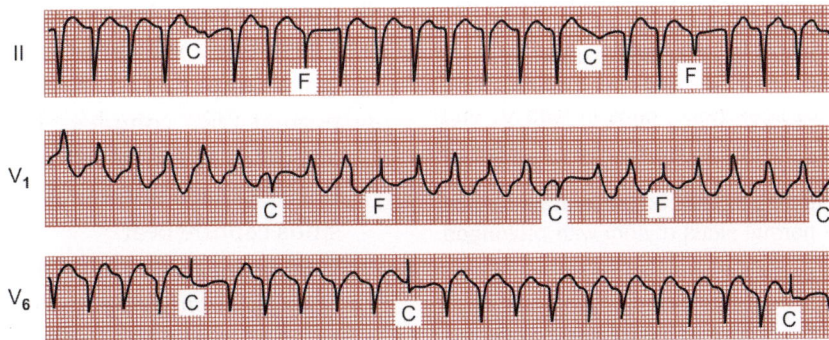

Fig. 35.29: Ventricular tachycardia showing fusion and capture beats. The electrocardiogram shows;
1. Upper rhythm strip (lead II) shows wide QRS complex tachycardia with superior axis of QRS. There are ventricular capture (C) and ventricular fusion (F) complexes. The rate is 165 bpm.
2. Middle rhythm strip (V_1) shows pattern of RBBB due to delayed ventricular activation. The focus of ventricular tachycardia being apical region of left ventricle will produce upright wide bundle branch type (monophasic R wave) pattern in V_1. There is associated ST segment depression and T wave inversion. Capture beats and fusion complexes are seen
3. Lower strip (lead V_6) shows wide QS pattern indicating the site of origin of tachycardia. The focus being in the apex of left ventricle, the excitation wave spreads towards right ventricle, hence, is away from the positive pole of V_6 resulting in QS complexes. The capture beats are seen.
   The fusion beats and ventricular capture complexes when present in wide QRS tachycardia invariably indicate it to be of ventricular origin

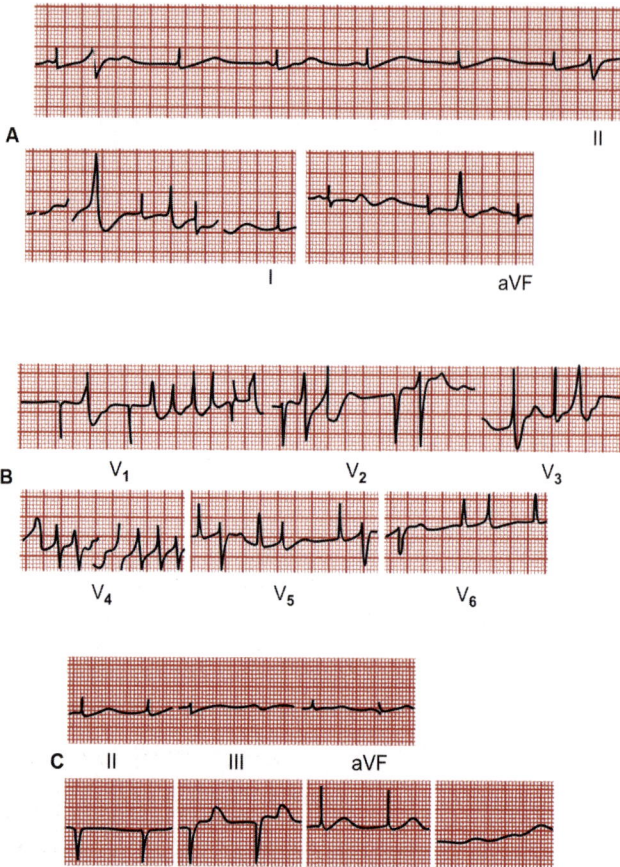

Fig. 35.30: Prolonged QT initiates ventricular tachycardia. The electrocardiogram shows;

A: The lead I, II and aVF are shown which reveal prolonged QT (QTc is 0.55 sec). Ventricular ectopics are seen which show R on T phenomenon, hence, are potentially malignant

B: The precordial leads (V₁-V₆) recorded from the same patient show non-sustained self-terminating polymorphic ventricular tachycardia seen twice, once in lead V₁ and then in V₄; while polymorphic VPCs are seen in most of precordial leads

C: After appropriate treatment, the electrocardiographic leads show restoration of normal sinus rhythm with prolonged QTc.

is unusual for VT. The onset may be paroxysmal or nonparoxysmal.

3. **The left axis deviation** with superior orientation ($-90°$ to $-180°$) is a characteristic feature and is manifested by positive deflection in lead 1 and negative deflection or rS complex in leads II and III. If the negative deflection is present in lead 1, then VT is unlikely.

4. **The run of ventricular ectopics**: There are at least *three successive ventricular ectopic* beats in a row.

5. **AV dissociation** (Fig. 35.27): It may appear sporadically, when this occurs, the sinus beats and ectopic ventricular impulses meet each other within AV node and interfere with each other's progress. The P waves, therefore, bear no relationship to the QRS complexes. AV dissociation has long been considered as a hallmark of VT, but now it has been seen that 25% cases do not exhibit AV dissociation in presence of ventricular tachycardia.

6. **Retrograde ventriculoatrial (VA) conduction**: It only occurs in about 25% cases and produces retrograde inverted P wave following each QRS complex in leads II, III and aVF. These P waves are pointed and dominantly positive in lead V₁.

7. **Fusion (Dressler's) beats**: They may, at times, appear in ventricular tachycardia. These beats indicate that ventricular depolarisation is being produced both by the sinus and ectopic beats, the proof of which is the shape of QRS which is blend of sinus and ectopic impulses in the same lead, and the abnormal focus is presumed to be in one of the ventricles. Therefore, presence of a fusion beat (s) in presence of wide QRS tachycardia supports the diagnosis of VT (Fig. 35.29).

8. **Sinus capture beats**: They occur occasionally. These beats indicate conduction of premature sinus impulses to the ventricles producing a normal QRS complex (Fig. 35.29). They may appear intermittently. In a run of wide QRS tachycardia, a normal QRS complex indicates a sinus capture beat.

9. **Concordant pattern of QRS in precordial leads**: The QRS complexes in chest leads V₁ through V₆ are sometimes either all positive or all negative in the presence of VT. An upright QRS complex in V₁ through V₆ also can occur due to conduction over left sided accessory pathway. About 25% cases of supraventricular tachycardia with aberrant conduction may show concordant pattern. Both these conditions must be excluded before labelling the patient having VT.

I II III aVR aVL aVF

V_1 V_2 V_3 V_5 V_6

VPC

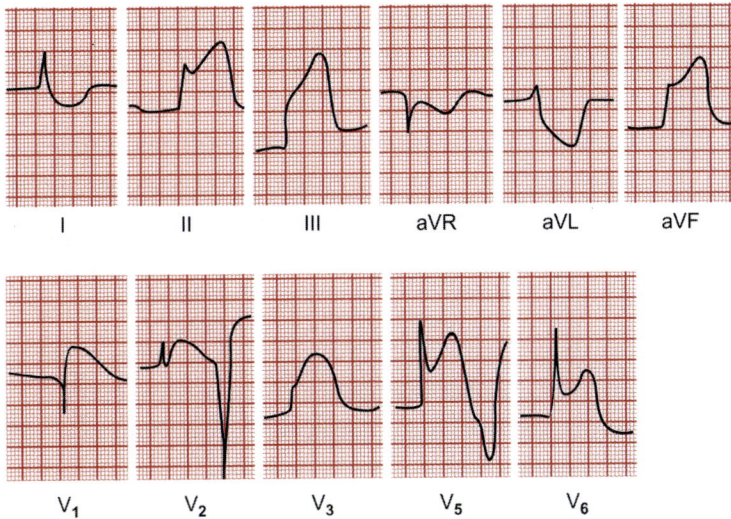

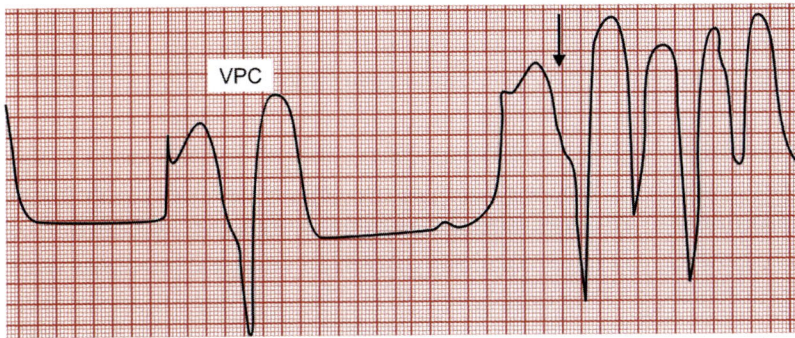

Fig. 35.31: Prinzmetal's angina with ventricular ectopics (R on T phenomenon) and ventricular tachycardia. The electrocardiogram shows;

i. The ST elevation in inferior leads (II, III and aVF) and precordial leads V_1-V_6 with reciprocal ST depression in leads I and aVL suggest Prinzmetal's variant angina

ii. The lower strip shows an ventricular ectopic falling on the R wave of sinus beat followed by another sinus beat after a compensatory pause. This next sinus beat is followed by a VPC which also falls on its R wave and triggers ventricular tachycardia (↓) evidenced by wide QRS complexes (4 complexes in a row including a VPc)

SECTION TEN

10. **A prolonged QT interval** (Fig. 35.30) and **ventricular ectopics with R on T phenomenon** (Figs 35.30 and 35.31) may trigger ventricular tachycardia.

11. **Initiation and termination**: Most commonly, very premature stimulation (early VPC) is required to initiate ventricular tachycardia electrically, while late coupled ventricular complexes usually initiate its spontaneous onset. Nonsustained VT (lasting for < 30 sec) terminates spontaneously (Fig. 35.31); while sustained VT (lasting for >30 sec) requires termination because of haemodynamic consequences.

Differential Diagnosis of Wide QRS Complex Tachycardias

Wide, bizarre QRS complexes only indicate that conduction through the ventricles is abnormal and such complexes can occur in;

1. *Supraventricular tachycardias with:*
   i) Aberrant intraventricular conduction (ventricular aberration)
   ii) Pre-existing bundle branch block
   iii) Conduction through an accessory pathway (reciprocating tachycardia).

2. *Ventricular tachycardia (ventricular ectopy)*: It is the most common cause of a wide QRS complex tachycardia, especially in the setting of a recent myocardial infarction.

The electrocardiographic distinction between supraventricular tachycardia with aberration and ventricular tachycardia is not only difficult but, at times, may be impossible and further electrophysiological studies may be required for confirmation.

During the course of tachycardia with wide QRS complexes, the presence of fusion beats and capture beats give maximum support for the diagnosis of ventricular tachycardia. A fusion beat implies activation of the ventricles from two different foci, and one of the foci presumed to be of ventricular origin. A capture beat, indicates that it has supraventricular origin, is slightly premature and is captured by the ventricles producing a normal configuration of QRS. AV dissociation once considered to be the hallmark of VT but nowadays it is not because; firstly, it does not occur in 25% cases where there may be retrograde ventriculo-atrial (VA) conduction. Secondly, even AV dissociation occasionally can occur in supraventricular tachycardia. Thirdly, even if P wave appears to be related to QRS complex, at times, it is difficult to determine whether the P wave is conducted antegradely to the next QRS (supraventricular tachycardia with aberrancy and a long P-R interval) or retrogradely from the preceding QRS complex (ventricular tachycardia). As a general rule, AV dissociation, if associated during a wide QRS tachycardia, is a strong presumptive evidence of ventricular tachycardia.

The differentiating features between ventricular aberrancy and ventricular tachycardia are discussed in details in chapter 39. However, the common electrocardigraphic features of ventricular tachycardia and supraventricular tachycardia with aberration are summarised in the Table 35.2.

Analysis of specific QRS contour can also be helpful in the diagnosis of VT and localising its site of origin. Mean frontal plane QRS axis (superior – 90° to –180°) and QRS duration >0.14 second with a QRS of normal duration during sinus rhythm supports ventricular tachycardia.

1. *Ventricular tachycardia with right bundle branch block pattern:* The following electrocardiographic features suggest it;

   i) The QRS complex is monophasic or biphasic in V_1 with an initial deflection different from that of sinus conducted QRS complex.

   ii) The amplitude of R wave in V_1 exceeds R′ wave (RSr′ or RR′ pattern).

   iii) A small r and a large S (rS complex) or a QS complex in V_6.

2. *Ventricular tachycardia having left bundle branch block pattern*: The following will be electrocardiographic findings;

   i) The axis is directed rightward producing negative deflections deeper in V_1 than in V_6.

   ii) A broad, prolonged R wave (>0.0.4 sec) in V_1.

   iii) A small q and large R (qR) or QS pattern in V_6.

   A discordant pattern can occur when the origin of VT from either ventricle is defined. A ventricular tachycardia arising from left ventricle produces wide QRS complexes that are upright in V_1-V_3 and downward in V_4-V_6. Similarly a VT arising from right ventricle produces upright, wide QRS complexes in V_4-V_6 and downward wide QRS complexes V_1-V_3. Variations in this pattern can also occur.

SECTION TEN

Table 35.2: Distinguishing features of ventricular aberrancy vs ventricular ectopy		
Feature with aberration	*Supraventricular tachycardia (ventricular ectopy)*	*Ventricular tachycardia*
• P wave	The QRS is preceded by a premature P wave except in junctional rhythm.	Not preceded by P wave.
• QRS morphology in V_1 and V_6	rSR′ in V_1; RS with wide S in V_6.	R, RR′ or QR in V_1; rS or qR in V_6
• Coupling interval	Not fixed	Fixed
• QRS duration	< 0.14 sec.	> 0.14 sec.
• R-R interval	Irregular	Regular, can be irregular
• Mean frontal plane QRS axis.	Depends on the pattern of bundle branch block, hence, can be right or left.	Left and superior
• QRS pattern in precordial leads (V_1-V_6)	Usually nonconcordant except conduction through left accessory pathway.	Mostly concordant
• AV dissociation	Not seen or uncommon	Common (75%)
• Fusion and capture beats	Not seen	Frequently seen
• Ashman's phenomenon	It can occur	Does not occur
• Vagal maneuver	Slowing or termination	No effect usually
• Bundle of His electrocardiography.	H-V interval is normal or short	Short or negative.

A concordant pattern (QRS complexes with similar configuration from V_1 to V_6 either all negative or all positive) and presence of 2:1 ventriculoatrial block favours VT.

A concordant pattern, a characteristic of VT, indicates anterior or posterior orientation of QRS forces originating from an ectopic ventricular focus

A heart rate more than 200 bpm does not favour VT. It raises the possibility of supraventricular tachycardia or atrial fibrillation with conduction over the accessory pathways. In the presence of pre-existing bundle branch block, a wide QRS tachycardia with configuration different from that occurred during sinus rhythm indicates VT.

Confirmation of VT can be done by certain electrophysiological studies (i.e. short or negative H-V interval on bundle of His electrocardiography), electrical induction of VT by premature ventricular stimulation and its termination by ventricular pacing.

Terms used in Reference to Ventricular Tachycardia

1. *Sustained VT :* Ventricular tachycardia lasting longer than 30 seconds is called *sustained VT*. It usually produces symptoms of weakness or syncope. It may degenerate into ventricular fibrillation if not controlled.
2. *Non-sustained VT* (Fig. 35.32): Ventricular tachycardia occurring in shorts brusts or paroxysms lasting only for less than 30 seconds is called *nonsustained VT*. It usually produces symptoms of light headedness or anginal pain.
3. *Monomorphic VT* (Fig 35.33): In this type, the configuration of all QRS complexes is similar and all look alike. All these complexes usually originate from single ectopic focus.
4. *Polymorphic VT* (Fig. 35.34): The configuration of QRS complexes varies. Changes in QRS configuration do not indicate different foci of origin of impulses but rather reflect different

SECTION TEN

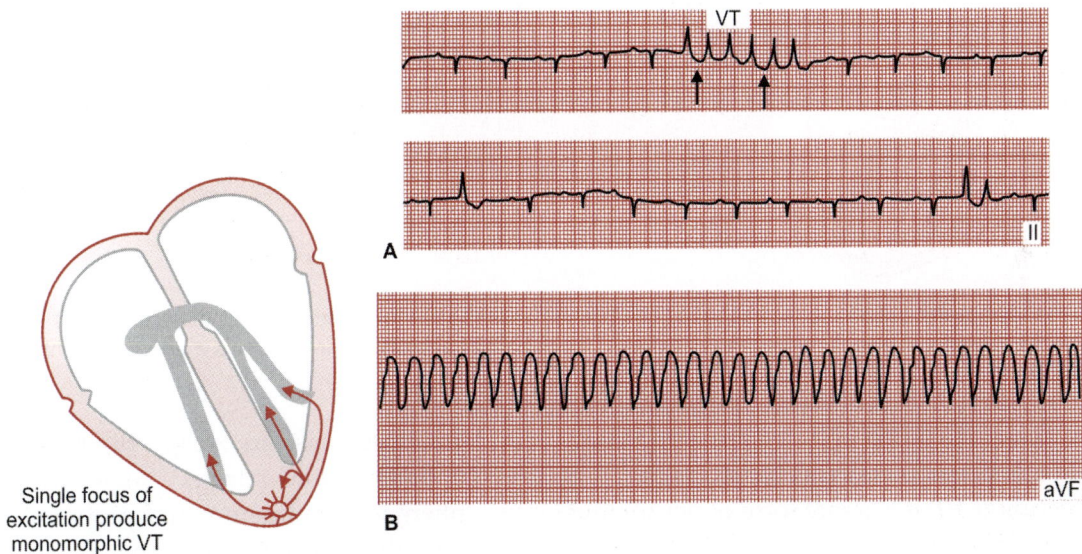

Single focus of excitation produce monomorphic VT

Fig. 35.32: Monomorphic ventricular tachycardia (VT).
A. Nonsustained VT. The electrocardiogram shows a short episode of monomorphic ventricular tachycardia at a rate of 170/min in the middle of upper strip. The retrograde P (P') waves are seen distorting the ST segment indicated by arrows (↑). The QRS complex are wide (>0.14 sec) and bizarre.
   In the lower strip, there is a VPC having same orientation as that of VT. At the end, there is a ventricular couplet which also has same orientation. All these features suggest nonsustained paroxysmal monomorphic VT.
B. The ECG (lead aVF) shows sustained monomorphic VT. Note the followings;
   i. Wide QRS complexes (>0.14 sec) look alike in the same lead
   ii. The heart rate is fast 250/min and is regular
   iii. There appears to be superior orientation of mean QRS axis
   iv. P waves are discernible

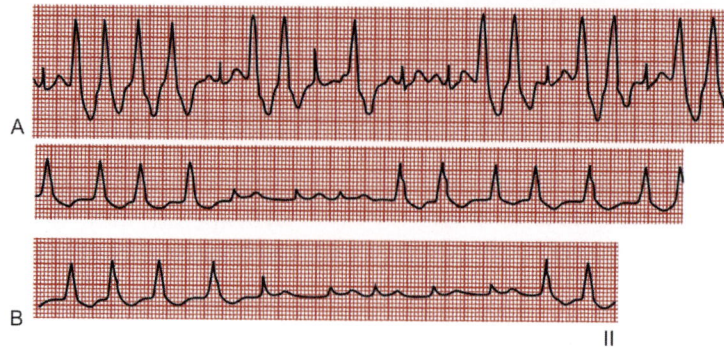

Fig. 35.33: Self-repetitive ventricular tachycardia.

A: The normal sinus rhythm is intermittently intercepted by ventricular tachycardia (two episodes, self terminating) and ventricular couplets. The continuous lead II shows;

  i. First beat in upper strip is sinus beat followed by an episode of self terminating nonsustained VT (four VPCs in a row). The episodes of tachycardia terminates followed by a sinus beat again, which, in turn, is followed by two VPCs.

  ii. Ventricular couplets. One sinus beat followed by two VPCs (a couplet) occurs in regular fashion at the end of the strip constituting a ventricular bigeminy rhythm

  iii. Sinus tachycardia. The sinus rate is > 100 bpm. This is due to sympathetic stimulation induced by nonsustained VT as well as continuous bigeminy rhythm

B: Self prepetuating repetitive VT. Lead II shows three episodes of monomorphic self-perpetuating VT (two in the upper and one in the lower). At the lower strip a ventricular couple is seen

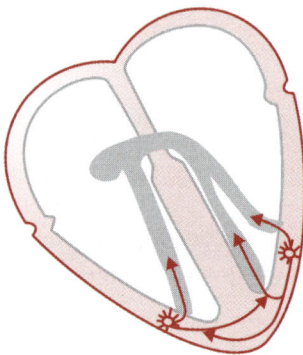

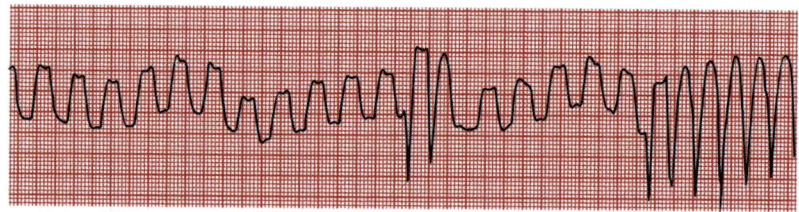

Fig. 35.34: Polymorphic ventricular tachycardia. The electrocardiogram shows wide QRS complexes (>0.14 sec) having different configurations indicating different pathways of myocardial activation. Heart rate is > 200/min slightly regular

pathways of activation of tachycardia impulses. It indicates a serious myocardial damage.

5. *Bidirectional VT:* It is a rare form of ventricular tachycardia in which the wide QRS complexes of varying amplitudes having right bundle branch block pattern alternate in opposite directions due to alternating left (–60° to –90°) and right (+120° to +130°) axis of QRS forces. The usual cause is digitalis (Read digitalis toxicity and see Fig. 45.5D). The ventricular rate is 140-200 bpm. Although the mechanism and site of origin of this tachycardia is controversial but most believe it to be of ventricular origin.

Treatment is to stop digitalis and use antiarrhythmic drugs such as lidocaine, phenytoin, potassium and propranolol to treat digitalis induced arrhythmia.

6. *Double tachycardia*: The simultaneous occurrence of an automatic atria tachycardia and a ventricular tachycardia is called double tachycardia.

7. *Torsades de pointes*: A particular type of polymorphic VT in which the QRS complexes of changing amplitudes appear to undulate or twist around an isoelectric line producing a *cork-screw appearance*. It occurs at rate of 200-250 bpm.

8. *Cardioversion:* It implies an application of a synchronised electric shock delivered precisely on the R wave. This is possible only if the ECG signal is transmitted to the cardioverter so that R wave sensing can occur.

9. *Defibrillation:* It implies an application of an unsynchronised electric shock. The current is delivered randomly during cardiac cycle. No ECG signal is used for defibrillation. It is used for emergency purpose for reversion of ventricular fibrillation (Fig. 35.40) which, if not treated, will lead to death within few minutes.

10. *Bundle branch re-entrant tachycardia:* This is characterised by wide QRS complexes due to circuit established over the bundle branches or fascicles. Retrograde conduction over the left bundle branch system and antegrade conduction over the right bundle branch produces LBBB pattern of QRS. Conduction in the opposite direction produces RBBB pattern which is less common. Re-entry also can occur over anterior or posterior fascicle (fascicular tachycardia). It is monomorphic sustained VT seen recently in patients of dilated cardiomyopathy or other structural heart diseases. Uncommonly, it can occur in the absence of a myocardial disease.

11. *Bundle branch or fascicular ectopic ventricular tachycardia:* This is a variety of slow ventricular tachycardia (HR <100 bpm) where the ectopic focus lies either in the one of bundle branch or a fascicle. If the focus lies in LBB, then RBBB pattern will appear in V_1 due to anterior and rightward direction of QRS forces. The wide rSR' pattern in V_1 (RBBB pattern) suggests one of the fascicles as the site of origin. The opposite will happen, in case, the ectopic focus lies in RBB. In the fascicular tachycardia, heart rate lies between 60-90/min.

12. **Parasystolic ventricular tachycardia**—Read Chapter 38 on Parasystole.

TORSADES DE POINTES

It is a variant of polymorphic ventricular tachycardia in which QRS complexes of changing amplitudes appear to twist around the baseline. *Torsades de pointes* (TdP) was originally described by Dessertenne as 'twisting of points'. The term 'torsades de pointes' is usually used to denote a syndrome and is not simply an ECG description of the QRS complex of tachycardia, is characterised by prolonged ventricular repolarisation with prolonged QTc interval (more than 0.44 sec). In this type of tachycardia, the U wave can also become prominent but its role is not clear. Long and short R-R cycles commonly precede the onset of torsades de pointes due to acquired causes. Although, often self-limiting, but can degenerate into ventricular fibrillation, hence, also called multiform ventricular flutter.

Causes

1. Class I antiarrhythmic drugs (quinidine, procainamide, disopyramide) and class III antiarrhythmic drugs such as amiodarone and sotalol.
2. Hypokalaemia, hypocalcaemia and hypomagnesaemia.
3. Psychotropic drugs (phenothiazines, tricyclic antidepressants), antihistaminics (astemizole, terfenedine), erythromycin, pentamidine and some antimalarials.
4. Acute myocardial infarction.
5. Liquid protein diets and starvation.
6. Romano-Ward syndrome, Jervell-Lange-Nielsen syndrome and other congenital disorders associated with prolonged Q-T interval.
7. Acquired prolonged Q-T syndrome due to any cause.
8. Central nervous system lesions.
9. Mitral valve prolapse.

Mechanisms

Electrophysiological mechanisms responsible for it are not well understood. Most data suggest that early afterdepolarisations are responsible for both prolonged Q-T syndrome and *torsades de pointes* or at least its initiation. Perpetuation may be due to a triggered activity, re-entry due to dispersion of repolarisation (QTd) produced by early afterdepolarisations or abnormal automaticity.

The Electrocardiogram (Fig. 35.35)

1. The polarity of QRS complexes alternates around the baseline. The QRS complexes tend to be bizarre, multiform, have sharply pointed apices and nadirs.

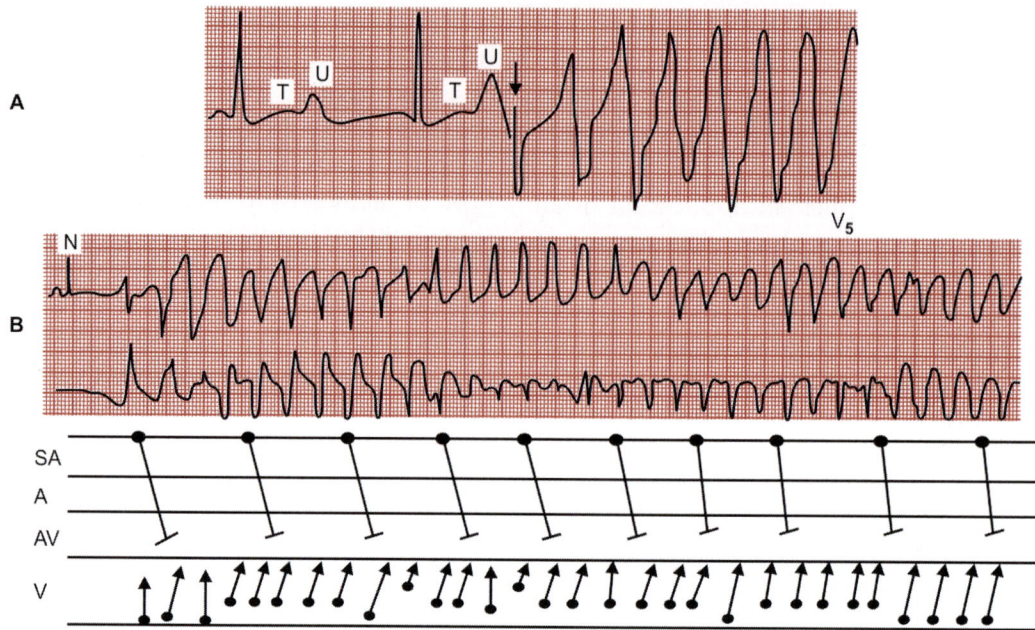

Fig. 35.35: *Torsades de pointes.*

A: Prolonged QT leading to development of polymorphic ventricular tachycardia (*torsades de pointes*)

B: The ECG lead II shows a normal complex (N) in the beginning with prolonged QT (p.44 sec) followed by a VPC with R on T phenomenon that triggers *torsade de pointes*. Note the variations in QRS complexes that twist both above and below the baseline

The QRS forms and axis undulate, thus, the sharp points of QRS complexes, for a short period of few seconds, may be directed upwards followed by sharp pointed QRS directed downwards for a short period of few seconds, hence, the name *'torsades de pointes'*. It is usually initiated by a VPC with prolonged QTc interval or VPCs with R on T phenomenon.

2. Torsades de pointes can terminate with progressive prolongation of cycle lengths with distinctly formed QRS complexes, or ending with a return to the basal rhythm, or to a period of ventricular standstill or to a new episode of torsades de pointes or to ventricular fibrillation.

3. The amplitude of QRS complexes may show waxing and waning.

4. The ventricular rate is extremely rapid (200-250 bpm).

5. The U wave can become prominant but its role is not clear.

This form of tachycardia, in particular, complicates the prolonged QTc interval because Q-T lengthening favours the relatively late premature ventricular complexes (R on T premature complexes) with short or long coupling to precipitate successive brusts of tachycardia during which the peaks of the QRS complexes appear successively on one side and then on the other side of isoelectric baseline, giving the typical twisting or cork screw appearance. Long-short R-R cycle sequences commonly precede the onset of *torsades de pointes* due to acquired causes.

Clinical Significance

1. Recently a tachycardia resembling *torsades de pointes* has been described in which Q-T interval is normal. In this type, premature VPCs with short coupling interval initiates the tachycardia.

2. Ventricular tachycardia morphologically similar to torsades de pointes without prolonged Q-T interval, whether spontaneous or induced, should be labelled as *'polymorphic ventricular tachycardia'* and not as torsades de pointes. This distinction has therapeutic implications.

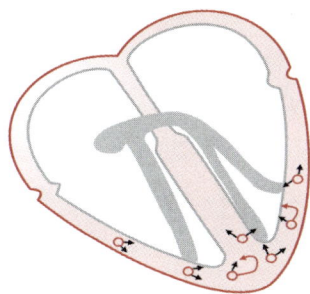

- Rapid re-entry of ventricular complexes
- Faster focus

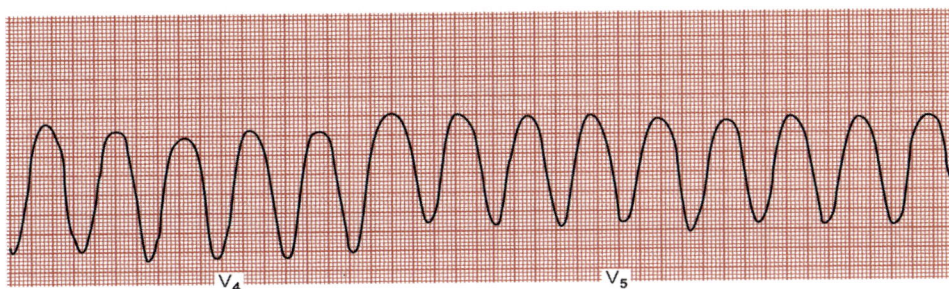

Fig. 35.36: Ventricular flutter. The electrocardiographic leads (V_4-V_5) show a ventricular rate of 210/min approx. The QRS complexes are discrete, wide, bizarre and blend imperceptibly with ST segment and T wave so that it is difficult to identify them separately. Large-amplitude waveforms appear contiguously (no baseline is visible between them) called 'sine-like' waveforms

VENTRICULAR FLUTTER

It is an expression of a very rapid and regular ectopic ventricular rhythm. It looks like a rapid ventricular tachycardia. Ventricular flutter is uncommon than tachycardia. On one hand, it looks like a rapid VT but is associated with haemodynamic disturbances, i.e. fall in BP and cardiac output and, on the other hand, it changes rapidly to ventricular fibrillation from which it differs in uniformity, constancy, regularity and by relatively large amplitude of QRS deflections.

Causes

These are the same as discussed under VT.

The Electrocardiographic Characteristics (Fig. 35.36)

1. The ventricular rate is 200-300 bpm and is regular.
2. Discrete QRS complexes, ST segment and T waves deflections are difficult to define and separate from each other. The large amplitude waveforms appear contiguously with no baseline between them. This results in a continuous 'sine-wave pattern'.

VENTRICULAR FIBRILLATION (VF)

Ventricular fibrillation is a catastrophic arrhythmia characterised by a rapid, irregular, disorganised ventricular rhythm resulting in lack of cardiac output, absent pulses and unrecordable BP. In the absence of ECG monitoring, ventricular fibrillation cannot be distinguished from ventricular asystole because both rhythm disturbances result in clinical cardiac arrest.

Causes or Predisposing Conditions

1. Myocardial ischaemia or acute myocardial infarction.
2. Cardiomyopathy.
3. Electrolytes disturbance (hypokalaemia, hypomagnesaemia).
4. Drug toxicity (digitalis and proarrhythmic drugs).
5. Failure to proper synchronisation during cardioversion.
6. Accidental electric shock across the heart (e.g. current leakage from electrical instruments, lightening injury, an improperly grounded equipment) and during competitive ventricular pacing to terminate the VT.
7. Atrial fibrillation and very rapid ventricular rates in the pre-excitation syndrome.
8. It is an terminal event in most of acute catastrophic events.
9. Ventricular fibrillation is probably the cause of death in cases of congenital long QT syndromes.
10. It occurs in severe hypothermia when the body temperature drops below 28°C.
11. Idiopathic ventricular fibrillation (Brugada syndrome).

Mechanisms

Ventricular fibrillation with in a variety of conditions, most commonly associated with ischaemic heart disease and usually a terminal event. Intracellular Ca^{++} accumulation, free radicals mediated

SECTION TEN

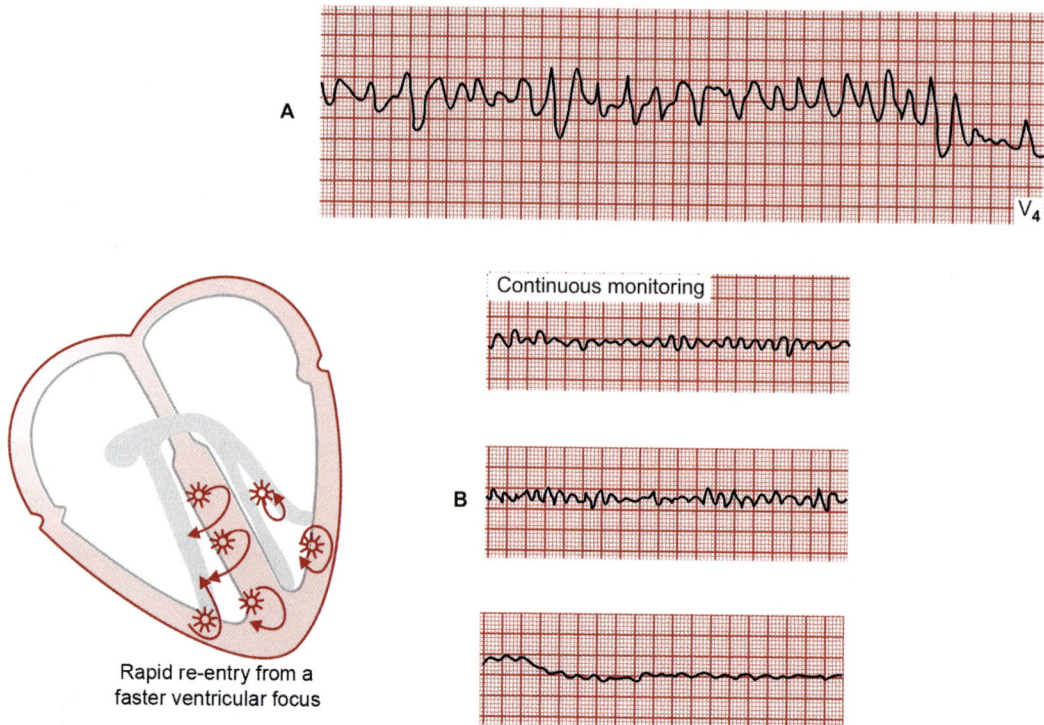

Rapid re-entry from a faster ventricular focus

Fig. 35.37: Ventricular fibrillation. The electrocardiogram shows;

A: Rhythm strip shows coarse ventricular fibrillation. There are large fibrillatory irregular non-identifiable waveforms and the baseline appears to undulate.

B: Fine ventricular fibrillation. The rhythm strips taken after several minutes of A show that fibrillatory waves have become smaller and smaller—called fine ventricular fibrillation. These changes are terminal, hence, called changes of dying heart that degenerate into ventricular asystole—a more or less straight line on ECG seen at the end of lower strip

cardiotoxicity, metabolic alterations and autonomic influences are important factors responsible for the development of ventricular fibrillation during ischaemia.

The Electrocardiogram (Fig. 35.37)

1. Ventricular fibrillation has no identifiable waveforms or patterns.
2. Undulating wavy baseline is composed of waveforms (QRS complexes) that vary in sizes and configurations. Early in the course of ventricular fibrillation, these fibrillatory waves become coarse and the rhythm is termed as *'coarse VF'*; after several minutes, these fibrillatory waves become smaller and smaller and the rhythm is termed as *'fine VF'*.

Classification of Ventricular Fibrillation

Clinically, it is of two types.

1. *Primary ventricular fibrillation:* It refers to ventricular fibrillation in a patient who does not have pre-existing or associated hypotension or

cardiac failure. It responds relatively well to electrical defibrillation, and resuscitation is usually successful.

2. *Secondary ventricular fibrillation:* It refers to ventricular fibrillation in a patient who has associated hypotension, respiratory or cardiac failure. Secondary VF is agonal and resuscitation usually fails.

VENTRICULAR ASYSTOLE

Definition: It is defined as complete absence of electrical activity of the heart. Asystole, also called cardiac standstill, represents the terminal cardiac event (dying heart) and cannot be distinguished from ventricular fibrillation without ECG monitoring.

Causes

1. Protracted episodes of VF.
2. Failure of pacemaker activity of the heart due to any cause such as drugs, acute myocardial infarction and so forth.

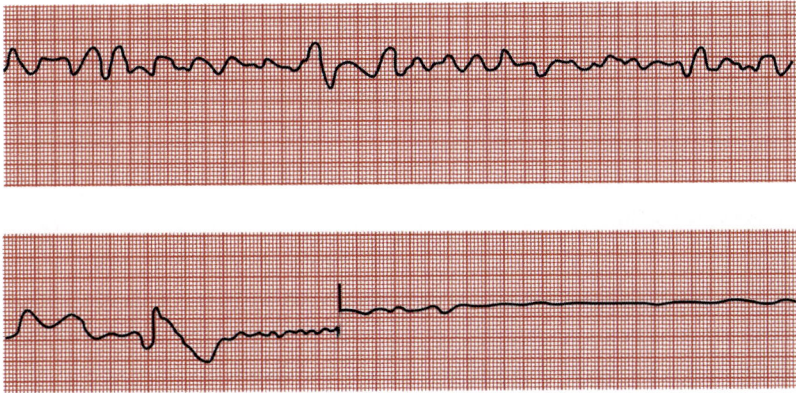

Fig. 35.38: Ventricular fibrillation degenerating into ventricular asystole

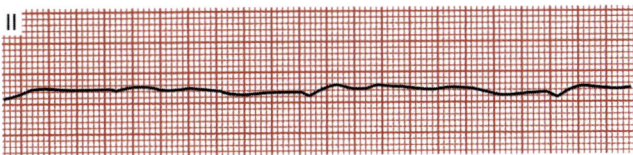

Fig. 35.39: Ventricular asystole. The rhythm strip shows no identifiable waveforms and baseline appears to be flat. It could well be fine VF degenerating into ventricular asystole—a terminal cardiac event

3. It is a terminal event in all acute catastrophic cardiovascular conditions.

The Electrocardiographic Characteristics (Figs 35.38 and 35.39)

1. No ECG waveforms are identifiable.

2. The baseline appears wavy or flat as a straight line. Before labelling it as asystole, a different lead must be recorded to show the baseline straight because a lead displacement can also produce a straight line. Electric main supply or power connections must be checked because electrical fault can also lead to straight line.

DYING HEART

It is an electrocardiographic expression of terminal cardiac events in which rapid ventricular tachycardia or ventricular flutter degenerates into ventricular fibrillation (first coarse and then fine) and finally into asystole (Fig. 35.39).

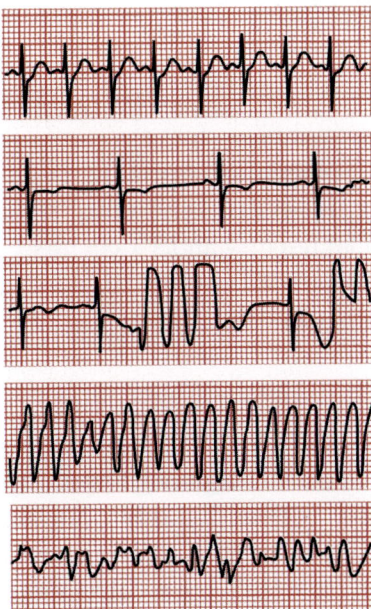

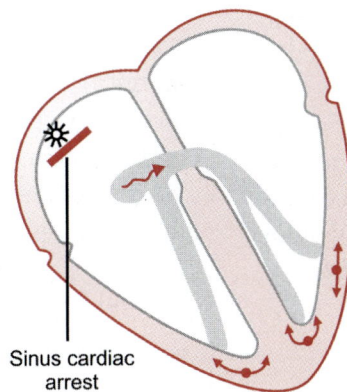

Sinus cardiac arrest

Fig. 39.40: Dying heart. Note the following on ECG; First strip shows sinus rhythm. Sinus bradycardia develops, with inversion of the T waves suggesting ischaemia. Short runs of ventricular tachycardia lead to polymorphic ventricular tachycardia and then to ventricular fibrillation which passed in to a systolic cardiac arrest

OTHER DIAGNOSTIC ELECTROCARDIO-GRAPHIC TECHNIQUES FOR ARRHYTHMIAS

1. Oesophageal electrocardiography
2. Cardiac mapping - body surface and direct cardiac mapping
3. Signal averaged electrocardiography.

1. Oesophageal Electrocardiography

It is a noninvasive method for diagnosis and analysis of atrial arrhythmias. A capsule electrode is used for this purpose which records electrical activity from back of the heart as oesophagus lies posterior to the atria. While analysing the rhythm, it is essential to search for the P waves. The P waves representing atrial activity are sometimes difficult to be seen on surface ECG. If P waves (or any atrial activity, flutter wave and so on) are not readily seen on conventional 12-lead ECG, transoesophageal leads may be used for this purpose. Bipolar recording is superior to unipolar recording. In addition, atrial and occasionally ventricular pacing can be attempted via a transoesophageal catheter electrode and both initiation and termination of tachycardias can be accomplished. No serious complications of transoesophageal pacing has been reported.

Uses

1. The oesophageal atrial electrocardiograms have been used to differentiate supraventricular tachycardia with aberrant intraventricular conduction from ventricular tachycardia.
2. To define the mechanism of supraventricular tachycardia. For example, if atrial and ventricular activation occurs simultaneously in a narrow QRS complex tachycardia, re-entry through an accessory AV pathway (WPW syndrome) can readily be excluded if retrograde P' waves do not follow QRS complexes and re-entry through AV node (AVNRT) becomes the most likely possibility.
3. For atrial pacing.

2. Cardiac Mapping

Cardiac mapping can be done from the body surface or directly from the heart. Actually, it is recording of the potentials or currents from the heart. The potential distributions are represented by contour lines of equal potentials (isopotentials) and each distribution is displayed instant by instant throughout activation, recovery or both. Although these methods are of academic interest, their clinical utility has not been established.

A. *Body surface mapping:* Isopotential body surface maps provide a complete picture of the effects of the currents from the heart on the body surface. These surface maps are used clinically:

1. To localise the site and areas of myocardial ischaemia.
2. To localise ectopic foci or accessory pathways.
3. To differentiate aberrant supraventricular conduction from ventricular ectopy.
4. To recognise the patients prone to develop arrhythmias and possibly the mechanisms involved.

B. *Direct cardiac mapping (recording potentials directly from the heart):* It is a method where potentials are recorded directly from the heart by utilising localising electrodes (epicardial, intramural or endocardial) and these potentials are depicted as a function of time in an integrated manner. The recording mode (bipolar or unipolar) and the method of display (isopotential or isochrone maps) are the problems under consideration.

Direct cardiac mapping via catheter electrodes or at the time of cardiac surgery can be used;

1. "To identify and localise the site of rhythm disturbance in patients with supraventricular and ventricular tachyarrhythmias for electrical or surgical ablation, isolation or resection of an accessory pathway in WPW syndrome, slow pathways in AV nodal re-entry and VT circuits."
2. To demarcate the anatomical course of His bundle to avoid injury during open heart surgery.

3. Signal Averaged Electrocardiogram (Fig. 35.41)

It is an independent noninvasive method used to predict those patients who are at high risk to develop ventricular tachycardia (VT) and sudden cardiac death. Signal averaging is a method that improves signal-to-noise ratio when signals are recurrent and noise is random. In conjuction with filtering and other methods of noise reduction, it can detect cardiac signals of low microvolts (mV) in amplitude by reducing noise amplitude from extraneous sources (noise produced by muscles, electronics and so on). With this method, electrical potentials generated by the sinus and AV node, bundle of His and bundle branches are detectable at the body surface.

Signal averaging is designed to detect signals called late ventricular potentials of 1 to 25 mV that are generated at re-entry sites within the heart. Re-entry is the mechanism most often implicated in VT. Signals recorded from re-entry sites are not visible on conventional 12 lead ECG because they are extremely small. The late ventricular potentials are waveforms continuous with the QRS complex probably corresponding to delayed and fragmented conduction in the ventricles.

Candidates for Signal Averaged ECG

1. *Myocardial infarction:* These late ventricular potentials have been recorded in 70-90% patients with sustained or inducible VT after myocardial infarction. In contrast to this, 0-6% normal individuals and 7-15% patients after myocardial infarction who do not develop ventricular tachycardia exhibit these late potentials. These late potentials can be detected as early as 3 hours following an acute myocardial infarction; its prevalence increases during first week and may disappear in some patients after one year.

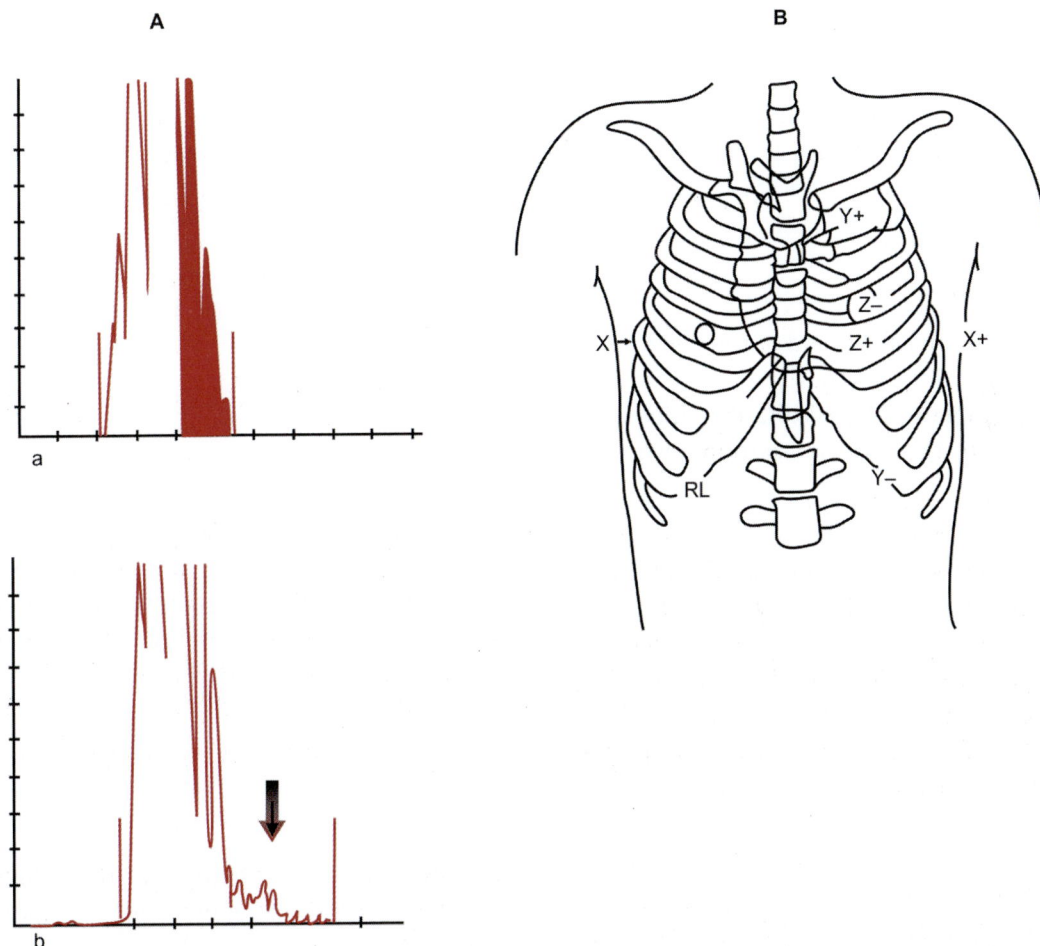

Fig. 35.41: Signal averaged electrocardiogram. **A:** (diagrammatic illustration) shows (a) SAE without late potentials and (b) SAE with late potentials (↓) when patient is at risk to develop VT. **B:** Orthogonal lead placement (X, Y and Z) for signal averaged ECG

SECTION TEN

The prognostic value of the signal averaged ECG is altered in the presence of bundle branch block, intraventricular conduction delay, paced rhythms and by selected antiarrhythmic drugs. Early use of thrombolytic agents may reduce the prevalence of late potentials after coronary occlusion.

2. *Cardiomyopathies:* Late potentials have been recorded in patients with VT due to dilated cardiomyopathy.

3. *Nonsustained VT or syncope:* It can be used to identify patients with non-sustained VT or syncope who may develop sustained VT at electrophysiological study.

Criteria Used for Analysis of Late Ventricular Potentials

1. *Total duration of filtered QRS* (greater than 114 msec is abnormal).

2. *Duration of terminal portion of QRS with amplitude < 40 mV.* Normally it remains for < 40 msec, therefore, duration > 40 msec is abnormal.

3. *Root mean square of terminal 40 msec* (less than 20 µV is abnormal).

Types of Analysis

1. Time domain analysis (filtered output corresponds in time with the input signal).

2. Frequency domain analysis. It provides useful information not available on time domain analysis.

Procedure

The patient lies supine and quiet to minimise muscle artifact during the test. The skin is shaved and prepared. The surface ECG electrodes are placed (Fig. 35.41) in orthogonal positions (X,Y,Z). At least 200 QRS complexes are computer averaged and the result is evaluated for the presence of late ventricular potentials by three parameters discribed above.

Suggested Reading

1. Ben-David J, Zipes DP: Torsades de pointes and pro-arrhythmia. *Lancet* **341**: 1578, 1993.
2. Blanck Z, Dhala A, Deshpande S, et al : Bundle branch re-entrant ventricular tachycardia. Cummulative experience in 48 patients. *J Cardiovas Electrophysiol* **4**: 253, 1993.
3. Brochier M, Motte G, Fauchier JP: Tachycardia ventriculare en torsades de pointes. *Actual Cardiol Vasc* **6**: 171, 1972.
4. Castellanos A, Lambert L, Arcebat AG: Mechanisms of slow ventricular tachycardia in acute myocardial. *Dis Chest* **56**:470, 1969.
5. Chung EK: Electrocardiography: Practical applications with Victorial Principles. Second edition, Hogerstown, Md, Harper and Row, 1980.
6. Dessertenne F: La tachycardie ventriculaire a deux foyers opposes variables. *Arch Mal Coeur* **59**: 263, 1966.
7. Dolara A: Early ventricular premature beats with repetitive ventricular fibrillation. *Am Heart J* **74**: 332, 1967.
8. Dubuc M, Nadeau R, Tremblay G, et al: Pace mapping using body surface potential maps to quide catheter ablation of accessory pathways in patients with WPW syndrome. *Circulation,* **87**: 135, 1993.
9. Epstein AE, Ideker RE: Ventricular fibrillation. In Zipes DP, Jalife J (Eds). Cardiac Electrophysiology. From cell to Bedside. 2nd edn, Philadelphia: WB Saunders company 927, 1994.
10. Fontaine G: A new look at torsades de pointes. *Ann NY Acad Science* **644**: 157, 1992.
11. Green LS, Lux RL, Ershler PR et al: Resolution of pace mapping stimulus site separation using body surface potentials. *Circulation* **90**: 462, 1994.
12. Griffith MJ, Garratt CJ, Mounsey P, et al: Ventricular tachycardia as default diagnosis in broad complex tachycardia. *Lancet* **343**: 386, 1994.
13. Grimm W, Marchlinski FE: Accelerated idioventricular rhythm, Bidirectional ventricular tachycardia. In Zipes DP, Jalife J (Eds): Cardiac Electrophysiology. From cell to Bedside. 2nd edn, Philadelphia: WB Saunders Company, 920, 1994.
14. Jazayeri, MR, Akhtar, M: Wide QRS complex tachycardia. Electrophysiological mechanisms and electrocardiographic features. In Zipes DP, Jalife J (Eds): Cardiac Electrophysiology. From cell to Bedside, Philadelphia, WB Saunders Company, 977, 1994.
15. Jervel A, Lange-Nielsen F: Congenital deaf-mutism, functional heart disease with prolongation of Q-T interval and sudden death. *Am Heart J* **54**: 59, 1957.
16. Katz A, Guetta V, Ovsyshcher, IA: Transoesophageal electrocardiography using a temporary pacing balloon-typed electrode in acute cardiac care. *Ann Emerg Med* **20**: 961, 1991.
17. Langendorf R, Pick A, Winternitz M: Mechanisms of intermittent ventricular bigeminy I. Appearance of etopic beats dependent upon the length of the ventricular cycle. "The rule of bigeminy". *Circulation* **11**:422, 1955.
18. Levine HD, Lown B, Streeper RB: The clinical significance of post-extrasystole T wave changes. *Circulation* **6**:638. 1952.
19. Meltzer LE, Kitchell JR: The incidence of arrhythmias associated with acute myocardial infarction. *Prog Cardiovac Dis* **9**: 50, 1966.

20. Miller JM: Recognition of ventricular tachycardia. In Zipes DP, Jalife J (Eds): Cardiac Electrophysiology. From cell to Bedside, 2nd edn. Philadelphia: WB Saunders Company 990, 1994.

21. Moser DK, Woo MA, Stevenson WG: Noninvasive identification of patients at risk for ventricular tachycardia with signal-averaged electrocardiogram. *Crit Care Nursing* **1**:80, 1990.

22. Motte G, Coumel P, Abitbol G, et al: Le syndrome Q-T long et syncope par 'torsades de pointes'. *Arch Mal Coeur* **68**: 831, 1970.

23. Murakawa Y, Inoue H, Koide T et al: Reappraisal of the coupling interval of ventricular extrasystoles as an index of ectopic mechanism. *Brit Heart J* **68**: 589, 1992.

24. Roden DM: Torsade de pointes. *Clin Cardiol* **16**: 683, 1993.

25. Rosenbaum MB: Classification of ventricular extrasystoles according to form. *J Electrocardiol* **2**:289, 1969.

26. Schamroth L: Idioventricular tachycardia. Editorial. *Dis Chest* **56**: 466, 1969.

27. Schamroth L: Idioventricular tachycardia. *J Electrocardiol* **1**: 205, 1968.

28. Schamroth L: Ventricular extrasystoles, ventricular tachycardia and ventricular fibrillation: Clinical electrocardiographic considerations. *Prog Cardiovas Dis* **23**:13, 1980.

29. Schamroth L: Concealed extrasystole and the rule of bigeminy. *Cardiologia* **46**: 51, 1965.

30. Shenasa M, Borggefe M, Havercamp W, et al: Ventricular tachycardia. *Lancet* **341**: 512, 1993.

31. Simson MB: Signal-averaged electrocardiography. In Zipes DP, Jalife J (Eds): Cardiac Electrophysiology: From cell to bed side. 2nd edn. Philadelphia WB Saunders Company 1038, 1994.

32. Sippens Groenewegen A, Spekhorst H, vanHemel NM, et al: Localisation of the site of origin of post-infarction ventricular tachycardia by endocardial pace mapping. Body surface mapping compared with 12 lead electrocardiogram. *Circulation* **88**: 2290, 1993.

33. Surawicz B, MacDonald MG: Ventricular ectopic beats with fixed and variable coupling: Incidence, clinical significance and factors influducing the coupling interval. *Am J Cardiol* **13**:178, 1972.

34. Surawicz B: Ventricular fibrillation. *Am J Cardiol* **28**:268, 1971.

35. Tye KH, Samant A, Dessler KB et al: R on T or R on R phenomenon. Relation to the genesis of ventricular tachycardia. *Am J Cardiol* **44**: 632, 1979.

36. Wang K, Hodges M: The premature ventricular complex as a diagnostic aid. *Ann Intern Med* **117**: 767, 1992.

37. Zipes DP: Genesis of arrhythmias and their electrophysiological consideration: In Braunwald Heart Disease - A text book of cardiovascular disease, 5th edn, Vol I Philadelphia, WB Saunders Company 548-85, 1997.

SECTION TEN

36

Reciprocal Rhythm and Reciprocal Tachycardia

- *Reciprocal rhythm—definition, preconditions and electrocardiographic manifestations*
- *WPW syndrome and reciprocating tachycardia as well as other forms of tachycardias.*

RECIPROCAL RHYTHM

Definition: It is a conduction sequence wherein an impulse originates from the conduction system (SA node, atria, AV node, bundle of His or ventricles), activates the atria if arises from atria or activates the ventricular if arises from the AV node or the ventricle but during or after it has traversed AV node, gains entry through an accessory pathway/ a bypass tract which enables it to reach atria or the ventricles again, so as to activate them once again. In this sequence, atria and ventricles are excited two or more times by the same impulse. This sequence is only possible when there are at least two conducting pathways within the AV node (junction) or around the AV node.

Mechanisms

Pre-requisites for reciprocating rhythm:
1. Existence of an accessory pathway or a bypass tract.
2. Presence of differential refractoriness within the two conducting pathways (AV node and accessory pathway), so that, there is a functional unidirectional block in the accessory pathway; whereas AV node is responsive to conduction.
3. A prolonged conduction time (long P-R interval), when a common AV nodal pathway is used for the reciprocating circuit. The long P-R interval provides the supraventricular impulse sufficient time and chance to get conducted again through another pathway not used during previous conduction.

1. Accessory Pathways or Bypass Tracts

The presence of an AV nodal bypass or an additional AV nodal pathway is must for reciprocating circuit.
   i. *Bundle of Kent:* It is a congenital tract connecting the atrium and the ventricle on either side (left or right), is situated ectopically anywhere along the AV ring. It completely bypasses the AV node and bundle of His, hence, called an atrioventricular bypass tract (Fig. 36.1). It is implicated in producing classic WPW syndrome.
   ii. *A Mahaim tract:* It is a congenital tract arising from either side of the AV node or bundle of His, ends blindly in the ventricle on the same side (Fig. 36.1).
   iii. *The James bundle :* A conduction pathway starts from the atrium, bypasses the upper part of AV node and ends in distal part of AV node on either side. It is implicated in producing Lown-Ganong-Levine syndrome.
   iv. *An intranodal pathway:* An additional intra-nodal pathway is present in the middle of AV node. The two pathways communicate with each other in upper part and the lower part as common upper and lower pathways (Fig. 36.1).

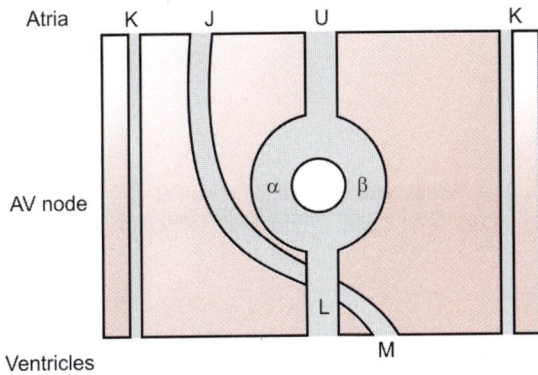

Fig. 36.1: Diagrammatic representation of accessory pathways around the AV node. J—James fibres, K—Kent bundle of fibres, M—Mahaim fibres, U—Upper common pathway of AV node, L—Lower common pathway of AV node, α and β = Two pathways in the middle of AV node indicating an additional intranodal accessory pathway

v. *Multiple accessory pathways*: It has been found that 10-15% patients have multiple accessory pathways and, on occassions, tachycardia can be due to a re-entrant loop conducting antegradely over one accessory pathway and retrogradely over the other.

The additional pathways may unite with AV nodal pathway at upper part (upper common pathway) or at lower part (lower common pathway) or at both upper and lower parts (upper and lower common pathways) or they may not unite at all and there is no common pathway.

2. Transient and Functional Unidirectional Antegrade Block in Reciprocating Circuit

Unequal refractoriness or responsiveness of two AV nodal pathways or AV nodal and accessory pathways is a basic condition for initiation of any reciprocal rhythm. This is necessary because an impulse arising, for example, in the ventricles, enters one pathway only and then returns to the ventricle in the opposite direction from another pathway to excite it again. If two pathways were equally responsive, then an impulse arising, for example, in the atria, or SA node would enter both pathways simultaneously and proceed in the same direction through both pathways, in such a situation, reciprocal mechanism is impossible. The above explained mechanism exists in classic WPW syndrome, where an atrial impulse enters two

AV nodal pathways simultaneously, gets conducted to the ventricles antegradely and excite the ventricles in sequential manner resulting in fusion complexes— a characteristic of WPW syndrome.

When, however, the refractory periods of the two pathways become unequal, the atrial impulse will enter through one pathway only, returns retrogradely through the another pathway, thereby, initiates the reciprocal rhythm. Therefore, functional transient unidirectional block in one of the conduction pathways is must to enable the development of reciprocal mechanism.

3. A relatively Prolonged Re-entry Period (Reciprocal Time)

An adequate or relatively prolonged time must elapse for the reciprocal impulse to initiate the reciprocal rhythm when a circuit includes an upper and/or a lower common AV nodal pathway. For example, in reciprocal rhythm of atrial origin, a relatively prolonged time must elapse to allow the atria and/or an upper common pathway to recover from their initial activation, so that, they become responsive again to allow the retrograde conduction of the beat producing an atrial echo or a reciprocal beat.

A prolonged reciprocal time may also be necessary in the case of AV nodal or ventricular reciprocal rhythm so as to allow the recovery of a lower common pathway and/or the ventricles.

The Electrocardiographic Manifestations

The reciprocal rhythm may occur with impulses of atrial, AV nodal and ventricular origin.

A. *Reciprocating Rhythm of Atrial Origin (Fig. 36.2)*

1. An atrial impulse activates the atria and passes antegradely to the ventricles through AV node and activates them. Reciprocal return of this impulse is possible if there is an accessory pathway in AV node (Fig. 36.2A) through which it enters while in transition in AV node or the ventricles. Now this impulse gets conducted retrogradely through this pathway to the atria once again and reactivates them producing an atrial *echo*. This is only possible when two AV nodal pathways (normal and accessory) have differential refractoriness.

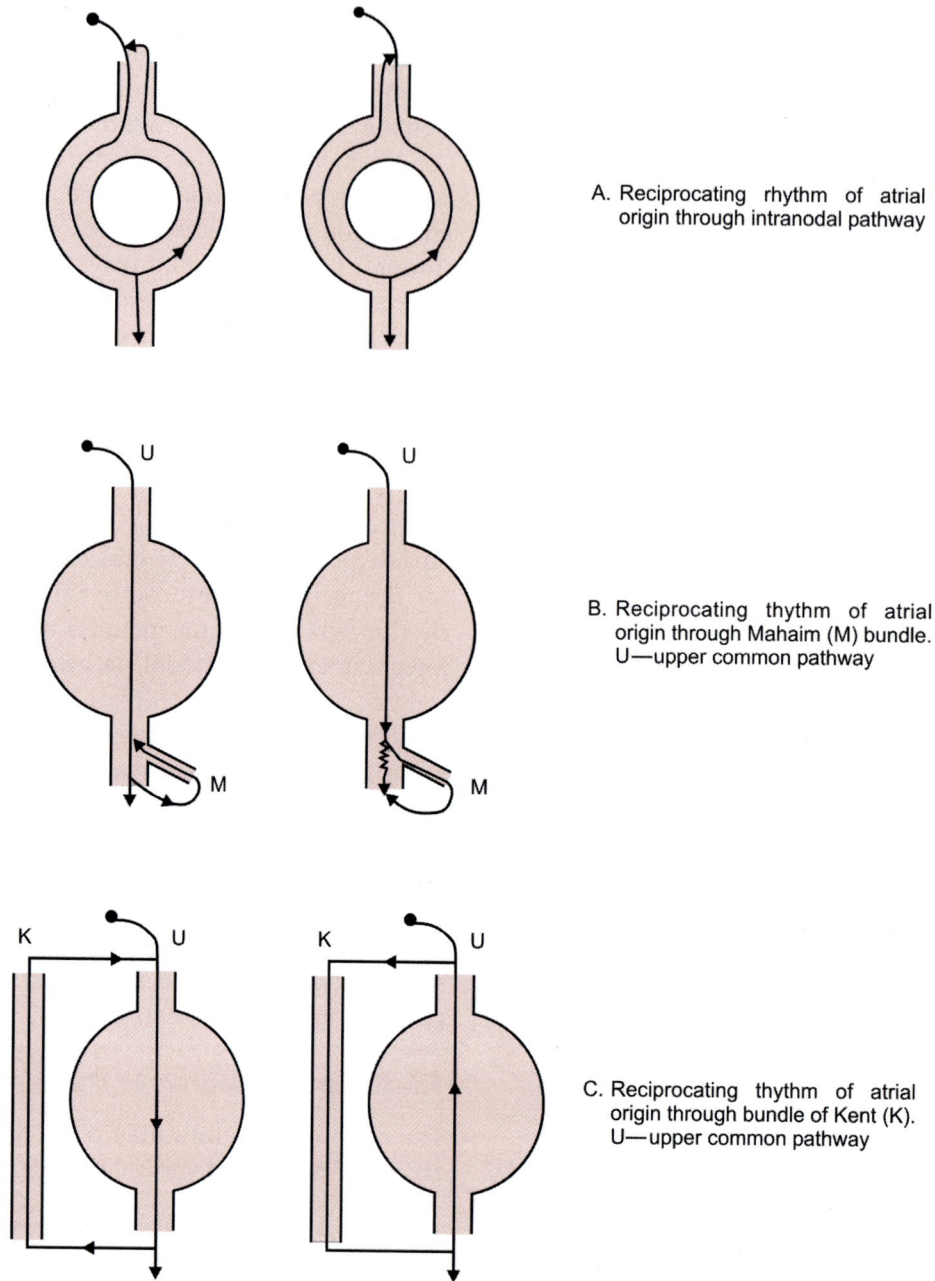

A. Reciprocating rhythm of atrial origin through intranodal pathway

B. Reciprocating thythm of atrial origin through Mahaim (M) bundle. U—upper common pathway

C. Reciprocating thythm of atrial origin through bundle of Kent (K). U—upper common pathway

Fig. 36.2: Mechanism of reciprocating rhythm of atrial origin through different accessory pathways

2. In another situation, the impulse, however, may get returned to the atria once it has reached the ventricles antegradely; the return of such an impulse will be facilitated by either Mahaim tract (Fig.36.2B) or a Kent pathway (Fig. 36.2C), in each case, it still has to traverse upper common pathway (U).

"In the presence of two pathways in AV node (normal and accessory) having differential refractoriness, an atrial ectopic impulse passes down through one of the pathways (usually normal pathway) towards the ventricles, but finding the other pathway responsive while the impulse is in the AV node or in its way to the ventricle or has reached the ventricle, enters

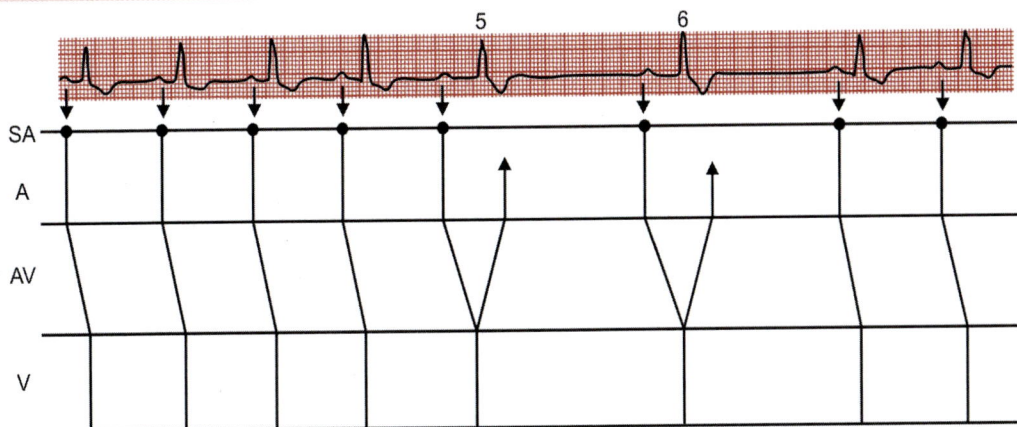

Fig. 36.3: Reciprocal atrial beats. The electrocardiogram (lead II) shows the first 4 beats are sinus conducted with P-R interval of 0.16 sec. The fifth and 6th beats are conducted with P-R interval of 0.28 and 0.26 sec, respectively. These beats with long P-R interval are followed by an inverted P (P') waves deforming the ST segments and forming P-QRS-P' complexes (labelled below in ladder diagram). This inverted P (P') wave is called an *atrial echo* and is linked to prolonged P-R interval of these beats resulting in reciprocal return of the sinus impulse through an additional intranodal pathway and an upper common pathway. If this sequence of reciprocal rhythm persists for sometime at a rate of > 100 bpm will result in reciprocal atrial tachycardial (Fig. 36.4)

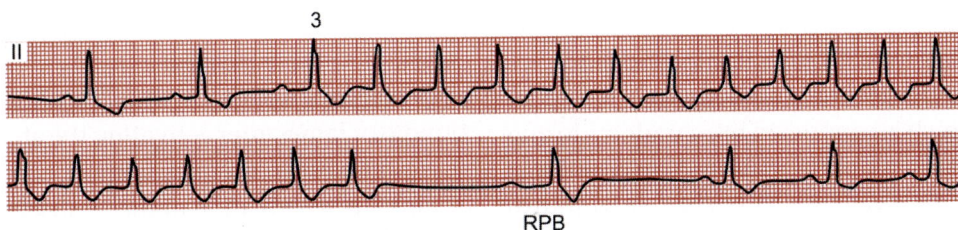

Fig. 36.4: Reciprocal atrial tachycardia. The ECG (leads II continuous strip) shows:
First two beats are sinus conducted with normal P-R interval of 0.16 sec and third beat is conducted with long P-R interval of 0.28 sec followed by an inverted P' wave (atrial echo) resulting in a run of tachycardia (>100 bpm) for some period called reciprocating atrial tachycardia which gets terminated in the middle of lower strip and is followed by a reciprocal beat (RPB) after a pause, then the normal sinus rhythm is restored as seen in last three beats of lower strip.
Note: The repetitive circuit between antegrade and retrograde pathways results in a reciprocating tachycardia

through the another pathway (usually accessary) and returns back to the atria and activates them for the second time producing an atrial echo."

The Electrocardiogram (Figs 36.3 and 36.4)

The basic pattern on ECG in reciprocal atrial rhythm will be "P-QRS-P' " sequence where:

"P wave is due to activation of the atria by sinus or an atrial impulse; the QRS complex is due to normal antegrade AV conduction and activation of the ventricles. The P' wave (inverted P wave) is reciprocal P wave (an atrial echo) due to retrograde conduction to the atria and their subsequent reactivation".

The retrograde P' is possible either through the intranodal re-entry or retrograde return through a Mahaim fibre or tract, therefore, the P-R interval of basic reciprocal sequence is prolonged which means the P-R interval of preceding P wave is prolonged. This is due to the fact that prolongation of antegrade conduction time is necessary for recovery of upper common pathway through which retrograde conduction becomes effective after traversing through the accessory pathway. This is a common finding that reciprocal beat occurs after prolonged P-R interval — a necessary pre-requisite for the reciprocal atrial rhythm.

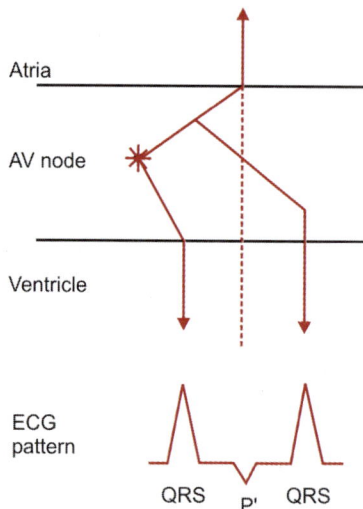

Fig. 36.5: Reciprocal rhythm of nodal origin

B. *The Reciprocal Rhythm of AV Nodal Origin*

In this type of reciprocal rhythm, the impulse arises in the AV node and spreads in two directions, i.e. antegradely (downward conduction) to the ventricles and retrogradely (upward conduction) to the atria. The impulse which is conducted retrogradely, during its passage through AV node, may enter an additional AV intranodal pathway, which enables it to return antegradely again to the ventricles and activates them for the second time (Fig. 36.5).

The Electrocardiogram (Fig. 36.6)

The basic pattern on ECG in reciprocal nodal rhythm will be "*QRS-P′-QRS*". This means P′ (inverted P) wave is sandwitched between two QRS complexes. The initial QRS is the result of an antegrade conduction of nodal impulse to the ventricles. The inverted P′ wave is due to retrograde conduction of nodal impulse to the atria. The second QRS is due to the reciprocal activation of the ventricles. The second QRS may be aberrantly conducted, hence, may be deformed.

C. *Reciprocating Rhythm of Ventricular Origin (Fig. 36.7)*

In this type, the impulse originates in the ventricles, activates them producing a wide and bizarre QRS complex, gets conducted retrogradely through the AV node to activate the atria. Reciprocal return of this impulse to the ventricles may occur either through AV node or through the bundle of Kent or through bundle of James after activating the atria, in each case, it would have to traverse a lower common pathway again. The reactivation of the ventricles by the return impulse constitute a reciprocal beat called '*return extrasystole*'.

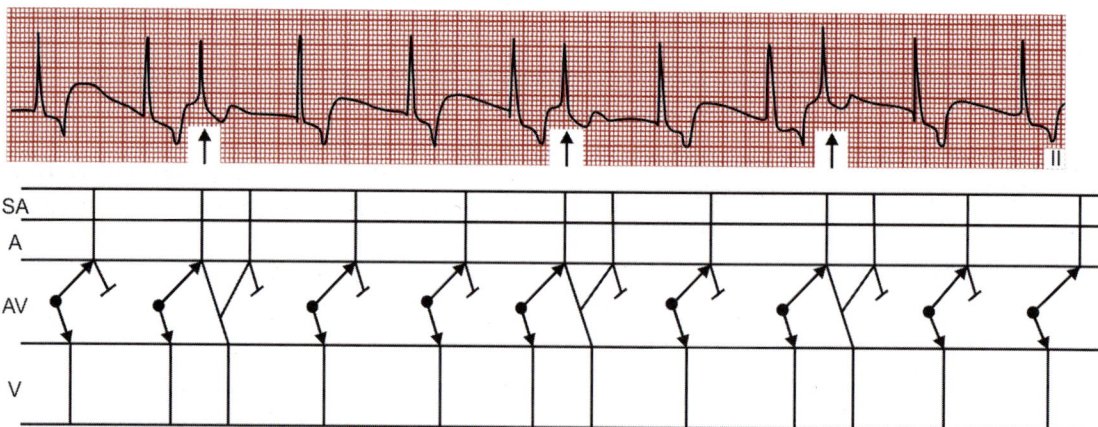

Fig. 36.6: The AV nodal reciprocal beats. The ECG (lead II shows);
  i. Basic AV nodal rhythm at a rate of 62 bpm
 ii. Wenckebach retrograde ventriculoatrial block. The first beat in upper strip is AV nodal beat with retrograde atrial activation (inverted P′ follows narrow QRS). This retrograde P is blocked and followed by another nodal ectopic (see the accompanying ladder diagram below)
iii. The second AV nodal beat with retrograde P′ is conducted again to the ventricles while passing through AV node producing a reciprocal beat (↑). The reciprocal sequence is QRS-P′-QRS, i.e. inverted P′ is sandwitched between two nodal beats, hence, there is reciprocating circuit in the AV node. The 3 nodal reciprocal beats shown by arrow (↑)

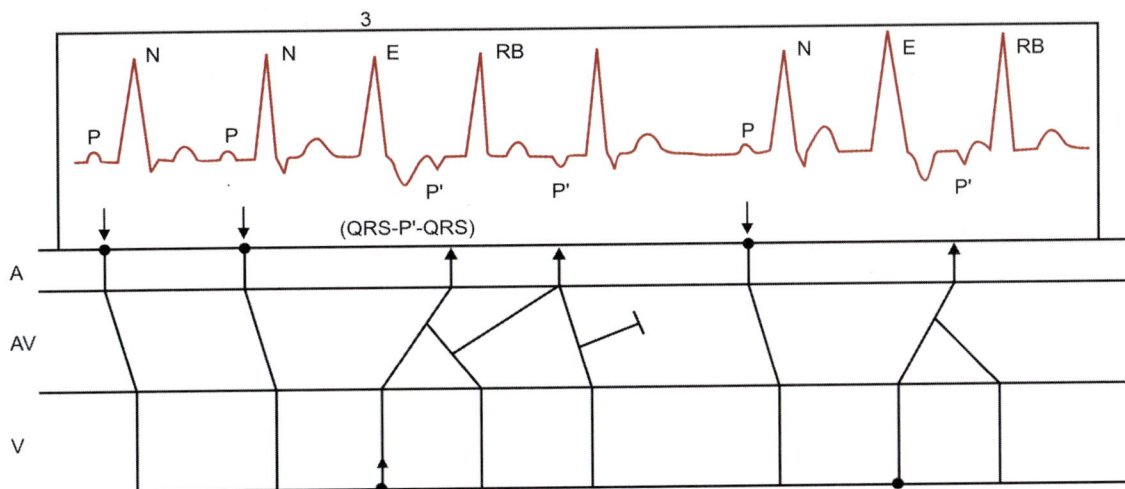

Fig. 36.7: Electrocardiographic recording (diagrammatic illustration) showing the following features of reciprocal rhythm of ventricular origin; The third QRS complex is wide and bizarre indicating ventricular extrasystole initiating the reciprocal rhythm. This is associated with an inverted P (P') wave due to retrograde conduction to the atria. This is followed by reciprocal return of the impulse to the ventricles resulting in reciprocal beat with normal QRS. This is followed by retrograde return to the atria (inverted P' wave) followed by another reciprocal beat with normal QRS complex. Retrograde conduction following this beat is blocked and, hence, circuit is broken (a bar in ladder diagram) and this is followed by a normal sinus beat. Again there is a ventricular extrasystole and further reciprocal beat indicating the reinitiation of reciprocal rhythm. If sequeuce does not get blocked and continues for sometimes, it will result in a reciprocating ventricular tachycardia.
A—Atria, AV—AV node, V—Ventricle, N—Normal sinus beat, RB—Reciprocal beat (a return extrasystole), E—Ventricular ectopic beat

The Electrocardiogram (Fig. 36.8)

The reciprocal rhythm of ventricular origin is reflected by "QRS-P´-QRS" sequence in which; "The initial QRS is due to activation of the ventricles by an extrasystolic ventricular impulse and is, therefore, wide and bizarre. The P´ (inverted P) wave is the result of retrograde activation of the atria. The second QRS of reciprocal sequence is the result of reciprocal activation of the ventricles by the returning impulse. The reciprocal impulse may follow normal intraventricular conduction pathway in which case the QRS complex (second QRS) will be of normal configuration. However, in second case, i.e. through an accessory pathway, the premature return of the impulse to the ventricles will give rise to abnormal ventricular activation, i.e. the resulting QRS complex is markedly different from the initial QRS complex. In both the situations, the second QRS will have different configuration than the first.

WPW SYNDROME AND RECIPROCATING RHYTHM/TACHYCARDIA

In WPW syndrome, there is an additional accessory pathway and the two pathways, i.e. normal and accessory are equally responsive to the impulse that would split and enter both the pathways simultaneously in the same direction with slight different speed, and both the beats stimulate the ventricles. Retrograde return through either pathway would become impossible if refractoriness of both the pathways is same. Therefore, simultaneous arrival of the two beats in the same direction to the ventricles results in their activation partly by both the beats producing a fusion complex, hence, in WPW syndrome, QRS is deformed due to fusion of these activations.

When, however, the refractoriness of the two pathways is different, the atrial or supraventricular impulse enters through one of the pathways, returns retrogradely through another pathway and thereby initiates reciprocal rhythm. Therefore, unidirectional antegrade block is prerequisite for development of reciprocal rhythm in WPW syndrome (as discussed ealier).

WPW Syndrome and Reciprocating Tachycardia (Kent Bundle Conduction, Fig. 36.9)

Even though the Kent bundle (accessory pathway) conducts more rapidly than does the AV node but has

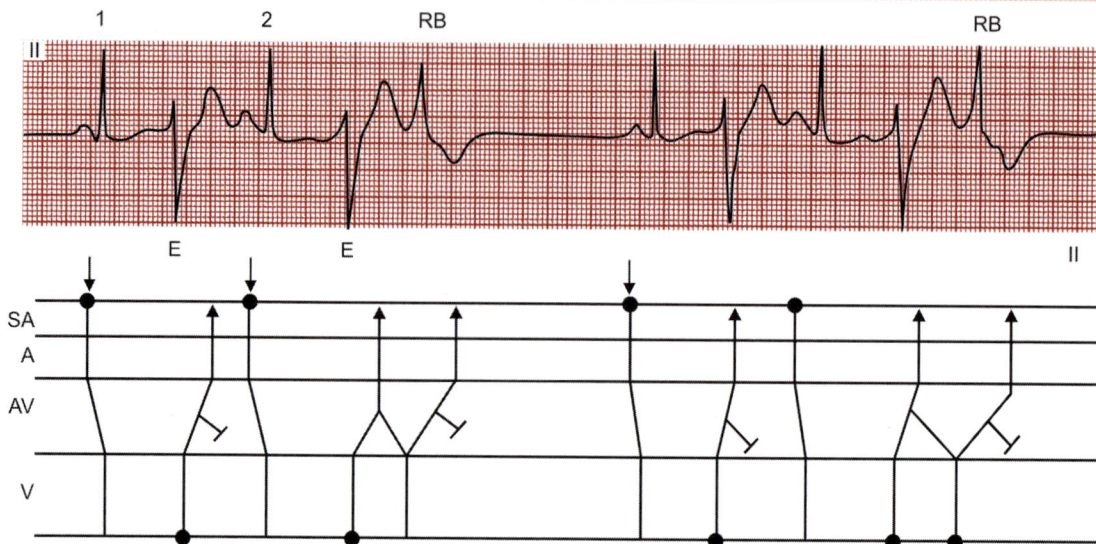

Fig. 36.8: Reciprocal rhythm of ventricular origin. The ECG lead II shows;

i. Basic sinus rhythm with normal P-QRS pattern

ii. First sinus beat is followed by an interpolated ventricular ectopic (bizarre QRS sandwitched between two sinus beats). The second beat has increased P-R interval as compared to first sinus beat, indicates increased AV conduction time. This second normal P-QRS complex is followed by an another ventricular ectopic (E) with retrograde atrial activation—the inverted P wave deforms the contour of ST segment due to its superimposition on ST segment. This second extrasystole (E) with retrograde atrial activation is followed by another QRS complex which resembles nodal QRS complex. This QRS is, in turn, conducted retrogradely to the atria, as reflected by superimposed inverved P' on the ST segment. The retrograde conduction to the atria penetrates the SA node, and resets its timing (indicated by a pause), which starts a fresh after an interval of 1.08 sec (duration of the pause). The cyclic arrhythmia is repeated.

NB: The ventricular couplet consisting of a ventricular ectopic beat which after retrograde conduction (inverted P) is conducted prematurily to the ventricles resulting in second QRS nodal complex. This sequence suggest the reciprocal sequence (QRS-P'-QRS)

a long refractory period during sinus rhythm, i.e. it takes longer for the accessory pathway to recover from excitation than does the AV node. Consequently, a premature atrial impulse occurring sufficiently early, gets blocked antegradely in the accessory pathway and is conducted to the ventricles through normal AV node-bundle of His pathway (Fig. 36.9A). The resultant H-V interval (on bundle of His electrocardiography) and QRS complexes are normal. This activation front (excitation wave) on reaching the ventricles, is conducted retrogradely back to the atria through the bypass tract or accessory pathway to activate the atria again resulting in a retrograde P' (inverted P) wave (Fig. 36.9B). The return of atrial premature impulse to the atria from ventricle through an accessory pathway is called 'reciprocating beat'; and rhythm maintained by such beats is called 'reciprocating rhythm. The classic ECG pattern of reciprocating rhythm will be inverted P waves (P'

waves) following QRS complexes in inferior oriented leads II, III and aVF due to deviation of excitation front superiorly through the accessory pathway.

Inverted P (P') wave follows QRS complex in inferior leads (II, III and aVF) in reciprocal tachycardia due to superior orientation of reciprocal impulse.

Such an event or rhythm can initiate the most common type of reciprocating tachycardia, which is characterised by antegrade conduction through the normal pathway and retrograde conduction through the accessory pathway (orthodromic AV reciprocating tachycardia). The accessory pathway blocking the atrial premature impulse in an antegrade fashion, recovers excitability in time to enable the impulse to pass retrogradely to atria, hence, an inverted P wave (P') follows normal QRS complex. This is classic (orthodromic) AVRT in which QRS complex is narrow and normal (Fig. 36.9C).

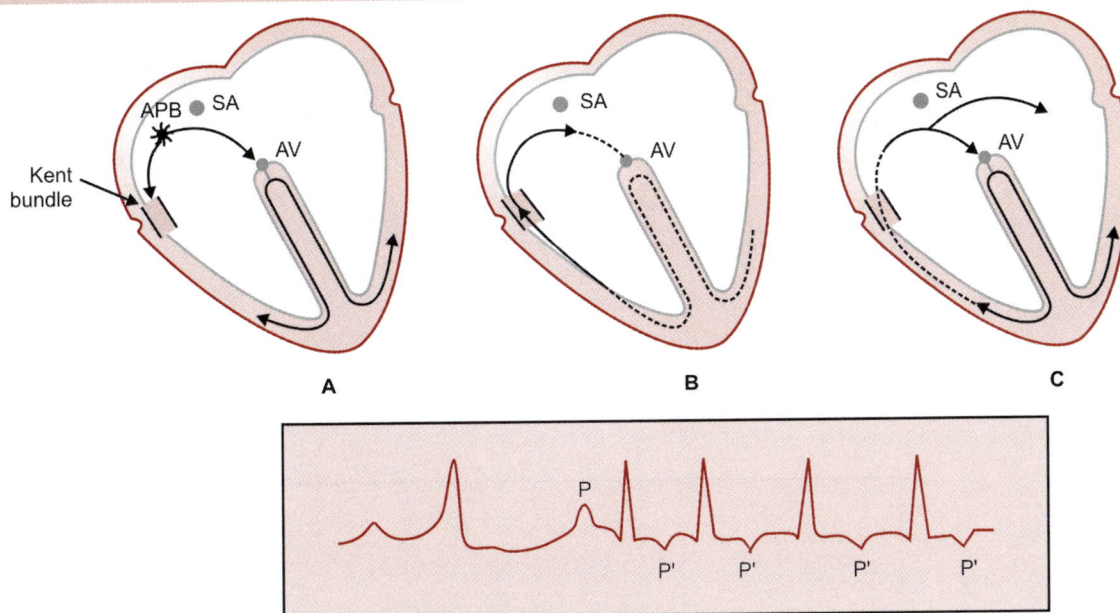

Figs 36.9A to C: Reciprocating tachycardia (orthodromic) in WPW syndrome with normal QRS (Diagram) initiated by an an atrial premature beat (APB)

A: The atrial premature beat (APB) is conducted to AV node antegradely, but APB is blocked in the anomalous pathway (Kent bundle). Now the same impulse is conducted to the ventricles via His-Purkinje system to produce narrow QRS. As pre-excitation does not occur, hence, short P-R interval and delta wave not recorded, i.e. WPW syndrome is concealed

B: The atrial impulse is conducted to the atria, retrogradely, to produce an inverted P' wave that follows narrow QRS

C: The same impulse is conducted clockwise to produce a reciprocating (re-entry) cycle; the same cycle now becomes self-perpetuating to produce reciprocal tachycardia in which narrow QRS complexes are followed by inverted P' wave (see the ECG drawn below). SA—sinus node, AV—atrioventricular node, P'—inverted P

Since antegrade conduction to the ventricular in above said mechanisms occurs through normal pathway only, pre-excitation does not take place and delta wave is not recorded, therefore, the WPW will not be evident electrocardiographically during this phase, hence, is said to be concealed WPW syndrome.

Much less frequently, there may be a tachycardia in which antegrade conduction occurs through the accessory pathway and retrograde conduction through the normal pathway (antidromic reciprocating tachycardia), the resultant QRS complex will be abnormal (pure delta wave will be recorded) in contrast to normal QRS in orthodromic tachycardia. This is due to total activation of ventricles by the impulse that has travelled over an accessory pathway (Figs 36.10A to C). Sometimes, two accessory pathways form the circuit in some patients with antidromic AVRT. In some patients, the accessory pathway conducts only in retrograde fashion (concealed conduction), but the circuit and mechanism of AVRT remain the same.

In both the tachycardias, the accessory pathway is an obligatory part of re-entrant circuit. In rare instances, bidirectional conduction over the accessory pathway can occur, in which, different fibres may be used for antegrade and retrograde conduction.

The Electrocardiographic Characteristics of Reciprocating Tachycardia (Fig. 36.11)

1. *A tachycardia with 1:1 (ventriculo-atrial) conduction:* The P wave is inverted in leads II, III and aVF. The inverted P wave usually follows QRS complex or may be merged with QRS.

2. Physiological or pharmacological vagotonic procedures or administration of other antiarrhythmic drugs (class I and III) do not induce second degree AV block and terminate it without preliminary disturbance of 1:1 relationship.

3. A rate of < 120 bpm is quite exceptional in reciprocating tachycardia. A rapid ventricular rate > 200 bpm with 1:1 conduction suggests reciprocating tachycardia.

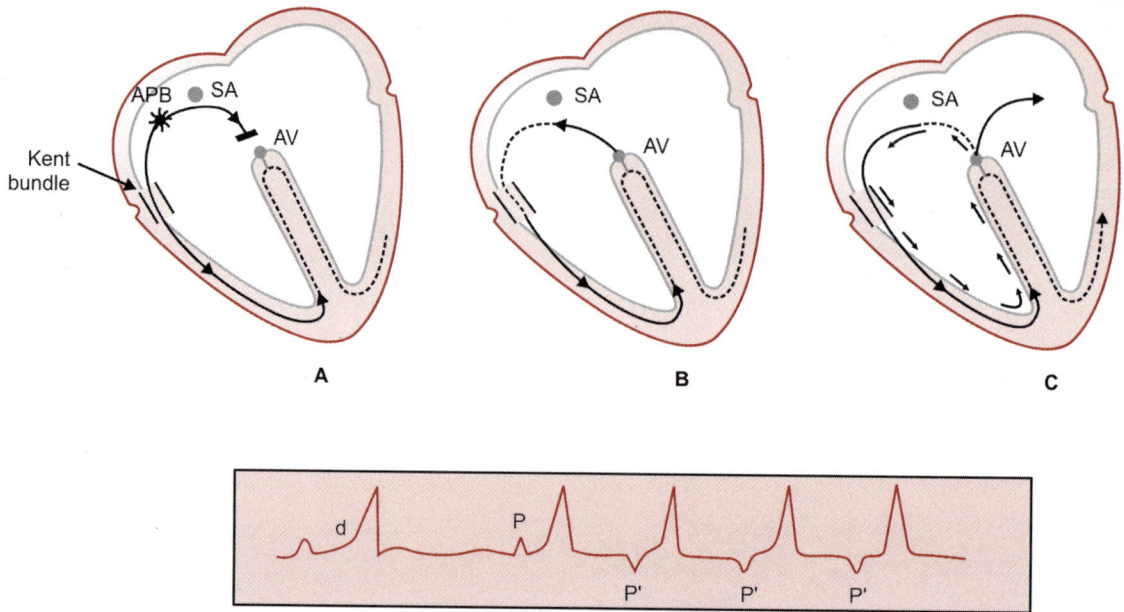

Figs 36.10A to C: Reciprocating tachycardia (antidromic) in WPW syndrome with abnormal QRS initiated by an atrial premature beat (APB)

A: Atrial premature beat (APB) finding the AV node refractory, gets conducted to the ventricles through anomalous pathway (Kent bundle) producing wide QRS and delta wave (d)

B: The atrial premature beat is conducted to the atria, in retrograde fashion, to produce an inverted P′ wave

C: The impulse is conducted counterclockwise to produce a reciprocating (re-entry) cycle, the same cycle is repeated indefinitely to produce reciprocating tachycardia. The ECG drawn below shows a WPW complex followed by a run of AVRT (wide QRS followed by an inverted P′)

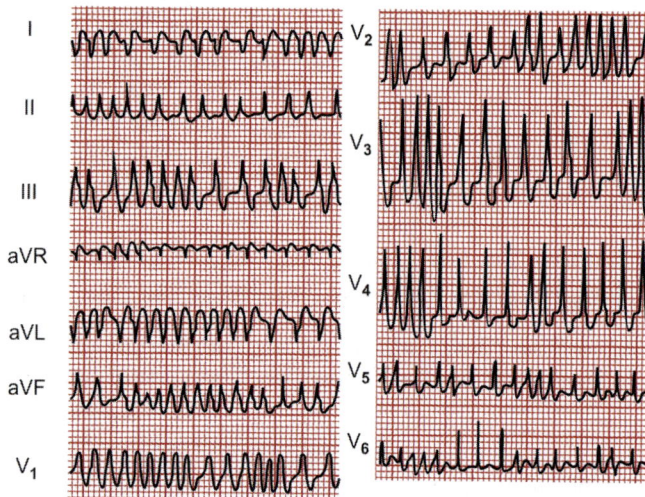

Fig. 36.11: Reciprocal tachycardia (1:1 conduction) in WPW syndrome with atrial fibrillation. The electrocardiogram shows;

i. Atrial fibrillation. There is irregular R-R intervals without visible fibrillatory 'f' waves. Ventricular rate is rapid > 200 bpm (200-300 bpm).

ii. The QRS complexes are wide and bizarre followed by retrograde P (inverted P′ waves) in leads II, III and aVF indicating that every beat is conducted to the ventricles with retrograde conduction to atria (1:1 conduction). The upright wide complexes in right precordial leads indicate type A WPW syndrome with reciprocating tachycardia

4. A tachycardia with wide, bizarre QRS complex if associated with 1:1 conduction strongly suggest reciprocal tachycardia. Conversely the association of second degree retrograde AV block effectively rules out reciprocating tachycardia and indicates the presence of PSVT.

5. A critically timed intracardiac electrical impulse or paired electrical stimuli will invariably terminate a reciprocating tachycardia, but this effect is unpredictable or uncertain in cases of focal tachycardia.

6. The precise origin of initiating impulse may be evident when the beginning of tachycardia is recorded, but may be difficult to determine during the course of actual tachycardia. Furthermore, a reciprocating tachycardia once initiated by a specific impulse origin may be interrupted and then continued by another impulse of different origin. For example: a reciprocating tachycardia initiated by a premature atrial impulse can be interrupted by an ectopic ventricular impulse. This interruption may terminate the tachycardia or may reset the cycle and continue the tachycardia.

WPW Syndrome with Bundle Branch Block

It is possible to have pre-excitation (WPW) syndrome and bundle branch block coexisting in the same patient. Bundle branch block can be diagnosed only when the anomalous bypass tract is contralateral, for example, if the bypass tract is situated on left side in a patient having right bundle branch block. In such a situation, the short P-R interval and delta wave suggest pre-excitation; while RBBB pattern reflecting terminal conduction delay by producing wide slurred S wave in V_5-V_6 will be apparent on ECG. These changes will only be seen when reciprocal tachycardia is not present.

The presence of short P-R interval, delta waves and left axis deviation in the presence of RBBB pattern in right precordial leads, shows coexistence of both WPW syndrome type A and RBBB.

The bundle branch block coexisting with pre-excitation syndrome cannot be diagnosed on ECG under following situations;
  (i) If ventricular excitation is continuously present and pre-excitation of the ventricles is entirely from the anomalous pathway.
  (ii) If bundle branch block is ipsilateral to the pre-excitation syndrome, i.e. both bundle branch block and bypass tract are present on the same side.
Under the conditions mentioned above, both ECG and vectorcardiography can be helpful.

Other Forms of Tachycardia in WPW Syndrome (Figs 36.12A and B)

Patients can have other types of tachycardias during which the accessory pathway is a bystander, i.e. uninvolved in the mechanism that leads to tachycardia such as AV nodal re-entrant or an atrial tachycardia that conducts to the ventricles through the accessory pathway. In patients with atrial flutter or atrial fibrillation, the accessory pathway is not a part of the mechanism responsible for the tachycardia, and the flutter or fibrillation occurs in the atrium unrelated to accessory pathway. Propagation of impulses to the ventricles during atrial flutter or fibrillation, therefore, can occur either through normal AV node - His bundle or an accessory pathway. Therefore, atrial fibrillation in WPW syndrome carries a potential risk of rapid ventricular tachycardia because of rapid conduction through the accessory pathway.

TACHYCARDIA THROUGH ATRIOHISTIAN PATHWAY (LOWN-GANONG-LEVINE SYNDROME WITH TACHYCARDIA)

Fibres that connect atrium to the bundle of His bypassing the AV node are called atriohistian tracts (James bundle), produce pre-excitation syndrome characterised by a short P-R interval and a normal QRS complex (Lown-Ganong-Levine syndrome). Although the tract has been defined anatomically, but tachycardia involving this bypass tract is not established and occurs infrequently (Figs 36.13A and B)

TACHYCARDIAS THROUGH MAHAIM FIBRES

Nodoventricular or nodofascicular fibres (Fig. 36.14): Since the nodoventricular or fascioventricular fibres connect the AV node or a fascicle with the ventricle, the conduction of impulses from SA node to AV node occurs normally with physiological delay in AV node, hence, P-R interval in this type of pre-excitation syndrome remains normal. The evidence of pre-excitation is reflected in wide, bizarre QRS with delta wave resembling QRS complexes of WPW syndrome. The ECG features of reciprocating tachycardias involving these fibres will simulate tachycardias in WPW syndrome, i.e. wide QRS complexes followed by inverted P′ waves in leads II, III and aVF, but it occurs rarely. It is after the reversion of tachycardia to normal sinus rhythm that the identity of nodofascicular or nodoventricular fibres will be established, i.e. wide QRS complexes with delta wave preceded by normal P-R interval instead of short P-R interval seen in WPW syndrome.

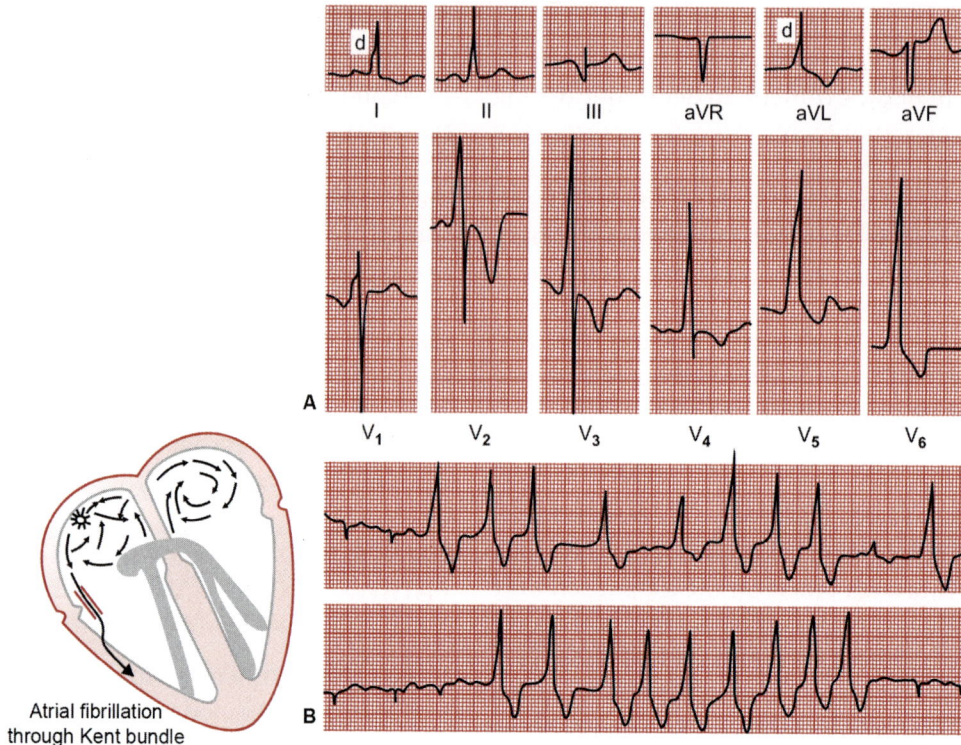

Fig. 36.12: WPW syndrome with an episode of reciprocal tachycardia and atrial fibrillation.

A: WPW syndrome. The electrocardiogram recorded during normal sinus rhythm shows characteristics of WPW syndrome;
  i. Short P-R interval (0.10 sec)
  ii. Wide QRS
  iii. Presence of delta wave (d) on the upstroke of R wave best seen in leads I, aVL and all precordial leads
      Note: He was a diagnosed case of WPW syndrome before developing atrial fibrillation and reciprocating tachycardia as shown in B.

B: WPW syndrome, atrial fibrillation and reciprocal tachycardia. The electrocardiogram shows;
  i. *Atrial fibrillation*: This is evident by undulating baseline due to fibrillatory (f) wave and variable R-R intervals seen in the beginning of upper and lower strips and at the end of lower strip. The QRS complexes are narrow with ventricular response of about 110 bpm indicating normal AV nodal conduction
  ii. *WPW syndrome*: It is characterised by wide, bizarre QRS complexes (fusion complexes) due to presence of delta wave on the upstroke of R wave (see 6th, 7th, 11th complex in upper strip). The shape of QRS complexes is different from other QRS complexes and are of low amplitude and they are variable in morphology due to the fact the shape of fusion complex in WPW syndrome depends on the contribution in activation process by pre-excitation wave that passes through the bypass tract and normal AV node. When the contribution is dominantly from the normal activation front conducted through the AV node, the QRS complex will resemble the pure normally conducted beat (QRS), i.e. 11th QRS complex in the upper strip indicated by a dot at the top. When the contribution is dominantly from the activation front conducted through by pass tract (anomalous tract) the fusion complex tends to resemble the pure anomalous complex, e.g. the 6th and 7th QRS complex in the top strip (indicated by dot at the top)
  iii. Reciprocating tachycardia. The other QRS complexes which are wide, abnormal followed by inverted P (P' waves) in both the strips indicate reciprocal tachycardia in a patient with WPW syndrome
      Note: The wide QRS complex tachycardia could be ventricular tachycardia, supraventricular tachycardia with aberration and reciprocating tachycardia. The wide QRS complex tachycardia in the presence of abnormal pathway (WPW complexes) with retrograde atrial activation suggest it to reciprocating tachycardia which is always 1:1 conduction

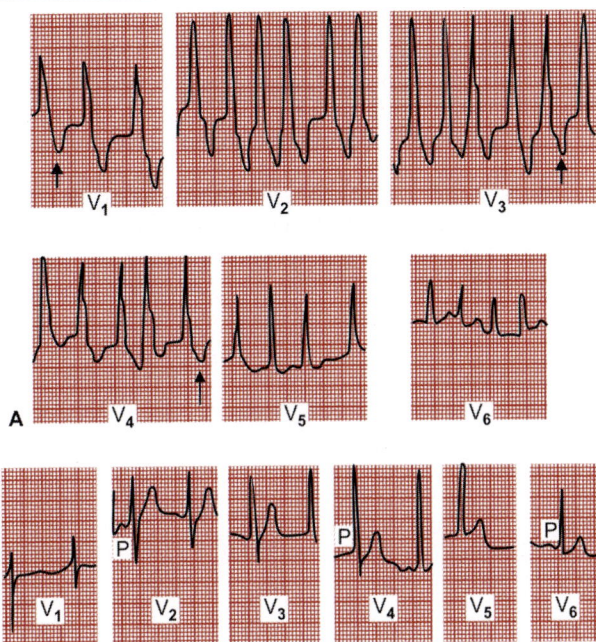

Fig. 36.13: Reciprocal tachycardia through Atriohistian (James bundle) pathway. The ECG shows;

A. There is wide QRS complex tachycardia with concordant pattern (upright QRS from V_1-V_6). Each QRS is followed by inverted P' wave indicated by arrows ($\uparrow$). There is irregular R-R interval. HR is > 200/min. All these features suggest reciprocal tachycardia rather than VT.

B. ECG recorded after reversion showed normal narrow QRS with short P-R interval < 0.12 sec with no delta wave. This is James bundle pre-excitation-*Lown-Ganong-Levine syndrome*

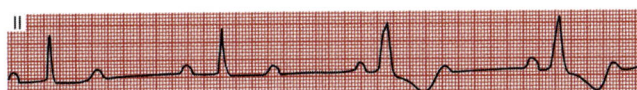

Fig. 36.14: Lead II shows 2:1 AV block. The P-R interval of sinus conducted (1st and 2nd) beats is 0.24 sec (Ist degree AV block), but the 3rd and 4th beats reflect normal P-R interval indicating accelerated conduction through infranodal accessory pathway (Mahaim fibre conduction)

Note: Mahaim type of conduction can be recognised only when some beats shows normal P-R interval; while basic sinus rhythm shows prolonged P-R interval. The tachycardia is rare in Mahaim type of conduction

Review at Glance

Reciprocal rhythm is a conducting sequence in which an impulse originating in the conducting system (SA node, atria, AV node or ventricle) passes antegradely, gets conducted retrogradely during transition in AV node or after reaching the ventricles, through an accessory pathway situated in AV node (intranodal) or outside the AV node (extranodal).

- Two pathways (normal and accessory) are must for reciprocal rhythm to occur.
- A functional unidirectional block of one of the conducting pathway is a precondition. This is due to differential refractoriness of two conducting pathways.
- When AV node is used as a pathway for reciprocal rhythm then preceding reciprocation, prolongation of P-R interval of preceding beat is must so as to allow the upper common pathway to recover from previous excitation so that it becomes responsive.
- The conduction sequence of various reciprocal rhythms is;
  (i) In atrial reciprocal rhythm, the sequence is *P-QRS-P'*
  (ii) In nodal reciprocal rhythm, the sequence is *QRS-P'-QRS*
  (iii) In ventricular reciprocal rhythm, the sequence is *QRS-P'-QRS* when ventricular extrasystole (QRS) initiates the reciprocal rhythm.

Suggested Reading

1. Burchell HB: Atrioventricular (AV) nodal (reciprocating) rhythm. *Am Heart J* **67**:391, 1964.
2. Dreifus LS, Nichols H, Morse D et al: Control of recurrent tachycardia in WPW syndrome by surgical ligation of the AV node. *Circulation* **38**:1030, 1968.
3. Durrer D, Schoo I, Suilenburg RM, Wellens HIJ: The role of premature beats in initiation and termination of supraventricular tachycardia in WPW syndrome. *Circulation* **36**:644; 1967.
4. Jackman W, Margolis D, Moulton K et al: Antegrade and retrograde pathway conduction over separate but close fibres. Evidence from RF catheter ablation. *Circulation* **(supple III)**: 317, 1990.
5. Kastor JA, Goldreyer BN: Reciprocal Rhythms in Schlant RC, Hurst JW (Eds). Advances in Electrocardiography, New York. Grune and Stratton Inc. 1972.
6. Kistin AD: Atrial reciprocal rhythm. *Circulation* **32**:687, 1965.
7. Langendorf R, Lev M, Pick R: Auricular fibrillation with anomalous AV excitation (WPW syndrome) initiating ventricular paroxysmal tachycardia. *Acta Control* **7**:241, 1952.

SECTION TEN

8. Moe GK, Mendez C: The physiological basis of reciprocal rhythm. *Prog Cardiovas Dis* **8**:461, 1966.

9. Pick A, Fisch C: Ventricular pre-excitation in the presence of WPW syndrome. *Am Heart J* **55**:504, 1958.

10. Schamroth L, Schamroth C: An introduction to electrocardiography, 7th edn, Blackwell Science Publication, 1990.

11. Schilnberg RM, Durrer D: Ventricular echo elicited by induced VPCs. *Circulation* **40**:337, 1969.

12. Shih HT, Miles WM, Klein LS, et al: Multiple accessory pathways in the permanent forms of junctional reciprocating tachycardia. *Am J Cardiol* **73**:361, 1994.

13. Wellens HJJ, Durrer D: The role of an accessory atrioventricular pathways in reciprocal tachycardia. Observations in patients with or without WPW syndrome. *Circulation* **36**:644, 1967.

14. deChillou C, Rodriguez LM, Schlapfer J, et al: Clinical characteristics and electrophysiologic properties of atrioventricular accessory pathways: Importance of the accessory pathway location. *J Am Coll Cardiol* **20**:666, 1992.

37

Atrioventricular Dissociation

- ■ *Definition, causes, mechanisms and electrocardiographic characteristics*
- ■ *AV dissociation with interference*
- ■ *AV dissociation versus complete heart block*

Definition: Atrioventricular dissociation is not a rhythm. It is a descriptive term used for any rhythm in which atria and ventricles are dissociated and are completely controlled by separate pacemakers. The atrial pacemaker is usually the sinus node and produces sinus rhythm but any atrial rhythm may be present. The ventricular pacemaker may originate from AV node, bundle of His, bundle branches or peripheral Purkinje tissue. The ventricular rate is faster than atrial rate.

Isorhythmic dissociation. It implies the same rate of discharge of both pacemakers resulting in synchronised dissociation (Fig. 37.1).

Double tachycardia. It refers to the presence of dual tachycardia—paroxysmal atrial tachycardia and tachycardia due to an acceleration of a subsidiary pacemaker, i.e. idionodal tachycardia (Fig. 37.2) present at the same time.

Aetiology: AV dissociation is not a primary disturbance, hence, is never a primary diagnosis. It is always secondary to another rhythm disturbance. Causes are tabulated (Table 37.1).

Mechanisms: Atrioventricular dissociation can arise due to:
1. A disturbance of impulse formation
2. A disturbance of impulse conduction.

1. A Disturbance of Impulse Formation

Slow sinus rates lead to emergence of a rhythm from a subsidiary pacemaker; for example, sinus bradycardia at a rate of 40 bpm will lead to emergence of an AV nodal rhythm at a rate of 50-55 bpm resulting

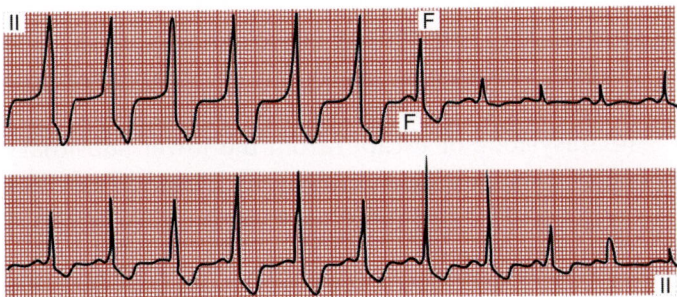

Fig. 37.1: Isorhythmic AV dissociation. Note the following characteristics on rhythm strip lead II.
  - i. There is accelerated idioventricular rhythm at a rate of 90 bpm in the beginning of the strip
  - ii. There is fusion complex (F) at the end of idioventricular rhythm followed by beginning of sinus rhythm generating narrow QRS complex for a short period at the end of upper strip
  - iii. The lower strip again shows idioventricular rhythm in which P waves are seen at the same rate as that of wide QRS complexes but are independent of it indicating AV dissociation of isorhythmic type. The cause may be haemodynamic modulation of the sinus rate via autonomic nervous system

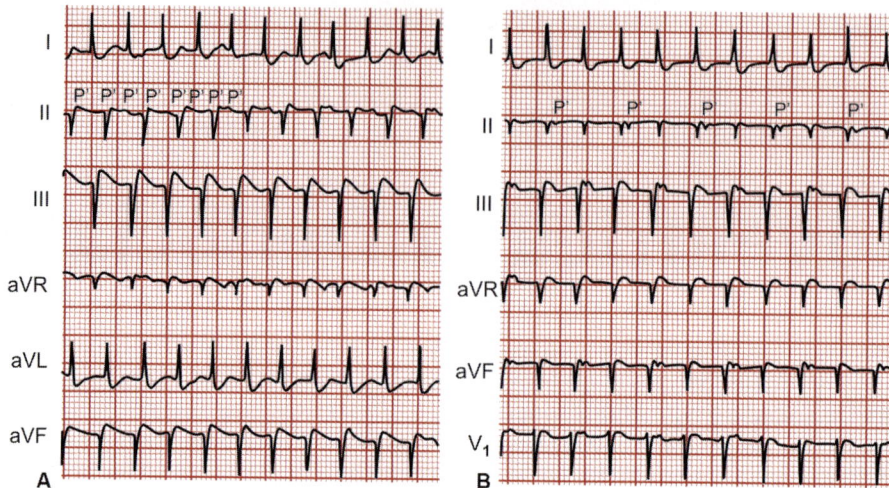

Fig. 37.2: Dual tachycardia (paroxysmal atrial and AV nodal tachycardia) induced by digitalis. The electrocardiogram shows;
A: Standard leads. There is paroxysmal atrial tachycardia (atrial beats are labelled as P' at a rate of 170-180 bpm and a junctional tachycardia with no visible P wave at a rate of 108 bpm. There no relationship between paroxysmal atrial tachycardia and junctional (AV nodal) tachycardia, hence, a diagnosis of dual supraventricular tachycardia with AV dissociation was made. As the patient was receiving digitalis, hence, it was inferred to be due to digitalis which was stopped and potassium chloride given.
B: After several hours, the ECG showed disappearance of paroxysmal atrial tachycardia but AV nodal tachycardia persisted at a slower rate (< 100 bpm). Now the P waves which were upright in lead II, III and aVF seen in A are inverted indicating retrograde conduction. These inverted P waves are seen (labelled P') after every second QRS complex indicating retrograde 2:1 block, therefore, in B there is junctional tachycardia with retrograde second degree AV block

Table 37.1: Causes of AV dissociation

1. *Slowing of sinus impulses resulting in emergence of a subsidiary pacemaker*
    - Sinus bradycardia with sinus arrhythmia
    - Sinoatrial exit blocks (SA blocks)
    - Sinus arrest
    - Vagotonaemia
    - Betablockers effect
    - Following cardioversion
    - Due to calcium channel blockers, i.e. verapamil, diltiazem.
2. *Acceleration of the subsidiary pacemaker*
    - Myocardial ischaemia
    - Digitalis intoxication
    - Catecholamine excess or atropine excess
    - Postoperative

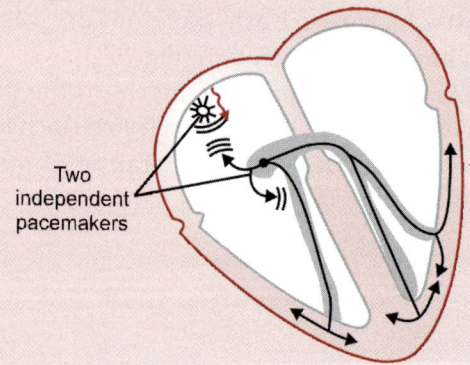

Two independent pacemakers

in AV dissociation. The atria are driven by the sinus pacemaker and the ventricles by the junctional or nodal pacemaker (Fig. 37.3). When this occurs, the impulses from these two independent pacemakers meet or collide—usually in the AV node and interfere with each other's conduction. The resulting dissociation is, hence, termed as *interference*

dissociation. This type of dissociation may be seen during ventricular or AV nodal escape beats or rhythms. In all these conditions, the beats (extrasystolic or escape) from the lower subsidiary pacemaker interfere with sinus discharge because they may occur at the same time as the delayed sinus discharge.

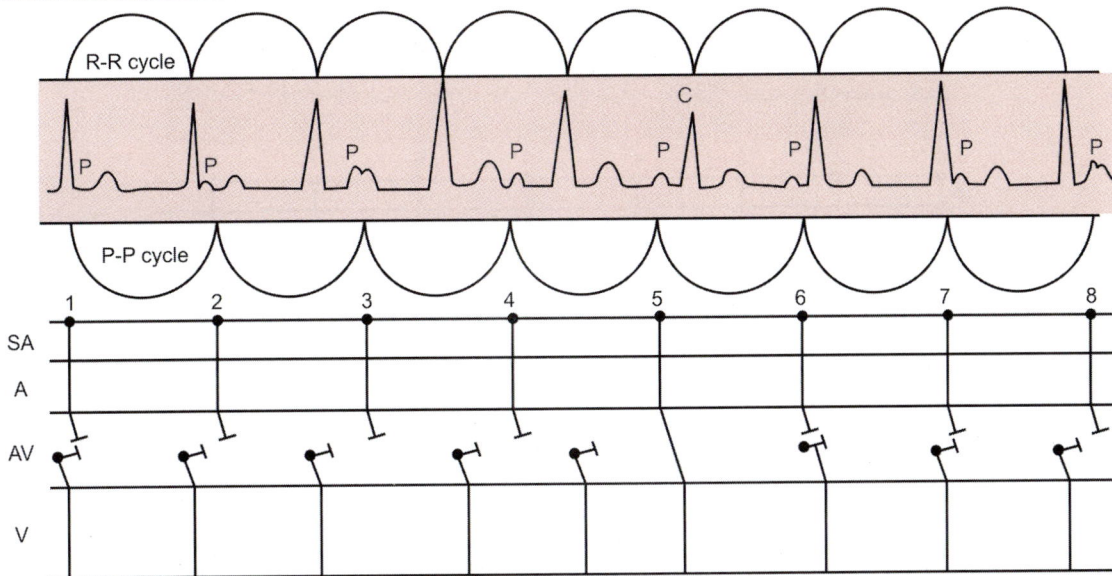

Fig. 37.3: Electrocardiogram (Diagrammatic illustration) showing AV dissociation with interference. The sinus discharge is slower than AV nodal discharge revealed by longer P-P intervals than R-R intervals, which leads to dissociation of P waves to QRS complexes. The first P wave is burried within QRS complex, the second P wave deforms the terminal part of R wave and then subsequent P waves are moving progressively further away from QRS complexes. The first four P waves of sinus discharge finds the AV node refractory; and the fifth sinus beat occurs at a relatively longer interval from the preceding QRS complex and thus finds the AV node responsive, hence, get conducted producing a *capture beat* (labelled C). The capture beats are hallmark of AV dissociation with interference. Below is drawn a ladder diagram. The black dots show the site of origin of the impulses. SA stands for sinoatrial level. A stands for atrial level, AV stands for Atrioventricular nodal level and V stands for ventricular level

SECTION TEN

AV dissociation with interference (Fig. 37.3): Interference dissociation occurs where there is;

a) Late or delayed impulse formation
b) Early or accelerated impulse formation

a. *Late or delayed impulse formation* : Late or delayed impulse formation in sinus bradycardia explains the interference. When sinus cycle length and cycle length of a subsidiary pacemaker (AV node, ventricles) approximate each other, then impulses from sinus and subsidiary pacemaker collide resulting in interference with each other's progress.

b. *Accelerated impulse generation*: Interference will also occur when there is premature or enhanced impulse generation from the subsidiary pacemaker (AV node or ventricle), such as, seen in ventricular ectopics, junctional or idionodal and ectopic ventricular tachycardia. This is due to the fact that during tachycardia there is shortening of cycle length of the subsidiary pacemaker which again approximates the sinus cycle length resulting in simultaneous arrival of both the impulses (sinus and ectopic) in the AV node resulting in interference with each other's progress.

In interference dissociation, two independent pacemakers (a supraventricular and a ventricular) having different rates of discharge, collide and interfere with mutual's progress, but a supraventricular beat may get conducted to the ventricles (ventricular capture) if a temporal opportunity is provided to do so.

The Electrocardiographic Characteristics (Figs 37.4 to 37.8)

1. Ventricular rate is faster than atrial rate.
2. P-P and R-R intervals are regular as both the pacemakers discharge regularly.
3. P wave has no relation to QRS complex. It may precede, fall on QRS or may follow it. This is because of fast ventricular and slow atrial rates.
4. P-R intervals become progressively shorter. This is most important diagnostic clue. As P-P intervals are longer (slow atrial rate) than R-R intervals (rapid ventricular rate), the P waves will overtake

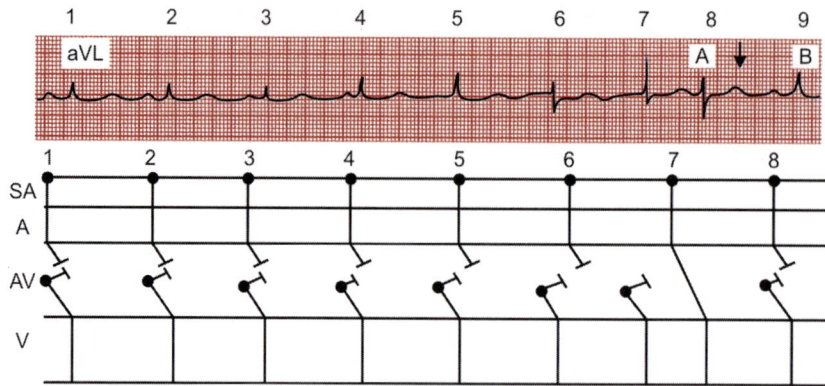

Fig. 37.4: The AV dissociation with interference. The electrocardiogram (lead aVL) shows the following characteristics:
  i. The sinus discharge is slower than AV nodal discharge, i.e. P-P intervals are longer than R-R intervals (there are eight P wave for nine QRS complexes)
  ii. There is complete dissociation of P wave from QRS complexes, i.e. P waves are unrelated to QRS complexes. The first P precedes QRS complex with a longer P-R interval, then P-R interval progressively shortens and fifth P wave gets burried within QRS complex, then subsequent P waves moves further away from QRS (sixth to eight P waves). The first six P waves of sinus discharge find AV node refractory, the seventh P wave occurs at a relatively longer interval from the preceding QRS complex and finds the AV node fully recovered and responsive, hence, gets conducted to the ventricles resulting in a premature QRS complex, called the *capture beat* (labelled as A). If this capture beat would not have occurred then next automatic nodal beat would have fallen after the usual R-R interval at the arrow, thus, the capture beat is a prematurely discharged beat, which on its way through AV node initiated the next automatic impulse at B instead of at the arrow. The capture beat, thus, doubly dissociates the ventricular rhythm. The *capture beats* are the hallmark of AV dissociation with interference
Below is drawn the ladder diagram to show the origin of impulses and their collision in AV node except the 7th sinus or atrial beat which is conducted to ventricle. SA—sinoatrial node, A—Atrial, AV—Atrioventricular nodal and V—Ventricular level

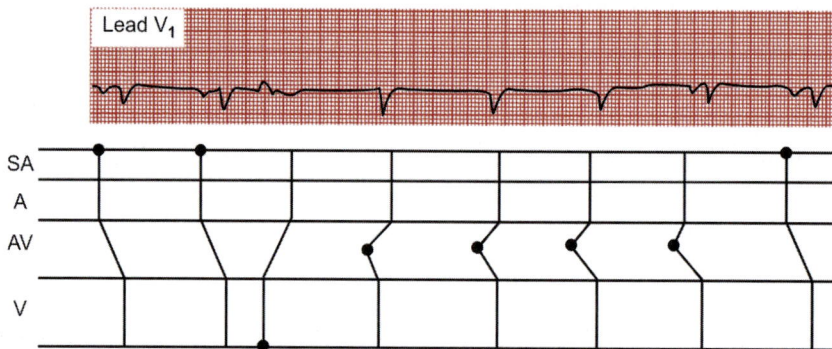

Fig. 37.5: AV dissociation triggered by a ventricular premature complex. The electrocardiogram (lead V_1) shows;
  i. The first two are sinus conducted beats with P-R interval of 0.16 sec. The P waves are biphasic
  ii. The third beat is ventricular premature complex, which temporarily suppressed the SA node, as a result of which AV node took the control of the rhythm for next four beats, until the SA node recovered and regained the overall control of the heart and pushed the sinus conducted beat, i.e. the last beat with P-R interval of 0.16 sec

QRS complexes and P-R intervals become progressively shorter. The P wave first becomes superimposed on the QRS complex and then eventually moves progressively away from the QRS complex. And when the P wave falls sufficiently behind the QRS complex, it may find an opportunity to get conducted to the ventricles resulting in an earlier QRS complex called a *'ventricular capture beat'*.

5. *Ventricular capture beats* commonly occur (Fig. 37.4.). Due to AV dissociation with interference within AV node; the ventricular or AV nodal

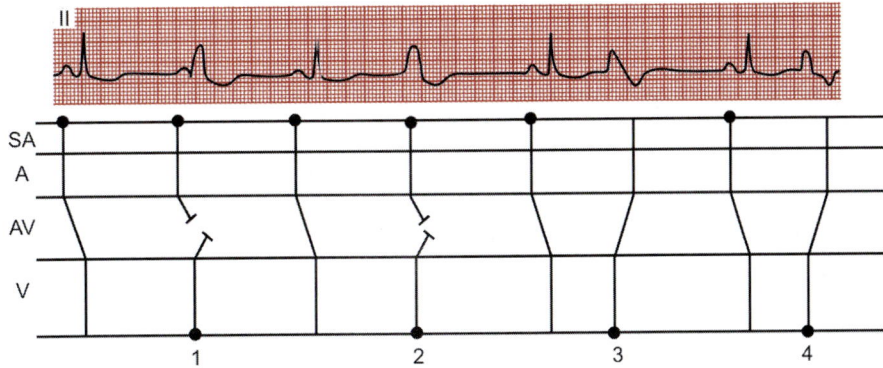

Fig. 37.6: Ventricular bigeminy rhythm with AV dissociation. The electrocardiogram (rhythm strip lead II) shows;
  i. Ventricular bigeminy rhythm—four couplets of bigeminy rhythm are seen
  ii. The first two ventricular ectopic beats (1,2) show AV dissociation and the last two ventricular ectopics (3,4) show retrograde conduction (inverted P' are seen following wide QRS complexes). The first ectopic beat is an end-diastolic VPC occurring after the sinus P wave. The next (second) VPC is earlier and the P wave is lost within it. The third and fourth ectopics are so much premature that the retrograde conduction is possible into the atria which have yet not been activated.

Note: Previously, it was thought that retrograde block is must for AV dissociation, otherwise, it was argued that faster beating AV node would take the full command of the heart. This is nowadays, considered not valid as shown in the above figure

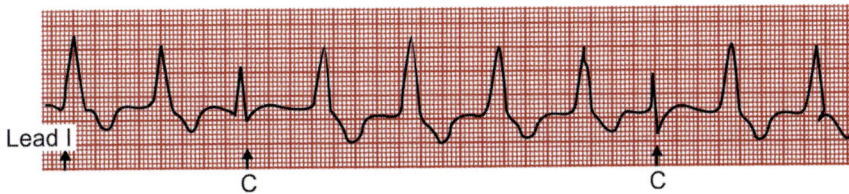

Fig. 37.7: Ventricular tachycardia with AV dissociation. The electrocardiogram (lead I) shows:
1. Wide QRS complex tachycardia at rate of 125 bpm
2. Two narrow QRS complexes are seen in between the wide QRS complex tachycardia. These are nothing but normally conducted sinus beats (↑) called *capture beats* (C). The presence of capture beats in ventricular tachycardia indicates AV dissociation because AV node was responsive to these two sinus beats and refractory to other

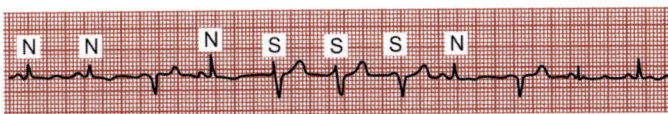

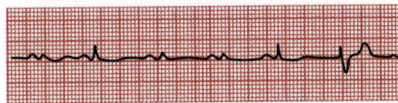

Fig. 37.8: Iatrogenic AV dissociation produced by pacemaker. The pacemaker triggered complexes (S) are seen with normal sinus complexes (N) indicating that spontaneous sinus discharge inhibited the pacemaker

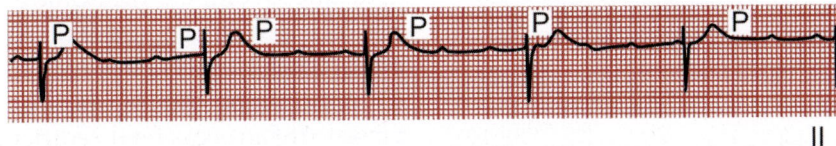

Fig. 37.9: AV dissociation without interference in complete heart block. The electrocardiogram shows;
1. Heart rate 25/min, regular. The QRS is slightly wider than normal
2. The atrial rate is 100/min regular. The P waves are well seen and do not have any relation to QRS
Note: In fact, this is not included in the ambit of AV dissociation, where interference is considered as must

impulses cannot be conducted retrogradely to the atria, as a result, sinus impulses cannot be conducted antegradely to the ventricles. However, as the two pacemakers discharge asynchronously (ventricular pacemaker is faster than atrial), the slower sinus discharge occurs later in relation to nodal or ventricular discharge, therefore, sinus P wave falls further and further away from QRS till a stage is reached when a sinus impulse may eventually reach the AV node when it is no longer refractory, gets conducted to the ventricles. This momentary activation of the ventricles by a sinus impulse during AV dissociation is called a *'capture beat'*. The capture beat is an early beat and is related to previous sinus P wave (Fig. 37.6). Long rhythm strips must be recorded in order to demonstrate their presence. Similar to ventricular capture by a supraventricular impulse, there can be retrograde atrial capture by a ventricular impulse in AV dissociation, in that situation, there will be inverted P' wave with long P-R interval.

6. When AV association is due to acceleration of the rate of subsidiary pacemaker, the P-R interval of the captured complex is often longer than expected. This is not first degree AV block but reflects depolarisation of the AV conducting tissue by immediately preceding QRS complex.

7. *Ventricular fusion complexes:* These complexes imply partial ventricular capture (Read Chapter 41), are produced by ventricular depolarisation partly by a supraventricular impulse and partly by an ectopic ventricular impulse originating from the focus of an accelerated escape ventricular pacemaker. Their shape is, thus, a blend or fusion of these two activation forces, hence, is intermediate between the supraventricular and ventricular complexes. They are hallmarks of AV dissociation.

AV nodal or ventricular extrasystoles/escape beats and AV nodal or ventricular tachycardia are the examples of AV dissociation with interference–simply called AV dissociation. Capture beats and fusion complexes are hallmarks of AV dissociation with interference. Ventricular capture or fusion indicates a brief period of break in AV dissociation for that beat.

2. A Disturbance of Impulse Conduction

AV dissociation without interference. Complete AV block or higher grades AV block lead to AV dissociation because both atria and the ventricles are controlled by two independent rhythms and they do not interfere with each other's affair. Hence, sinus rhythm and a ventricular escape rhythm in complete heart block is an example of AV dissociation without interference. In complete heart block, the sinus impulse has no opportunity to get conducted to ventricles due to complete barrier in AV node.

AV dissociation with interference is simply called AV dissociation, hence, complete AV block is an AV dissociation without interference from which it has to be differentiated.

Complete heart block versus AV dissociation: AV dissociation is present in complete heart block, called complete AV dissociation without interference (Read Chapter on AV block). In some situations when fusion or capture beats are not seen, we have to differentiate AV dissociation from complete heart block. The following points may help.

1. In complete heart block, atrial rate is more than ventricular rate (number of P waves are more than number of R waves); while in AV dissociation, ventricular rate is more than atrial (more R waves than P waves).

2. In complete heart block, no P wave gets conducted to the ventricles due to complete barricade between atria and ventricles. However, in AV dissociation, some P waves may get conducted producing capture beats or fusion beats. This is explained in Figure 37.5.

Conventionally, complete AV block is complete AV dissociation because the impulses are not conducted further from either side and they do not collide in AV node due to complete barricade between them, hence, not included in the ambit of AV dissociation with interference-simply called AV dissociation. Therefore, AV dissociation differs from complete AV block by presence of an occasional ventricular capture (capture beats and fusion complexes). This is due to the fact that a supraventricular impulse, if given an opportunity at proper time, may get conducted to ventricles in AV dissociation but such a temporal opportunity does not exist in complete heart block.

Suggested Reading

1. Castellanos A, Azan L, Calvino JM: Dissociation with interference between pacemakers located within AV conducting system. *Am Heart J* **56**:562, 1958.
2. Levy MN, Ederstein J: The mechanism of synchronisation in isorhythmic AV dissociation. II. Clinical studies. *Circulation* **42**:689,1970.
3. Marriott HJJ: A-V dissociation. A re-appraisal. *Am J Cardiol* **2**: 586, 1988.
4. Pick A: AV dissociation. A proposal for comprehensive classification and consistent terminology. *Am Heart J* **66**: 147,1963.
5. Schott A: Atrioventricular dissociation with or without interference. *Prog Cardiovasc Dis* **2**: 444, 1959.
6. Schubart AF, et al: Isorhythmic dissociation : Atrioventricular dissociation with synchronisation. *Am J Med* **24**: 209, 1958.

38

Parasystole

Definition: It is a form of dual rhythm, wherein, two pacemakers; one usually in the SA node and the other either in the atrium or AV node or a ventricle, discharge concurrently and independently to control the rhythm of the heart. Therefore, depending on the site of parasystolic focus, the second rhythm may be atrial, nodal or ventricular—called *atrial, nodal* or *ventricular parasystole* respectively. The ventricular parasystole is the commonest.

Causes

1. May occur in normal individual
2. Myocardial disease
3. Cardiac pacemakers and transplanted heart are examples of iatrogenic parasystole.

Mechanism (Fig. 38.1)

Parasystole is an abnormal rhythm produced by two independent pacemakers, one in the SA node, is the dominant pacemaker, and the other called para-systolic pacemaker lies in the atrium, or AV node or the ventricle.

There is a fundamental rule in cardiac electro-physiology that the fastest or dominant pacemaker governs the heart rate. All other subsidiary pace-makers are prematurely discharged by the impulses from the dominant pacemaker, thus, the sinus pacemaker silences the slower subsidiary pacemakers. In other words, lower pacemakers normally are not protected from the dominant pacemaker. *'Protection' here means freedom from the dominant pacemaker.*

Occasionally, a subsidiary pacemaker acquires the property of protection and operates all the time without fail at its inherent rate of discharge. Therefore, the rate of parasystolic focus varies depending on the site of focus. The protective mechanism lies in the vicinity of parasystolic focus due to which neither the sinus impulses are able to penetrate the ectopic pacemaker focus nor ectopic impulses are able to leave the focus and activate the surrounding myocardium. In other words, the parasystolic focus demonstrates both the *'entrance'* and *'exit'* block. The block is in the form of unidirectional block and usually of higher grade but, occasionally, first and second degree entrance or exit blocks can be demonstrated, and explain the occasional variation in the regular parasystolic rate.

Parasystolic focus enjoys freedom from the dominant pacemaker, hence, is a protected zone.

Parasystolic ventricular beats differ from the coupled ventricular premature beats in that the discharge from the parasystolic focus does not require a triggering impulse except the initial ventricular premature contractions in intermittent episodes of parasystole. Instead, come what may, the parasytolic pacemaker fires off automatically, rhythmically and at its own inherent rate of impulse formation. The parasystolic focus has to produce an impulse whether it is conducted or blocked.

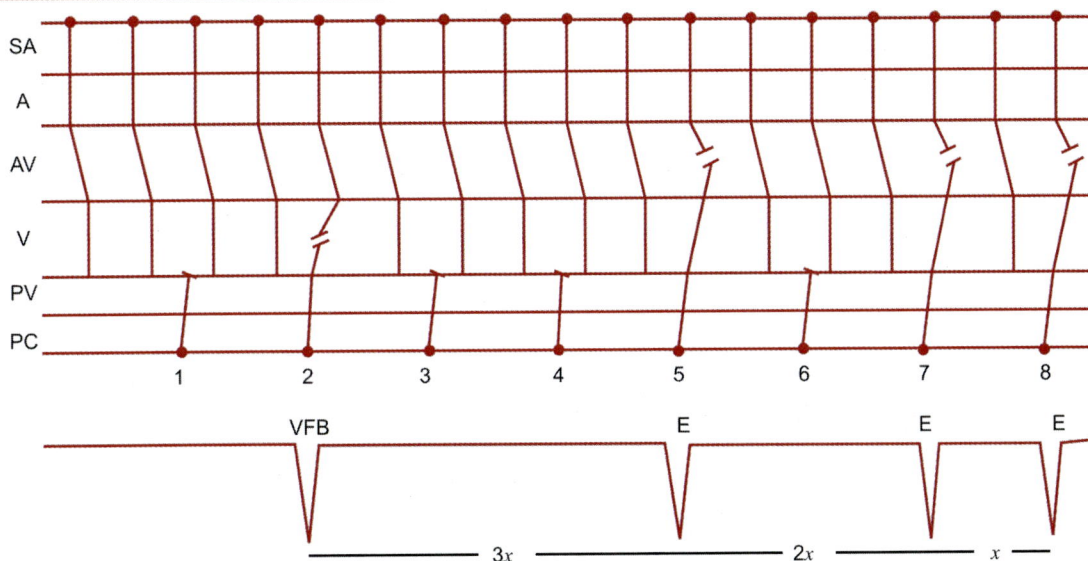

Fig. 38.1: Mechanism of ventricular parasystole (diagram). The SA node discharges regularly but its impulses cannot penetrate the parasystolic ventricular area (PV) because it is protected area. The parasystolic centre discharges regularly but at a slower rate than SA node. The parasystolic impulses 1,3,4,6 find the paraventricular myocardium (PV) refractory as a result of prior stimulation by the sinus impulse; these parasystolic impulses do not manifest electrocardiographically. On the other hand, ectopic impulses 2,5,7, and 8 find the myocardium responsive, hence, express electrocardiographically. The parasystolic discharges and sinus discharges bear no relationship as evidenced by variable coupling intervals between sinus and parasystolic impulse. As the ectopic discharge is regular, the longer manifest interectopic interval between a ventricular fusion beat (2nd) and an ectopic beat (5th) is multiple (3x) of the shortest interectopic interval between 7th and 8th ectopic beats (x). The other interectopic interval between 5th and 7th ectopics is twice (2x) of the short interectopic interval between 7th and 8th ectopic beats (x)

Two pacemakers exist in the heart in parasystole, each discharging at its own inherent and independent rate, and each activating the heart when it finds myocardium sensitive.

Electrocardiographic Characteristics of Ventricular Parasystole (Fig. 38.2)

There are four characteristics on ECG.
1. Variable coupling intervals.
2. The longer interectopic intervals are multiple of a shortest interectopic interval
3. Appearance of fusion or combination beats.
4. The conduction of parasystolic impulse whenever the myocardium is excitable.

1. *Variable coupling intervals :* Coupling interval is the interval between an ectopic (parasystolic) complex and the preceding sinus conducted complex. In contrast, ventricular ectopics or extrasystoles show a fixed coupling interval because they are forced or triggered by the preceding sinus beat. The parasystolic

pacemaker is autonomous, i.e. *the king of his own empire*, beats independently of sinus pacemaker and beat gets conducted if surrounding myocardium is responsive. These two pacemakers beat asynchronously and do not have any relation with each other. This is the reason behind the variable coupling intervals. Marked variations in coupling intervals is a cardinal sign of parasystole.

The two pacemakers in parasystole beat independently and bear no relation to each other and produce variable coupling intervals

2. *Interectopic intervals:* The longer interectopic intervals, i.e. the intervals between two manifest ectopic parasystolic discharges on ECG are multiple of the shortest interectopic interval. When there is an exit block (an exit block means a block around the ectopic beat), the expected parasystolic impulses are not conducted to the ventricles, hence, a long interectopic interval is produced.

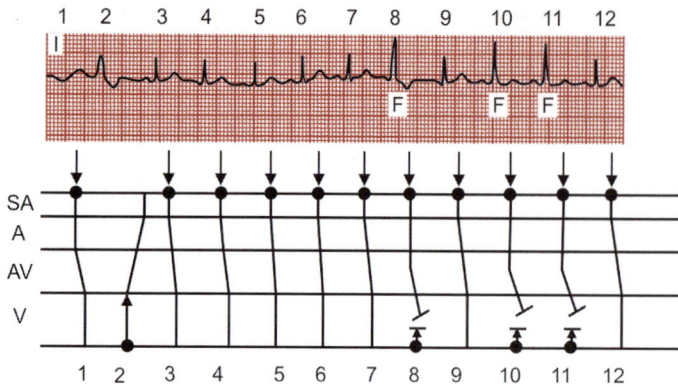

Fig. 38.2: Ventricular parasystole. The majority of QRS complexes except 2nd, 8th, 10th and 11th are sinus conducted and are preceded by P waves. The 8th, 10th and 11th QRS complexes are also preceded by P waves but the configuration of their QRS is different from sinus conducted beat. It is intermediate between a pure sinus conducted beat and a pure ventricular ectopic (2nd beat), hence, these are fusion beats (F). The interval between ventricular fusion beats and the preceding normal sinus conducted beats are not fixed coupled. The interectopic interval between 2nd and 8th complex is 3.9 sec (see ladder diagram below), between 8th and 10th is 1.3 sec and between 10th and 11th is 0.65 second. All these intervals are multiple of 0.65 seconds indicating a parasystolic discharge at a rate of about 92/min

Mechanism: In parasystole, the ectopic discharges are autonomous but all of them do not manifest because some of them may occur when the ventricles are refractory following activation by sinus pacemaker. The ectopic discharge becomes manifest finding the surrounding ventricular myocardium responsive. Since the ectopic discharges are regular, whether they manifest or not, therefore, longer interectopic intervals become multiple of shortest interectopic interval (Fig. 38.2). This feature on ECG is a diagnostic sign of parasystole.

> *The longer interectopic intervals are always multiple of the shortest interectopic interval*

3. Fusion beats : Occasionally, synchronous or near synchronous discharge of both pacemakers (sinus and parasystolic) occurs resulting in activation of the ventricles by both the impulses, i.e. each activating a part of the ventricles. The QRS complex of fusion beat is, thus, blend of these discharges, hence, has a configuration intermediate between pure sinus and pure ventricular or parasystolic beat. The characteristics of fusion beat has been discussed in respective section (Chapter 41).

> *Fusion beat means discharges from both the foci fuse or merge and produce a complex which has an intermediate configuration between the pure complexes produced by each of them.*

4. The conduction of parasystolic impulses whenever the myocardium is excitable : The parasystolic focus

is protected and its timing is not altered by the dominant rhythm, produces depolarisation of the myocardium whenever it is excitable. Constant or intermittent complete entrance block insulates and protects the parasystolic focus from surrounding electrical events. Occasionally, the *exit block* may occur during which it may fail to depolarise even the excitable myocardium. Parasystole with exit block is suspected when the parasystolic focal discharge fails to appear even though the cardiac tissue is responsive. The analogy commonly invoked to represent parasystole is the behaviour of a fixed-rate nonsensing (VOO) pacemaker. In parasystole, the ectopic ventricular discharge appear intermittently during normal sinus rhythm.

> *All parasystolic impulses do not excite the myocardium. Some impulses finding the myocardium responsive, excite it and get manifested electrocardiographically.*

PARASYSTOLIC VENTRICULAR TACHYCARDIA

The usual rate of parasystole irrespective of its origin is relatively slow ranging from 30-60 bpm. Ventricular parasystole is the most common parasystolic rhythm, whereas atrial or AV nodal parasystole is encountered occasionally in clinical practice. Rarely, ventricular parasystole may produce a tachycardia (three or more successive parasystolic beats) called a *parasystolic ventricular tachycardia.* Parasystolic ventricular tachycardia has slower ventricular rate than ordinary ventricular tachycardia, hence, resembles an accelerated idioventricular rhythm.

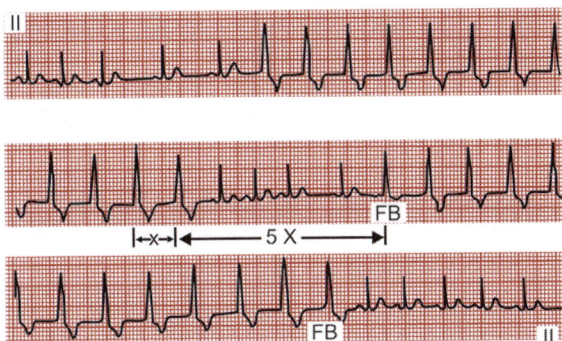

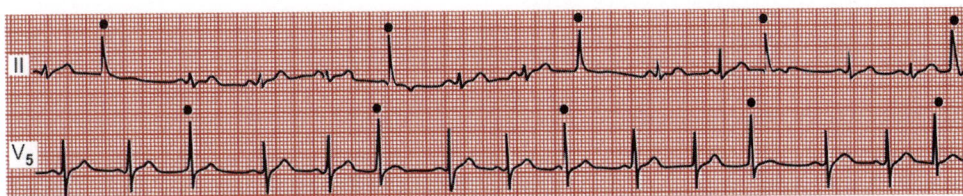

Fig. 38.3: Parasystolic ventricular tachycardia. The electro-cardiogram (lead II) shows;

i. *Intermittent sinus rhythm.* The basic sinus rhythm (normal P-QRS-T) is seen in intermittently at a rate of 92 bpm.

ii. *Long and short parasystolic intervals.* There are runs of ventricular discharges from a parasystolic focus at a rate of 83 bpm interspersed between normal sinus rhythm. The longest interectopic interval (labelled as 5x) is multiple of a shortest interectopic interval, i.e. between two consecutive beats (labelled as x).

iii. *Fusion complexes.* The fusion beats or complexes are seen randomly at the initiation or at the termination of ventricular rhythm (labelled as FB)

iv. *An idioventricular rhythm or tachycardia.* The wide QRS complexes occur at a rate of 83 bpm which indicate parasystolic ventricular tachycardia rather than ventricular tachycardia (HR > 100/min)

Fig. 38.4: Atrial parasystole with 2:1 conduction simulating second degree AV block. Note the following characteristics on electrocardiogram (lead V_1);

i. There are two types of P waves one with upright deflection labelled as P' and other with biphasic deflection labelled as P wave which is normal sinus conducted P. The P' waves are parasystolic in origin.

ii. The sinus P wave occur at a rate of 77/min, while parasystolic P' wave occur at a rate of 150/min producing arial parasystole with 2:1 conduction. This is not a case of 2nd degree AV block because (i) the shape of all P wave is not same because all are not sinus conducted (ii) two types of P wave indicated their dual origin, hence indicate two pacemakers in atria instead of one (iii) the P waves have no fixed P-R interval or fixed relationship to QRS

The Electrocardiogram (Fig. 38.3)

1. The ventricular rate is slow <100 bpm. The QRS complexes are wide and bizarre (> 0.14 sec) with no visible P waves.

2. Due to presence of exit block, there will be short and long interectopic intervals. The longer inter-ectopic intervals will always be multiple of shortest interectopic interval (interval between two successive ectopics).

3. Fusion complex: Since parasystole is an independent rhythm to the basic rhythm, ventricular fusion complex or complexes frequently occur.

ATRIAL PARASYSTOLE AND PARASYSTOLIC ATRIAL TACHYCARDIA

This is less common than ventricular parasystole. Atrial parasystolic pacemaker discharges regularly independent of sinus pacemaker and produces manifest abnormal P' waves whenever the atrial myocardium is sensitive.

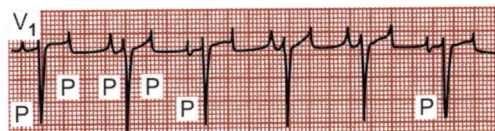

Fig. 38.5: AV nodal parasystole. The ECG (lead II, V_5) shows;

i. There is regular sinus rhythm at a rate of 90 bpm

ii. In between sinus complexes are AV nodal ectopics indicated by black dots at the top occurring at regular rate and do not have P waves.

iii. The sinus beats and AV nodal ectopic beats have no relationship to each other, i.e. they are independent of each other as indicated by varying coupling intervals. The longer interectopic intervals are multiple of shorter interectopic intervals indicating parasystolic focus in AV node. The shorter interectopic interval is twice the presumed shortest interectopic interval while longer interectopic interval is thrice the presumed shortest interectopic interval

NB: The shortest interectopic interval is not evident as there are no two consecutive AV nodal ectopics, hence is presumed.

The Electrocardiogram (Fig. 38.4)

1. There will be two types of P waves in the same lead, i.e. one normal P wave produced by the sinus pacemaker and other is abnormal P' wave produced by parasystolic atrial pacemaker.
2. There will be variable coupling intervals.
3. The longer interectopic P'-P' intervals are multiple of the short interectopic P'-P' interval.
4. In parasystolic atrial tachycardia, atrial rate is more than 100 bpm.

Clinical Significance

1. Although parasystole is more commonly found in cardiac patients than in healthy individuals, but the arrhythmia is benign and self-limited. Treatment is needed in symptomatic patients whose symptoms are directly related to parasystole.
2. Parasystole has a tendency to be refractory to various antiarrhythmic agents.
3. It is not a digitalis induced arrhythmia, hence, in a digitalised patient, an arrhythmia must be interpreted correctly, otherwise, it may be interpreted as digitalis induced VPCs.

Suggested Reading

1. Chung EK: Parasystole. *Prog Cardiovas Dis* **11**: 64, 1968.
2. Kinoshita S: Mechanism of ventricular parasystole. *Circulation* **35**: 304, 1967.
3. Lagendorf R, Pick A: Parasystole with fixed coupling. *Circulation* **35**: 304, 1967.
4. Langendorf R, Pick A: Mechanisms of intermittent ventricular bigeminy: II Parasystole, and parasystole or re-entry with conduction disturbance. *Circulation* **11**: 431, 1955.
5. Pick A: Parasystole, *Circulation* **8**:243, 1953.
6. Watanabe Y: Reassessment of parasystole. *Am Heart J* **81**: 451, 1971.

39

Ventricular Aberrancy or Aberrant Intraventricular Conduction

■ *Definition, causes, mechanisms and electrocardiographic characteristics*
■ *Differential diagnosis of a wide QRS tachycardia*
■ *Atrial fibrillation with ventricular aberration—Ashmann phenomenon*
■ *Aberrant intraventricular conduction during atrial flutter—mimicking extrasystolic ventricular bigeminy*
■ *Ventricular aberrancy versus intermittent bundle branch block*

PHASIC ABERRANT INTRAVENTRICULAR CONDUCTION

A sinus or a supraventricular ectopic beat having a narrow QRS complex is considered to be conducted without aberrancy. However, when there is an isolated, bizarre, wide QRS complex, then it is considered either an aberrantly conducted supraventricular impulse or a ventricular ectopic beat (ventricular ectopy). The rapid succession of such beats produces a wide QRS complex tachycardia.

Definition: Ventricular aberrancy means an abnormal intraventricular conduction of a supraventricular beat or beats. This abnormal conduction through the ventricles usually occurs via one of the bundle branches or a fascicle producing a bundle branch block or a fascicular block pattern-wide QRS complex; which may resemble a ventricular extrasystole. The ventricular aberrancy may be temporary or phasic, and, occasionally, may be permanent. The phasic aberrancy producing wide QRS complexes may occur during supraventricular rhythms which otherwise reveal normal intraventricular conduction, hence, may mimic extrasystolic ventricular tachycardia (ventricu-lar ectopy), therefore, the differentiation between the two (Table 39.1) is of utmost importance because both have different treatment and prognosis.

A supraventricular beat which gets aberrantly conducted through the ventricles produces a pattern of one of the bundle branch blocks (triphasic pattern); the succession of such beats results in a wide QRS complex tachycardia.

Mechanisms of Ventricular Aberrancy

Any supraventricular beat or rhythm, i.e. sinus rhythm, nodal rhythm, atrial and nodal ectopic beats, paroxysmal atrial or nodal tachycardia, atrial flutter and atrial fibrillation, etc may be complicated by aberrant intraventricular conduction. The aberrancy depends on;

1. Unequal Refractoriness of Bundle Branches and Critically Timed Impulses

Depending on the refractoriness of bundle branches and timing of incoming impulses, there can be three situations;

a) *When the refractory period of bundle branches are equal.* An impulse which comes early and finds both the bundle branches refractory, gets blocked and there is no intraventricular conduction, results in blocked 'P' wave. On the other hand, if the impulse comes late and finds both the bundles recovered from previous excitation, gets conducted with normal intraventricular conduction producing a narrow normal QRS complex.

b) *When the refractory period of both the bundle branches is unequal and there* is differential recovery of these bundles from previous excitation, then an impulse which comes early, may find both bundles refractory, gets blocked. On the other hand, when an impulse comes late, will find both bundles recovered, gets conducted with normal intraventricular conduction.

c) *When the refractory period of the bundle branches is unequal as in situation (b),* but the impulse is neither too early nor too late, finding one of the bundle branches fully recovered when other is still refractory; gets conducted down to the ventricles via the recovered bundle branch producing a wide QRS due to blocked or unrecovered other bundle branch (RBBB or LBBB). When there is differential recovery of the bundles, left bundle recovers first, hence, the aberrant intraventricular conduction, though not invariably, but commonly, results in right bundle branch block pattern (rSR' or rsR'). Therefore, essential conditions for aberrant intraventricular conduction are given in the box and explained by the diagram (Figs 39.1A and B).

> *Unequal refractory periods of bundle branches with differential recovery favour the critically timed impulses to get conducted aberrantly through the ventricles.*

2. Heart Rate (Long and Short Cycle Lengths)

The phenomenon of unequal refractoriness of the bundle branches applies to the heart rate also. At slow heart rate (between 60-75/min), the extrasystoles or sinus impulses find both the bundle branches fully recovered, hence, get conducted normally. With an increase in heart rate (>90/min), the sinus or atrial extrasystolic impulses may, sometimes,

Refractory period of bundle branches

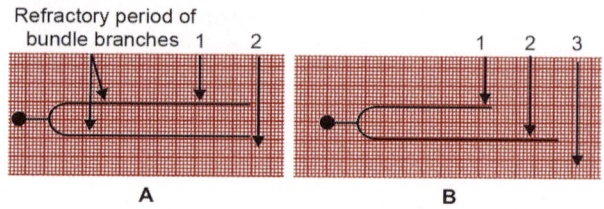

Fig. 39.1: Diagram reflecting the refractory period of bundle branches (dark parallel lines)
A: With equal refractory periods, an early supraventricular impulse (1) is blocked; while late (2) is conducted
B: With unequal refractory periods, an early supraventricular impulse (1) is blocked, while late (3) gets conducted. The supraventricular impulse which is neither too late nor too early, i.e. critically timed impulse (2) finds one bundle branch refractory and the other responsive, gets conducted through recovered (responsive) bundle branch-called intraventricular aberration

find the left bundle branch recovered and right bundle branch refractory, therefore, right bundle branch block pattern due to aberrant ventricular conduction of such impulses may occur. This is summarised in the box and represented in Figure 39.2.

> ### Cycle lengths and aberrant conduction
>
> * *Cycle lengths (R-R intervals) change from long to short, such as, in atrial fibrillation, predisposes to aberrant intraventricular conduction.*
> * *Short cycle lengths (rapid heart rate) of sinus arrhythmia, may be associated with aberrant intraventricular conduction.*
> * *Long cycle lengths (slow heart rate) are usually associated with normal ventricular conduction.*

3. The Ashmann Phenomenon

The preceding R-R interval determines the duration of refractory period, hence, with long preceding R-R interval, the refractory period will be relatively longer; and shorter R-R intervals will have subsequently short refractory periods. This can be translated to heart rates. At rapid heart rates (short R-R intervals), the refractory period is short; while at slow heart rates (long R-R intervals), the refractory period will be long. The effect of heart rate on aberrancy has already been discussed above.

The aberrant complex usually appears when a long cycle length (or R-R interval) is followed by a shorter cycle length. The shorter cycle length terminates with

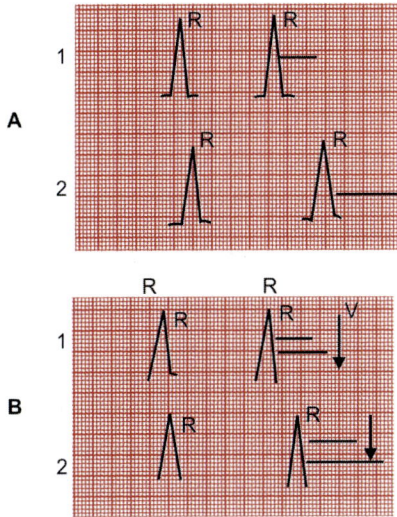

Fig. 39.2: Effect of long and short cycle lengths (R-R interval) on the ensuing refractory period denoted by parallel lines (diagram)

A: 1. With shorter preceding R-R interval, subsequent refractory period will be relatively shorter
 2. With longer preceding R-R interval, subsequent refractory period will be longer

B: 1. With short R-R interval (short refractory period), an early beat (V) is conducted normally without aberration
 2. When there is long R-R interval (a long refractory period) the same early impulse (V) is conducted with aberration because it finds one bundle branch refractory but other is responsive due to unequal recovery of bundle branches

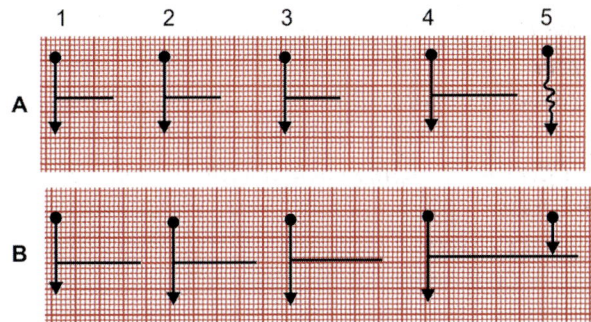

Fig. 39.3: The Ashmann phenomenon (diagram). The continuous transverse line represents the effective refractory period following each conducted impulse. At regular rhythm (first three beats in A and B), the refractory period remains constant. With sudden change in cycle length (between 3 and 4 in A and B), the refractory period lengthens. When the basic refractory period is already long or is relatively long (as in B), the further lengthening resulting from change in cycle length, i.e. long cycle length (Ashmann phenomenon) may result in a block (in B) or aberrant conduction (in A) of the ensuring impulse 5

the aberrant complex. This may be referred to as long-short intervals leading to aberrant conduction called the *Ashmann phenomenon*. This phenomenon may be observed during atrial fibrillation due to variable (long and short) R-R intervals and following a blocked or nonconducted atrial ectopic. The phenomenon is diagrammatically repesented (Fig. 39.3). The Ashmann phenomenon during atrial fibrillation is discussed towards the end of this chapter.

The Ashmann phenomenon

Aberrant intraventricular conduction is facilitated by a long preceding cycle length followed suddenly by a short cycle length. The shorter cycle length terminates with the aberrant complex.

Conditions Associated with Ventricular Aberration

1. Premature excitation. Conduction will fail or be delayed if the stimulus is premature and falls during

the effective refractory period of AV node. When the premature impulse falls during the relative refractory period of a single bundle branch, the unilateral delay results in the bundle branch block pattern of the premature beat. Duration of refractory period depends on the basic heart rate and preceding cycle length. Normally, the effective refractory period shortens with an increase in heart rate and lengthens with slowing of heart rate. Irrespective of heart rates or cycle lengths, the degree of aberration depends on premature excitation.

The morphology of QRS in aberration is determined by the length of refractory period of AV node, bundle of His and bundle branch system. Normally, at slow heart rates, the right bundle has the longest refractory period, followed by AV node and left bundle; and the bundle of His has the shortest refractory period. At rapid heart rates, the duration of the refractory period of the left bundle exceeds that of right bundle, hence, aberrancy at rapid rates results in LBBB pattern.

At slow heart rates, the descending order of the effective refractory period is;
Right bundle > AV node and left bundle > bundle of His.
Therefore, a supraventricular premature impulse falling during the effective refractory period of one of

the bundles, is conducted through the other bundle producing a pattern of BBB (RBBB pattern is commoner than LBBB).

2. Effect of changing cycle lengths on refractoriness

(Ashmann's phenomenon). Since the duration of the refractory period depends on the preceding cycle length (R-R interval), the longer the length of the preceding cycle, the longer is the refractory period that follows, hence, at constant heart rate, sudden prolongation of preceding cycle length may result in aberration. Therefore, this aberrancy, due to changes in the preceding cycle length is known as *Ashmann's phenomenon*. The Ashmann's phenomenon type of aberrancy results in morphology of QRS usually of RBBB pattern or left anterior or left posterior fascicular block pattern and may persist for a number of cycles.

Recognition of aberrancy during irregular supraventricular rhythms During irregular supraventricular rhythms (atrial fibrillation, repetitive atrial tachycardia or atrial tachycardia with Wenckebach AV block), aberrancy due to Ashmann's phenomenon (Fig. 39.4) is recognised by:

1. A comparatively long cycle (R-R interval) precedes the aberrant QRS.
2. RBBB aberrancy is common in which the initial QRS vector is normally oriented.
3. Irregular coupling of the aberrant QRS.
4. Absence of compensatory pause following the aberrant QRS.

3. Tachycardia-dependent aberrancy (phase 3 aberrancy)

Aberration, often does not appear at relatively slow heart rates frequently below 75/min, however, at certain critical heart rates >90/min, aberrancy may occur due to impaired intraventricular conduction called tachycardia–dependent aberration or phase 3 aberrancy. Supraventricular tachycardia with aberrant conduction is an example of phase 3 aberrancy (Figs 39.5 and 39.6).

The appearance and disappearance of aberration depends on very small change in cycle lengths, a change frequently difficult or impossible to detect on ECG. For this, a reasonable long continuous recording must be available to reveal a comparison of the earliest available cycle length terminated by a normal QRS with cycle length terminated by the first aberrantly

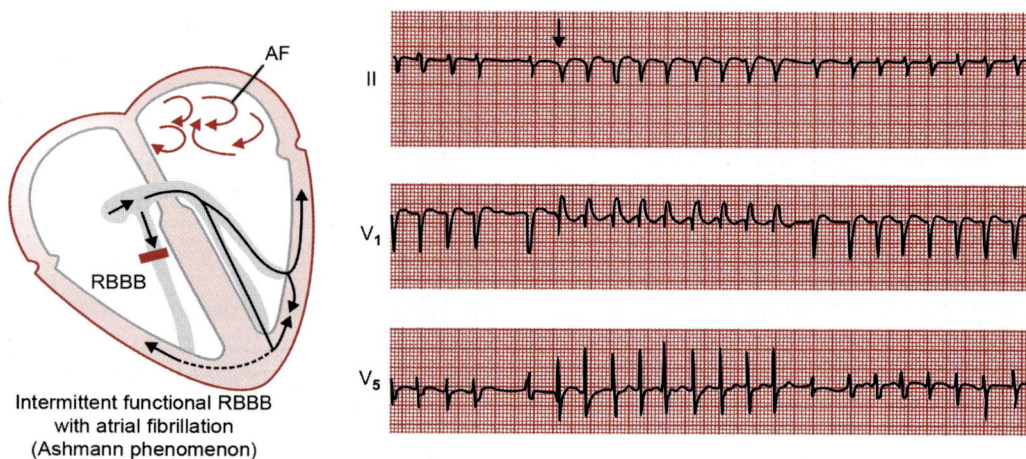

Fig. 39.4: Ashmann's phenomenon in atrial fibrillation. The basic rhythm on electrocardiogram is atrial fibrillation with rapid ventricular response of about 160 bpm. In leads V_1 and V_5 there is a short run of wide QRS complex tachycardia following a long R-R cycle.

In lead II, there is also a short run of wide QRS complexes of variable shape and size in the middle following a long R-R interval (arrow). Both these episodes of wide QRS tachycardia indicate atrial fibrillation with phasic aberrant intraventricular conduction (Ashmann's phenomenon) due to following reasons.
1. The basic rhythm is AF which produces long and short cycle lengths due to variable ventricular response
2. The wide QRS tachycardia is initiated by preceding long R-R cycle
3. The wide QRS complexes have RBBB in lead V_1 and V_6

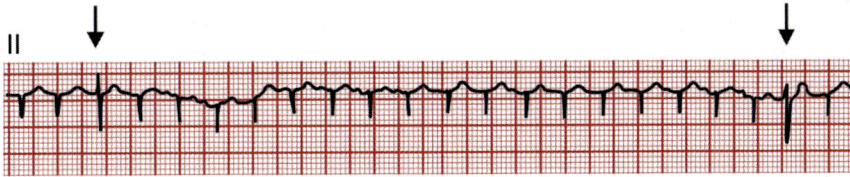

Fig. 39.5: Sinus tachycardia with aberrantly conducted beats. The electrocardiogram shows the third and last but one (indicated by arrows) complexes conducted with aberration with superior orientation of their mean QRS, hence, there is rS pattern of anterior fascicular block. These complexes are not atrial premature complexes because they are conducted with normal P wave and P-R interval, and there is no compensatory pause

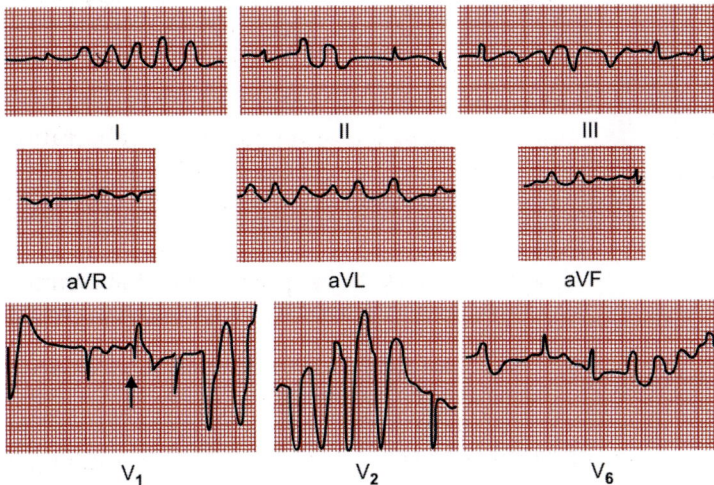

Fig. 39.6: Tachycardia induced LBBB type of aberrancy. The basic rhythm is sinus at rate of 160/min. The wide QRS complexes are seen intermittently interspersed in between sinus complexes. The wide QRS have left bundle branch block pattern (wide R in V_6, lead I and aVL and wide QR pattern in V_1-V_2)

This appears to be rate dependent LBBB aberrancy

One complex in lead V_1 shows rSR' pattern ($\uparrow$) indicating RBBB type of aberrancy.

Note: It could well be intermittent bundle branch block but because of its appearance at certain critical heart rate and rapid change in normal sinus to aberrant conduction irrespective of cycle length and variations in QRS morphology favour aberrant conduction

conducted beat. This comparison will aid in the diagnosis of tachycardia–dependent aberrancy. The difference in the duration of two such cycle lengths is often less than 0.04 sec.

The characteristics of tachycardia dependent aberrancy are:

1. It appears at certain critical heart rates.
2. QRS pattern is LBBB type.
3. It is independent of preceding cycle length.
4. Occasionally may appear without or with a slight change in the cycle length.
5. It occurs in the presence of a heart disease.

4. Bradycardia-dependent aberrancy (phase 4 aberrancy): A prolonged cycle may be terminated by an aberrant QRS and forshortening of the cycle may normalise the QRS. Slow diastolic depolarisation (phase 4) of transmembrane action potentials during prolonged cycle is implicated as the cause of this type of aberrancy (Fig. 39.7).

5. Concealed conduction: Conduction in the bundle branches may be impaired by concealed penetration of a supraventricular impulse or by trans-septal activation from the contralateral bundle.

6. Myocardial depression (Fig. 39.8): Drugs, metabolic and electrolyte disorders are frequent causes of QRS aberrancy. The severity of depression of conduction varies, and the QRS may exhibit pattern of RBBB or LBBB or fascicular block or any other combination. Myocardial diseases may sometimes be associated with aberrantly conducted beats, in addition to bundle branch blocks or fascicular blocks, from which they have to be differentiated.

Note: The aberrancy can be differentiated from BBB by the presence of distortions in the initial and terminal portions of QRS. The appearance of aberration is usually rate-dependent while BBB is rate-independent.

7. Post-extrasystolic aberration: Rarely, a compensatory pause following an atrial or nodal extrasystole may be terminated by an aberrantly conducted sinus

SECTION TEN

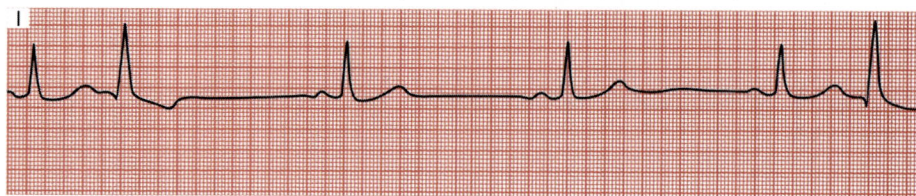

Fig. 39.7: Decceleration related aberrancy. The ECG (lead I) shows sinus bradycardia (43 bpm) with aberrantly conducted supraventricular nodal ectopic beats. The second and the last complexes in the rhythm strip are premature nodal complexes with no visible P wave, wide QRS complex (<0.14 sec) having orientation similar to sinus beats and followed by a long compensatory pause, indicate rate-dependant intraventricular aberrancy

Note: These are not nodal escape beats as they occur earlier than anticipated time and are followed by a compensatory pause.

SECTION TEN

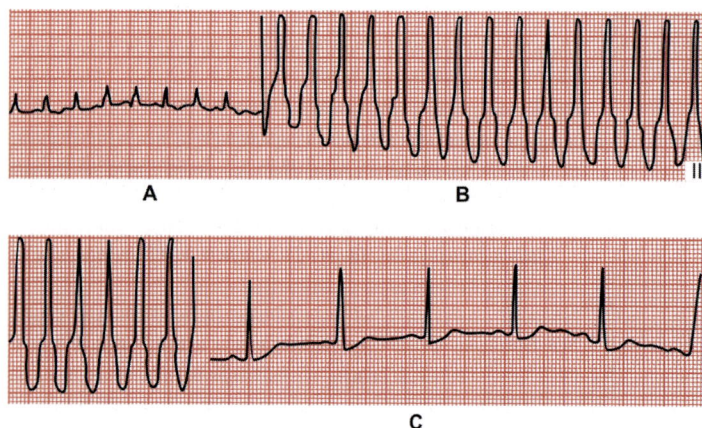

Fig. 39.8: Myocardial depression induced aberrancy. The ECG lead I shows;

A: Supraventricular tachycardia at a rate of 200/min

B: Phasic aberrant conduction in supraventricular tachycardia (LBBB type)

C: The restoration of normal sinus rhythm after termination of tachycardia.

The ST segment depression may be an evidence of myocardial disease

beat or an escape beat; the two have to be differentiated. The cause of post-extrasystolic or post-pausal aberrancy is attributed to slow diastolic depolarisation, unequal recovery of conducting tissue or increased diastolic volume.

8. *Sinus arrhythmia*: Physiological aberrancy observed in a normal heart during sinus arrhythmia is due to short and long cycle lengths. This has to be differentiated from rate-related aberrancy.

> *Sinus rhythm, AV nodal rhythm, atrial and AV nodal ectopics, paroxysmal atrial and AV nodal tachycardias, atrial fibrillation and atrial flutter may be complicated by aberrant ventricular conduction.*

ECG Characteristic of an Aberrantly Conducted Beat or Beats (Figs 39.9 and 39.10)

To diagnose an aberrant supraventricular beat or beats; proceed as follows ;

1. To diagnose an aberrant conduction, take a long strip of that lead which shows ventricular aberrancy, and sinus conducted impulses. The lead selected is usually V_1 or V_6 or any standard lead. The lead V_1 or V_6 is selected specifically to define the pattern of bundle branch block.

2. Examine the sinus conducted beats, i.e. morphology of P wave, P-R interval and morphology of QRS.

3. Now select a beat with wide QRS. Examine whether it is preceded by a normal or an abnormal P wave, if preceded by an abnormal P wave, then it is supraventricular beat conducted with intraventricular aberration. Depending on its timing, it may or may not be followed by a compensatory pause. An early occurring atrial premature beat with ventricular aberration may be followed by a compensatory pause, while an interpolated atrial premature beat with ventricular aberration will not have a compensatory pause. Similar will be the situation with nodal ectopics with inverted P wave preceding wide QRS or embedded P wave within QRS.

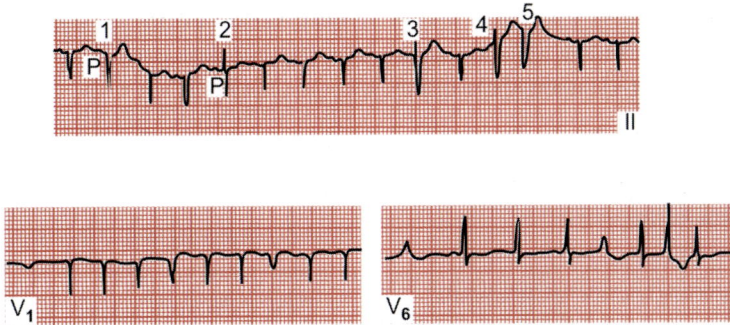

Fig. 39.9: Aberrantly conducted supraventricular beats. The electrocardiogram shows;
1. Upper strip (lead II). The first, third and fourth (labelled as 1,3,4) ectopics have short P-R interval, come early and find one of the bundle branch refractory and get conducted through the other bundle branch producing aberration. Similarly, the 5th ectopic (5) beat is successively aberrantly conducted with much more aberration. All these atrial ectopics have rS pattern with wide slurred S wave resembling anterior fascicular block pattern. On the other hand the 2nd atrial ectopic (2) comes slightly late gets conducted with less degree of intraventricular aberration
2. Lower strip (lead V_1, V_6). The aberrantly conducted beats have LBBB pattern (slurred R in V_6 and slurred S in V_1). Confirms the pattern of aberrantly conducted beat in lead II to be from left anterior fascicle. Last but one complex in V_6 is ventricular ectopic

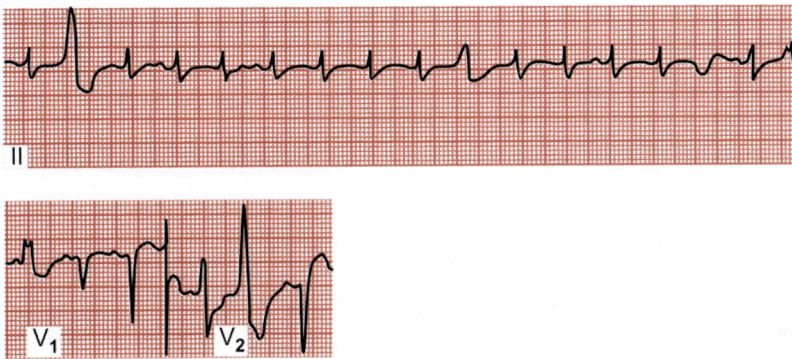

Fig. 39.10: Ventricular ectopy as well as ventricular aberrancy. The leads II (continuous recording) shows a normal sinus rhythm intercepted by ventricular ectopics and atrial premature beats conducted with various types of aberrancy.
  i. In the upper strip (lead II), there are two VPCs (2nd and 15 beats). First VPC has wide QRS and second has QS pattern. Both are interposed between two sinus beats, hence, are interpolated VPCs. There are two aberrantly conducted APCs (10th and 17th) having abnormal P wave, short P-R interval and a bundle branch block pattern. There is no compensatory pause.
  ii. The lower strip (lead V_1) shows first beat as an APC (abnormal P wave, short P-R interval and RBBB pattern of QRS) with aberrant conduction followed by two sinus beats. The lead V_2 next shows again first as an APC with aberrant conduction. This APC has RS pattern which is wide and is followed by a VPC. The last beat is sinus conducted beat. The electrocardiographic leads show that both ventricular ectopy and aberrancy can coexist in the same lead

4. To decide which bundle is refractory and which is responsive, study the pattern of QRS of the aberrant conducted beat. If the aberrant conducted beat has rSR′ pattern in V_1, it indicates that right bundle was refractory and left bundle only was responsive; and if the pattern is wide qR or qRS or RR′ in V_1, then it is left bundle branch block pattern which means right bundle was responsive and left bundle was refractory to conduction. Sometimes, anterior fascicular block pattern may occur in which an aberrant conducted beat has rS pattern in leads, II, III and aVF.

5. Now examine the initial orientation (0.04 sec) of QRS in the lead showing aberrantly conducted supraventricular beats. For example, initial orientation of 0.04 sec in V_1 is normally reflected by

SECTION TEN

r wave of normal rS complex in this lead; if the wide QRS has similar orientation (rSR' pattern), then it is an aberrantly conducted supraventricular impulse.

ECG Clues to an Aberrantly Conducted Supraventricular Impulse

- It is preceded by an abnormal P wave or a normal P wave (aberrantly conducted sinus beat)
- The QRS complex is wide but its initial orientation is similar to the sinus conducted beats
- There may or may not be a compensatory pause following wide QRS
- It has a pattern of one of the bundle branch blocks
- QRS duration is usually < 0.14 sec.

A supraventricular impulse with wide QRS may, at times, mimics ventricular ectopic from which it has to be differentiated from therapeutic point of view. A wide QRS complex tachycardia following an aberrantly conducted supraventricular impulse is presumed to be of supraventricular origin and treated accordingly. The differences between an aberrantly conducted supraventricular impulse and a ventricular ectopic are tabulated (Table 39.1).

VENTRICULAR ABERRANCY

A ventricular ectopic beat produces a wide QRS complex due to delayed and abnormal ventricular conduction; the succession of such beats produces a wide QRS complex tachycardia called *extrasystolic ventricular tachycardia.*

Differentiation Between a Supraventricular Tachycardia with Aberration and a Ventricular Tachycardia (Table 39.2)

The distinction between the two is necessary from clinical point of view.

The differentiation of an ectopic ventricular tachycardia from a supraventricular tachycardia with aberrant ventricular conduction is based on the following principles;

1. The relationship of abnormal QRS complex to the preceding P or P' wave
2. Identification and configuration of a capture beat or beats.
3. Presence or absence of a ventricular fusion beat or beats.
4. Morphology of QRS complexes.
5. The presence or absence of an attempt at a compensatory pause.

ATRIAL FIBRILLATION WITH VENTRICULAR ABERRATION

In atrial fibrillation, a large number of fibrillatory waves randomly and irregularly bombard the AV node, most of them finding the AV node and bundle branches responsive, get conducted to the ventricles producing normal QRS complexes at irregular intervals. As there is variations of cycle lengths (variable R-R intervals) in atrial fibrillation, aberrances can occur following a long-short cycle lengths—called Ashmann's phenomenon as already discussed. In

Table 39.1: Differences between an aberrantly conducted supraventricular beat and a ventricular ectopic	
An aberrantly conducted supraventricular beat	*A ventricular ectopic*
• It is preceded by a normal or an abnormal P wave	• It is usually not preceded by P wave which is burried within QRS, i.e. concealed conduction,
• Pattern of QRS is either of RBBB(rSR') or LBBB (qRS or RR'), hence, is triphasic	• It has usually Rs pattern (biphasic pattern)
• Initial vector of QRS does not change	• There is change in initial QRS vector
• Wide QRS is due to differential refractoriness of bundle branches, i.e. one bundle branch is refractory and other is responsive	• Wide QRS is due to delayed and abnormal conduction of ventricular beat arising from an ectopic focus in one of the ventricles
• QRS duration is <0.14 sec	QRS duration is usually >0.14 sec

Table 39.2: The differentiating features between a supraventricular tachycardia with aberrant conduction and a ventricular tachycardia

Feature	Supraventricular tachycardia with aberrant ventricular conduction (Figs 39.11 to 39.15)	Ventricular tachycardia (Read Chapter 35)
1. The relationship between abnormal QRS and preceding P or P′ waves;		
(i) When the P or P′ waves are visible on ECG	Wide QRS complexes preceded by abnormal P′ waves favour supraventricular tachycardia with aberration because atrial event is undisturbed and precedes ventricular event	Wide QRS complexes are not preceded by abnormal P′ waves. The P′ waves either get merged within QRS due to simultaneous antegrade activation of the ventricles and retrograde atrial activation or, abnormal P′ (inverted P′) waves may follow them if there is delayed retrograde atrial activation.
(ii) When P or P′ waves not visible	The P or P′ waves may not be visible in paroxysmal atrial tachycardia or AV nodal tachycardia In such a situation, examine the beginning of paroxysm; if initiated by an atrial ectopic or AV nodal ectopic with aberrant conduction, then it is SVT with aberrant conduction. Similarly, in atrial fibrillation, if 'f' waves are not visible, tachycardia following a long cycle length (R-R interval), indicates it to be SVT with aberrant conduction. If in the rhythm strip, there are isolated atrial or nodal ectopics with aberrant conduction preceding or following tachycardia, then it is most likely SVT with aberrant conduction.	Ventricular tachycardia may be preceded by ventricular ectopics or a ventricular ectopic or ectopic(s) with R on T phenomenon. If wide QRS complex tachycardia occurs in a patient with prolonged QTc syndrome, it is invariably ventricular in origin. Similarly, if bidirectional or polymorphic VPCs are seen in the rhythm strip preceding or following the paroxysm, it is ventricular tachycardia rather than supraventricular.
(iii) AV dissociation	AV dissociation does not occur because each supraventricular beat is conducted with aberration	It is common. There are two pacemakers in VT (one in SA node and other in the either ventricle), the impulses from both of them collide in AV node and interfere with each other's progress, hence, AV dissociation with interference is common.
2. QRS morphology characteristics		
(i) Initial vector of QRS	Does not change. Aberrant ventricular conduction is dominated by pattern of RBBB which does not interfere with the initial vector of QRS	Initial vectors are markedly changed. VT is dominated by abnormal and delayed ventricular activation that interferes with the initial vectors.

Contd...

SECTION TEN

Contd...

Feature	Supraventricular tachycardia with aberrant ventricular conduction	Ventricular tachycardia
(ii) The QRS configuration	Triphasic pattern of bundle branch block (rSR' in V$_1$ or qRS in V$_6$). As the initial vectors producing normal rS in V$_1$ and qR in V$_6$ does not change, therefore, addition of terminal R' wave in V$_1$ and S in V$_6$ due to anterior and rightward QRS axis due to RBBB makes typical rSR' in V$_1$ and qRS in V$_6$-a characteristic of SVT with aberrant conduction	Monophasic or diphasic configuration of QRS in V$_1$ and V$_6$ which is not only wide but bizarre also. These complexes are either dominantly upright or dominantly negative with notched apex or nadir in the same lead. (Fig. 39.11)

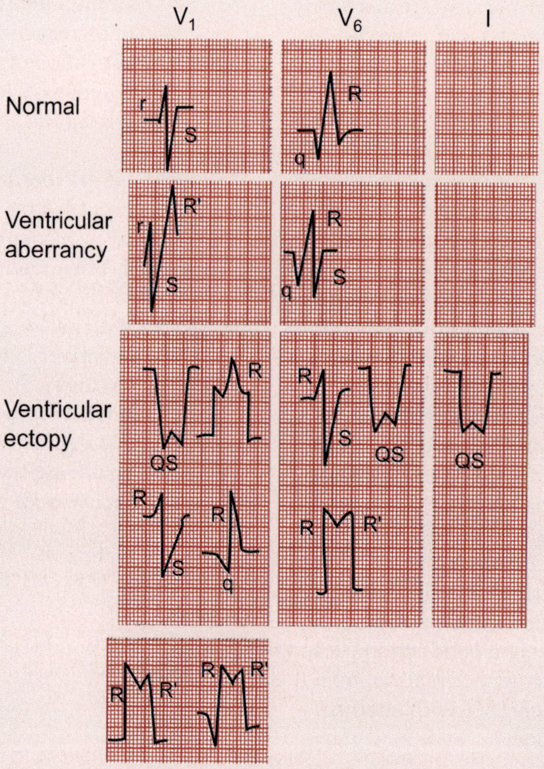

Fig. 39.11: Electrocardiographic patterns of ventricular aberrancy *vs* ectopy in different leads

Feature	Supraventricular tachycardia with aberrant ventricular conduction	Ventricular tachycardia
(iii) Relative amplitude of R and R' deflection	There is usually RBBB pattern in lead V$_1$ where initial r is smaller than terminal R' wave (Fig. 39.11)	The lead V$_1$ if reflects a bizarre dominantly upright biphasic QRS (RR' pattern); then initial deflection of the QRS (R wave) is larger than the terminal deflection of QRS–the R' wave. The notched upright QRS complex resembles to a pair of rabbit's ears (Fig. 39.11).
(iv) Initial small q wave followed by R wave (qR complex)	Less common	More common

Contd...

Contd...

Feature	Supraventricular tachycardia with aberrant ventricular conduction	Ventricular tachycardia
(v) Concordant pattern. It means either all positive or all negative deflections in precordial leads (V_1-V_6)	Nonconcordant pattern in precordial leads. Rhythm is mostly regular.	Concordant pattern is common in which series of bizarre QRS complex are either positive or negative. This is due to the fact that QRS axis in VT has either dominant anterior or posterior orientation. Rhythm may be slightly irregular.
(vi) QRS pattern in V_1-V_4	In LBBB type of aberrancy, there will be QS pattern in leads V_1-V_2 with deepest QS in V_2	If the QS complex is deepest in V_4 than V_2 or V_3, then ventricular ectopy is most likely
(vii) QRS complex in V_6	There is either an rS or RS complex in V_6 due to RBBB where S wave is deep and widened. This pattern is also seen in bifascicular block (RBBB with LAH), RVH and true dextrocardia, hence these conditions must be excluded	There is either a wide notched positive QRS (RR') deflection or a negative QRS (QS) deflection
(viii) Changes in lead I	There is always a positive QRS deflection in lead I. This may involve the whole QRS (LBBB type of aberrancy) or an initial part producing rS pattern (RBBB type of aberrancy).	A QS pattern in lead I is highly suggestive of VT. A positive QRS deflection in lead I usually excludes VT.
(ix) Variations in QRS amplitude and shape	Multiform QRS complexes with fine gradations in the beginning or at the end. This is due to the fact that different degrees of prematurity of the supraventricular beats with different coupling intervals result in varying degrees of aberration	There is uniform QRS configuration because all the complexes arise from a single ectopic ventricular focus. Fine gradations of QRS are absent, hence, QRS complexes are smooth
(x) Duration of QRS	< 0.14 sec	> 0.14 sec
(xi) Mean frontal plane QRS axis	Normal or near normal frontal plane QRS axis, i.e. in the range of 0° to + 90° or +100°.	A superiorly oriented QRS in the region of –0° counterclockwise to –180°. A frontal plane QRS axis in north-west zone of -90° counterclockwise to -180° is highly suggestive of VT
3. The identification and configuration of capture and fusion complexes. (A capture beat is normally conducted sinus impulse; whereas fusion complex is a blend of normal and abnormal QRS complexes)	As there is no AV dissociation, hence, capture beats and fusion complexes do not occur	Due to AV dissociation with interference, capture and fusion beats are common, occur intermittently and even may terminate VT. The presence of capture and fusion beat forms an important diagnostic clue to VT.

SECTION TEN

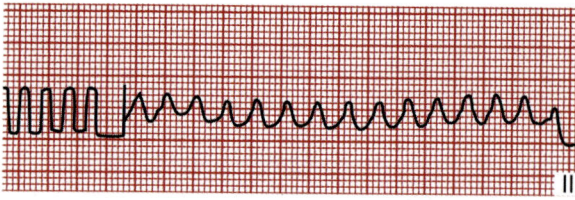

A

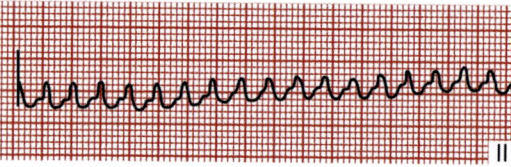

B

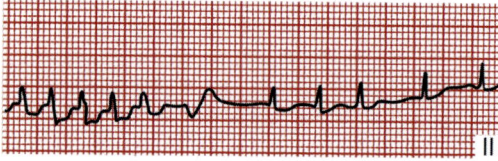

C

Fig. 39.12: Paroxysmal supraventricular tachycardia (PSVT) with aberration:

A: The electrocardiogram (lead II) recorded in emergency department revealed wide QRS tachycardia (PSVT with aberration). There is wide QRS pattern with invisible P waves in either lead of ECG, hence, relation of P wave to QRS was difficult to ascertain, therefore, it was labelled as PSVT with aberrant intraventricular conduction.

B: Carotid massage was done because it can differentiate AV nodal re-entry tachycardia which may either be abolished or there may be no effect, but atrial ectopic or automatic tachycardia does not respond to it. The electrocardiogram recorded after carotid massage shows no response, hence, still could be either of them

C: IV adenosine was tried to disallow re-entry of the tachycardia impulses within AV node. The electrocardiogram showed the beginning of reversion to sinus rhythm (terminal portion of ECG)

D: Restoration of normal sinus rhythm with visible normal P wave, P-R interval and normal QRS complex with tachycardia induced ST depression.

The reversion to normal sinus rhythm by drugs which block the re-entry through AV node suggested it to be supraventricular tachycardia with aberrant intraventricular conduction.

Note: Adenosine may be useful to differentiate wide QRS tachycardias, since it terminates many supraventricular tachycardias with aberrancy or reveals the underlying atrial mechanism by slowing AV conduction, but neither it affects the conduction over accessory pathway not it terminates most ventricular tachycardia–hence, a useful therapeutic test for differentiation in situations where it is difficult to establish the origin of wide QRS tachycardia. Remember it can terminate occasionally a VT

Fig. 39.13: Paroxysmal supraventricular tachycardia (PSVT) with aberrant conduction. The electrocardiogram shows;

i. Regular heart rate (regular R-R interval) of 165 bpm approx.

ii. P wave are visible preceding wide QRS in leads I, aVL and V$_6$

iii. A discordant QRS pattern in precordial leads (V$_1$-V$_6$)

iv. The wide QRS shows pattern of LBBB (wide R wave or Rs pattern in leads V$_6$, I and aVL with wide S in V$_1$)

v. The duration of QRS is <0.14 sec

vi. Left axis deviation of QRS. The upright deflection in lead I and aVL with negative deflection in lead III indicates left axis >−30° which virtually rules out VT and favours PSVT with aberrant conduction through left anterior fascicle

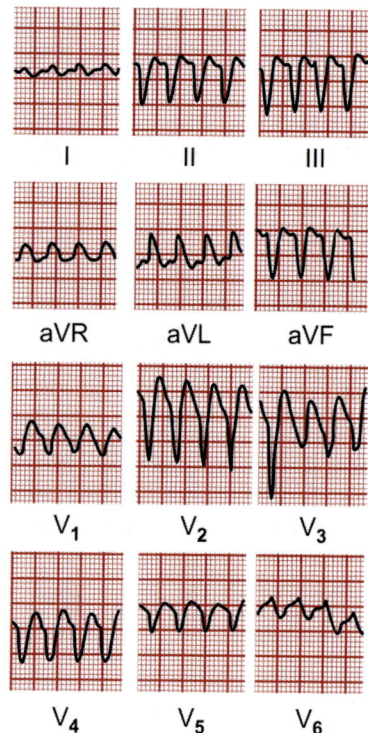

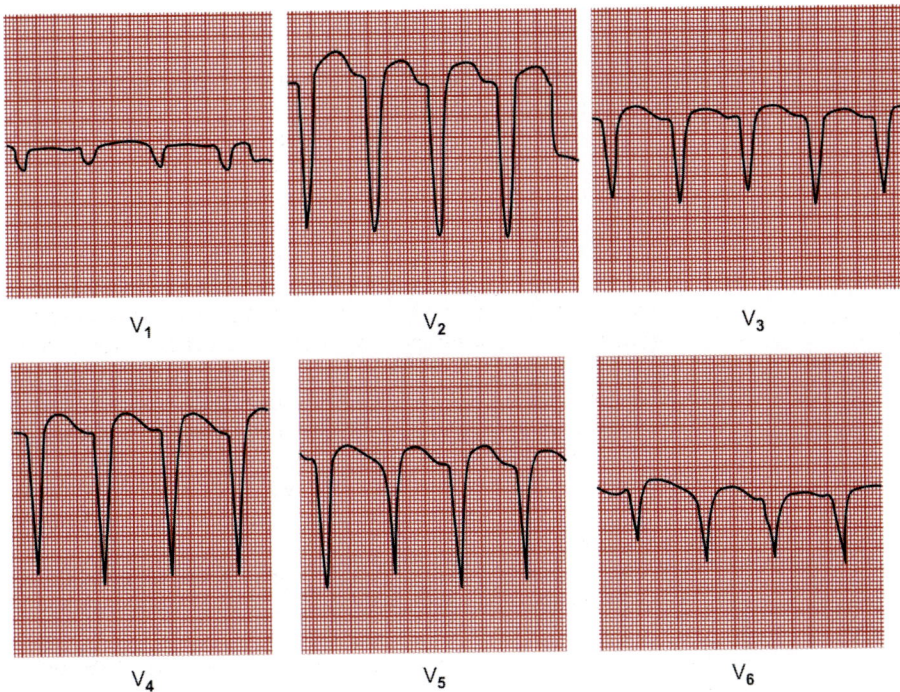

V₁   V₂   V₃

V₄   V₅   V₆

Fig. 39.14: Concordant pattern of QRS in supraventricular tachycardia with aberration. The precordial leads show wide QRS (<0.14 sec) with ventricular rate of 164/min. There is evidence of electrical alternans of QRS seen in most of the leads. There are negative QRS complexes from V₁-V₆ (concordant pattern). The ECG was recorded from a patient without any evidence of a heart disease. After reversion of tachycardia with adenosine, normal ECG was recorded (not displayed). It is not only difficult but impossible to rule out VT in this case, hence, patient was referred for detailed electrophysiological studies

long-short cycle lengths phenomenon, long cycle length poses to aberrancy and short cycle length terminates with an aberrant complex.

In atrial fibrillation, in addition to aberrant complexes, ventricular extrasystoles or ectopics also can occur. These ectopics have no relation to previous cycle length. As QRS complexes are wide and bizarre both in aberrant conduction and in ventricular extrasystoles, they have to be differentiated from clinical point of view because aberrantly conducted supraventricular complexes require no treatment; while frequent ventricular extrasystoles need treatment, otherwise, they may initiate a ventricular tachycardia.

The Analysis of Electrocardiogram (Figs 39.16 and 39.17)

1. Atrial fibrillation is characterised by a wavy or undulating baseline with visible or invisible fibrillatory (f) waves; conducted with irregular R-R intervals. Normal intraventricular conduction produces QRS complexes that are narrow.
2. An abnormal wide QRS complex or complexes; if seen, may be due to aberrantly conducted fibrillatory waves or ventricular ectopics.

3. An aberrantly conducted beat can be recognised by the following characteristics.
   (i) It may have a wide and bizarre QRS simulating a ventricular ectopic or extrasystole or may be just abnormal and wider than other normal conducted beats in the same lead.
   (ii) It will have a pattern of one of bundle branch blocks, commonly RBBB, best seen in lead V₁. This is in contrast to the monophasic or diphasic QRS complex of a ventricular extrasystole.
   (iii) The initial vector of an aberrantly conducted beat will be similar to other conducted beats having normal QRS; while initial vector will be different in ventricular extrasystole (Fig. 39.18).
   (iv) There will be no compensatory pause following an aberrantly sinus conducted beat because it occurs on an anticipated time of other conducted beats but atrial or nodal ectopics with aberrant conduction may be followed by a compensatory pause (Fig. 39.7), while, there is a pause or a tendency to creat a pause following a ventricular extrasystole.
   (v) Short and fixed coupling interval is a characteristic of a ventricular extrasystoles because they occur prematurely at a fixed interval due

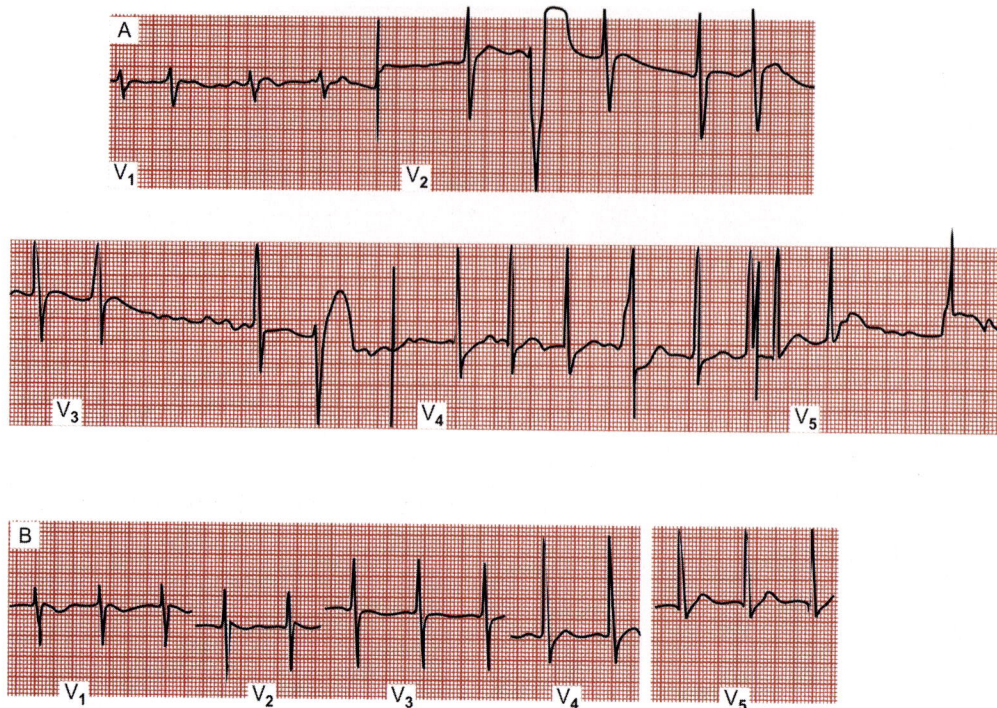

Fig. 39.15: Toxic myocarditis (aluminium phosphide intoxication) induced aberrance and ventricular ectopy. The electrocardiogram (V_1-V_5) recorded from a patient with aluminium phosphide poisoning shows atrial fibrillation with aberrant ventricular conduction as well as VPCs.

A. i. Atrial fibrillation is evidenced by undulation of baseline due to fibrillatory wave (f waves) seen in leads V_1, V_3 and V_5 and irregular R-R intervals

   ii. Aberrant ventricular conduction. The 4th complex in V_4 is aberrantly conducted due to the following reasons;
      a. The initial vector of aberrant conducted beat is same as that of sinus conducted beats
      b. There is no attempt at compensatory pause

   iii. Ventricular premature complexes (VPCs). There is an interpolated VPC in lead V_2. Another VPC in lead V_3 comes after a long R-R cycle length–a phenomenon called "Rule of bigeminy".

B. Restoration of normal rhythm in the same patient after appropriate treatment and recovery indicates reversible nature of ECG changes.

Note: Aberrancy in this patient may be due to toxic myocarditis or due to atrial fibrillation or both. It is difficult to pinpoint its underlying mechanism. Ventricular ectopy is due to myocarditis.

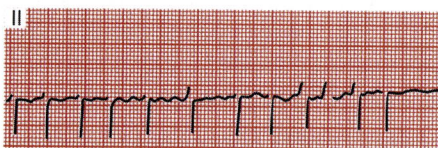

Fig. 39.16: Aberrantly conducted beats in atrial fibrillation (Ashmann's phenomenon). The electrocardiogram (lead II) shows;

i. Atrial fibrillation is evident by wavy irregular baseline due to fibrillatory waves with fast irregular ventricular response

ii. At the end of the strip, there are 4 aberrantly conducted beats. These beats have initial vector similar to normally conducted beats, i.e. R wave. There is an S wave (RS pattern) seen in these 4 beats. The RS pattern in lead II indicates anterior fascicular block pattern; it means conduction is occurring through the posterior fascicle which is responsive. Aberrant conduction in atrial fibrillation is due to alternation of long and short cycle lengths–Ashmann's phenomenon

to constant rate of discharge of an ectopic focus. In contrast, an aberrantly conducted beat or beats do not show such phenomenon—a feature that distinguishes between the two.

(vi) *Rule of bigeminy:* In atrial fibrillation there is change in cycle lengths (short and long cycle lengths). The longer R-R intervals may, at times, followed a ventricular extrasystoles—a phenomenon called rule of bigeminy (Figs 39.15 and 39.18)

ATRIAL FLUTTER WITH VENTRICULAR ABERRATION

The QRS complexes are normal in atrial flutter unless there is coincidental bundle branch block or a

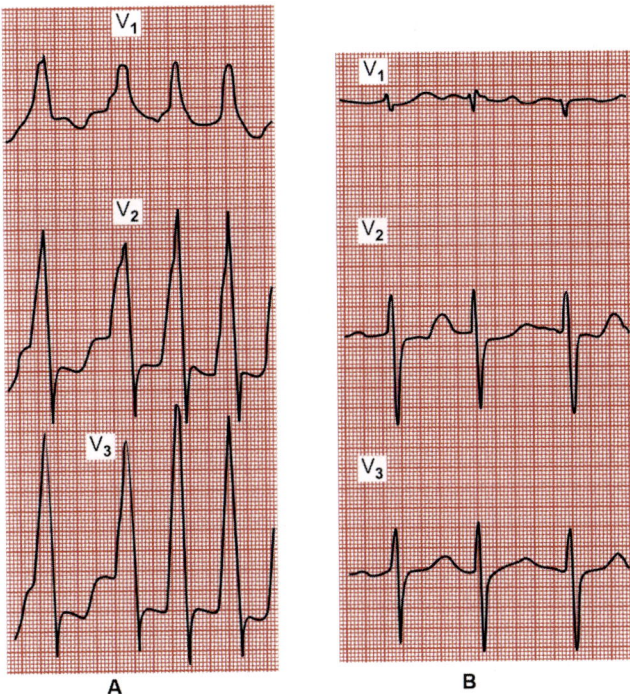

Fig. 39.17: Atrial fibrillation with phasic aberrant intraventricular conduction.

A: Leads V_1-V_3 show tall wide R wave, variable R-R intervals and no P wave indicating atrial fibrillation with aberrant conduction

B: Restoration of sinus rhythm with normal pattern in V_1-V_2 with visible P waves

complicating phasic aberrant intraventricular conduction. Atrial flutter with a fixed conduction ratio usually does not show aberrancy, but when there is alternation from slow conduction to rapid conduction, then relatively early occurring beats may be conducted with intraventricular aberration. The best example of ventricular aberrancy may be seen when there is atrial flutter with alternating 4:1 and 2:1 conduction.

Pathogenesis of Ventricular Aberrancy

When atrial flutter with 4:1 conduction alternates with 2:1 conduction; then the 2:1 conducted beats may show an aberration since the 2:1 AV block results in inscription of two beats in quick succession and aberration occurs due to a long pause created by 4:1 AV block. Furthermore, the conducting impulses in 2:1 AV block are relatively premature; and long pause of 4:1 AV block results in ensuing prolongation of refractoriness of the bundles that favours the ensuing aberration.

The Electrocardiogram (Figs 39.20 and 39.21)

For diagnosis of atrial flutter with phasic aberrant intraventricular conduction, a long strip of one of the leads, e.g. II, III or aVF is necessary because these are best leads to show atrial flutter. The other lead to be chosen is either V_1 or V_2. Examine the long continuous lead strip stepwise.

1. Ascertain that continuous lead strip shows atrial flutter with 4:1 conduction block.
2. Now look for any phasic alternation of 4:1 AV conduction with 2:1 AV conduction.
3. Remember that 2:1 AV conduction in atrial flutter without 4:1 AV block does not show aberration. Otherwise also, in alternating 4:1 AV block and 2:1 AV block in atrial flutter may not show aberration if the impulses in 2:1 AV conduction are not too premature to face refractoriness of the conduction tissue.
4. Only early conducted beats in 2:1 AV block following a sequence of 4:1 AV block may show aberrant conduction simulating extrasystolic ventricular bigeminy (Fig. 39.20). The aberrancy of conduction can be made out if;

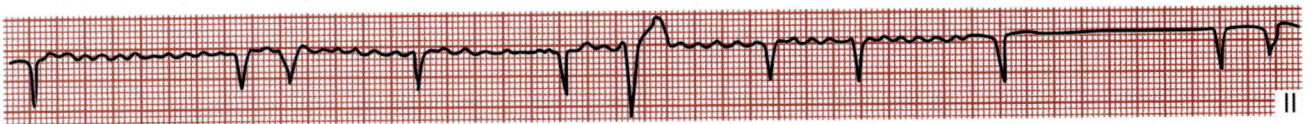

Fig. 39.18: Atrial fibrillation with ventricular ectopic beats. The electrocardiogram (lead II) shows;

i. Atrial fibrillation is evidenced by irregular baseline due to distortion produced by fibrillatory waves and there is irregular ventricular response (variable R-R intervals)

ii. Ventricular premature complexes (VPCs). The 3rd, 6th and 11th complexes are ventricular premature complexes as they occur earlier than anticipated time and are followed by a compensatory pause. All the VPC's occur following a long R-R interval—a phenomenon called "Rule of bigeminy" (see also Fig. 39.13).

SECTION TEN

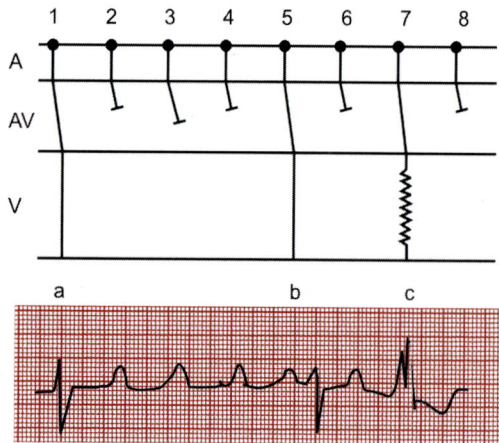

Fig. 39.19: Ladder diagram illustrating flutter with alternating 4:1 and 2:1 AV blocks. The conducted impulses with 2:1 AV block show aberration following 4:1 conduction sequence. This may mimic extrasystolic ventricular bigeminy

i) The initial vector of an abnormal QRS complex of ventricular bigeminy is the same as that of normal conducted QRS complex. This does not occur in extrasystolic ventricular bigeminy.

ii) The QRS complex with aberrant conduction will have triphasic pattern (rSR') instead of biphasic pattern of ventricular extrasystolic bigeminy.

iii) The pause following an abnormal QRS is identical to the pause created by the 4:1 AV conduction with normal QRS complex which confirms the change of sequence of conduction from 4:1 to 2:1.

Fig. 39.21: Atrial flutter with variable conduction. The electrocardiogram (lead II) shows;
  i. The flutter (F) waves are clearly seen without undulation of baseline forming a 'saw-toothed' appearance. The atrial rate is about 300/min
  ii. The R-R interval is irregular with variable conduction ratio 2:1, 3:1, 4:1
  iii. The QRS complex are normal and narrow indicating normal ventricular conduction
  iv. At an arrow (↓), there is a complex showing different mode of ventricular conduction (rS complex) instead of pure R wave seen throughout the strip. This could be an aberrant conduction through left anterior fascicle as duration of QRS is normal

  The saw-toothed appearance, atrial rate of 300 bpm, normal QRS configuration, an aberrant conducted beat favours it to be an atrial flutter

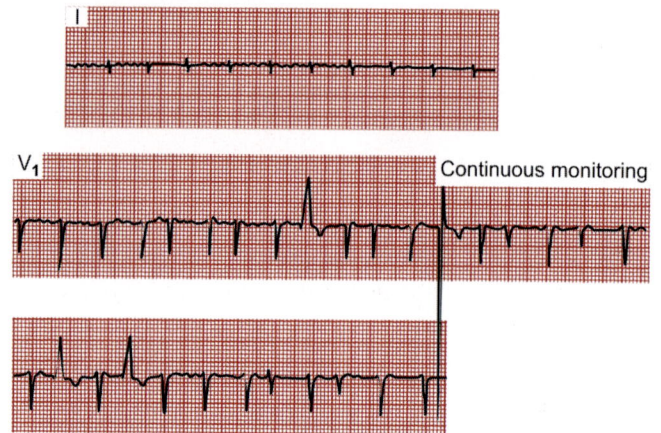

Fig. 39.20: Atrial flutter with fixed alternate 4:1 and 2:1 conduction showing supraventricular beats (flutter waves) conducted with aberration simulating ventricular bigeminy. The electrocardiogram shows;
  i. Upper strip (lead I) shows atrial flutter with 4:1 block
  ii. Middle and bottom strip V_1, show a period of 4:1 AV conduction alternating with 2:1 AV conduction. Note the variable block that is associated with normal intraventricular conduction—last 8 complexes of the bottom strip
  iii. The bigeminal pattern in the beginning of the lower strip reflects two wide bizarre QRS complexes alternating with normal QRS complexes. This stimulates ventricular bigeminy. Critical and close analysis reveals that these are not ventricular ectopics but are aberrantly conducted flutter impulses which terminate the cycles of 2:1 AV conduction. The evidence in favour of aberrancy of these beats include the similar initial vector of normal and abnormal QRS complexes, triphasic pattern (rSR') and variability in degree of aberration and lastly the pause following these wide QRS complexes is same to the pause created by 4:1 AV block
  iv. Similarly two isolated aberrantly conducted flutter waves (wide rSR' complexes) are seen terminating the 4:1 conduction in upper strip of lead V_1

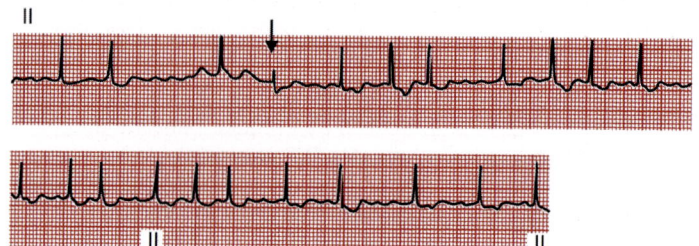

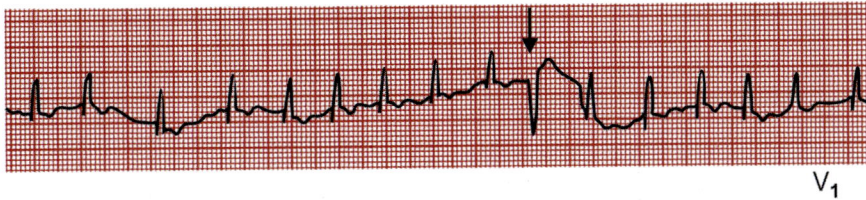

V_1

Fig. 39.22: Atrial fibrillation with right bundle branch block. The electrocardiogram (lead V_1) shows;
  i. Atrial fibrillation. It is evident by wavy irregular undulating baseline between QRS complexes. There are fine fibrillatory waves seen between the complexes. The R-R interval is irregular at a rate of 110/min approx. indicating fast ventricular response.
  ii. The QRS complexes have right bundle branch block (rSR') pattern which is wide (>0.12 sec)
     Atrial fibrillation may show aberrant intraventricular conduction (Ashmann's phenomenon due to alternation of long/short cycle lengths); in that situation, few beats may show bundle branch pattern especially right bundle branch block pattern but here every beat has rSR' pattern which indicates that basic rhythm is right bundle branch block type, hence, this ECG demonstrates the presence of atrial fibrillation with RBBB rather than atrial fibrillation with aberrant conduction
  iii. VPC. These is a right ventricular VPC (↓) characterised by different configuration of wide QRS and a compensatory pause. The ECG was recorded from a patient with cardiomyopathy.

Clinical Significance

When there is an alternation of 4:1 conduction with 2:1 conduction, there will be a ventricular bigeminy rhythm which mimics extrasystolic ventricular bigeminy. The accurate differentiation between ventricular bigeminy due to intraventricular aberration and extrasystolic ventricular bigeminy becomes more important from clinical and therapeutic point of view. The atrial flutter with phasic intraventricular aberration is an indication to begin with digitalis and to increase its dose if patient is already on digitalis, whereas an extrasystolic ventricular bigeminy is an indication to stop digitalis, if patient is already taking, therefore, the history of intake of digitalis becomes an important clue.

VENTRICULAR ABERRANCY VERSUS INTERMITTENT BUNDLE BRANCH BLOCK

Both ventricular aberrancy and intermittent bundle branch block produce wide, bizarre QRS complexes mimicking one of the bundle branch block pattern, i.e. RBBB pattern (rSR' in V_1) or LBBB pattern (QRS or RR' in V_6); that may appear transiently or intermittently for a brief period on ECG. The two have to differentiated from clinical and therapeutic point of view, because the ventricular aberrancy, on one hand, is always a functional disturbance related to refractoriness of the bundle branches and is of no consequence;

while, on the other hand, intermittent bundle branch block is invariably organic in origin, may adversely influence the cardiac disease. On the basis of ECG alone, it is not only difficult, but, at times impossible to differentiate the two. The RBBB type of aberrancy, being more common, has to be differentiated from intermittent RBBB which in itself is less common. The ECG, if interpreted in the light of clinical setting, one may be able to distinguish between the two keeping in mind the followings;

  (i) The ventricular aberration is rate-dependent phenomenon; while intermittent bundle branch block is rate-independent.
  (ii) Ventricular aberrancy can occur normally during sudden acceleration and deceleration of the heart rate; but intermittent bundle branch block does not occur under normal conditions. The congenital RBBB, if present, will produce a fixed and continuous pattern rather than intermittent complexes.
  (iii) Intermittent bundle branch block is associated with acute myocardial events such as acute MI, but ventricular aberrancy is related commonly to tachycardias or bradycardias.

Transient, wide, bizarre QRS complexes mimicking a bundle branch block, if appear at normal heart rates, indicate invariably intermittent bundle branch block (Fig. 39.22) rather than ventricular aberrancy.

SECTION TEN

Suggested Further Reading

1. Fisch C: Electrocardiography and vectorcardiography. In: Braunwald E (Ed): *Heart Disease* 2nd edn. Philadelphia: WB Saunders, 155, 1984.

2. Goldman EJ: *Principles of Clinical Electrocardiography* 12th edn. Los Altos, California. Lange Medical Publishers, 1986.

3. Gouaux JH, Ashmann R: Auricular fibrillation with aberration simulating ventricular paroxysmal tachycardia. *Am Heart J* **34**: 366, 1947.

4. Langerdorf R: Aberrant ventricular conduction. *Am Heart J* **41**:700, 1951.

5. Marriott HJL, Fogg E: Constant monitoring for cardiac dysrhythmias and blocks. *Mod Conc Cardiovasc Dis* **30**: 103, 1970.

6. Marriott HJL, Sandler IA: Criteria, old and new, for differentiating between ectopic ventricular beats and aberrant ventricular conduction in the presence of atrial fibrillation. *Prog Cardiovasc Dis* **9**:18, 1966.

7. Marriott HJL: Practical electrocardiography, 4th ed. Baltimore : William and Wilkins 1972.

8. Marriott HJL: Workshop in electrocardiography. Oldmar, Florida. Tampa, Tracings, 1972.

9. Sandler A, Marriott HJL: The differential morphology of anomalous ventricular complexes of right bundle branch block type in lead V_1-Ventricular ectopic versus aberration. *Circulation* **31**: 551, 1965.

10. Schamroth L, Chesler E: Phasic aberrant ventricular conduction. *Br Heart J* **25**: 219, 1963.

11. Schamroth L, Schamroth C: An introduction to electrocardiography. 7th edn, Blackwell Science Ltd. 1990.

12. Wellens HJJ, Bar FW, Lie KI: The value of electrocardiogram in the differential diagnosis of a tachycardia with a widened QRS complex. *Am J Med* **64**: 27, 1978.

40

Escape Rhythm

- ■ *Definition, causes or clinical conditions associated with escape beats or escape rhythm*
- ■ *Pathogenic mechanisms*
- ■ *Electrocardiographic manifestations and graphic representation of escape beats*
- ■ *Clinical significance*

ESCAPE BEATS AND ESCAPE RHYTHM

Definition : The spontaneous discharge from a slower subsidiary pacemaker (e.g. atrial, AV nodal or ventricular) that has escaped from the control of dominant SA node pacemaker is called an *'escape beat"*. The escape beat or beats occur when the SA node and / or AV node is diseased or is at fault.

When the subsidiary pacemaker is able to discharge two or more consecutive beats, the rhythm is called an *'escape rhythm'*.

Escape rhythm is a secondary phenomenon rather than a primary rhythm disorder

Pathogenic Mechanisms

The heart has a dominant (SA node) pacemaker which maintains the normal continuous heart rhythm. In addition, the heart has potential sites for pacemaker activity, e.g. the atria , AV node and the ventricles. These sites contain pacemaker cells which generate pacemaker activity when dominant pacemaker is at fault, hence, called subsidiary pacemakers. Each pacemaker whether dominant or subsidiary, has its own inherent rate of discharge and a cycle length. The inherent rate of discharge decreases as we move from the SA node to atria, to AV node and to the ventricles, hence, the maximum rate of discharge is the property

of the SA node; while the subsidiary ventricular pacemaker has the lowest rate of discharge.

The normal heart rhythm is maintained by the sinus node who is *'the king of his own empire'*, does not allow the subsidiary pacemaker to discharge normally. This is due to the fact that impulses from fast sinus node reach the lower subsidiary site earlier than its anticipated inherent discharge, suppress its activity and abolish the immature impulses from the subsidiary pacemaker prematurely. The cycle of subsidiary pacemaker begins a fresh as soon as its passive discharge is suppressed or abolished by the fastest pacemaker. This reset ectopic cycle from a subsidiary pacemaker will again be anticipitated and abolished by the next sinus discharges and this process continues. This phenomenon leads us to think that there is only one pacemaker that lies in the SA node.

When the sinus node is at fault, i.e. it is not able to form the impulses temporarily or they are formed at a slower rate than the inherent rate of discharge of lower subsidiary pacemaker, or when there is some type of conduction block from SA node to atria or in AV node, then a slower subsidiary pacemaker (having next higher rate of discharge) has an opportunity to fire and is thus able to discharge spontaneously. This spontaneous discharge of a subsidiary pacemaker is known as an *escape beat*. Escape beats arise from the atria or AV node when SA node is at fault, and arise from a ventricle when both the SA node and AV node are at fault (dual nodal disease).

The discharges from the slower subsidiary pacemaker reach maturity and fire spontaneously only and if the fastest pacemaker is at fault, i.e. escape beat/rhythm occurs secondarily by default.

Causes

Therefore, the common causes include two types of disorders;

1. *Suppression or slowing of sinus pacemaker:* The temporary suppression of sinus pacemaker or slow formation of impulses by it, for example, sinus bradycardia results in escape beats or an escape rhythm.

2. *Conduction defects:* Failure of the sinus impulses to reach the lower subsidiary pacemaker, for example in SA blocks, results in escape beats from AV node—a subsidiary pacemaker having an inherent property of next higher rate of discharge of 40-60 bpm.

When both the SA node and the AV node, or the AV node fail to conduct the impulses; for examples SA blocks or/and AV blocks (second degree and complete AV block) result in ventricular escape beats. The ventricle is the lowest and slowest pacemaker having an inherent property to discharge at a rate of 15-40 bpm.

The situations that are associated with atrial or nodal escape beat/beats or escape rhythm include;

i) *Sinus arrest or sinus pause:* One or more AV nodal or junctional beats may arise and often terminate the prolonged period of sinus arrest or sinus pause.

ii) *An atrial ectopic beat:* Frequently, premature suppression of the SA node discharge by an atrial ectopic beat is followed by a prolonged interval of sinus node inhibition, during which one or more nodal or junctional escape beat or beats may be recorded.

iii) *Sinus arrhythmia with profound bradycardia:* Escape beats may occur during sinus arrhythmia with bradycardia if the rate of discharge of the sinus pacemaker momentarily falls below the inherent rate of impulse formation in the AV node.

iv) *Delayed arrival of sinus impulses:* Delayed arrival of sinus impulses to AV node may also result in the nodal escape beat or beats. The ECG in such a situation will show :

a) The interval between the last sinus beat and the nodal escape beat exceeds the basic sinus cycle length (i.e. sinus P-P interval) and corresponds to the cycle length of nodal or junctional pacemaker.

b) In the given lead, the interval preceding each of the several nodal beats is essentially the same which indicates constant rate of discharge of AV node, but this may not always be true, because some variation in the length of the pause preceding a nodal escape beat is, sometimes, encountered in the presence of AV nodal arrhythmia similiar to sinus arrhythmia. This explains the slight variation in R-R intervals seen occasionally in nodal escape rhythm.

c) Ordinarily, the nodal or junctional escape beat fails to reach the atria and is not accompanied by a retrograde or inverted P' wave. The reason for this is that junctional or nodal escape beats are more or less discharged at the rate which is more or less equal to the sinus rate, hence, these impulses meet and cancel each other's progress in AV node (AV interference). In such a situation, the nodal escape beat either obscures a superimposed sinus P wave or is immediately preceded by a non-conducted P wave. During nodal escape beats, there is in fact, a transient AV dissociation.

v) *AV blocks:* During a short period of blocked impulses at AV node, AV nodal or ventricular escape beats may appear before the conduction is restored. During marked depression of rhythmicity of AV node such as in complete AV block, the secondary pacemaker situated in the ventricle or bundle of His is permitted to escape resulting in ventricular escape beats or rhythm, called *idioventricular rhythm.* The shape of QRS in idioventricular rhythm depends on the site of pacemaker;

(i) When the pacemaker is situated above the bifurcation of the common bundle, the QRS is narrow resembling AV nodal beats/rhythm.

(ii) When the pacemaker lies in the ventricle, then QRS complexes are wide and bizarre resembling ventricular ectopics. The idioventricular rhythm (escape rhythm) is discussed in Chapter 35.

Graphic Representation of an Escape Beat or Beats

The escape beat arising from the AV node or ventricle does not get conducted retrogradely to the atria because of synchronous or near synchronous discharge of P wave with QRS complex, hence, the P is either buried within QRS or just precedes the QRS with short P-R interval.

The intracardiac conduction of an escape beat may be conveniently represented graphically by a ladder diagram in which ordinate represents the anatomical levels of SA node, atria, AV node and ventricles; the abscissa represents time (Fig. 40.1). The course of conduction is represented by continuous line.

Artificial Escape Beats or Rhythm

A demand electrical pacemaker in fact produces an artificial escape rhythm as it is so designed that it fires when it does not sense any electrical activity, i.e. the QRS is not sensed for a set period.

The Electrocardiographic Manifestations

The escape beat always occurs late, i.e. it follows an interval which is longer than the normal dominant sinus cycle length. The escape beat may arise from atria (atrial escape) or AV node (nodal escape) or ventricles (ventricular escape). In fact, an escape beat is an ectopic beat with the exception that pre-ectopic interval is slightly longer than post-ectopic interval as it occurs later than anticipated sinus beat. There is

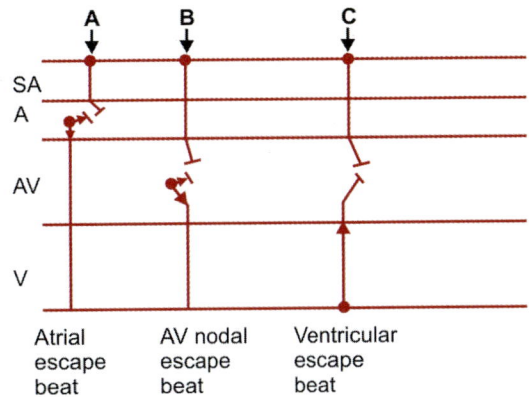

Fig. 40.1: Ladder diagram showing the escape beats (atrial, AV nodal and ventricular). The ordinate reflects the anatomical levels and the abscissa represents time. The black dot represents the impulse origin.
A: Atrial escape beat. It interferes with sinus beat in atria
B: AV nodal escape beat. There is interference between a sinus impulse and an AV nodal escape beat at the level of AV node
C: Ventricular escape beat. There may be synchronous or near synchronous discharge of a sinus impulse and a ventricular escape beat leading to interference with AV dissociation at the level of AV node

no compensatory pause following an escape beat—a feature that distinguishes it from an extrasystole.

1. *An atrial escape beat* (Fig. 40.2): It is characterised by the late inscription of an abnormal P' wave (Read Chapter 32).
2. *AV nodal escape beat* (Figs 40.3 to 40.5). It is characterised by the late inscription of an AV nodal beat (Read Chapter 33).
3. *A ventricular escape beat* (Figs 40.6 to 40.8). It is characterised by the late inscription of a bizarre QRS complex of an ectopic ventricular beat.

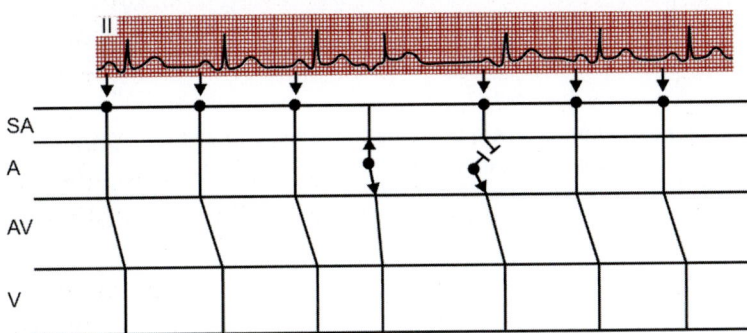

Fig. 40.2: An atrial premature beat with an escape beat occurring immediately after the compensatory pause: The ECG (lead II) shows;
  i. There is sinus rhythm at a rate of 75 bpm
  ii. There is an atrial premature complex (4th complex) having an inverted P wave followed by a narrow QRS
  iii. Following the compensatory pause of APC, there is an atrial escape beat (x) with abnormal upright low amplitude P wave preceding QRS
Below is drawn the ladder diagram to show an atrial ectopic and AV nodal escape beat. SA—Sinoatrial, A—Atrial, AV—AV nodal and V—Ventricle

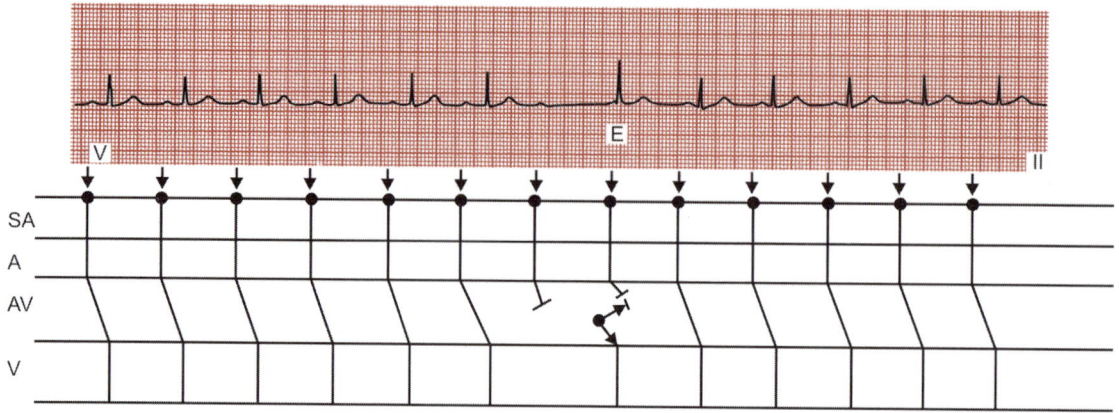

Fig. 40.3: AV nodal escape beats in Wenckebach type of AV conduction. The lead II (continuous strip) shows progressive lengthening of P-R interval followed by a nonconducted P wave which results in AV nodal escape beat (E).

Below the strip, a ladder diagram is drawn to represent the AV node escape beat and Wenckebach type of AV conduction. The black dots represent the origin of impulses.

SA—sinoatrial node, A—atria, AV—AV node V—ventricles

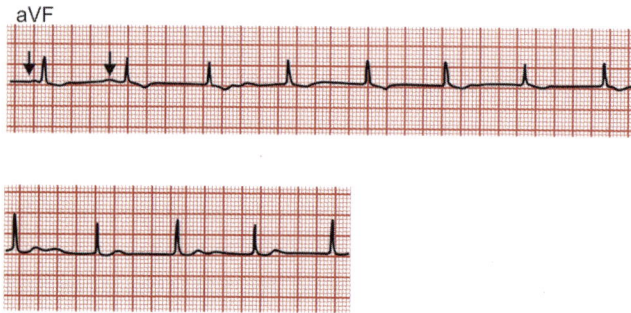

Fig. 40.4: AV nodal escape rhythm. The electrocardiographic lead II (upper strip) shows first two beats as sinus conducted beats preceded by P-R interval of 0.12 sec and 0.16 seconds respectively. The ventricular rate is just 56 bpm. The second beat (↓)then is followed by a run AV nodal complexes (no visible P wave with narrow QRS) at a rate of 60 bpm indicating nodal escape rhythm. It appears that sinus rate following the first two sinus beats has fallen further leading to an emergence of nodal escape rhythm. The lower strip (lead II) shows just continuation of nodal rhythm. The sagging ST segment of sinus beats as well as nodal beats could be due to inferior wall ischaemia leading to sinus node dysfunction

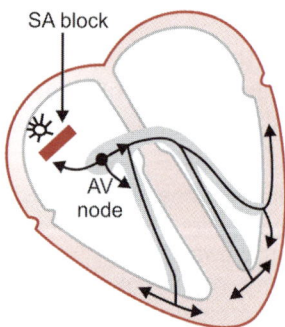

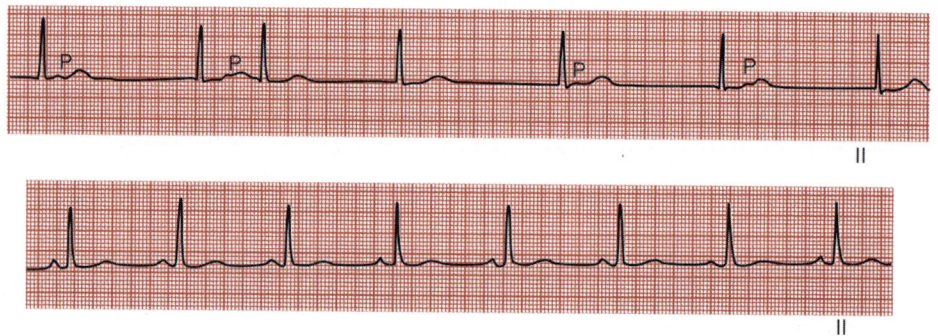

Fig. 40.5: Nodal rhythm. The upper strip (lead II) shows nodal rhythm at a rate of 50/min. There is one atrial ectopic also. The lower strip shows disappearance of nodal rhythm with acceleration of the heart rate

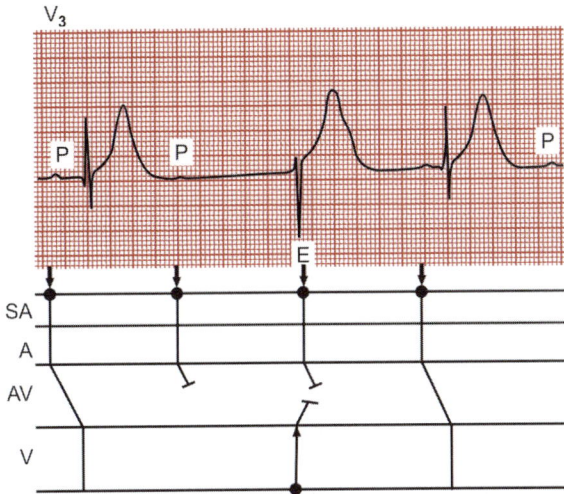

Fig. 40.6: Ventricular escape beat. The electrocardiogram (V$_3$) shows;
  i. AV block. The first P wave is conducted with P-R interval of 0.20 sec and second P is blocked
  ii. Ventricular escape beat. The third complex is ventricular escape beat (E) which has narrow QRS complex having orientation opposite to sinus conducted QRS complexes. The P wave falls on the ascending limb of rS complex. The narrow QRS complex indicates its site of origin below the bundle of His, may be from the fascicle of a bundle branch

Below is drawn a ladder diagram to show second degree AV block and an ventricular escape beat

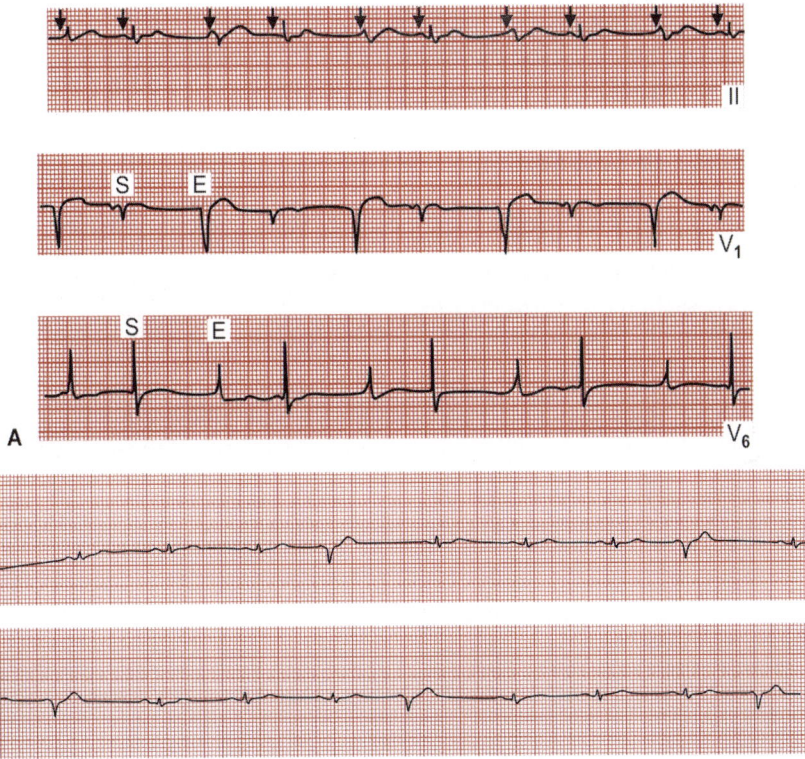

Fig. 40.7: A: Ventricular escape bigeminy in the presence of Wenckebach 3:2 SA block in a patient with structural nodal disease. The ECG shows;
  i. Lead II shows each narrow QRS complex has either a preceding P wave or a superimposed P waves (↓). There is alternation of short and long R-R intervals. The long R-R interval is less than the twice of short R-R interval, indicates intermittent sinus pauses due to 3:2 Wenckebach SA block
  ii. Leads V$_1$ and V$_6$ show a sinus conducted beat(s) followed by a ventricular ectopic (E) occurring regularly in an alternate manner constituting bigeminy rhythm. This bigeminal rhythm is an escape bigeminy because the ventricular extrasystole shows a late inscription (pre-ectopic interval is longer than post-ectopic) and occurred whenever there was slowing of heart rate due to SA block.

B: Ventricular escape quadrigeminy

Note: Ventricular bigeminy or trigeminy/quadrigeminy occurs whenever both SA node and AV node are diseased. Normally, in the presence of SA block, there should be nodal escape beats or rhythm but presence of ventricular escape beats (bigeminy or quadrigeminy pattern in this case) indicates indirectly that AV node might also be diseased. The ECG was recorded from a patient with sick sinus syndrome—a structural nodal disease. The presence of SA block is a proof of sinus nodal disease

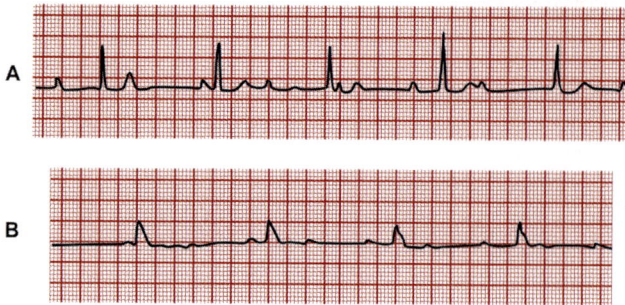

Fig. 40.8: Complete (third degree) heart block with AV nodal (A) and ventricular (B) escape rhythm. The electrocardiogram shows;

A. AV nodal escape rhythm. There is complete heart block (P-P, R-R inervals are regular, atrial rate is more than ventricular rate, hence, P waves are unrelated to QRS complexes) in which QRS complexes are narrow indicating AV nodal escape rhythm at a rate of 44/min

B. Ventricular escape rhythm. The QRS complexes are wide and ventricular rate is 38/min regular

---

Diagnostic clues to escape beat/rhythm
- There must be a cause to explain the emergence of an escape beat/rhythm.
- The escape beat occurs late, i.e. it occurs at an interval which is longer than the normal sinus cycle, i.e. R-R interval between a sinus beat and an escape beat is longer than R-R interval between two consecutive sinus beats.
- There is no compensatory pause following an escape beat.

Clinical Significance

1. Escape beat or beats occur secondary to some cause, hence, the significance of escape beat/rhythm lies in the primary cause/event such as sinus bradycardia, SA blocks or AV blocks.
2. Escape beat/rhythm specifically does not require treatment except the removal/treatment of the underlying cause.

Suggested Reading

1. Kistin AD: Atrioventricular junctional premature and escape beats with altered QRS and fusion. *Circulation* **34**:740, 1966.
2. Walsch TJ: Ventricular aberration of AV nodal escape beats. Comments concerning the mechanism of aberration. *Am J Cardiol* **10**:217, 1962.

41

Ventricular Fusion Beats

- Definition and causes
- Variations in configuration of QRS complexes
- Pathogenesis of ventricular fusion beats

VENTRICULAR FUSION COMPLEXES OR BEATS

Normally, a ventricular complex is recorded when the sinus impulse invades the ventricles. A ventricular fusion beat or complex is defined as 'the complex produced by two impulses invading the ventricles simultaneously and taking part in their activation, i.e. a part of activation is done by one impulse followed by activation by the other impulse to complete the process of activation'. Therefore, a fusion beat is a blend of activation by two impulses—a sinus and an ectopic ventricular impulse, hence, its configuration will be 'in-between' that of "pure QRS complex" resulting from sinus beat and the "pure QRS complex" initiated by an ectopic ventricular beat. Thus, a fusion beat is also called a summation beat or a combination beat. To diagnose a fusion beat, a long continuous lead must record;

  i) The pure ectopic ventricular complex.
  ii) The pure sinus ventricular complex.
  iii) The intermediate fusion complex.

In fact, the timing of the two impulses (one normal and other ectopic) is such that they discharge synchronously to produce a fusion complex on ECG at a time when a normal sinus beat is expected. The R-R interval between sinus beat and fusion beat is equal to R-R interval between two sinus beats. Therefore, the main features of a fusion beat (Figs 41.1 and 41.2) are;

1. The configuration is 'in-between' a normal beat and an ectopic ventricular beat.
2. It must coincide with the sinus beat in timing.

Variations in Configuration of Ventricular Fusion Beats

The configuration of a ventricular fusion beat (VFB) will depend on the relative contribution of the sinus or atrial, and ventricular impulse to ventricular activation. If dominant contribution is by atrial or sinus impulse, the resulting QRS configuration of fusion beat will resemble pure sinus QRS complex; if dominant contribution results from an ectopic ventricular impulse, the resulting QRS configuration will mimic pure ectopic QRS. If ventricular activation is contributed equally by both (a sinus beat and an ectopic ventricular beat) then configuration will be more or less 'in-between' the pure ectopic and pure sinus QRS complexes. Thus, in a tracing, there is always a tendency to variability in the shape of ventricular fusion complexes. Marked variations in shape of fusion QRS complexes is a characteristic and diagnostic feature.

Variations in configuration of QRS on ECG is a characteristic feature of ventricular fusion beats because shape of fusion complex depends on the relative contribution to ventricular activation by the sinus impulse and the ectopic impulse.

The Pathogenesis of Ventricular Fusion

There are two possible groups of causes of ventricular fusion beats.

1. *Interference dissociation at the ventricular level* (Fig. 41.3): When the ventricles are invaded simul-

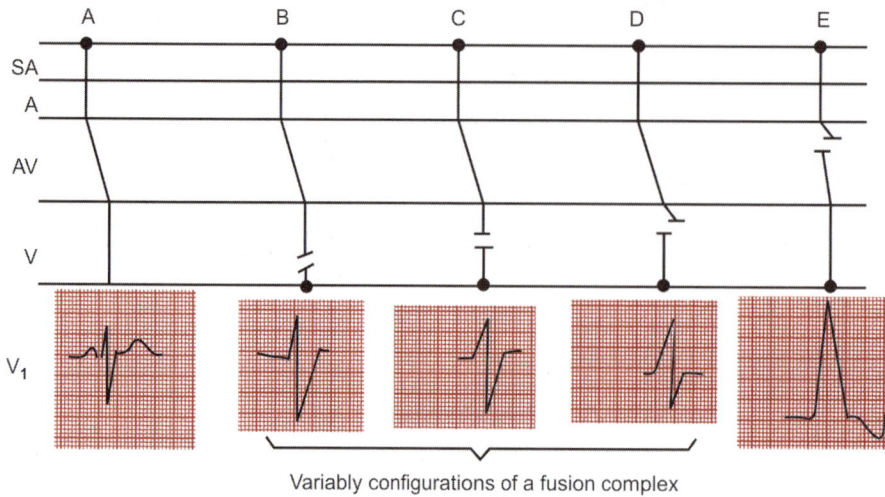

Variably configurations of a fusion complex

Fig. 41.1: Fusion complex (ladder diagram). **A:** The normal sinus conducted beat. **B, C** and **D:** Ectopic ventricular beats with dissociation and interference from the near synchronous sinus discharge within the ventricle resulting in variability of the fusion complexes. **E:** Pure ventricular ectopic with dissociation and interference at AV nodal level by near synchronous sinus discharge

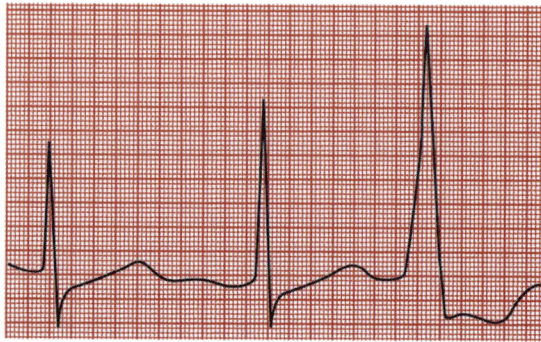

Fig. 41.2: A fusion complex. The ECG lead shows three complexes, first a sinus complex, the second is a fusion complex and the third is a ventricular premature complex (VPC).

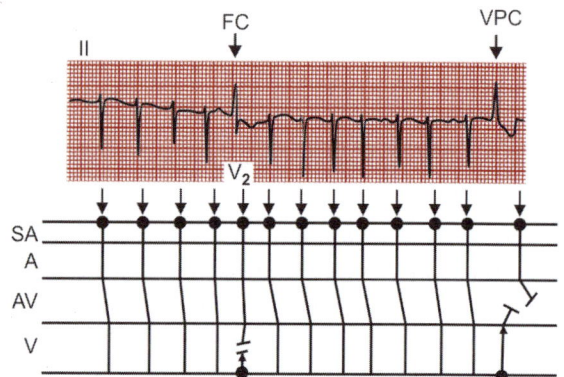

Fig. 41.3: Marked sinus arrhythmia with a fusion complex (FC) and a ventricular premature complex (VPC). The electrocardiogram (lead II) shows;
i. *Sinus arrhythmia* : It is revealed by variablity in the R-R intervals of sinus conducted beats. There is variability in the amplitude of QRS complexes
ii. The last beat in the strip is a ventricular ectopic with wide QRS complex and associated ST-T changes
iii. The fifth beat in the strip has narrow QRS complex, comes at a time of expected sinus beat, has configuration in-between normal beat and ventricular ectopic and the R-R interval with preceding sinus beat and with the next sinus beat is equal, hence, it is fusion beat.

Note: A fusion complex denotes that the ventricles have been depolarised by both the sinus beat and an ectopic beat, hence, is a blended complex.

Below is drawn ladder diagram showing the pathway of conductions of sinus beats, fusion complex and a VPC
SA—SA node, A—Atria, AV—AV node, V—Ventricles

taneously by a sinus and an ectopic ventricular impulse resulting in the interference at ventricular level, a fusion beat results. A fusion beat (partial ventricular capture) is a premature supraventricular beat since it reaches the upper part of the ventricles before the ventricular ectopic impulse, and takes part in the initiation of ventricular activation. The causes of fusion complexes by this mechanism include;
a) Ventricular parasystole (Fig. 38.1).
b) Ventricular tachycardia (Chapter 35, Fig. 35.29). The onset and offset of accelerated ventricular rhythm occurs via the fusion complexes (Fig. 35.24B).
c) End-diastolic ventricular extrasystoles (Fig. 41.4)
d) AV dissociation (See Chapter 37, Fig. 37.1)

2. *Fusion due to Wolff-Parkinson–White syndrome* In WPW syndrome, activation front splits into two; one gets conducted through an accessory pathway and the other through normal pathway into the

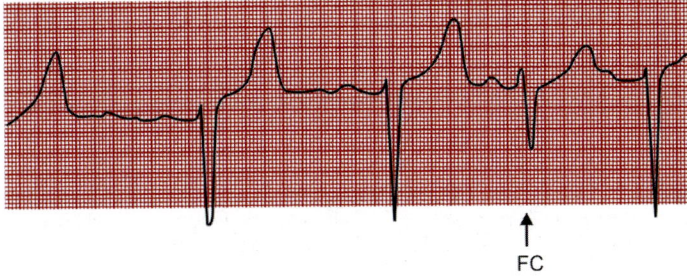

FC

Fig. 41.4: A fusion complex due to end-diastolic VPC. The ECG shows;

Sinus arrhythmia: The first R-R interval (not clearly visible) appears to be longer than next R-R interval. The first visible QRS has been produced at P-R interval of 0.18 second and next complex has P-R interval of 0.20 sec, i.e. there is variability in P-R intervals. The third visible QRS complex has short P-R interval of 0.16 sec and its shape is different than other three QRS complexes. The 4th beat is again conducted at P-R interval of 0.20 sec. The third visible beat appears to be a fusion complex due to end-diastolic VPC

ventricles resulting in activation of different parts of the ventricles. The fusion complexes (wide QRS with delta wave) in WPW have been discussed in Chapter 22.

Clinical Significance

Their presence in ventricular tachycardia differentiates it from supraventricular tachycardia. Similarly a fusion complex in AV dissociation differentiates it from complete heart block.

42

Ventricular Capture Beats

- ■ *Definition, causes and its mechanisms*
- ■ *The electrocardiographic characteristics*
- ■ *Significance*
- ■ *Differentiation between a capture beat and a fusion beat*

Normally, a ventricular complex is recorded when a sinus impulse invades the ventricles and activates them simultaneously. Usually during an interference AV dissociation between a sinus pacemaker (sinus impulses) and a faster subsidiary pacemaker (AV nodal or ventricular impulse), both of them have more or less same rate of discharge; neither the sinus impulse is conducted antegradely nor the impulses from the subsidiary pacemaker get conducted retrogradely. This is due to refractoriness of AV node consequent to partial penetration by the sinus impulses.

"At times, however, a sinus impulse having a critical timing, i.e. arrives at a time when AV node has recovered from refractoriness and is responsive, gets conducted to the ventricles through AV nodal pathway and momentarily excites the ventricles. As this beat has captured the ventricle, hence, called a capture beat."

Definition: In the presence of AV dissociation between a sinus pacemaker and a subsidiary pacemaker, an isolated sinus impulse that gets conducted to the ventricles and momentarily activates them is called a *'ventricular capture beat'*. The capture beat is an example of complete ventricular capture by a sinus impulse, which is possible in AV dissociation but impossible in complete heart block—a point of distinction between the two.

Types of Ventricular Capture

Ventricular capture may be complete or incomplete (partial).

1. *The complete ventricular capture:* A sinus impulse that captures the ventricles completely and solely activates them is conventionally called - an *capture beat*.

2. *Incomplete (partial) ventricular capture:* A sinus beat that reaches the ventricles more or less concomitantly with the ventricular ectopic impulse and takes part in their activation is called a *beat with an incomplete ventricular capture*. In fact, when two pacemakers (a sinus and a subsidiary) discharge impulses that invade the ventricles simultaneously with the result, the ventricular activation occurs partly by the sinus impulse and partly by the ectopic ventricular impulse. The complex so produced is a blend or fusion of activations by the sinus impulse and a ventricular ectopic impulse—hence called a *'fusion complex'* has already been discussed in Chapter 41.

Causes: The causes of capture beats (complete capture) and fusion beats (incomplete capture) are more or less same (Read Chapter 41).

Mechanism: The ventricular capture beats occur mostly in AV dissociation with interference, due to presence of two pacemakers; one situated in the SA node and other is a subsidiary pacemaker situated in the AV node or ventricle; and the subsidiary pacemaker discharges at a higher rate (accelerated nodal or ventricular rhythm). Due to slower rate of discharge of SA node, the P waves occur progressively later in relation to the QRS complex of faster ectopic rhythm. Consequent to it, the sinus impulse that arrives at the AV node slightly later, but still falls within the refractory period of ectopic cycle (cycle of ectopic rhythm), is not conducted to the ventricles. But when the same sinus impulse arrives sufficiently late at a critical time when the AV node has recovered from the previous excitation, gets conducted to the ventricles—captures the ventricles completely and solely activates them is called a *capture beat*. The capture beats occur as an isolated phenomenon.

Timing and Conduction of Capture Beats

As the ventricular ectopic impulses occur faster than the sinus impulses, hence, a sinus impulse cannot capture the ventricle. Due to slow sinus discharge, P waves march ahead of QRS complexes progressively till a time that a sinus impulse finds AV node responsive and gets conducted to the ventricles. The critical timing of the sinus impulse is thus a decisive factor for ventricular capture.

The sinus impulse that captures the ventricles (capture beat) may be conducted as follows:
1. With normal AV nodal and intraventricular conduction.
2. With prolonged P-R interval (first degree AV block).
3. With aberrant intraventricular conduction.
4. With concealed AV nodal conduction.

The Electrocardiographic Characteristics of a Capture Beat (Fig. 42.1)

The following characteristics of a capture beat help in its recognition.

1. *The P wave*

The capture beat is always preceded by a P wave

2. *The QRS*

The shape and size of QRS complex depends on the site of subsidiary pacemaker.

A. *When the subsidiary pacemaker is in the ventricle*. In this situation, the QRS complex of the capture beat is quite different from the QRS of ventricular ectopic impulse and varies as follows:
   (i) The QRS complex of the capture beat may be normal with normal intraventricular conduction.
   (ii) The QRS complex of capture beat may be wide and bizarre due to phasic aberrant ventricular conduction.

B. *When the subsidiary pacemaker is in the AV node*, then;
   (i) A capture beat may have normal QRS. The QRS of the capture beat will be exactly same as the basic AV nodal rhythm.
   (ii) An abnormal QRS with phasic aberrant ventricular conduction. The QRS complex will be of right bundle branch block pattern.

Significance

1. *Resetting of AV Nodal or Ventricular Rhythm*

A capture beat reaches the AV nodal or ventricular pacemaker and discharges it prematurely, thus, resets the AV nodal or ventricular rhythm, with the result, the nodal or ventricular cycle starts a fresh from the moment the sinus impulse reaches and discharges the AV nodal or ventricular rhythm. A capture beat is a

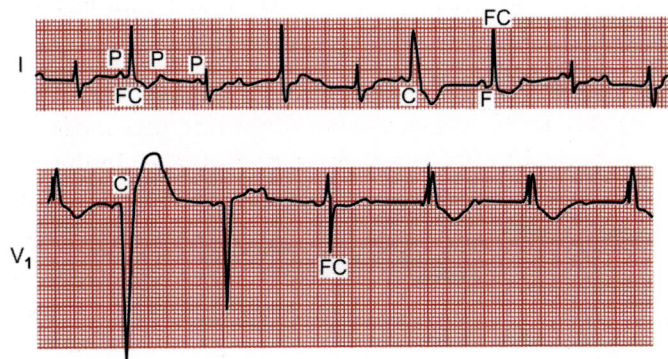

Fig. 42.1: Idionodal rhythm with capture beats and fusion complexes. The rhythm strips (lead I and V_1) show:
   i. *Sinus tachycardia* at a rate of 100/min (P-P interval is 0.60 sec)
   ii. *Idionodal rhythm.* It is characterised by rSR' pattern in V_1 and wide slurred S wave in lead I. The rate is 50/min
   iii. Capture beats (C): The 6th beat in lead I and second beat in V_1 are capture beats wtih P-R interval of 0.16 sec
   iv. Fusion beats/complexes (FC): The 2nd and 7th narrow QRS complexes in lead I and 4th complex with wide QRS (> 0.12 sec) in V_1 are fusion complexes

Note: Idionodal or idioventricular rhythm or tachycardia can give rise to ventricular capture if there is a suitable condition for the the sinus beat to get conducted

Table 42.1: Differentiating features between a capture and a fusion beat	
A ventricular capture beat	*A ventricular fusion beat*

• It is a sinus impulse that reaches the ventricles and activates them, i.e. there is complete ventricular capture
• A capture beat may be conducted
   (i) With normal AV nodal and intraventricular conduction (normal QRS)
   (ii) With aberrant ventricular conduction (wide and bizarre QRS)
   (iii) With concealed AV nodal conduction (No QRS)
• A capture beat reaches the subsidiary pacemaker (AV node or ventricle) and resets its timing
	• It is a sinus impulse that reaches the ventricle simultaneously with the ectopic impulse, takes part in their activation partly, i.e. there is partial ventricular capture
	• A fusion beat is conducted through normal pathways and blends with ventricular ectopic impulse, hence, the QRS of fusion beat is intermediate between sinus complex and ventricular ectopic complex
	
	• It does not reach the ventricular pacemaker, hence, consequently has no effect on the ventricular ectopic rhythm

SECTION TEN

premature beat with short coupling interval but the post-capture beat interval remains the same as that of AV nodal or ventricular cycle.

In contrast to a capture beat, a fusion beat (sinus beat wth incomplete ventricular capture), does not reach the ventricular pacemaker, hence, has no effect on the ventricular rhythm. However, the onset and offset of idioventricular rhythm may occur through a fusion complex.

2. Concealed AV Nodal Capture

During AV dissociation between sinus and AV nodal rhythm, the capture impulse may penetrate the AV node without traversing it completely - a phenomenon called concealed conduction. No QRS complex is therefore recorded in relation to this capture beat. This is because the capturing impulse reaches the AV nodal pacemaker and discharges it prematurelly thereby resetting and postponing its cycle. The rhythm is consequently interrupted by an inordinate and unexpected long R-R interval. The concealed penetration of the capturing impulse into AV node is thus recognised by the postponement of AV nodal cycle.

3. Paired Capture Beats

Usually capture beats occur in isolation but, occasionally, they may manifest with paired or consecutive capture beats. The conduction time of first capture beat in paired capture beats is longer than the second capture beat because the first capture beat is more premature than the second.

Differentiation between a ventricular capture beat and a ventricular fusion beat: These are listed in the Table 42.1.

Suggested Reading

1. Schamroth L, Friedberg HD: Significance of retrograde conduction in AV dissociation. *Brit Heart J* **6**: 896, 1965.

Artificial Pacemakers

SECTION ELEVEN

43

Artificial Pacemakers

■ Definition, indications, components of pacemaker and methods of pacing
■ Functions of pacemaker, identification of coding system and physiology of pacemakers
■ Methods of pacing and ECG patterns in relation to the site of pacing
■ Malfunctions of pacemaker and their remedial measures and pacemaker pearls

Definition: An electronic device which generates and transmits an electrical signal to the atria, ventricles or both, is called *an artificial pacemaker*. These pacemakers actually constitute an electrical back-up systems that keep the heart rate fast enough to prevent the symptoms due to slow heart rate, hence, are used in symptomatic patients. There are two types of pacemakers, i.e. *temporary* and *permanent;* that are used depending on the clinical situation. Most complex devices are incorporated in some sophisticated pacemakers to abolish rapid dysarrhythmias such as ventricular tachycardias and fibrillation.

Types of Pacing

1. *Temporary:* It is a done during emergency situations. The indications are:
   1. Ventricular asystole
   2. Symptomatic bradycardia due to transient atrioventricular block following cardiac surgery, myocardial ischaemia or drug toxicity.

   It follows that temporary pacing is used to tide over the crisis in those situations which are usually transient and reversible. This means that every temporary pacing is not to be followed by permanent pacing.

   Temporary pacing is used in situations/conditions that are transient and reversible.

2. *Permanent:* Permanent pacing does not automatically follow temporary pacing. The indication to

permanent pacing is individualised after careful analysis of each patient's clinical condition.

Indications: The following indications have been recommended by American Heart Association Task Force Committee on pacemaker implantation, 1991.

1. **Acquired AV blocks**
   - Complete AV block (acquired)
   - Symptomatic bradycardia due to second degree AV block
   - Atrial fibrillation or atrial flutter associated with advanced or complete heart block (unrelated to drugs known to impair AV conduction).

2. **AV blocks associated with myocardial infarction**
   - Persistent advanced second degree AV block or complete heart block or block in the His-Purkinje system (alternating bilateral bundle branch block) following acute myocardial infarction.
   - Transient AV block with associated bundle branch block.

3. **Chronic bifascicular or trifascicular block**
   - Bifascicular block with intermittent complete heart block and symptomatic bradycardia.
   - Bifascicular or trifascicular block with intermittent type II second degree AV block (symptoms not necessary).

4. **Sick sinus syndrome**
   - Sinus node dysfunction (sinus bradycardia, sinus arrest, sinoatrial block) accompanied by symptoms of dizziness or syncope.
5. **Hypersensitive carotid sinus:** Recurrent syncope provoked by carotid sinus stimulation (asystole longer than 3 seconds in the absence of drugs that depress SA node or AV node conduction).
6. **Newer unconventional indications:** The third update on recent guidelines of American Heart Association (AHA) and American College of Cardiology (ACC) have mentioned several newer indications in certain specific situations but they have kept them under class II (a or b) indications of AHA/ACC guidelines. They encompass either single or multisite pacing. They are:
   - Hypertrophic cardiomyopathy
   - Dilated cardiomyopathy
   - Vasovagal syncope (malignant)
   - Atrial fibrillation to prevent recurrence and maintain sinus rhythm
   - The long QT syndrome—high risk patients
   - Symptomatic bradycardia/chronotropic incompetence after cardiac transplantation.

Note: Class II means divergence of opinion regarding need for transplantation.

Components of a Pacemaker

All the pacemakers have:
1. A pulse generator
2. A pacing catheter

1. ***The pulse generator:*** It contains batteries that generate the electrical signals. Two types of generators are used depending on the type of pacing.

Temporary generators have removable batteries contained in generator house. Controls on the face of the unit allow the operator to manipulate pacing parameters.

Permanent generators are run on long lasting system of batteries. Most generators use lithium batteries that last 2-10 yrs. Pacing parameters are set during the implantation procedure or by a programmer placed directly on the generator.

2. ***The pacing catheter:*** It is also called the lead or the electrode. It forms the link between the pulse generator and the myocardium. It has a two way

transmission line that (i) delivers the electrical stimulus to the heart and (ii) also conduct the information about the intrinsic activity of the heart back to the generator for processing. Most of the permanent pacing catheters have fixation devices, e.g. screws, tines, or barbs; that help to maintain long-term contact with the heart. Temporary pacing catheters are constructed without any fixation device so that they can be removed when pacing is no longer required (Fig. 43.1).

Methods of Pacing

Temporary pacing: The temporary catheter is commonly passed through a large vein (transvenous approach) and is advanced under fluoroscopy until the right atrial or right ventricular endocardium is reached. The catheter is connected to the external generator. Temporary pulse generators are controlled by manipulating dials provided on the face of the unit. Pacing parameters are set by manipulations and the unit is turned on Figure 43.2.

> *Note: In emergency conditions, transthoracic pacing or pacing by insulated wires may be done;*
>
> *In transthoracic pacing, a special pacing catheter is threaded into the ventricle through a large bore needle inserted directly into the heart through anterior chest wall.*
>
> *Insulated pacing wires may be attached to the outer surface of the atrium or ventricle, or both, during cardiac surgery. These wires are taken to the surface through the anterior chest wall and connected to the generator set if pacing is required. When pacing is no longer required, the wires are gently pulled through the wound.*

Permanent pacing (Fig. 43.3): A subcutaneous space or pocket is created surgically in the infraclavicular region or in the abdominal wall for placement of the pulse generator. One end of the pacing catheter is interfaced with either the epicardial or endocardial surface of the heart; the other end is attached to the source of electrical energy (generator). Pacing parameters are set, the unit is turned on and the wound is closed surgically. The procedure for (1) endocardial and (2) epicardial pacing is as follows:
1. The catheter is inserted through a big vein, e.g. saphenous vein, and advanced into the right

A. Temporary pacing catheter

B. Permanent pacing catheter

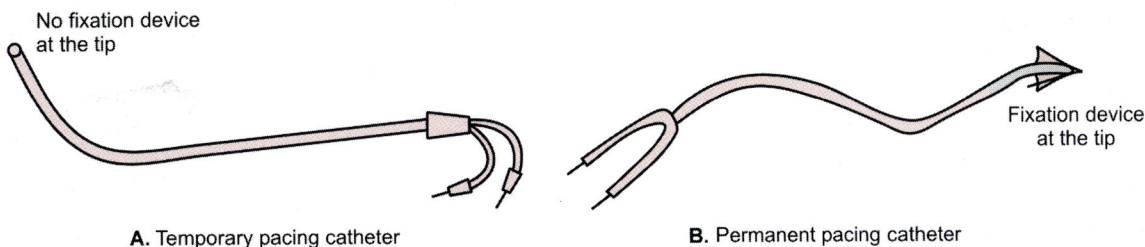

Fig. 43.1: Diagram of two types of catheters for pacing

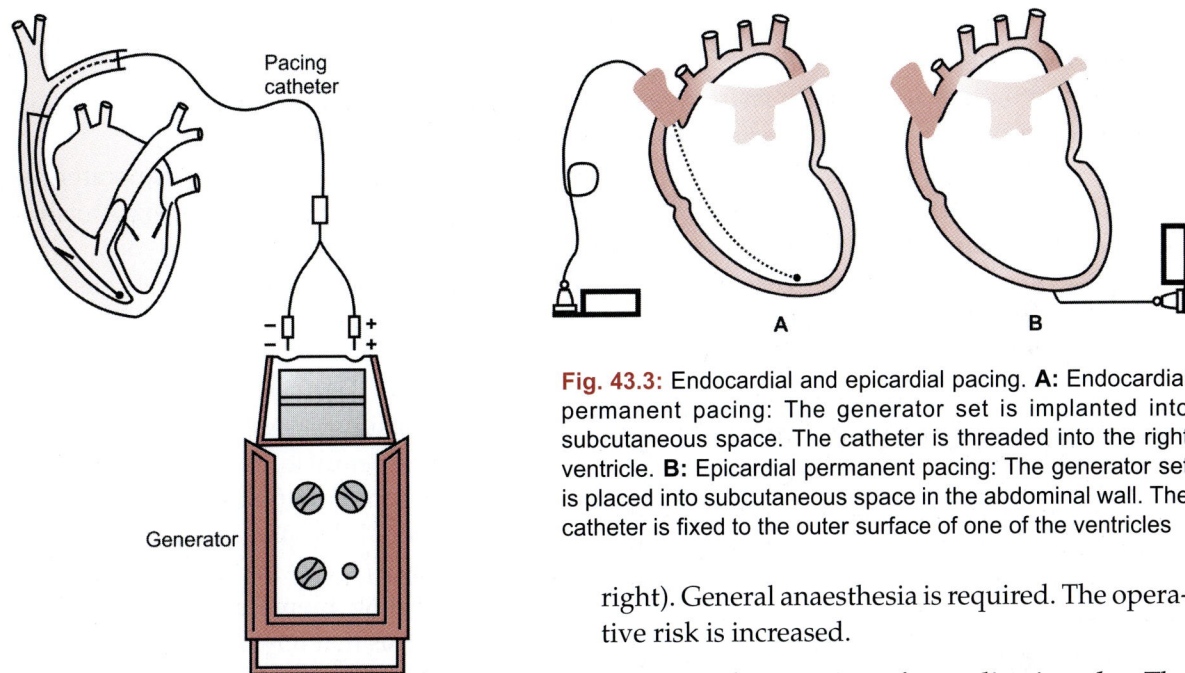

Fig. 43.2: Temporary pacing (diagram). A pacing catheter is connected to a temporary generator. A bridging cable or pacemaker extension cord (not shown) can be used between the generator and the catheter

Fig. 43.3: Endocardial and epicardial pacing. **A:** Endocardial permanent pacing: The generator set is implanted into subcutaneous space. The catheter is threaded into the right ventricle. **B:** Epicardial permanent pacing: The generator set is placed into subcutaneous space in the abdominal wall. The catheter is fixed to the outer surface of one of the ventricles

atrium or the ventricle until the catheter tip touches the endocardium (endocardial pacing). The procedure is simple and without any risk. General anaesthesia is not needed. This is called *conventional endocardial pacing*.

2. The other mode of pacing (epicardial pacing) is complex. It is used in situations where conventional pacing cannot be achieved successfully. The pacing catheter is passed surgically through *transthoracic or transxiphisternal approach*. The pacing catheter is commonly passed through abdominal approach and is attached to the epicardial surface of one of the ventricles (left or

right). General anaesthesia is required. The operative risk is increased.

Mechanism of generation of a cardiac impulse: The impulse is produced by sequential depolarisation of the ventricles, e.g. one ventricle is depolarised first followed by depolarisation of the other. The ECG pattern will depend on the ventricle paced. If pacing stimulus is delivered to the left ventricle (epicardial or transthoracic pacing), the depolarisation wave travels from the left ventricle to the right ventricle, hence, the resulting QRS with resemble a right bundle branch block (RBBB) pattern (wide rSR' pattern in V_1). This is due to delayed depolarisation of right ventricle. If the pacing stimulus is delivered to the right ventricle (endocardial or transvenous pacing) then reverse will happen. The excitation wave travels from the right ventricle to the left leading to delayed depolarisation of left ventricle, hence, the QRS complex will resemble pattern of LBBB (wide QRS complexes which are negative in V_1). If monitoring lead is V_1, then positive wide QRS indicates left ventricular pacing and negative wide QRS complex indicates right ventricular pacing.

Monitoring lead: Lead V_1 or MCL_1 is commonly recommended for continuous monitoring of ECG in patients with artificial pacemakers.

External or Transcutaneous Pacing

The external (transcutaneous or transchest) pacing refers to the delivery of a pacing stimulus through electrodes applied to the chest wall. It is designed for emergency situations (asystole or resistant sympto-matic bradycardia). The external pacing is either the demand or fixed rate pacing and can be achieved quickly. Successful transcutaneous pacing requires a higher current output than conventional endocardial pacing. Delivery of the stronger current causes skin burn or pain which can be minimised by using large pacing pad electrodes.

There are several models available for external pacing. Some models have defibrillator/monitors incorporated with external pacing capabilities; while others use a special pacing cassette inserted into a box or receptacle on the defibrillator, still others display the pacing control on the face of the unit along with defibrillation control.

The procedure is simple. The large pacing pads are attached across the chest of the patient (one on the front and other on the back) or on the front of chest (anterior-anterior positions). A pacing cable runs from the electrodes (pads) to the defibrillator/monitor. ECG leads are attached to the patient at conventional sites and the ECG signal is delivered to the machine directly through a special patient cable. Pacing parameters include current output (in ampere), pacing rate and pacing mode, which are set and the unit is turned on. The ECG is observed for proper sensing. Current output initially used is small but increased slowly and ECG observed for evidence of capture (spike followed by wide complex). The method to use pads is given in the box. It is, however, a temporary measure and should be followed by the insertion of a transvenous temporary pacemaker as soon as circumstances allow.

Instructions for use of the pads
- Remove the hair from the chest by shaving so as to maximise contact with the skin surface.
- The coloured ends of the pacing pads must match the coloured ends on the cable, e.g. red with red and black with black.

Functions of Artificial Pacemakers

1. Sensing
2. Firing
3. Capturing

1. ***Sensing:*** Ability to process the intrinsic electrical signals is called sensing.
2. ***Firing:*** It means the pulse generator has delivered a stimulus to the heart. Firing is visible on ECG as pacemaker spike.
3. ***Capturing:*** It means heart has captured the stimulus and has responded to it, which is detected on the ECG as a waveform (P wave or QRS complex). If pacing catheter is in the atrium, then pacemaker spike will be followed by 'P' wave; if it is in the ventricle, then spike is followed by a wide QRS complex (widening of QRS is due to sequential depolarisation of ventricle as already discussed). As the QRS complexes are wide resembling premature complexes, therefore, no diagnosis that rely on the morphological changes in QRS (for example, infarction, ischaemia or ventricular hypertrophy) can be made from the appearance of the paced QRS complexes.

Key Pacing Parameters

It includes:

1. ***Automatic interval*** *(escape or demand interval):* An interval between two paced beats is called automatic interval (Fig. 43.4). It determines the pacing rate. It is set either in milliseconds (msec) or in beats per minute (bpm).
2. ***Escape interval*** (Fig. 43.4): It is same as automatic or demand interval unless hysteresis is present. The pacing interval may be atrial (interval between two atrial beats, i.e. P waves) or ventricular (interval between two ventricular paced events, i.e. QRS), which may be reset by premature beats (intrinsic activity).

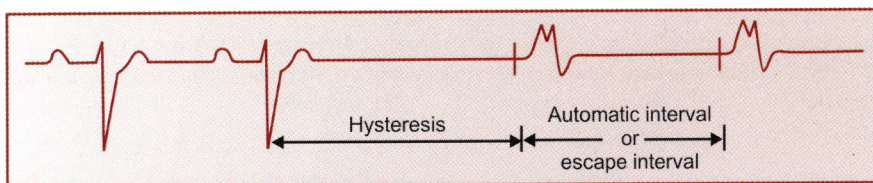

Fig. 43.4: Various intervals. The automatic interval is measured between two paced beats. The diagram shows hysteresis, i.e. the distance between last intrinsic beat and the first paced best is longer than the automatic or escape or demand interval

3. *Hysteresis* (Fig. 43.4): It is a feature incorporated into single chamber permanent generators. It refers a longer interval between a sensed intrinsic beat and the first paced beat. It is slightly longer than automatic interval. Hysteresis allows the artificial pacemaker to delay firing a little later than automatic interval with the hope that the patient's sinus pacemaker will fire. If sinus pacemaker takes over the rhythm, the pacemaker will not fire. Hysteresis preserves the life of the battery.

4. *Amount of the current:* The minimum amount of the current required to evoke a response is called 'threshold' and determined during the insertion of pacemaker. The milliamperes (mA) reflect the strength of the output signal. The signal should normally be strong enough to produce capture or depolarisation, but not so strong as to cause diaphragmatic or phrenic nerve palsy or unnecessary exhaustion of the pacemaker battery.

5. *Pacemaker sensitivity:* It means the ability of generator to process and to programme the incoming cardiac signals of varying voltages into millivolts (mV). Sensitivity is manipulated easily on a temporary generator; when the sensitivity or millivolt dial is turned to the lowest number, this means the generator will sense virtually all intrinsic activity even at the low-voltage signals. When the millivolt dial is turned to highest number, this means the generator is instructed to ignore virtually all intrinsic activity even the high-voltage signals.

The lower number on the dial correlates with demand mode of pacing, whereas the higher numbers correlate with asynchronous or fixed rate mode of pacing.

Note: Over a period of days or weeks after permanent pacing, the inflammation and fibrosis of tissue around the tip of pacing lead may raise the stimulation threshold. Therefore, threshold in the permanent generator is set higher than the initial stimulation threshold to compensate for the initial increase in the threshold that accompanies the lead placement. Later on, the threshold usually comes down.

Programmability of Pacemaker

This allows for modification of pacing function after implantation and for adaptation to changes according to clinical needs. Pacemaker programming is accomplished by activation of the programming head positioned over the implanted pulse generator after making desired changes in the programmable parameters given in the box. A radiofrequency system is routinely used to communicate the programme to the pacemaker.

Programmable pacemaker functions	
• Rate	• Energy output
• Sensitivity	• Lead polarity
• Hysteresis	• Refractory period
• Mode of function	• AV delay

Identification of Coding System (see the box)

The coding system of artificial pacemakers refers to the functions available with the pacemaker generators. This is developed because of complexity of the pacemakers design. A five letter coding system is universally accepted. The first three letters describe the fundamental operations; while the other two refer to more sophisticated devices incorporated into some permanent pacing generators.

1. The first letter stands for the chamber(s) paced, e.g. atrium (A), ventricle (V), or both or double (D) and none (O).

SECTION ELEVEN

Pacemaker identification code (Recommend by North American Society of Pacing and Electrophysiology and British Pacing and Electrophysiology Group)				
Chamber (s) paced	Chamber (s) sensed	Mode of responses (sensing function)	Programmable functions	Special anti-tachyarrhythmia functions
V = Ventricle	V = Ventricle	T = Triggered	P = Programmable	P = Pacing (anti-tachyarrhythmia)
A = Atrium	A = Atrium	I = Inhibited (demand)	M = Multi-programmable	S = Shock
D = Double (dual A + V)	D = Double (dual A + V)	D = Double (dual function; T + I)	O = None (permanent pacemaker only)	D = Double (P + S)
O = None		O = None	C = Communicating	
		R = Reverse	R = Rate modulation	

2. The second letter denotes the chamber(s) sensed. If the sensing of electrical signal occurs in the atria, it is denoted as A; if sensing occurs in the ventricle, then letter 'V' is used. The letter 'D' indicates sensing of both the chambers and letter 'O' means no sensing facility or sensing is absent.

3. The third letter refers to mode of response of the generator to a sensed signal. The inhibited (I) mode means the pacemaker fires on demand because it is inhibited by intrinsic electrical signals and will not fire if these signals are sensed within the escape interval. The triggered (T) mode means the pacemaker is triggered to fire when it senses a specific intrinsic event (a P wave or QRS complex). The designation 'D' means both modes (inhibited and triggered) are operative. The designation 'O' means sensing is absent. The type of pacing without sensing is called asynchronous or fixed rate pacing. The generators fire at fixed rate without sensing the intrinsic activity. The asynchronous or fixed rate pacing is rarely used nowadays.

4. The fourth letter stands for programmability rate or energy output only or both. The designation 'P' indicates programmable; 'M' indicates multiprogrammable, 'O' stands for non-programmable, 'C' for communicating and 'R' stands for rate modulation.

5. The fifth letter stands for the ability of the pulse generators to sense tachycardias and reflects that anti-tachycardia function is available in the pacemaker generator. The letter P stands for pacing, D stands for double function P and S. The letter S stands for shock and E stands for none.

The pacemaker coding examples using first three letters (commonly used) are depicted in the Figure 43.5.

Physiology of the Pacemakers

The pacemakers are designed to maintain or increase cardiac output in a physiological manner. The recent pacemakers represent a significant advancement in pacemaker technology when compared with earlier units.

First generation pacemakers: They were single chamber units designed to deliver impulses into one chamber (usually a ventricle). Their purpose was simply to maintain heart rate. For examples; VOO, AOO pacemakers were earlier models, produced asynchronous pacing and are no longer used. They are used when dual chamber pacemakers are not indicated such as in patients with atrial fibrillation, atrial flutter or multifocal atrial tachycardia. This is because all dual chamber devices depend upon a stable atrial rhythm for proper functioning.

Second generation pacemakers: These are dual chamber pacemakers designed to stimulate the normal sequence of depolarisation in the heart. Dual chamber pacemakers stimulate the atria and the ventricles in sequence, thereby preserving normal AV synchrony. These pacemakers have more physiological approach than earlier ones. Dual chamber pacing units use two catheters, one in the right atrium and the other in the right ventricle. These pacemakers may have inhibited mode of response or triggered mode of response. Their

A. AAI pacemaker

B. VVI pacemaker

C. DDD pacemaker

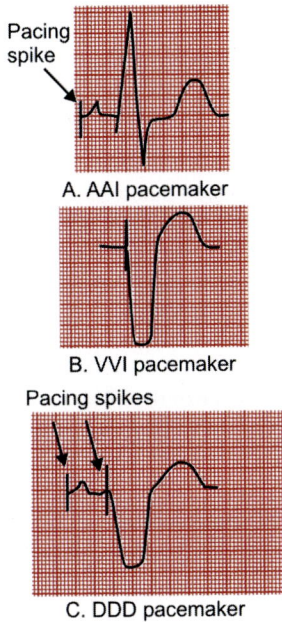

1: AAI pacemaker
A—stands for a single chamber (atrium) paced.
A—stands for a single chamber (atrium) sensed.
I—stands for inhibited mode of response.
Working: This single chamber pacemaker looks for P wave and fires into the atrium if no P wave is sensed. The pacing spike is followed by a 'P' wave.

2: VVI pacemaker
V—stands for single chamber (ventricle) paced.
V—stands for single chamber (ventricle) sensed.
I—stands for inhibited mode of response.
Working: This single chamber pacemaker looks for 'QRS' complex, fires into the ventricle if no 'QRS' is sensed. The pacing spike is followed by a wide QRS.

3: DDD pacemaker
D—stands for dual (both) chambers (atrium and ventricle) paced.
D—stands for both atrium and ventricle sensed.
D—stands for dual mode of response operative.
Working: The dual chamber pacemaker looks for a 'P' wave; if no 'P' is sensed, the pacemaker delivers a stimulus to the atrium. After a prolonged AV delay (P-R interval), if no QRS is sensed, a second stimulus is delivered into the ventricle. The first pacemaker spike is followed by P wave and the second spike is followed by QRS.

Fig. 43.5: Pacemaker code examples. 1—AAI pacemaker, 2—VVI pacemaker and 3—DDD pacemaker

advantage is that AV synchrony is preserved. These are commonly used nowadays.

Third generation pacemakers: These are *rate-responsive pacemakers.* This is a major advancement in pacemaker technology. These single-chamber or dual chamber units allow the rate of pacing to increase in response to physiologic demand. They are *biosensor,* programmed to respond to variations in activity, respiration, blood temperature, blood pH and other parameters that are under investigations.

Candidates for dual-chamber pacing include patients who cannot tolerate the loss of AV synchrony associated with conventional single-chamber pacemaker (VVI). Loss of synchrony or loss of atrial boost in single-chambered ventricular demand pacemaker (VVI) produces the pacemaker syndrome consisting of dizziness, weakness and lethargy as a major disadvantage.

Types of Cardiac Pacing

The various types of pacing provided by the pacemakers include:
1. Asynchronous pacing (VOO, AOO, and DOO)
2. Demand single chamber pacing (VVI, AAI, VVT and AAT)
3. P-synchronous pacing (VAT and VDD)
4. AV pacing (DVI)
5. Universal pacing (DDD)
6. Unipolar and bipolar pacing.

1. ***Asynchronous or fixed rate pacing** (VOO, AOO, and DOO):* Asynchronous pacemakers do not sense any electrical signals, hence, the main disadvantage is emergence of competitive rhythms due to interference by any spontaneous electrical activity occurring within the heart. Asynchronous pacing occurs whenever a magnet is placed over the implanted generator in order to evaluate pacing function. Asynchronous pacing and concomitant occurrence of patient's spontaneous rhythm result in iatrogenic parasystole (Fig. 43.6).

2. ***Demand or synchronous single chamber pacing** (VVI, AAI, VVT and AAT):* Both sensing and pacing circuits are incorporated. Some generators (VVI, AAI) have inhibited (demand) mode or response, hence, no pacemaker artifact will appear. The triggered response generators (VVT and AAT) deliver an output impulse at the *precise time of sensing* the intracardiac signal, and thus falls within the sensed complex and does not contribute to activation of the cardiac chamber. A pacing artifact will appear within QRS, which does not mean ventricular activation but only indicates that ventricular complex is sensed.

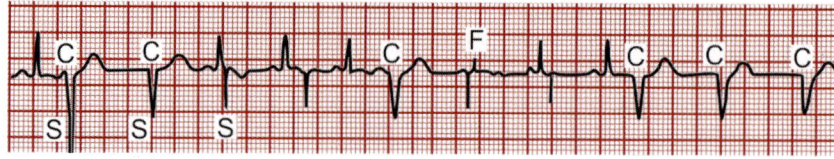

Fig. 43.6: Asynchronous ventricular pacing (VOO): This is produced by placing the magnet over the implanted pulse generator. Pacing stimulus (S) is delivered to the ventricles at rate of 60/min (magnet rate). Pacing stimuli are delivered at regular intervals indicating sensing of spontaneous QRS does not occur. Ventricular capture (C) occurs when the ventricular tissue is responsive. A fusion complex (F) is seen, which indicates ventricular activation both by pacing stimulus and transmission of sinus impulse through nodal—His pathway system

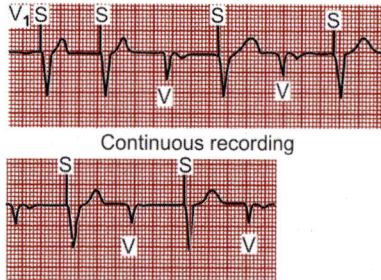

Continuous recording

Fig. 43.7: Ventricular inhibited pacing (VVI): Pacing is programmed at rate of 75/min (interstimulus distance between first and second paced beats is = 20 × 0.04 = 0.8 sec). Spontaneous QRS complexes (V) inhibited the pacing discharge. When no spontaneous QRS complexes are sensed, ventricular pacing at the programmed rate (0.8 sec) occurs as denoted by 'S'

Triggered pacing might be confused with the failure to sense unless mode of function of generator is known (Fig. 43.7).

The demand pacemakers (VVI, AAI) units are not only inhibited by intrinsic cardiac signals but may be inhibited also, both by extraneous (electro-cautery, diathermy, microwave ovens, etc) or extrinsic (patient's muscle potentials) electrical signals which are sensed by them. Such sensed signals will produce pauses in the paced rhythm. Triggered response (VVT and AAT) generators do not have this problem. Newer generator design and programmability have helped to reduce these 'over-sensing' problem.

The pacing functions of demand pacemaker cannot be evaluated if patient's spontaneous activity overwhelms the programmed rate of the generator, since the pulse generator output will be inhibited. Application of a magnet over the generator makes its mode of function asynchronous, hence, capture of atria or ventricles by the pacemaker, can be confirmed

provided that pacing stimuli fall outside the refractory period of the cardiac tissue as shown in Figure 43.6 of asynchronous pacing.

3. *P-synchronous pacing (VAT and VDD):* This is dual-chamber pacing in which an electrode is placed both in atrium and ventricle, when the atrial electrode senses an electrical signal, a P wave is produced. A ventricular pacing stimulus is delivered after a programmable *AV delay*, which corresponds to the P-R interval (Fig. 43.8). VAT generators are nowadays obsolete as they do not sense ventricular activity. Newer devices (VDD) are used as they sense both atrial and ventricular activity. These devices usually provide atrial and ventricular rhythm in a 1:1 ratio (one P wave for each QRS); allowing for an increase in the ventricular paced rate concomitant with increase in the sinus rate. The pulse generators are so designed not to allow rapid ventricular paced rates to occur should the atrial rate becomes too fast. If atrial activity is not sensed, even then these pulse generators pace the ventricles on demand at the programmed back-up rate.

AV pacing (DVI): DVI pacemaker generators pace dual chambers (atrium and ventricle) but sense only the ventricular electrical activity. Since atrial sensing does not exist and atrial stimulus is always emitted, hence, there is possibility of existence of competitive atrial rhythms if an atrial pacing stimulus falls in the atrial vulnerable period. These units work after a programmed AV interval after an atrial pacing stimulus has been delivered. If spontaneous sinus P wave occurs and stimulates a spontaneous QRS complex, the generators behave differently. Some generators respond by inhibition of ventricular

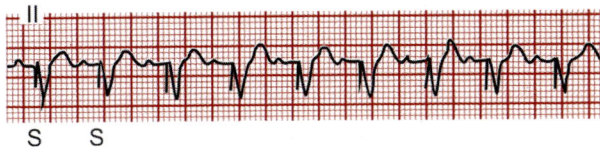

Fig. 43.8: P-asynchronous pacing (VDD): The atrial rhythm is sinus. After programmed AV delay, a ventricular stimulus (S) is delivered, hence ventricular pacing rate is same as the sensed atrial rate, i.e. 72/min. The AV delay is set at 0.25 sec. The P-to-stimulus(S) interval is 0.28 sec indicating that P wave was sensed 0.03 sec later after its inscription on ECG. The precise time of sensing a P wave depends upon the conduction time within the atria, quality of intracardiac signal and location of atrial or ventricular electrode (S)

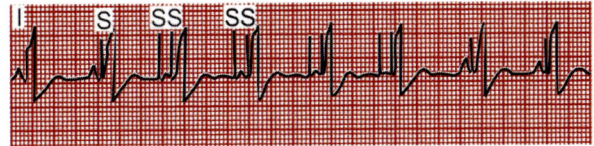

Fig. 43.9: DDD pacing (atrial and ventricular pacing). The first two P waves are sinus conducted and inhibited the atrial pacing output circuit, while the ventricular output circuit is intact and discharged(S). After this, the P waves and QRS complexes are paced at programmed rate of 72/min since no spontaneous QRS complex occurs during this period. Had a spontaneous QRS been stimulated by either a sinus or a paced P wave, then the ventricular output circuit would have been inhibited similar to atrial circuit

output, others deliver output impulse within the refractory period of ventricular tissue at the end of programmed AV delay; and still others deliver output impulse within the AV interval.

4. *Universal pacing (DDD):* Both atrium and ventricle (dual chamber device) are paced and sensed on demand in this type of pacing (Fig. 43.9). Thus, they are more or less physiological pacemakers as they approach the physiology of normal AV conduction. The disadvantage of these pacemaker devices include:
1. *Pacemaker mediated re-entrant tachycardia (Fig. 43.10):* This is due to their ability to sense retrograde atrial activity and stimulate the ventricles in response.

2. They are not useful in patients with disturbance in atrial rhythm (atrial fibrillation, flutter, choatic atrial rhythm). These pacemakers require stable atrial rhythm for proper functioning. Actually dual chamber device of any type is not useful in such patients with atrial instability where VVI pacemaker is implanted. *Biosensors* are nowadays being evaluated in such situations. Some biosensors currently being investigated include right ventricular temperature, right ventricular pH, QT interval and muscular activity. Changes in these biological parameters reflect physiologic needs resulting in changes in the paced rate. These pacing systems are termed *'rate-adaptive'*.

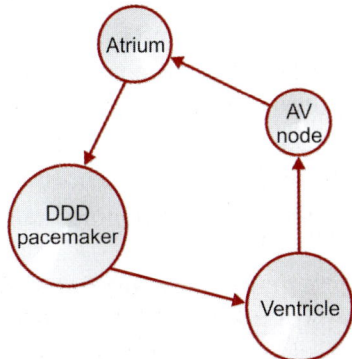

SECTION ELEVEN

Fig. 43.10A: Diagrammatic illustration of the sequence of events in endless loop tachycardia (Pacemaker induced tachycardia by DDD pacemaker)

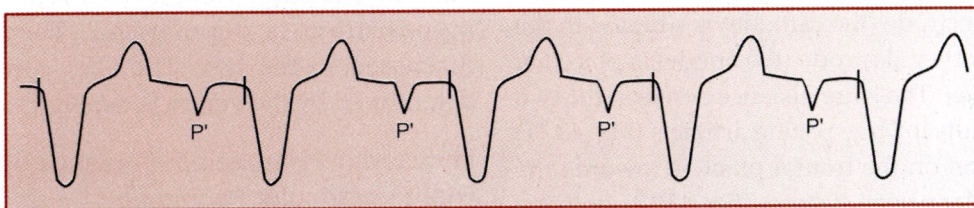

Fig. 43.10B: Pacemaker mediated re-entrant tachycardia (Diagram). Note the retrograde P' (inverted) visible on the ECG after T wave. Each time a retrograde P' is sensed and is followed by a wide QRS. If this cycle perpetuates, tachycardia will result

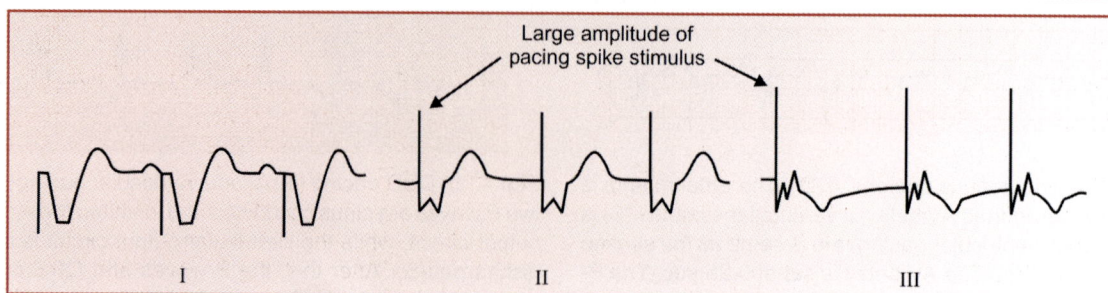

Fig. 43.11A: Unipolar ventricular pacing system (diagram). The large amplitude of the pacing stimulus indicates that this is unipolar system. The axis of the pacing artifacts, i.e. duration of current flow, is inferiorly oriented, indicates that generator lies inferior to heart, i.e. lies in the upper abdomen. The paced QRS have a right bundle branch block pattern (wide downward complex in lead I) indicating that the pacemaker is implanted on the left ventricular epicardial surface

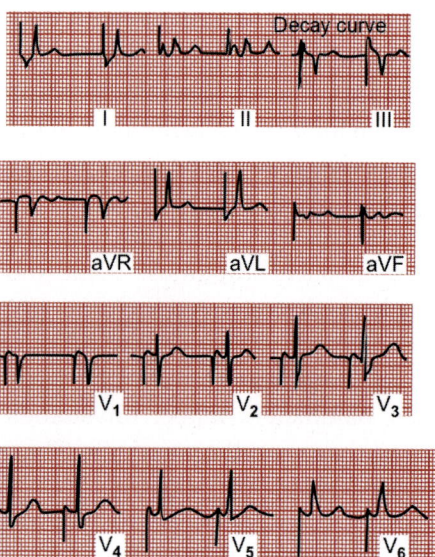

Fig. 43.11B: Transvenous atrial pacing with AV conduction (unipolar pacing): The large artifacts are the result of unipolar pacing due to an atrial electrode. The large artifact and its associated *decay curve* often obscures the contour of paced 'P' waves. This tracing shows upright P wave in II, III and aVF and negative in leads I and aVL which means P wave vector is directed inferiorly and rightwards and the site of atrial electrode is right atrium

5. *Unipolar and bipolar pacing:* In unipolar pacing system, one electrode (the cathode) is situated in the heart and the other electrode (the anode) is placed at the generator set. The large distance between the two electrodes results in large pacing artifacts (Fig. 43.11) whose direction on the frontal plane is towards the anode. In bipolar pacing systems (Fig. 43.12), both the electrodes are placed within the heart at a distance of 1-2 cm apart. Either of two electrodes may serve as

cathode. The pacing artifacts are small due to short interelectrode distance and its direction in the frontal plane reflects the direction of current flow.

In these pacing systems, if ECG is recorded on digital ECG machines instead of analog ones, may show marked variation in the amplitude and polarity of pacing impulse. This is because digital machine samples the pacing stimulus at a specific intervals, and then recreates it on the paper, thus, the inscribed stimulus artifact is not seen in real time. In some instances, the pacing stimulus may be entirely invisible giving the wrong impression of failure of generator output. Recognition of this artifact of recording in patients with these types of pacemakers is important, so as, to avoid erroneous impression of pacemakers malfunction.

There is little to choose between two systems; the unipolar is more sensitive but is also more susceptible to interference by external stimuli (e.g. electrical interference, skeletal muscle potentials).

ELECTROCARDIOGRAPHIC PATTERNS OF PACED COMPLEXES

The shape of paced complex will depend on how the myocardium is depolarised. They are briefly discussed in the box. The QRS configuration is determined by the ventricle depolarised late.

Myocardial Infarction in Presence of Right Ventricular Pacing

Myocardial infarction can occur in a patient who has an implanted pacemaker (right ventricular pacing).

Electrocardiographic patterns in relation to the site of pacing

Site of pacing	Electrocardiographic pattern
• Right atrium (appendage or any portion)	Paced atrial complexes will have variable shapes of paced 'P' waves since atrial electrodes may be placed in the atrial appendage or recrewed into any portion of the atrium.
• Right ventricle (endocardial or epicardial area)	This will produce left bundle branch block (LBBB) pattern (wide QRS) in leads I, aVL, V_5 and V_6 since right ventricle is getting depolarised ahead of left ventricle (Fig. 43.13). Sometimes, leads V_5-V_6 show deep S waves because the main electrical forces may be moving away from the horizontal level where V_5-V_6 are recorded (Fig. 43.14). Mean frontal plane axis will be superior away from the inferior leads as apex of heart is depolarised before the base.
• Right ventricular outflow tract	Same as above, i.e. LBBB pattern. The mean frontal plane axis will be inferior (left lower quadrant) as base of heart is depolarised ahead of apex.
• High interventricular septum	The paced QRS complexes have either indeterminate delayed pattern or have near normal QRS. This is due to activation of both sides of septum simultaneously.
• Left ventricular (epicardium or endocardial)	QRS complexes have right bundle branch block (RBBB) pattern (rSR') because left ventricle is depolarised ahead of right ventricle.

The pattern of ECG reflects ventricle being depolarised late. The mean frontal plane QRS axis will depend on the location of epicardial electrodes relative to each other (bipolar system) or to the pulse generator (unipolar system).

Note: Spontaneous QRS complexes in paced patients show marked T wave inversion, the cause of which is not understood.

Uncomplicated right ventricular pacing produces LBBB pattern in leads I, aVL, V_5 and V_6, therefore, the diagnosis of acute myocardial infarction in paced patient is based on the same criteria as used for complete LBBB with myocardial infarction. Large unipolar stimuli mask Q waves. As already discussed in LBBB, the initial QRS forces in LBBB remain unchanged, therefore, the presence of R or QR complex (but not QS) following pacing stimuli in leads I, aVL, V_5-V_6 suggest anterior myocardial infarction. Although the sensitivity of qR complex is low, but its specificity is 100% because qR complex is never seen during the uncomplicated right ventricular pacing. Second diagnostic criteria is notching of ascending limb of QRS in these leads. Similarly qR complex in leads II, III and aVF is diagnostic of inferior wall infarction.

The ST-T wave abnormalities occur more commonly during acute myocardial infarction than the qR complex or QRS notching as described above. Pronounced primary ST segment elevation with convex configuration in the anterior or inferior leads is highly suggestive of infarction in addition to qR pattern. The diagnosis, further, becomes certain when the polarity of T wave is opposite to that of ST segment elevation. The ST segment depression concordant with QRS, occasionally, can occur in V_3-V_6 during uncomplicated right ventricular pacing. Conse-

quently, obvious ST segment depression in V_1-V_2 should be considered as abnormal and indicative of anterior infarction or ischaemia.

Inhibition of pacemaker by chest wall stimulation or by reduction of pacing rate or output may allow the emergence of spontaneous rhythm and reveal diagnostic infarction Q waves.

MALFUNCTIONING OF PACEMAKERS

All pacemakers are not alike. Therefore, before diagnosing a pacemaker malfunction, its specific functions and parameters, must be known. Pacemaker malfunction results from abnormalities in sensing, firing and/or capturing. Most of these problems can be traced to component failure, battery failure, or problems at the interface between the tip of the catheter and the heart. Some problems may be due to an error in interpretation (pseudo-malfunction) rather than actual malfunction. The error in interpretation is common with newer DDD pacemakers.

I. ABNORMALITIES IN SENSING

These are of three types:
a. Undersensing
b. Oversensing
c. Inappropriate sensing

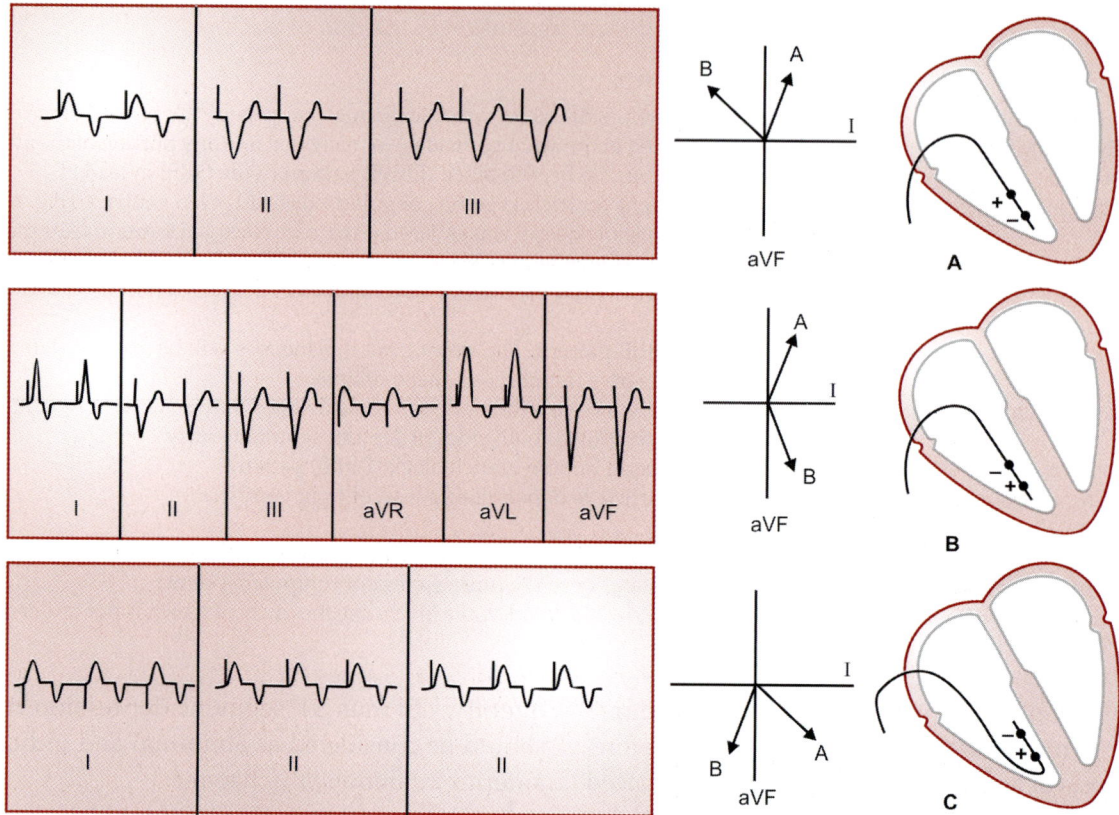

Fig. 43.12: Bipolar pacing systems (diagram)

A: The pacing catheter is in the apex of right ventricle. The tip (distal) electrode is cathode and ring (proximal) electrode is anode. The interelectrode distance is small, hence pacing artifact will also be small. As the current flows from cathode to anode, the pacing artifact axis will be oriented rightwards and superiorly (↑B), producing small negative deflections in leads I, II and III. Since myocardium is depolarised leftward and superiorly (↑A), there will be upright QRS in lead I and negative QRS in leads II and III

B: The tip (distal) electrode is anode and the ring is the cathode. The pacing artifact axis is leftwards and inferiorly (↑B) and the myocardium is depolarised leftward and superiorly (QRS axis is toward ↑A), hence, both pacing artifact and QRS complexes are upright in lead I and aVL and negative in II, III and aVF

C: The pacing catheter lies in the outflow tract of right ventricle. The current flows from cathode to anode (tip to ring), hence, pacing artifact axis is directly inferiorly (arrow B) resulting in upward deflections in leads II and III, and from the left to right producing pacing artifact negative in lead I. Since the myocardium is depolarised from base to apex (the QRS axis is towards ↑A) resulting in upright QRS in leads II and III

A. Undersensing: It is the most common cause of failure to sense. This occurs when generator sensitivity (mV) may be set too high (it is not sensitive enough to sense the incoming signals), the voltage of incoming signals may be too low due to myocardial disease or the lead is out of position. Also, oversensing (T waves, muscle artifact, etc) may allow undersensing of appropriate QRS signals.

Diagnosis: Paced beats appear too early, too late or not at all (Fig. 43.15).

Remedial Measures

1. Increase the sensitivity of a temporary generator by turning the sensitivity or millivolt dial to a lower number, (e.g. from 10 to 2), then observe the paced beats that appear on time.

2. Reprogramme a permanent generator to increase the sensitivity, e.g. lower the mV setting.

3. Take overpenetrated chest X-ray to check the lead position, reposition the lead if displaced.

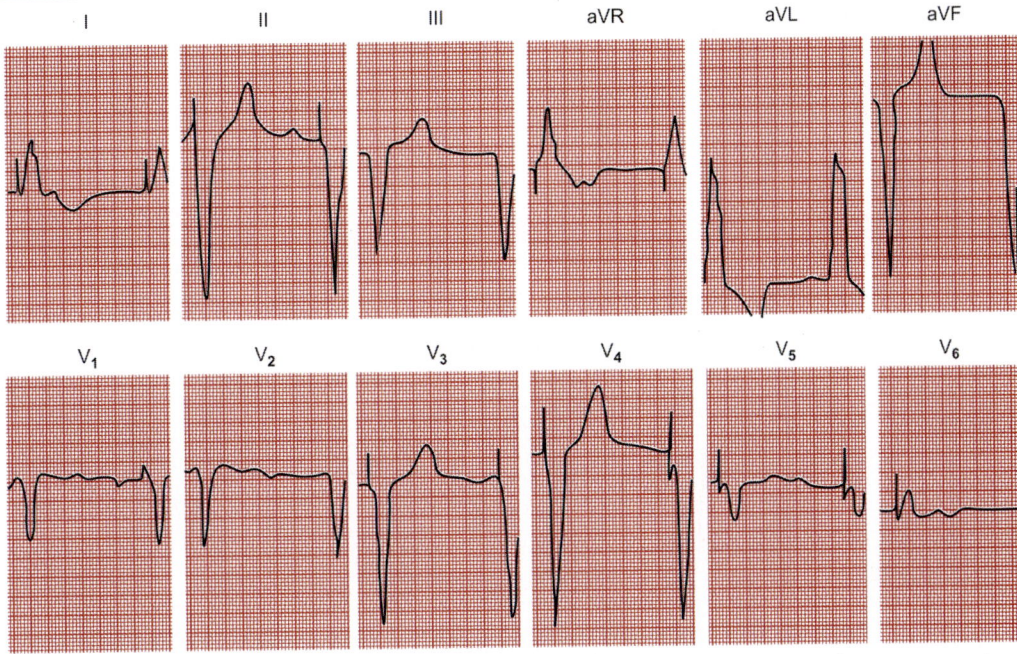

Fig. 43.13: Pacemaker rhythm (62 bpm) with consistent ventricular capture and *left atrial enlargement:* The ECG is taken from an old male patient with complete heart block. A temporary transvenous catheter was placed in right ventricle. The pacing stimulus precedes each QRS complex. The presence of LBBB indicates that pacemaker is in right ventricle. The negative QRS complexes in leads II, III and aVF signifies the catheter is placed in the apex of right ventricle. There is sinus rhythm of 62 bpm with complete heart block. The broad, late, negative component of P wave in lead V_1—typical of left atrial enlargement are also seen

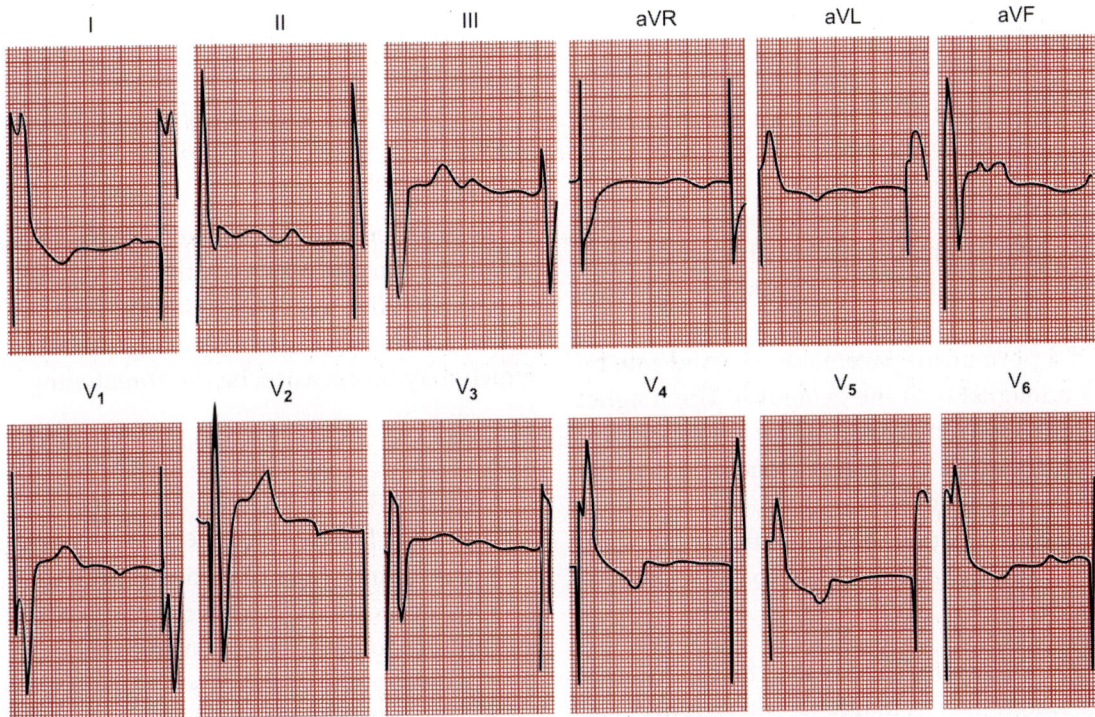

Fig. 43.14: Unipolar ventricular pacing. Right ventricular pacing has been done in a patient with complete AV block. Note pacemaker firing is fixed at a rate of 60 bpm with consistent ventricular capture. A pacing stimulus precedes each QRS. A LBBB pattern identifies that the pacing catheter is in the right ventricle. The P wave in lead II and III is 2.5 mm in amplitude which indicates right atrial enlargement

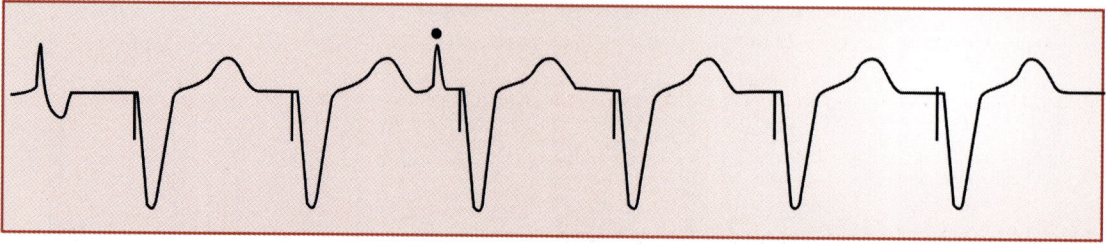

Fig. 43.15: Undersensing (diagrammatic illustration). The pacemaker fires earlier than expected time because it has not sensed the QRS complex *(asterisk)*

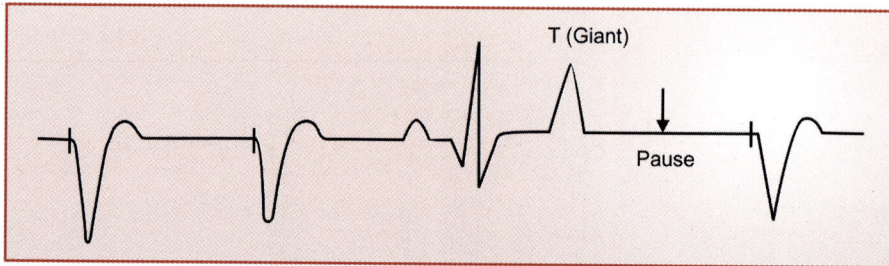

Fig. 43.16: Oversensing (diagrammatic illustration). Giant T wave has inhibited the pacemaker to fire in time *(asterisk)*. The pacemaker has fired later than it should be (at ↓) producing a pause

B. *Oversensing:* It means the generator is too sensitive and is sensing wrong signals (muscle activity and T waves instead of QRS). Oversensing can cause inhibition of pacemaker impulse (Fig. 43.16).

Diagnosis: Paced beats either do not appear in time or not at all producing a pause.

Remedial Measures

1. Decrease the sensitivity of a temporary generator set by turning the millivolt dial to a higher number, e.g. from 2 to 5 until the unit starts to sense properly.
2. Convert a permanent pacemaker to fixed rate by placing a magnet over the generator. The magnet will blind the sensing circuits. This is a temporary measure designed to preserve pacing until the underlying problem is corrected.
3. Reprogramme a permanent generator to decrease the sensitivity, or rarely, change to the asynchronous mode.

C. *Inappropriate sensing:* It may lead to inhibition of the output signal. Electromagnetic interference, e.g. microwaves ovens, electrocautery devices, MRI may result inappropriate or intermittent inhibition of output signal (Fig. 43.17).

Remedial Measures

1. Avoid sources of electromagnetic interference.
2. Include information about potential sources of electromagnetic interference in the discharge planning instructions. Refer to the manufacturer's instructions regarding environmental hazards (e.g. over-head transmission lines and welding equipment).

D. *Loss of sensing:* Pacemaker fails to recognise the incoming signals, results in the delivering of pacing stimulus earlier than expected (Fig. 43.18). This may cause competitive atrial and ventricular rhythm, which may on occasion be life-threatening.

Causes

1. Pacemaker malfunction
2. Normally functioning pacemaker
   - Low amplitude of intrinsic QRS
   - Inappropriate intrinsic QRS vector perpendicular to pacemaker sensing axis
   - Improper position of sensing electrode
   - Electromagnetic interference
   - Intrinsic QRS appearing in pacemaker refractory period
   - Intraventricular conduction defects (Fig. 43.19).

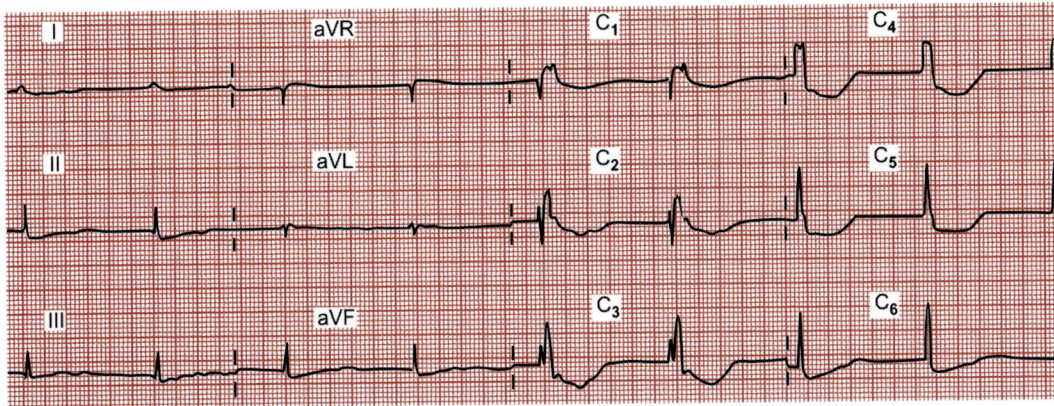

Fig. 43.17: Pacemaker malfunction following transthoracic cardioversion. There is inhibition of pacemaker output signal—pacemaker spikes are not seen. The intrinsic idioventricular rhythm at a rate of 50/min is visible. The patient had VVI pacemaker for complete heart block with pacing rate adjusted to 60/min. The DC shock was given to this patient for ventricular tachycardia, which resulted in temporary inhibition of output signals which was resumed after sometimes

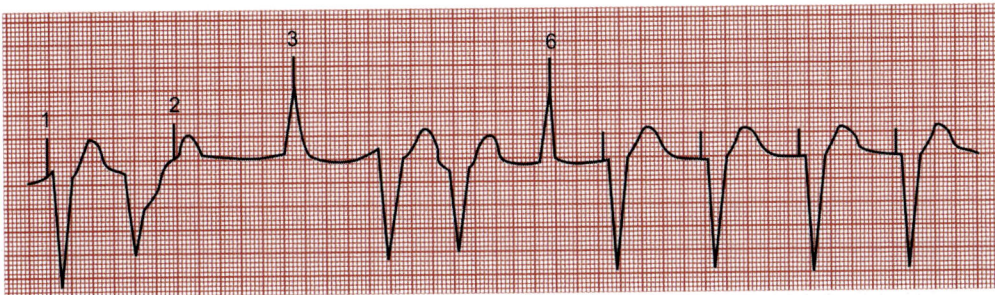

Fig. 43.18: Intermittent failure to sense (diagram). Pacing stimulus are delivered earlier than expected (QRS complexes 2,3, 6 are not sensed) indicating failure to sense these complexes probably due to their poor quality. The delivery of pacing stimulus, if occurs during vulnerable period, may result in repetitive ventricular rhythms

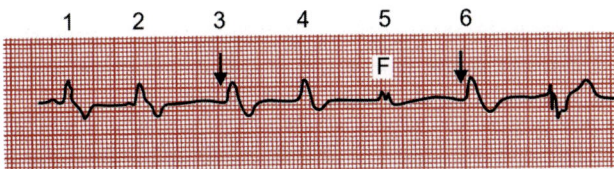

Fig. 43.19: *Sensing artifact due to LBBB:* Left ventricular epicardial pacing. The pacing was done in a patient with LBBB. The last QRS of the tracing is pure paced complex. The first 6 complexes are spontaneous complexes. The fifth is a fusion complex (F). Pacing artifact (↓) appear within two of the spontaneous QRS complexes (3,6) suggesting that QRS was not sensed. Sensing function was normal. This rhythm strip illustrates that LBBB delayed the depolarisation wave-front from reaching the epicardial electrodes in time to inhibit the output of pulse generator programmed at 60/min

II. ABNORMALITIES OF FIRING

Failure of firing means failure of appearance of pacing spike on ECG in time when it should be. Failure to fire results from depletion of pacemaker battery, fracture of the pacing catheter or its insulation, a disconnection within the system or oversensing.

Remedial Measures

1. Tighten all the connections of a temporary pacemaker.
2. Replace the battery in a temporary generator set.
3. Overpenetrated X-ray chest to detect lead wire fracture. Sometimes, it may be difficult to detect.
4. Replace the pacing catheter.
5. Replace the battery in a permanent generator.
6. Evaluate for oversensing.
7. Newer technology allows for impedence and/or ECG to be evaluated through the pacing lead utilising a special analyser.

Continuous recording

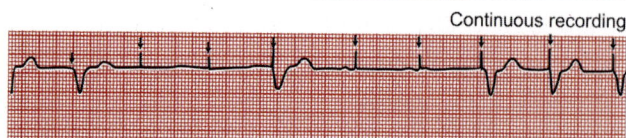

Fig. 43.20: Intermittent failure to capture. Pacing spikes are represented by arrows. On many occasions pacemaker spikes are not followed by wide QRS indicating failure to capture

III. ABNORMALITIES OF CAPTURING

Failure to capture means failure of expected waveform (P or QRS) to appear after the pacing spike (Fig. 43.20). Failure to capture is a major disadvantage of temporary pacemakers and results often from the migration of catheter tip within the heart or loss of contact of the catheter with the myocardium. In permanent pacemakers, the failure to capture is either due to lead fracture or fibrosis at the tip of lead causing exit block, i.e. impulses do not enter the myocardium. The causes of failure to capture are given in the box.

Causes of failure to capture

1. Pacemaker malfunction (e.g. battery failure, electrode wire fracture, etc)
2. Normally functioning pacemaker.
   - Poor electrode-endocardium contact (fibrosis, inflammation or oedema around the tip of electrode).
   - Advanced heart diseases.
   - Electrolyte imbalance (hyperkalaemia or hypokalemia)
   - Drugs (procainamide, quinidine, propranolol, etc)
   - Hypoxia, acidosis or alkalosis

Remedial Measures

1. Increase the milliamperes (voltage) on a temporary generator until effective capture is achieved.
2. Take an overpenetrated X-ray chest to know the position of catheter.
3. If catheter is out of position, then shift the patient to her or his left side. The effect of gravity in this position may re-establish the contact of the catheter to endocardium.
4. Reposition the pacing catheter.
5. Use a bridging cable (or extension cable) to reduce traction on externalised pacing wires.

6. Reprogramme a permanent generator.
7. Teach the patients about recommended post-insertion activity.
8. Correct the acid-base or electrolyte disturbance, if found to be the cause.

IV. ABNORMAL PACING RATE

A change in the pacing rate (acceleration or deceleration) or erratic/irregular pacing can occur due to normal function. Causes due to pacemaker malfunction are often found by exclusion. A constantly changing spike to spike interval during pacing often is caused by oversensing and/or a problem with the electrode rather than component failure. Cause of changes in the pacing rate are given in the box.

Causes of change in the pacing rate

I. *Normal function*
   - Low programmed rate
   - Application of a magnet
   - Inaccurate speed of ECG machine
   - Apparent malfunction in special function pulse generators, e.g. triggered mode (AAT, VVT)
   - Reversion to interference rate with either a faster or a slower rate than the spontaneous free running or magnet rate (according to manufacturer)

II. *Abnormal function*
   - Deceleration pacing rate due to battery failure
   - Runaway pacemaker: Either spontaneous or due to therapeutic radiation or electrocautery
   - Component failure (e.g. irregular delivery of pacing stimulus). Spontaneous or due to therapeutic radiation, electrocautery or defibrillation
   - Change in mode after therapeutic radiation, electrocautery or defibrillation. If functionally reset from electromagnetic interference, the device can be reprogrammed to its original mode.
   - Phantom programming (done without documentation) or misprogramming.
   - Oversensing.

SECTION ELEVEN

The Electrocardiogram

(i) The pacing spikes appear either at fast rates or slow rates than the fixed set rate of the pacemaker. As a rule, a failure to capture almost always occurs when the pacing rate is accelerated markedly, is a manifestation of abnormal functioning pacemaker.

(ii) *"Runaway pacemaker"* Pacemaker spikes appear at very fast rate > 600/min but life-threatening rates of stimulation are now rare but can still occur. At extremely rapid rates, stimulation is either ineffectual (rapid pacing spikes without producing tachycardia) or can occur intermittently, producing bursts of tachycardia.

Remedial Measures

1. Runaway pacemaker requires immediate disconnection and removal of the pacemaker.
2. Do not attempt to revert the tachycardia due to 'runaway' pacemaker as it is resistant to all antiarrhythmics.

PACEMAKER RE-ENTRANT TACHYCARDIA (ENDLESS LOOP TACHYCARDIA)

Dual chamber pacemakers (DDD) have two leads implanted; one each in the atrium and the ventricle, produce, sometimes, re-entrant ventricular tachycardia. One of the most common precipitating event is a premature ventricular complex (VPC). As long as the retrograde conduction is intact (the impulses from the ventricles can pass to atria through AV node), the abnormal impulse may be conducted retrogradely to the atria, to produce an inverted P′ wave. If the atrial lead senses the retrograde P (inverted P′) wave, the ventricular pacing via the ventricular lead will produce a QRS automatically after a programmed AV delay. Each subsequent event (QRS followed by an inverted P′ wave) perpetuates the cycle, a vicious cycle set up in this way leads to tachycardia (Fig. 43.10). Sometimes, an intrinsic proxysmal ventricular tachycardia may occur due to myocardial disease from which it has to be differentiated from therapeutic point of view (Fig. 43.20).

Initiating events: Any condition capable of separating the sinus P wave from QRS complex, coupled with retrograde ventriculoatrial conduction can initiate endless loop tachycardia. These include a ventricular premature complex (VPC), loss of atrial capture, myopotential sensing by the atrial channel of unipolar devices, undersensing of sinus P waves with preserved sensing of retrograde P waves, a prolonged AV interval and application and removal of the magnet.

Remedial Measures

1. The tachycardia can usually be abolished acutely by placing a magnet over the generator which converts it to asynchronous mode.
2. Long-term prevention of tachycardia includes drugs to decrease the atrioventricular conduction and reprogramming certain parameters of the pacemakers.

Pacemaker syndrome: It consists of fatigue, dizziness syncope and distressing pulsations in the neck and chest. These symptoms are due to adverse haemodynamic effects of ventricular pacing. The contributory mechanisms to pacemaker syndrome include; (i) loss of atrial contribution to ventricular systole due to AV asynchrony, (ii) vasodepressor reflex initiated by cannon 'a' waves and (iii) systemic and pulmonary regurgitation due to atrial contractions against a closed AV valve.

Remedial Measures

1. Maintain AV synchrony by dual chamber pacing.
2. In the case of a ventricular demand pacemaker, symptoms can be abolished by programming an escape rate of 15-20 bpm below that of the paced rate.

Pacemaker Pearls

1. *Be prepared to intervene with drugs or countershock or both, if arrhythmias are produced during insertion of a temporary pacing catheter.*
2. *For defibrillation, turn off a temporary pacemaker to eliminate the risk of generator damage. If there is permanent implant, then avoid placement of defibrillator paddles over the generator or close to it.*
3. *Insulate exposed metal by wearing unpowered rubber gloves.*

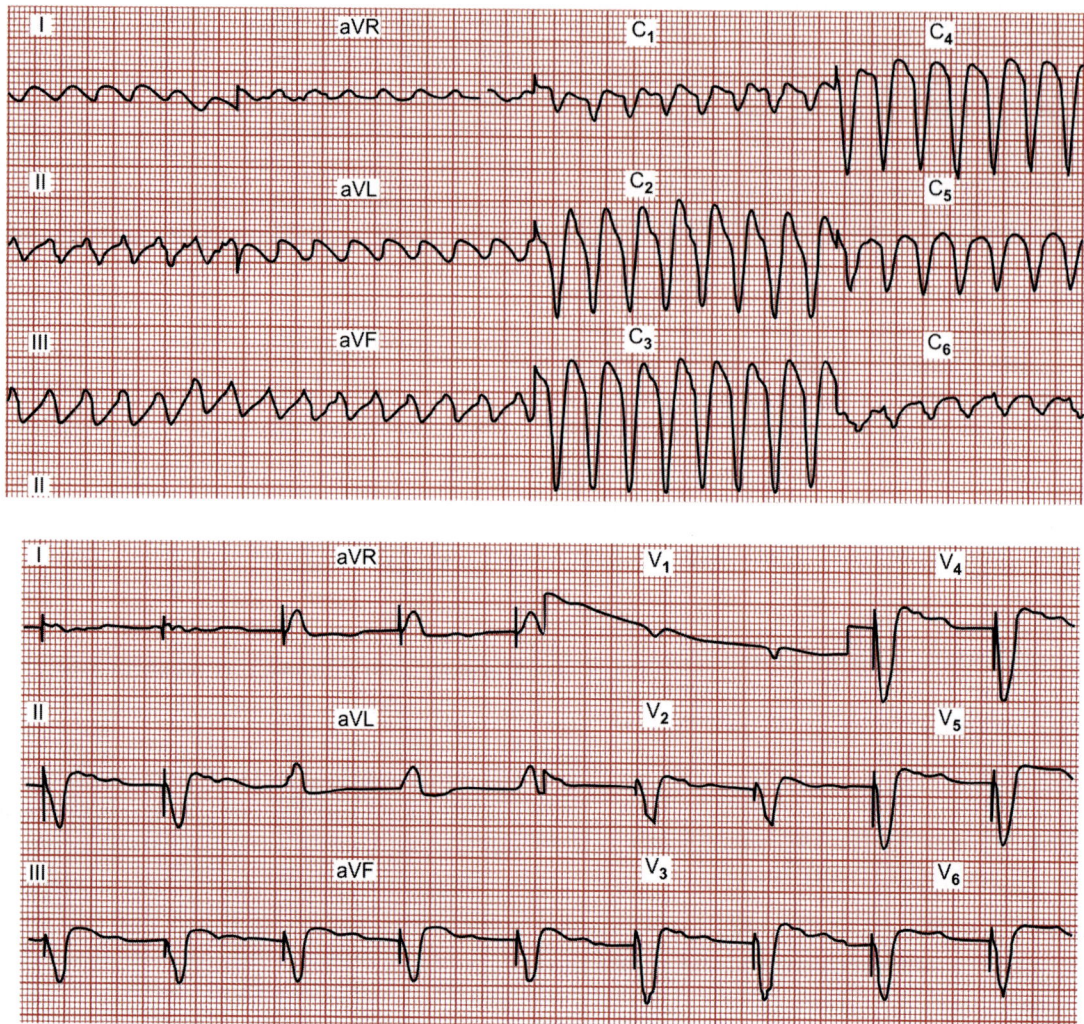

Fig. 43.21: A: Paroxysmal ventricular tachycardia in a patient with demand artificial VVI pacemaker. The patient got pacemaker for complete AV block with syncopal attacks. Demand pacemaker was implanted at a preset rate of 60 bpm. This type of tachycardia was recorded immediately after pacemaker also, was treated and pacemaker continued function normally. A second episode of paroxysmal ventricular tachycardia is depicted which was recorded when patient complained of palpitation. This type of tachycardia may occur either due to;

   i. Malfunctioning of pacemaker (run away pacemaker): In this type of VT, there is acceleration of preset rate of pacemaker. The pacemaker spikes indicating firing will be visible, but here they are not seen, hence, is not due to pacemaker malfunction.

   ii. In this ECG, the QRS complexes are wider (>140 msec against preset QRS of 108 msec). There is concordant pattern of the tachycardia, i.e. All QRS are negative in all precordial leads with superior QRS axis. This paroxysm of tachycardia appears to originate from the diseased heart rather than pacemaker induced because QRS is wider > 140 msec against the preset rate of 108 msec. The rapid rate of tachycardia (168/min) continuously inhibited the pacemaker from firing, hence, pacemaker spikes are not seen

B: After termination of episode of ventricular tachycardia. The ECG shows normal functioning pacemaker at a preset rate of 60 bpm. The P waves are seen in between, not preceding paced QRS indicating that demand pacemaker has been implanted for complete AV block. The paced QRS is negative in V_1 indicating it to be in right ventricle

   4. *Use a plastic cover for temporary generator to minimise the risk of damage if liquid is spilled on the controls.*

   5. *Electrical equipment should be properly grounded to minimise the electrical hazard.*

   6. *Protect exposed surgical wires by protective sleeves or plastic tube.*

7. *The patient with a pacemaker should not undergo MRI.*

8. *Use a bridging cable between generator and the external ends of a temporary pacemaker to minimise the risk of catheter displacement.*

9. *Suspect perforation of right ventricular wall by the pacing catheter if patient develops repeated hic-cough or a pericardial rub is audible. Take an overpenetrated X-ray chest to confirm the position of the catheter and reposition it at proper site, if diaphragm is being irritated.*

10. *Perforation of interventricular septum by a rigid pacemaker catheter will cause a sudden change in the polarity of the paced QRS complexes. This will manifest with wide upward QRS complex in lead V_1 following the pacing spike in case the right ventricle is being paced. Reverse will happen in left ventricular pacing.*

11. *Thrombosis and embolisation from a pacing catheter is rare, but if it occurs, can be fatal. Consider this possibility in case if patient develops sudden tachycardia, perspiration, shortness of breath, or chest pain.*

12. *Teach the patient how to take the radial pulse, when to notify the physicians (i.e. if the pulse falls below the present pacing rate), what environmental hazards to avoid, and why postimplant follow-up is necessary.*

13. *Disconnect the pacemaker in case tachycardia is being produced by 'runaway' pacemaker.*

Review at Glance

- Pacemakers are mostly used when heart rate is too slow (symptomatic bradycardia). Antitachycardia pacemakers are occasionally used to slow or terminate the rate when it is too fast.
- The pulse generators use replaceable batteries that generate the artificial electric signals. The pacing catheter delivers the signal to the heart.
- Permanent pacemakers have fixation devices so as to ensure long-term contact with the heart muscle.
- Endocardial pacing refers to insertion of the catheter through intravenous route into the heart until it makes a close contact with the endocardium. Epicardial pacing means the pacing catheter is inserted via a transthoracic (or transxiphisternal) route and is attached to the pericardium.

- Paced QRS complex is wider than normal because depolarisation of the ventricles is sequential and prolonged by the pacing stimulus delivered to one of the ventricles.
- Sensing refers to ability of the pacemaker to process the incoming signals.
- Firing means ability of the pacemaker to discharge a stimulus. Firing is recognised as a pacing spike (vertical line) on ECG.
- Capturing is the heart's ability to respond to a pacing stimulus. Capturing results in a P wave or QRS complex immediately after the pacing stimulus.
- The automatic interval is the pacing rate. The escape interval is the time between two paced events and is usually the same as automatic interval.
- Hysteresis is a programmable feature of single chamber pacemakers that allows a slightly longer interval between a sensed intrinsic event and the first paced event.
- Threshold is the minimum amount of current needed to cause depolarisation and milliamperes (mA) represent the output signal.
- Sensitivity (mV) is the ability of the generator to process or "see" incoming signals.
- The inhibited mode of pacing means that the pacemaker fires "on demand", or only when it does not sense a QRS complex.
- The triggered mode of pacing means that the pacemaker is cued to fire after it senses an event.
- The asynchronous mode of pacing means sensing is absent and the pacemaker fires at preset fixed rate.
- Physiological pacemakers (e.g. DDD) preserve normal AV synchrony. Nonphysiological pacemakers (VVI) are unable to preserve normal AV synchrony.
- Rate-responsive pacemakers control the rate in response to physiologic demand by sensing selected parameters such as activity and blood pH.
- Failure to sense means that the paced beats appear too early or too late or not at all.
- Pacemaker re-entrant tachycardia is associated with dual chamber pacing systems due to sensing of retrograde P´ waves.
- Failure to fire is recognised by the absence of a scheduled pacing spike on ECG.

- Failure to capture means that pacing spike is not followed by a P wave or QRS complex.
- Abnormal pacing rates (acceleration or deceleration or irregular pacing spikes) can occur during normal and abnormal pacemaker function (malfunction).

Suggested Reading

1. A report of the American College of Cardiology. American Heart Association Task Force on assessment of diagnostic and therapeutic cardiovascular procedures (committee on pacemaker implantation). *J Am Coll Cardiol* **18**:1, 1991.
2. ACC/AHA Task Force on practice. Guidelines for implantation of cardiac pacemakers. *JACC* **31**:175, 1998.
3. Barold SS, Falkoff MD, Ong LS, Heinle RA: Electrocardiography of contemporary DDD pacemakers: Basic concepts, upper rate response, retrograde ventriculoatrial conduction and differential diagnosis of pacemaker tachycardias. In Saksena S, Goldschalger N (Eds): Electrical Therapy for Cardiac Arrhythmias, Pacing, Antitachycardia Devices, Catheter Ablation. Philadelphia, WB Saunders Compnay, 1990.
4. Barold SS: Timing cycles and operational characteristics of pacemakers. In Ellenbogen KA, Kay GN, Wilkoff BL (Eds): Clinical Cardiac Pacing. Philadelphia, WB Saunders Company, 1995.
5. Beare PG, Myers JL: Principles and Practice of Adult Health Nursing. CV Mosby, St Louis, 1990.
6. Chung EK: Artificial Cardiac Pacing: Practical Approach. Williams and Wilkins, 1979.
7. Furman S, Hayes DL, Holmes DR Jr: A Practice of Cardiac Pacing. Futura 1986.
8. Goldschlager N (Editor): Cardiac pacemaker. Cardiol Clin **3**:1, 1985.
9. Goldschlager N, Goldman MJ: Principles of Clinical Electrocardiography. Prentice Hall International, 1989.
10. Hayes DL, Vliestra RE: Pacemaker malfunction. *Ann Int Med* **119**:828, 1993.
11. Kern LS: Cardiac Critical Care Nursing. Aspen Publishers, 1988.
12. Lipman BC, Cascio T: ECG assessment and interpretation. FA Davis, 1994.
13. Mond HG: Cardiac pacemaker: Function and malfunction. Grune and Stratton, 1983.
14. Raitt MH, Stelzer KJ, Larmore GE et al: Runaway pacemaker during high energy neutron radiation therapy. *Chest* **106**:955, 1994.
15. Souliman SK, Christie J: Pacemaker failure induced by radiotherapy. *PACE* **17**:270, 1994.
16. Visant MO, Spence MI: Common-sense approach to coronary care: A program, 5th edn, CV Mosby:St Louis, 1989.
17. Furman S: Newer modes of cardiac pacing. Description of pacing modes. *Mod Concepts Cardiovasc Dis* **52**:1, 1983.
18. Kudmer PL, Goldschlager N: Cardiac pacing in 1980's. *N Engl J Med* **311**:1671, 1984.
19. Personett V et al: Indications for dual chamber pacing. *PACE* **7**:318, 1984.
20. Zoll PM et al: External noninvasive temporary cardiac pacing. Clinical trials. *Circulation* **71**:937, 1985.

Miscellaneous Disorders

SECTION TWELVE

44

Heart in Endocrine Disorders and Injuries

- ■ *The electrocardiogram in various endocrinal disorders–hyper and hypothyroidism, acromegaly, Cushing's syndrome and Addison's disease, pheochromocytoma*
- ■ *The electrocardiogram in physical injuries—hypothermia and trauma to the heart*
- ■ *The electrocardiogram in electrical injuries*
- ■ *The electrocardiogram in cardiac tumours*

HYPERTHYROIDISM (THYROTOXICOSIS)

Cardiovascular findings in hyperthyroidism (thyrotoxicosis) include; a wide pulse pressure, sinus tachycardia, a collapsing pulse, atrial arrhythmias especially atrial fibrillation, cardiac enlargement and precipitation of angina, and at times an overt heart failure. A *'to and fro'* high pitched sound (Lerman scratch) may be audible in the pulmonary area. The cardiovascular manifestations depend on the severity of hyperthyroidism but mild hyperthyroidism on the other hand, may precipitate cardiac failure or cause irregularity in rhythm especially atrial fibrillation. Patients with atrial fibrillation without underlying heart disease should be screened for thyrotoxicosis specifically old persons. ECG changes are characteristically seen during thyroid crisis or storm or severe uncontrolled hyperthyroidism.

The Electrocardiogram (Figs 44.1 and 44.2)

Usually, the ECG changes in hyperthyroidism include sinus tachycardia, high voltage of QRS complexes and nonspecific ST-T abnormalities. Atrial fibrillation with rapid ventricular rate is common. Arrhythmias associated with hyperthyroidism are listed in the box. Atrial and nodal arrhythmias are attributed to shortening of AV conduction time and functional refractory period. Intra-atrial conduction disturbances manifested by prolongation or notching of P waves and prolongation of P-R interval can occur uncommonly. Ocassionally, second and third degree AV block can occur, the cause of which is not clear. Intraventricular conduction disturbances, most commonly right bundle branch block pattern can occur in 15% patients without associated heart disease of any aetiology. These changes resolve with treatment of hyperthyroidism. Normalisation of ECG changes takes longer time, i.e. weeks and months.

HYPOTHYROIDISM (MYXOEDEMA)

Cardiovascular findings in myxoedema include; slow pulse rate (bradycardia), cardiomegaly (primary hypothyroidism), conduction disturbances and pericardial effusion. These changes are due to hypometabolism and myxoedematous infiltration into the heart and pericardium.

The Electrocardiogram (Fig. 44.3)

1. *Slow heart rate:* Majority of the patients have bradycardia (HR < 60 bpm).
2. *Low voltage* of P-QRS-T complexes especially in the standard limb leads is common, but if there is an

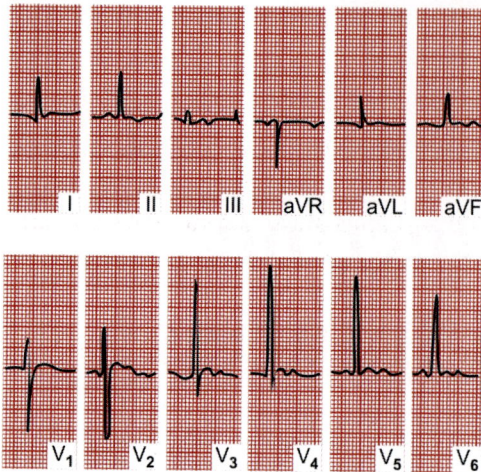

Fig. 44.1: Grave's disease (exophthalmic goitre with hyper-thyroidism). The electrocardiogram recorded from a 28 yr female shows;

  i. High voltage of QRS in precordial leads. The sum total of $RV_6 + SV_1$ of 36 mm in a young patient of thyrotoxicosis does not indicate left ventricular hypertrophy, suggest it to be due to thyrotoxicosis and young age
  ii. Heart rate is 115 min regular (lead III shown)
  iii. The T wave inversion in leads II, III, aVF, V_2-V_6

Arrhythmias associated with hyperthyroidism

- Sinus tachycardia
- Atrial ectopics or extrasystoles
- Paroxysmal atrial fibrillation is common. Atrial fibrillation with 1:1 conduction producing high ventricular rate can occur (Fig. 44.2)
- Paroxysmal atrial tachycardia (rare)
- Paroxysmal atrial flutter (rare)
- Idionodal tachycardia (nonparoxysmal AV nodal tachycardia)
- Paroxysmal AV nodal tachycardia.

associated pericardial effusion then there is generalised low voltage graph. The T waves may become flat.

3. *Conduction disturbances,* i.e. prolongation of P-R interval or first degree AV block may occur. Other conduction blocks are less common. Incomplete or complete right bundle branch block has been observed.

4. Prolongation of QTc interval.

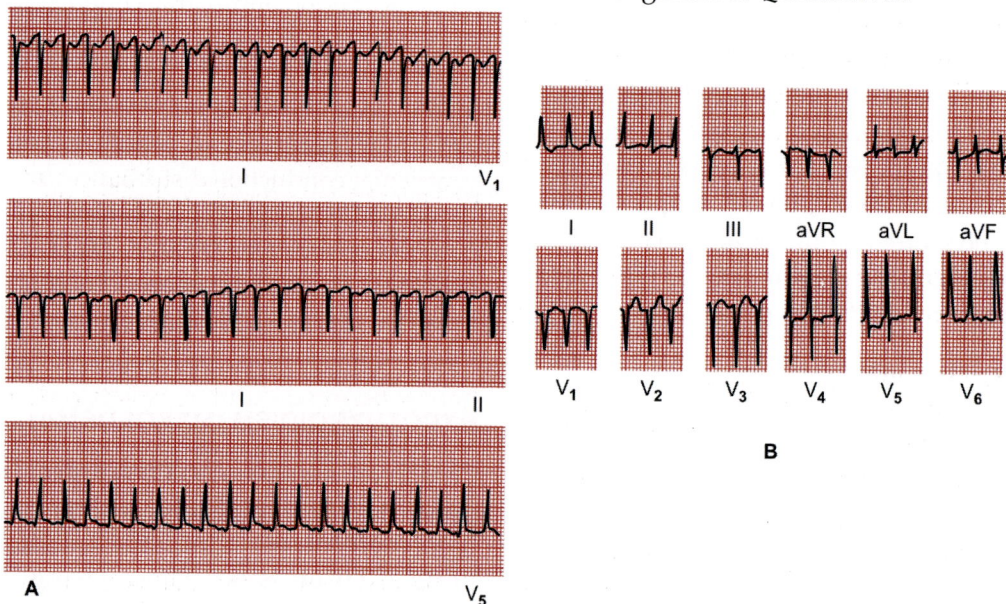

Fig. 44.2: A: Atrial fibrillation with 1:1 conduction in hyperthyroidism. The electrocardiogram shows;
  i.   Ventricular rate is fast, i.e. 250 bpm and regular
  ii. The QRS complexes are narrow
  iii. Atrial fibrillation with 1:1 conduction will not show fibrillation waves, hence, difficult to diagnose and is otherwise rare. The conditions that lead to it are:
      i.   Hyperthyroidism
      ii. WPW syndrome
      iii. Phaeochromocytomas
      iv. Major cardiac surgery
B: Atrial fibrillation in thyrotoxicosis with myocardial ischaemia. Atrial fibrillation with a ventricular rate of about 200 per minute. The T waves are inverted in the anterior and lateral leads, indicating probable ischaemia

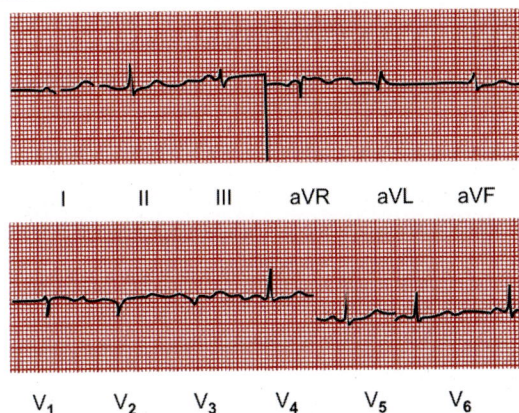

Fig. 44.3: Hypothyroidism. The electrocardiogram shows;
  i. Low voltage graph. None of standard lead records complex more than 5 mm and precordial leads more than 10 mm
  ii. The patient had slow heart rate (<60/min) as revealed by lead V_6
  iii. T waves are flat in leads III, aVL, aVF and of low amplitude in V_5-V_6

5. *The ST-T changes* suggestive of ischaemic heart disease or a primary myocardial abnormality may be seen in older patients.
6. It is possible that hypothermia in association with hypothyroidism may contribute to ventricular re-entrant arrhythmias.

All these changes resolve with successful treatment of myxoedema but complete resolution takes longer time.

ACROMEGALY

The cardiovascular manifestations include; cardiomegaly which is out of proportion than generalised organomegaly. In addition, the frequency of a number of cardiovascular disorders is increased in acromegalics; hypertension, premature coronary artery disease, congestive heart failure and cardiac arrhythmias, especially frequent ventricular premature complexes and intraventricular conduction defects. Indeed, because of frequent occurrence of congestive heart failure and cardiac arrhythmias in patients who otherwise have no predisposing factors (e.g. no hypertension, coronary artery disease or atherosclerosis), it has been suggested that a specific *acromegalic cardiomyopathy* exists.

The Electrocardiogram

1. ST segment depression with or without T wave abnormalities.
2. Intraventricular conduction disturbances. Bundle branch block is common.
3. Rhythm disturbances, supraventricular and ventricular ectopic rhythms, complex ventricular premature complexes are common.
4. Changes of left ventricular hypertrophy appear in acromegalics.

All these characteristic features on ECG have been attributed to the existence of cardiomyopathy in acromegaly.

CUSHING'S SYNDROME

The electrocardiographic manifestations in patients with Cushing's syndrome, if seen are, in general, as a result of hypertension or hypokalaemia. The P-R interval tends to be shorter than normal.

HYPERALDOSTERONISM

Many of the cardiovascular effects of hyperaldosteronism are nonspecific, being related to the effects of aldosterone on arterial pressure and potassium balance. Hypertension, hypokalaemia and metabolic alkalosis are common.

The Electrocardiogram

The electrocardiogram may show the effects of hypokalaemia as well as effects of hypertension in long standing cases.

1. *Effects of hypokalaemia:* The T wave flattening, prominence of U waves, premature ventricular complexes, prolonged QTc and arrhythmias may be observed (Read also ECG changes in hypokalaemia).
2. *Effects of hypertension:* They are revealed by left ventricular hypertrophy and myocardial ischaemia.

These ECG changes are similar to hypertension treated with potassium losing diuretics (loop diuretics) producing hypokalaemia.

ADRENAL INSUFFICIENCY

The most common cardiovascular manifestation in adrenal insufficiency (Addison's disease) is arterial hypotension with postural accentuation and syncope in significant number of patients.

The Electrocardiogram

1. Low voltage graph
2. Sinus bradycardia
3. Prolonged QTc intervals
4. Low or interval T waves
5. Conduction defects. First degree AV block may occur in 20% patients
6. Changes due to hyperkalaemia are not uncommon.

PHEOCHROMOCYTOMA (CATECHOLAMINES EXCESS)

The cardiovascular manifestations of pheochromocytoma include; paroxysmal attacks of palpitations, hypertension and headache, signs of hypermetabolism and sympathetic overstimulation. Many of the features are similar to hyperthyroidism.

The Electrocardiogram

The electrocardiogram is abnormal in as many as 75% of patients with pheochromocytoma. The changes consists of T wave inversion, left ventricular hypertrophy, sinus tachycardia, frequent supraventricular ectopics or paroxysmal supraventricular tachycardia. An occasional patient may have short P-R interval and a narrow QRS complex suggesting that catecholamines are modifying AV conduction (accelerated AV conduction).

With marked elevation of blood pressure, changes suggestive of myocardial damage may appear. These include transient ST elevation or marked diffuse T wave inversion and depression of ST segment. All these changes are reversible and revert to normal after removal of the tumour or following pharmacological blockade.

However, a specific catecholamine induced myocarditis or cardiomyopathy has also been suggested in pheochromocytoma based on the above mentioned electrocardiographic findings and histopathological evidence of myocarditis.

PARATHYROID DISORDERS

Disordered parathyroid secretion is associated with two cardiovascular disturbances—cardiac arrhythmias and hypertension. Changes in calcium metabolism as well as direct effect of parathyroid hormone on the cardiovascular system appear to be responsible for ECG changes.

The electrocardiogram (Read changes due to hypercalcaemia and hypocalcaemia)

PHYSICAL INJURIES

HYPOTHERMIA

The clinical conditions associated with hypothermia are tabulated (Table 44.1).

Table 44.1: Clinical conditions associated with hypothermia
1. *Accidental hypothermia:* This is a well known complication of cold exposure and has been reported in winter months. It is seen in older or inebriated individuals.

• Myxoedema	• Wernicke's encephalopathy
• Pituitary insufficiency	• Myocardial infarction
• Addison's disease	• Cirrhosis of the liver
• Hypoglycaemia	• Pancreatitis
• Cerebrovascular disease	• Ingestion of drugs or alcohol

2. *Hypothermia secondary to acute illness*

• Congestive heart failure	• Drugs overdosage
• Uraemia	• Acute respiratory failure
• Diabetes mellitus	• Hypoglycaemia

3. *Immersion hypothermia*
   • Deep cold water swimmers

The Electrocardiogram (Fig. 44.4)

The electrocardiogram is usually distorted by muscular tremors. The typical ECG findings include:

i. Sinus bradycardia (often extreme slow heart rates).
ii. Slow atrial fibrillation.
iii. Escape rhythms due to bradycardia. Atrial and ventricular ectopics may occur.
iv. Prolongation of P-R interval (1st degree AV block). In severe cases, 2nd degree AV block can occur.
v. Prolongation of QTc interval (Fig. 44.5).
vi. The ST segment depression with low to inverted 'T' waves are seen in profound hypothermia.

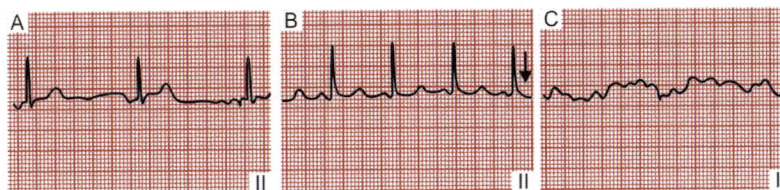

Fig. 44.4: Hypothermia. The electrocardiogram (A, B, C) shows;
A: Sinus bradycardia (HR 43/min)
B: Osborne 'J' waves are seen at the terminal portion of QRS (best seen in last complex ↓). The ST segment depression is also seen
C: Ventricular fibrillation recorded from a patient with severe hypothermia

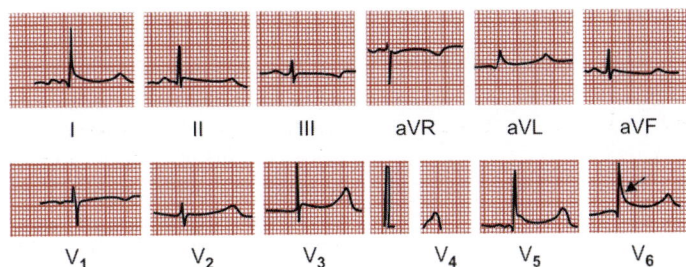

Fig. 44.5: Hypothermia. The electrocardiogram was recorded from a 50 years female with acute cold exposure (rectal temperature 94°F). Note the following characteristics of hypothermia;
i. There is J point elevation best seen in lateral precordial leads V_4, V_5 and V_6. This is a characteristic feature
ii. Sinus bradycardia was present (not shown)
iii. There is prolongation of QT interval
iv. The Osborne 'J' waves are seen in leads V_5-V_6 (indicated by an arrow)

vii. *The Osborne 'J' waves.* The 'J' waves are seen at the terminal portion of QRS complexes before the ST segment. Although their genesis is not fully understood, they probably occur due to differential sensitivity of cellular Na^+ and Ca^{++} depolarising currents to temperature. The J waves are neither the part of QRS complex nor the ST segment, but are separated waveforms.

viii. Ventricular fibrillation may occur in severe hypothermia.

ELECTRICAL INJURIES

For an electric current to flow, there must be a closed circuit and an electrical potential difference must exist between two points in the completed circuit. The pathway of the current through the body is crucial. An accident involving passage of a current between a point of contact on the leg and other point being the ground is likely to be less injurious than one in which passage of current is between the hand and the foot, and the heart lies between two poles of the closed circuit. Therefore, heart is involved only when it lies between the two points which complete the circuit.

The Electrocardiogram

- Sinus tachycardia
- The ST segment depression and T wave inversion
- Arrhythmias-usually ventricular; both benign and malignant arrhythmias (ventricular fibrillation) can occur
- Sudden death.

DROWNING

Cardiovascular manifestations in drowning are due to asphyxia, hypoxia and metabolic acidosis.

The Electrocardiogram

- Sinus tachycardia
- Supraventricular arrhythmias are common. They resolve with treatment of hypoxia and acidosis.

SECTIONTWELVE

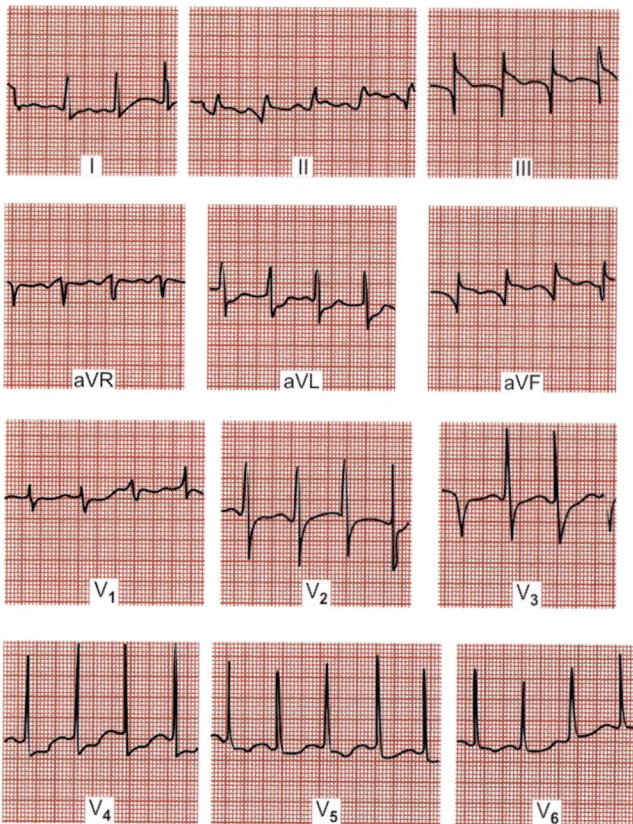

Fig. 44.6: Myocardial contusion or concussion simulating acute inferior wall infarction. The ECG was recorded from a young 26 yrs male patient with nonpenetrating chest injury in accidental and emergency department. The ECG shows narrow deep Q waves in leads II, III, aVF simulating inferior wall infarction. There is slight depression of ST segment in V_4-V_6 suggesting associated lateral wall ischaemia. There is sinus tachycardia (HR > 100 bpm). All these changes are known to occur in nonpenetrating chest injury producing myocardial contusion/concussion, but infarction cannot be ruled out easily. The CPK (MB) estimation was normal. Echocardiogram did not reveal an akinetic or hypokinetic segment. Follow-up of the patient and subsequent advise for coronary angiography was not possible as patient succumbed to his injuries

- The ST segment depression and T wave inversion due to myocardial ischaemia. It also resolves with treatment of hypoxia and acidosis.

TRAUMA TO THE HEART

Trauma to the heart may lead to myocardial contusions, traumatic pericarditis, coronary artery laceration and can produce coronary artery thrombosis.

The Electrocardiogram (Fig. 44.6)

- The ECG pattern of acute myocardial ischaemia or acute myocardial necrosis leading to pathological Q waves may be present.
- ECG pattern of pericarditis—The ST segment elevation with concavity upwards, is also common in traumatic pericarditis and myocardial contusion.
- Supraventricular and ventricular arrhythmias may occur, and at times, may be life-threatening. In addition, both atrioventricular and intraventricular conduction defects as well as sinus node dysfunction are seen.
- In case, there is hemopericardium leading to cardiac temponade—a low voltage graph may be recorded.

TUMOURS OF THE HEART

Primary myocardial or metastatic tumours involve the heart by infiltration of myocardial tissue and produce the characteristic ECG changes due to disturbance of conduction and rhythm, the precise nature of which is determined by location of the tumour.

The Electrocardiogram (Fig. 44.7)

- Low voltage of QRS complexes due to infiltration of the walls of the ventricles or due to concomitant pericardial effusion. This is common with intramural tumours.
- Intraventricular conduction defects are common with tumours situated in the areas of AV node

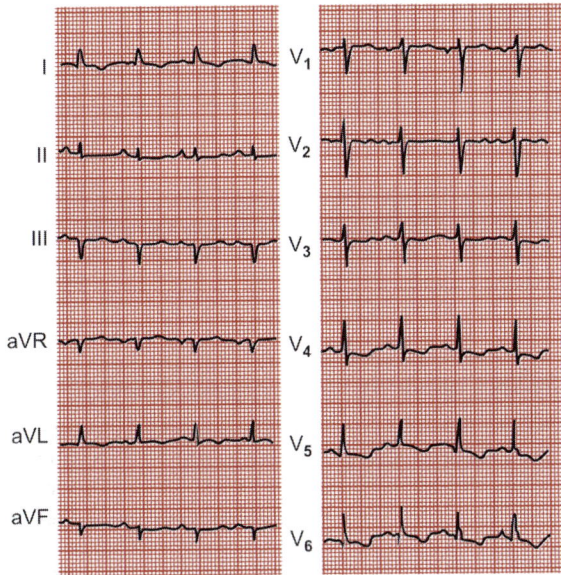

Fig. 44.7: Metastatic infiltrative myocardial disease. The ECG was recorded from a patient of lung carcinoma with metastatic infiltration into the myopericardium leading to pericardial effusion. The pericardial fluid showed malignant cells and ECG recorded shows;

  i. Low voltage graph due to associated pericardial effusion

  ii. There is q wave in V_5-V_6 with ST segment depression and T wave inversion, height of the R wave is reduced and equal in both the leads. There is also ST segment depression with T wave inversion in leads V_3-V_4. These changes indicate infiltration of the myocardium by an electrically inert substances, i.e. tumour

(angiomas, mesotheliomas). They include complete heart block, asystole and can lead to sudden death.

- Q wave resembling acute myocardial infarction may be observed. These are due to inert myocardial areas created by a metastasising tumour.
- *Arrhythmias:* A wide variety of arrhythmais may be produced including atrial fibrillation or flutter, paroxysmal atrial tachycardia with or without block, nodal rhythm, ventricular premature complexes, ventricular tachycardia and ventricular fibrillation.

Suggested Reading

1. Bognolo DA, Rabow FI, Vijayanagar RR et al: Traumatic sinus node dysfunction. *Ann Emerg Med* **11**:319, 1982.
2. Ciaccheri M, Cecchi F, Arcangeli C et al: Occult thyrotoxicosis in patients with chronic and paroxysmal isolated atrial fibrillation. *Clin Cardiol* **7**:413, 1984.
3. Cooperman Y, Low S, Laniado S: Traumatic heart block. *PACE* **12**:25, 1989.
4. Emslie-Smith D, Sladden GE, Striling GR: The significance of changes in electrocardiogram in hypothermia. *Br Heart J* **21**:343, 1959.
5. Fazio S, Cittadini A, Cuocolo A et al: Impaired cardiac performance is a distinct feature of uncomplicated acromegaly. *J Clin Endocrinol Metab* **79**:441, 1994.
6. Goel BC, Hanson CS, Hans J: AV conduction in hyper and hypothyroid dogs. *Am Heart J* **83**:504, 1972.
7. Harvey WP: Clinical aspects of cardiac tumours. *Am J Cardiol* **21**:328, 1968.
8. Khaleeli AA, Memon N: Factors affecting resolution of pericardial effusions in primary hypothyroidism. A clinical, biochemical and echocardiographic study. *Postgrad Med J* **58**: 1073, 1982.
9. Kumar A, Bhandari AK, Rahimtoola SH: Torsade de pointes an marked QT prolongation in association with hypothyroidism. *Ann Intern Med* **106**:712, 1987.
10. McLean RF, Devitt JH, McLellan BA et al: Significance of myocardial contusion following blunt chest trauma. *J Trauma* **33**:240, 1992.
11. Olshausen K, Bischoll S, Kahaly G et al: Cardiac arrhythmias and heart rate in hyperthyroidism. *Am J Cardiol* **63**:930, 1989.
12. Osborn JJ: Experimental hypothermia. Respiratory and blood pH changes in relation to cardiac function. *Am J Physiol* **175**:389, 1953.
13. Sacca L, Cittadini A, Fazio S: Growth hormone and the heart. *Endocr Rev* **15**:55, 1994.
14. Schwab RH et al: Electrocardiographic changes occurring in rapidly induced deep hypothermia. *Am J Med Sci* **248**:290, 1964
15. Strauss WE, Asinger RW, Hodges M: Mesothelioma of atrioventricular node. Potential utility of pacing. *PACE* **11**:1296, 1988.
16. Strenson G, Swedber K: QRS amplitudes, QT intervals and ECG abnormalities in pheochromocytoma patients before, during and after treatment. *Acta Med Scand* **224**:231, 1988.
17. Surawicz B, Mangiardi ML: Electrocardiogram in endocrine and metabolic disorders. In Rios JG (Eds): Clinical Electrocardiogram Correlations. Philadelphia, FA Davis Co., 1977.

45

Drugs, Poisons and the Heart

- The electrocardiogram in different drugs toxicity—digitalis, antiarrhythmics, phenothiazines and tricyclic antidepressants, quinine, L-dopa, emetine, etc
- Heart in systemic poisonings—organophosphorus and aluminium phosphide, etc
- Heart in envenomations—scorpion bite

DRUGS AND THE HEART

Drugs affect the eletrocardiographic events through their effects on the intracellular and extracellular ionic movements and action potentials. Their effects can be seen in alterations in morphology of P-QRS-T; and P-R, QRS and QTc intervals. They also produce alterations in heart rate and rhythm.

Digitalis

It is a water soluble cardiac glycoside having an half life of 1-6 days and is highly concentrated in the myocardium after administration.

Actions

1. *Positive inotropic effect:* It is exhibited in normal, nonfailing hypertrophied as well as failing heart. It augments contractility of the heart by inhibiting transmembrane sodium and potassium movements by inhibiting the monovalent cation transport enzyme—*coupled Na^+, K^+, ATPase,* the latter is localised to sarcolemma, acts as a receptor for cardiac glycoside whose action results in increased intracellular sodium content, which in turn, results in an increase in intracellular calcium concentration. The increased myocardial intake of calcium evokes a positive inotropic response.

2. *Negative chronotropic effect:* A clinical significant negative chronotropic action occurs only in the setting of heart failure. In the nonfailing heart, the effect is negligible, hence, digitalis should not be used for the treatment of sinus tachycardia unless heart failure is present. Large doses of digitalis may result in sinoatrial blocks due to depression of impulse conduction out of sinus node. It does not suppress impulse formation by the SA node.

3. *Augments automaticity and ectopic impulse activity:* Low concentrations of glycoside produce a little effect on the action potentials; while high concentrations result in reduction in phase 4 of resting potential and augment the rate of diastolic depolarisation. These two effects lead to an enhanced automaticity and ectopic impulse activity. With reduction in rate of rise of action potential, there is slowing of conduction velocity which predisposes to development of re-entry. This explains the arrhythmogenic potential of digitalis. Digitalis induces arrhythmias by re-entry and increased automaticity.

4. *Prolongation of effective refractory period:* Due to vagotonic effect, digitalis prolongs the effective refractory period of AV node. Due to vagolytic action, it shortens the refractory period of atrial and ventricular muscle. Due to these effects, most of small action potential beats do not react the ventricles due to refractoriness of AV node, thus, explains the slowing of heart rate in supraventricular tachycardia by digitalis. In atrial fibrillation, the slowing of the heart rate is explained by prolongation of an effective

refractory period of AV node and increased concealed conduction with fewer impulses penetrating the AV junction owing to both vagal and direct effect of digitalis on junctional tissue.

The Electrocardiographic Manifestations

Digitalis Effect (Figs 45.1 and 45.2A and B)

Therapeutic serum levels of digitalis may produce subtle alterations in the electrocardiogram called the *digitalis effect.* The therapeutic-to-toxic ratios are identical for all glycosides. The radioimmunoassay for digoxin and digitoxin made possible the correlation of serum glycosides levels with the presence of toxicity. In patients receiving standard maintenance dose of digoxin or digitoxin, and in whom no signs of intoxication are present, their serum concentration approximates to 1.0-1.5 ng/1 and 20-25 ng/1 respectively. The effects on ECG at these concentrations are called *digitalis effects.* The digitalis does not affect QRS, i.e. ventricular depolarisation. The ECG manifestations of digitalis effect include:

1. *Inverse check mark configuration of ST segment (Fig. 45.1):* The ST segment is usually straight, reflecting neither a convexity nor concavity, develops a downward course (downsloping) with a sharp terminal rise that may cross the baseline before it blends with T wave. This type of ST segment resembles inverse check mark sign (mirror image of check mark sign)–a characteristic feature of digitalis effect, is seen in leads depicting dominantly upright QRS complexes, i.e. in leads with tallest R waves. If this type of ST segment also appear in leads with negative QRS, though rare phenomenon, indicates digitalis toxicity rather than effect.

Digitalis in therapeutic dosage does not depress the proximal part of ST segment, therefore; if inverse check mark sign is associated with depression of proximal ST segment, then either digitalis toxicity or associated myocardial involvement due to ischaemia or coronary insufficiency may be suspected

2. *The T wave:* Therapeutic doses of digitalis diminish the amplitude of T wave without any change in its direction. The T wave inversion indicates digitalis toxicity rather than effect. Therefore, if inverse check mark configuration of ST segment is associated with T wave inversion, then digitalis

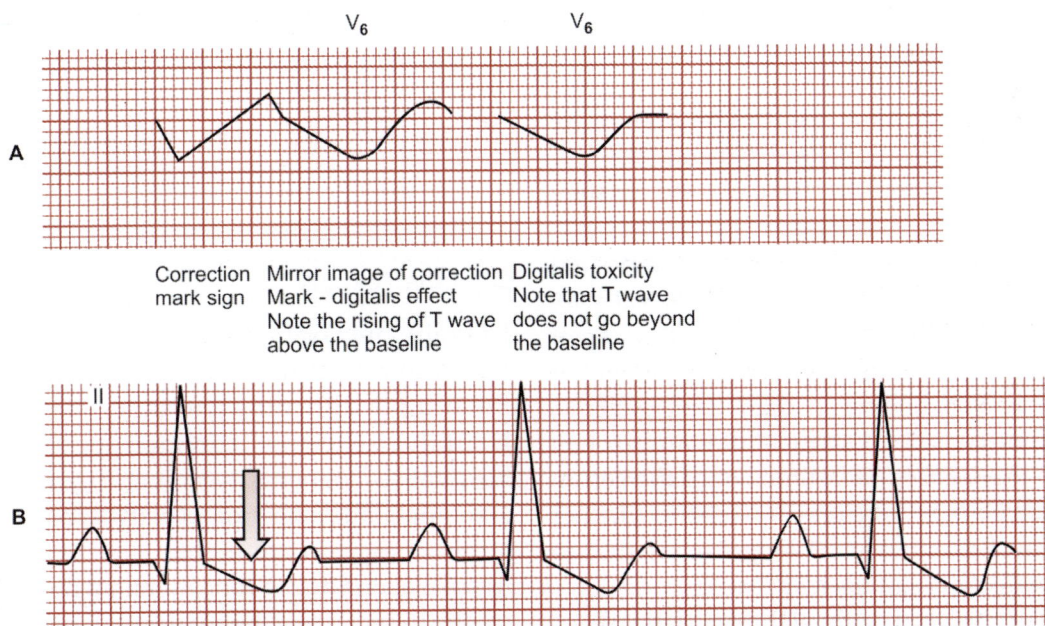

| Correction mark sign | Mirror image of correction Mark - digitalis effect Note the rising of T wave above the baseline | Digitalis toxicity Note that T wave does not go beyond the baseline |

Fig. 45.1: Digitalis effect (diagram). **A:** Note the straight downward sloping ST segment with steep terminal rise of T wave beyond the baseline—a characteristic of digitalis effect (inverse checkmark sign). **B:** The QT is shortened (0.28 sec). The QTc is 0.35 sec, R-R interval is 0.64 sec

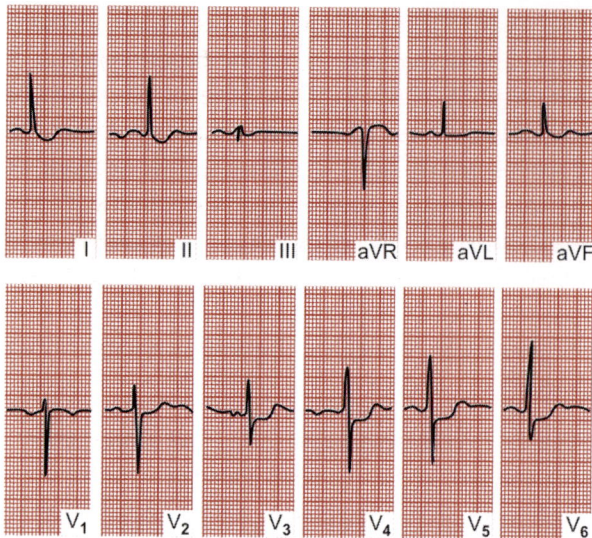

Fig. 45.2A: Digitalis effect. The electrocardiogram shows;
i. Scooped out ST segment producing mirror image of a *tick mark* (correct mark) sign. This is seen in leads I, II, III, aVF, V$_3$-V$_6$
ii. The QT interval is short (0.34 sec)
iii. The ST segment is convex in leads aVR and V$_1$
iv. The P-R interval is 0.16 sec

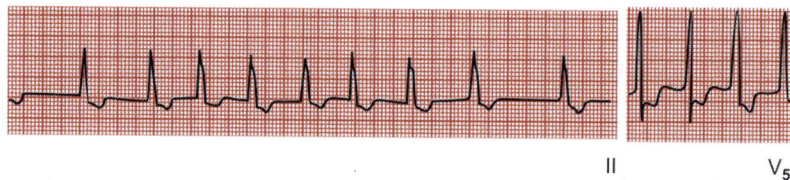

Fig. 45.2B: Digitalis effect. The electrocardiogram (leads II and V$_5$) shows atrial fibrillation (irregular R-R intervals) for which patient was receiving digoxin. The atrial fibrillation with a ventricular rate of about 100 bpm is still present. The ST segment is depressed with mirror image (inverse) of a check mark sign indicating digitalis effect. The wide QRS complexes in lead II indicates aberrant intraventricular conduction

toxicity should be suspected provided there was no pre-existing T wave inversion before the administration of digitalis.

3 *Short QTc interval:* As a result of shortening of electrical systole in digitalised patients, the Q-T interval also shortens. This is an early and constant effect.

4. There is prolongation of P-R interval as compared to pretreatment baseline. The P-R interval may lengthen by 0.04 to 0.08 sec or more, but does not go beyond 0.22 seconds at heart rate of 60/min. It is an occasional finding in digitalised patients, hence, some consider it a sign of digitalis toxicity rather than an effect. Measurement of the serum digitalis levels may be helpful in assessing whether or not the P-R interval prolongation is due to digitalis effect or digitalis toxicity.

5. Slowing of the heart with slight prolongation of P-R interval is digitalis effect rather than toxicity. First degree AV block (P-R interval > 0.24 sec at heart rate of ≤ 60 bpm) is a sign of digitalis toxicity rather than effect.

Digitalis effect is characterised by slowing of the heart rate, inverse tick mark shape of ST segment, shortening of QTc and lengthening of P-R interval. Some physicians consider first degree AV block as digitalis effect while others consider it as a toxic effect.

Digitalis Toxicity

Digitalis preparations have a narrow therapeutic range, so maintaining the desirable serum levels of the drug is difficult even under ideal conditions. Digitalis toxicity is common, occurs in 20% of hospitalised patients receiving digoxin. When the symptoms and signs of toxicity appear, the serum levels of digoxin are higher than 2.0-3.0 ng/l. The hypokalaemia due to concommitant diuretics therapy or due to secondary hyperaldosteronism is the most common precipitating factor. In addition, old age, hypoxaemia, acute myocardial infarction, magnesium depletion, renal insufficiency, hypercalcaemia, electrical cardioversion and hypothyroidism reduce the tolerance of the patient to digitalis therapy and may provoke latent digitalis toxicity.

Chronic digitalis intoxication is insidious in onset and is characterised by exacerbation of heart failure, weight loss, cachexia, neuralgias, gynaecomastia, yellow vision, gastrointestinal symptoms and deliriums. Digitalis induced arrhythmias (Table 45.1) precede extracardiac toxic manifestations in about 50% cases.

Table 45.1: Digitalis induced arrhythmias and conduction disturbances

1. *Automatic arrhythmias*
   - Nonparoxysmal atrial tachycardia with second degree AV block is a common arrhythmia. Atrial ectopics and/or atrial bigeminy are common.
   - Accelerated junctional rhythm with AV dissociation
   - Junctional (idionodal) tachycardia with AV dissociation
   - Ventricular premature complexes (VPCs); ventricular bigeminy, trigeminy, VPCs with R on T phenomenon and multiform ventricular complexes.
   - Ventricular tachycardia (multifocal or bidirectional) occurs with advanced heart disease.
   - Ventricular fibrillation
2. *SA block*–They manifest occasionally.
3. *AV block*
   - Second degree—Wenckebach's (Mobitz's type I)
   - High grade
   - Complete. It is infrequent.

Most common arrhythmias are atrial (nonparoxysmal atrial tachycardia with second degree AV block) and ventricular (V. bigeminy, trigeminy, etc). Bundle branch block is not expected with digitalis use. Sinus bradycardia due to SA exit block may occur. Atrial fibrillation and flutter are uncommon. When the digitalis is being given for atrial fibrillation to slow heart rate, the digitalis toxicity is suggested by the following features:

1. Regular QRS complexes reflecting complete AV block and a subsidiary pacemaker rhythm with its origin in AV junction, bundle branches or Purkinje system.
2. Regular QRS rhythm with episodic type II (2:1, 3:1) AV block.
3. Regular QRS rhythm with periodic type I (Wenckebach) AV block.
4. Ventricular arrhythmias.

The common toxic effects of digitalis on ECG include atrial arrhythmias (atrial ectopics, atrial tachycardia with AV blocks), ventricular arrhythmias (V bigeminy is commonest), ectopics with R on T phenomenon, multiform ventricular ectopics, bidirectional VT or ectopics and AV blocks. The effects of digitalis during its toxicity will also be present.

The Electrocardiogram (Figs 45.3 and 45.4A to E)

The ECG manifestations of digitalis toxicity include:
1. Scooping of ST segment with T wave inversion or inverse check mark sign type of ST segment—an expression of digitalis effect, is present along with frank inversion of T waves in leads registering upward QRS complexes, may even be seen in leads with negative QRS complexes–a rare occurrence.
2. Significant lengthening of P-R interval but not beyond 0.22 sec (Fig. 45.3) is common. First degree AV block (P-R > 0.24 sec at heart rate of 60/min) may be present.
3. Supraventricular arrhythmias, e.g. extreme sinus bradycardia, atrial ectopics, sinoatrial (SA) exit block, junctional ectopics, junctional escape rhythm, accelerated junctional rhythm (Fig. 45.4A), junctional tachycardia (Fig. 45.5B), paroxysmal atrial tachycardia with AV block (Fig. 45.5A) and supraventricular bigeminy (Fig. 45.4E).
4. Ventricular arrhythmias, e.g. ventricular bigeminy (Fig. 45.4B), trigeminy, multiform or bidirectional VPCs (Fig. 45.5C), ventricular tachycardia, ventricular fibrillation, bidirectional ventricular tachycardia (alternation of polarity of QRS complexes) (Fig. 45.4D).

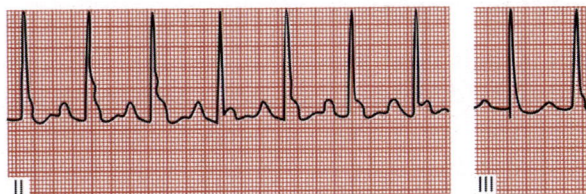

Fig. 45.3: Digitalis toxicity. The ECG shows first degree AV block (P-R interval is 0.24 sec) due to digitalis toxicity. Note the short QT interval and scooping of ST segment in the form of mirror sign of tick mark

AV nodal rhythm	Ventricular bigeminy	Second degree AV block (2:1)

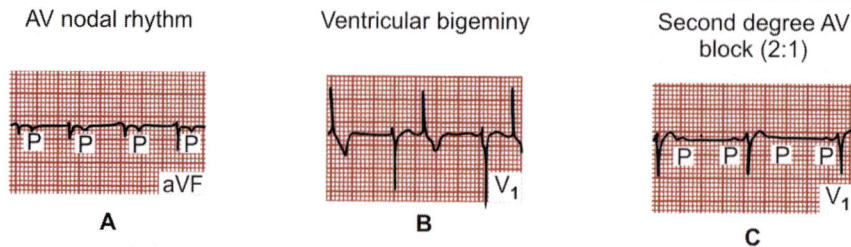

A　　　　　**B**　　　　　**C**

Figs 45.4A to C: Digitalis induced arrhythmias and conduction disturbances. The electrocardiogram shows;

A: AV nodal rhythm (lead aVF). There are invered P waves (labelled) that follow each QRS complex at heart rate of 70/min regular

B: Ventricular bigeminy (lead V₁): Each sinus conducted beat is followed by a ventricular ectopic regularly

C: Second degree (Mobitz type II) AV block (lead V₁). There is fixed 2:1 AV conduction. The P waves are labelled

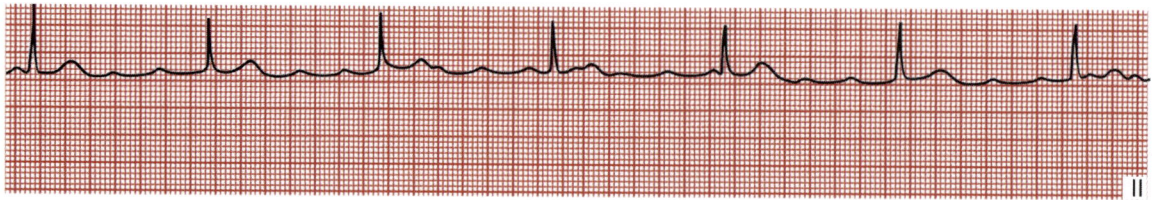

Fig. 45.4 D: Complete AV block with paroxysmal atrial tachycardia and idioventricular escape rhythm (digitalis toxicity). The P-P intervals are regular at a atrial rate of 150/min. The ventricular rate is about 38/min regular (R-R intervals are regular). The P waves have no relation to QRS. The QRS complexes are slightly wider. The third QRS appear more wider because of fortuitous superimposition of P wave on QRS, otherwise P waves are well clear of QRS. The last QRS is immediately followed by an upright P wave distorting the ST segment

5. Atrioventricular blocks—an atrial tachycardia with AV block, second degree AV block (Wenckebach type I) or Mobitz type II (Fig. 45.4C) and complete AV block (Fig. 45.4D).

6. Digitalis toxicity precipitated by loop diuretics, may at times, cause prominent U waves.

> • *Prolongation of P-R interval not exceeding 0.22 second suggests digitalis effect.*
> • *Prolongation of P-R interval ≥ 0.24 second suggests digitalis toxicity rather than its effect.*

Clinical Significance

1. In a digitalised patient, it is pertinent to differentiate digitalis effect from digitalis toxicity because the former requires continuation of maintenance dose of digitalis; while the latter needs discontinuation of digitalis and diuretics (if being used).

2. Due to narrow range between therapeutic to toxic levels, in case of doubt, serum digitalis levels should be done.

3. Worsening of congestive hear failure, at times, may suggest digitalis toxicity.

4. In digitalised patients, appearance of ventricular ectopics (unifocal, multifocal, bigeminy rhythm) could either be due to primary disease for which digitalis is being used or digitalis toxicity. It is pertinent to differentiate the two, because the former requires continuation, while the latter needs discontinuation of digitalis. In such a situation, the clinical symptoms and other ECG changes of digitalis toxicity may help. In case of doubt, serum level of digoxin must be done.

5. There is no correlation between clinical signs and symptoms of digitalis toxicity with its electrocardiographic findings.

Antiarrhythmic Drugs

Antiarrhythmics are classified according to their electrophysiological effects. The widely used Vaughan William system places all antiarrhythmics into 4 groups; majority of them fall in class I; which is further subdivided into Ia, Ib and Ic (Table 45.2). Drugs in

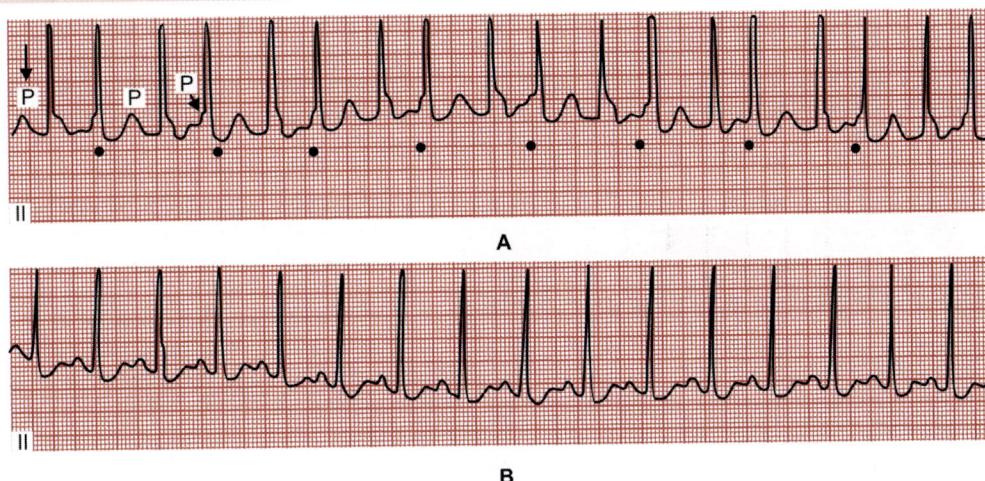

Fig. 45.4E: Supraventricular bigeminy rhythm induced by digitalis. The electrocardiogram (lead II) was recorded from a patient with cardiomyopathy who was receiving digitalis and came with symptomatic digitalis toxicity (nausea, vomiting, etc). The slurring or notching of QRS complexes is due to myocardial disease itself.

A: The electrocardiogram recorded during digitalis toxicity shows first degree AV block with supraventricular bigeminy. At the beginning of the strip, the first beat is sinus conducted with P-R interval of 0.28 sec (indicated by an arrow) followed by an atrial (supraventricular) ectopic (denoted by dot below) with P′ (abnormal P) wave on upstroke of R wave followed by a compensatory pause. After this, similar group beating (one normal and one supraventricular premature beat) occurs regularly and supraventricular premature beats have been denoted by dots below. It appears that P wave of sinus conducted beats falls on the T wave of ectopic beats, hence, tip of T wave instead of being round is peaked. This is occurring regularly due to rapid heart rate with first degree AV block. The P′ wave of supraventricular beats is small and has negligible P-R interval (one of P′ is labelled). The ST segment of sinus and ectopic beats is scooped out due to digitalis effect. This scooping is very well seen in ST segment of ectopics which is wide as compared to normal sinus beat which show inverse tick mark sign which is also a digitalis effect

B: After stopping digitalis. There is diappearance of first degree AV block and supraventricular bigeminy. Now P-R interval is 0.16 sec. The rhythm is regular sinus with rate of 100/min. The P waves are nicely seen preceding normal QRS complexes. The ST segment still resembles more or less inverse *tick mark* sign indicating persistence of digitalis effect

All these features noted in rhythm strip A appears to be digitalis induced, hence, disappeared after stoppage of digitalis

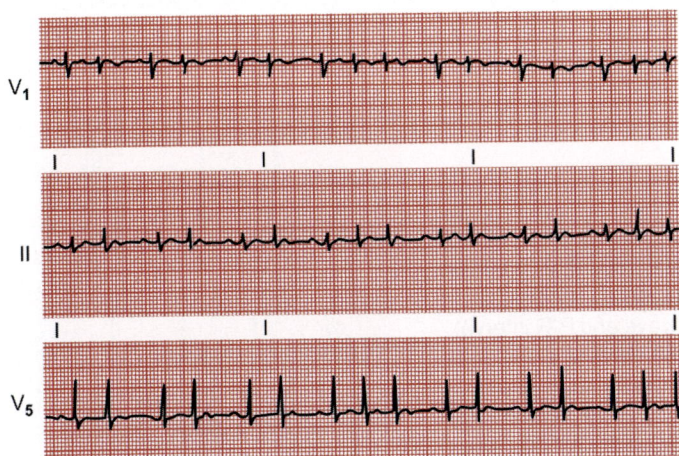

Fig. 45.5A: Tachyarrhythmias induced by digitalis. Non-paroxysmal atrial tachycardia with second degree (Mobitz type II) AV block. The ECG leads show atrial rate of 150 bpm with varying second degree AV block (Mobitz type II—3:2 and 4:3) causing irregular ventricular response. Some complexes are bizarre due to phasic aberrant intraventricular conduction (Ashman's phenomenon). This was produced by digitalis and disappeared after discontinuation of digitalis

class I exert effects primarily by blocking the fast sodium channels altering depolarization and to some extent repolarisation. The class II drugs are beta-blockers, class III drugs prolong repolarisation by blocking K+ channels and class IV drugs include calcium channel blockers (Fig. 45.6).

SECTION TWELVE

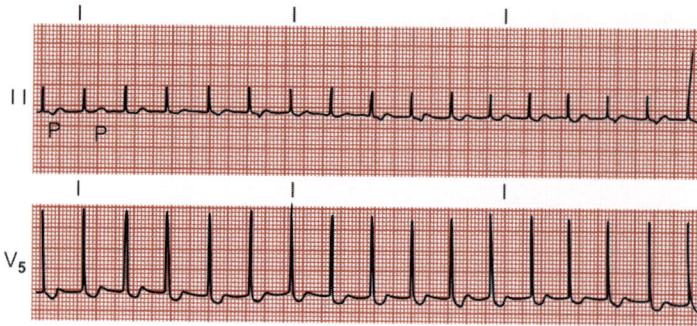

Fig. 45.5B: Tachyarrhythmias induced by digitalis. Nonparoxysmal AV nodal tachycardia (digitalis toxicity). The patient was having digitalis for rheumatic heart disease with valvular lesions. The electrocardiogram (leads II, V_5) shows;

i. *AV junctional (nodal) tachycardia.* The heart rate is 106 bpm. Each QRS complex is followed by a retrograde P (inverted P) and R-R interval is regular. These ECG findings also occur in reciprocating tachycardia through an anomalous accessory pathway. The reciprocating tachycardia can be excluded by electrophysiological studies only

ii. Left ventricular hypertrophy is present by voltage criteria, i.e. R in V_5 > 27 mm

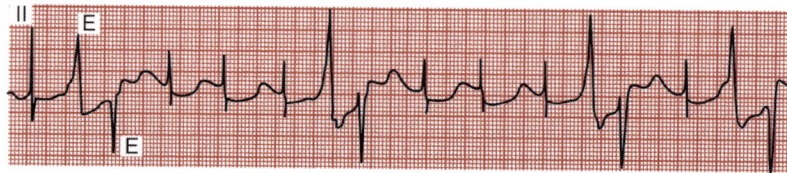

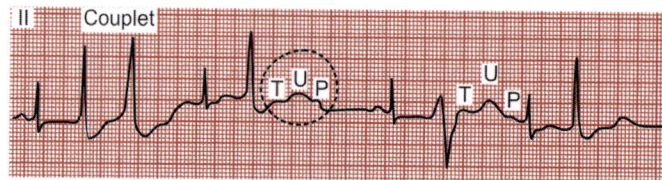

Fig. 45.5C: Digitalis induced arrhythmias. The ECG was recorded from a patient receiving digitalis developed toxicity in the presence of hypokalaemia (serum K^+ 2.3 mEq). Note the following characteristics;

i. Top strip (lead II). There are bidirectional VPC's (alternating polarity) seen in couplets. The two consecutive VPCs having opposite orientation in a couplet are labelled as 'E'

ii. Bottom strip (lead II). On continuous monitoring, a monomorphic couplet was recorded in the beginning followed by frequent ventricular polymorphic ectopics

iii. The QTc is prolonged which indicates hypokalaemia. Remember that digitalis shortens the QTc. The wide T wave are actually 'TUP' complex (encircled) seen in hypokalaemia due to superimposition of P and U on T-a characteristic sign of hypokalaemia

iv. Post-extrasystolic 'U' wave are seen clearly (see the encircled labelled complex) which are highly suggestive of hypokalaemia

v. The P wave of encircled complex is blocked due to hypokalaemia

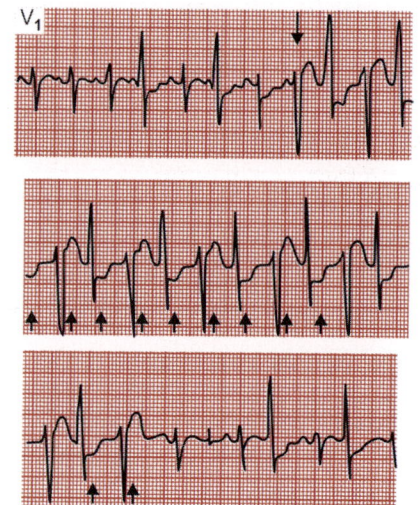

Fig. 45.5D: Digitalis induced bidirectional tachycardia. The electrocardiogram was recorded from a patient with symptomatic digitalis toxicity (nausea, vomiting, etc). The first 3 beats of top strip are sinus conducted with normal P wave and P-R interval. The 4th and 6th beats are VPCs with short P-R interval. At arrow, there is a VPC with short P-R interval, which triggers the onset of bidirectional ventricular tachycardia—two types of QRS configuration of VPCs alternate with each other. In the middle strip, two QRS configurations have different orientations of P waves; one QRS complex precedes by an upright P wave while other QRS complex is followed by inverted P (P') wave (Both upright and inverted P are represented by an arrow ↑ below) indicating retrograde conduction (ventriculo-atrial conduction). The tachycardia terminates with stopping of digitalis and restoration of sinus rhythm with VPCs (uni-directional) is seen in the end of lower strip

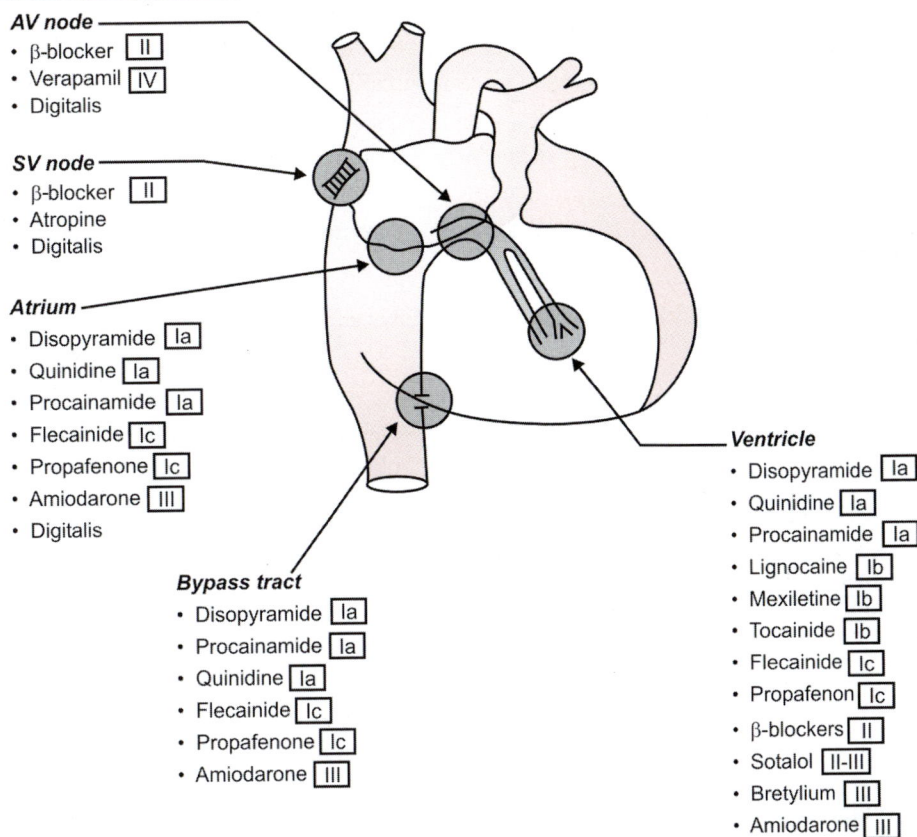

AV node ——
- β-blocker [II]
- Verapamil [IV]
- Digitalis

SV node ——
- β-blocker [II]
- Atropine
- Digitalis

Atrium ——
- Disopyramide [Ia]
- Quinidine [Ia]
- Procainamide [Ia]
- Flecainide [Ic]
- Propafenone [Ic]
- Amiodarone [III]
- Digitalis

Bypass tract
- Disopyramide [Ia]
- Procainamide [Ia]
- Quinidine [Ia]
- Flecainide [Ic]
- Propafenone [Ic]
- Amiodarone [III]

Ventricle
- Disopyramide [Ia]
- Quinidine [Ia]
- Procainamide [Ia]
- Lignocaine [Ib]
- Mexiletine [Ib]
- Tocainide [Ib]
- Flecainide [Ic]
- Propafenon [Ic]
- β-blockers [II]
- Sotalol [II-III]
- Bretylium [III]
- Amiodarone [III]

Fig. 45.6: Drugs that affect different sites of heart (diagram). The class of drug according to Vaughan William classification is given in the small boxes (□)

Class IA drugs (Fig. 45.8): These are given to treat both supraventricular and ventricular arrhythmias. Despite their proven efficacy and usefulness, these drugs can be proarrhythmic and can be associated with side effects. The electrophysiological actions of this class of drugs are given in the Table 45.2 and their effect on ECG is diagrammatically represented in Figure 45.7.

Class IB drugs: These are given to treat ventricular arrhythmias. Phenytoin is used frequently in digitalis induced arrhythmias. Tocainide and mexiletine are oral agents but lidocaine is a parenteral preparation only. The electrophysiological actions of these drugs are tabulated (Table 45.2) and their effects on ECG are diagrammatically represented in Figure 45.7.

Class IC drugs: They may be used to treat both supraventricular and ventricular arrhythmias. These drugs are also proarrhythmic.

PHENOTHIAZINES AND OTHER ANTIPSYCHOTIC DRUGS

The phenothiazines, i.e. chlorpromazine and related compounds affect the cardiovascular system directly and indirectly through CNS and autonomic nervous system. The effects with normal dosage are:
1. They depress myocardial contractility.
2. They impair AV and intraventricular conduction.

The Electrocardiogram (Fig. 45.9)

The electrocardiographic findings with excessive dosage include:
1. ST segment depression.
2. Flattening or inversion of T waves
3. Prolongation of Q-T (QTc) interval
4. Prominent U waves
5. Prolongation of P-R interval, widening of QRS complexes similar to class I antiarrhythmics. Ventricular tachycardia is uncommon.

Table 45.2: Classification of antiarrhythmic drugs (Vaughan William)

Class	Drugs	Electrophysiological effects (Fig. 45.7)					Comment
	Fast Na$^+$ channels	Action potential duration	Slow Ca^{++} channels	Effect on phase 4 repolarisation			Comment
IA	• Quinidine • Procainamide • Disopyramide	Block	Prolong	No effect	Depress	They reduce V$_{max}$, and prolong action potentials
IB	• Phenytoin • Lidocaine • Tocainide • Mexiletine	Block	Shorten	No effect	Depress	They do not reduce V$_{max}$ They shorten action potentials duration
IC	• Flecainide • Encainide • Propafenone	Block	No effect/ shorten	No effect/ block	Depress	They reduce V$_{max}$, slow conduction and can prolong refractoriness
II	Beta blockers, e.g. propranolol, metoprolol atenolol, timolol, nodolol sotalol, etc.	No effect/ block	No effect/ shorten	No effect	depress	They block beta-adrenergic receptors
III	• Bretylium • amiodarone • Sotalol	Block	Prolong	No effect	Depress	They block K$^+$ channels and prolong repolarisation
IV	Calcium channels blockers, e.g. nifedipine, verapamil diltiazem, others	No effect	Prolong	Block	Depress	They block slow Ca^{++} channels

ANTIDEPRESSANTS

1. **Amitryptyline:** The ECG manifestations (Fig. 45.10) include;
   (i) Mild sinus tachycardia probably as a consequence of both inhibition of norepinephrine uptake and blockade of muscarinic receptors.
   (ii) Prolongation of P-R, QTc, QRS intervals because conduction at all levels is delayed by the drug.
   (iii) Dangerous ventricular arrhythmias can be precipitated particularly when bundle branch block is present.

2. **Lithium:** The prolonged use causes a benign and reversible inversion of T waves on ECG which disappear after discontinuation of therapy.

Antimalarial Drug

Quinine Toxicity

The quinine is widely used as an antimalarial drug. It is drug of choice in treatment of cerebral malaria. The electrocardiographic effects of quinine and quinidine are similar (Fig. 45.11). Thus, when the patient is on quinine therapy, blood pressure and ECG monitoring are mandatory for continuation of therapy for long time.

Antiparkinsonian Drug

Levodopa: Cardiac arrhythmias, otherwise, are not uncommon in old aged patients of parkinsonism but chances get increased in patients receiving L-dopa for treatment. However, the β-adrenergic action of levodopa on the heart, as well as direct β-adrenergic receptors stimulation by other metabolites of the drug present a potentially serious side effect of L-dopa. Fortunately, incidence of arrhythmias is low. Sinus tachycardia, atrial and ventricular ectopics, atrial flutter, atrial fibrillation and ventricular tachycardia have been reported. These cardiac arrhythmias, also common during old age and in patients with ischaemic heart disease receiving levodopa, can easily be controlled by beta blockers.

Class 1A

Class 1B

Class 1C

• Notching of P wave
• Shortening of PT interval
• Widening of QRS
• Depression of ST segment
• Prolongation of QT (QTc)

• No effect on P wave
• QRS normal
• No ST segment depression
• Shortening of QT (QTc)

• Prolongation of P-R interval
• Prolongation of QT interval
• Widening of QRS

Class II

Class III

• Sinus bradycardia
• Flat P wave
• First degree AV block
• Ascending ST elevation
• Tall, tented T waves

• Sinus bradycardia
• Marked prolongation of QT interval
• No change in QRS
• No change in ST segment

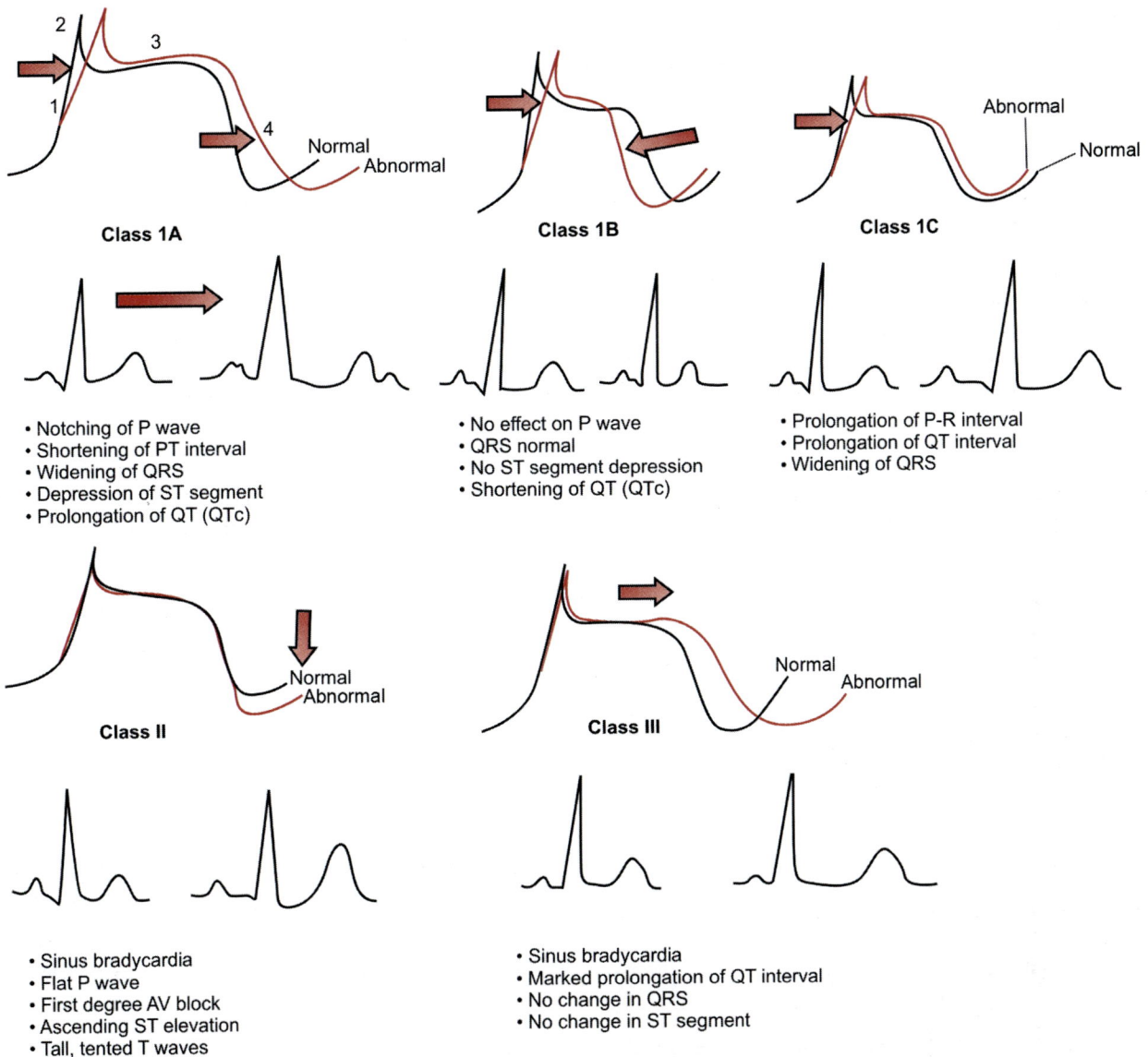

Fig. 45.7: The electrocardiographic effects of some antiarrhythmias (class I, II and III)

Tissue Amoebicide

Emetine: It is an alkaloid derivative of Epecac. When given intramuscular, it is highly effective in destroying the trophozoites in tissues including those in the walls of intestine and in the liver. Previously, it is was a commonly employed drug in amoebic liver abscess, but nowadays, other potent amoebicidal drugs, i.e. metronidazole, tinidazole, secnidazole, etc have replaced it. The common ECG changes include; T waves inversion and prolongation of QTc interval. Rarely arrhythmias and prolongation of QRS

complexes are seen. However, if used, blood pressure and ECG should be monitored.

HEART IN SYSTEMIC POISONINGS

Organophosphorus

Organophosphorus compounds (OPC) being anti-ChE (anticholinesterase) agents produce three types of clinical effects—muscarinic, nicotinic and CNS. The cardiac involvement is due to excitation of parasympathetic system, hence, sinus bradycardia is an

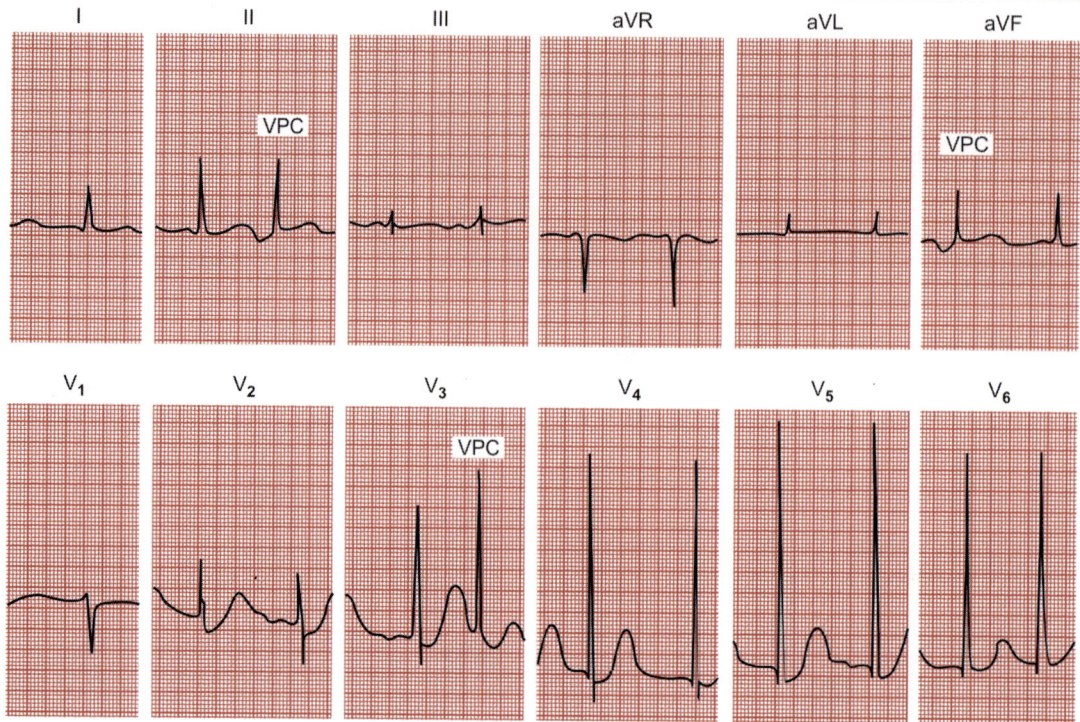

Fig. 45.8: The prolongation of QTc due to quinidine toxicity (class IA antiarrhythmic drug). The ECG shows the following characteristics;

  i. The rhythm is sinus. A VPC is seen in leads II, aVF and V_3 which suggest that patient was taking quinidine for an arrhythmia
  ii. P-R interval is 0.14 sec
  iii. Left ventricular hypertrophy is evident from voltage criteria (R wave in V_6 > 26 mm and in V_5 > 27 mm and RV_6 + SV_1 > 35 mm) with associated ST-T changes
  iv. The ST segment depression in leads V_2-V_3 is due to quinidine as this is not a features of LVH
  v. The Q-T interval is 0.40 sec. The QTc = $\dfrac{QT}{\sqrt{R\text{-}R}}$ = 0.51 sec which is prolonged due to quinidine

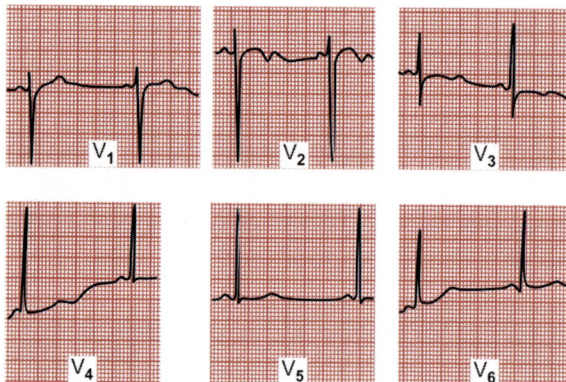

Fig. 45.9: Haloperidol (an antipsychotic drug) toxicity. The electrocardiogram was recorded from a psychiatric patient receiveing haloperidol, who on one day ingested a high dose and become semiconscious. The findings include;

  i. *Slow heart rate.* There is sinus bradycardia (HR is just 60/min regular). This is due to parasympathomimetic effect of the drug
  ii. *ST-T changes.* There is minimal ST depression with T inversion V_2-V_4. Low amplitude of T waves in V_5-V_6
  iii. *Prolonged QTc.* The QTc is 0.48 sec
    The (ii) and (iii) findings suggest its quinidine like effect

important sign of cardiotoxicity. Excitation followed by inhibition also is produced by ACh (acetylcholine) at the medullary vasomotor and cardiac centres, therefore, at times, sinus tachycardia may be noted in late stages of poisoning due to parasympathetic inhibition as well as due to hypoxaemia resulting from bronchoconstriction and collection of secretions. Most of the conduction disturbances are due to slowing of

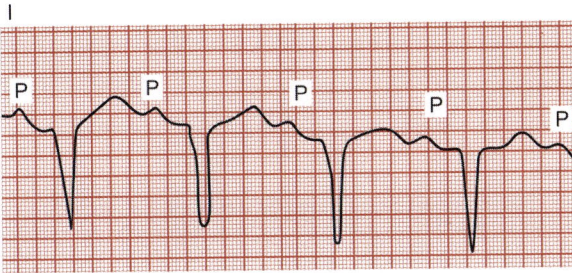

Fig. 45.10: Toxicity due to an antidepressant (amitryptyline). The patient of depression receiving amitryptyline, took a large dose one day for which he was referred to us by psychiatrist with ECG for interpretation. The lead I reveals;
 i. Prolongation of P-R interval of 0.24 sec
 ii. There is widening of QRS complexes >0.12 sec
 iii. Prolongation of QTc (0.53 sec)
  All there electrographic effects suggest amitryptyline toxicity

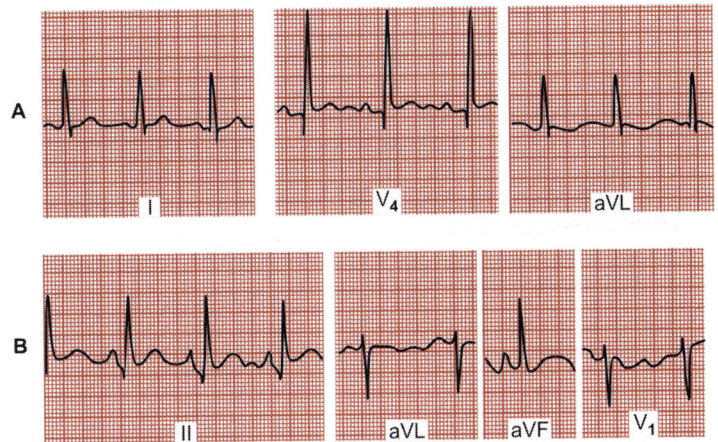

Fig. 45.11: Quinine toxicity. The patient of cerebral malaria was being treated with quinine. The electrocardiogram recorded shows;
A: *At the start of therapy.* The QT is 0.32 sec and QTc = 0.41 sec. These intervals are within normal limits.
B: *After few days of therapy:* The QT is 0.36 sec and QTc is 0.45 sec. There is prolongation of QTc due to quinine therapy and needs further continuous monitoring if therapy is to be continued

conduction throughout the heart which may result in escape beats and rhythms.

The Electrocardiogram

The electrocardiographic features are due to muscarinic and nicotinic effects (early effects) and hypoxaemia (late effect). These include:
1. Sinus bradycardia
2. AV blocks (Ist degree AV block is commoner than second degree and complete AV block).
3. Sinus tachycardia.
4. Supraventricular premature complexes, AV nodal rhythm, etc.
5. Bundle branch block—RBBB has been observed infrequently.
6. ST-T changes.
   - ST depression has been reported in about one third patients.
   - T wave—low voltage or inversion of T wave is common. Dome-shaped low to flat T waves have been observed due to hypokalaemia.
7. Ventricular premature beats, fusion complexes, etc. Idioventricular escape rhythm can occur due to

slowing of the sinus discharge, which may become accelerated producing idioventricular tachycardia.

Metal (Aluminium, Zinc) Phosphide Poisoning

Metal phosphides (Al, Zn) are used in agriculture as pesticides, insecticides and rodenticides. Out of these, the aluminium phosphide (AlP) is a commonly used solid fumigant pesticide for preservation of stored grains in grain silos, warehouses and at homes. The Zn_3P_2, on the other hand, is used as rodenticide in the form of baits. The toxic effects of these metal phosphides are due to liberation of a toxic phosphine (PH_3) gas. The phosphine acts as a protoplasmic poison, inhibits certain enzymes such as cytochrome-C-oxidase and catalase similar to cyanide and produces hypoxic organ toxicity. The hallmark of this poisoning is cardiotoxicity that includes shock, myocarditis (toxic) and all types of arrhythmias and conduction disturbances.

The Electrocardiographic Manifestations

The electrical activity of the heart is affected in many ways but exact mechanism of its pathogenesis is still

SECTIONTWELVE

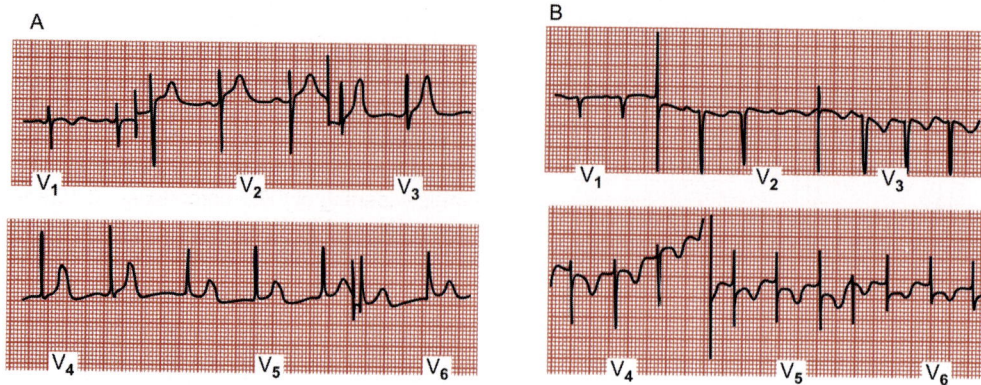

Fig. 45.12: Evolution of ST-T changes in aluminium phosphide poisoning. The ECG (V_1-V_6) taken at different intervals shows;
A: The ECG taken at admission shows normal sinus rhythm at a rate of 75 bpm. The T waves are upright with normal ST segment
B: The ECG taken after several hours shows sinus tachycardia (HR is 125 bpm) with ST segment depression and T wave inversion in leads V_2-V_6.

   All these ECG changes suggest global myocardial ischaemia due to aluminium phosphide poisoning. These changes simulate subendocardial ischaemia but are widespread and do not conform to any fixed coronary artery disease

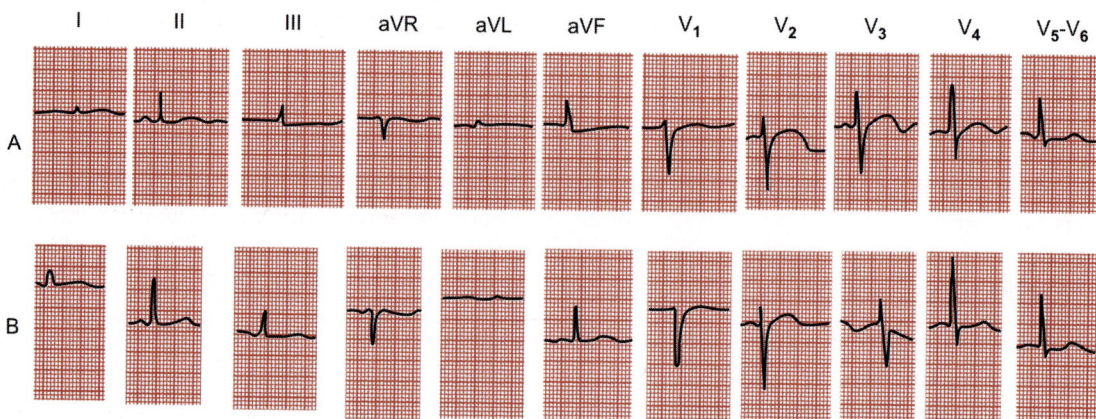

Fig. 45.13: Reversible ischaemic pattern in acute aluminium phosphide poisoning. The electrocardiogram recorded from a patient during acute aluminium phosphide poisoning (A) and after recovery (B) shows;
A: Note the coving ST segment in leads V_1-V_6 with inversion of T wave V_1-V_4. There is low voltage graph (QRS < 5 mm) in standard leads I, II, III, aVR, aVL and aVF. T wave is flat in all these leads.
B: Following recovery from poisoning (72 hours after poisoning), the ECG reverted to normal with improvement in voltage in standard and precordial leads and disappearance of ST-T changes in precordial leads, indicating reversible myocardial injury in a patient with this poisoning

unclear. The toxic myocarditis, electrolyte disturbances and cellular hypoxia contribute to most of these manifestations. The electrocardiographic manifestations mostly simulate the electrocardiographic patterns seen in acute myocardial infarction and acute myocarditis; the basic difference being that these changes are non-inflammatory and non-ischaemic, arise as a disturbance due to cellular metabolism induced by cellular hypoxia. The ECG patterns include:

1. *Ischaemic patterns* (Figs 45.12 to 45.15): The ischaemic patterns characterised by ST elevation/depression in more than two leads may frequently be seen in this poisoning. They simulate ischaemic myocardial injury.
2. *Conduction defects:* The various conduction defects of SA node, AV node and bundle branches (Fig. 45.15) may be seen in this poisoning, the pathogenesis of which is not known, but may be due to hypoxia and autonomic disturbances.

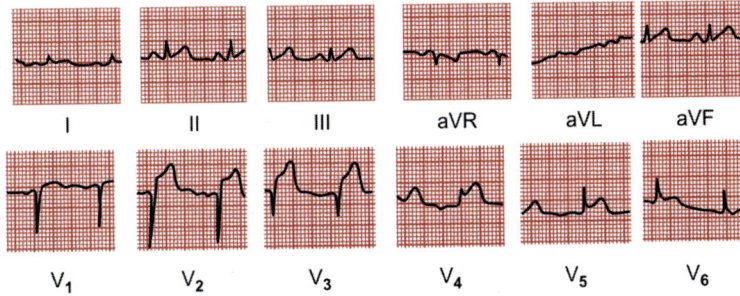

Fig. 45.14A: Pattern of acute myocardial injury in acute aluminium phosphide poisoning simulating acute anterior wall infarction. There is low voltage graph. There is ST segment elevation leads I, II, III, aVL, aVF, V_2-V_6 with upright T wave which is draggred upwards in V_2-V_6. All these changes reversed with recovery of the patient

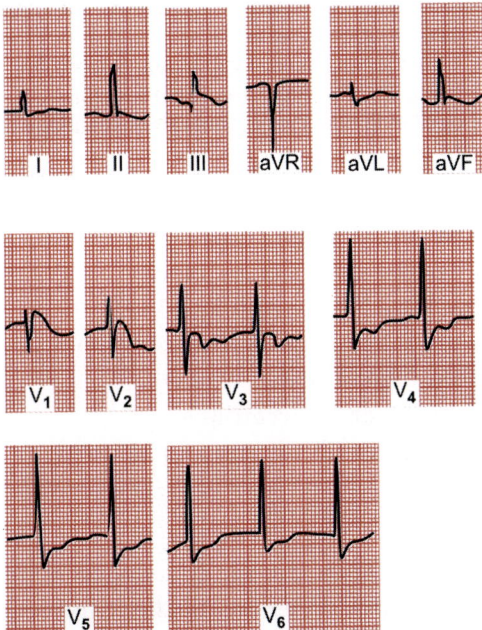

Fig. 45.14B: Acute myocardial injury simulating acute inferior wall infarction and anterior wall ischaemia. There is ST elevation with T wave inversion in leads II, III and aVF. Simultaneously there is ST segment elevation in leads V_1-V_2 with coving ST segment in V_3-V_4 and depressed ST segment in V_5-V_6. The T is dragged upward in leads V_1-V_2, symmetrically inverted in V_3-V_4 and biphasic in V_5-V_6

3. *Rhythm disturbances:* The rhythm of the heart is disturbed in aluminium phosphide poisoning mostly due to direct as well as free radicals mediated cardiotoxicity. All sorts of arrhythmias that occur in a setting of acute myocardial infarction may be seen in this poisoning. They may include

(i) *Disturbance of sinus rhythm* (Fig. 45.16)
   - Sinus arrhythmias (varied R-R intervals)
   - Sinus bradycardia
   - Sinus tachycardia
   - Sinus arrest or sinoatrial blocks

(ii) *Atrial arrhythmias:* They are frequent than ventricular, probably due to the fact that atria are more vulnerable to hypoxia:
   - Atrial ectopics, atrial escape beats
   - Atrial bigeminy
   - Wanderning atrial pacemaker and multifocal atrial tachycarida (Fig. 45.17)
   - Paroxysmal atrial tachycardia
   - Atrial fibrillation
   - Vagotonic block-atrial standstill

(iii) *AV nodal disturbances*
   - AV nodal ectopics
   - Junctional rhythm (Fig. 45.18)

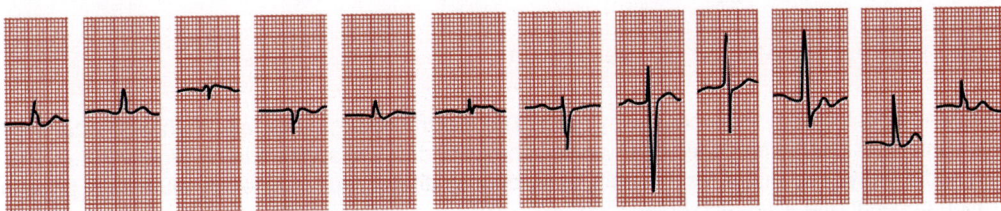

Fig. 45.15: Incomplete left bundle branch block pattern in acute aluminium phosphide poisoning. The ECG shows loss of q wave in leads I, aVL, V_5-V_6. The QRS is wider and is slurred (R-R' pattern) in these leads. There is left axis deviation

SECTIONTWELVE

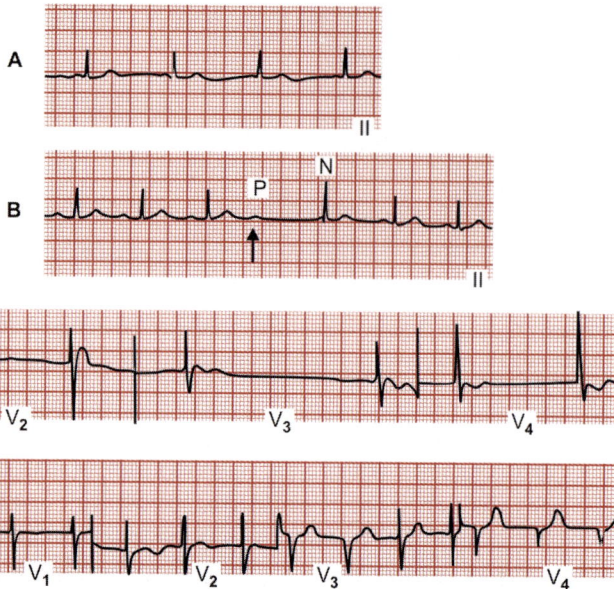

Fig. 45.16: Sinus node dysfunction in acute aluminium phosphide poisoning:
A: Sinus bradycardia (HR < 60/min)
B: Blocked P wave with nodal escape beat. First three complexes are sinus followed by a blocked P wave (↑), which led to nodal escape beat (N), then normal sinus rhythm is restored
C: Upper strip shows long sinus pauses the longest being 2.8 sec, indicates vagotonaemia
Lower strip shows disappearance of sinus pauses

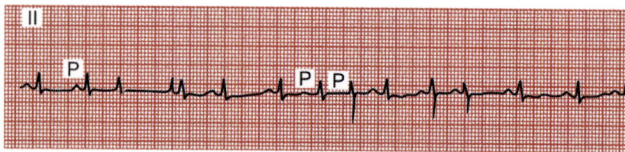

Fig. 45.17: Multifocal atrial tachycardia recorded from a patient with aluminium phosphide poisoning. The electrocardiogram shows variable shapes of P waves (some of P waves are labelled), variable P-R intervals and variable R-R intervals. The atrial rate is >100 bpm. This is not wandering atrial pacemaker because of its high atrial rate. This is not atrial fibrillation because some of P waves are nicely seen and labelled; and there no undulation of baseline, i.e. isoelectric baseline is seen between P waves

- AV nodal tachycardia
- Various grades of AV block
4. *Ventricular arrhythmias* (Fig. 45.19)
   - Ventricular ectopics (monomorphic, polymorphic, bigeminy, etc)
   - Ventricular tachycardia
   - Ventricular fibrillation and asystole

Clinical Significance

1. The electrocardiographic changes in aluminium phosphide poisoning are transient and reversible

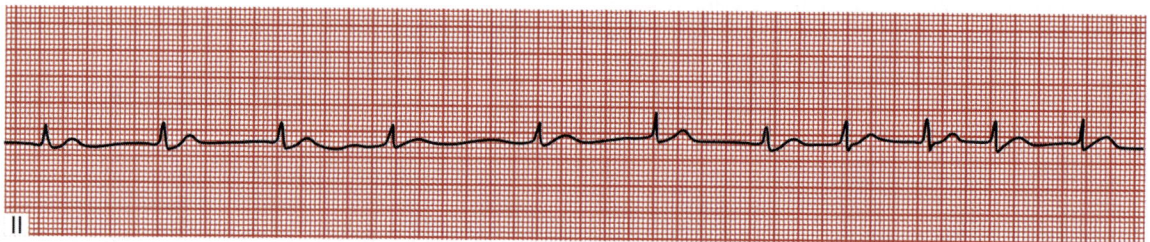

Fig. 45.18: Accelerated nodal rhythm with nodal arrhythmia. The electrocardiographic lead II shows nodal rhythm at a rate of 75 bpm. The QRS complexes are not preceded by P waves. The QRS duration appears to be slightly wider. The R-R interval is variable indicating nodal arrhythmia under the influence of autonomic disturbance induced by aluminium phosphide poisoning. There is acceleration of nodal rate at the end of the strip
Note: AV node can also exhibit nodal arrhythmia similar to sinus node arrhythmia

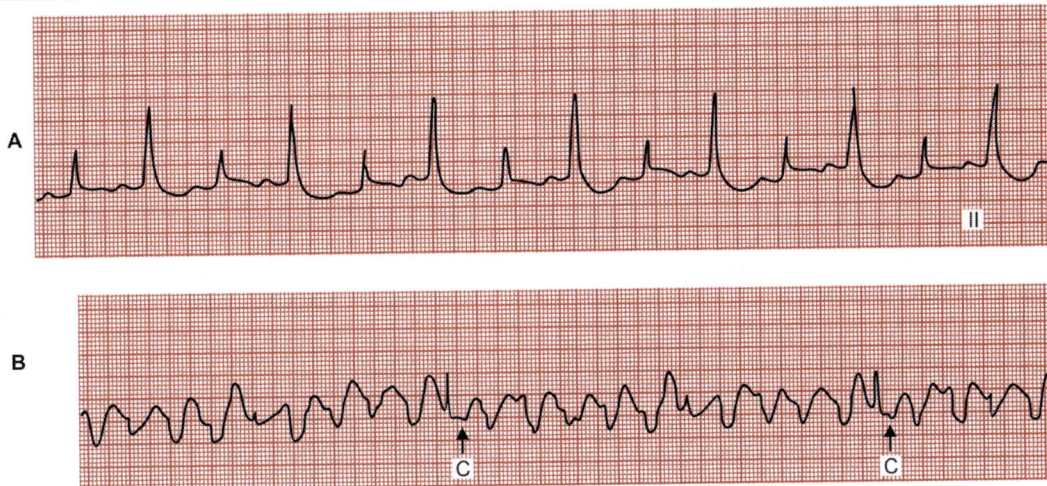

Fig. 45.19: Ventricular arrhythmias in aluminium phosphide poisoning. The ECG (lead II) shows;
A: Ventricular bigeminy. A narrow normal QRS alternates with wide QRS of end-diastolic interpolated VPCs
B: Polymorphic ventricular tachycardia. There is wide QRS tachycardia of variable QRS configurations. Capture beats (C) are seen in between

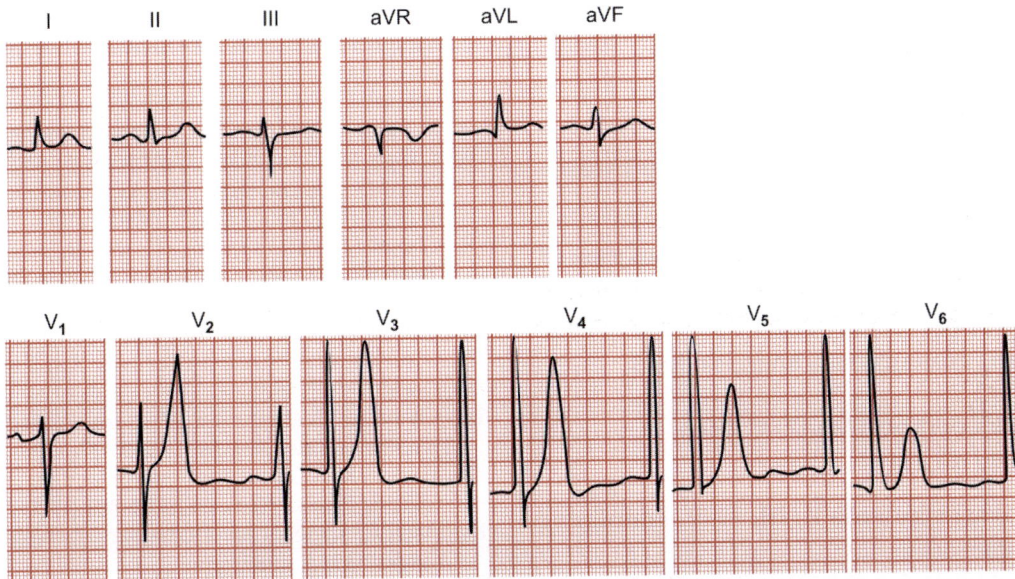

Fig. 45.20: Probable scorpion envenomation. The electrocardiogram was recorded from a young female bitten by scorpion (as detailed by the patient) while working in the field. There were sting marks but exact identity of scorpion could not be established. Note the falling heart rate (62/min) with tall tented T waves in leads II, III, aVF and V_2-V_6. This could be due to cholinergic effect of scorpion bite. These tall tented T waves can simulate;
  i. Posterior wall infarction
  ii. Hyperkalaemia
  iii. Cerebrovascular accidents
  iv. Early repolarisation syndrome (a normal variant)

in most of the cases within few days to few weeks, occasional case may take longer time to recover from these changes.

2. There is no antidote to this poisoning. The most of electrocardiographic manifestations neither influence the course or prognosis of the patients nor require any specific management except malignant ventricular arrhythmias where magnesium sulphate or amiodarone (class III antiarrhythmic) have been found effective.

SECTIONTWELVE

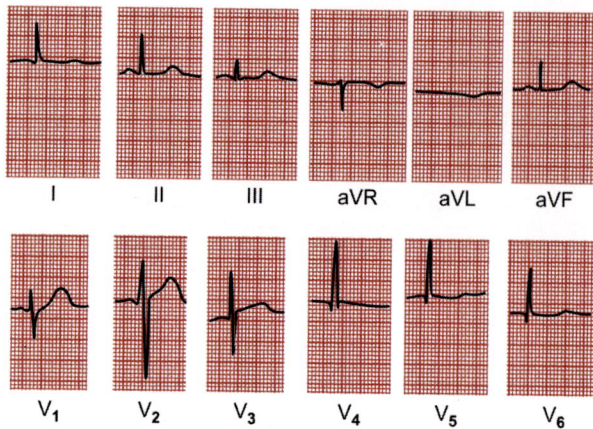

Fig. 45.21: Scorpion sting bite. The ECG shows prolongation of QTc and sagging ST segment and low amplitude of T waves in leads V_4-V_6

3. There is no residual cardiac damage following this poisoning if the patient survives; otherwise, mortality is very high (37-100%) in this poisoning.

HEART IN ENVENOMATION

Scorpion Envenomation (Scorpion Sting Bite)

Envenomation by an Indian red scorpion (M. tamulus) is a dangerous than other scorpion envenomation (P. greavinomous, black scorpion), evokes a potent autonomic response characterised by both transient cholinergic and prolonged adrenergic effects.

The Electrocardiographic Manifestations (Figs 45.20 and 45.21)

1. Tented T waves in leads II, III, V_2-V_6 simulating early repolarisation.
2. ST-T changes stimulating myocardial infarction may occur.
3. Transient VPCs and ventricular bigeminy pattern may be seen.
4. Supraventricular tachycardia.
5. Left anterior hemiblock.
6. Left ventricular hypertrophy pattern.
7. Transient prolongation of QTc (0.42 to 0.56 sec) can be seen in first 24-48 hrs of envenomation.
8. Fatal cases may show marked tachycardia, low voltage of QRS, bundle branch block pattern with widened QRS complexes and P-QRS-T alternans. All these changes suggest the evidence of myo-

carditis due to scorpion envenomation. Occasionally, myocarditis by severe envenomation, may progress to dilated cardiomyopathy.

Suggested Reading

1. Aggarwal SB: A clinical, biochemical, neurobehavioural and sociopsychological study of 190 patients admitted to hospital as a result of acute organophosphorus poisoning. *Enviorn Res* **62**:63-70, 1993.
2. Amara CFS, Lopes JA, Magalhaes RA et al: Electrocardiographic evidence of myocardial damage after serrulatus scorpion poisoning. *Am J Cardiol* **67**:655, 1991.
3. Bardagi A, Vidal F, Richart C: T waves alternans associated with amiodarone. *J Electrocardiol* **26**: 155, 1993.
4. Basset AL, Hoffman BF: Antiarrhythmic drugs: Electrophysiological actions. *Annu Rev Pharmacol* **11**:143, 1971.
5. Bawaskar HS, Bawaskar PH: Cardiovascular manifestations of severe scorpion sting in India (Review of 34 children. *Ann Trop Paediatric* **11**:381-87, 1991.
6. Bawaskar HS: Diagnostic cardiac premonitoring signs and symptoms of red scorpion sting. *Lancet* **11**:552-54, 1982.
7. Chugh SN, Chugh K, Sant Ram et al: Electrocardiographic abnormalities in aluminium phosphide poisoning with special reference to its incidence, pathogenesis, mortality and histopathology. *J Ind Med Assoc* **89**:32-35, 1991.
8. Chugh SN, Dushyant, Sant Ram et al: Incidence and outcome of aluminium phosphide poisoning in a hospital study. *Ind J Med Res* **94**:232, 1991.
9. Chugh SN: Alluminium phosphide poisoning. In API Textbook of Medicine, 6th edn, published by Association Physicians of India, Mumbai, 1999.
10. Chung EK: Electrocardiography: Practical applications with Victorial Principles 3rd edn. Appleton and Lange, Norwalk, CT, 1985.
11. Elkayam U, Frishman W: Cardiovascular effects of phenothiazines. *Am Heart J* **100**:397, 1980.
12. Fisch C, Knoebel SB: Recognition and therapy of digitalis toxicity. *Prog Cardiovasc Dis* **12**: 383, 1970.
13. Fisch C, Knoebel SB: Digitalis cardiotoxicity. *J Am Coll Cardiol* 5191A, 1985.
14. Gueron M, Sofer S: Cardiac dysfunction and pulmonary oedema following scorpion envenomation. *Chest* **102**: 1307-09, 1992.
15. Gueron M, Ilia R, Sofer S: Scorpion venom cardiomyopathy. *Am Heart J* **123**:725, 1993.
16. Herin SE, Jurca M, Vichim FL et al: Reversible cardiomyopathy in patients with severe envenoming by T typus serrulatus: Evaluation of enzymatic, electrocardiographic and echocardiographic alterations. *Ann Trop Paediatric* **13**:173-82, 1993.
17. Langer GA: Effects of digitalis on myocardial ionic exchange. *Circulation* **46**:180, 1972.
18. Marriott HJL, Conover MB: Advanced concepts on arrhythmias, 2nd edn. CV Mosby Company. St Louis, 1989.
19. Marriott HJL: Practicol Electrocardiography, 7th edn. William and Wilkins Baltimore, 1983.

20. Poojking T: Myocarditis from scorpion sting. *Br Med J* **3**:374-7, 1964.

21. Singh BN, Hauswirth O: Comparative mechanism of action of antiarrhythmic drugs. *Am Heart J* **87**: 367, 1974.

22. Singh S, Balkishan, Singh S et al: Parathion poisoning in Punjab. A clincial and electrocardiographic study of 20 cases. *J Assos Phy Ind* **17**:185, 1969.

23. Smith TW, Antman EM, Friedman FL et al: Digitalis glycosides–mechanisms and manifestations of toxicity. *Prog Cardiovasc Dis* **26**:413, 1984.

24. Surawicz B, Lasseter KC: Effect of drugs on the electrocardiogram. *Prog Cardiovasc Dis* **13**:26, 1970.

25. Vaughan Williams EM: A classification of antiarrhythmic action reassessed after a decade of new drugs. *J Clin Pharmacol* **24**: 129-147, 1984.

26. Warroll DA: Envenomation by snakes and venomous arthropodes. In API Textbook of medicine 6th edn; Ed. GS Sainani. Association of physicians of India Mumbai 1320-1, 1999.

46

The Electrolytes and the Heart

- *The potassium disturbance (hypo and hyperkalaemia): causes and electrocardiographic characteristics*
- *The calcium disturbance (hyper and hypocalcaemia): causes and electrocardiographic characteristics*
- *The magnesium disturbance (hypo and hypermagnesaemia): causes and electrocardiographic characteristics*

THE ELECTROLYTE DISTURBANCES

The common electrolytes disturbances which influence electrocardiographic changes are:
1. Hypokalaemia and hyperkalaemia
2. Hypocalcaemia and hypercalcaemia
3. Hypomagnesaemia and hypermagnesaemia

HYPOKALAEMIA

Potassium is the principal intracellular cation, takes part in depolarisation and repolarisation of cardiac cells membrane. Normal serum potassium level is 3.5-5.5 mEq/l. Hypokalaemia is said to be present if serum potassium level is less than 3.0 mEq/l.

Causes

The causes of potassium depletion are tabulated in Table 46.1.

The Electrocardiographic Manifestations (Fig. 46.1)

The electrically active tissues of the heart are particularly sensitive to changes in the extracellular concentration of K^+ and dramatic ECG changes may accompany abrupt changes in potassium. The ECG changes appear when serum K^+ level falls below 3.0 mEq/l but are marked when concentration falls below 2.0 mEq/l.

Table 46.1: Causes of potassium depletion and hypokalaemia

1. Gastrointestinal
   - Low dietary·intake
   - Gastrointestinal loss due to repeated vomiting, diarrhoea, fistulas, ureterosigmoidostomy, etc.
2. Renal
   - Metabolic alkalosis
   - Diuretics (loop diuretics)
   - Hyperaldosteronism (primary or secondary due to malignant hypertension, Barter's syndrome, juxtaglomerular cell tumour).
   - Liquorice ingestion
   - Glucocorticoids excess (iaterogenic, Cushing's syndrome, ectopic ACTH production)
   - Renal tubular acidosis
   - Renal tubular defects due to leukaemia, Liddle's syndrome and antibiotics
3. Conditions causing intracellular shift of potassium
   - Hypokalaemic periodic paralysis
   - Insulin effect
   - Alkalosis

A progressive decrease in the extracellular K^+ results in a progressive decrease in the duration of phase 2 and a progressive increase in the duration of phase 3 and total action potential (Fig. 46.1). These changes in action potential are reflected in progressive depression of the ST segment, a decrease in the amplitude of T wave and an increase in the amplitude of U wave. In net shell, there is prolongation of ventricular depolarisation giving rise to a slight

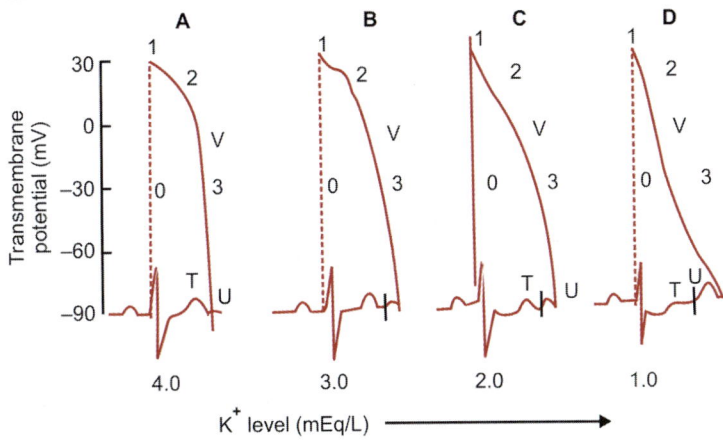

Fig. 46.1: The effect of hypokalaemia on action potential curve (diagram). The ventricular (V) action potential curve is superimposed on ECG deflections. The vertical axis represents transmembrane action potential (mV) and the horizontal axis represents extracellular concentration of potassium (K+ in mEq/l).
A. It represents the normal phases of action potentials (0,1,2,3)
B, C, and D: Note the progressive decrease in duration of phase 2 and progressive increase in the duration of phase 3 and total action potential duration with progressive decline in extracellular K+ levels. Note also the increase in action potential and resting membrane amplitudes

increase in duration of QRS by 0.02 second, and a prolonged and delayed ventricular repolarisation giving rise to prominent U waves. As the prominent U wave becomes fused to T wave, hence QT-U interval instead of QT interval becomes measurable, which is prolonged, while QT (actual) remains presumably normal.

The Electrocardiogram (Figs 46.2 to 46.4)

1. *Progressive diminution of the amplitude of T wave and increase in the amplitude of U wave.* There is progressive decrease in the height of T waves which may become low to flat. There is increase in the amplitude of U waves which are so near to the T waves that it is impossible to separate them. Prominent U wave, sometimes, caused confusion during calculation of Q-T interval when it is in fact the Q-U interval that is being measured and led to incorrect diagnosis of long Q-T interval. Therefore, it is necessary to differentiate U wave from T wave. The only differentiating feature is that U wave is more round than T wave (Fig. 46.3). The appearance of U wave is not diagnostic of hypokalaemia as they also occur in the course of therapy with

antiarrhythmic drugs-amiodarone, phenothiazines, tricyclic antidepressants and hereditary long Q-T syndrome. However, post-extrasystolic giant U wave is highly suggestive of hypokalaemia.

The low amplitude of T wave and prominent U waves are probably due to prolonged Purkinje system repolarisation induced by hypokalaemia.

The causes of prominent U waves other than hypokalaemia are given in the box.

Causes of prominent U waves

I. *Normal—sinus bradycardia*
II. *Abnormal*
   - *Drugs—type I antiarrhythmics, amiodarone, phenothiazines, tricyclic antidepressants.*
   - *Hereditory long Q-T syndrome*
   - *Left ventricular hypertrophy.*
   - *Acute and chronic ischaemic heart disease.*
   - *Hypokalaemia*

2. *QRS duration:* Due to prolonged depolarisation, the QRS duration is slightly increased by 0.02 second but its total duration does not exceed 0.1 sec.

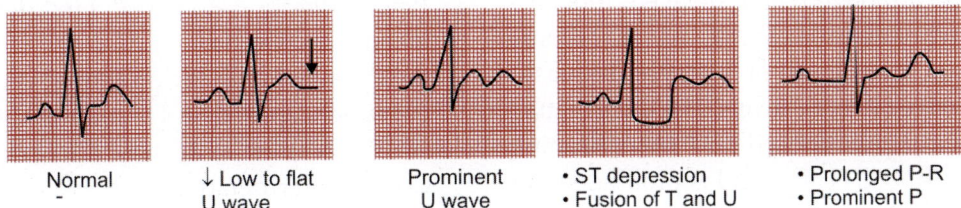

Normal — | ↓ Low to flat U wave | Prominent U wave | • ST depression • Fusion of T and U | • Prolonged P-R • Prominent P

Fig. 46.2: The effects of hypokalaemia on ECG deflections (diagram)

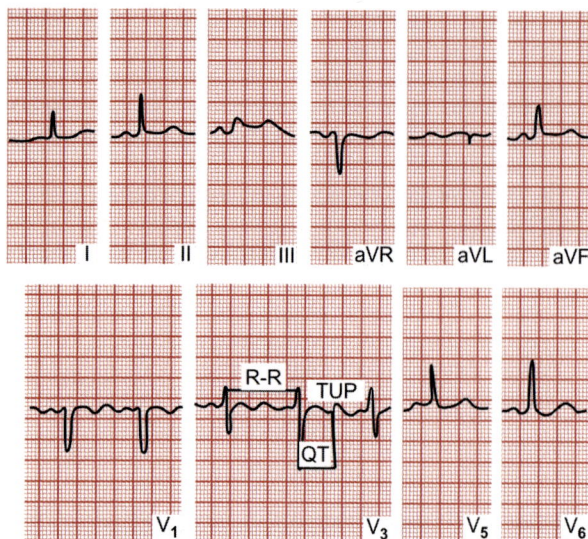

Fig. 46.3A: Hypokalaemia (serum K$^+$ 2.0 mEq/L). The electrocardiogram shows;

i. Prominent U wave equivalent to T wave is seen in leads V$_1$-V$_3$ (one of the complex labelled). The T and U waves are separately seen

ii. The P wave and P-R interval are normal

iii. The QTc and QTU is prolonged, i.e. 0.55 sec (Q-T = 0.44 sec, R-R = 0.64 sec)

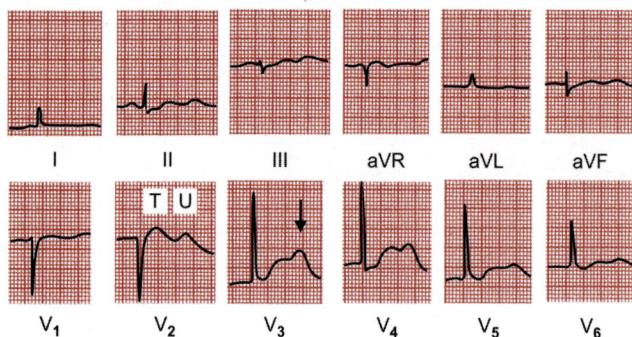

Fig. 46.3B: Giant 'U' wave in hypokalaemia. The electrocardiogram shows prominent U wave in precordial leads, which is taller than T in the same complex—called *giant 'U'* wave (↓), are seen in leads V$_2$-V$_5$

3. *Prolonged QTU interval, while QT interval remains normal* (Figs 46.4A and B): A prominent U wave on ECG reflects prolonged and delayed repolarisation. In hypokalaemia, the U waves become prominent and amplitude of T waves decreases with progressive fall in K$^+$ levels. The U wave may sometime gets superimposed on T wave forming 'TU' complex and QTU interval is prolonged but QT interval remains normal. The QTc may also get prolonged.

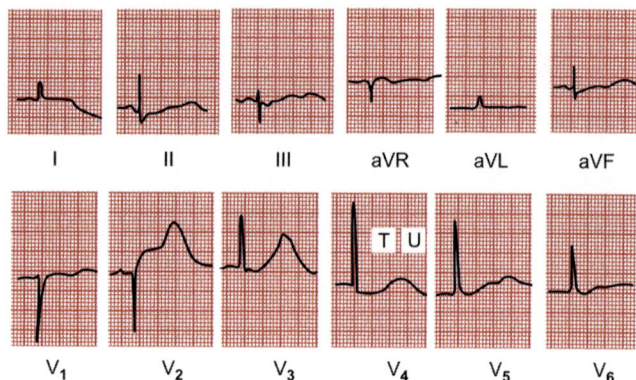

Fig. 46.4A: Prolonged QTU interval in hypokalaemia (serum K$^+$ 1.8 mEq/L). The T and U waves are visible in lead V$_2$; while in other leads (II, III, aVF, V$_3$-V$_6$) the T wave is broadened due to superimposition of U wave to form *TU* wave. The QTU interval is 0.76.sec

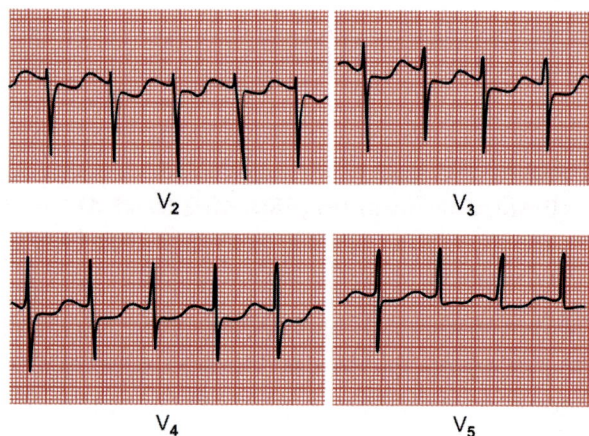

Fig. 46.4B: TUP complex in hypokalaemia (serum K$^+$ 1.8 mEq/L). The electrocardiogram ((lead V$_2$-V$_5$) shows;

i. Prolongation of QT or QTc interval, i.e. QT = 0.42, QTc = 0.53 sec

ii. The T wave is wide due to merger of U and P wave (TUP complex)

iii. The P wave are not seen as they are merged with T wave (TUP complex)

iv. The ST segment is depressed but not horizontally which occurs in hypocalcaemia

4. *Prolongation of P-R interval:* First degree AV block is common. The prolongation of P-R interval brings the P wave near to the preceding U wave and may get superimposed on TU complex forming a wide 'TUP' complex, and may also cause confusion. Correct interpretation is necessary. Second degree Wenckebach type of AV block may also be associated with low potassium level.

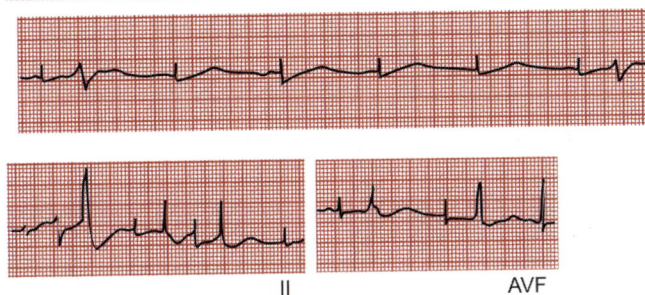

Fig. 46.5: Hypokalaemia with VPCs.
1. Upper strip (lead II) shows prolonged QT interval of 0.67 second (QTc is 0.56 second) due to hypokalaemia. Two monomorphic VPCs (2nd and 8th complexes) are seen
2. Lower strip (leads II and aVF) shows polymorphic VPCs in lead II and ventricular bigeminy in aVF

5. *ST segment depression*: There is ST segment depression in all leads. The depression may be horizontal or concave upwards.
6. *Arrhythmias:* A variety of atrial and ventricular arrhythmias may occur, especially in patients receiving digitalis. Digitalis induces supraventricular and ventricular ectopics (Fig. 46.5) and rhythms because of enhanced automaticity and re-entry secondary to slowing of conduction and shortening of effective refractory period. Hypokalaemia produces arrhythmias due to delayed and prolonged repolarisation and prolonged QTc; ventricular tachycardia (*torsade de pointes*) and ventricular fibrillation may occur in severe hypokalaemia with prolonged QTc interval.

HYPERKALAEMIA

An increase in the serum potassium level above upper limit of the normal (>5.5 mEq/l) is termed *hyperkalaemia*. The ECG findings make their appearance when potassium level rises beyond 6.0 mEq/l.

It is not necessary to have ECG changes in all patients with hyperkalaemia.

Aetiology: The causes of hyperkalaemia are given in the Table 46.2.

The Electrocardiographic Manifestations— Pathogenesis and Correlation with Potassium Levels (Fig. 46.6)

As extracellular K^+ is increased to 6.0 mEq/L, the action potential duration shortens because of

Table 46.2: Causes of hyperkalaemia
1. Inadequate excretion
A. Renal failure (uraemia)
• Acute renal failure
• Chronic renal failure
• Renal tubular disorders
B. Adrenal insufficiency
• Hypoaldosteronism
• Addison's disease
C. Potassium sparing diuretics
• Spironolactone
• Triameterene
• Amiloride
2. A. Shift of potassium from tissues into circulation
• Crushed muscles
• Haemolysis
• Internal bleeding
B. Drugs
• Succinylcholine
• Digitalis poisoning may cause rise in K^+ if potassium sparing diuretics are being used.
• Beta-adrenoreceptor antagonists
C. Acidosis
D. Hyperosmolality
E. Insulin deficiency
F. Hyperkalaemic periodic paralysis
3. Excessive potassium intake in the form potassium salts or fruit juices.

decreased phase 2, and the velocity of repolarisation increases. These changes in action potential are probably responsible for shortening of QT (QTc) interval and peaking of T waves on ECG. Peaking of T waves is the earliest electrocardiographic manifestation of hyperkalaemia.

As the extracellular K^+ further increases, resting membrane potential progressively decreases (Fig.46.6), the decrease in the rate of depolarisation of action potential slows intraventricular conduction and increases the duration of QRS complex. These changes are present at serum K levels of 6.5 mEq/L or more.

Where K^+ level exceeds 7.0 mEq/L, the amplitude of P wave decreases and the duration of P wave increases because of slow conduction in the atria. The P-R interval is frequently prolonged as a result of slow AV conduction. The P waves are usually not seen when serum potassium level exceeds 8.0 mEq/L but QRS complexes are seen indicating that excitibility of ventricular fibres is retained even at high K^+ levels. The secondary ST-T changes may be seen, and are due to delayed intraventricular conduction.

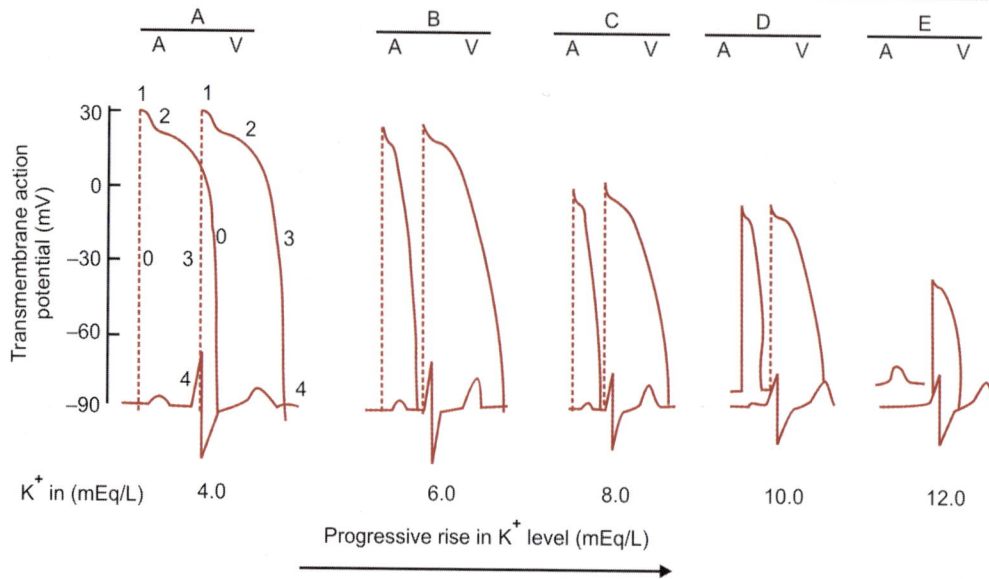

Fig. 46.6: The effect of hyperkalaemia on action potential curve; atrial (A) and ventricular (V). An atrial (A) and ventricular (V) action potential curves are superimposed on ECG deflections (diagram). The vertical axis represents transmembrane potential (mV) and horizontal axis represents the extracellular K^+ in mEq/L. The various phases (0,1,2,3,4) of action potential curve are depicted in (A). The rate of depolarisation of the action potential is indicated in AP by the *broken vertical lines*. The decreasing space between dashes indicating a slowing of upstroke velocity due to slowing of rate of depolarisation. The slowest upstroke is shown by a *continuous line* (atrial AP in D and ventricular AP in E). Note the decreasing upstroke velocity and increasing duration of the QRS complex with increasing levels of K^+ indicated by arrow ($\rightarrow$). In (A) and (B) the atrial and ventricular AP have same amplitude of transmembrane resting potential, where as in (C) and (D), the transmembrane resting potential of atrial AP is less negative than that of ventricular AP, and the amplitude of the atrial AP is lower than that of corresponding ventricular AP. AP = Action potential curve

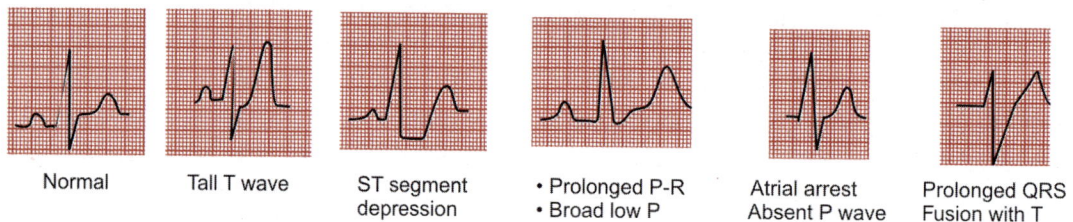

Fig. 46.7: The effects of hyperkalaemia on ECG deflection (diagram)

Ectopic ventricular rhythms, such as extrasystoles, tachycardia, flutter and fibrillation may also be encountered in the advanced stages of hyperkalaemia. Ventricular arrhythmias presage terminal ventricular standstill.

The Electrocardiogram (Figs 46.7 and 46.8)

There is good correlation between rise in serum potassium levels and ECG changes. ECG actually reflects the gradient between myocardial intracellular and extracellular potassium ions. The abnormality involves the P wave, the QRS complex, the T wave and the ST segment.

(i) *The P wave:* With increase in K^+ levels, there is decrease in the amplitude and increase in the duration of the P waves, which progressively become smaller and ultimately may disappear (atrial standstill).

(ii) *The P-R interval:* It is normal in initial stages but becomes prolonged with marked rise in K^+ levels. At higher levels, even AV blocks can occur.

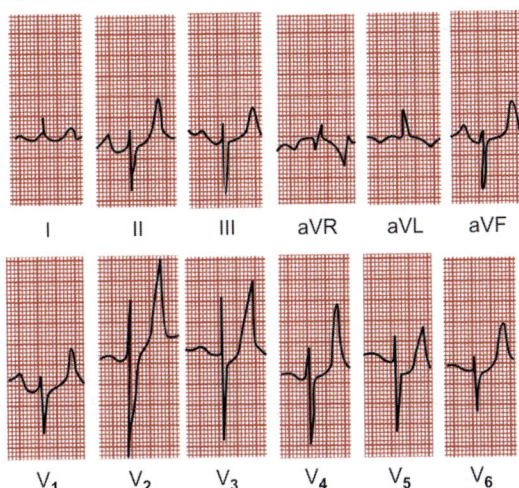

Fig. 46.8: Hyperkalaemia (serum K⁺ 6.6 mEq/L). The electrocardiogram shows;
  i. P waves are normal with normal P-R interval
  ii. Tall, slender, tented T waves are seen in leads II, III, aVF, V₁-V₆
  iii. Q-T interval is 0.28 sec. This is an effect of high K⁺ level on repolarisation of myocardial cells

(iii) *The QRS complex:* The amplitude of R wave decreases and the total duration of QRS increases with increasing K⁺ levels. At higher levels, the QRS complexes become wide and bizarre indicating delayed intraventricular conduction.

(iv) *The T wave:* The earliest electrocardiographic manifestations of hyperkalaemia (> 6.0 mEq/L) is high peaked, tall tented T waves, seen in all the leads especially precordial leads. With the further rise in K⁺ levels, its amplitude and peaking character decreases but width increases. At markedly high levels, the T waves become broad with wide, bizarre QRS resembling *sine-wave* pattern.

The tall T waves are by no means diagnostic of hyperkalaemia, since normal persons, patients with posterior wall infarction and bradycardia may have similar T waves. However, peaking of T waves is highly suggestive of hyperkalaemia.

(v) *The QT (QTc) interval:* The QT (QTc) interval shortens with rise in K⁺ levels, bringing the T wave near to QRS complex.

(vi) *The ST-T changes:* There is marked ST depression with upright T waves due to delayed intra-ventricular conduction. These are called secondary ST-T changes and do not indicate ischaemia.

(vii) *Arrhythmias:* Atrial standstill may occur. Ventricular arrhythmias–extrasystoles, tachycardia, flutter, fibrillation occur with increasing level of K⁺. At very high levels, cardiac standstill may develop as a terminal event.

HYPERCALCAEMIA

The normal plasma calcium level is 4.5 to 5.0 mEq/l (9.0 to 10.5 mg/dl), levels > 10.5 mg/dl, i.e. higher than upper limit of the normal indicate hypercalcaemia. The ionised calcium is more important in clinical setting as this fraction is associated with neuromuscular excitability. The plasma level of ionised calcium is 2.3 to 2.8 mEq/l or 4.5 to 5.6 mg/dl (1.1-1.4 mmol/l). Hypercalcaemia may be symptomatic or asymptomatic. Symptoms generally appear at calcium levels above 11.5 mg/dl, but some patients even at this levels are asymptomatic. Severe hypercalcaemia is defined as a serum calcium level at or above. 15 mg/dl and is a medical emergency. When serum calcium is 15 to 18 mg/dl or higher, coma and cardiac arrest may occur.

Aetiology: Causes of hypercalcaemia are given in the Table 46.3.

Hypercalcaemia from any cause can result in fatigue, depression, mental confusion, anorexia, nausea, vomiting, constipation, polyuria, renal tubular defects, alterations in electrocardiogram and cardiac arrhythmias.

The Electrocardiogram (Fig. 46.9)

A high calcium concentration shortens the phase 2 and, decreases the duration of action potential and the effective refractory period of the heart, resulting in shortening of repolarisation producing changes in ST segment and QT interval.

Elevation of serum calcium levels above 12.0 mg/dl results in shortening of Q-T interval. This shortening is inversely proportional to serum calcium levels. The shortening is entirely due to outward bowing of ST segment which is a characteristic manifestation. Sometimes, the ST segment may virtually disappear after becoming incorporated into T waves.

SECTION TWELVE

Table 46.3: Causes of hypercalcaemia

1. Parathyroid related
   - Primary hyperparathyroidism due to solitary adenoma or multiple endocrine neoplasia
   - Lithium therapy
   - Familial hypocalciuric hypercalcaemia.
2. Malignancy related
   - Solid tumours with bone metastases
   - Nonmetastatic complications of malignancy (lung, kidneys)
   - Haematological malignancies (leukaemia, lymphoma, multiple myeloma).
3. Vitamin D related
   - Vitamin D intoxication
   - Sarcoidosis and other granulomatous diseases
   - Idiopathic hypercalcaemia of infancy.
4. High bone turnover
   - Hyperthyroidism
   - Immobilisation
   - Thiazides diuretics
   - Vitamin A intoxication.
5. Associated with renal failure
   - Secondary hyperparathyroidism
   - Aluminium intoxication
   - Milk-alkali syndrome.

At serum levels of 16 mg/dl or higher, the T waves become prolonged or widened, thereby, try to counteract the shortening of Q-T intervals. The T wave at this level may even become inverted or flattened.

A "J" wave has also been described rarely. Arrhythmias are uncommon.

HYPOCALCAEMIA

Chronic hypocalcaemia is less common than hypercalcaemia. Critically ill patients may have transient hypocalcaemia in association with disorders, such as sepsis, burn, acute renal failure or after extensive transfusion of citrated blood. Hypocalcaemia is said to be present, if serum calcium levels are below the lower limit of normal. The blood for calcium estimation should be taken without the help of the tourniquet.

Aetiology: The causes are given in the Table 46.4.

The Electrocardiogram (Fig. 46.10)

Low calcium concentration prolongs the phase 2 of action potential of most of the different cardiac fibres.

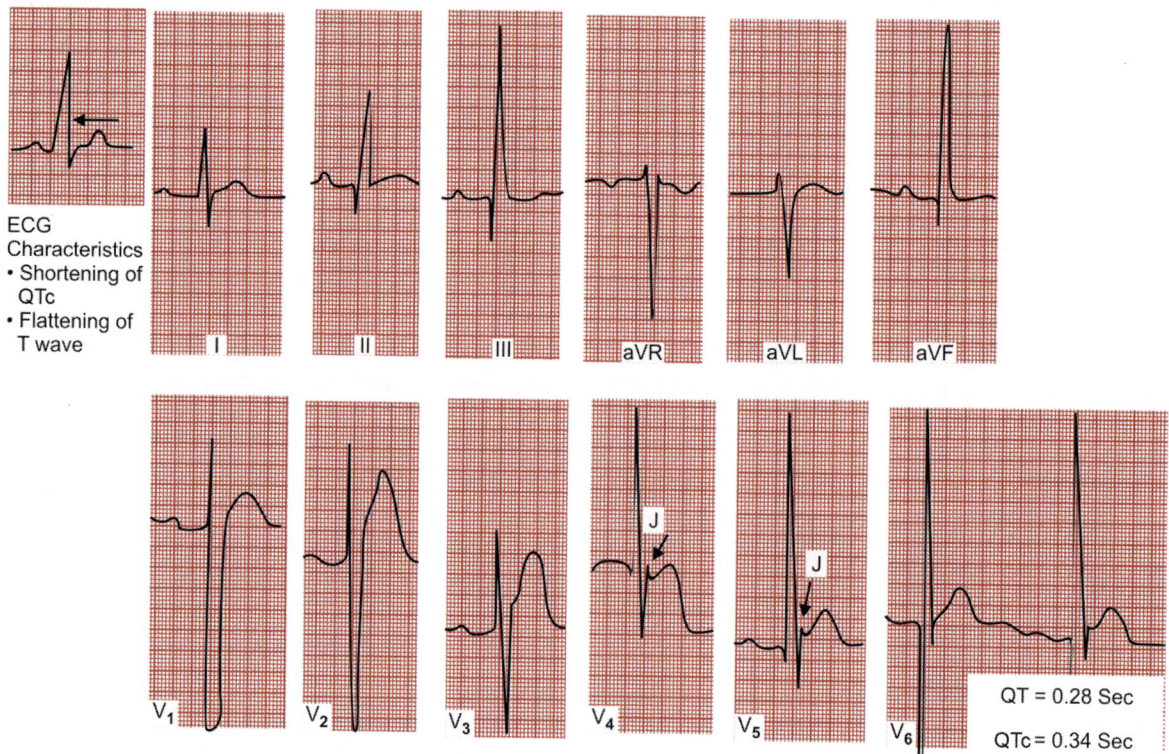

Fig. 46.9: Hypercalcaemia due to hyperparathyroidism (serum calcium 16.0 mEq/L). The electrocardiogram shows;
i. The Q-T and QTc intervals are shortened (labelled) due to virtual absence of ST segment which is hardly discernible
ii. There is widening of T wave to counteract the short Q-T interval—an effect of hypercalcaemia
iii. 'J' waves (labelled) are also seen. These 'J' wave or osborn's waves are also seen in hypothermia

Table 46.4: Causes of hypocalcaemia

1. Absent PTH (parathormone)
   - Hereditary hypoparathyroidism (DiGeorge's syndrome)
   - Acquired hypoparathyroidism
   - Hypomagnesaemia
2. Ineffective PTH
   - Chronic renal failure
   - Lack of active vitamin D metabolism, i.e. decreased dietary intake, insufficient exposure to sunlight, anticonvulsants and vitamin D dependent ricket-type I.
   - Vit. D ineffective i.e. malabsorption, vitamin D dependent ricket-type II.
3. PTH overwhelmed
   - Severe acute hyperphosphataemia due to tumour lysis, acute renal failure or rhabdomyolysis.
   - Osteitis fibrosa after parathyroidectomy
4. Alkalosis

Prolongation of phase 2, in turn, increases the duration of the total action potential and that of the effective refractory period.

Low levels of calcium produce lengthening of QT interval (QTc interval). This is, in fact, due to prolongation of ST segment that has increased horizontally and in duration, so that the ST segment tends to hug the base line. The QT interval may be prolonged in the range of 0.50 to 0.60 sec out of which more than half of prolonged QT is contributed by lengthening of the ST segment. Unlike hypokalaemia, the ST segment is not displaced from the baseline, i.e. it is straight. In hypocalcaemia, true QT interval is prolonged while in hypokalaemia it is QTU rather than actual QT that is prolonged due to appearance of prominent U wave—a distinguishing feature on ECG between the two.

The T waves are normal in duration, configuration and amplitude, and are somewhat asymmetrical. The P wave, QRS complex and U wave are not affected by hypocalcaemia. Arrhythmias are uncommon than hypokalaemia.

> *Hypocalcaemia can usually be recognised on ECG by prolonged QT (QTc) provided other conditions responsible for prolonged QT are excluded.*

HYPOMAGNESAEMIA

The electrocardiographic manifestations of hypomagnesaemia are similar to hypokalaemia. This fact is further strengthened by the fact that if potassium supplementation fails to normalise the QTc interval, hypomagnesaemia must be suspected.

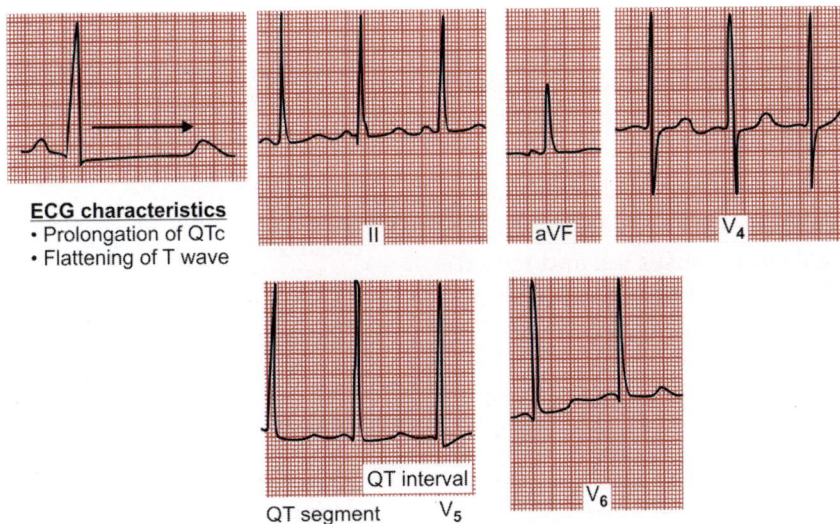

ECG characteristics
- Prolongation of QTc
- Flattening of T wave

Fig. 46.10: Hypocalcaemia. The electrocardiogram shows the lengthening of QTc interval (0.52 sec; QT = 0.42 and R-R = 0.64 sec). The Q-T segment is prolonged (0.32 sec) which is mainly contributing to prolonged QTc where T wave is small and upright. This is in contrast to hypokalaemia where QT segment does not lengthen but QTc gets prolonged due to abnormality of T wave or appearance of U wave

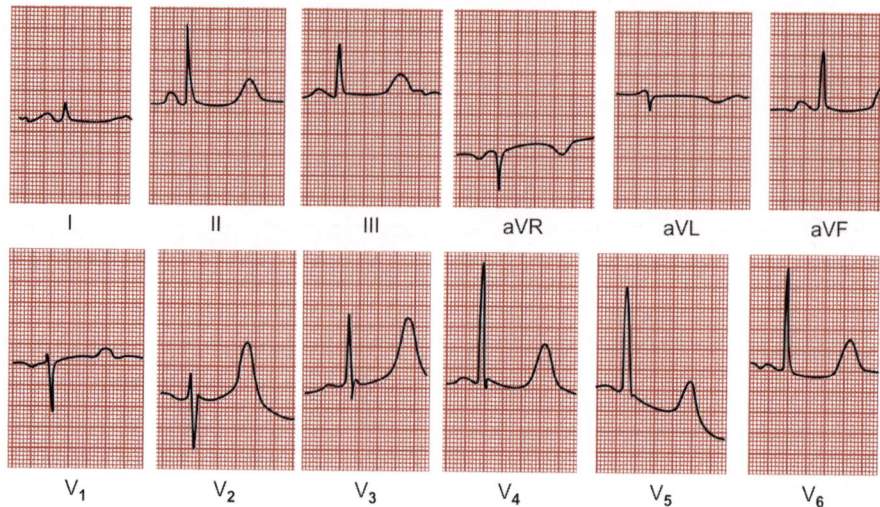

Fig. 46.11: Uraemia with hypocalcaemia (serum Ca^{++} 6.6. mEq/l) and hyperkalaemia (serum K^+ 6.6 mEq/l). The electrocardiogram shows;
   i. *Hypokalaemic effect:* There is straightening and prolongation of ST segment. The QTc interval is prolonged
   ii. *Hyperkalaemic effect:* There are tall tented T waves in precordial leads and inferior leads
      Note: Hypocalcaemia *per se* does not affect T waves

HYPERMAGNESAEMIA

The electrocardiographic effects of hypermagnesaemia are similar to hyperkalaemia. The QRS complex may be widened and the P-R interval is prolonged. No definite ECG criteria has been evolved to separate the two conditions with certainty.

URAEMIA

Uraemia is characterised by hypocalcaemia, hyperkalaemia and acidosis, therefore, electrocardiographic manifestations are either a blend of hypocalcaemia and hyperkalaemia or may be of hyperkalaemia alone. The hypocalcaemia produces prolongation of QTc interval, while hyperkalaemia causes tall and tented T waves, therefore, both types of ECG changes may be seen in uraemia (Fig. 46.11).

Suggested Reading

1. Ahmed R, Yano K, Mitsuoka T et al: Changes in T wave morphology during hypercalcaemia and its relation to the severity of hypercalcaemia. *J Electrocardiol* **22**:125, 1989.
2. Bashour T et al: Atrioventricular and intraventricular condition in hyperkalaemia. *Am J Cardiol* **35**:199, 1975.
3. Douglas PS, Carmichael KA, Palevsku PM: Extreme hypercalcaemia and electrocardiographic changes. *Am J Cardiol* **54**:674, 1984.
4. Fisch C: Relation of electrolyte disturbances to cardiac arrhythmias. *Circulation* **47**:408, 1973.
5. Helfmant RH: Hypokalaemia and arrhythmias. *Am J Med* **80**:13, 1986.
6. Lind L, Ljunghall S: Serum calcium and the ECG in patients with primary hyperparathyroidism. *J Electrocardiol* **27**:99, 1994.
7. Loeb HS, Pietras RJ, Gunnar RM: Paroxysmal ventricular fibrillation in two patients with hypomagnesaemia. *Circulation* **47**:210, 1968.
8. O'Neil JP, Chung EK: Unusual electrocardiographic findings-bifasicular block due to hyperkalaemia. *Am J Med* **61**: 537, 1976.
9. Surawicz B, Kunin AS, Sims EAH: The effects of haemodialysis and glucose insulin administration on plasma potassium and the electrocardiogram. *Circ Res* **12**:145, 1963.
10. Surawicz B: Electrolytes and the electrocardiogram. *Am J Cardiol* **12**:656,1963.
11. Surawicz B: Relationship between electrocardiogram and electrolytes. *Am Heart J* **73**:814, 1967.

47

Heart in Cerebrovascular and Neuromuscular Disorders

- The electrocardiogram in cerebrovascular accidents
- The electrocardiogram in hypokalaemic periodic paralysis
- The electrocardiogram in neuromuscular disorders (muscular dystrophies, myotonic dystrophies and Friedreich's ataxia)

CEREBROVASCULAR ACCIDENT (CVA)

Cerebrovascular accidents (CVA) may be accompanied by ECG abnormalities in approximately 90% patients reflecting changes in the autonomic nervous system. These ECG changes are observed during acute episode, more commonly in cerebral haemorrhage than cerebral thrombosis. These changes primarily affect the repolarisation and the cardiac rhythm; and usually resolve over time.

The Electrocardiogram (Figs 47.1 to 47.4)

The electrocardiographic changes associated with CVA are quite variable and may include:

1. Sinus bradycardia due to raised intracranial tension especially seen in subarachnoid haemorrhage
2. Prolongation of QTc interval (Fig. 47.1).
3. Tall, peaked and symmetric inversion of T waves resembling T wave inversion of subendocardial infarction (Fig. 47.2). The ST segment may be dramatically elevated and T waves dramatically inverted.
4. Abnormally wide T waves and prominent U waves (Fig. 47.3).
5. Tall and upright T waves due to rapid and prolonged ventricular repolarisation (Fig. 47.4).

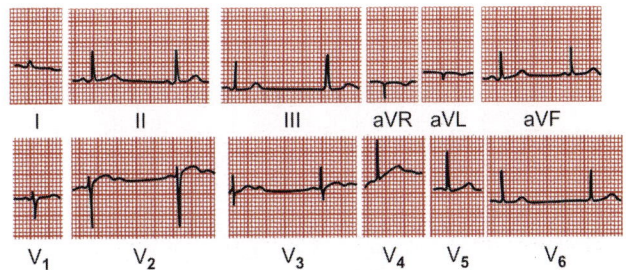

Fig. 47.1: The electrocardiogram recorded from a patient with subarachnoid haemorrhage shows;
  i. Sinus bradycardia (HR is <60/min)
  ii. QTc is variable from 0.40 to 0.44 sec. In such a situation, QT dispersion should be calculated
  iii. Prominent 'U' waves are seen in leads V_2-V_4

CVA may cause repolarisation changes (ST-T changes) on ECG

6. Arrhythmias. Atrial arrhythmias (ectopics, fibrillation, supraventricular tachycardia), junctional rhythms and ventricular arrhythmias (ectopics, ventricular tachycardia or *torsade de pointes* and fibrillation) can occur.
7. Conduction disturbances include first, second or third degree AV block.

SECTIONTWELVE

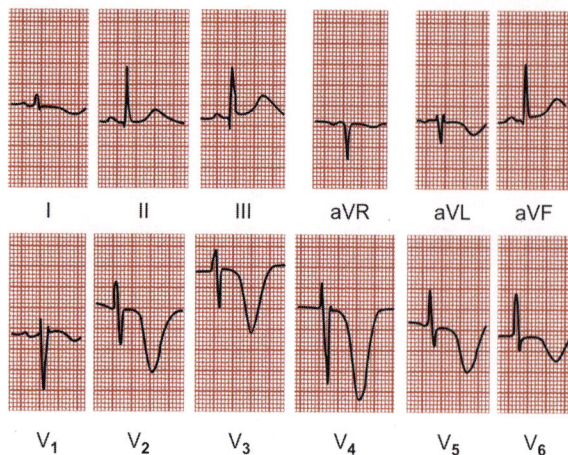

Fig. 47.2: Deep symmetric T wave inversion in intracerebral bleed. The ECG recorded from a young patient with deep intracerebral haemorrhage shows wide, deep symmetric T wave inversion in leads I, aVL, V_2-V_6 simulating subendocardial infarction or ischaemia. The QT interval is prolonged >0.44 second

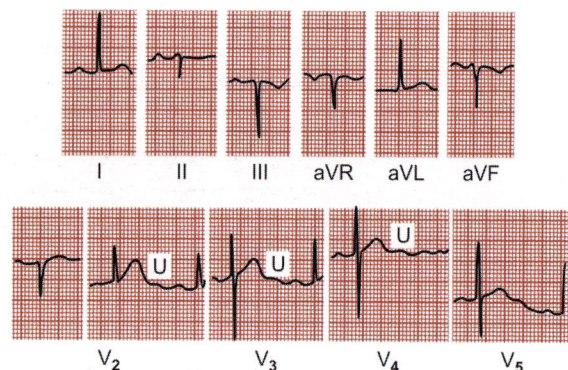

Fig. 47.3: Abnormally wide upright T waves and prominent U waves recorded from a patient with cerebral haemorrhage proved on CT scan. The electrocardiogram shows;
  i. Heart rate is slow at a rate of 60/min regular. This is due to raised intracranial tension leading to vagotonaemia.
  ii. P-R interval is prolonged 0.28 sec indicating first degree heart block
  iii. Wide upright T waves are seen in leads I, V_2 to V_6 indicating delayed and prolonged repolarisation—a characteristic feature of CVA
  iv. Prominent upright U wave follows wide T wave in leads V_2-V_6 indicating delayed late repolarisation of ventricles
  v. QTc is 0.40 sec. It is not prolonged.

HYPOKALAEMIC AND HYPERKALAEMIC PERIODIC PARALYSIS

Hypokalaemic periodic paralysis occurs as an autosomal dominant condition in two-thirds of cases

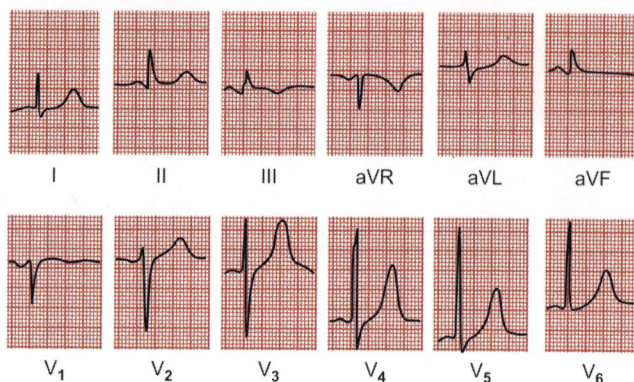

Fig. 47.4: Tall upright T waves in subarachnoid haemorrhage. The electrocardiogram recorded from a 58 yrs male without any evidence of previous organic heart disease, admitted with subarachnoid haemorrhage proved on CT scan. The ECG at admission showed tall positive T wave simulating hyperkalaemia in precordial leads (V_2-V_6). There are small insignificant q waves in leads II, III and aVF which may be mistaken for inferior wall infarction but other changes of infarction are absent

and as a sporadic condition in rest one-third. The males are commonly and severely affected. It occurs in attacks during which proximal limb muscles are usually involved. Bulbar and respiratory muscles are rarely involved and if involved, may prove fatal. Hyperkalaemic periodic paralysis is similar to hypokalaemic type except that attacks of flaccid paralysis occur in younger age, occur more frequently, are milder and tend to be shorter (minutes or hours).

The Electrocardiogram (Fig. 47.5)

The electrocardiographic manifestations occur due to hypokalaemia which precipitates the attack, hence, the abnormalities on ECG (prolonged QT interval and cardiac arrhythmias) occur during acute episode and may disappear during recovery. The electrocardiographic changes noted are similar to hypokalaemia due to any cause. (Read ECG manifestations of hypokalaemia).

The electrocardiogram in hyperkalaemic variety shows tall peaked T waves during an attack. (Read ECG manifestations of hyperkalaemia).

NEUROMUSCULAR DISORDERS

The neuromuscular disorders that are associated with cardiac involvement and abnormal electrocardiograms are:

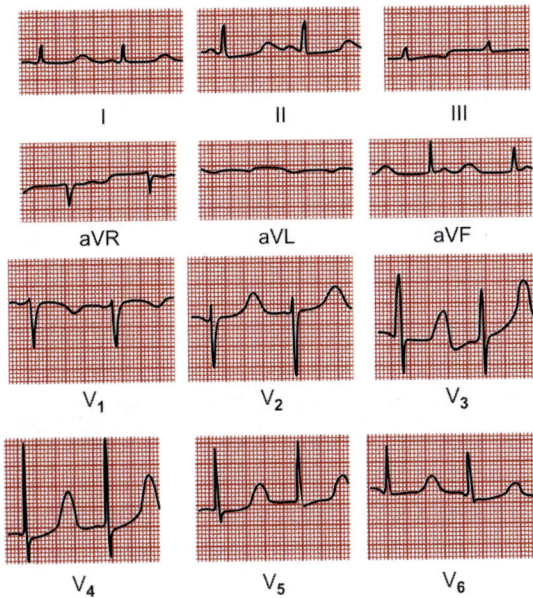

Fig. 47.5: Hypokalaemic periodic paralysis. The electrocardiogram recorded from a 20 years male patient during an attack shows prolongation of QT (QTc). The QT is 0.52 sec and QTc = $0.52 \div \sqrt{80}$ = 57 sec. There is tendency to ST segment depression in leads I, II, III, aVL, aVF and V_2-V_6

1. Duchenne's or pseudohypertrophic muscular dystrophy
2. Becker's-muscular dystrophy
3. Limb-girdle dystrophy
4. Emery-Dreifuss muscular dystrophy
5. Myotonic muscular dystrophy
6. Friedreich's ataxia
7. Guillain-Barré syndrome
8. Kugelberg-Welander syndrome
9. Poliomyelitis

1. DUCHENNE'S MUSCULAR DYSTROPHY

It is an X-linked recessive disorder, manifests in young boys. Duchenne's dystrophy is a myopathic disorder that involves striated muscle fibres (skeletal, cardiac), smooth muscle fibers (vessels) and nervous system. The existence of cardiomyopathy has been reported in almost all the cases but death due to it is uncommon. Congestive heart failure rarely occurs except during severe stress. The electrocardiographic abnormalities that have been documented in Duchenne's dystrophy are expressed as rhythm and conduction disturbances.

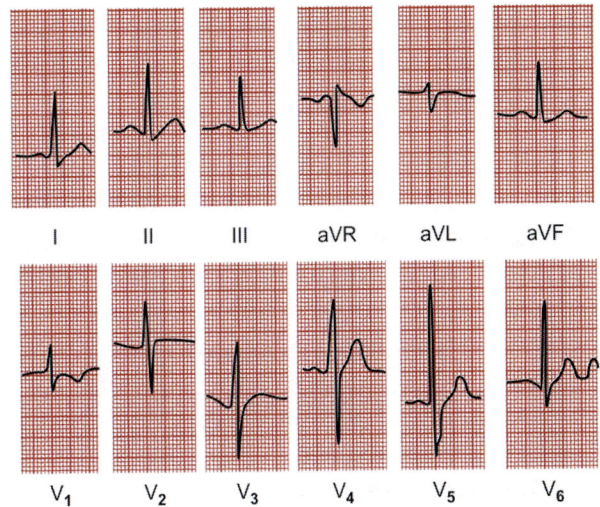

Fig. 47.6: Duchenne's type of myopathy. ECG shows right ventricular dominance—R wave is larger than S wave with T inversion in lead V_1 with persistence of S wave in V_5-V_6 in a 24 years old man

The Electrocardiogram (Fig. 47.6)

1. *Ventricular hypertrophy pattern:* Tall R waves in leads V_1-V_2 and increased R/S amplitude ratio, together with deep Q waves in leads I, aVL and V_5-V_6 are characteristics of rapidly progressive Duchenne's dystrophy. Female carriers even, sometimes, reflect electrocardiographic abnormalities in the form of large R/S ratio in leads V_1-V_2 as compared to normal adult women.

   Mechanisms: A reduction and loss of electrical forces caused by myocardial dystrophy in the postero-basal region and lateral walls of left ventricle results in anterior shift of the QRS forces.

2. *Rhythm disturbances:* The most common rhythm disturbance is inappropriate sinus tachycardia which may be persistent or labile (occurs during waking hours or sleep), is common in children below 12 years of age. The mechanism of sinus tachycardia has not been established but is attributed to autonomic dysfunction (e.g. increase in sympathetic activity and/or a decrease in parasympathetic activity).

   The supraventricular rhythm disturbances observed include; atrial ectopics, intermittent atrial ectopic rhythms, AV nodal rhythm and sustained supraventricular tachycardia. Atrial flutter, a rare tachyarrhythmia in children, is seen as a common preterminal tachyarrhythmia associated with atrial fibrillation.

The incidence of ventricular instability is increased especially in older patients with depressed left ventricular function (cardiomyopathy). Ventricular ectopic rhythms occur commonly in patients with cardiomyopathy and include; premature ventricular complexes, couplets and nonsustained VT. The pathogenesis of ventricular arrhythmias is not clear, but is attributed to left ventricular wall motion abnormalities and left ventricular dysfunction.

3. *Conduction disturbances:*
   (i) *Accelerated AV conduction:* Short P-R intervals are common due to an accelerated conduction. Earlier reports of increased P-R intervals due to delayed conduction has now been confirmed to occur only in late stages of the disease.
   (ii) *Intraventricular conduction delay:* The fascicular blocks (anterior or posterior), right bundle branch block (RBBB) and exceptionally a bifascicular block have been observed in late stages of the disease and are attributed to fibrosis and vascular degeneration involving AV node and the peripheral conduction system.

2. BECKER'S MUSCULAR DYSTROPHY

Becker's muscular dystrophy is considered as a milder allelic variant of Duchenne's muscular dystrophy, but the clinical expression—both the phenotype and the presence and degree of cardiac involvement are much more variable. Becker's dystrophy is later in onset and slow in progression than Duchenne's dystrophy. Cardiac involvement can occur at any age and is unrelated to the extent of skeletal muscle involvement. X-linked dilated cardiomyopathy without clinical signs of skeletal myopathy is believed to be genetic in origin (Becker gene on short arm of X-chromosome). Severe familial dilated cardiomyopathy can occur in Becker's progressive muscular dystrophy. Becker's dystrophy expresses on ECG as a conduction disturbance (common) and/or rhythm disturbance.

The Electrocardiogram

1. *Conduction disturbances:* Fascicular blocks, bundle branch blocks (right or left) and AV blocks—

complete heart block, occur due to abnormalities of the His bundle and infranodal conduction.

2. *Rhythm disturbances:* They are uncommon. Ventricular arrhythmias have been documented in patients with Becker's dystrophy and are believed to be a cause of sudden death.

3. LIMB-GIRDLE DYSTROPHY

(i) *Erb type:* Intraventricular conduction defects and fascicular blocks have been reported.

(ii) *Fascioscapulohumeral type (Landouzy-Dejerine type):* The electrophysiological abnormalities of atria (atrial paralysis), AV node and His-Purkinje conduction system have been described.

(iii) *Emery-Dreifuss muscular dystrophy:* The cardiac involvement is commoner than other two types. The electrocardiographic abnormalities include:
   a. Atrial standstill has been reported in adults, rarely in children, is characterised by absence of P waves on 12 lead ECG and oesophageal electrocardiograms. Atrial tachycardia, atrial flutter or fibrillation are common.
   b. Conduction disturbances in the form of slow junctional rhythms or complete heart block may warrant the use of permanent pacemaker.

4. MYOTONIC MUSCULAR DYSTROPHY

Because specialised cardiac tissue and the myocardium have intimate embryological origin, hence, both are affected commonly and cardiac involvement is, therefore, an integral part of myotonic dystrophy. The conduction tissue is more commonly involved than myocardium. The electrocardiographic abnormalities are limited to conduction system, occur due to fibrosis, fatty infiltration and atrophy involving the sinus node, AV node and His-Purkinje system. Myocardial dystrophy is responsible for atrial and ventricular arrhythmias.

The Electrocardiogram

(i) *Conduction disturbances:* The most common ECG changes include; prolongation of P-R interval, left anterior fascicular block, wide QRS complexes (intraventricular conduction defect of His-Purkinje system) and sinus bradycardia. AV blocks also can occur and may lead to Stokes-Adams attacks.

(ii) *Arrhythmias*
   - Atrial—premature atrial complexes, atrial flutter, atrial fibrillation, etc.
   - Ventricular—premature ventricular complexes and ventricular tachycardia. Ventricular tachycardia has also been responsible for sudden death.

5. FRIEDREICH'S ATAXIA

The incidence of cardiac involvement is more than 90% in patients with Friedreich's ataxia. The most common cardiac abnormality is hypertrophic (common) or dilated cardiomyopathy (less common). The electrocardiographic features are due to cardiomyopathies.

The Electrocardiogram (Fig. 47.7)

(i) *Features suggestive of hypertrophic cardiomyopathy:* Asymmetric septal hypertrophy or hypertrophy of free walls of ventricles or both, may manifest electrocardiographicaly singly or in combination. The Q waves in leads II, III and aVF may be seen due to septal hypertrophy and may simulate inferior wall infarction. Pattern of left ventricular hypertrophy with or without septal hypertrophy may present in the form of large amplitude of R waves in precordial leads (V_5-V_6). There may be, occasionally, a pattern of right ventricular hypertrophy (large R wave more than S wave in lead V_1), with right axis deviation (for details read ECG features of hypertrophic cardiomyopathy).

(ii) *Features suggestive of dilated cardiomyopathy* in the form of low voltage graph, ST-T wave changes, pattern of either ventricular hypertrophy, conduction disturbances (fascicular or bundle branch blocks) may be seen (For details read ECG features of dilated cardiomyopathy).

(iii) *Arrhythmias:* Atrial flutter or fibrillation or ventricular arrhythmias are commonly seen in patients of Friedreich's ataxia with dilated cardiomyopathy rather than hypertrophic cardiomyopathy.

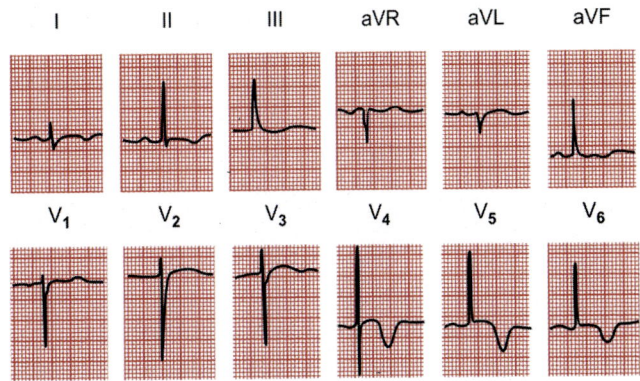

Fig. 47.7: Friedreich's ataxia with cardiomyopathy. The ECG recorded from a 14 yrs boy shows symmetric T wave inversion with cove-plane configuration of ST segment in leads I, II, aVL and V_4-V_6. In addition, there is ST segment depression and T wave inversion in inferior leads (III and aVF)

These ST-T changes in inferior and lateral leads in young boy with Friedreich's ataxia indicate associated cardiomyopathy

6. GUILLAIN-BARRÉ SYNDROME

It is a common neurologic disorder characterised by flaccid paralysis of the limbs with paraesthesias; and is acquired due to post-infective demyelinating polyneuropathy. The syndrome may remain limited to the peripheral parts or may ascend to involve respiratory and bulbar muscles (Landry's ascending paralysis). Autonomic dysfunctions especially sympathetic overactivity may occur and may contribute to electrocardiographic abnormalities.

The Electrocardiogram

1. *Heart rate and rhythm:* There may be wide fluctuations in heart rate and R-R intervals due to dysautonomia. Tachycardia is common.
2. *Arrhythmias:* Both bradyarrhythmias (sinus arrest, complete heart block) and tachyarrhythmias (atrial and ventricular ectopics) are common. Idioventricular rhythm may occur. The chances of arrhythmias are increased in patients who are put on ventilatory support.

7. KUGELBERG-WELANDER SYNDROME

This is childhood proximal spinal muscular atrophy of autosomal recessive transmission. There are a few reports of cardiac involvement in the Kugelberg-Welander syndrome producing atrial fibrillation, atrial standstill, conduction defects (AV blocks) and dilated heart failure.

The Electrocardiogram

(i) *Rhythm disturbances:* Disturbances of rhythm take the form of premature beats (atrial and ventricular), atrial fibrillation, atrial flutter or multifocal atrial tachycardia.

(ii) *Conduction disturbances:* Disturbances in conduction are manifested by impaired AV conduction (first, second and third degree AV block), and abnormalities of infranodal conduction (left anterior fascicular block—left axis deviation, and a bundle branch block)

Suggested Reading

1. Caponnetto S, Patorini C, Tirelli G: Persistent atrial standstill in a patient affected with fascioscapulohumeral muscular dystrophy. *Cardiologia* **53**:341, 1968.
2. Carruth JE, Silverman ME: Torsade de pointes-atypical ventricular tachycardia complicating subarachnoid haemorrhage. *Chest* **78**:886, 1980.
3. Child JS, Perloff JK, Bach PM et al: Cardiac involvement in Friedreich's ataxia. *J Am Coll Cardiol* **7**:1370, 1986.
4. Effendy FN, Bolognesi R, Bianchi G et al: Alteration of partial and total atrial standstill. *J Electrocardiol* **12**:121, 1979.
5. Emery AEH: X-linked muscular dystrophy with early contractures and cardiomyopathy (Emery-Dreifuss type). *Clin Genet* **32**:360, 1987.
6. Gascon P, Ley TJ, Toltzis RJ et al: Spontaneous subarachnoid haemorrhage simulating acute transmural myocardial infarction. *Am Heart J* **105**:511, 1983.
7. Gottdiener JS, Sherber HS, Hawley RJ et al: Cardiac manifestations in polymyositis. *Am J Cardiol* **41**:1141, 1978.
8. Gould L, Reddy RC, Kollali M et al: Electrocardiographic normalisation after cerebrovascular accident. *J Electrocardiol* **14**:191, 1981.
9. Greenland P, Griggs RC: Arrhythmic complications in Guillain-Barré syndrome. *Arch Int Med* **140**:1053, 1980.
10. Hawlay RJ, Milner MR, Gottdiener JS et al: Myotonic heart disease. A clinical follow-up. *Neurology* **41**:259, 1991.
11. James TN, Cobbs BW, Coghlan HC et al: Coronary disease, cardioneuropathy and conduction system abnormalities in cardiomyopathy of Freidreich's ataxia. *Br Heart J* **57**:446, 1987.
12. Kimura S, Yokota H, Tateda K et al: A case of the Kugelberg-Welander syndrome complicated with cardiac lesions. *Jpn Heart J* **21**:417, 1980.
13. Mikolich JR, Jacobs WC, Fletcher GF: Cardiac arrhythmias in patients with acute cerebrovascular accidents. *JAMA* **246**:1314, 1981.
14. Oppenheimer SM, Hachinski VC: The cardiac consequences of Stroke. *Neurol Clin* **10**:167, 1992.
15. Perloff JK, Roberts WC, deLeon AC et al: The distinctive electrocardiogram of Duchenne's progressive muscular dystrophy. *Am J Med* **42**:179, 1967.
16. Perloff JK, Moise NS, Stevenson WG et al: Cardiac electrophysiology in Duchenne's muscular dystrophy: From basic science to clinical expression. *J Cardiovasc Electrophysiol* **3**:394, 1992.
17. Perloff JK: Cardiac rhythm and conduction in Duchenne's muscular dystrophy. *J Am Coll Cardiol* **3**:1263, 1984.
18. Persson A, Solders G: R-R variations in Guillain-Barré syndrome. A test of autonomic dysfunction. *Acta Neurol Scand* **67**:294, 1983.
19. Sluca C: The electrocardiogram in Duchenne's muscular dystrophy. *Circulation* **38**:933, 1968.
20. Stevenson WG, Perloff JK, Weiss JN et al: Fascioscapulohumeral muscular dystrophy: Evidence for selective, genetic, electrophysiologic cardiac involvement *J Am Coll Cardiol* **15**:592, 1990.
21. Stober T, Amstatt T, Sen S et al: Cardiac arrhythmias in subarachnoid haemorrhage. *Acta Neurochir* **93**: 37, 1988.
22. Yamour BJ, Sridharan MR, Rice JF et al: Electrocardiographic changes in cerebrovascular haemorrhage. *Am Heart J* **99**:294, 1990.

Appendices

Appendix A

Cardiac Drugs—Oral and Intravenous

Table: Cardiac drugs—their mechanism of action, dose, uses and special remarks

Drug	Mechanism of action	Dose	Uses	Special remarks
Adrenaline (Epinephrine)	• β_1 (beta 1) and β_2 (beta 2) agonist. • Positive inotropic and chronotropic effects. • Vasoconstrictive and bronchodilator.	For VF/Asystole—1 mg (1:10,000 solu) *IV bolus* (if given peripherally follow with 20 ml NS flush) repeat after 3-5 min as required. *Maintenance dose* is 1-4 µg/min (titrate it to the response).	• Ventricular fibrillation (VF) or asystole. • Hypotension. • Anaphylaxis.	• If IV access delayed in cardiac arrest, can be given via ET route (dilute in 10 ml NS or sterile water, use 2 to 2½ times IV dose). Central route is preferred. • Avoid mixing it in alkaline solutions.
Amiodarone	Class III anti-arrhythmic drug; prolongs action potential and refractory period, inhibits adrenergic stimulation and depresses V_{max}	*Oral:* Loading dose-800 to 1600 mg/day for 1 to 3 weeks. *Maintenance* 600-800 mg/day for 4 weeks then 200/400 mg/day. *IV:* 15 mg/min for 10 min, 1 mg/min for 360 min, 0.5 mg/min thereafter.	• Potentially dangerous or life-threatening ventricular arrhythmias not responding to conventional drugs. • Supraventricular arrhythmias associated with WPW syndrome	• Half life is 13-107 days, may be proarrhythmic, may cause photosensitivity, neuropathy, liver damage, hyperthyroidism and lung fibrosis. • Monitor ECG for bradycardia and prolongation of P-R, QRS and QTc intervals. • Drug interaction may increase serum levels of digoxin, warfarin and class I drugs.
Atenolol	Class II anti-arrhythmic drug (cardioselective beta blocker), decreases HR and BP.	*Oral:* 25-150 mg/day	• Hypertension • Angina pectoris • Postmyocardial Infarction angina.	• Monitor for bradycardia, hypotension and/or CHF. • Avoid it in patients with CHF, asthma, diabetics on hypoglycaemia agents, COPD, sick sinus syndrome and AV blocks
Adenosine	Slows conduction through AV node, interrupts re-entry pathways in AV node.	*IV bolus:* 6 mg over 1-3 min (follow with 20 ml NS flush); If no response within 2 min, then 12 mg rapid IV bolus. For primary poulmonary hypertension: constant IV infusion in doses of	• Narrow QRS complex PSVT. • To judge the effectiveness of ablation of accessory pathway • Useful in paediatric patients for diagnosis and treatment of tachyarrhythmias (PSVT)	• Short half life (5 min). • Flushing, dysphonia, chest pressure are common side effects: • May produce transient bradycardia, sinus arrest, AV blocks and ventricular ectopy as tachycardia terminates

Contd...

APPENDICES

Table Contd...

Drug	Mechanism of action	Dose	Uses	Special remarks
		50 µg/kg/min and increased every 2 min until side effects develop	• Used for stress myocardial perfusion imaing • Primary pulmonary hypertension	• Can be used to determine the origin of wide QRS complex trachycardia, i.e. if ineffective then tachycardia is ventricular rather than supraventricular. It can also, sometimes, reverts VT
Amrinone	Positive inotropic effect (increases CO), vasodilator agent (decreases preload and afterload)	*IV:* Loading dose: 0.75 mg/kg over 2-3 min, may be repeated after 30 min. *Maintenance infusion:* 5-15 µg/kg/min (dose titrated according to response). Do not exceed 10 mg/kg in a day.	CHF	• Avoid mixing it in dextrose; • Incompatible with fursemide; • May exacerbate myocardial ischaemia or worsen ventricular ectopy.
Amlodipine	Class IV antiarrhythmic agent (calcium channel blocker)	Oral 2.5 to 10 mg daily	• Hypertension • Angina • Coronary vasospasm	• Side effects include tachycardia, flushing, GI disturbance, oedema and hyperkalaemia
Atropine	Parasympatholytic agent (increases HR)	*IV:* 0.5-1.0 mg as bolus, repeat every 3-5 min as needed (max. dose 3 mg).	• Symptomatic bradyarrhythmias. • Cardiac asystole.	• If IV access is delayed during asystolic cardiac arrest, may be given via ET route (dilute in 10 ml of NS or sterile water, use 2 × IV dose (twice of IV dose). • Not effective in transplanted heart, hence, use alternative drugs. • May increase myocardial O_2 demand. • May cause urinary retension in old persons.
Bretylium tosylate	Class III antiarrhythmic drug, inhibits release of norepinephrine and is vasodilator.	*IV in VF:* 5 mg/kg as bolus (undiluted), if no response repeat 10 mg/kg IV bolus. Maintain infusion at 1-2 mg/min (Do not exceed 30-35 mg/kg/day).	VF, VT and other potentially life-threatening arrhythmias resistant to conventional therapy.	• Rapid IV administration may cause nausea, vomiting. • In conscious and alert patient, give IV bolus over 8-10 min. • May cause hypotension. Monitor BP. Avoid its use in digitalis toxicity.
Captopril	ACE inhibitor (decreases BP)	• *Oral:* 6.25-100 mg t.i.d. to q.i.d.	• Hypertension • CHF • Prevention of extension of infarction	• Do not give with food or antacid, may cause orthostatic hypotension, cough, rash, fever, angioedema and ARF in bilateral renal artery stenosis.
Carvedilol	A cardioselective beta blocker	• *Oral:* 3.125 mg to 12.5 mg once daily for CHF; 6.25-30 mg daily for hypertension.	• Hypertension • CHF	• Monitor for bradycardia and AV conduction • Monitor for hypotension • To be withdrawn graduallly • Monitor renal functions.

Contd...

Table Contd...

Drug	Mechanism of action	Dose	Uses	Special remarks
Digoxin	Parasympathomimetic action (slows HR and AV conduction); positive inotropic effect (increases cardiac output) It enhances excitability, automaticity and ectopic impulse formation	*Oral:* Loading dose: 0.25-0.5 mg stat then 0.25 mg every 4 hour × 2 doses. *Maintenance*—variable (0.25 mg dose on alternate days or 5 days in a week, etc.) *IV:* Loading dose: 0.25-0.5 mg slow IV bolus, then 0.25 mg IV after 2-4 hours.	• CHF • To slow the ventricular response in atrial fibrillation and atrial flutter • To terminate PSVT.	• Avoid administration within 2 hours of antacid. • May be proarrhythmic. • Monitor K⁺ level and correct hypovolaemia. • Its serum level increases with verapamil, quinidine, amiodarone.
Digoxin immune Fab.	This is an antibody that binds with free (unbound) digoxin. So that it cannot bind to cellular receptors.	*IV:* Unknown digoxin dose—800 mg Known digoxin dose—total body load × 66.7 = dose in mg (infuse through a filter over 30 min except in life-threatening situations; then give IV bolus).	*Overdose* of digitalis preparation (especially in presence of digitalis induced arrhythmias).	Digoxin level rises after its use; indicates digoxin bound to antibody fragments, so levels may be misleading.
Diltiazem	Class IV antiarrhythmic; calcium channel blocker, slows conduction through AV node and is a vasodilator.	*Oral:* 30-120 mg t.i.d. or q.i.d. *IV:* Loading dose: 0.25 mg/kg IV over 2 min, then after 15 min 0.35 mg/kg IV over 2 min. Maintenance dose: 5-15 mg/hr.	• Angina pectoris, • Coronary vasospasm • Hypertension • Non-Q wave MI • Control of ventricular rate in atrial flutter and fibrillation and reverts PSVT • Hypertrophic cardiomyopathy.	• Watch for bradycardia or CHF when used orally. • Watch for hypotension.
Disopyramide	Class IA antiarrhythmic	*Oral:* 100-200 mg 6 hourly or as a long acting prep (200 –400 mg after 12 hr).	• Ventricular arrhythmias • Supraventricular arrhythmias (terminates and prevent recurrent episodes due to AV nodal re-entry)	• Give on an empty stomach. • Monitor for CHF. • May cause torsade de pointes. • May cause dry mouth, constipation, blurred vision, and urinary retention in old persons. • Torsade de pointes
Dobutamine	Adrenergic agonist (simulates β₁-receptors; positive inotropic effect). At low doses increases CO without increase in HR	*IV:* 2-20 µg/kg/min (dose titrated according to response)	• CHF • Cardiogenic shock • For stress myocardial perfusion imaging	• Correct hypovolaemia. • Avoid extravasation into tissues.
Dopamine	Adrenergic agonist; effects dose specific, i.e. i. Low dose enhances renal flow ii. Moderate dose produces positive inotropic effect. iii. High dose produces vasoconstriction.	*IV:* 2-20 µg/kg/min (dose titrated according to response). The dose is tapered gradually.	• CHF • Hypotension	• Correct hypovolaemia. • It is inactivated in alkaline solutions. • If dose required is > 20 µg/kg/min to maintain BP, then use it with dobutamine or norepinephrine.

Contd...

APPENDICES

APPENDICES

Table Contd...

Drug	Mechanism of action	Dose	Uses	Special remarks
Enalapril	ACE inhibitor, reduces BP.	*Oral:* 2.5-40 mg/day in divided doses.	• Hypertension • CHF • To reduce infact size in MI.	• May produce first dose hypotension, hence, monitor BP. • Leucopenia, pancytopenia, cough, rash, fever, angioedema, loss of taste, ARF in bilateral renal artery stenosis and hyperkalaemia
Encainide	Class IC antiarrhythmic drug; suppresses automaticity; and increases refractory period.	*Oral:* 25-50 mg after every 8 hours.	• Supraventricular arrhythmias • Ventricular arrhythmias.	• May be proarrhythmic.
Esmolol	• Short acting β-blocker (decreases HR, BP, Contractility) • Slows conduction through AV node.	*IV:* Loading dose: 500 µg/kg over 1 min. followed by 500 µg/kg/ min infusion over 4 min; may repeat sequence after 5 min with an increase in maintenance infusion dose (do not exceed 200 µg/kg/min).	• Supraventricular tachycardia (SVT) • Hypertension associated with surgical procedures.	• Monitor for hypotension • Monitor for redness, swelling, burning at injection site.
Flecainide	• Class IC antiarrhythmic drug (slows conduction; suppresses automaticity and increases refractory period)	*Oral:* 50 to 100 mg every 12 hr up to 400 mg/day.	• Ventricular arrhythmias • Supraventricular arrhythmias.	• May be proarrhythmic.
Isoproterenol	• β1 and β2 agonist (increases HR and CO) • Vasodilator	*IV:* For asystole and arrhythmias: 2-10 µg/min (titrate the dose according to response)	• Symptomatic bradyarrhythmias unresponsive to atropine. • Temporary control of haemodynamically significant bradycardia in denervated heart. • Refractory torsade de pointes.	• May increase myocardial O₂ demand, hence avoid in acute MI.
Lidocaine (xylocaine)	Class IB antiarrhythmic drug (suppresses automaticity)	*IV:* Loading dose: 1-1.5 mg/kg as bolus, may repeat 0.5-1.5 mg/kg/IV bolus every 5-10 min, maximum to a total of 3 mg/kg. Maintenance infusion at 1-4 mg/min (titrate according to response)	• Ventricular tachyarrhythmias. • Its prophylactic use in AMI is disputed	• If IV access is delayed in cardiac arrest, give it via ET route (dilute in 10 ml NS or sterile water) • Do not use it to suppress ventricular escape beats. • Monitor for mental confusion, delirium, stupor • Rarely, malignant hyperthermia
Labetalol	α and β receptors blocker	*Oral:* 100-600 mg bid *IV:* 2 mg/min	• Hypertension • Phaeochromocytoma	• Similar to β-blocker with more postural effects

Contd...

Table Contd...

Drug	Mechanism of action	Dose	Uses	Special remarks
Lisnopril	ACE inhibitor, reduces BP	*Oral*: 5-40 mg/day in individual doses	Uses similar to Enalapril	Same as with Enalapril
Losartan and Irbesartan	Angiotensin receptors blockers	*Oral*: Losartan 25-50 once or twice a day • Irbesartan 150-300 mg/day	• Hypertension • HT in diabetic nephropathy	• Monitor BP and K⁺ levels • Avoid in pregnancy and bilateral renal artery stenosis
Magnesium	Important cation for heart, plays a role in initiation and maintenance of cardiac contraction.	*IV*: for refractory VT/VF: 1-2 g diluted in 100 ml dextrose (5%), infuse over 1-2 min. *Post MI*: 1-2 g (8-16 mEq) in 50-100 ml dextrose (5%), infuse over 5-60 min, follow with 0.5-1 g/hr. IV over 24 hr.	• Hypomagnesemia in acute MI • Precipitated tachyarrhythmias and pump failure. • Post MI arrhythmias. • Torsade de pointes.	• May cause hypotension, hence monitor BP. • May cause asysole (high doses).
Moricizine HCl	Class IC antiarrhythmic drug (slows conduction; suppresses automaticity and increases refractory period).	*Oral*: Loading dose-300 mg 8 hourly Maintenance dose—100-400 mg 8 hourly.	• Ventricular tachyarrhythmias.	• Proarrhythmic effect • CNS efīcts, i.e. tremors, headache vertigo, nystagmus, etc. • Nausea, vomiting
Metoprolol	Class II antiarrhythmic. (selective β-blocker); decreases HR and CO.	*Oral*: 25-400 mg/day in divided doses. *IV*: For acute MI; 5 mg as bolus,then after every 2 min for 3 doses; then 50 mg orally after 6 hours for 8 doses; then 100 mg oral b.i.d.	• Angina pectoris • Hypertension • Supraventricular arrhythmias. • Acute MI • Hypertrophic cardiomyopathy.	• Give with food • Monitor for bradycardia, hypotension and CHF. • Contraindications are similar to atenolol • Side effects—dizziness, depression, bronchospasm, GI symptoms, hypertriglyceridemia, Raynaud's phenomenon • Sudden withdrawal may precipitate angina or CHF
Mexiletine	Class IB antiarrhythmic drug (decreases duration of action potential and refractory period)	Oral: 200-400 mg tid upto 1200 mg/day	• Ventricular tachyarrhythmias.	• Give with food. • Monitor for liver dysfunction. • Monitor for hypotension and bradycardia • May cause CNS effects (tremors, dysarthria, diplopia, dizziness, nystagmus, etc)
Nadolol	Class II antiarrhythmic drug (nonselective β-blocker)	*Oral*: 40-120 mg (max. dose upto 240 mg)	• Angina pectoris • Hypertension • Supraventricular arrhythmias.	• Monitor for bradycardia and CHF. • Drug level increases with renal failure. • Contraindications and side effects are same as with other β-blockers
Nifedipine	Class IV antiarrhythmic drug (calcium channel blocker)	*Oral*: 10-40 mg tid or qid (max 160 mg/day) *Sublingual*: 5-10 mg (titrate	• Angina pectoris • Coronary vasospasm • Hypertension.	• Monitor for CHF • May cause peripheral oedema, flushing, tachycardia,

Contd...

APPENDICES

APPENDICES

Table Contd...

Drug	Mechanism of action	Dose	Uses	Special remarks
		the dose according to response). It lowers the BP in accelerated or malignant hypertension or hypertensive emergency.		hyperkalaemia and GI disturbances
Nitroglycerin	Vasodilator (venodilation, reduces preload and improves collaterals formation to ischaemic myocardium	*IV:* 5-20 µg/min and titrate higher dose according to response. Sublingual: 0.4 mg dose upto 3 doses. Local ointment (transdermal)	• Unstable angina • Acute MI • Preload reduction in CHF • Hypertension associated with surgical procedures. • Sublingual for relief of anginal pain • Locally used for anginal pain and to prevent thrombophlebitis	• Prepare admixture in glass bottle and protect from sunlight. • Use nonpolyvinyl chloride tubing (as drug may be absorbed into conventional polyvinyl chloride tubing). • Monitor for hypotension. • Correct hypovolaemia.
Nitroprusside	Vasodilator (arterio-dilator, reduces afterload)	*IV:* 0.5-10.0 µg/min (titrate it according to the response)	• Hypertensive crisis or Hypertensive encephalopathy. • Afterload reduction in CHF.	• Protect from light • Monitor serum cyanate and the thiocyanate levels; may cause weakness, diaphrosis and muscle twitchings. • Monitor for hypotension and metabolic acidosis. • May exacerbate myocardial ischaemia.
Norepinephrine (noradrenaline)	• α and $β_1$ agonist • Vasoconstrictor, raises BP. • Some positive inotropic effect (increases CO)	*IV:* 0.5-1 µg/min up to 30 µg/min (titrate according to response)	• Hypotension or shock.	• Avoid extravasation (causes tissue necrosis on extravasation) • Do not infuse in alkaline solution. • Correct hypovolaemia.
Phenylephrine	α-agonist (vasoconstriction) raises BP.	*IV:* Loading dose: 0.1-0.18 mg/min. Maintenance: 0-04-0.06 mg/min (titrate dose according to response).	• Hypotension.	• Avoid extravasation.
Phenytoin	• Class IB antiarrhythmic drug (suppresses automaticity and enhances conduction through AV node) • Antiepileptic drug	*Oral:* 100 mg tid or qid. *IV:* Loading dose: 50-100 mg after 10-15 min with max. upto 1 gm.	• Ventricular tachyarrhythmias especially digitalis induced. • Torsade de pointes.	• Give it with food. • Avoid administration within 2 hour of antacid ingestion. • Monitor for blood dyscrasias. • Gum hypertrophy and bleeding. • Monitor calcium. • Avoid administration in dextrose as infusion (precipitate will form) • Rapid IV administration may cause CNS depression and hypotension. • May cause cerebellar dysfunction, i.e. nystagmus, ataxia, etc

Contd...

Table Contd...

Drug	Mechanism of action	Dose	Uses	Special remarks
Procainamide	Class IA antiarrhythmic drug (suppresses automaticity and excitability)	*Oral:* 250-1000 mg after 3-6 hours; long acting prep. 500-1000 mg after 6 hrs. *IV:* 25-50 mg over 1 minute, then repeat every 5 min. until arrhythmia is controlled or hypotension results or QTc is prolonged. Dose of constant rate infusion is (2-6 mg/min) (Total IV dose is 1000-2000 mg)	• Ventricular tachyarrhythmias. • Supraventricular tachyarrhythmias. (converts AF to sinus rhythm)	• To be taken empty stomach. • May be associated with torsade de pointes. • Drug induced SLE, hypersensitivity reactions. • Monitor for hypotension during IV use. • Widening of QRS and prolongation of QTc. • CNS side effects (psychosis, hallucinations, depression, etc)
Propafenone	• Class IC antiarrhythmic drug (blocks fast Na$^+$ channels, prolongs conduction through AV node; suppresses automaticity and triggered activity) • Some beta blocker activity.	*Oral:* 150 mg tid upto 300 mg tid. (Do not exceed 1200 mg/day)	• Ventricular tachyarrhythmias.	• May be proarrhythmic. • Dizziness, disturbance in taste and blurred vision are common side effects • Bronchoconstriction
Propranolol	Class II antiarrhythmic drug (nonselective β-blocker) decreases HR, BP and slows conduction through AV node.	*Oral:* 10-80 mg tid or qid upto 320 mg/day *IV:* 0.5-3 mg as bolus, may repeat in 2 min; then after every 4 hours.	• Angina pectoris • Hypertension • Supraventricular arrhythmias. • AMI • Hypertrophic cardiomyopathy • Thyrotoxic heart disease	• Give with food • Monitor for bradycardia, AV block and CHF. • Side effects–dizziness, depression, bronchospasm, fatigue and raised lipids levels • Sudden withdrawal may precipitate angina and MI
Quinidine	Class IA antiarrhythmic drug (decreases automaticity and excitability)	*Oral for APC/VPC:* 200-300 mg after every 6-8 hours. *For PSVT:* 400-600 mg after every 2-3 hrs until reverted, then 200-300 mg after every. 6-8 hours.	• Supraventricular arrhythmias • Ventricular arrhythmias.	• To be taken empty stomach • Monitor for GI disturbance • May be associated with torsade de pointes and cardiac syncope • Monitor QRS and QTc. • Phenobarbitone and phenytoin shortens its action by enzyme induction. It elevates serum digoxin levels
Ramipril	ACE inhibitor, reduce BP	*Oral:* 2.5-20 mg daily in one or two doses	Uses similar to Enalapril and Lisinopril	Same as with Enalapril and Lisinopril
Sotalol	Class II (beta-blocker) and Class III (lengthens action potential duration) antiarrhythmic properties.	*Oral:* 80 to 160 mg bid upto 320 mg/day (rarely upto 640 mg/day)	• Ventricular tachyarrhythmias	• Watch for any arrhythmia (proarrhythmic effect). • Monitor QTc interval • Reduce the dose in renal insufficiency (clearance is through kidneys)

Contd...

APPENDICES

Table Contd...

Drug	Mechanism of action	Dose	Uses	Special remarks
Timolol	Class II antiarrhythmic drug (nonselective β-blocker); decreases HR and BP; and slows conduction through AV node.	*Oral:* 10-20 mg bid to maximum of 60 mg/day.	• Angina pectoris • Hypertension • Supraventricular arrhythmias • Acute MI • Hypertrophic cardiomyopathy	• Monitor for bradycardia and CHF • Contraindications and side effects are similar to atenolol and Metoprolol
Trimethaphan	• Sympathetic and autonomic ganglion blocker. • Vasodilator (decreases BP).	*IV:* 0.5-6.0 mg/min, and titrate slowly for response.	• Hypertensive crisis • Aortic dissection	• May cause respiratory arrest, postural hypotension, dry mouth, visual symptoms, constipation, urinary retention, impotence, etc.
Tocainide	Class IB antiarrhythmic drug (supresses automaticity)	*Oral:* 400-600 mg 8 hourly upto 2400 mg/day.	• Ventricular tachyarrhythmias.	• Give with food • CNS side effcts
Verapamil	(i) Class IV antiarrhythmic drug (calcium channel blocker); slows conduction through AV node, slows HR and decreases BP. (ii) Vasodilator effect	*Oral:* 40-120 mg tid or qid upto 480 mg/day *IV:* 2.5-5.0 mg IV bolus over 2 min; may repeat after 10-15 min as 5-10 mg over 2 min to a total of 20 mg.	• Angina pectoris • Hypertension • Controls ventricular rate in atrial fibrillation and atrial flutter and may revert it. • Terminates narrow QRS complex PSVT.	• Give it with food • Monitor for bradycardia and CHF • Do not give in presence of VT.

Abbrev: HR = Heart rate, BP = Blood pressure, MI = Myocardial infarction, CHF = Congestive heart failure, AV = Atrioventricular, SVT = Supraventricular tachycardia, PSVT = Paroxysmal supraventricular tachycardia, ACE = Angiotensin converting enzyme, CO = Cardiac output, ECG = Electrocardiogram, IV = Intravenous, APC = Atrial premature complex, VF = Ventricular fibrillation, VT = Ventricular tachycardia, ET = Endotracheal tube, NS = Normal saline. IV use is limited to emergency situations
Note: This is brief account of antiarrhythmic drugs and is applicable to adult patient only and the doses described are for arrhythmias unless otherwise stated. For in-depth knowledge and indications, contraindications, dosages, route of administration and side effects, always consult pharmacology reference book.

Appendix B
Normal 12-Lead Surface ECG and Its Variations in Adults

An understanding of the normal range of electrocardiographic deflections and its variation in adults depends on the basic understanding of normal and abnormal electrophysiology of the heart. Many of the configurations which may appear normal but may represent abnormalities when interpreted in the light of clinical findings. Therefore, the information given in the table is to be used as a guide to the interpretation of ambiguous and barderline graphs. It is stressed that for proper interpretation, a good electrocardiogram reflecting these deflections is must.

Lead	P wave	Q wave	R wave	S wave	ST segment	T wave
I	Upright 1 mm in amplitude 3 mm (0.12 sec) in width	Small 0.04 sec and less than 25% of R wave	Dominant, largest deflection out of QRS.	Small, less than R or negligible	Usually isoelectric, may vary from + 1 to –0.5 mm	Upright
II	Upright, 2 mm in amplitude and 3 mm in width	Small or none	Dominant	Less than R wave or none.	Usually isoelectric may vary from +1 to –0.5 mm	Upright
III	Upright, flat, biphasic or inverted depending on frontal plane axis; 2 mm in amplitude and 3 mm in width.	Small or none may be large 0.04 sec and 25% of R wave depending on frontal plane axis.	None to small or dominant depending on frontal plane axis.	None to dominant depending on frontal plane axis.	Usually isoelectric may vary from +1 to – 0.5 mm.	Upright, flat, biphasic or inverted depending on frontal plane axis.
aVR	Inverted	Small, none or large (QS complex)	None or small depending on frontal plane axis.	Usually QS complex (cavity pattern)	Usually isoelectric, may vary from +1 to –0.5 mm	Inverted
aVL	Upright, flat, biphasic or inverted depending on frontal plane axis.	Small, none or large depending on frontal plane axis.	Small, none or large depending on frontal plane axis.	None to dominant depending on frontal plane axis.	Usually isoelectric may vary from +1 to –0.5 mm	Upright, flat, biphasic or inverted depending on frontal plane axis.

Contd...

APPENDICES

Table Contd...

Lead	P wave	Q wave	R wave	S wave	ST segment	T wave
aVF	Upright	Small, or none	Small none or large depending on frontal plane axis.	None to dominant depending on frontal plane axis.	Usually isoelectric, may vary from +1 to –0.5 mm.	Upright, flat, biphasic or inverted depending on frontal plane axis.
V_1	Biphasic, upright, flat or inverted	None or may be QS	Less than S, or none (QS complex) small r' may be present	Dominant sometimes, QS pattern	0 to +3 mm	Upright flat or biphasic or inverted.
V_2	Upright, biphasic or inverted	None, may be QS complex	Less than S or none (QS) or small r' may be present	Dominant or may be QS complex	0 to +3 mm	Upright flat, biphasic or inverted
V_3	Upright	None	R less than or equal to or greater than S.	S greater than or equal to or less than R	0 to 3 mm	Upright
V_4	Upright	None	R>S	S<R	Usually isoelectric or may vary from +1 to –0.5 mm	Upright
V_5	Upright	Small	Dominant < 27 mm	S wave is less than S wave in V_4, and S < R	Same	Upright
V_6	Upright	Small	Dominant < 26 mm	S less than S wave of V_5, and S < R	Same	Same

Appendix C
Analysis of an Arrhythmia

1. **The atrial rhythm:** Look for the P wave in leads II, III, aVF and V₁, or rhythm strip showing any one of the leads. For accurate analysis of arrhythmia, a long strip of at least 1 minute should be recorded.

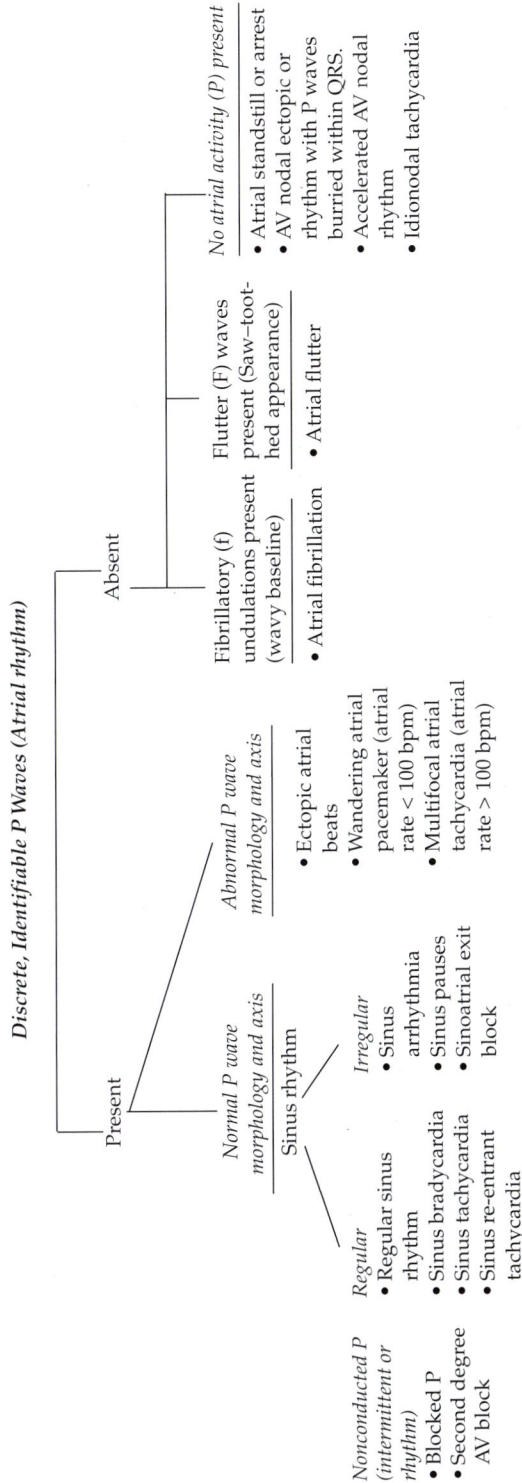

Discrete, Identifiable P Waves (Atrial rhythm)

Present

Normal P wave morphology and axis
Sinus rhythm

Regular
- Regular sinus rhythm
- Sinus bradycardia
- Sinus tachycardia
- Sinus re-entrant tachycardia

Irregular
- Sinus arrhythmia
- Sinus pauses
- Sinoatrial exit block

Nonconducted P (intermittent or rhythm)
- Blocked P
- Second degree AV block

Abnormal P wave morphology and axis
- Ectopic atrial beats
- Wandering atrial pacemaker (atrial rate < 100 bpm)
- Multifocal atrial tachycardia (atrial rate > 100 bpm)

Absent

Fibrillatory (f) undulations present (wavy baseline)
- Atrial fibrillation

Flutter (F) waves present (Saw-toothed appearance)
- Atrial flutter

No atrial activity (P) present
- Atrial standstill or arrest
- AV nodal ectopic or rhythm with P waves burried within QRS.
- Accelerated AV nodal rhythm
- Idionodal tachycardia

APPENDICES

APPENDICES

2. **The QRS rhythm:** Look for the relation of P waves to QRS. Note whether basic atrial rhythm is associated with or dissociated from QRS.

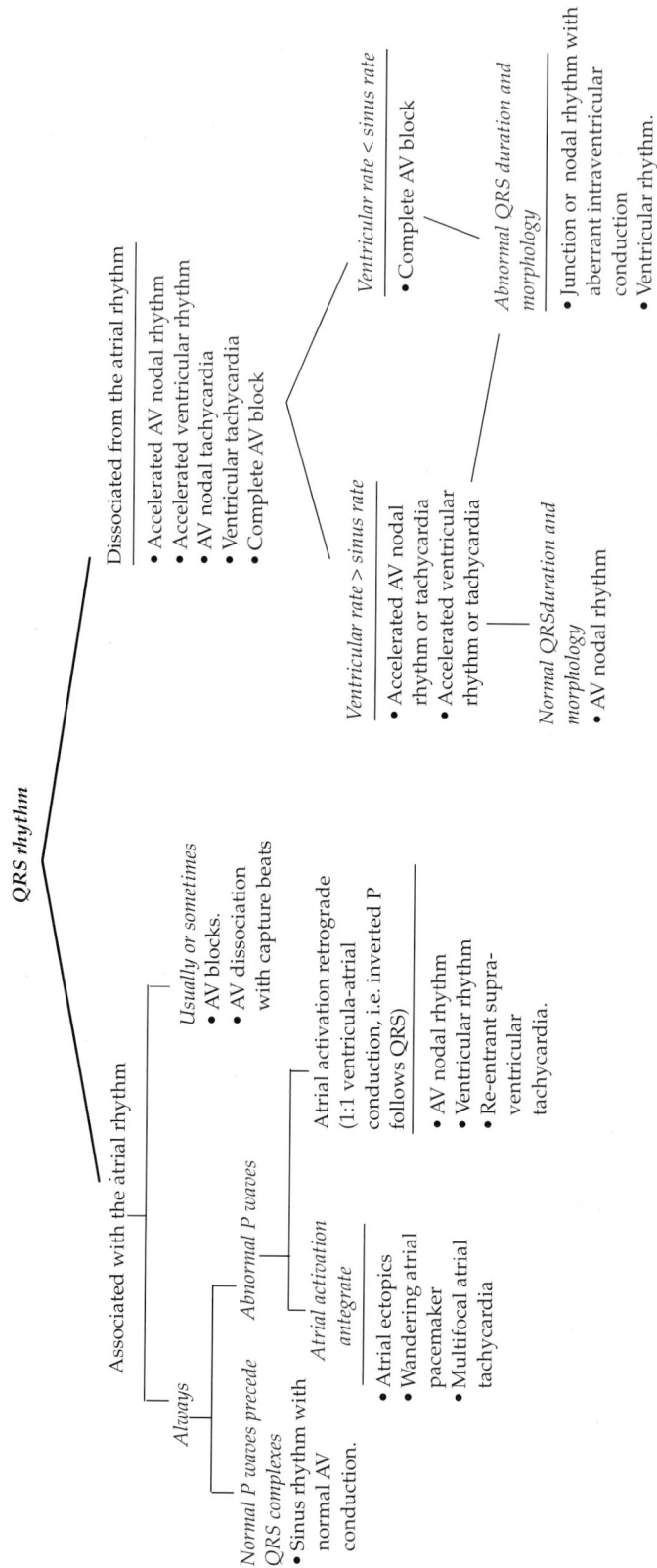

QRS rhythm

- **Associated with the atrial rhythm**
  - *Always*
    - *Normal P waves precede QRS complexes*
      - Sinus rhythm with normal AV conduction.
    - *Abnormal P waves*
      - *Atrial activation antegrate*
        - Atrial ectopics
        - Wandering atrial pacemaker
        - Multifocal atrial tachycardia
      - Atrial activation retrograde (1:1 ventricula-atrial conduction, i.e. inverted P follows QRS)
        - AV nodal rhythm
        - Ventricular rhythm
        - Re-entrant supraventricular tachycardia.
  - *Usually or sometimes*
    - AV blocks.
    - AV dissociation with capture beats

- **Dissociated from the atrial rhythm**
  - Accelerated AV nodal rhythm
  - Accelerated ventricular rhythm
  - AV nodal tachycardia
  - Ventricular tachycardia
  - Complete AV block

  - *Ventricular rate > sinus rate*
    - *Normal QRS duration and morphology*
      - AV nodal rhythm
    - *Abnormal QRS duration and morphology*
      - Accelerated AV nodal rhythm or tachycardia
      - Accelerated ventricular rhythm or tachycardia

  - *Ventricular rate < sinus rate*
    - Complete AV block
    - *Abnormal QRS duration and morphology*
      - Junction or nodal rhythm with aberrant intraventricular conduction
      - Ventricular rhythm.

Appendix D
Proforma for ECG Reporting

Name   Age and Sex   OPD/CR No.

Drug if being taken   Bed No._____

Standardisation

Voltage

Heart rate

Rhythm

Rotation of heart

Position of heart

P wave
- Amplitude
- Width/duration

P-R interval (second)_____

QRS complex
- Axis_____
- Duration_____

- Configuration_____

Normal_____
or
Abnormal: Deep Q waves in leads_____
R= S complex in leads_____
Deep S wave in leads_____

ST segment e.g.:
- Coved_____
- Raised_____
- Plane depression_____

In leads_____

T wave
- Low to inverted
- Tall and symmetrical

Throughout or in leads_____

U wave
- Inverted_____
- Prominent_____

In leads_____

QT or QTU and QTc (seconds)_____

Abnormalities detected: List the abnormalities
                             1.
                             2.
                             3.
                             4.
                             5.
                             6.

Conclusions

Terminology to be used   1. Normal electrocardiogram
                             2. Electrocardiogram within normal limits
                             3. Borderline electrocardiogram (List questionable features and
                                 give suggestion if needed)
                             4. Abnormal electrocardiogram suggestive/diagnostic of . . . .
                             5. Abnormal electrocardiogram consistent with . . . .
                             6. Nonspecific electrocardiographic changes

FURTHER SUGGESTION/ADVICE WHENEVER NECESSARY

1. Suggest serial records.
2. Suggest recording of additional leads or long strip of a lead.
3. Record leads III and aVF in deep inspiration and deep expiration.
4. Advise exercise/stress test or Holter monitoring.

Signature of Physician

APPENDICES

Appendix E
The ABCs of Cardiopulmonary Resuscitation

Basic life support implies the maintenance of an airway and, the support of breathing and the circulation without the use of equipment other than a simple airway device is called cardiopulmonary resuscitation (CPR). The CPR- a combination of expired air ventilation and chest compressions forms the basis of modern basic life support. The term *cardiac arrest* means a sudden arrest of cardiac output, which may be reversible with appropriate management. It does not include the stoppage of respiratory activity as terminal event in serious illness; in these situations, the techniques of basic life support are usually appropriate.

Survival from cardiac arrest is most likely when it is of recent onset and is witnessed; when the bystander summons help from the emergency services and starts immediate resuscitation without any further loss of time; for example cardiac arrest in VF; and when defibrillation and advanced life support measure are instituted at an early stage.

Basic life support is the emergency treatment of any acute condition in which the brain suddenly fails to receive enough O_2. It involves assessment followed by action of the ABC. A stands for *airway*, B but *breathing* and C for *circulation.*

ASSESSMENT

Immediately assess any danger to the victim and yourself from such hazards as falling masonry electricity wire, gas or traffic. Establish whether the victim is conscious or unconscious by shaking his/her shoulders and asking loudly "Hello; Are you OK? Be careful not to aggravate any existing injury, particularly of the cervical spine.

If victim is unresponsive, shout loudly for help or send a onlooker or bystander to telephone for an ambulance. Complete your assessment by opening the airway, checking for breathing and feeling the pulse.

Loosen the tight clothes around the victim's neck and remove any obvious obstruction from the mouth; leave the tight fitted denture in place. Extend but do not hyperextend the neck thus lifting the tongue off the posterior wall of pharynx. This is achieved by placing one hand on the forehead of victim and exerting pressure to tilt the head, at the same time placing two fingers under the point of the chin to lift it forwards (Fig. 1). This will often allow the breathing to restart

Look for chest movements; listen for breath sounds and feel for air with your cheek; spend about 5 seconds for these procedures before deciding that breathing is absent

Feel the pulse. The best pulse to feel in an emergency situation is the carotid (Fig. 1B), but if the neck is injured, the pulse may be felt at the femoral artery. Spend atleast 5 second before deciding that pulse is absent.

ACTION

If the victim is unconscious but pulse is present and he/she is breathing, place his/her in the recovery position, if necessary, supporting the chin to maintain a patent airway; in this position the tongue will clear the posterior pharyngeal wall and any vomit or secretion will dribble out of the angle of the mouth rather than obstructing the airway, or later on, cause risk of aspiration pneumonia

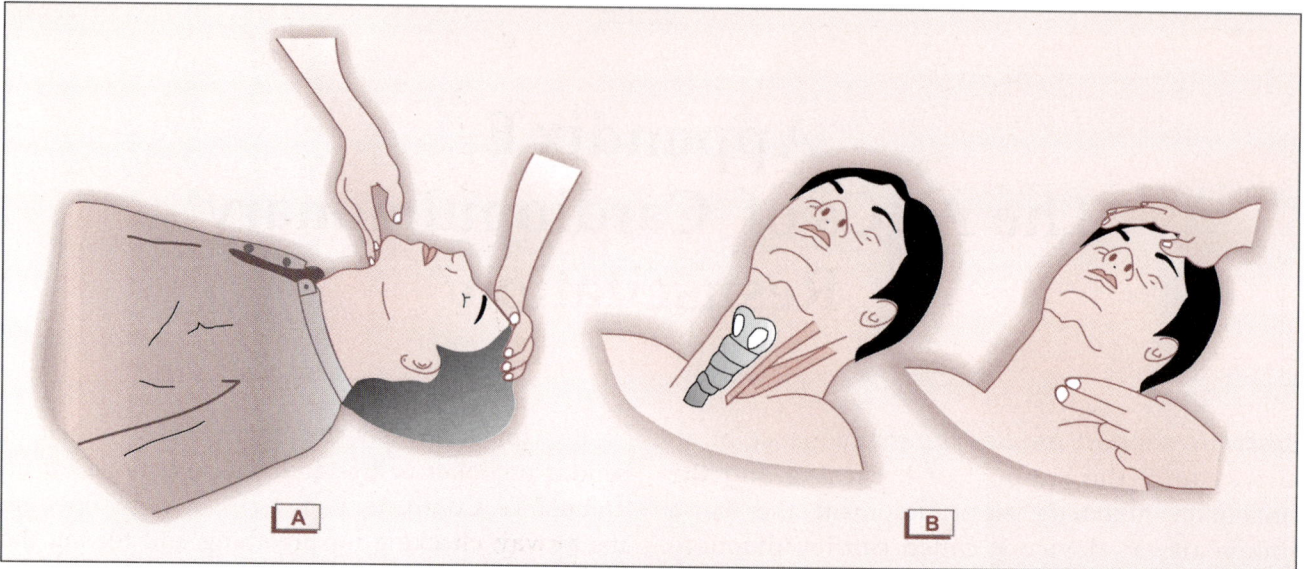

Fig. 1: (A) Head tilt and chin lift (B) Checking the pulse

Go or telephone for help if you do not have any other rescuer.If the pulse or breathing is absent your immediate action will be to follow ABC of Cardiopulmonary Resuscitation.

A. AIRWAY

Clearing the airway is critical step in preparation for cardiac resuscitation. If tilting the head and lifting the chin do not clear the airway, then it seems that a foreign body might be obstructing the airway. First try to remove it by sweeping the fingers in the mouth. If desired result is not achieved, give five firm blows between the scapulae, this may dislodge a foreign body by compressing the air that remains in the lungs thereby producing an upward thurst of force behind the obstructing material and dislodging it and leading to its subsequent expulsion (Fig. 2).

If both fingers sweep and back blows are not able to clear the airway, then try five abdominal thrust (Fig. 3B). If person is unconscious, then kneel over the victim, make a fist of one of your hand and place it immediately below the victim's xiphisternum (Fig. 3A).

The Heimlich' Maneuver (Abdominal Thrust)

Grasp your fist with your other hand and push firmly and suddenly upwards and backwards (Fig. 4).

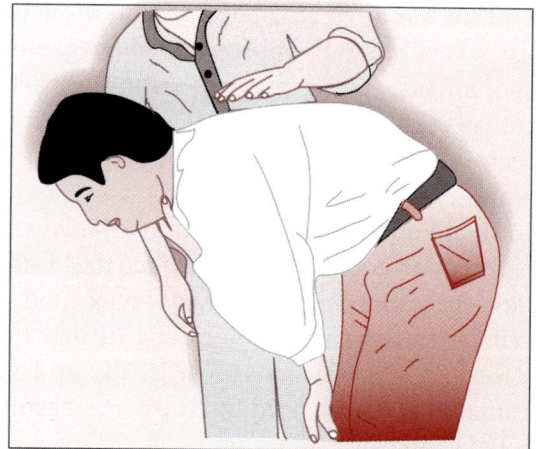

Fig. 2: Choking and back blows

Discharge alternate abdominal thrust with back slaps (Fig. 5). The Heimlich maneuver is not entirely benign. Ruptured abdominal viscera in the victim have been reported.

Note: It there is strong suspicion that respiratory arrest precipitates cardiac arrest, particularly in the presence of a mechanical airway obstruction, a second precordial thump should be delivered after the airway is cleared.

B. BREATHING (Fig. 6)

When there is no breathing but pulse is present then make the victim to lie on his/her back and deliver 10

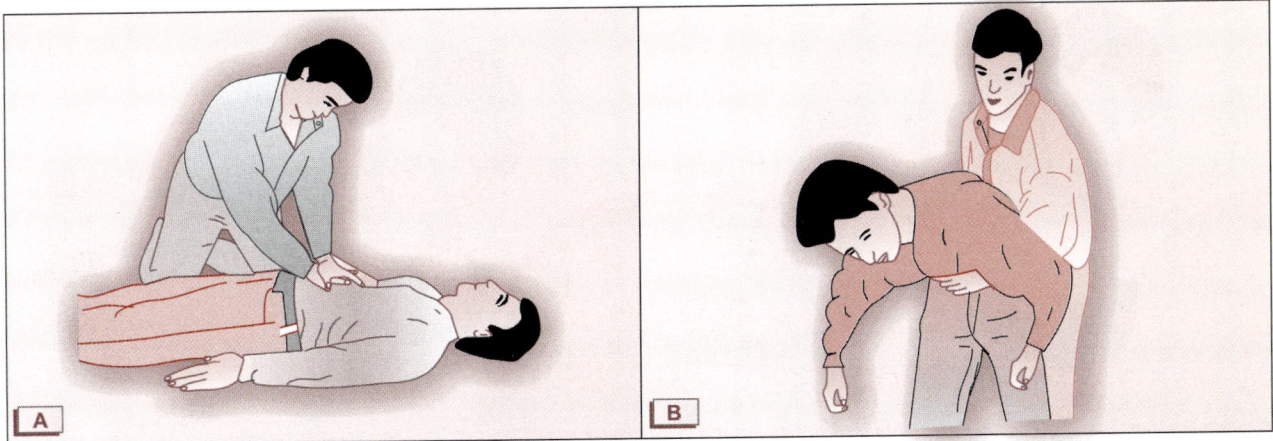

Fig. 3: Abdominal thrust. (A) In unconscious patient state, (B) Conscious patient

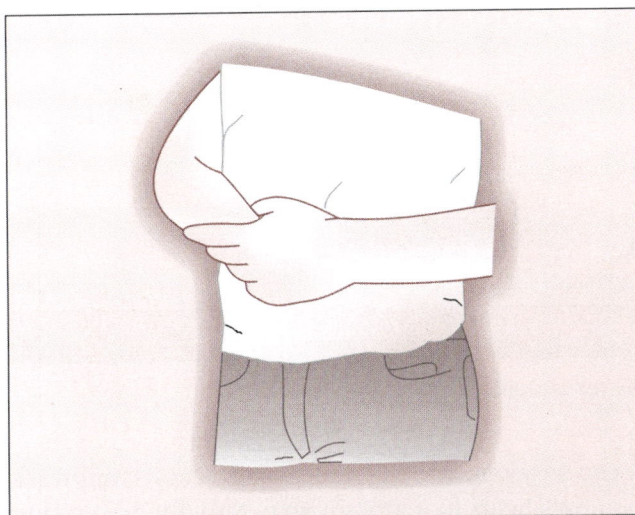

Fig. 4: Heimlich's maneuver in conscious patient

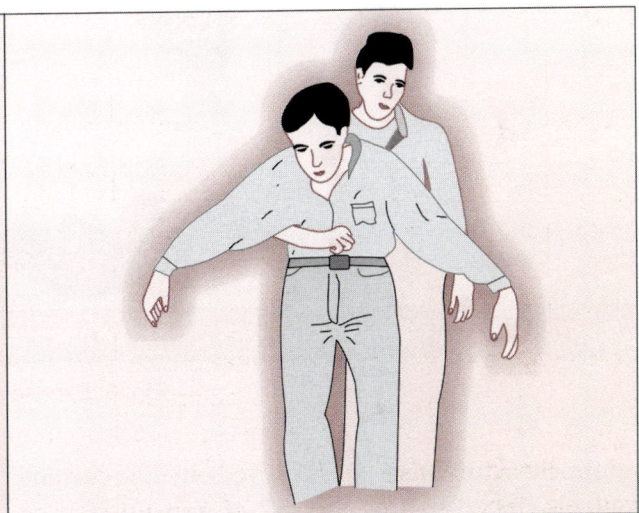

Fig. 5: Alternate abdominal thrust with back slaps

breaths of expired air ventilation. Maintain the patent airway by tilting the head and lifting the chin. Close the nose with fingers of your hand on the forehead. Take a deep breath, seal your lips formally around those of victim, and breath out until your see the victim's chest clearly rising taking about 2 seconds for a full ventilation. Move your head away, observe the victim's chest fall and take another deep breath and breath out the air; the chest should rise as you blow in and fall when you take your mouth away. Each breath must visibly expand the victim's chest but not cause overinflation as this may cause entry of air into oesophagus and stomach causing gastric distension and vomiting but passive regurgitation into

the lungs may often goes undetected. After 10 ventilations if victim's spontaneous breathing does not take place and help is not available then, make arrangement to shift the patient to the hospital. Till arrangements are made, reassess consciousness, breathing and the pulse, and continue ventilation as necessary, rechecking the pulse after every ten breaths.

In hospital setting, a variety of devices are available including plastic oropharyngeal airways, oesophageal obturators, the masked AMBU bag and endotracheal tube. Intubation is the procedure of choice but time should not be wasted even in the hospital setting, therefore temporary support with AMBU bag ventilation is the usual method until

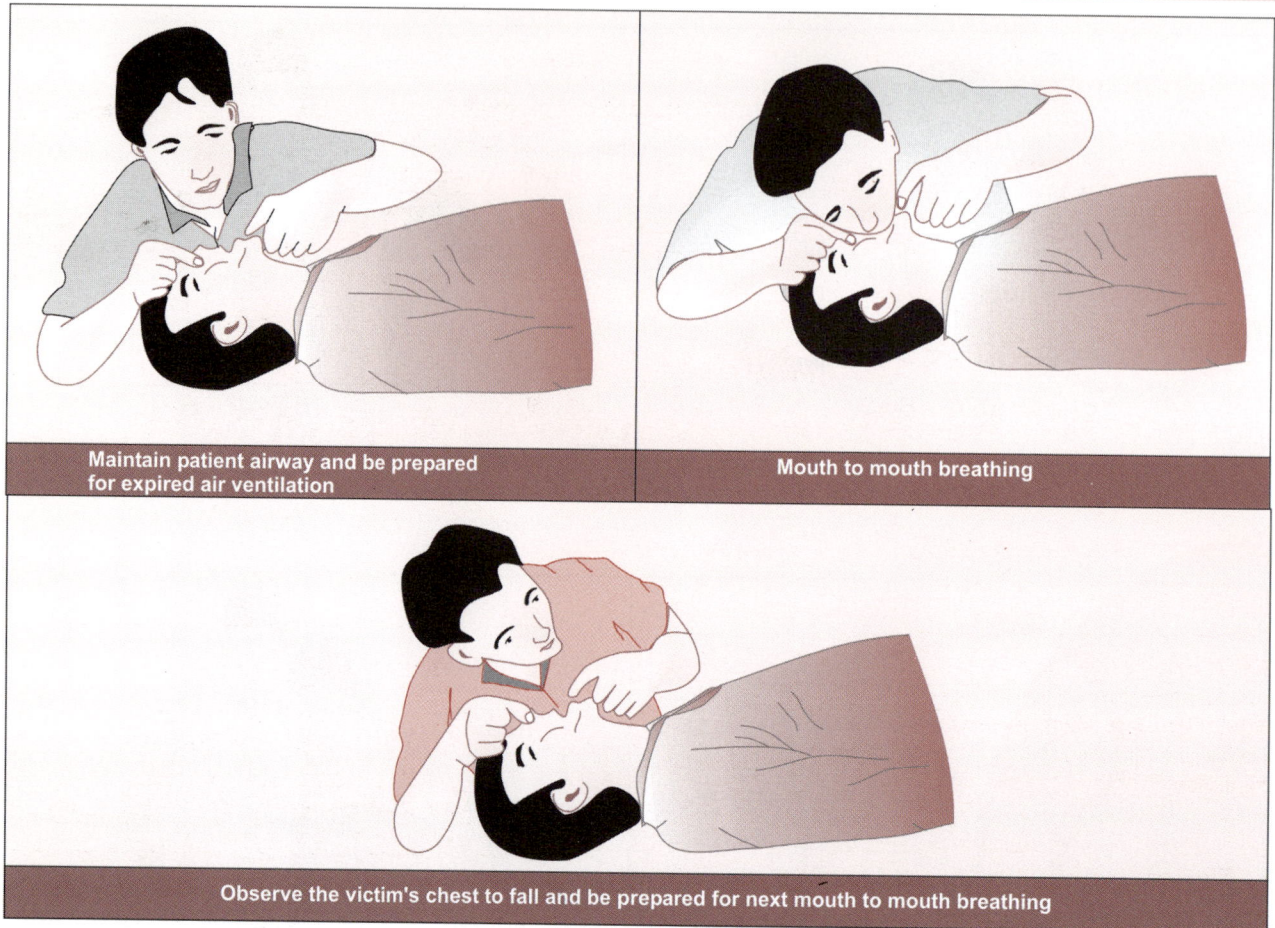

Maintain patient airway and be prepared for expired air ventilation

Mouth to mouth breathing

Observe the victim's chest to fall and be prepared for next mouth to mouth breathing

Fig. 6: Expired air resuscitation

endotracheal tube insertion is carried out. The current available data assessing the risk of transmission of AIDS and hepatitis B infection during mouth to mouth breathing is minimal and risk predicted is very low.

Conventional CPR ventilatory techniques require that the lungs be inflated 10 to 12 times/ minute whether one or two rescuers are present. In one rescuer resuscitation, a pause for ventilation (two breaths) is taken after every 15 chest compressions; for two rescuers one breath is administrated after every fifth compression. The techniques of CPR are based on the hypothesis that increased intrathoracic pressure is prime mover of the blood, rather than cardiac compression itself.

C. CIRCULATION

This element of basic life support is intended to maintain blood flow, i.e. circulation until definite steps can be taken. The rationale behind chest compression allows heart to maintain an externally driven pump action by sequential emptying and filling of its chambers with competent valves favoring the forward flow.

If no breathing and no pulse, ask for help immediately to transfer the patient to a hospital nearby.

If the pulse is absent (cardiac arrest), the victim is unlikely to recover as a result of cardiopulmonary resuscitation (CPR) alone; defibrillation and other advanced life support is urgently required. If you are alone, call for help to shift the patient and telephone for an ambulance. In the mean time, make the victim lie on his/her back on the firm surface (floor), open the airway by tilting the head and lifting the chin, and give two breaths of expired air ventilation and start chest compressions (2 breaths after every 15 chest compressions).

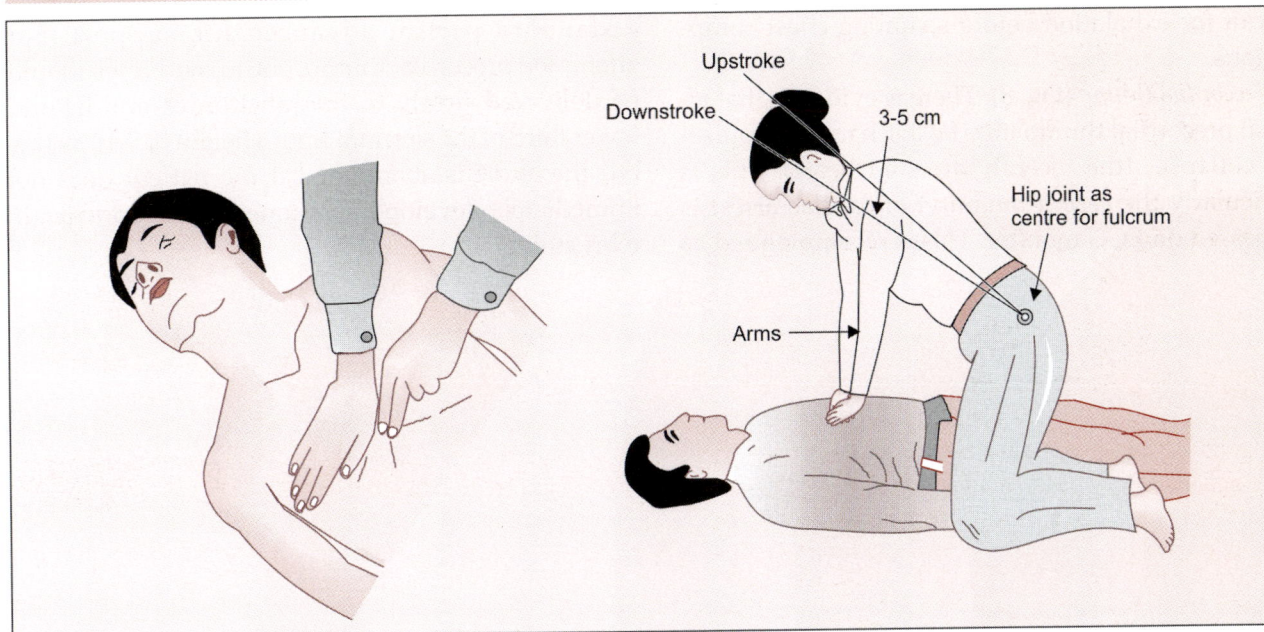

Fig. 7: External chest compression
Left: locating the correct hand position on lower half of the sternum
Right: Proper position of rescuers. Shoulders are directly over the victim's sternum and elbows are locked.
Sufficient force to be used to depress the sternum by 1 to 2" (3-5 cm) with abrupt relaxation at a rate of 80-100
compressions / min

The correct place to compress the chest is the centre of the lower half of the sternum. Locate the xiphisternum by feeling along the rib margin, place your middle finger on the xiphisternum and index finger on the bony sternum above. Slide the heel of your other hand down to these fingers and leave it there. Remove your first hand, place it on the dorsum of lower hand (second). Depress the sternum firmly by keeping your arm straight and elbows locked so as to provide a less tiring and more forceful fulcrum at the junction of the shoulders and back (Fig. 7), using this technique in an adult, compress the sternum about 3-5 cm keeping the pressure firm, controlled and applied vertically, with abrupt relaxation, and the cycle is carried out at a rate of 80 compressions in a minute.

After each 15 compressions, give two breaths of expired air ventilation. Return your hands immediately to the sternum and give 15 further compressions, and continue compressions and ventilation in a ratio of 15:2.

In case two rescuers are present, one should assume the responsibility for ventilation and the other

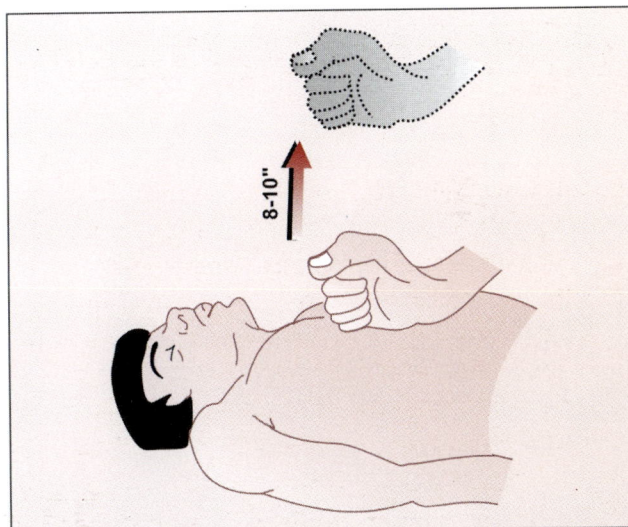

Fig. 8: Precordial thump. A firm blow with closed fist to be discharged at the junction of middle and lower third of sternum

for chest compression. The compression rate will remain same as 80 compression in a minute, but now there will be a pause after every 5 compressions to allow a single ventilation in a ratio of 5:1. Provided the victim's airway is maintained it is not necessary to wait for exhalation before resuming chest compressions.

Precordial thump (Fig. 8): There is evidence that an initial precordial thump may be discharged in pulseless collapse (the recently arrested heart). This is particularly the case if the onset of cardiac arrest is witnessed on ECG monitor. This is recommended as a standard part of advanced life support. For attempted precordial thump, one to two blows should be delivered firmly to the junction of middle and lower third of the sternum from a height of 8-10 inches, but the effort is abandoned if the patient does not immediately develop a spontaneous pulse and begin rebreathing.

Index

Note: Symbol *f* denotes for figure and *t* denotes for table.

A

Aberrant intraventricular conduction 503
Action potential 13, 14 *f*
    clinical importance of 14
    generation in pacemaker cell 13
Acute rheumatic carditis 339
Adrenal insufficiency 560
Angina pectoris 217
Antiarrhythmic drugs 15
Aorto-Pulmonary communication
        (WINDOW) 310
Arrhythmia, analysis of 609
Arrhythmias, classification of (t) 398
Arrhythmogenesis 399
    abnormal automaticity 400
    anatomical re-entry 402 *f*
    concealed conduction 405
    graphic representation for intracardiac
        conduction 400 *f*
    mechanism of arrhythmogenesis 401 *f*
    parasystole 405
    phenomenon of concealed conduction
        404 *f*
    QT dispersion 405
    re-entry (circus movement) mechanism
        403 *f*
    single focus of subthreshold activity
        (Wedensky facilitation) 405
    supernormal conduction 402
    tachyarrhythmias due to re-entry 403
    triggered activity 400
Atrial activity, unconventional leads 11
    intra-atrial leads 11
    lewis lead 11
    oesophageal leads 11, 12 *f*
Atrial arrhythmias 412
Atrial bigeminy 415
Atrial bigeminy rhythm 415 *f*
Atrial ectopics 412
    abnormal P wave morphology 412
    atrial premature beats with normal and
        short P-R intervals 413 *f*
    atrial premature complexes (APCs) 413
        with retrograde conduction 413 *f*
    clinical significance 415
    compensatory pause 414
    conduction 414
    deformity of T wave 415
    fixed coupling interval 413

heart rate and rhythm 412
    multifocal atrial ectopics 413 *f*
    P-R interval 414
    shape of QRS 414
    wenckebach's conduction 414 *f*
Atrial escape beat 415
Atrial fibrillation (AF) 425
    aberration in atrial fibrillation 428
    Ashman's phenomenon 428
    causes 426
    electrocardiogram 426
    mechanisms 425
    slow atrial fibrillation 426
Atrial flutter 422
    with alternating 4:1 and 2:1 conduction
        424
    clinical significance of 425
    differential diagnosis 424
    electrocardiogram of 422
        atrial rate 422
        flutter waves 422
        morphology of QRS complexes 423
        pattern produced by atrial flutter 424
        second degree AV block 422
        ventricular rate 422
    flutter fibrillation 425 *f*
    impure flutter 425 *f*
    mechanism of 422
    types of 423
Atrial interpolated beat 415
Atrial parasystole 416
Atrial septal defect (ASD) 288
    common atrium 294
    corrected transposition of great vessels
        302, 303 *f*
    dextrocardia 294
        technical dextrocardia 300 *f*
        true (mirror image) dextrocardia
            299 *f*
    Eisenmenger's syndrome 292
    endocardial cushion defect 291 *f*
    haemodynamic alterations 300
    Lutembacher's syndrome 289
    malposition, malformation of the heart
        294
    ostium primum type 289
    ostium secundum type 288, 290 *f*
    patent ductus arteriosus (PDA) 299,
        301 *f*, 302 *f*
    patent foramen ovale 289

sinus venosus type 288
    ventricular septal defect 294, 296 *f*, 297 *f*
    with pulmonary hypertension 293 *f*
    with reversed shunt 292
Atrial tachycardias 417
    atrial re-entrant tachycardia 420
    automatic ectopic 418
    causes of 417
    digitalis induced non paroxysmal 417
    electrocardiogram 419
    mechanisms of 418
    multifocal atrial tachycardia 421
Atrioventricular dissociation 491
    aetiology of 491
    causes of 492 *t*
    complete heart block versus AV
        dissociation 496
    disturbance of impulse conduction 496
    electrocardiographic characteristics of
        493, 499
    Iatrogenic 495 *f*
    mechanism of ventricular parasystole
        499 *f*
    mechanisms of 491
    triggered by a ventricular premature
        complex 494 *t*
    ventricular bigeminy rhythm with 495 *f*
    ventricular tachycardia with 495 *f*
    with interference 493 *f*
    without interference 495 *f*
Atrioventricular block 122
    analysis, first degree AV block 124 *f*
    AV blocks, diagnosing at glance 133
    bundle of his electrocardiography 122 *f*
    classification 122
    clinical significance 130
    complete (third degree) AV block 128
    in acute MI with idioventricular escape
        rhythm of RBBB pattern. 131 *f*
    with idionodal escape rhythm 131 *f*
    congenital and acquired complete AV
        block 132
    high-grade AV block and complete AV
        block 133 *t*
    incomplete AV blocks 122
    measurement, intervals and site of block
        124 *t*
    mobitz type I (wenckebach) AV block
        125, 127 *f*
    mobitz type II AV block 127, 128 *f*, 129
    stokes Adams attacks 132
    typical wenckebach period 126 *f*

Automaticity 52
Axial reference systems 26, 27 *f*
   conventional labelling 27 *f*
   hexaxial reference system 26, 27 *f*, 30 *f*
   triaxial reference systems 26
Axis 31
   causes of axis deviation 32, 34, 34 *t*, 228
   electrical axis 25
   lead axis 25
   mean manifest electrical axis 28
   mean QRS axis 36 *f*
   methods for determination of 31
      calculation of mean QRS axis 31 *f*
      quadrant method 31, 32 *f*
      visual impression method 32
   QRS-T axes angle 36
   ST segment axis 37, 39 *f*
   T wave axis 36

B

Bundle branch blocks 135
   bundle branch block alternans 151, 152 *f*
   causes of 137
      branch block pattern 139
      Brugada syndrome 143
      incomplete right bundle 139
      intermittent 142
      intraventricular conduction in 138
      with left ventricular hypertrophy 141
      with persistent ST segment
         elevation 143
      with right ventricular hypertrophy
         142
   complete pattern 136
   incomplete pattern 137
   intermittent bilateral bundle branch
      block 151
   left bundle branch block (LBBB) pattern
      144
      complete 144
      effect of deep respiration on 147
      incomplete left 147
      intermittent 150
      with AV conduction delay 149
      with left anterior fascicular block 148
      with left posterior fascicular block
         148
      with left ventricular hypertrophy 150
   masquerading bundle branch block 151
   right bundle branch block pattern 137
      with bifascicular block 162 *f*
      with left posterior fascicular block
         164 *f*

C

Cardiac rhythm, analysis of 399
Cardiomyopathies 359
   amyloid heart disease 362
   arrhythmogenic right ventricular
      dysplasia 364
      clinical significance 364
      ECG 364

carcinoid syndrome 363
dilated (congestive) 359
   arrhythmias 361
   atrial enlargement 359
   conduction disturbances 361
   QRS abnormalities 359
   QRS-T angle 361
   ST segment and T wave
      abnormalities 361
endomyocardial fibrosis (EMF) 363
   biventricular EMF 364
   left ventricular EMF 363
   right ventricular 363
haemochromatosis 362
haemodynamic alterations 362
hypereosinophilic syndromes 363
restrictive 362
   causes of 362
   classification of 362 *t*
sarcoid heart disease 362
Cardiopulmonary resuscitation 613
Cerebrovascular accident (CVA) 591
   deep symmetric T wave inversion in
      intracerebral bleed 592 *f*
   subarachnoid haemorrhage 591 *f*
   tall upright T wave in subarachnoid
      haemorrhage 592 *f*
   upright T waves and prominent U
      waves, cerebral haemorrhage 592 *f*
Chronic cor pulmonale 380
   causes of 385 *t*
   ECG characteristics in acute and chronic
      cor pulmonale due to COPD 386 *f*
   right atrial and right ventricular hyper-
      trophy in 385 *f*
   right atrial and right ventricular hyper-
      trophy in COPD with 384 *f*
   right bundle branch block in a patient
      with 387 *f*
Chronic obstructive pulmonary disease 382
   electrocardiogram 382
      nonprogression of R wave and low
         voltage graph in 383 *f*
      P wave abnormality 382, 383 *f*
      the T wave abnormality 383
   without obstructive disease of the
      airways 384
Chronic rheumatic valvular heart disease 340
   aortic regurgitation 348, 349 *f*
      with aortic stenosis 349 *f*
   aortic stenosis 346
   double mitral valve lesions, ECG clues
      to 347
   floppy mitral valve syndrome 351, 352
      f, 353 *f*
   mitral regurgitation 343, 346 *f*
      combined mitral stenosis and
         regurgitation 345
      rheumatic mitral regurgitation 344 *f*
      rheumatic mitral regurgitation with
         atrial fibrillation 345 *f*
   mitral stenosis 346 *f*
      rheumatic heart disease with mitral
         stenosis 341 *f*

rheumatic heart diseases with
   severe mitral stenosis 342 *f*
rheumatic mitral stenosis with atrial
   fibrillation 343 *f*
rheumatic mitral valve disease 346 *f*
tricuspid stenosis 349
   rheumatic mitral and tricuspid
      stenosis 350 *f*
   tricuspid stenosis, ECG clues to 351
Conduction, basic concepts 109
   cardiac conduction defects 108
   conduction block 110
   conduction system 397
   conduction through AV node 109
   conduction tissue, heart 4
   formation of impulse in SA node 109
   intracardiac conduction 110 *f*, 399
   intracardiac conduction defects,
      anatomical sites of 107 *f*
   intraventricular conduction defect 151,
      152 *f*
      causes of nonspecific 153
   intraventricular conduction, disorders of
      135
   re-entry mechanism 110
Congenital aortic stenosis 311
Congenital pulmonary stenosis 285, 286 *f*,
   287 *f*
Continuous ambulatory (Holter) monitoring
   197
   artifacts and errors 201
   indications of 199
   interpretation of ambulatory electro-
      cardiographic recording 200 *t*
   methods of analysis of 201
   recording systems of 197
   superiority over exercise testing 201
Continuous monitoring system 11
   five electrodes monitoring system 11
   in coronary care unit 11
   three electrodes monitoring system 11
Cushing's syndrome 559

D

Depolarization 13
   action potential 14 *f*
   atrial depolarization wave 16, 109
   depolarization dipole 15
   depolarization of septum 18 *f*
   process, ventricular depolarization 20 *f*,
      27, 110
   ventricular activation 21 *f*
Double tachycardia 492
Drowning 561
Drugs 564, 594
   antiarrhythmic drugs 568
   antidepressants 572
      amitryptyline 572
      lithium 572
   antimalarial drug 572
      quinine toxicity 572
   antiparkinsonian drug 572
      levodopa 572

antipsychotic drugs 571
digitalis 564
  clinical significance of 568
  digitalis effect 565
  digitalis toxicity 565
  electrocardiographic manifestations
    of 565
heart in envenomation 580
  electrocardiographic manifestations
    of 580
  scorpion envenomation 580
heart in systemic poisonings 573
  clinical significance of 578
  electrocardiographic manifestations
    575
  metal (aluminum zinc) phosphide
    poisoning 575
  organophosphorus 573
phenothiazines 571
tissue amoebicide 573
  emetine 573

E

Ebstein's anomaly 307, 308 f
Einthoven triangle 26 f, 27 f
Eisenmenger's syndrome 301
Electro-cardiogram 3, 16
  abnormalities among asymptomatic
    population 223
  calculation of heart rate on 51
  ECG complex 4
  effect of muscular contractions/tremors
    53 f
  electrocardiographic intervals 59
    causes of widening of QRS 60 t
    characteristics of QT or QTc 61
    JT interval 63
    long and short QT or QTc, causes of
      62 t
    measurement of QT 61
    mechanism of widening of QRS 60 f
    P-P interval 63
    P-R interval 59
    prolongation of VAT 60 f
    QRS interval 59
    QT derived from different heart rates
      62 t
    QT dispersion 62
    QT interval 60
    QU interval 63
    R-R interval 63
    ventricular activating time (VAT) 60
    wide QTd, conditions associated 63 t
    widening of QRS complex 60
  electrical activity 3
  electrocardiographic paper 49
  heart rate on 50
  in adults 53
  in children 65
  in infants 65
  normal components of 54

normal P-QRS-TU characteristics 55 f
of an athlete 73
pre-requisite for good recording 53
segments and junctions on ECG 64
  R-S junction 64
  ST segment 64
  PR segment 64
  TP segment 64
standardization of 49
usefulness of 3
variations during standardization 50
waveforms of 16
Electrical activity 4
Electrical field, heart 25
Electrical injuries 561
Electrocardiographic variants 67
  anxiety neurosis 72 f
  athlete's heart 70, 72 f
  athletic heart syndrome 72
  change after heavy carbohydrate meal 72
  counterclockwise rotation 71 f
  early repolarisation syndrome 73
  effect of heavy carbohydrate meal 70
  effect of obesity on ECG changes 71 f
  juvenile pattern in adult 68
  nonprogression of R wave 71 f
  persistent juvenile pattern 72 f
Electrodes 7
Electrolyte disturbances 582
  effect of hyperkalaemia on action
    potential curve 586 f
  effect of hypokalaemia on action
    potential curve 583 f
  effects of hypokalaemia on ECG
    deflections 583 f
  giant 'U' wave in hypokalaemia 584 f
  hyperkalaemia 585, 587-590
  hyperkalaemia due to hyperparathy-
    roidism 588 f
  hyperkalaemia on ECG deflection 586 f
  hypokalaemia 582
  hypokalaemia with VPCs 585 f
  hypokalaemic and hyperkalaemic
    periodic paralysis 592
  lengthening of QTc interval 589 f
  prolonged QTU interval in hypokalaemia
    584
  TUP complex in hypokalaemia 584 f
  uraemia 590
  uraemia with hypocalcaemia 590 f
Emphysema 380
Escape beats 521
  artificial escape beats 523
  AV nodal escape beats in 524 f
  AV nodal escape rhythm 524 f
  causes of 522
  clinical significance of 526
  diagnostic clues to 526
  electrocardiographic manifestations of
    523
  nodal rhythm 524 f
  pathogenic mechanisms of 521
  ventricular escape beat 525 f
  ventricular escape bigeminy 525 f

Escape rhythm 52, 521
Exercise electrocardiography 173
  arrhythmias, exercise induced 188
  exercise testing 173
    basis of 173
    indications of 173
    pre—requisites for 178
    safety and risks of 175
    standardized methods for 175
  false negative exercise ECGs, causes of 180
  flase positive exercise ECGs, causes of 179
  Master's two steps 176
    bicycle ergometer 176
  pharmacological agents and actions 190
  stress test 186
    contraindications to stress testing 175
    pharmacological methods of 189
  treadmill test 176
    Bruce protocol 177, 185 f, 186 f, 187 f,
      191
    Cornell protocol 177
    Naughton protocol 177
  various exercise, ECG patterns 184 f

F

Fascicular blocks 154
  applied anatomy 154
  bifascicular blocks 162
  combined fascicular blocks 161
  left anterior fascicular block 155, 156 f,
    157 f
    hemiblock (LAH) block with left
      ventricular hypertrophy 158
    with left ventricular hypertrophy 159 f
  left posterior hemiblock 158, 160 f
  left septal fascicular block 161
  peri—infarction block 161
  physiology 154
  trifascicular block 163, 165 f
Frontal plane QRS axis 28, 33 f
  determination of 28
    adjustment method 30
    bisector method 29
    perpendicular method 29

H

Hyperaldosteronism 559
Hyperthyroidism 557
Hypertrophic cardiomyopathy 330
  aetiology of 330
  clinical significance of 335
  electrocardiogram of 332
    arrhythmias 334
    atrial hypertrophy 334
    conduction defects 334
    with atrial fibrillation 335 f
    with short P-R interval 334 f
    left ventricular hypertrophy 332
    prolonged QT and increased QT
      dispersion 334
    right ventricular hypertrophy 333

short P-R interval 334
WPW syndrome 334
macroscopic subtypes 331
sites of hypertrophy 331 *f*
Hypertrophy 75
atrial hypertrophy 76, 85
aetiology 76
characteristics of normal P wave 77
electrocardiographic criteria 77
biatrial and biventricular hypertrophy
103 *f*
biatrial with right ventricular hypertrophy in mitral stenosis 83 *f*
biventricular hypertrophy 102
aetiology 102
electrocardiographic patterns 102
mechanisms 102
combined right and left atrial hypertrophy 82
aetiology 82
ECG characteristics 83
left atrial hypertrophy 78
clinical significance 79
electrocardiogram 78
left ventricular hypertrophy 89, 96
abnormalities of QRS 89
abnormalities of U wave 92
associated left atrial enlargement 92
diastolic or volume overload 90
effect of rotation on 95
electrocardiographic criteria 89
left ventricular strain 95
pattern 89
scoring system for 96
ST-T changes 91
wide QRS-T angle 92
with horizontal heart 92
with vertical heart 95
right atrial hypertrophy 79, 81 *f*, 82 *f*
'qR' complex in V$_1$
abnormalities of the P wave axis 80
direct 79
indirect 80
P Pulmonale 79
QRS complex amplitude in lead V$_2$ 81
QRS deflection in V$_1$ 81
right ventricular hypertrophy 97
abnormalities of QRS 98
aetiology 97
associated atrial hypertrophy 99
electrocardiographic criteria 97
electrocardiographic patterns 98
extremities leads 99
major sites of 97 *f*
mechanisms 97
precordial leads 99
standard leads 99
ST-T,U changes 99
vector analysis 101
voltage criteria of 101
ventricular hypertrophy 87
causes of systolic/diastolic overload
on left ventricle 87 *f*

changes in repolarisation 88 *f*
ECG criteria for 89
mechanisms of ECG changes in 82
normal versus delayed conduction 88 *f*
R wave in normal and hypertrophied
ventricle 88 *f*
ventricular strain 89
voltage criteria of RVH 101
Hypothermia 560
Hypothyroidism 557

I

Idioventricular rhythm 52
Intrinsicoid deflection 22 *f*
Isorhythmic dissociation 492

J

Junctional or nodal rhythm 52

K

Katz-Wachtel phenomenon 294

L

Lead system 7, 11
chest electrodes 8, 10 *f*
chest leads 8
significance of recording 8
classification of 7
lead axis 9
limb lead system 7, 8, 9 *f*
placement of six chest electrode 10 *f*

M

Modes, activation of atria and ventricles 6 *t*
Modes, activation of the heart 5
Myocardial infarction 225
atrial infarction 268
ECG features of 268
chronic established changes 245
differential electrocardiographic,
diagnosis of 262
electrocardiographic patterns 226
epicardial, subendocardial (B) injury 232 *f*
evolution of acute MI 237, 265 *f*, 271 *f*
hyperacute myocardial infarction 235
absent Q wave 236
clinical significance of 237
increased height of 'R' wave 235
increased ventricular activation time
(VAT) 235
slope elevation of ST segment 236
tall and wide 'T' wave 236
infarction at combined locations 258
infarction of left ventricle 248
anterior left ventricular infarction 248

ECG changes of inferoposterolateral
infarction 255
inferior wall infarction 248
inferolateral infarction 249
inferoposterolateral myocardial
infarction 251
nontransmural myocardial infarction
251
posterior wall myocardial infarction
249
inferior wall infarction 261, 266 *f*, 269 *f*,
277 *f*, 276 *f*
localization, by electrocardiographic
patterns 247
localizing, site of coronary artery
occlusion 260
noninfarction Q waves 230
pattern of infarction 238
Q waves and related QRS abnormalities
in 229 *f*
Q waves, QR complex or QS complex of
R wave 230 *f*
QRS complex abnormalities 226
right ventricular infarction 264, 266 *f*
serial ECGs and its significance during 244
site, coronary artery occlusion 261
ST segment changes 231
subendocardial infarction 267
systolic and diastolic currents of injury
234 *f*
'T' wave changes 234
U wave changes 235
ventricular aneurysm 277, 278 *f*, 279 *f*
with bundle branch blocks 269, 271 *f*,
272 *f*, 274 *f*, 275 *f*, 278 *f*
with conduction disturbance 268
Myocardial ischaemia 207
abnormalities of U wave 215
abnormalities, ST segment 208
abnormalities, T wave in 212
acute coronary insufficiency 210 *f*, 211 *f*
clinical significance, ST segment
depression 210
electrocardiographic manifestations of
207 *f*
genesis, ST segment depression 208 *f*
global T wave inversion 214 *f*
inferolateral ischaemia 214 *f*
nonspecific ST segment and T wave
changes 216
pseudodepression and pseudoelevation,
ST segment 212 *f*
QRS—T angle 213
reversible ST segment depression 216 *f*
ST segment alternans in acute transmural
ischaemia 212 *f*
ST segment and T wave changes, causes
of 217
ST segment elevation in transmural
ischaemia 211 *f*
T wave inversion, various forms of 214 *f*
true ST depression and elevation 212 *f*
types and forms, ST segment depression
210

Myocarditis 355
  aetiology of 355
  causes of 355
  Chagas' myocarditis 358
  electrocardiogram 356
    abnormalities or QRS 356
    arrhythmias/AV blocks 357
    prolongation of QTc 357
    ST segment change 357
    T wave change 357
  evolution of 358
  pathogenic pathophysiology of 356
Myxoedema 557

N

Neuromuscular disorders 592
  Becker's muscular dystrophy 594
  Duchenne's muscular dystrophy 593
  Friedreich's ataxia 595
  Guillain-Barre syndrome 595
  hypokalaemic periodic paralysis 593 f
  Kugelberg-Welander syndrome 595
  limb-girdle dystrophy 594
  myotonic muscular dystrophy 594
Nodal rhythm/beats 430
  acceleration of AV nodal rhythm 436, 438 f
  AV nodal (junctional) escape beats 432, 434
  AV nodal (junctional) rhythm 435
  AV nodal beats 431
  AV nodal beats/rhythm 432 f, 436 f
  AV nodal disturbance, type of 431
  AV nodal ectopic beat 435 f
  AV nodal ectopics 433 f
  AV nodal escape rhythm 437 f
  causes of 432
  differential diagnosis of 438
  idionodal tachycardia 439 f
  idionodal tachycardia with AV dissocia-tion 438 f
  nodal impulse 430
  paroxysmal AV nodal extrasystolic tachycardia 439 f
  premature AV nodal complexes/AV 434
  wenckebach conduction with AV nodal escape beats 434 f
Normal 12-leads surface ECG and variations 607
Normal QRS complex, characteristics of 55
Normal QRS-T complex/deflection 55

P

P wave 5, 38
  abnormalities of P waves 83
  characteristics in retrograde (ventriculo-atrial) conduction 83
  characteristics of 54
  coronary sinus rhythm 85f

genesis of P wave 16
  junctional rhythm with retrograde atrial activation 84 f
  left atrial rhythm 85 f
  normal P waves in different leads 17 f
  P wave axis 37
    associated clinical conditions 38
    determination of 37
    normal and abnormal P wave axes 38 f
  P wave vector 16
Pacemakers 535
  artificial pacemaker 535
  artificial pacemaker, paroxysmal ventricular tachycardia 552 f
  asynchronous ventricular pacing (VOO) 542 f
  bipolar pacing systems 546 f
  components, pacemaker 536
  DDD pacing 543 f
  electrocardiographic patterns of paced complexes 544
  electrocardiographic patterns, site of pacing 545
  endocardial and epicardial pacing 537 f
  external or transcutaneous pacing 538
  functions of artificial pacemakers 538
  key pacing parameters 538
  malfunctioning, pacemakers 545
    abnormalities in sensing 545
    abnormalities of capturing 550
    abnormalities of firing 549
    oversensing 548 f
    undersensing 548 f
  methods of pacing 536
  natural pacemaker 52
  pacemaker code 541 f
  pacemaker identification code 540
  pacemaker re-entrant tachycardia 543 f, 551
  pacemaker rhythm 547 f
  pacemaker sites in the heart 52 f
  P-asynchronous pacing (VDD) 543 f
  physiology of 540
  potential pacemakers 397
  programmability of pacemaker 539
  temporary pacing 537 f
  transvenous atrial pacing with AV conduction 544 f
  types of cardiac pacing 541
  types of pacing 53
  unipolar ventricular pacing 547 f
  unipolar ventricular pacing system 544 f
  ventricular inhibited pacing 542 f
  wandering atrial pacemaker rhythm 416
Parasystole 498
  atrial parasystole 501
  parasystole ventricular tachycardia 500
  parasystolic atrial tachycardia 501
Pentalogy of fallot 306
Pericarditis 366
  aetiology of 366
  cardiac temponade due to massive pericardial effusion 372 f

causes of 366 t
chronic constrictive pericarditis 371
evolution of electrocardiographic changes during 367
  changes in P-R segment 369
  ST segment and T wave changes 367
idiopathic acute pericarditis myocardial ischaemia 369 f
pericarditis effusion with cardiac temponade 371 f
pericarditis with effusion 370
pericarditis with effusion and atrial fibrillation 373 f
Persistent truncus arteriosus 309
Pheochromocytoma 560
Physiology, R wave progression 22
  clinical significance 23
  progression of R wave 23 f
Positions, heart 40
  around horizontal or oblique axis 43
  horizontal position 41
  intermediate heart position 42
  semihorizontal position 42
  semivertical position 42
  vertical position 41
Primary pulmonary hypertension 287, 288 f
Prinzmetal's angina 218
  abnormalities, QRS complex 222
  abnormalities, T wave 221
  asymptomatic electrocardiographic abnormalities 223
  atrioventricular block 222
  clinical significance of 220
  complex ventricular arrhythmias 222
  coronary vasospasm 221 f
  electrocardiogram of 219
  elevation, ST segment 219
  hall mark of 220
  intraventricular conduction defects 222
  inversion, U wave 222
  types, ST segment elevation 220 f
Prolonged Q-T syndrome 313
  acquired prolonged Q-T syndrome 314
  clinical significance 315
  congenitally prolonged QTc syndrome 314 f
  Jervell-Lange-Nielsen syndrome 313
  QT dispersion with prolonged QTc syndrome 315
  Romano-Ward syndrome 313
Pulmonary embolism 374
  differential diagnosis 377
  electrocardiographic manifestations 374
    acute corpulmonale due to thrombo-embolism 376 f
    frontal plane leads 374
    horizontal plane leads 376
    in acute pulmonary thromboembolism 378
    right atrial hypertrophy due to acute embolism 377 f
  S_I, Q_{III}, T_{III} syndrome in acute 375
  pathogenesis 374

Q

QRS amplitude, factors affecting 56
QRS complex, factor governing 5, 56
QRS deflection 57
QRS-T angle 58

R

R wave in precordial leads, progression of
  56 f
R wave progression, abnormalities of 56
Reciprocal rhythm 478
  accessory pathways 478
  AV nodal reciprocal beats 482 f
  electrocardiographic manifestations 479
  mechanism of reciprocating rhythm 478,
    480 f
  of nodal origin 482 f
  of ventricular origin 483 f, 484 f
  prolonged re-entry period 479
  reciprocal atrial beats 481 f
  transient and functional unidirectional
    antegrade block in 479
Reciprocating tachycardia 483
  Lown-Ganong-Levint syndrome with
    tachycardia 487
  reciprocal atrial tachycardia 481 f
  reciprocal tachycardia through
    atriohistian (James Bundle) pathway
    489 f
  reciprocating tachycardia (antidromic) in
    WPW syndrome 486 f
  reciprocating tachycardia (orthodromic)
    in WPW syndrome 485 f
  reciprocating tachycardia(1:1 conduction)
    in WPW syndrome 486 f
  tachycardia through atriohistian pathway
    487
  tachycardias through mahaim fibres 487
  WPW syndrome with bundle branch
    block 487
Repolarisation 13
  phases of repolarisation 14 f
  repolarisation dipole 16 f
  ventricular repolarisation 18
Rotation, heart 40
  anteroposterior axis 40
  clockwise rotation 43, 44 f
  counterclockwise rotation 43, 44 f
  effect of deep respiration on rotational
    patterns 44
  effect of respiration on rotation of heart 45
  longitudinal or oblique axis 40

S

S_I, S_{II}, S_{III} syndrome 167
  aetiology 168
  in chronic obstructive pulmonary disease
    168 f
  mean frontal plane QRS axis in 167 f
  mechanisms 167

straight back syndrome 168
  with anterior wall MI 168 f
Sinus arrhythmia 408
  diagnostic clues to 408
  types of 498
    nonrespiratory 408
    respiratory 408
    ventriculophasic 408
Sinus bradycardia 408
  causes of 409
  electrocardiogram of 409
Sinus nodal re-entrant tachycardia 410, 411 f
  electrocardiogram of 410
  mechanisms of 410
  probable sinus node re-entrant tachycardia
    411 f
Sinus node dysfunction 111 116 f
  diagnostic clues, sick sinus syndrome
119
  disorders of 111
  distinguishing features SA and AV block
    113 t
  dual nodal disease (f) 117
  hemiblock 118
  hypersensitive carotid sinus syndrome 120
  physiology of 111
  second degree SA block 113
  sick sinus syndrome 115
  sinoatrial blocks 112
  sinus arrest 111
  sinus bradycardia 115 f
  sinus node recovery time 119
  tachycardia syndrome 118
Sinus rhythm 407
  electrocardiogram 407
  normal sinus rhythm 408 f
Sinus tachycardia 409
  causes of 410
  electrocardiogram of 410
  mechanism of 409
Supraventricular tachycardias 440
  atrioventricular nodal tachycardias 441
    accessory pathway 445 f
    atrioventricular re-entrant
      tachycardia (AVRT) 444
    AV nodal conduction pattern in
      AVNRT 442
    AV nodal re-entrant tachycardia 441
    differential diagnosis of 446
    mechanisms of 442 f
    mode of conduction 441
    narrow QRS complex tachycardia 447
    paroxysmal AV nodal re-entrant
      tachycardia (AVNRT) 444 f
    paroxysmal supraventricular re-entrant
      tachycardias 443 f
    pathogenesis 441
    P-R and R-P relationship 446
  paroxysmal supraventricular tachycardia
    440
Systemic hypertension 389
  arrhythmia/AV blocks 392
  biatrial and biventricular hypertrophy
    with COPD and systemic
    hypertension 392 f
  effect of treatment 392

hypertension associated with other
  conditions 392
inferior wall infarction in a patient with
  390 f
left atrial enlargement 389
left axis deviation 392
left ventricular hypertrophy 389
myocardial ischaemia/infarction pattern
  392
with first degree AV block 391 f
with myocardial ischaemia and atrial
  fibrillation 391 f

T

Tetralogy of fallot 304
Thyrotoxicosis 557
Trauma to the heart 562
Tricuspid atresia 310
Trilogy of fallot 307
Tumours, heart 562

V

Vectors
  calculation of QRS vector 34
    on both frontal and horizontal plane 35
    on horizontal plane 34
  cardiac vector 25
  mean QRS vector 36
  mean spatial QRS vector 35 f
  QRS vectors 28 f
  vectors on lead aVF 28
Ventricular aberrancy 503
  aberrantly conducted beats in atrial
    fibrillation 516 f
  aberrantly conducted supraventricular
    beats 509 f
  Ashmann's phenomenon in atrial
    fibrillation 506 f
  atrial fibrillation with 510
  atrial fibrillation with phasic aberrant
    intraventricular conduction 517 f
  atrial fibrillation with right bundle
    branch block 519 f
  atrial fibrillation with ventricular ectopic
    beats 517 f
  atrial flutter with 516
  atrial flutter with variable conduction
    518 f
  conditions associated with 505
  deceleration related aberrancy 508 f
  ECG characteristic aberrantly conducted
    beat 508
  electrocardiographic pattern, ventricular
    aberrancy vs ectopy 512 f
  mechanisms of 503
    Ashmann's phenomenon 504, 505 f
    heart rate 504
    unequal refractoriness 503
  myocardial depression induced
    aberrancy 508 f
  paroxysmal supraventricular tachycardia
    with aberrant conduction 514

paroxysmal supraventricular tachycardia with aberration 514 *f*

pathogenesis of 517

QRS in supraventricular tachycardia with aberration 515 *f*

sinus tachycardia with aberrantly conducted beats 507 *f*

tachycardia induced LBBB type of aberrancy 507 *f*

toxic myocarditis induced aberrance and ventricular ectopy 516 *f*

ventricular aberrancy versus intermittent bundle branch block 519

ventricular ectopy and ventricular aberrancy 509 *f*

Ventricular activation complex 16

activation of both ventricles 17

activation of posterobasal portions 18

activation right and left ventricles, QRS forces 19 *f*

cavitary lead 21

cavitary pattern 21

dominance of left ventricle 17

genesis of QRS complex 16

left ventricular epicardial complex 20

pulmonary conus 18

right ventricular epicardial complex 19

septal depolarization 17

types of QRS complex 19

uppermost part of interventricular septum 18

Ventricular arrhythmia/dysarrhythmia 448

accelerated idioventricular rhythm 459, 460 *f*

accelerated idioventricular rhythm with incomplete RBBB pattern 460 *f*

accelerated ventricular rhythm 460 *f*

analysis of late ventricular potentials 476

compensatory pause, VPC 451 *f*

diagnostic electrocardio-graphic techniques for 474

dying heart 473

end-diastolic VPC 450 *f*

indioventricular rhythms 458

interpolated ventricular premature complex 452 *f*

left ventricular premature complexes 457 *f*

monomorphic ventricular premature complexes 456 *f*

monomorphic ventricular tachycardia (VT) 467 *f*

multiform ventricular premature complexes 453

origin of ventricular premature complexes 456

polymorphic ventricular premature complexes 456 *f*

polymorphic ventricular tachycardia 468 *f*

post-extrasystolic T wave change 458 *f*

prinzmetal's angina with ventricular ectopics 465 *f*

right ventricular premature complexes 456 *f*

rule of ventricular bigeminy 454 *f*

self-repetitive ventricular tachycardia 468 *f*

signal averaged ECG 475

torsades de pointes 469, 470 *f*

unifocal ventricular premature complexes 453 *f*

ventricular asystole 472

ventricular bigeminy 454 *f*

ventricular couplet 453 *f*

ventricular ectopics 448, 450 *f*

ventricular ectopics, significance of 457

ventricular escape rhythm in complete heart block 459 *f*

ventricular fibrillation 471, 472 *f*

ventricular fibrillation degenerating into ventricular asystole 473 *f*

ventricular flutter 471

ventricular pentageminy 455 *f*

ventricular premature complex 449 *f*

ventricular premature complexes with R on T phenomenon 452 *f*

ventricular premature complexes, conduction of 457

ventricular premature complexes, variants of 451

ventricular quadrigeminy rhythm 455 *f*

ventricular tachycardia 461 *f*, 462 *f*, 463 *f*, 464 *f*

ventricular trigeminy 454 *f*

ventricular triplet 454 *f*

wide QRS complex tachycardias, differential diagnosis of 465

Ventricular capture 530

causes of 530

electrocardiographic characteristics, capture beat 531

incomplete (partial) ventricular capture 530

mechanism of 530

significance of 531

the complete ventricular capture 530

timing and conduction of capture beats 531

Ventricular capture beat 530

Ventricular escape rhythm 52

Ventricular fusion complexes 527

clinical significance of 529

fusion complex 528 *f*

fusion complex due to end-diastolic VPC 529 *f*

pathogenesis of 527

sinus arrhythmia with a fusion complex and VPC 528 *f*

variations in configuration 527

Voltage measurement 64

W

Wolff-Parkinson-White syndrome 313, 334, 483

(Type C) simulating posterolateral infarction 321 *f*

conduction through the right postero-septal accessory pathway 324 *f*

congenital mahaim fibres with pre-excitation 326 *f*

differential diagnosis, on ECG 325

electrocardiographic pattern-bundle or kent 313

intermittent WPW syndrome 323

intermittent WPW syndrome, continuous ECG leads 324 *f*

leads and parameters, localization of accessory tract 322

localization of accessory pathway 323 *f*

Lown-Ganong-Levine syndrome 313, 327, 487

mechanisms of pathogenesis 317

pathogenesis 318 *f*

pre-excitation through a James bundle 328 *f*

Rosenbaum classification of 320

variants 326

variations in ECG pattern of 319

various accessory pathways 321

with atrial fibrillation 325 *f*